Register Now for On[...]
to Your Boo[...]

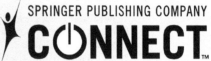

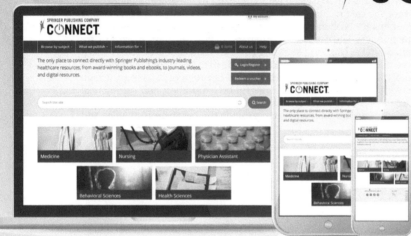

Your print purchase of *Neonatal Nurse Practitioner Certification Intensive Review* **includes online access to the contents of your book**—increasing accessibility, portability, and searchability!

Access today at:

**http://connect.springerpub.com/content/book/978-0-8261-8032-2
or scan the QR code at the right with your smartphone
and enter the access code below.**

*Scan here for
quick access.*

BE8GMX19

SPRINGER PUBLISHING COMPANY
View all our products at springerpub.com

Amy R. Koehn, PhD, NNP-BC, received her PhD in nursing from Indiana University in 2014 and joined the University of Tennessee Health Science Center (UTHSC) nursing faculty in 2015 as the concentration coordinator for the DNP NNP program. She received her MSN from the University of Colorado at Colorado Springs in 2001 and her BSN from Bethel College in North Newton, Kansas, in 1993. She has over 20 years' experience as a neonatal nurse practitioner (NNP) in a variety of level III and IV NICUs in roles both at the bedside and as a team member for neonatal air and ground transports. From the beginning of her NNP career, Dr. Koehn was expected to engage in quality improvement projects within the NICU, which led to the habit of seeking evidence-based best practices for the care of our fragile patients. She has developed continuing education programs for both nursing staff and APRN practitioners. As a mentor for novice practitioners, she developed orientation and education programs for newly graduated NNPs. Her long-standing clinical and recent academic experiences serve as evidence of the qualification to guide in maintaining the relevance of the ever-evolving NNP role. Dr. Koehn shares her love of learning through lectures at the local, state, and national levels for both academic and commercial purposes. These activities promote continued sharing, learning, and participation in the camaraderie that is the basis to provide the best care for babies and their families!

NEONATAL NURSE PRACTITIONER CERTIFICATION INTENSIVE REVIEW

Fast Facts and Practice Questions

Amy R. Koehn, PhD, NNP-BC

EDITOR

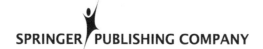

SPRINGER PUBLISHING COMPANY

Springer Publishing Company, LLC
11 West 42nd Street
New York, NY 10036
www.springerpub.com
http://connect.springerpub.com

Acquisitions Editor: Elizabeth Nieginski
Compositor: Diacritech

ISBN: 978-0-8261-8021-6
e-book ISBN: 978-0-8261-8032-2
DOI: 10.1891/9780826180322

20 21 22 / 5 4 3 2

The author and the publisher of this Work have made every effort to use sources believed to be reliable to provide information that is accurate and compatible with the standards generally accepted at the time of publication. Because medical science is continually advancing, our knowledge base continues to expand. Therefore, as new information becomes available, changes in procedures become necessary. We recommend that the reader always consult current research and specific institutional policies before performing any clinical procedure. The author and publisher shall not be liable for any special, consequential, or exemplary damages resulting, in whole or in part, from the readers' use of, or reliance on, the information contained in this book. The publisher has no responsibility for the persistence or accuracy of URLs for external or third-party Internet websites referred to in this publication and does not guarantee that any content on such websites is, or will remain, accurate or appropriate.

Library of Congress Cataloging-in-Publication Data
Library of Congress Control Number: 2019917096

Contact us to receive discount rates on bulk purchases.
We can also customize our books to meet your needs.
For more information please contact: sales@springerpub.com

Amy R. Koehn: https://orcid.org/0000-0003-4025-5959

Publisher's Note: **New and used products purchased from third-party sellers are not guaranteed for quality, authenticity, or access to any included digital components.**

Printed in the United States of America.

*This book is dedicated to the advanced practice nurses
who devote their time, talents, and hearts to caring for
and protecting the tiniest and most fragile of the human
population, the babies. It is a calling from the heart, which
cannot be ignored when heard. We, at the highest level of
the nursing profession, are obligated to remain informed,
educated, and knowledgeable about information that impacts
their care, as it is ever-evolving. This book provides but a
stepping stone on your journey in this frequently joyous
and occasionally heartbreaking service to infants and their
families. May you never stop learning, and may you actively
serve by taking time to pass on what you have learned to those
who come after you. It is by this legacy that we ensure these
precious beings receive care, ensuring their ability to reach the
potential that is limitless in each new life.*

CONTENTS

CONTRIBUTORS

Ana Arias-Oliveras, MSN, CRNP, NNP-BC
Children's Hospital of Philadelphia
Philadelphia, Pennsylvania

Debra Armbruster, PhD, APRN, NNP-BC, CPNP-BC
Nationwide Children's Hospital
Columbus, Ohio

Jodi M. Beachy, MSN, NNP-BC
Ohio Health
Dublin, Ohio

Amanda D. Bennett, DNP, PNP, NNP-BC, VA-BC
University of Illinois at Chicago, College of Nursing
Chicago, Illinois

Elena Bosque, PhD, ARNP, NNP-BC
Seattle Children's Hospital
Seattle, Washington

Cheryl A. Carlson, PhD, APRN, NNP-BC
Medical University of South Carolina
Charleston, South Carolina

Rebecca Chuffo Davila, DNP, NNP-BC, FAANP
University of Iowa, College of Nursing
Iowa, City, Iowa

Jennifer Etheridge, MS, APRN-CNP, NNP-BC
Nationwide Children's Hospital
Columbus, Ohio

Kim Friddle, PhD, APRN, NNP-BC
Primary Children's Hospital, Intermountain
Health Care
Salt Lake City, Utah

Courtney Grassham, MSN, NNP-BC
Pediatrix Medical Group of New Mexico
Albuquerque, New Mexico

Pauline D. Graziano, MS, APRN, NNP-BC
Bernard and Millie Duker Children's Hospital
Ghent, New York

Tosha Harris, DNP, NNP-BC
North Mississippi Medical Center Women's Hospital
Tupelo, Mississippi

Carolyn J. Herrington, PhD, RN, NNP-BC
Wayne State University, College of Nursing
Detroit, Michigan

Jacqueline Hoffman, DNP, ARNP, NNP-BC
Rush University, College of Nursing
Chicago, Illinois

Antonette Hurst, APRN, NNP-BC
Nationwide Children's Hospital
Columbus, Ohio

Lisa R. Jasin, DNP, NNP-BC
Wright State University College of Nursing
Dayton, Ohio

Denise Kirsten, DNP, NNP-BC
Rush University, College of Nursing
Chicago, Illinois

Amy Koehn, PhD, NNP-BC
University of Tennessee Health Science Center, College of
Nursing
Memphis, Tennessee

Kimberly Horns LaBronte, PhD, APRN, NNP-BC, FAANP
Primary Children's Hospital, Intermountain Health Care
Salt Lake City, Utah

Carrie Lewis, APRN, NNP-BC
Nationwide Children's Hospital
Columbus, Ohio

Vivian Lopez, MSN, RN-NIC, PNP, NNP-BC
Maimonides Medical Center
Glendale, New York

Valerie Marburger, MS, APRN-CNP, NNP-BC, CPNP-PC
Nationwide Children's Hospital
Columbus, Ohio

Karen Q. McDonald, DNP, APRN, NNP-BC, PCLC
CHG Healthcare
Midvale, Utah

Hope McKendree, MSN, CRNP, NNP-BC
The John's Hopkins Hospital
Baltimore, Maryland

Leanne M. Nantais-Smith, PhD, RN, NNP-BC
Wayne State University, College of Nursing
Detroit, Michigan

Christi Olsen, MSN, APRN, NNP-BC
Mednax Physician Group
Phoenix, Arizona

Yvette Pugh, MS, CRNP, NNP-BC
Holy Cross Hospital
Silver Spring, Maryland

Cheryl B. Robinson, DNS, MS, NNP-BC
Curriculum Design Resources (CDR)
Fort Payne, Alabama

Lori Baas Rubarth, PhD, APRN, NNP-BC
Creighton University, College of Nursing
Omaha, Nebraska

Terri Schneider-Biehl, MN, RN, NNP-BC
Rady Children's Hospital
San Diego, California

Sandra L. Smith, PhD, APRN, NNP-BC
University of Louisville School of Nursing
Louisville, Kentucky

Barbara Snapp, DNP, ARNP, NNP-BC
Children's National Hospital
Washington, District of Columbia
Mary Washington Hospital
Fredericksburg, Virginia

Karen Stadd, DNP, CRNP, NNP-BC
The Johns Hopkins Hospital
Baltimore, Maryland

Shawn Sullivan, MSN, NNP-BC
Le Bonheur Children's Hospital
Memphis, Tennessee

Kelly Sulo, DNP, NNP-BC
Rush University Medical Center
Chicago, Illinois

Patricia E. Thomas, PhD, NNP-BC, CNE
University of Texas at Arlington, College of Nursing
Arlington, Texas

Ke-Ni Niko Tien, DNP, CRNP, NNP-BC
The Johns Hopkins Hospital
Baltimore, Maryland

Tami Wallace, DNP, APRN, NNP-BC
Nationwide Children's Hospital
Columbus, Ohio

Mary Walters, MS, CRNP, NNP-BC
Mercy Medical Center
Baltimore, Maryland

Julie E. Williams, DNP, CRNP, NNP-BC
The Johns Hopkins Hospital
Baltimore, Maryland

Janice Wilson, DNP, CRNP, NNP-BC
University of Maryland School of Nursing
Baltimore, Maryland

Karen Wright, PhD, NNP-BC
Rush University College of Nursing
Chicago, Illinois

FOREWORD

If you are reading this book, you are most likely preparing to take the neonatal nurse practitioner (NNP) certification exam. *Congratulations!* You have completed your NNP education and are ready to demonstrate mastery of your didactic and clinical education. Why is certification so important, and why do most states require national board certification to practice as an NNP? At any point in time, there are 30 to 35 NNP programs in the United States. All NNP programs have common curriculum and clinical requirements, but there are many differences. Obtaining certification as an NNP demonstrates to families and the public that you have achieved a level of knowledge to safely provide quality care and management to their babies.

This book has been a long time coming! Over the years, many students and NNPs have wondered why there is not a textbook dedicated to preparing graduates to take the NNP board certification. Finally, Amy Koehn decided it was time to find a way to get a certification preparation textbook ready for NNP graduates. Amy organized and edited the textbook, recruited nationally known neonatal educators and clinical practice NNP experts to write the chapters and test questions, and helped prepare a sample certification exam. This book is well organized, presents in-depth information on systems and common problems of the newborn, and discusses the importance of safety, quality, research, and evidence-based practice to provide the best care for newborns and their families. The book chapter authors used readily available information and references that are commonly used to develop questions for the certification exam.

Although this book is primarily meant for new NNP graduates, it is useful for experienced, certified NNPs as well. After reading some of the chapters, my first thought was, "Surely, I knew that at one time, and I just forgot it." It is impossible to know everything, and the amount of information in the world is projected to double again by 2020. Personally, I found the book well written and very useful. NNP graduates should find this book helpful in preparing for the certification exam. It is important that we demonstrate our knowledge and readiness to provide care to our small, ill, and vulnerable patients. After all, providing excellent care to our babies and their families is not just a job or profession, it is our calling! Good luck on your certification exam.

Bobby Burrell Bellflower, DNSc, NNP-BC, FAANP
Associate Professor/DNP Program Director
University of Tennessee Health Science
Center College of Nursing
Memphis, Tennessee

PREFACE

This book, *Neonatal Nurse Practitioner Certification Intensive Review: Fast Facts and Practice Questions*, is designed as an in-depth study guide for the National Certification Corporation (NCC) certification exam for neonatal nurse practitioners (NNPs). It is appropriate for graduates at both at the master of science in nursing (MSN) and doctor of nursing practice (DNP) degree levels. The book may also be used as a comprehensive review for NNPs with existing certification prior to taking the NCC continuing competency assessment exam for certification renewal. This book, unique in the market for neonatal content review, synthesizes the knowledge necessary to assist the reader with passing the certification exam for an NNP to become board certified (i.e., NNP-BC). It follows the outline provided by the NCC of exam content and text references within both its Candidate Guide and Core NP Examination Registration Catalog found on their website. It uses the same textbook references recommended by the NCC in the creation of the certification exam. The book is organized in an outline format, highlighting key content information from the reference texts in precise and succinct statements. Single topics with multiple references are combined into each chapter to provide a broad perspective. References are included so that the reader may go directly to the primary textbook source for a more in-depth review. The book does not need to be read sequentially as a whole—rather, the chapters may be read individually, based on an individual's learning needs.

Amy R. Koehn

A 175-question simulated Final Practice Exam is available as an e-Chapter at https://connect.springerpub.com/content/book/978-0-8261-8032-2/chapter/ch32.

ACKNOWLEDGMENTS

First and foremost, I would like to acknowledge each contributor who donated their time, talent, and energy to make this book come to life. This group project was indeed a demonstration of the best of efforts by all those involved. I am honored and humbled to serve my part, and, from the heart, I thank those who participated.

I want to thank Elizabeth Nieginski with Springer Publishing Company for taking a chance on an unproven editor and selling the dream so that it could become a reality. Thanks, too, to Hannah Hicks, for consistently and joyously answering my thousands of emails.

I owe a debt to my friends and colleagues, especially Dr. Bobby Bellflower, Dr. Laura Reed, Dr. Laura Melaro, and Mary Martin-Hemphill, for being always willing to offer advice, prop me up, push me forward, and on occasion listen to me whine.

Finally, I want to acknowledge my husband, Matt. In our 28 years together, he has supported me through three undergraduate programs, two graduate nursing programs, and the transition from expert clinician to novice academic faculty. I say "thank you" for being my partner in life. I would not be who I am today without you.

BACKGROUND AND INFORMATION ON CERTIFICATION

Barbara Snapp, DNP, APRN, NNP-BC

The neonatal nurse practitioner (NNP) is a registered nurse with a special interest in infants, premature infants, and toddlers through the age of 2, and their families and caretakers (NANN #3059, 2014). NNPs have acquired, at minimum, a graduate-level education in neonatal care and are routinely found in the NICU or newborn care units. The NNP role encompasses a wide range of activities, including the care of critically ill infants, both term and preterm, delivery room management, discharge planning, developmental follow-up, family care, research, quality improvement, and education (National Association of Neonatal Nurses [NANN] #3058, 2013). Although the role is influenced by individual state practice acts (Barton Associates, 2019), the core competencies and educational requirements to take the certification exam remain the same for all NNPs.

EARLY HISTORY OF PRIMARY CARE NURSE PRACTITIONERS

Recognizing a serious gap in healthcare accessibility, in 1965, a nurse named Loretta Ford and a pediatrician, Henry Silver, created what is credited as the first nurse practitioner (NP) program at the University of Colorado. Following the establishment of these hospital-based programs, within a decade there were 65 pediatric and primary care NP programs operating in the United States (Honeyfield, 2009). Aided by the educational funds made available through the Nurse Training Act of 1984, by the early the 1980s there were 15,000 NPs and over 200 NP programs (Honeyfield, 2009).

DEVELOPMENT OF THE NNP ROLE

The NNP role evolved in the early 1970s following the growth of ICUs dedicated to infants. One of the earliest newborn ICUs was created by Dr. Louis Gluck at Yale-New Haven Hospital. Found in large, university-affiliated hospitals, these early NICUs were staffed with medical interns and residents. However, the time residents spent in specialty areas was curtailed, and then overall residency hours were limited by graduate medical education (GME) guidelines (Hutter, Kellogg, Ferguson, Abbott, & Warshaw, 2006). With a proliferation of NICUs around the country, the promotion of regionalization, and the need for transport teams, additional neonatal-specialized personnel were required (Hutter et al., 2006; Samson, 2006).

In 1972, Patricia Johnson created a curriculum for an advanced practitioner but with a focus on neonatal management. Similar to the pediatric practitioner programs, the neonatal in-hospital programs flourished with little oversight or basic nursing education. Each institution created a curriculum to address its specific hospital needs and then awarded the NNP a certificate upon completion (Honeyfield, 2009).

EDUCATIONAL CHANGES

Neonatal educators recognized the need to shift the NNP educational programs from hospital-based certificates to university-affiliated graduate programs. It is interesting to note this shift was originally met with resistance from the academic leaders as promoting a medical-based education model that required physician involvement but minimal nursing input. Ultimately, the success of the NNP role resulted in a move to graduate education for nurse practitioners and acceptance of medical practice knowledge enveloped in a nursing model (Honeyfield, 2009). Curriculum oversight was initially conducted by the American Nurses Association (ANA; 1975–2001) but shifted to the NANN in 2002 when the first Education Standards and Guidelines for NNP Programs was published (Honeyfield, 2009; NANN # 3059, 2014).

In 2000, the American Academy of Pediatrics Committee on the Fetus and Newborn endorsed master's-level preparation for NNP (Samson, 2006). The early part of that decade saw the formation of Licensure, Accreditation, Certification, and Education (LACE), a collaborative group of over 40 key stakeholders representing NPs, nurse midwives, nurse anesthetists, and clinical specialists, created to examine and coordinate LACE for APRNs. The purpose of this collaborative was "to provide a structure for dialogue, debate, and consensus" for an APRN model (Goudreau, 2011; see Table A.1).

TABLE A.1 Governing Components of LACE

Licensure	Accreditation	Certification	Education
NCSBN	NLN	ANCC NCC	Education Standards and Curriculum Guidelines for Neonatal Nurse Practitioner Programs (established by NANN)

Source: National Council for State Boards of Nursing. (2019). *APRN consensus model.* Retrieved from https://www.ncsbn.org/aprn-consensus.htm.

ANCC, American Nurses Credentialing Center; NANN, National Association of Neonatal Nurses; NCC, National Certification Corporation; NCSBN, National Council of State Boards of Nursing; NLN, National League for Nursing.

Although state practice acts vary, most states require board certification and/or a graduate degree and specialty certification for entry into practice. The APRN Consensus Model (National Council of State Boards of Nursing [NCSBN], 2019) allows for more fluidity between states and increased consistency on licensure requirements throughout the United States. An ever-increasing number of states are legislating independent NP practice and NP prescriptive authority (Barton Associates, 2019).

SPECIALTY ORGANIZATIONS

The 1980s saw the development of women's and children's specific supportive organizations. One of the earliest (1969) was the nursing arm of the American Congress of Obstetrics and Gynecologists (ACOG), the Nursing Association of ACOG (NAACOG), which eventually morphed into the Association of Women's Health, Obstetric, and Neonatal Nursing (AWHONN; Honeyfield, 2009; Samson, 2006; Wohlert, 1979; see Table A.2).

In 1984, the NANN was established and began publishing *Neonatal Network*, a neonatal nursing journal. *Neonatal Network* eventually became the journal of the subsequently formed Academy of Neonatal Nurses (ANN), and NANN began publishing *Advances in Neonatal Care* (ANC; Samson, 2006). In 2007, the National Association of Neonatal Nurse Practitioners (NANNP) was developed under the aegis of the NANN. To this day, the NANNP remains the only organization dedicated exclusively to the practice of NNPs (NANN # 3059, 2014).

BOARD CERTIFICATION

It was recognized in the early 1970s that neonatal nurses lacked a specialty examination such as those already available for nurse anesthetists and nurse midwives. Originally operating on simultaneous and parallel paths to develop a certification examination, ultimately the ANA and NAACOG jointly developed a standardized certification examination. Unfortunately, early results revealed widely disparate passing rates. Recognizing that sharing the responsibility was not adequately serving the target nursing population, the National Certification Corporation (NCC) was created and is now the board-certifying organization for NNPs (NANN # 3059, 2014; Honeyfield, 2009; Hutter et al., 2006; Wohlert, 1979). Dorothy Telega, RN, 1974 NAACOG president, stated, "By achieving formal recognition for superior performance in nursing practice, the certified nurse will serve as a role model and will be identified with excellence in clinical practice" (Wohlert, 1979, p. 17).

Passing the NCC board certification exam to earn the title of "NNP-BC" is the initial step after graduation toward building a career. Recertification occurs every 3 years and requires an assessment exam that will guide an education plan for tested areas needing improvement (NCC, 2019). Once the areas for improvement are identified, there are many ways to earn continuing nursing education (CNE) to fulfill NCC educational plan requirements. Conferences paired with an accrediting organization may offer CNE and will often designate the appropriate specific specialty codes: general management, pharmacology, physical assessment, physiology and pathophysiology, or professional practice. Continuing education can also be obtained in other ways, such as precepting students, making continuing education

TABLE A.2 Abbreviations

ANN	Academy of Neonatal Nurses
AANP	American Association of Nurse Practitioners
AAP	American Academy of Pediatrics
ACEN	Accreditation Council for Education in Nursing
ACOG	American Congress of Obstetricians and Gynecologists
ANA	American Nurses Association
ANCC	American Nurses Credentialing Center
APRN	Advanced Practice Registered Nurse
AWHONN	Association of Women's Health, Obstetric, and Neonatal Nurses
CCNE	Commission on Collegiate Nursing Commission
LACE	Licensure, Accreditation, Certification, Education
NAACOG	Nurses Association of American Congress of Obstetricians and Gynecologists
NANN	National Association of Neonatal Nurses
NAPNAP	National Association of Pediatric Nurse Practitioners
NANNP	National Association of Neonatal Nurse Practitioners
NCC	National Certification Corporation
NCSBN	National Council of State Boards of Nursing
NLN	National League for Nursing
NNP	Neonatal Nurse Practitioner
NONPF	National Organization of Nurse Practitioner Faculties

presentations, or authoring a book or journal article (NCC, 2019). The NCC website provides details on maintenance certification: https://www.nccwebsite.org/maintain-your-certification/subspecialty-certification-maintenance. (See Table A.3).

Neonatal Nurse Practitioner Certification Intensive Review: Fast Facts and Practice Questions is intended for use by the new graduate as well as the experienced practitioner. The content is arranged as topic snapshots for a timely review. Should a topic need further investigation, each section and chapter includes references and page numbers to guide the reader to the original sources.

An NNP is a well-respected member of the healthcare team. Achieving board certification is the expectation of a subject-matter expert and competent clinician. Dr. Koehn (Ed.) and the contributing authors offer *Fast Facts* as a thorough overview of NNP practice for board certification as a "NNP-BC."

TABLE A.3 Requirements to Sit for NCC Board Certification Examination

Requirements	Time Frame	Additional Requirements	Testing	Maintenance
Current U.S. licensure	Must be taken within 8 years of graduation date	Documentation of course completion	General assessment: 21%	Assessment test
Successful completion of accredited master's, post-master's, or DNP program (certificate programs no longer accepted)		Application fees	General management: 22%	Education plan for up to 45 continuing education hours
Minimum 600 clinical and 200 didactic hours		Complete application checklist	Disease process: 55%	
			Professional practice: 2%	

Source: National Certification Corporation. (2019). *Certification examination core.* Retrieved from https://www.nccwebsite.org/content/documents/cms/exam-np-bc.pdf

REFERENCES

Barton Associates. (2019). *Nurse practitioner scope of practice laws.* Retrieved from https://www.bartonassociates.com/locum-tenens-resources/nurse-practitioner-scope-of-practice-laws

Goudreau, K. (2011). Editorial: LACE, APRN consensus . . . and WIIFM (what's in it for me)? *Clinical Nurse Specialist, 25*(1), 5–7.

Honeyfield, M. E. (2009). Neonatal nurse practitioners: Past, present, and future. *Advances in Neonatal Care, 9*(3), 125–128.

Hutter, M. M., Kellogg, K. C., Ferguson, C. M., Abbott, W. M., & Warshaw, A. L. (2006). The impact of the 80-hour resident workweek on surgical residents and attending surgeons. *Annuals of Surgery, 243*(6), 864–875.

National Association of Neonatal Nurses. (2013). *Neonatal nurse practitioner workforce. Position statement #3058.* Retrieved from http://nann.org/uploads/About/PositionPDFS/NNP_Workforce_Position_Statement_01.22.13_FINAL.pdf

National Association of Neonatal Nurses. (2014). *Advanced practice registered nurse: Role, preparation, and scope of practice. Position statement #3059.* Retrieved from http://nann.org/uploads/Membership/NANNP_Pubs/APRN_Role_Preparation_position_stateet_FINAL.pdf

National Certification Corporation. (2019). *Certification examination core.* Retrieved from https://www.nccwebsite.org/content/documents/cms/exam-np-bc.pdf

National Council for State Boards of Nursing. (2019). *APRN consensus model.* Retrieved from https://www.ncsbn.org/aprn-consensus.htm

Samson, L. F. (2006). Perspectives on neonatal nursing: 1985–2005. *Journal of Perinatal and Neonatal Nursing, 20*(1), 19–26.

Wohlert, H. (1979). NAACOG–The first 10 years. *Journal of Obstetric, Gynecologic, and Neonatal Nursing, 8*(1), 9–22.

STUDY AND TEST-TAKING TIPS

Cheryl B. Robinson, DNS, MS, NNP-BC

INTRODUCTION

From the first day you decided to accept a position in the NICU, you have been working toward this day. Everything about caring for such a vulnerable population forces each of us to be our best and understand as much as possible about neonatal-specific development, diseases, and responses to the care we provide. We also become experts at keying in on the wordless cues the most immature of the population screams at us. Certification as a neonatal nurse practitioner (NNP) allows us to demonstrate we have achieved a level of more expert skills and fine-tuned knowledge, further enhancing our ability to care for neonates and their families. The acronym P.A.S.S.—Prepare, Assess, Study, Succeed—has been utilized by a veteran NNP educator to help students pass the National Certification Corporation (NCC) NNP exam and is offered here for your benefit.

PASS

Prepare · Assess · Study · Succeed

Prepare

OVERVIEW

The NCC is the certifying body for all NNPs in the United States. Before or during your educational program, be sure to download the latest versions of NCC materials regarding the certification process (www.nccwebsite.org). Each year the NCC updates its exam catalogs, and regardless of your graduation date, the year in which you test will be the exam catalog you will need to follow. Download the most current Candidate Guide while still in your educational program. Familiarize yourself with exam fees and eligibility requirements, testing methods, American Disabilities Act (ADA) requests for testing accommodations, policies and procedures, and certification exam content.

The NCC does not provide any review courses or study materials; however, upon acceptance of your application, you will be provided with a detailed outline of the test and suggested study resources (www.nccwebsite.org/certification-exams/how-to-study). At present, NCC does provide a preview test that you can purchase on their website as well as a detailed content test map.

DURING YOUR PROGRAM

For those who purchase this book during their program, there is a variety of information contained in the chapters that will be helpful as you travel through your academic journey. Once you start the specialized didactic and clinical portion of your studies, every class, every assignment, and every quiz/exam/case study needs to be viewed as part of your preparation for the NCC exam. Required readings will be assigned. Determine the time you can set aside to read, and for that time be intentional. The goal is that you do not return to the same pages twice. The second time you read something, you only retain a fraction of what you can ascertain the first time. Even if you get through only several pages per session, get the most out of the reading. You may want to make notecards of the most important points; you may want to draw a figure or a concept map to capture the content. Rereading material will not guarantee retention success (Miyatsu, Nguyen, & McDaniel, 2018).

Whether your program teaches content from a disease standpoint or from a body system standpoint, you can start to organize your didactic content according to the categories outlined by a certification test map (Figure B.1). The content areas

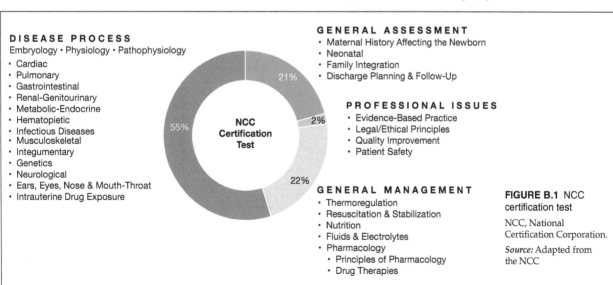

DISEASE PROCESS
Embryology • Physiology • Pathophysiology

- Cardiac
- Pulmonary
- Gastrointestinal
- Renal-Genitourinary
- Metabolic-Endocrine
- Hematopietic
- Infectious Diseases
- Musculoskeletal
- Integumentary
- Genetics
- Neurological
- Ears, Eyes, Nose & Mouth-Throat
- Intrauterine Drug Exposure

GENERAL ASSESSMENT
- Maternal History Affecting the Newborn
- Neonatal
- Family Integration
- Discharge Planning & Follow-Up

PROFESSIONAL ISSUES
- Evidence-Based Practice
- Legal/Ethical Principles
- Quality Improvement
- Patient Safety

GENERAL MANAGEMENT
- Thermoregulation
- Resuscitation & Stabilization
- Nutrition
- Fluids & Electrolytes
- Pharmacology
  - Principles of Pharmacology
  - Drug Therapies

NCC Certification Test — 55%, 21%, 2%, 22%

FIGURE B.1 NCC certification test

NCC, National Certification Corporation.

Source: Adapted from the NCC

outlined by the NCC will be fair game for testing. Note, the Disease Process section is broken into embryology, physiology, and pathophysiology. You will need to know all three aspects for every disease process covered in test map.

Make your notes now: Do *not* depend on your memory. You will not remember rationales from the exam or quiz you took last week. Do not memorize specific questions and answers, as you will not see that exact question or the same set of answers again. For questions to which you have access to for review, note the topic of the question: What was the question asking you to consider? As per the NCC outline, place the question topic in either of the following:
• General Assessment
• General Management
• Disease Process
• Professional Issues

After determining the general topic of the question, decide which part of the detailed outline the topic matter is addressing. Keep up with what you are covering and what content you are receiving while you are progressing through the program. Be sure to pay attention to the content you test well on and the content you struggle with on tests. You will want to visit your document later as you begin the concentrated study for the certification exam.

WHEN SHOULD I TAKE THE NCC?

Every student and every certified NNP will have a different answer to this specific question. The literature, albeit from medicine and not graduate nursing, provides a majority of evidence for testing as soon as you are eligible after graduation. For MD candidates who voluntarily delayed taking the pediatric board certification exam, the result was fewer people successfully pass the exam (Du, Althouse, Tan, & 2016). The following conclusions were determined by the authors:
• Essential knowledge weakened with the passage of time between school and certification exam.
• Candidates who delayed examination were, overall, less confident of their knowledge at the time of graduation.
• Weak clinical students often felt discouraged at graduation, so they delayed examination.
• All candidates, regardless of status at graduation, need to certify as soon as possible to maximize their chances to successfully pass the board examination.

Studies conducted on other specialties, such as emergency medicine, general surgery, preventive medicine, and internal medicine, also reported that a delay in taking the appropriate certification exam resulted in more failures (Malangoni et al., 2012; Marco et al., 2014).

CAN I BE SUCCESSFUL?

Do you possess the qualities and traits to successfully complete your specialty certification exam? If you have successfully completed your program . . . Yes! You do! Qualities and traits outlined in the medical literature associated with successful testing include the following:
• Distinctive intellectual capabilities composed of subject knowledge, diagnostic reasoning abilities, and test-taking skills (Marco et al., 2014)
• Naturally ambitious, intellectually curious, intensely interested in the subject material, and enthusiastic about learning (Zakarija-Grkovic, Bosnjak, Buljan, Vettorazzi, & Smith, 2019)

Assess

Quinn, Smolinski, and Peters (2018) determined from interviews with successful NCLEX-RN® candidates that using practice questions, taking practice tests, making a test review plan, and having appropriate review materials were instrumental to their success. Conversely, Claudette (2014) reported candidates' reasons for their failure on the NCLEX-RN exam, which included "distraction, not knowing what to expect, poor test-taking skills, and overall inadequate preparation" (p. 12). Unsuccessful candidates also falsely concluded that since they had performed better in their program than others who had already been successful on the exam, they should pass as well (Claudette, 2014). You need to judge your performance only against the standard of the course and not fellow students.

Assessment is the starting place for all nursing care, and preparing for the NCC exam is no different. There are a few areas of assessment you will need to address:
• What do you know right now?
• How do you manage test anxiety?
• When do you plan on studying?

WHAT DO YOU KNOW RIGHT NOW?

You need to assess your knowledge base as it stands after completing your program. One way to do this is to take as many practice quizzes or exams as you can find. An excellent tool to assess your areas of strengths and areas needing additional review is the exam offered by the Center for Certification Preparation and Review (CCPR). The company is not affiliated with the NCC, but for a small fee you can purchase the NNP exam and receive the rationales for questions you answered incorrectly. The test is set up exactly as the NCC is set up, so if you have not been tested in this manner in your program, you will be able to experience how the NCC exam is formatted.

Take the CCPR exam from start to finish—all 175 questions at one time. Set yourself up in a testing environment that resembles what you will experience when taking the actual NCC exam. Use the timer provided to gauge your progress through the exam. You will then have either a quantifiable testing time frame to be satisfied with or an assessment of where you need to trim time.

Review your exam. You will be provided rationales for the questions you did not correctly answer. Use the information to fill in your NCC Certification Test Map (Exhibit 1).

Wait a week, and then retake the exam. Pay close attention to the questions you do not answer correctly and mark your checklist provided at the end of the chapter. The topic areas will set your NCC Certification Test Map.

See Appendix A for information on accessing the CCPR exam.

A second online NNP certification prep course is offered via Pediatrix University (www.pediatrix.com/CertificationPrep). The registration is free, and depending on module updates on the website, you will have access to a 50-item self-assessment quiz, module materials, and a 125-item posttest. As with the CCPR, use a checklist to record the content areas of the questions you did not answer correctly. The exam also mirrors the NCC exam to help prepare you for what to expect.

As stated earlier, the NCC website contains a preview test as a detailed content test map you may purchase and take. Again, mark your checklist with the content areas of the questions you do not answer correctly. The point is to

EXHIBIT 1

• PREPARE • ASSESS • STUDY • SUCCEED •

— NCC CERTIFICATION TEST MAP —

GENERAL ASSESSMENT - 21% (~37 Q)

	Passed	Study More
Maternal History Affecting the Neonate	☐	☐
Neonatal Physical Assessment	☐	☐
Family Integration	☐	☐
Discharge Planning & Follow-up	☐	☐

GENERAL MANAGEMENT - 23% (~40 Q)

	Passed	Study More
Thermoregulation	☐	☐
Resuscitation & Stabilization	☐	☐
Nutrition	☐	☐
Fluids & Electrolytes	☐	☐
Pharmacology		
Principles of Pharmacology	☐	☐
Drug Therapies	☐	☐

PROFESSIONAL ISSUES - 2% (~34 Q)

	Passed	Study More
Evidence-Based Practice, Legal/Ethical Principles, Quality Improvement, Patient Safety	☐	☐

THE DISEASE PROCESS - 55% (~96 Q)

	Embryology		Physiology		Pathophysiology	
	Passed	Study More	Passed	Study More	Passed	Study More
Cardiac	☐	☐	☐	☐	☐	☐
Respiratory	☐	☐	☐	☐	☐	☐
Renal-Genitourinary	☐	☐	☐	☐	☐	☐
Metabolic-Endocrine	☐	☐	☐	☐	☐	☐
Hematopietic	☐	☐	☐	☐	☐	☐
Infectious Disease	☐	☐	☐	☐	☐	☐
Musculoskeletal	☐	☐	☐	☐	☐	☐
Integumentary	☐	☐	☐	☐	☐	☐
Genetics	☐	☐	☐	☐	☐	☐
Neurological	☐	☐	☐	☐	☐	☐
Ears, Eyes, Nose, & Mouth-Throat	☐	☐	☐	☐	☐	☐
Intrauterine Drug Exposure	☐	☐	☐	☐	☐	☐

develop a study plan concentrating on materials on which you do not already have a firm grasp. Studying what you already know will make you feel smart, but at this point in your preparation, know you are smart! Success on the NCC will be determined by taking what you already know well and adding not-so-well-known content at the end of your program.

HOW DO YOU MANAGE TEST ANXIETY?

First, you have to recognize whether or not you have test anxiety. Everyone has some anxiety related to test-taking, and some anxiety is positively correlated with an improved performance (Rana & Mahmood, 2010). Test-taking anxiety has been identified by both students and faculty as strongly impacting success rates on the NCELX-RN (Quinn & Peters, 2017). Some students are motivated by the pressure of performing well on an exam, while others experience the pressure as a fear of failure and are overwhelmed (Gibson, 2014).

Test anxiety may affect cognitive aspects such as forgetfulness, disorganization, or irrelevant thinking (LeBeau et al., 2010). Other empirical referents for test anxiety include cognitive impairment, which measures concentration, focus, fear of failure, lack of confidence in skills, feeling unprepared for tests, forgetfulness, or test-irrelevant thinking (Driscoll, 2007). In some situations, a student's self-worth may be linked to the outcome of the exam, and fear of failure may result in clinical depression (Anxiety and Depression Association of America [ADAA], 2012). Cognitive test anxiety (CTA) occurs when the student becomes consumed with worry about test-taking and is mentally stressed in addition to the physiological or emotional responses, such as a pounding heart, sweating, nausea, headache, or crying (Johnson, 2019).

See Appendix B for articles related to combating test anxiety.

There is a strong positive correlation between high test anxiety and poor test performance (Cassady & Johnson, 2002). Recognizing test anxiety and applying appropriate interventions will improve learning outcomes and in effect increase the chances of success on certification. Those students who believe they can be successful (self-efficacy) actually perform better, and controlling test anxiety is one way to add control in the testing environment (Onyeizugbo, 2010).

WHEN DO YOU PLAN ON STUDYING?

Urban legends exist concerning the power of cramming before an exam. The academic literature does not support the process. Your entire program has provided you information about when to study for an exam. The NCC exam is just that, an exam. The NCC will notify you of an exam window so that you can realistically identify on a calendar the days you will have available to study. Make an appointment with yourself for a "study date." Put the date on the calendar, and do not miss the day!

Study

You now have your study exam outline. Studying for the NCC cannot be separated from testing for the NCC. You will be given a maximum of 3 hours to take the exam, and if you take an average of 1 minute per question, you will be sitting for 2 hours and 55 minutes. Therefore, *before* you get to the testing day, you need to structure your study time around 3-hour blocks. Do not let the first time you work intensively be the

day of the exam. Think about being in training—you do not run a 10K on the same morning you decide to run a 10K. You must build up your stamina, and in the case of the NCC exam, you will need the ability to keep your mind sharp for all 175 questions. Do not consider reading or rereading (mentioned earlier) as study. Reading is what you do prior to studying. You will need to actively engage with content material. Some examples might include the following:

- Become the teacher and prepare the content to share with someone else.
- Tie the content to a clinical situation or find an example from practice to apply the content.
- Draw a concept map to capture all the areas with associated content (see Figure B.2).

One successful study strategy will be to gather a few texts for review purposes only. At this point, learning something new for the first time will not be an efficient use of your time. Some examples of texts for study review might include the following:

- Tappero, E. P., & Honeyfield, M. E. (2018). *Physical assessment of the newborn: A comprehensive approach to the art of physical examination* (6th ed.). New York, NY: Springer Publishing.
- Eichenwald, E., Hanson, A. R., Martin, C., & Stark, A. R. (2018). *Cloherty and Stark's manual of neonatal care* (8th ed.). Philadelphia: PA: Lippincott, Williams, & Wilkens.

Other good resources are question-and-answer texts such as:

- Polin, R. A., & Spitzer, A. R. (2014). *Fetal and neonatal secrets* (3rd ed.). Philadelphia: PA: Elsevier Saunders.
- Morton, S., Ehret, D., Ghanta, S., Sajti, E., & Walsh, B. (2015). *Neonatology review: Q&A*. D. Brodsky & C. Martin (Eds.). Brodsky & Martin Publishing.

Successful study habits include taking practice exams, scheduling study time, and spending some time studying with others. Strategies not helpful include recopying notes,

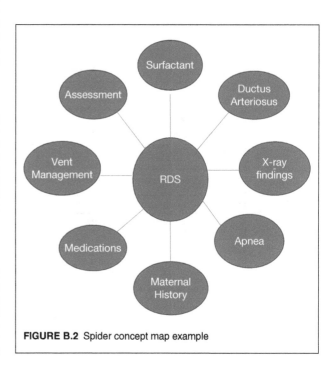

FIGURE B.2 Spider concept map example

intensive studying the night before the exam, and making outlines (Zakarija-Grkovic et al., 2019).

We have a tendency to want to study what we already know or what we get right on a quiz. Whatever you do, avoid continuing to study and take exams on your best topics of knowledge. Completing more questions on what you already know will not necessarily correlate with a higher score on the exam. You will get those questions correct on the NCC exam without any further study. Plan to study material on which you do not already have a firm grasp.

Make sure you build in structure during your study time and avoid multitasking, distractions in the environment, and using your computer (Downs, Tran, McMenemy, & Abegave, 2015). Research has demonstrated writing by hand to be associated with better retention of materials (Patterson, 2016).

QUESTION STRUCTURE

All questions on the NCC certification exam are written to reflect entry-level NNP practice. There are two types of questions: those that have been pretested and statistically analyzed, and those that are being pretested to ensure the item meets the statistical threshold set by the NCC for test items.

You should only practice with items that mirror the certification exam. You may have experienced this question format within your program, but if not, that is more reason to avail yourself of one or more of the practice exams previously mentioned.

Questions on the NCC exam contain three parts:

1. #1 a Stem . . . (you may think of this as the question)
   a. #2 a Key (correct answer)
   b. #3 Distractors (incorrect answer)
   c. Distractors (incorrect answer)

An example of this is the following:
Crowley, M. A. (2015). Neonatal respiratory disorders. In R. Martin, A. Fanaroff, & M. Walsh (Eds.), *Fanaroff and Martin's neonatal-perinatal medicine: Diseases of the fetus and infant* (10th ed., pp. 374–390). Philadelphia, PA: Elsevier.

Practice Question

> Aspiration of meconium will:
> A Decrease surface tension
> B Displace natural surfactant
> C Increase pulmonary vasodilation
> • Correct Answer: **B**
>   Rationale: Meconium displaces surfactant, thereby increasing surface tension and causing pulmonary vasoconstriction

THE PLAN OF ATTACK

1. Read the stem of the question first and answer the question *before* looking at the distractors.
2. Then look at the distractors.
   a. If you see a distractor matching your initial answer, choose the distractor and move to the next question.
   b. If you do not see your initial answer to the question, return to the stem of the question and reread slowly followed by reading each of the distractors with the stem.

The correct answer should be grammatically correct in line with the stem.
   c. If all the distractors match grammatically, then look for key words in the stem and see if those same key words appear in one of the distractors.
      i. One technique to determine the answer is to use the answer choices make a question: In the example: Does aspiration of meconium cause increased pulmonary vasodilation? Does aspiration of meconium cause a decrease in surface tension? Does meconium displace surfactant? The one to which the answer is "yes" is the correct answer.
3. If you are still unsure, mark the question to return to when you finish the remaining questions. Sometimes a later question will contain helpful information to trigger a correct response.
4. If you must completely guess, the literature supports choosing "b." Test writers, even when they are fully cognizant of the "edge avoidance" phenomenon, tend to bury the answer in the middle (Attali & Bar-Hillel, 2003).

Succeed

Success comes in the form of preparation, and a great way to do this is to prepare checklists.

The first checklist you will need to make:
- You have viewed all the NCC documents regarding certification. Locate the Guide to Testing Methods (www.ncc website.org/content/documents/cms/ncc-testing-guide.pdf), *before* you submit your application to the NCC. The comprehensive guide will provide you details about testing.
- You have completed your NNP certification application and mailed application with fee to the NCC.
- You have received your eligibility letter from the NCC via email.
- You have located an approved testing center and have scheduled a testing day within the 90-day window of the date on the eligibility letter you received from the NCC.
- You have purchased a basic calculator (battery operated, noiseless, nonprogrammable, nonprinting). In some instances, the testing center will provide a calculator, but do not leave this item to chance.
- You have learned as much as possible about the exam.
- You have completed at least one trip to the testing center during the same time of day when you will have to arrive for testing.

Drive by the location several times: once to locate and then several times during the time of day you will need to arrive on your testing day. Traffic patterns are important since you will not be able to take your exam if you are 15 minutes late arriving at the site. If late, you will not be able to reschedule, not have your money refunded, and will have to submit a completely new application packet to the NCC. You should determine an alternate route to the testing site in case of traffic problems. Determine, in realistic time, how long the commute will be, what parking entails, cost either in cash/coin or by credit card, and how long you can park. Once you begin the test, you will not be able to return to your car, so allot yourself a minimum of 4 hours parking time.

Go into the testing site on one of your visits. Determine the location of the bathroom and whether there are snack or drink machines. Visit the actual testing room if possible. You may need to arrange this opportunity with the testing site prior to your exam date. You want to go into the room and sit at one of the computer terminals. Visualize yourself sitting in the chair and looking at the computer screen. Determine whether there are any smells that are disturbing. You may need to wear a favorite scent on your clothes or place an essential oil on your wrist. Studies have supported the use of aroma therapy to increase concentration when students are testing (Johnson, 2019).

Make a folder that contains all the materials you will need to supply at the testing center.

Next checklist—be sure you have:
- Email from the NCC
- Two forms of identification. One must be an approved photo ID. Both must have your current name (the *same* as provided to the NCC with your application) and your signature.

If you are getting married, think carefully of the logistics of having the same name on your diploma or equivalent, the name on your application packet to the NCC, the name on your eligibility letter from the NCC, and the name on the two IDs you will take to the testing center.

The night before, be sure to be as physically ready as possible. Get a good night sleep and get hydrated (be sure to go to bathroom before you start exam).

CERTIFICATION TEST DAY

Before you leave your home/hotel:
- Do you have a copy of your NCC eligibility letter?
- Do you have an approved photo ID and another approved ID?
- Do you have proper payment for parking?
- Do you have your preferred snack and/or drink that you will have available to you when you get back to your car after testing?

At the testing center:
- You only have your wallet and keys.
- You only have your eligibility letter.
- You secure your personal items with the test administrator.

Before starting the exam:
- Familiarize yourself with the computer monitor, keyboard, and mouse.
- Determine whether you will want to use the built-in timer on the computer screen.
- Gather the available piece of paper and pencil from the test administrator.
- Take advantage of the practice questions made available by the NCC. You will not lose any time by completing the questions.
- Read over the instructions one more time before you begin.
- Take a few cleansing breaths before you begin.

During the exam:
- Use your scratch paper to write down any equation, lab value, mnemonic, and so on. Do not wait until you are in the exam to try and remember.
- Read over each question carefully.
- Answer every question. An unanswered question is considered a wrong answer. Give yourself the benefit of completing all items.

CONCLUSION

As we say to the families of our precious patients, discharge planning begins on the day of admission. So much the same goes for you: Preparation for the NCC certification exam begins on day 1 of your academic program.

Every class, every assignment, every quiz/exam/case study needs to be recorded as part of your preparation in order to develop a study plan concentrating on materials on which you do not already have a firm grasp. You have been working toward this day for years now—*you can do it*! Just remember to *pass*!

REFERENCES

Anxiety and Depression Association of America. (2012). *Test anxiety.* Retrieved from http://www.adaa.org/living-with-anxiety/children/test-anxiety

Attali, Y., & Bar-Hillel, M. (2003). Guess where: The position of correct answers in multiple choice test items as a psychometric variable. *Journal of Educational Measurement, 40*(2), 109–128. doi:10.1111/j.1745-3984.2003.tb01099.x

Cassady, J. C., & Johnson, R. E. (2002). Cognitive test anxiety and academic performance. *Contemporary Educational Psychology, 27,* 270–295. doi:10.1006/ceps.2001.1094

Claudette, M. (2014). Lived experiences of failure on the National Council Licensure Examination-Registered Nurse (NCLEX-RN): Perceptions of registered nurses. *Journal of International Nursing, 6*(1), 10–14. doi:10.5958/j.0974-9357.6.1.003

Downs, E., Tran, A., McMenemy, R., & Abegave, N. (2015). Exam performance and attitude toward multitasking in six, multimedia-multitasking classroom environments. *Computers & Education, 86,* 250–259. doi:10.1016/j.compedu.2015.08.008

Driscoll, R. (2007). *Westside test anxiety scale validation. Education Resources Information Center.* Retrieved from http://www.eric.ed.gov/PDFS/ED495968.pdf

Du, Y., Althouse, L., & Tan, R. (2016). Voluntarily postponing testing is associated with lower performance on the Pediatric Board Certifying Examination. *Journal of Pediatrics, 177,* 308–312. doi: 10.1016/jpeds.2016.06.030

Gibson, H. A. (2014). A conceptual view of test anxiety. *Nursing Forum, 49*(4), 267–277.

Johnson, C. E. (2019). Effect of inhaled lemon essential oil on cognitive test anxiety nursing students. *Holistic Nursing, 33*(2), 95–100. doi:10.1097/HNP.0000000000000315

LeBeau, R. T., Glenn, D., Liao, B., Wittchen, H. U., Beesdo-Baum, K., Ollendick, T., & Craske, M. (2010). Specific phobia: A review of the DSM-IV specific phobia and preliminary recommendations for DSM-V. *Depression and Anxiety, 27*(2), 148–167. doi:10.1002/da.20655

Malangoni, M. A., Jones, A. T., Rubright, J., Biester, T. W., Buyske, J., & Lewis, F. R. (2012). Delay taking the American Board of Surgery qualifying examination affects examination performance. *Surgery, 152*(4), 738–743. doi:10.1016/j.surg.2012.07.001.

Marco, C. A., Counselman, F. L., Korte, R. C., Purosky, R. G., Whitley, C. T., & Reisdorff, E. J. (2014). Delaying the American Board of Emergency Medicine qualifying examination is associated with poorer performance. *Academic Emergency Medicine, 21,* 688–693. doi:10.1111/acem.12391.

Miyatsu, T., Nguyen, K., & McDaniel, M. A. (2018). Five popular study strategies: Their pitfalls and optimal implementations. *Perspectives on Psychology, 13*(3), 390–407. doi:10.1177/1745691617710510

Onyeizugbo, E. U. (2010). Self-efficacy and test anxiety as correlates of academic performance. *Educational Research, 1*(10), 477–480.

Patterson, M. C. (2016). A naturalistic investigation of media multitasking while studying and the effects on exam performance. *The Teaching of Psychology, 44*(1), 51–57. doi:10.1177/0098628316677913

Quinn, B. L., & Peters, A. (2017). Strategies to reduce nursing student test anxiety: A literature review. *Journal of Nursing Education, 56*(3), 145–151. doi:10.3928/01484834-20170222-05

Quinn, B., Smolinski, M., & Peters, A. B. (2018). Strategies to improve NCLEX-RN success: A review. *Teaching and Learning in Nursing, 13,* 18–26. doi:10.1016/j.teln.2017.09.0021

Rana, R. A., & Mahmood, N. (2010). The relationship between test anxiety and academic achievement. *Bulletin of Education and Research, 32*(2).

Zakarija-Grkovic, I., Bosnjak, A. P., Buljan, I., Vettorazzi, R., & Smith, L. J. (2019). The IBLCE exam: Candidate experience, motivation, study strategies used and predictors of success. *International Breastfeeding Journal, 14*(2), 1–13. doi:10.1186/s13006-018-0197-2

1 MATERNAL HISTORY IN THE ANTEPARTUM

Courtney Grassham
Lisa R. Jasin

INTRODUCTION

The impact of the maternal history on the outcome to the neonate cannot be overstated. There is a direct correlation between what affects the mother and what affects the neonate. The ability to understand the links between maternal history and neonatal presentation is the key to the initial stabilization of any neonate. This chapter covers maternal hypertension disorders, diabetes, pulmonary conditions, cardiovascular conditions, infectious conditions, hematological conditions, substance exposure, pharmaceutical exposure, and fetal testing.

HYPERTENSION IN PREGNANCY

- Hypertension is the most common complication in pregnancy and cause of most of the morbidity/mortality for both maternal and neonatal. Hypertension-related complications are a leading cause of maternal death in the United States (Jeyabalan, 2015, p. 250; Moore, 2018, p. 119; Poole, 2014, p. 124).
- Types of hypertension are outlined in Table 1.1.

Chronic Hypertension

- Chronic hypertension, diagnosed when hypertension is present before pregnancy or recorded before 20 weeks' gestation, affects up to 5% of pregnant women.
- The majority of cases of chronic hypertension seen in pregnancy are idiopathic, also called essential hypertension. However, women should also be evaluated for secondary hypertension as pregnancy outcomes are worse for women with secondary hypertension.
- Severity of maternal and fetal complications depends on the severity of hypertension.
  - ○ When chronic hypertension is secondary to maternal chronic renal disease, there are significantly elevated odds of preeclampsia (PE), premature delivery, small for gestational age, and pregnancy failure.
  - ○ Women with untreated severe chronic hypertension are also at increased risk for stroke and other cardiovascular complications during pregnancy.
- Women with chronic hypertension are at increased risk of slowing of fetal growth and of superimposed PE.
  - ○ Routine ultrasounds, nonstress tests, amniotic fluid index (AFI), and biophysical profiles (BPPs) are recommended (Moore, 2018, pp. 121–122).
- Treatment of chronic hypertension is often a balancing act between lowering maternal blood pressure and lessening the potential for harm to fetus from medications.
- The medications most commonly used to manage hypertension include methyldopa, labetalol, and nifedipine

TABLE 1.1 Types of Hypertension in Pregnancy

Chronic hypertension	Present before pregnancy. Diagnosed before 20 weeks. Hypertension that persists more than 12 weeks after delivery.
Gestational hypertension	New hypertension after 20 weeks with absence of proteinuria. Onset before 36 weeks can progress rapidly to preeclampsia. Normalizes after pregnancy.
Preeclampsia–eclampsia	New hypertension after 20 weeks with new-onset proteinuria OR in the absence of proteinuria, new-onset hypertension with the new onset of any of the following (severe features of preeclampsia): Thrombocytopenia Elevated liver transaminases or severe right upper quadrant pain Renal insufficiency/oliguria Pulmonary edema New-onset cerebral or visual disturbances that do not respond to treatment
Chronic hypertension with superimposed preeclampsia	Preeclampsia that occurs in someone who has hypertension before pregnancy. The outcomes are typically more severe for women and infants.

Sources: Data from Moore, T., (2018). Hypertensive complications of pregnancy. In C. Gleason & S. Juul (Eds.), *Avery's diseases of the newborn* (10th ed., pp. 120–124). Philadelphia, PA: Elsevier; Harper, L., Tita, A., & Karumanchi, S. (2019). Pregnancy-related hypertension. In R. Resnik, C. Lockwood, T. Moore, M. Greene, J. Copel, & R. Silver (Eds.), *Creasy and Resnik's maternal-fetal medicine: Principles and practice* (8th ed., p. 810). Philadelphia, PA: Elsevier; Jeyabalan, A. (2015). Hypertensive disorders of pregnancy. In R. Martin, A. Fanaroff, & M. Walsh (Eds.), *Fanaroff and Martin's neonatal-perinatal medicine: Diseases of the fetus and infant* (10th ed., p. 251). Philadelphia, PA: Elsevier; Poole, J. (2014). Hypertensive disorders of pregnancy. In K. Simpson & P. Creehan (Eds.), *Perinatal nursing* (4th ed., p. 122). St. Louis, MO: Lippincott Williams & Wilkins.

(Harper, Tita, & Karumanchi, 2019, p. 833; Moore, 2018, p. 121; Poole, 2014, p. 123).
  - ○ Medications avoided during pregnancy due to risk for fetal damage include angiotensin-converting enzyme inhibitors, angiotensin receptor blockers, renin inhibitors, and mineralocorticoid receptor antagonists (Moore, 2018, p. 121).
- Monitoring women with chronic hypertension includes daily blood pressure checks, routine growth ultrasounds, and BPP testing, with nonstress testing if there is concern for fetal status (Moore, 2018, p. 121).

Preeclampsia–Eclampsia

- The presentation of PE can be mild to severe.
  - PE is defined as blood pressure >140 mmHg/90 mmHg with proteinuria or severe features.
  - Severe features are defined as blood pressure >160 mmHg/110 mmHg; or other criteria as listed in Table 1.1 (Harper et al., 2019, p. 825).
- There are a multitude of risk factors that predispose to development of PE, including race, obesity, and number of fetuses. The combination of any of these factors increases the incidence of PE.
  - Potential race disparities tend to affect more severity than incidence of PE, and may be due to rates of chronic hypertension in these populations. The populations include African American and Native American women (Harper et al., 2019, p. 813).
  - Women who are obese prior to pregnancy have a higher risk of developing PE, with increased risk as obesity worsens.
  - Women who are having a multiple gestation tend to develop PE sooner and more severely than singleton pregnancies (Harper et al., 2019, p. 813; Jeyabalan, 2015, p. 253; Moore, 2018, p. 124).
- Eclampsia, a "severe feature," of PE, is the occurrence of generalized tonic–clonic seizures in association with PE. It affects approximately 1 in 2,500 deliveries in the United States.
- If eclampsia is left untreated, status epilepticus may develop, which causes repetitive seizures that are more frequent and of longer duration. If the seizures occur while the patient is remote from medical care, maternal and fetal mortality are as high as 50% in severe cases.
  - Almost half of the seizures in the pregnant woman occur before the patient's admission to the labor and delivery department, approximately 30% occur during the intrapartum stage, and the remainder occur postpartum.
  - There is a considerable drop in the risk of eclampsia by 48 hours postpartum, with seizures occurring in less than 3% of women beyond that time.
- Drug of choice for treatment of eclampsia is intravenous (IV) magnesium sulfate. Secondary treatment with anticonvulsants may be necessary in severe cases.
- During future pregnancies, women are at higher risk for reoccurrence of PE if they needed to be delivered before 28 weeks gestation. However, emerging evidence exists that the subsequent cases of PE are not necessarily worse (Harper et al., 2019, p. 832).
- A low daily dose of aspirin, 81 mg/day, has been shown to reduce the frequency of diagnosis of PE and preterm delivery before 34 weeks gestation in those women who are at high risk for reoccurrence of PE or who have multiple risk factors and in their first pregnancy (Harper et al., 2019, p. 832).

Neonatal Outcomes in Maternal Hypertension

- Severe intrauterine growth restriction (IUGR) is common in the fetus of women who have any form of hypertension in pregnancy secondary to uteroplacental insufficiency. However, the rate and severity do increase if women develop PE superimposed on chronic hypertension (Harper et al., 2019, p. 826; Jeyabalan, 2015, p. 253; Moore, 2018, p. 125).

- Although stillbirth rates associated with PE have declined, neonates born of affected pregnancies maintain a higher risk of neonatal death or morbidities. These risks are inversely related to gestational age (Harper et al., 2019, p. 826; Jeyabalan, 2015, p. 253).
- Infants have higher risk of postnatal complications secondary to frequent hypoxemic insults due to uteroplacental insufficiency (Moore, 2018, p. 125).
- Neonates born to mothers with PE may also have thrombocytopenia or neutropenia, which further complicates their newborn course; however, these usually resolve spontaneously (Moore, 2018, p. 124).
- The gestational age at onset and severity of maternal symptoms determines the need for intervention. If the infant less than 28 weeks of age, the effort will be to manage maternal symptoms and allow infant to mature. If the infant is older than 28 weeks, the course may move to elective delivery after administration of antenatal cortical steroids (Harper et al., 2019, p. 825; Moore, 2018, p. 125).

CARDIAC DISEASE IN PREGNANCY

The occurrence of cardiac disease in pregnancy includes both congenital and acquired forms of cardiac disease. The number of pregnancies affected by congenital cardiac disease continues to increase as medical advances have resulted in more survivors to adulthood. Understanding the impact of cardiac disease on pregnancy is vital because the maternal cardiovascular system is responsible for meeting the needs of both the mother and the fetus.

Cardiac adaptations of pregnancy are outlined in Table 1.2.

TABLE 1.2 Cardiac Adaptations of Pregnancy

Increased	Total blood volume Plasma volume Red cell volume Cardiac output Heart rate Uterine blood flow Myocardial contractility
Decreased	Diastolic blood pressure Systemic vascular resistance Pulmonary circulation
Unchanged	Systolic blood pressure Central venous pressure Pulmonary capillary wedge pressure Ejection fraction Left ventricular stroke work index

Sources: Data from Arafeh, J. (2014). Cardiac disease in pregnancy. In K. Simpson & P. Creehan (Eds.), *Perinatal nursing* (4th ed., p. 226). St. Louis, MO: Lippincott Williams & Wilkins; Blackburn, S. T. (2018). Cardiovascular system. In *Maternal fetal & neonatal physiology: A clinical perspective* (5th ed., p. 253). Elsevier.

Signs of Potential Cardiac Disease in the Pregnant Woman

Pregnancy may elicit many signs or symptoms that may be confused with cardiac complications. These include dizziness, dyspnea, orthopnea, fatigue, syncope, systolic murmurs, dysrhythmias, and cardiomegaly.

It can be difficult, then, to determine whether maternal symptoms are changes found in pregnancy or an indication of an existing or developing maternal cardiovascular disease process (Arafeh, 2014, p. 227).

- Signs concerning for maternal cardiovascular disease:
  ○ Severe dyspnea
  ○ Orthopnea
  ○ Paroxysmal nocturnal dyspnea
  ○ Syncope with exertion
  ○ Chest pain with exertion
  ○ Systemic hypotension
  ○ Persistent jugular venous distention
  ○ Sinus tachycardia >15% normal heart rate
  ○ Pulmonary edema, with or without hemoptysis
  ○ Pleural effusion (Arafeh, 2014, p. 228)

Effect of Cardiovascular Disease on Pregnancy

The World Health Organization (WHO) has developed a risk classification system for cardiovascular risk that helps to define and provide guidelines for the treatment of cardiovascular disease in pregnancy. Many congenital heart defects are classified in the system. There are six cardiac complications that carry the classification of high risk: aortic valve stenosis, coarctation of the aorta, Marfan syndrome, peripartum cardiomyopathy, severe pulmonary hypertension, and Tetralogy of Fallot (TOF). The estimated maternal mortality risk ranges from 5% to 60%. Table 1.3 details the modified WHO classification system for identifying risk of mortality or morbidity in pregnant patients with cardiovascular disease.

There are a set of cardiovascular disorders that may fall into the WHO risk classification of II or III depending on the individual. These defects include those with mild left ventricular impairment, hypertrophic cardiomyopathy, Marfan syndrome not associated with aortic root dilation, repaired coarctation of the aorta, and aortic dilation less than 45 mm in individuals with a bicuspid aortic valve (Blanchard & Daniels, 2019, p. 921).

ACYANOTIC CONGENITAL HEART DEFECTS

- Atrial septal defect (ASD):
  ○ The most common heart defect in pregnancy
  ○ Risk category depends on the size of shunt (larger defect equals greater risk).
  ○ If there is no maternal pulmonary hypertension, there is likely to be minimal effect on the fetus (Arafeh, 2014, p. 230; Blanchard & Daniels, 2019, p. 927).
- Ventricular septal defect (VSD):
  ○ Size of defect is again the most important indicator for pregnancy outcome. Larger defects are associated with increased risk of congestive heart failure (CHF) and pulmonary hypertension development.
  ○ If pulmonary hypertension exists, there is high risk for both maternal and fetal death (Arafeh, 2014, p. 230; Blanchard & Daniels, 2019, p. 928).
- Pulmonic stenosis:
  ○ The degree of obstruction is more important than the location of the obstruction in determining the risk of pregnancy (Arafeh, 2014, p. 230).
  ○ Moderate pulmonary stenosis usually will not influence the woman or fetus. Severe pulmonary stenosis will require treatment with a valvuloplasty and typically has minimal effect on the fetus (Blanchard & Daniels, 2019, p. 932).

TABLE 1.3 World Health Organization Maternal Cardiovascular Risk Classification

Risk Class	Principle	Application
I	No increased risk for maternal mortality and no/mild increase in morbidity	Uncomplicated/mild Pulmonary stenosis Patent ductous arteriosus Mitral valve prolapse Repaired simple lesions Atrial septal defect Ventricular septal defect PDA Anomalous pulmonary venous drainage Ectopic beats Isolated atrial or ventricular
II	Small increased risk of maternal mortality or moderate increase in morbidity	Unrepaired septal defect Atrial or ventricular Repaired tetralogy of Fallot Most arrhythmias
III	Significantly increased risk of maternal mortality/severe morbidity Requires expert counseling Pregnancy will require intensive cardiac specialty and obstetric monitoring	Mechanical valve Systemic right ventricle Fontan circulation Unrepaired cyanotic heart disease Complex congenital heart disease Aortic root dilation of 40 mm to 45 mm in those with Marfan syndrome Aortic root dilation of 45 mm to 50 mm in those with bicuspid aortic valve
IV	Extremely high risk of maternal mortality or severe morbidity Pregnancy contraindicated Termination should be offered If pregnancy continues, same care as level III	Pulmonary artery hypertension regardless of cause History of peripartum cardiomyopathy with any residual left ventricular function impairment Severe mitral stenosis Severe symptomatic aortic stenosis

PDA, patent ductus arterioles.

Source: Data from Blanchard, D., & Daniels, L. (2019). Cardiac diseases. In R. Resnik, C. Lockwood, T. Moore, M. Greene, J. Copel, & R. Silver (Eds.), *Creasy and Resnik's maternal-fetal medicine: Principles and practice* (8th ed., p. 921). Philadelphia, PA: Elsevier.

- Aortic stenosis:
  ○ Maternal aortic stenosis may be congenital or acquired.
  ○ The degree of obstruction is more important than the location of the obstruction in determining the risk of pregnancy.
  ○ The presence of a mechanical aortic valve will require continuous anticoagulation (Arafeh, 2014, p. 230; Blanchard & Daniels, 2019, p. 931).

CYANOTIC CONGENITAL HEART DEFECTS

- TOF:
  ○ There is minimal maternal risk if the defect has been corrected and there are no subsequent limitations.
  ○ Pregnancy should be avoided if the defect is corrected, but there is a history of CHF, cardiomegaly, decreased right ventricular pressure or current peripheral hypoxia, or polycythemia.

- TOF that is uncorrected is associated with higher rate of maternal morbidity and poor prognosis for infant (Arafeh, 2014, p. 230).
  - Infants born to women with TOF have a 5% to 10% chance of inheriting the defect (Blanchard & Daniels, 2019, p. 932).
- Aortic congenital heart defects
  - Coarctation of the aorta
    - Maternal risk for PE is increased in women with coarctation.
    - The pregnancy will be most affected if it is an uncorrected coarctation.
    - This risk is significantly higher if it is a complicated coarctation (Arafeh, 2014, p. 231; Blanchard & Daniels, 2019, p. 934).
- Marfan syndrome
  - The outcome depends on the presence and degree of aortic root involvement, which is determined by the dilation of the aorta.
  - The type of delivery is largely dependent on the degree of aortic root dilation. Women with no dilation may deliver vaginally; however, women with dilation >4 cm should be delivered via cesarean section.
  - Women with Marfan syndrome should have extensive preconception counseling; there is a 50% risk of transmission of Marfan syndrome to the fetus.
  - Increased estrogen levels present in pregnancy put pregnant women at higher risk for aortic dissection (Arafeh, 2014, p. 231; Blackburn, 2018, p. 266; Blanchard & Daniels, 2019, p. 943).

Cardiomyopathy in Pregnancy

Dilated Cardiomyopathy
- This is diffuse dilation of the cardiac muscle that causes a decrease in cardiac output and an increase in cardiac filling pressures, resulting in dyspnea, edema, and fatigue.
- These patients are at increased risk for pulmonary embolism or stroke.
- The analysis of serum levels of B-type natriuretic peptide (BNP) may identify those pregnant women with cardiomyopathy who are at highest risk for cardiac events.
- Treatment includes the use of both ACE inhibitors and beta-adrenergic blocking agents to slow the deterioration of left ventricular function (Blanchard & Daniels, 2019, p. 939).

Peripartum Cardiomyopathy
- This occurs in the last portion of pregnancy or first months postpartum in women with no previous cardiac disease.
- The cause of peripartum cardiomyopathy is not fully known, there is increasing evidence that there may be a genetic component.
- There has also been an identified increased incidence of peripartum cardiomyopathy in pregnant women who have been diagnosed with PE.
- Other identified risk factors include increased maternal age, chronic hypertension, multiple gestation, or multiparity.
- The treatment of peripartum cardiomyopathy is like that of other patients with CHF. The vasodilator of choice in pregnancy is hydralazine.
- If cardiac dysfunction is severe, anticoagulation may be indicated. Warfarin is not recommended for anticoagulation in pregnancy. Low molecular weight heparin is preferred to unfractionated heparin for anticoagulation.

- This may reoccur in future pregnancies, even if full recovery is noted as evidenced by a normalized ejection fraction (Blackburn, 2018, p. 266; Blanchard & Daniels, 2019, pp. 939–940).

Idiopathic Hypertrophic Cardiomyopathy
  - Although hypertrophic cardiomyopathy is usually inherited in an autosomal dominant fashion, there have been spontaneous mutations identified.
  - Outflow tract obstruction may be increased by:
    - Physiological decrease in peripheral vascular resistance in pregnancy
    - An increase in circulating catecholamines during the labor process
    - The use of the Valsalva maneuver in labor
  - Goals of treatment include:
    - Avoiding hypovolemia
    - Maintaining venous return
    - Avoiding anxiety, excitement, and strenuous activity (Blanchard & Daniels, 2019, pp. 939–940)

PULMONARY DISEASE IN PREGNANCY

The cardiorespiratory system needs to be functioning correctly in order to achieve the proper oxygenation of both maternal and fetal tissues. Pulmonary changes and conditions that may affect maternal oxygenation also affect the fetus.

Pulmonary changes in pregnancy are summarized in Table 1.4.

TABLE 1.4 Pulmonary Changes in Pregnancy

Increased	Minute ventilation Alveolar ventilation Tidal volume Oxygen consumption PaO_2 Arterial pH
Decreased	Functional residual capacity Residual volume $PaCO_2$
Unchanged	Respiratory rate

Sources: Data from Arafeh, J. (2014). Cardiac disease in pregnancy. In K. Simpson & P. Creehan (Eds.), *Perinatal nursing* (4th ed., p. 226). St. Louis, MO: Lippincott Williams & Wilkins; Whitty, J., & Dombrowski, M. (2019). Respiratory diseases in pregnancy. In R. Resnik, C. Lockwood, T. Moore, M. Greene, J. Copel, & R. Silver (Eds.), *Creasy and Resnik's maternal-fetal medicine: Principles and practice* (8th ed., p. 1043). Philadelphia, PA: Elsevier.

Pneumonia

- The most common nonobstetrical infectious cause of morbidity and mortality in the peripartum period is pneumonia.
- Pneumonia can be associated with poor fetal growth, preterm delivery, and perinatal loss, with preterm delivery being the leading complication (Whitty & Dombrowski, 2019, pp. 1045–1046).

BACTERIAL PNEUMONIA

- The two identifiable organisms most commonly causing pneumonia are pneumococcus and *Haemophilus influenzae*. Most cases of bacterial pneumonia are not able to be identified (Whitty & Dombrowski, 2019, p. 1046).

- Pregnant women are at higher risk for influenza-associated pneumonia. Of the subtypes of influenza, type A is more likely to cause infection (Whitty & Dombrowski, 2019, p. 1048).
- All pregnant women should be vaccinated with the influenza vaccine during pregnancy; those at higher risk should be vaccinated earlier in pregnancy. The vaccine helps to confer antibodies on the newborn as well that have detectable levels in cord blood (Whitty & Dombrowski, 2019, p. 1049).
- Women at high risk for pneumonia, such as those with sickle cell disease, with a splenectomy, or who are immunocompromised should receive the pneumococcal vaccine to protect the woman and the fetus (Whitty & Dombrowski, 2019, p. 1048).

Viral Pneumonia

- Viral pneumonia could be the primary cause or be associated with a secondary bacterial infection. Thus, hospitalized women with viral symptoms should also be treated for most common organisms that could cause a secondary bacterial infection (Whitty & Dombrowski, 2019, p. 1046).

VARICELLA

- Varicella is safe to be treated with acyclovir during pregnancy to aid in prevention of varicella pneumonia. Varicella infection has not been associated with increased risk of birth defects (Whitty & Dombrowski, 2019, p. 1049).
- Varicella vaccine is not indicated in pregnancy; however, knowing maternal antibody status aids in identifying women most at risk for infection during pregnancy.
  - Administration of varicella vaccine in pregnancy or within 3 months of conception has been associated with increased risk of birth defects (Whitty & Dombrowski, 2019, p. 1050).

Tuberculosis

- Pregnancy complicates the multidrug treatment of tuberculosis (TB) because many of the drugs in the regimen are not safe during pregnancy.
  - The initial treatment for pregnant women with TB is isoniazid, also known as isonicotinylhydrazide (INH) and rifampin.
  - Despite concern for treating TB, at-risk women should be screened as it can be vertically and laterally transmitted. Women with a positive purified protein derivative (PPD) can be screened with a chest x-ray after the first trimester.
- Neonates born to women who are taking medications for TB but who have inactive TB need a PPD screen at birth and at 3 months.
- Active TB at the time of delivery is an indication to separate woman and child after delivery to prevent transmission to newborn.
  - Neonates who are born to women with active TB should receive prophylactic treatment until women have negative disease for 3 months (Whitty & Dombrowski, 2019, p. 1054).

Asthma

- Asthma is the most common respiratory complication in pregnancy and preexisting asthma is worsened by pregnancy.
- Women with preexisting asthma should continue to take their control medications and avoid triggers. They are also at higher risk for PE, premature birth, low birth weight, IUGR, and perinatal mortality. Fetal risks are proportionate to the control of asthma during pregnancy (Nodine, Hastings-Tolsma, & Arruda, 2016, p. 19; Whitty & Dombrowski, 2019, p. 1055).
- Treatment with any medication during pregnancy is better than hypoxia in the mother.
  - Inhaled corticosteroids are the preferred method of treatment (Nodine et al., 2016, p. 19; Whitty & Dombrowski, 2019, p. 1057).
  - Oral decongestants used in the first trimester have been associated with gastroschisis development, so inhaled decongestants or inhaled corticosteroids are preferred.
  - Women who are receiving immunotherapy prior to pregnancy may continue during pregnancy; however, it should not be initiated during pregnancy (Whitty & Dombrowski, 2019, p. 1059).
- Labor management should include IV corticosteroids during labor and 24 hours postdelivery if women are currently on systemic corticosteroids or have had several short courses of steroids during pregnancy (Whitty & Dombrowski, 2019, p. 1061).

Cystic Fibrosis

- Increased survival in cystic fibrosis (CF) patients has resulted in more pregnancies affected by CF. Women with CF who have preconception counseling had better maternal and neonatal outcomes (Nodine et al., 2016, p. 19; Whitty & Dombrowski, 2019, p. 1063).
  - Preconception counseling should include discussion that the pregnancy may shorten the mother's life span and result in a preterm infant with multiple complications. The counseling should also include paternal testing, as all infants will be at least heterozygous carriers for CF (Nodine et al., 2016, p. 19; Whitty & Dombrowski, 2019, p. 1065).
- Maternal patients with CF are at increased risk for vitamin K deficiency, so prothrombin time should be monitored, and women given parenteral vitamin K as indicated (Nodine et al., 2016, p. 19; Whitty & Dombrowski, 2019, p. 1066).

DIABETES IN PREGNANCY

Pathophysiology of Diabetes

- Early pregnancy: There is beta-cell hyperplasia caused by increased insulin production. The relative hyperinsulinism allows for increased fat deposition. The combination of the hyperinsulinism and nausea/vomiting associated with early pregnancy increases the risk for hypoglycemia (Daley, 2013, p. 206).
- Later pregnancy: During this time there is accelerated growth and increasing levels of diabetogenic hormones. These hormones include cortisol, estrogen, progesterone, prolactin, and human placental lactogen (Daley, 2013, p. 206). Hepatic glucose production also increases during this stage to compensate for periods of maternal fasting.

Classification of Diabetes

- All women who are diagnosed at their first prenatal appointment and/or before 24 weeks' gestation should be considered as undiagnosed diabetics.
- There are now more women in pregnancy affected by type 2 than type 1 (Daley, 2013, p. 206).

TYPE 1 DIABETES

- Type I diabetes is a result of absolute insulin deficiency from autoimmune action directed at the pancreas (Brown & Chang, 2018, p. 90; Daley, 2013, p. 206).
  - ○ Exogenous insulin needs in the first half of pregnancy may decrease and the risk for hypoglycemic incidents increases, compared to later in pregnancy when the insulin requirement may be as many as two to three times higher than prepregnancy requirements (Brown & Chang, 2018, p. 97).
  - ○ The risk of stillbirth has been demonstrated to be higher in type 1 diabetic women compared to type 2 diabetic women; however, both are significantly higher than non-diabetic women (Brown & Chang, 2018, p. 95; Moore, Hauguel-De Mouzon, & Catalano, 2019, p. 1067).
    - ■ Preexisting diabetes that is poorly controlled can result in a threefold increase in congenital malformations when compared to women who do not have diabetes prior to pregnancy.
    - ■ A prepregnancy hemoglobin A1C (HbA1c) level of greater than 10% puts the embryo at highest risk. The risk may be compounded if the woman has associated medical conditions that also require medications (Brown & Chang, 2018, p. 93).

TYPE 2 DIABETES

- This is a result of insulin resistance and relative insulin deficiency (Brown & Chang, 2018, p. 90; Daley, 2013, p. 204; Moore et al., 2019, p. 1068).

Gestational Diabetes

- Gestational diabetes cases are divided into those that are controlled by diet and those that need insulin for control (Moore et al., 2019, p. 1067).
- Table 1.5 outlines possible maternal and fetal complications of diabetes in pregnancy.

TABLE 1.5 Complications of Diabetes in Pregnancy

Maternal Complications of Hyperglycemia	Infant Complications of Hyperglycemia
Polyhydramnios Hypertension Urinary tract infections Pyelonephritis Monilial vaginitis Retinopathy Nephropathy Increased risk for gestational hypertension, preeclampsia, and vascular disease	Increased incidence of respiratory distress syndrome due to inhibiting release of surfactant Excessive fetal growth and subsequent LGA status Congenital malformations Spontaneous abortion Neonatal metabolic disorders (hypoglycemia, hypocalcemia, hypomagnesemia) Prematurity Hypertrophic and congestive cardiomyopathy Polycythemia Hyperbilirubinemia Birth injury

LGA, large for gestational age.

Sources: Data from Daley, J. (2014). Diabetes in pregnancy. In K. Simpson & P. Creehan (Eds.), *Perinatal nursing* (4th ed., p. 207). St. Louis, MO: Lippincott Williams & Wilkins: Nodine, P., Hastings-Tolsma, M., & Arruda, J. (2016). Prenatal environment: Effect on neonatal outcome. In Gardner

et al. (Eds.), *Handbook of neonatal intensive care* (8th ed., p. 12). St. Louis, MO: Elsevier; Brown, Z., & Chang, J. (2018). Maternal diabetes. In C. Gleason & S. Juul (Eds.), *Avery's diseases of the newborn* (10th ed., p. 102). Philadelphia, PA: Elsevier; Moore, T., Hauguel-De Mouzon, S., & Catalano, P. (2019). Diabetes in pregnancy. In R. Resnik, C. Lockwood, T. Moore, M. Greene, J. Copel, & R. Silver (Eds.), *Creasy and Resnik's maternal-fetal medicine: Principles and practice* (8th ed., pp. 1073–1083). Philadelphia, PA: Elsevier.

- Table 1.6 lists possible congenital anomalies associated with diabetes in pregnancy.

TABLE 1.6 Types of Fetal Congenital Anomalies Associated With Diabetes

Organ System	Anomalies
Central nervous system	Spina bifida Anencephaly Hydrocephalus
Cardiovascular system—these defects account for 40%–50% of congenital anomalies associated with diabetes	Ventral septal defect Tetralogy of Fallot Transposition of the great arteries Hypoplastic left heart syndrome Coarctation of the aorta Atrial septal defect Pulmonic stenosis Double outlet right ventricle Truncus arteriosus
Genitourinary tract	Hydronephrosis Renal agenesis Ureteral duplication Hypospadias
GI tract	Intestinal atresias Anal atresia

GI, gastrointestinal.

Source: Data from Brown, Z., & Chang, J. (2018). Maternal diabetes. In C. Gleason & S. Juul (Eds.), *Avery's diseases of the newborn* (10th ed., p. 93). Philadelphia, PA: Elsevier.

Medical Treatment of Diabetes

- Diet and nutrition counseling are always considered first line of treatment (Brown & Chang, 2018, p. 97; Daley, 2013, p. 215).
- Insulin has been studied extensively in pregnancy and is known to be safe, as it does not cross the placental barrier.
- Oral medications have become increasingly popular as more studies have been published demonstrating safety. Metformin and glyburide are the most commonly used oral agents. Infants of women treated with glyburide should have frequent monitoring for hyperbilirubinemia (Brown & Chang, 2018, p. 97; Nodine et al., 2016, p. 12).
- Table 1.7 describes overall practices for fetal surveillance in women who have diabetes during pregnancy.

Timing of Delivery

- This depends on glycemic control and results of fetal surveillance. It is no longer recommended to deliver automatically before 40 weeks (Brown & Chang, 2018, p. 98; Daley, 2013, p. 216; Nodine et al., 2016, p. 12).

TABLE 1.7 Fetal Surveillance for Diabetes

Gestational Age	Poorly Controlled—Type 1 or 2 Diabetes	Well-Controlled Type 1 or 2 Diabetes	GDMA1	GDMA2
6–8 weeks	Ultrasound estimation of gestational age	Routine care	Not applicable	Not applicable
11–13 weeks	NT measurement	Routine care	Routine care	Routine care
15–20 weeks	Maternal serum alpha-fetoprotein level	Routine care	Routine care	Routine care
20–22 weeks	High-resolution ultrasound and fetal echocardiograph	Routine care	Routine care	Routine care
26–28 weeks	Ultrasound measurement of interval growth	Routine care	Routine care	Routine care
28 weeks	Twice daily FMC and weekly NST	Twice daily FMC	Twice daily FMC	Twice daily FMC
32 weeks	Twice weekly NST or weekly biophysical profile, ultrasound assessment of interval growth	Weekly NST		Weekly NST
34–36 weeks		Twice weekly NST		Twice weekly NST
36–38 weeks	Ultrasound estimation of fetal weight	Ultrasound estimation of fetal weight	Ultrasound estimation of fetal weight Weekly NST	Ultrasound estimation of fetal weight
39–40 weeks	Elective birth	Elective birth	Elective birth if cervix favorable or LGA	Elective birth if cervix favorable or LGA

GDMA1; Diet-Controlled Gestational Diabetes; FMC, fetal movement count; GDMA2, Insulin-Controlled Gestational Diabetes; LGA, large for gestational age; NST, nonstress test; NT, nuchal translucency.

Sources: Data from Daley, J. (2014). Diabetes in pregnancy. In K. Simpson & P. Creehan (Eds.), *Perinatal nursing* (4th ed., p. 216). St. Louis, MO: Lippincott Williams & Wilkins; Brown, Z., & Chang, J. (2018). Maternal diabetes. In C. Gleason & S. Juul (Eds.), *Avery's diseases of the newborn* (10th ed., p. 98). Philadelphia, PA: Elsevier; Moore, T., Hauguel-De Mouzon, S., & Catalano, P. (2019). Diabetes in pregnancy. In R. Resnik, C. Lockwood, T. Moore, M. Greene, J. Copel, & R. Silver (Eds.), *Creasy and Resnik's maternal-fetal medicine: Principles and practice* (8th ed., pp. 1094–1096). Philadelphia, PA: Elsevier.

COMMON INFECTIOUS DISEASES IN PREGNANCY

Bacterial Infections

BACTERIAL VAGINOSIS
- The primary symptom of bacterial vaginosis (BV) is a malodorous, thin, gray discharge.
- Diagnosis is based on having three of the four following symptoms:
  - Amine-like or fishy odor after intercourse or administration of KOH prep
  - Thin homogenous gray discharge
  - Elevated pH of secretions
  - Presence of clue cells on wet mount
- BV is consistently associated with preterm delivery, clinical chorioamnionitis, and endometritis.
- Treatment is typically metronidazole twice a day for 7 days or clindamycin twice a day for 7 days (Duff, 2019, pp. 865–866).

GONORRHEA
- Gonorrhea is the oldest known sexually transmitted infection (STI) and is caused by *Neisseria gonorrhoeae*, and may cause:
  - Gonococcal ophthalmia neonatorum usually onsets within 4 days after birth; incubation can be up to 21 days. If the condition is untreated, it can cause corneal ulceration, scarring, and blindness.
  - Disseminated gonococcal infection
  - Preterm premature rupture of membranes
  - Chorioamnionitis
  - Preterm delivery
  - IUGR
  - Fetal/neonatal septicemia
- All infections should be treated, and ideal treatment of uncomplicated infection is single dose of ceftriaxone (Rocephin) given intramuscularly (IM). Pregnant women should not be given quinolones or tetracyclines. It is also important for sexual partners to be treated (Duff, 2019, pp. 866–868).

CHLAMYDIA
- This is the most common bacterial sexually transmitted disease (STD) infection in the United States and is caused by *Chlamydia trachomatis*.
- Infection during pregnancy is associated with:
  - Premature prolonged rupture of membranes
  - Low birth weight
  - Preterm delivery

○ Neonatal conjunctivitis—50% of exposed infants develop it in first 2 weeks of life

○ Neonatal pneumonia—up to 20% develop pneumonia within 4 months of birth

- The preferred drug of choice for pregnant women is a single dose of azithromycin, due to increased compliance (Duff, 2019, pp. 869–871).

SYPHILIS

- Syphilis is caused by *Treponema pallidum* and is efficiently transmitted sexually, and frequently is transmitted with only a single encounter.
- Diagnosis can be made on either microscopic examination or with serologic testing.
  ○ There are nonspecific serologic tests, such as the venereal disease research laboratory (VDRL) and rapid plasma reagin (RPR) test, that will typically become nonreactive once treatment is completed.
  ○ The treponema-specific tests remain positive despite treatment.
- Parenterally administered penicillin is the preferred treatment for syphilis regardless of the stage of disease (Duff, 2019, pp. 907–908).

URINARY TRACT INFECTIONS (UTIS)

- UTIs complicate one in five pregnancies, and as such are the most common medical complication.

ASYMPTOMATIC BACTERIURIA

- Diagnosed in the presence of 1,000 or more colonies of bacteria per milliliter of urine.
- Multiple metanalyses confirm the link between asymptomatic bacteriuria (ASB) and preterm delivery and low-birth-weight infants.
- Factors that increase risk of ascending infection:
  ○ Increased excretion of bicarbonate
  ○ Glycosuria
  ○ Increased urinary excretion of estrogen (Duff, 2019, p. 873)
- The bacteria responsible are typically normal flora from gastrointestinal tract and vaginal and periurethral areas. Most common bacteria involved include:
  ○ *Escherichia coli*—Resistance is present in 30% of strains in the United States
  ○ *Klebsiella*
  ○ *Proteus*
  ○ *Staphylococcus saprophyticus*
  ○ *Group beta streptococcus (GBS)*
  ○ *Enterobacter species*
- Diagnosis is by a culture of the urine.
- Short courses of antibiotic are preferred treatment in pregnancy to minimize the risk to the fetus, to have increased patient compliance, and to minimize the emergence of resistant bacteria and associated costs.
  ○ Commonly used antibiotics are ampicillin (Omnipen), amoxicillin (Amoxil), cephalexin (Keflix), and nitrofurantoin (Macrobid).
- Because many cases of UTI predate pregnancy, there is no identified prevention strategy; however, frequent monitoring in identified women with ASB is recommended (Duff, 2019, pp. 874–875).

CYSTITIS IN PREGNANCY

- Cystitis is a distinct syndrome characterized by urinary urgency, frequency, dysuria, and suprapubic discomfort without systemic symptoms such as fever and costovertebral angle (CVA) tenderness.
- The reoccurrence risk is lower than for ASB or pyelonephritis and, unlike ASB, there are no implications for preterm birth or low birth weight.
- The responsible organisms are the same as those for ASB.
- Cystitis is diagnosed by a midstream collection of urine that has more than 100 colonies of bacteria per milliliter in women who have dysuria.
- Immediate antibiotic therapy should be started and last for 3 days on initial infection and 7 to 10 days on subsequent infections. Treated women should also get a test of cure urine culture 1 to 2 weeks after treatment is completed.
- Women who have more than three infectious episodes in a year need chronic suppressive therapy (Duff, 2019, p. 876).

ACUTE PYELONEPHRITIS

- The most common risk factors for acute pyelonephritis are the presence of ASB or a previous case of acute pyelonephritis.
- The most common strains of bacteria involved include *E. coli, Klebsiella,* and *Enterobacter* species.
- Pyelonephritis is suspected when there is a high fever, chills, flank pain, dysuria, frequency, and urgency.
  ○ Most pregnant women with pyelonephritis are initially monitored in the hospital for 12 to 24 hours secondary to the need for aggressive fluid resuscitation, need for monitoring for pulmonary overload, and need to have fetus monitored.
  ○ If pregnant patients respond to initial IV antibiotics, they may be released and continue 2 weeks of oral antibiotics (Duff, 2019, p. 878).
- Pyelonephritis can increase the risk of preterm labor and delivery. Close to one-fifth of pregnant patients with pyelonephritis go on to develop multisystem organ involvement.
- Suppression therapy is highly recommended due to the high incidence of reoccurrence (Duff, 2019, pp. 877–879).

Viral Infections

HUMAN PAPILLOMAVIRUS INFECTION

- Human papillomavirus infection (HPV) is a DNA virus that has more than 100 different types, and is the most common STI in the United States.
- Neonatal implications include respiratory papillomatosis.
- Treatment is limited to women with multiple lesions near the vaginal introitus (Duff, 2019, p. 872).

CYTOMEGALOVIRUS

- Cytomegalovirus (CMV) is a member of the herpes virus family. It is the most common congenital viral infection and may remain dormant in the host for many years.
  ○ The typical incubation period is 28 to 60 days (Duff, 2019, p. 888; Schleiss & Marsh, 2018, p. 494).
- The first-time or primary exposure of a woman in pregnancy is associated with the highest transmission risk and more serious complications for the fetus. The presence of congenital CMV infection in neonates of previously exposed women may represent reinfection with a different strain of the CMV virus (Schleiss & Marsh, 2018, p. 494).
  ○ Congenital infection risk is highest if the pregnant patient is infected in the third trimester. Conversely, the risk of congenital infection is lowest when pregnant women have a recurrent infection (Duff, 2019, p. 889).

- Serial monitoring of immunoglobulin titers can distinguish between acute and recurrent infection.
- The damage to the fetus in congenital CMV infection may represent infection of the placenta and its sequelae, as opposed to actual infection of the fetus.
- Diagnosis is made by viral culture or polymerase chain reaction (PCR). PCR is the process used in the laboratory to make copies of DNA segments. The highest concentration of the virus is in plasma, urine, seminal fluid, saliva, and breast milk.
- Testing of the neonate is important to determine when the infant was exposed. Positive test results prior to 3 weeks of age represent an in utero infection, while positive test results after 3 weeks of age can represent infection from the birth canal or via breast milk (Schleiss & Marsh, 2018, p. 497).
- Maternal treatment may be indicated in primary or recurrent infections and can decrease the incidence of symptomatic infants.
    - Maternal treatments include the use of IV hyperimmune globulin specific for CMV, or high-dose valacyclovir (Duff, 2019, p. 890; Schleiss & Marsh, 2018, p. 497).
- CMV prevention includes the use of safe sex practices, good handwashing when encountering children's diapers or toys, and avoidance of CMV-positive blood products (Duff, 2019, p. 890).

HERPES SIMPLEX VIRUS (HSV)
- HSV 1 and HSV 2 can equally cause infection in the oral cavity, skin, and anogenital areas.
- Primary infection late in pregnancy places the fetus at highest risk of transmission (Baley & Gonzalez, 2015, pp. 782–783; Duff, 2019, p. 894; Schleiss & Marsh, 2018, p. 485). The risk for neonatal transmission is lower in those women who are experiencing recurrent infection.
- Diagnosis of primary presentation is evidenced by visible painful vesicles and ulcers.
- Recurrent presentations have a shorter duration and typically less systemic symptoms.
- The gold standard for testing continues to be the viral culture; however, PCR testing is quicker and more sensitive than cultures.
- Acyclovir is the treatment of choice for outbreaks and suppressive therapy (Duff, 2019, p. 895).
- Prevention of transmission to infant is achieved by primary cesarean section if there are active genital lesions (Baley & Gonzalez, 2015, p. 786).

Viral Hepatitis

- Hepatitis A is not associated with perinatal transmission.
- Hepatitis E is only rarely associated with perinatal transmission; however, it is associated with high maternal mortality in developing countries.
- Hepatitis B, D, C, and G are associated with perinatal transmission.
    - Hepatitis A, E, C, and G are diagnosed by antibody detection.
    - Hepatitis B is diagnosed by the detection of the hepatitis B surface antigen.
    - Hepatitis D is diagnosed by antigen detection.
- Maternal antenatal therapy with tenofovir (Viread) is effective in reducing rates of perinatal transmission.

- Hepatitis A, E, and B are all prevented with specific vaccination.
- Hepatitis D is prevented by the hepatitis B vaccine.

Protozoal Infections

TRICHOMONIASIS
- Trichomoniasis is a common cause of vaginitis with characteristic intense itching, strong odor, and discharge. However, many women will have minimal to no symptoms (Duff, 2019, p. 863). The incidence of trichomoniasis may be as high as 50% of pregnancies, depending on population.
- Cultures are more sensitive than wet prep for diagnostic purposes.
- Premature rupture of membranes occurs more frequently in culture-positive pregnancies.
- Gold standard of treatment is a single dose of metronidazole.
- Routine screening is not recommended in absence of symptoms (Duff, 2019, p. 864).

TOXOPLASMOSIS
- Toxoplasmosis is a protozoan that is dependent on cats and is excreted in the cat's feces.
- Most human infections are asymptomatic, unless an immunocompromised human is involved.
    - Congenital infection is most likely to occur when the maternal infection occurs in the third trimester.
- Testing is done by PCR and detection of the antibody to toxoplasmosis.
- Treatment consists of oral sulfadiazine; treatment duration may be as long as 6 weeks.
- As a preventative measure, pregnant women should avoid encountering cat litter. If contact is necessary, litter should be changed daily and gloves always worn (Duff, 2019, pp. 910–911).

Fungal Infections

CANDIDIASIS
- Vulvovaginal candidiasis is most commonly caused by *Candida albicans*. Increased colonization can occur during pregnancy, in women with diabetes, or in those who have recently taken antibiotics or steroids (Duff, 2019, p. 862).
- Diagnosis is made by KOH wet prep/gram stain or culture of vaginal secretions. If a woman is having recurrent infections, the species of Candida can be genetically subtyped (Duff, 2019, p. 863).
- Congenital infection can manifest within the first 24 hours as superficial skin infections, oral infections, or systemic disease with involvement of multiple organs (Duff, 2019, p. 863).

COMMON HEMATOLOGIC DISEASES

Coagulation Disorders

ANTIPHOSPHOLIPID SYNDROME
- Antiphospholipid syndrome (APS) is the most common acquired thrombophilic disorder. Antibodies are produced that promote thrombosis. Women with APS are at increased risk of arterial and venous thrombosis, autoimmune thrombocytopenia, miscarriage, and fetal loss. Treatment during pregnancy is with unfractionated or low-molecular weight heparin with or without low-dose aspirin (Blackburn, 2018, p. 229; Rodger & Silver, 2019, p. 955).

- Numerous obstetrical complications increase the risk of medically indicated preterm birth:
  - Abruption
  - Fetal death
  - PE
  - IUGR
  - Recurrent pregnancy loss
- Of women with APS who reach viability in pregnancy, 50% develop PE and one-third of pregnancies have IUGR. Abnormal fetal heart rate tracings that result in cesarean delivery are common (Rodger & Silver, 2019, p. 955).

DISSEMINATED INTRAVASCULAR COAGULATION

- The risk of disseminated intravascular coagulation is higher in pregnancy in association with placental abruption, severe PE, eclampsia, intrauterine fetal death, amniotic fluid embolism, or septic abortion (Blackburn, 2018, p. 229).

INHERITED THROMBOPHILIAS

- Inherited thrombophilias are associated with venous thromboembolism (VTE). VTE includes both deep vein thrombosis and pulmonary emboli (Rodger & Silver, 2019, p. 956).
  - The risk of VTE increases up to sixfold in pregnancy. Greater than 80% of deep vein thromboses (DVTs) occur on the left because of compression of the left iliac vein by the right iliac and ovarian veins. Three-fourths of DTVs occur during the antepartum period and one-fourth during postpartum. Most pulmonary emboli occur postpartum and are associated with cesarean section (Blackburn, 2018, p. 228).
  - Unfractionated or low-molecular weight heparin is considered the drug of choice for thromboembolic disorders during pregnancy because the molecular weight of both prevents placental transfer.
    - Coumarin derivatives inhibit vitamin K-dependent coagulation factors because of their abilities to cross the placenta, whereas vitamin K-dependent coagulation factors do not. This may impair fetal coagulation and increase the risk of fetal and neonatal hemorrhage.
    - Warfarin, when given during the first 11 to 13 weeks of pregnancy, has been associated with a syndrome involving the face, eyes, bones, and central nervous system. Warfarin has also been associated with an increased risk of abortion (Blackburn, 2018, p. 228).

FACTOR V LEIDEN

- Factor V Leiden (FVL) is the most common of the serious inheritable thrombophilias and is the leading cause of activated Protein C resistance.
- FVL thrombophilia is associated with approximately 40% of VTE events in pregnant women.
- FVL thrombophilia is associated with early and late pregnancy loss (Rodger & Silver, 2019, pp. 956–957).

ANTITHROMBIN DEFICIENCY

- More than 250 mutations have been identified in the antithrombin (AT) gene. AT deficiency is the least common of the heritable thrombophilias, but can also be acquired secondary to liver impairment, sepsis, or disseminated intravascular coagulation, or due to severe nephrotic syndrome.

- Both inherited and acquired AT deficiencies are associated with VTE. AT deficiency is associated with increased risk of stillbirth after 28 weeks gestation, fetal growth restriction, abruption, and preterm delivery (Rodger & Silver, 2019, p. 960).

ACQUIRED PLATELET DISORDERS
PRIMARY IMMUNE THROMBOCYTOPENIA

- Primary immune thrombocytopenia is also known as idiopathic thrombocytopenic purpura (ITP) or autoimmune thrombocytopenia purpura, defined as a platelet count less than 100,000 cell/dL. IgG antibody binds to the platelets and makes them more susceptible to destruction. The goal of maternal treatment is to achieve a platelet count of greater than 30,000 during pregnancy and greater than 50,000 at the end of pregnancy. Treatment includes glucocorticoid drugs, IV immune globulin, rhesus immune globulin, platelet transfusion, and splenectomy.
- The fetus is at risk for thrombocytopenia due to maternal antiplatelet IgG crossing the placenta. This can lead to purpura, ecchymoses, hematuria, and melena, as well as, in rare cases, intracranial hemorrhage resulting in severe neurologic impairment or death. There is no clear evidence that cesarean delivery prevents neonatal intracranial hemorrhage.
- Delivery should be attended by a neonatologist or pediatrician who can treat possible hemorrhagic complications. Platelets, fresh frozen plasma, and IV immunoglobulin should be readily available (Rodger & Silver, 2019, pp. 966–967).

ANEMIA

- The most common anemias in pregnancy are iron deficiency anemia, megaloblastic anemia of pregnancy (folic acid deficiency), and alpha and beta thalassemia (Blackburn, 2018, p. 226).
- Maternal anemia (hemoglobin less than 8.5 g/dL) in early pregnancy is related to preterm birth, but not small-for-gestational-age infants. In women with severe anemia (hemoglobin less than 6 to 8 mg/dL), maternal arterial oxygen content and oxygen delivery to the fetus are decreased.
  - Elevated hemoglobin (greater than 14.5 g/dL) in early pregnancy is associated with stillbirth and small-for-gestational-age infants (Blackburn, 2018, p. 226).
- Fetal attempts to adapt to maternal anemia include:
  - Increased placental blood flow
  - Redistribution of blood within the fetal organs
  - Increased red blood cell (RBC) production (to increase the total oxygen-carrying capacity)
  - Decrease in diffusing distance for oxygen across the placenta
- Fetal effects from maternal anemia include:
  - Decreased growth
  - Increased mortality due to the lack of an adequate oxygen supply and nutrients (Blackburn, 2018, p. 226)

IRON DEFICIENCY ANEMIA

- The most common cause of anemia during pregnancy is iron deficiency (Blackburn, 2018, p. 226). Generally, iron deficiency anemia is preventable or easily treated with iron supplements. Even if the mother has low iron levels and is anemic, the fetus will usually not suffer. The placenta continues to transport iron to meet fetal needs (Blackburn, 2018, pp. 225–226).

- When a pregnant woman experiences severe iron deficiency and anemia, the fetus may have decreases in RBC volume, hemoglobin, iron stores, and cord ferritin levels. This may carry over to cause a worsening iron deficiency during infancy.
  - Iron deficiency anemia before midpregnancy is associated with an increased risk of low birth weight, preterm birth, and perinatal mortality (Blackburn, 2018, pp. 226–227).

MEGALOBLASTIC ANEMIA

- Folic acid deficiency is the most common cause of megaloblastic anemia in the pregnant woman. Vitamin B12 deficiency is less common in pregnancy. Severe folic acid deficiency has been associated with:
  - Maternal PE and abruptio placenta
  - Fetal malformations, including an increased risk of neural tube defects and cleft lip and palate
  - Premature birth and low birth weight
- Supplementation with folic acid is recommended for women of childbearing age to reduce the risk of neural tube defects. Supplementation should occur before pregnancy because neural tube defects occur early in the first trimester.
- In later pregnancy, the fetus has higher levels of folate and elevated folate-binding protein, which protects against fetal folate deficiency. Even with low maternal folate levels, neonatal cord levels are usually within normal limits (Blackburn, 2018, p. 227).

SICKLE CELL DISEASE

- Sickled cells can obstruct blood flow in the microvasculature. The areas most susceptible to obstruction are those characterized by slow flow and high oxygen extraction, such as the spleen, bone marrow, and placenta. Obstruction leads to venous stasis, further deoxygenation, platelet aggregation, hypoxia, acidosis, further sickling, and eventually infarction (Blackburn, 2018, p. 227).
- A woman with sickle cell anemia normally has a lower hemoglobin level and oxygen-carrying capacities. Women may become slightly more anemic as plasma volume increases during the pregnancy and may experience an increased risk of sickling attacks.
- Fetal and neonatal complications of prematurity and fetal growth restriction arise secondary to placental infarction and fetal hypoxia. Fetal hypoxia is a result of decreased oxygen transport due to abnormal biochemistry of the maternal hemoglobin and loss of placental tissue for gas and nutrient exchange caused by the infarctions (Blackburn, 2018, p. 227).

THALASSEMIA

- Thalassemia leads to alterations in the RBC membrane and decreased RBC life span due to a disorder in the synthesis of the alpha or beta-peptide chains of the hemoglobin molecule.
- *Alpha thalassemia* is an alteration in the production of alpha chains. The severity of presentation is dependent on how many of the four genes on chromosome 16 that are involved in alpha chain production are nonfunctional or have altered function. Pregnant women with alpha thalassemia with one or two genes affected have mild anemia or "silent presentation." If all four alpha genes are missing, the fetus is able to synthesize neither normal fetal hemoglobin nor adult hemoglobin. These infants develop high output cardiac failure and hydrops fetalis, and are often stillborn or die shortly after birth.

- Treatments for the fetus and newborn include intrauterine transfusions (decreased perinatal mortality and morbidity), lifelong transfusion therapy, and stem cell transplants (Blackburn, 2018, p. 227).
- *Beta thalassemia major* often results in females dying in childhood or adolescence. If females survive, they are often infertile. Women with *Beta thalassemia minor* have a mild hypochromic, microcytic anemia, and generally do not have an increased maternal or infant morbidity if their condition is stable (Blackburn, 2018, p. 228).

FETAL ASSESSMENT

The goal of fetal assessment is to identify fetuses that are adequately oxygenated or at risk for hypoxia, reduce perinatal morbidity and mortality, and decrease stillbirth and long-term neurologic injury (Cypher, 2016, p. 135; Hackney, 2015, p. 181). Table 1.8 identified indications for fetal surveillance.

TABLE 1.8 Indications for Fetal Surveillance

Indications for Fetal Surveillance	
Maternal Conditions	**Pregnancy Related or Fetal Conditions**
Antiphospholipid syndrome Cyanotic heart disease Systemic lupus erythematosus Chronic renal disease Diabetes requiring medication Hypertension Cholestasis Hyperthyroidism (poorly controlled) Hemoglobinopathies (hemoglobin SS, SC, or S-thalassemia)	Hyertension (gestational or preeclampsia) Gestational diabetes requiring medication Decreased fetal movement Amniotic fluid volume disorders (oligo- or polyhydramnios) Intrauterine growth restriction Postterm pregnancy Isoimmunization Previous intrauterine fetal demise Multiple gestation Previous fetal demise Preterm premature rupture of membranes Unexplained third-trimester bleeding

Sources: Data from Cypher, R. L. (2016). Antepartum fetal surveillance and prenatal diagnosis. In S. Mattson & J. E. Smith (Eds.), *Core curriculum for maternal-newborn nursing* (5th ed., pp. 135–136). St Louis, MO: Saunders Elsevier; Hackney, D. N. (2015). Estimation of fetal well-being. In R. Martin, A. Fanaroff, & M. Walsh (Eds.), *Fanaroff and Martin's neonatal-perinatal medicine: Diseases of the fetus and infant* (10th ed., p. 182). Philadelphia, PA: Elsevier.

- Other indications for prenatal screening include advanced maternal age, a parent or previous fetus/infant with a chromosomal abnormality, and an increased risk of chromosomal or structural anomaly based on noninvasive screen results (Cypher, 2016, p. 136).
- Methods of antenatal testing are either screening or diagnostic:
  - Antenatal screening methods are not definite, are reported as a ratio of the likelihood the fetus will be abnormal, and include measurements of

maternal serum analytes, ultrasound evaluations, or both. Screening methods evaluate for risk of structural abnormalities (open neural tube defects or ventral wall defects), fetal aneuploidy (Trisomy 21, 13, and 18), and placental abnormalities (Cypher, 2016, p. 148).

○ In a best case scenario, diagnostic testing will determine if the fetus is affected or not affected. However, no test is 100% effective or correct. Some fetal anomalies can be diagnosed with ultrasound. Fetal tissue samples may be required for diagnosis of fetal karyotype abnormalities. Chorionic villous sampling or amniocentesis is used to obtain fetal samples, each with its own limitations and risks (Cypher, 2016, p. 148).

Fetal Fibronectin

• Fetal fibronectin (fFN) is a protein secreted by the trophoblast and is thought to play a role in the placental–uterine attachment. fFN is normally present in vaginal or cervical fluid prior to 20 weeks. After 20 weeks, fFN may be an indication of imminent labor.

• The fFN is used to evaluate women with premature contractions when diagnosis or premature labor is uncertain.

○ A negative fFN test with other reassuring signs, such as no sign of infection, abruption, or progressive cervical change, can be used to avoid more invasive interventions, such as admission, tocolysis, or glucocorticoid administration (Barron, 2014, p. 112).

Nonstress Test

• The nonstress test (NST) is the most common antepartum screen (Barron, 2014, p. 113; Cypher, 2016, p. 139) performed after 32 weeks gestational age. Fetal heart rate is monitored as well as uterine activity. Results are given as reactive, nonreactive, or inadequate.

○ A reactive NST: heart rate between 110 and 160 beats per minute (bpm), normal beat-to-beat variability (5 bpm), and two accelerations of at least 15 bpm lasting at least 15 seconds within 20 minutes.
  ▪ A reactive NST is reassuring with a decreased risk of fetal demise in the following week (Barron, 2014, p. 113) of approximately 3 in 1,000 (Dukhivny & Wilkins-Haug, 2017, p. 8).

○ A nonreactive test is defined as less than two accelerations in 40 minutes (Barron, 2014, p. 113; Cypher, 2016, p. 139; Hackney, 2015, p. 182; Kaimal, 2014, p. 551; Dukhivny & Wilkins-Haug, 2017, p. 8).
  ▪ A nonreactive NST is typically repeated later the same day or another test of fetal well-being is performed (Dukhivny & Wilkins-Haug, 2017, p. 8), such as ultrasound (Barron, 2014, p. 113; Cypher, 2016, p. 139; Hackney, 2015, p. 183; Kaimal, 2014, p. 551).

• The NST is commonly performed weekly, although twice-weekly testing is recommended for high-risk conditions (Cypher, 2016, p. 140; Dukhivny & Wilkins-Haug, 2017, p. 9; Hackney, 2015, p. 186).

Biophysical Profile

• The BPP provides an indication of fetal well-being when there is risk for altered oxygenation (Cypher, 2016, p. 142).

• The BPP combines an NST with amniotic fluid volume (vertical fluid pocket >2 cm), fetal breathing movements, fetal activity, and normal fetal musculoskeletal tone. A score of 0 to 2 is assigned to each category.

○ Reassuring tests, with a score of 8 to 10, are repeated weekly.

○ Less reassuring results, with a score of 5 to 6, are repeated the same day.

○ Very low scores of 0 to 4 may indicate need for delivery (Barron, 2014, p. 114; Cypher, 2016, p. 143; Dukhivny & Wilkins-Haug, 2017, pp. 9–10; Hackney, 2015, p. 183; Kaimal, 2014, p. 551).

• The likelihood a fetus will die in utero within 1 week of a reassuring BPP is approximately 0.6 to 0.7 per 1,000. The negative predictive value for a stillbirth within 1 week of a reassuring BPP is >99.9% (Dukhivny & Wilkins-Haug, 2017, p. 10).

Ultrasound

• Ultrasound can be used for dating confirmation, early detection of anomalies, and assessment of fetal well-being (Barron, 2014, p. 111; Cypher, 2016, p. 151) as well as a screening tool for detection of aneuploidy in the second semester. When combined with first-trimester screening for aneuploidy, the use of ultrasound (US) has been shown valuable in decreasing the risk assessment for trisomy 21 (Dukhivny & Wilkins-Haug, 2017, p. 4).

• Doppler flow studies assess maternal–fetal blood flow in the umbilical artery, middle cerebral artery, umbilical vein, and ductus venosus, and provide information regarding fetal adaptation and reserve (Cypher, 2016, p. 144; Kaimal, 2014, p. 557). Changes in blood flow represent systolic and diastolic shifts during the cardiac cycle (Cypher, 2016, p. 144; Hackney, 2015, p. 184).

○ Absent end-diastolic flow (AEDF) indicates elevated placental resistance leading to no blood flow in diastole (Cypher, 2016, p. 144; Kaimal, 2014, p. 556).

○ Reversed diastolic flow (REDF) indicates absent end-diastolic flow that has continued for a prolonged period and is more indicative of a poor outcome, which includes fetal or neonatal death (Cypher, 2016, p. 144; Kaimal, 2014, p. 557).

○ Findings of absent or reversed end-diastolic flow indicate a need to prepare for delivery (Kaimal, 2014, p. 557).

Amniocentesis

• Amniocentesis is performed under ultrasound guidance and can be performed as early as 10 to 14 weeks gestation. It is typically performed in the second trimester at 15 to 20 weeks (Barron, 2014, p. 112; Cypher, 2016, p. 150; Stark, 2017, p. 5).

○ Amniocentesis performed earlier than 13 weeks is associated with an increased incidence of club foot as well as an increased pregnancy loss rate of 1% to 2%, compared to 0.5% to 1% when performed during the second trimester (16–20 weeks; Dukhivny & Wilkins-Haug, 2017, p. 5).

• Amniotic fluid can be analyzed for alpha-fetoprotein (AFP), acetylcholinesterase (AchE), bilirubin, and pulmonary surfactant (Barron, 2014, p. 112; Cypher, 2016, p. 150; Dukhivny & Wilkins-Haug, 2017, p. 5). Increased AFP in combination with AChE in amniotic fluid has a sensitivity of >98% for identification of neural tube defects (Dukhivny & Wilkins-Haug, 2017, p. 5).

- Fetal cells can be analyzed for chromosomes and genetic makeup (Cypher, 2016, p. 150; Dukhivny & Wilkins-Haug, 2017, p. 5). Fluorescence in situ hybridization (FISH) can detect second-trimester karyotype abnormalities of chromosomes 13, 18, 21, X, or Y with approximately 90% sensitivity (Dukhivny & Wilkins-Haug, 2017, p. 5).

ALPHA FETOPROTEIN/TRIPLE OR QUAD SCREENS
- Alpha fetoprotein (AFP) is a fetal-specific molecule synthesized by the fetal yolk sac, fetal GIT, and fetal liver.
  - The maternal serum AFP (MSAFP) is usually significantly lower than the AFP in the fetal plasma or in the amniotic fluid (Bajaj & Gross, 2015, p. 140).
- MSAPF is drawn between 15 and 25 weeks (Bajaj & Gross, 2015, p. 140; Stark, 2017, p. 2). MSAFP is included in second-trimester testing as a triple screen or quad screen.
  - The triple screen includes MSAFP, human chorionic gonadotropin, and unconjugated estriol.
  - The quad screen includes the aforementioned in addition to inhibin (Cypher, 2016, p. 148).
- MSAFP testing should be offered to all women. MSAFP levels elevated above 2.5 multiples of the median for gestational age are considered abnormal (Bajaj & Gross, 2015, p. 140; Dukhivny & Wilkins-Haug, 2017, p. 2). Elevated MSAFP occurs in 70% to 85% of fetuses with open spina bifida and 95% of fetuses with anencephaly (Dukhivny & Wilkins-Haug, 2017, p. 2). Elevated MSAFP is also associated with ventral wall defects (Bajaj & Gross, 2015, p. 140).
- Clinicians may opt to repeat MASFP testing after the first moderately elevated result. On repeat analysis, one-third is below the threshold. A repeat test that is below the threshold after an elevated test has not been associated with an increase in false-negative results (Bajaj & Gross, 2015, p. 140).

ULTRASOUND AS FOLLOW-UP TO ELEVATED MASFP
- The next step in the face of a repeat elevated MSAFP, or if a repeat MSAFP is not done, is an ultrasound (Bajaj & Gross, 2015, p. 140). In half of women with elevated levels, ultrasonic examination reveals another cause. This is most commonly an error in the estimate of gestational age (Dukhivny & Wilkins-Haug, 2017, p. 2). Ultrasound that incorporates changes in head shape (lemon sign) or cerebellar deformity (banana sign) increases the sensitivity of ultrasound for visual detection of open spinal defects (Dukhivny & Wilkins-Haug, 2017, p. 2).

AMNIOCENTESIS AS FOLLOW-UP TO ELEVATED MASFP
- The option of amniocentesis should also be discussed with the patient (Bajaj & Gross, 2015, p. 140).
- The two main analytes measured in amniotic fluid are amniotic fluid AFP and amniotic fluid AChe. Elevated amniotic fluid AFP and AChe predict an open fetal neural tube defect (NTD) with 96% accuracy, and have a false-positive rate of 0.14% (Bajaj & Gross, 2015, p. 140). Contamination of the amniotic fluid sample with blood accounts for half of false-positive results. A fetal karyotype should also be performed on the amniotic fluid obtained (Bajaj & Gross, 2015, p. 140).

OUTCOMES
- An elevated MSAFP in the second trimester that cannot be explained by fetal structural abnormality or underlying maternal conditions is associated with poor fetal outcomes, including increased risk of intrauterine fetal demise, placental abruption, and PE (Bajaj & Gross, 2015, p. 140).

CONCLUSION

The healthy development of the fetus is dependent on the health status of the mother. Alterations in the cardiorespiratory, hematologic, or endocrine systems may adversely affect the fetus by either their presence or treatments needed to correct these alterations. Close monitoring of both maternal and fetal well-being is vital to ensure a positive outcome to the pregnancy.

REVIEW QUESTIONS

1. The most common complication in pregnancy is gestational:
   A. Anemia.
   B. Diabetes.
   C. Hypertension.

2. Changes to the maternal pulmonary system during pregnancy include a decrease in the woman's:
   A. Alveolar minute ventilation.
   B. Functional residual capacity.
   C. Overall oxygen consumption.

3. Administration of the varicella vaccine within 3 months of conception has been associated with a/an:
   A. Absence of fetal varicella infection.
   B. Decreased risk of maternal pneumonia.
   C. Increased risk of birth defects.

4. Pregnant women should be cautioned against allowing infections with *N. gonorrhoeae* to go untreated due to effects on the fetus, including the:
   A. Complications of chorioamnionitis.
   B. Potential for neonatal presbyopia.
   C. Likelihood of experiencing a birth injury.

5. The biophysical profile (BPP) antenatal screening combines a nonstress test (NST) with measurements of amniotic fluid volume, fetal breathing movements, fetal musculoskeletal tone, and fetal:
   A. Femur length.
   B. Motor activity.
   C. Velocity flow.

REFERENCES

Arafeh, J. (2014). Cardiac disease in pregnancy. In K. Simpson & P. Creehan (Eds.), *Perinatal nursing* (4th ed., pp. 224–245). St. Louis, MO: Lippincott Williams & Wilkins.

Bajaj, K., & Gross, S. J. (2015). Genetic aspects of perinatal disease and prenatal diagnosis. In R. Martin, A. Fanaroff, & M. Walsh (Eds.), *Fanaroff and Martin's neonatal-perinatal medicine: Diseases of the fetus and infant* (10th ed., pp. 130–146). Philadelphia, PA: Elsevier.

Baley, J., & Gonzalez, B. (2015). Perinatal viral infections. In R. Martin, A. Fanaroff, & M. Walsh (Eds.), *Fanaroff and Martin's neonatal-perinatal medicine: Diseases of the fetus and infant* (10th ed., pp. 782–833). Philadelphia, PA: Elsevier.

Barron, M. L. (2014). Antenatal care. In K. R. Simpson & P. A. Creehan (Eds.), *Perinatal nursing* (4th ed., pp. 89–121) Philadelphia, PA: LWW.

Blackburn, S. T. (2018). *Maternal fetal & neonatal physiology: A clinical perspective* (5th ed.). Philadelphia, PA: Elsevier.

Blanchard, D., & Daniels, L. (2019). Cardiac diseases. In R. Resnik, C. Lockwood, T. Moore, M. Greene, J. Copel, & R. Silver (Eds.), *Creasy and Resnik's maternal-fetal medicine: Principles and practice* (8th ed., pp. 920–948.e3). Philadelphia, PA: Elsevier.

Brown, Z., & Chang, J. (2018). Maternal diabetes. In C. Gleason & S. Juul (Eds.), *Avery's diseases of the newborn* (10th ed., pp. 90–103). Philadelphia, PA: Elsevier.

Cypher, R. L. (2016). Antepartum fetal surveillance and prenatal diagnosis. In S. Mattson & J. E. Smith (Eds.), *Core curriculum for maternal-newborn nursing* (5th ed., pp. 135–158). St Louis, MO: Saunders Elsevier.

Daley, J. (2014). Diabetes in pregnancy. In K. Simpson & P. Creehan (Eds.), *Perinatal nursing* (4th ed., pp. 203–223). St. Louis, MO: Lippincott Williams & Wilkins.

Dukhivny, S., & Wilkins-Haug, L. E. (2017). Fetal assessment and prenatal diagnosis. In E. C. Eichenwald, A. R. Hansen, C. R. Martin, & A. R. Stark (Eds.), *Cloherty and Stark's manual of neonatal care* (8th ed., pp. 1–14) Philadelphia, PA: Lippincott, Williams & Wilkins.

Duff, P. (2019). Maternal and fetal infections. In R. Resnik, C. Lockwood, T. Moore, M. Greene, J. Copel, & R. Silver (Eds.), *Creasy and Resnik's maternal-fetal medicine: Principles and practice* (8th ed., pp. 862–919.e8). Philadelphia, PA: Elsevier.

Hackney, D. N. (2015). Estimation of fetal well-being. In R. Martin, A. Fanaroff, & M. Walsh (Eds.), *Fanaroff and Martin's neonatal-perinatal medicine: Diseases of the fetus and infant* (10th ed., pp. 1181–195). Philadelphia, PA: Elsevier.

Harper, L., Tita, A., & Karumanchi, S. (2019). Pregnancy-related hypertension. In R. Resnik, C. Lockwood, T. Moore, M. Greene, J. Copel, & R. Silver (Eds.), *Creasy and Resnik's maternal-fetal medicine: Principles and practice* (8th ed., pp. 810–838.e9). Philadelphia, PA: Elsevier.

Jeyabalan, A. (2015). Hypertensive disorders of pregnancy. In R. Martin, A. Fanaroff, & M. Walsh (Eds.), *Fanaroff and Martin's neonatal-perinatal medicine: Diseases of the fetus and infant* (10th ed., pp. 250–264). Philadelphia, PA: Elsevier.

Kaimal, A. J. (2019). Assessment of fetal health. In R. Resnik, C. Lockwood, T. Moore, M. Greene, J. Copel, & R. Silver (Eds.). *Creasy and Resnik's maternal-fetal medicine: Principles and practice* (8th ed., pp. 549–563.e3). Philadelphia, PA: Elsevier.

Moore, T., Hauguel-De Mouzon, S., & Catalano, P. (2019). Diabetes in pregnancy. In R. Resnik, C. Lockwood, T. Moore, M. Greene, J. Copel, & R. Silver (Eds.), *Creasy and Resnik's maternal-fetal medicine: Principles and practice* (8th ed., pp. 1067–1097.e5). Philadelphia, PA: Elsevier.

Moore, T., (2018). Hypertensive complications of pregnancy. In C. Gleason & S. Juul (Eds.), *Avery's diseases of the newborn* (10th ed., pp. 119–125e2). Philadelphia, PA: Elsevier.

Nodine, P., Hastings-Tolsma, M., & Arruda, J. (2016). Prenatal environment: Effect on neonatal outcome. In S. Gardner, B. Carter, M. Hines, & J. Hernandez (Eds.), *Merenstein & Gardner's handbook of neonatal intensive care* (8th ed., pp. 11–31). St. Louis, MO: Elsevier.

Poole, J. (2014). Hypertensive disorders of pregnancy. In K. Simpson & P. Creehan (Eds.). *Perinatal nursing* (4th ed., pp. 122–142). St. Louis, MO: Lippincott Williams & Wilkins.

Rodger, M., & Silver, R. M. (2019). Coagulation disorders in pregnancy. In R. Resnik, C. Lockwood, T. Moore, M. Greene, J. Copel, & R. Silver (Eds.), *Creasy and Resnik's maternal-fetal medicine: Principles and practice* (8th ed., pp. 1309–1333.e8). Philadelphia, PA: Elsevier.

Schleiss, M., & Marsh, K. (2018). Viral infections of the fetus and newborn. In C. Gleason & S. Juul (Eds.), *Avery's diseases of the newborn* (10th ed., pp. 482–526.e19). Philadelphia, PA: Elsevier.

Whitty, J., & Dombrowski, M. (2019). Respiratory diseases in pregnancy. In R. Resnik, C. Lockwood, T. Moore, M. Greene, J. Copel, & R. Silver (Eds.), *Creasy and Resnik's maternal-fetal medicine: Principles and practice* (8th ed., pp. 1043–1066.e3). Philadelphia, PA: Elsevier.

2 MATERNAL HISTORY IN THE INTRAPARTUM

Cheryl B. Robinson

INTRODUCTION

Every pregnancy, whether complicated or not, can be drastically altered during intrapartum. For the fetus, intrapartum places additional physiological stressors. Depending on the fetus' tolerance of labor and delivery, the Neonatal Nurse Practitioner (NNP) must be ready to intervene as the neonate makes the transition to life outside of the womb. An understanding of the intrapartum period, and the events that transpire prior to the actual delivery, is requisite knowledge for successful resuscitation and stabilization.

INTRAPARTUM

- Intrapartum covers the period of time from onset of labor to generally 1 hour after delivery of the neonate. The intrapartum period can be considered high risk based on medical conditions of the mother either present prior to pregnancy or as a complication of the pregnancy, or due to events occurring during the labor process placing the mother and/or fetus at risk for morbidity or mortality.
- The appropriate timing of labor and subsequent birth is strongly associated with positive perinatal outcomes. Infants born prior to 37 0/7 weeks are considered preterm, and those born after 42 0/7 weeks, or 294 days after the first day of the last menstrual cycle, are considered post-term (Norwitz, Mahendroo, & Lye, 2019).
- There is no one theory adequately explaining why labor begins. Combined maternal–fetal processes are initiated to decrease uterine quiescence and increase uterine activity (Simpson & O'Brien-Abel, 2014). Although the communication pathways between mother, fetus, and placenta requires a sequential initiation, redundancy in positive feedforward and negative feedback loops prevent any one single factor to be responsible for the onset of labor (Simpson & O'Brien-Abel, 2014, p. 343).
- Intrapartum has been divided into four stages and is summarized in Table 2.1.

The Placenta

- The uterine extracellular matrix is signaled to remodel as the blastocyst adheres to endometrial uterodomes and is eventually surrounded by maternal circulation. The embryonic yolk sac develops a vein system to enhance nutrient transport and an acceleration of cellular differentiation results in the embryo attachment to the primitive placenta.

TABLE 2.1 The Four Stages of the Intrapartum

First Stage—progression measured by cervical changes	Latent: 0–3 cm Active: 4–7 or 6 cm for nulliparous women and 5 cm for multiparous women Transition: 8–10 cm
Second Stage—complete cervical dilation and ends with the birth of the baby	Initial latent phase (passive fetal descent) Active pushing phase
Third Stage—begins with the birth of the baby and ends with the delivery of the placenta	
Fourth Stage—begins with delivery of the placenta and ends with stabilization of mother in the immediate postpartum period	

Source: Data from Simpson, K. R., & O'Brien-Abel, N. (2014). Labor and birth. In K. Simpson & P. Creehan (Eds.), *Perinatal nursing* (4th ed., pp. 343–444). St. Louis, MO: Lippincott Williams & Wilkins.

Placenta Previa

PATHOGENESIS

- The underlying pathogenesis of placenta previa is unknown. It is described as painless third-trimester bleeding. All women presenting with painless vaginal bleeding after 20 weeks' gestation should be assumed to have a placenta previa until proven otherwise (Hull, Resnik, & Silver, 2019, pp. 786–787).
- Vital to the definition is the exact location of the placenta in relation to the internal cervical os. Two terms are recommended: placenta previa and low-lying placenta. A transvaginal ultrasound (TVUS) after 16 weeks' gestation can have the following results:
  - ○ Normal—Placental edge is 2 cm or more from the internal cervical os.
  - ○ Low lying—Placental edge is <2 cm from internal cervical os.
  - ○ Placenta previa—Placental edge covers the internal cervical os (Hull et al., 2019, p. 787).
- Bleeding prior to labor results from the lower uterine segment development, effacement of the cervix with increasing gestational age, prelabor uterine contractions, intercourse, and vaginal examination. Bleeding during labor is due to cervical dilatation and the forces separating the placenta from the underlying decidua (Hull et al., 2019, p. 787).

- Low lying and placenta previa should be delivered by cesarean section even though there is a risk of intraoperative hemorrhage.
- Risk factors for placenta previa include the following:
  - Prior pregnancy complicated by placenta previa
  - Prior cesarean section
  - Advanced maternal age (>35 years of age)
  - Multiparity
  - Prior suction curettage
  - Smoking (Hull et al., 2019, p. 786)

FETAL/NEONATAL COMPLICATIONS

- Due to the risk of postpartum hemorrhage, neonatal resuscitation may depend on the amount of maternal blood loss (Hull et al., 2019, p. 788).

Vasa Previa

PATHOGENESIS

- Although rare, vasa previa occurs with the improper insertion of the umbilical cord into the placenta and can have grave consequences for a fetus. In vasa previa, the insertion of the umbilical cord into the placenta is velamentous, with the umbilical vessels coursing through the fetal membranes before inserting into the placental disk and the unsupported vessels then overlying the cervix (Hull et al., 2019, p. 791).
  - Unrecognized or overlooked, the fetal mortality rate is almost 60% because at rupture of membranes (ROM), there is tearing of fetal vessels. Because the entire fetal cardiac output passes through the cord, it can take <10 minutes for total fetal exsanguination to occur (Hull et al., 2019, p. 791).
- Risk factors for vasa previa include the following:
  - A low-lying placenta
  - Multiple gestation
  - In vitro fertilization (Hull et al., 2019, p. 791)

Fetal/Neonatal Complications

- Exsanguination of the fetus, and, if born alive, the neonate will present with profound hypoxia, acidemia, hypovolemic shock, and severe respiratory and cardiovascular compromise (Hull et al., 2019, p. 791)

Abruptio Placentae

PATHOGENESIS

- Abruptio placentae is the premature separation of a normally sited placenta before birth, after 20 weeks' gestation. Incidence peaks between 24 and 26 weeks' gestation. The degree of abruption ranges across a broad clinical spectrum, from minor degrees of placental separation, with little effect on maternal or fetal outcome, to major abruption, associated with fetal death and maternal morbidity (Hull et al., 2019, p. 793).
- Abruption results from bleeding between the decidua and placenta with the hemorrhage dissecting the decidua apart. When this happens, there is loss of the corresponding placental area for gaseous exchange and provision of fetal nutrition.
- Although the process may sometimes be self-limited, there can be ongoing further dissection of the decidua.

Dissection can lead to external bleeding if it reaches the placental edge and tracks down between the fetal membranes; circumferential dissection leading to near-total separation of the placenta can occur, particularly with concealed abruption.
- The underlying event in many cases of abruption is thought to be vasospasm of abnormal maternal arterioles, but abruption may also occur due to trauma, such as motor vehicle accident. The trauma causes acute shearing forces affecting the placenta–decidua interface. The sudden decompression of an overdistended uterus (such as occurs with membrane rupture in polyhydramnios) or delivery of a multiple-gestation pregnancy can also lead to abruption (Hull et al., 2019, p. 794).
- Risk factors for abruption include the following:
  - A history of a previous abruption
  - Maternal hypertension
  - Smoking
  - Preeclampsia
  - Substance abuse (cocaine or crack cocaine) causing vasospasm or abrupt increases in blood pressure
  - Multiparity
  - The presence of uterine fibroids (Hull et al., 2019, p. 794)

FETAL/NEONATAL COMPLICATIONS

- Infant outcomes are associated with increased rates of perinatal asphyxia, intraventricular hemorrhage, periventricular leukomalacia, and cerebral palsy (Hoyt & Pages-Arroyo, 2015; Hull et al., 2019, p. 793).

AMNIOTIC FLUID

Fluid Volume

- The rate of change of amniotic fluid (AF) volume depends on the gestational age. AF volume increases progressively between 10 and 30 weeks of gestation. After 30 weeks the increase slows, and AF volume may remain unchanged until 36 to 38 weeks of gestation, when it tends to decrease (Ross & Beall, 2019, p. 62).
  - At 12 weeks' gestation, the amount of AF is approximately 50 mL and continues rising throughout pregnancy to a high of about 1000 mL between 36 and 38 weeks' gestation. After 38 weeks' gestation, the amount of AF starts to decrease. AF contains 98% to 99% water, with its solute composition changing throughout gestation (Dubil & Magann, 2015, p. 340).
- Throughout gestation, amniotic fluid volume (AFV) is highly regulated, gradually increasing in the first trimester, stabilizing in the second trimester, and decreasing late in the third trimester while remaining in a relatively narrow range of volumes (Dubil & Magann, 2015, p. 343)
- AFV is determined by the amniotic fluid index (AFI), which is measured by ultrasound. In each quadrant of the uterus, the vertical measure of the fluid pockets that do not include the umbilical cord are added together (Rezaee, Lappen, & Gecsi, 2013, p. 24).
- Sonographic techniques to estimate AFV include subjective (qualitative) estimation, which includes designations of normal, increased, decreased, or absent; and semiquantitative methods: measurement of a two-diameter pocket (2×2), maximum vertical or single deepest pocket (SDP), and the AFI (Dubil & Magann, 2015, p. 341).

Functions

- AF is necessary for normal human fetal growth and development. The fluid volume cushions the fetus, protecting both the fetus and umbilical cord from mechanical trauma or external injury, and its bacteriostatic properties may help to maintain a sterile intrauterine environment and steady temperature. The space created by the AF allows fetal movement, aids in the normal development of both the lungs and the limbs, and prevents amnion from adhering to the fetus. Finally, AF offers convenient access to fetal cells and metabolic by products, and it has been used for fetal diagnosis more often than any other gestational tissue (Ross & Beall, 2019, p. 62).

Production and Composition of AF

- Fetal swallowing, urination, pulmonary secretions, nonkeratinized skin, intramembranous (IM) movement between fetal blood and the placenta, and transmembranous movement across the amnion and chorion account for the movement of AF and solutes.
  - Swallowing in the fetus is demonstrated between 8 and 11 weeks' gestation, with increasing volumes noted as gestational age increases (Dubil & Magann, 2015, p. 341). Near-term fetal swallowed volume is subject to periodic increases as mechanisms for thirst and appetite develop functionality. However, despite the fetal ability to modulate swallowing, this modulation is unlikely to be responsible for AF volume regulation (Ross & Beal, 2019, p. 64).
  - Renal nephrons are formed at 9 to 11 weeks, at which time fetal urine is excreted into the AF. The amount of urine produced increases progressively with advancing gestation, and it constitutes a significant proportion of the AF in the second half of pregnancy (Ross & Beall, 2019, p. 63) Renal agenesis is therefore associated with low AF levels (Dubil & Magann, 2015, p. 340).
  - Driven by chloride ion exchange across the pulmonary epithelium, approximately 300 to 400 mL of fluid is excreted from the fetal pulmonary system (Dubil & Magann, 2015, p. 340). Under physiologic conditions, half of the fluid exiting the lungs enters the AF and half is swallowed; therefore, although total lung fluid production approximates one third that of urine production, the net AF contribution made by lung fluid is only one sixth that of urine Ross & Beall, 2019, p. 63).
  - Since fetal skin remains nonkeratinized until week 22 to 25, surface exchange is a main factor contributing to fluid dynamics in early pregnancy (Dubil & Magann, 2015, p. 340). It is thought that early AF arises as a transudate of plasma, either from the fetus through nonkeratinized fetal skin or from the mother across the uterine decidua or the placenta surface or both; however, the actual mechanism is unknown (Ross & Beall, 2019, p. 63).
  - Because the volume of AF does not greatly increase during the latter half of pregnancy, another route of fluid absorption is likely. The most likely route is the IM pathway: the route of absorption from the amniotic cavity directly across the amnion into the fetal vessels. Studies have demonstrated a continuous, bidirectional flow of water and solutes from AF to the fetal circulation in vivo (Ross & Beall, 2019, pp. 64–65).

- Transmembranous movement across the amnion and chorion involves discussion of fluid dynamics and water permeability of the biologic membranes. This process may involve any or all of the following:
  - Simple diffusion
  - Diffusion of hydrophilic substances
  - Facilitated diffusion
  - Active transport
  - Receptor-mediated endocytosis (Ross & Beall, 2019, p. 65)
- See Figure 2.1

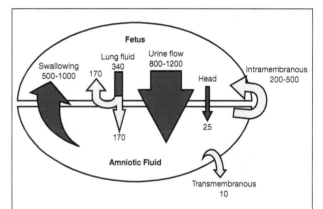

FIGURE 2.1 Pathways between the fetus and amniotic fluid (in milliliters)

Source: Reproduced with permission from Gilbert, W. M., Moore, T. R., Brace, R. A. (1991). Amniotic fluid volume dynamics. *Fetal and Maternal Medicine Review, 3,* 89. Cambridge University Press.

Oligohydramnios

PATHOPHYSIOLOGY

- Oligohydramnios has been defined as an AFV that is <200 mL: and occurs in 1% to 2% of pregnancies. A sonograph assessment of a single deepest pocket (SDP) <2 cm and an AFI <5 cm, or a qualitative assessment of a low-volume can also lead to a diagnosis of oligohydramnois (Dubil & Magann, 2015, p. 345). Additional assessment findings include estimated fetal size less than maternal dates.
- Low AF can be caused by underproduction or loss, or can be idiopathic. Underproduction can be the result of absent or dysfunctional kidneys, urinary tract obstruction, uteroplacental insufficiency, maternal medications, or maternal dehydration. Loss is also caused by ROM (Dubil & Magann, 2015, p. 345).
- If oligohydramnios is prolonged and occurs during the canalicular phase of alveolar proliferation (16–18 weeks' gestation), severe pulmonary hypoplasia associated with a high perinatal mortality can occur. Although the exact physiologic cause of pulmonary hypoplasia is unclear, any maternal or fetal complication leading to the inhibition of fetal breathing, any lack of a trophic function of AF within the airways, or any simple mechanical compression of the chest are proposed as causes (Dubil & Magann, 2015, p. 348).
  - Associated with postmature infants, renal agenesis, polycystic kidneys, and fetal urinary tract obstructions.
  - Leakage of AF

Fetal/Neonatal Complications

- The NNP should expect with a maternal diagnosis of oligohydramnios for there to be close medical and nursing supervision, with associated fetal monitoring. The labor will likely be induced and there may be the presence of amnioinfusion during labor.
- Preparation for an emergent cesarean section, along with an intensive resuscitation and stabilization, should be anticipated. The neonate will likely have wrinkled, leathery skin, and may have skeletal deformities or experience fetal hypoxia.
- If oligohydramnios is present in a postdate pregnancy, the loss of AF may be from leaking membranes. The possibility of perinatal/fetal infection should be assessed.

Polyhydramnios

PATHOPHYSIOLOGY

- The exact cause of polyhydramnios is unknown. Risk factors include multiple gestations, Rh-sensitized pregnancies, and fetal gastrointestinal obstructions and atresias.
- Polyhydramnios is generally defined as an AF level >20 or a volume of 2000 mL of fluid. Fluid pockets can be >8 cm and the condition can have a chronic or rapid onset (Dubil & Magann, 2015, p. 350).
- The etiology of an increased AF level falls into three categories: decreased absorption, overproduction, or idiopathic. Fetal swallowing is the predominant mechanism of AF removal, so congenital abnormalities associated with the gastrointestinal track (tracheal atresia, duodenal atresia, tracheal or bowel obstruction) or the neurologic system (anencephaly, trisomy 18, trisomy 21) are often present (Dubil & Magin, 2015).
- Other factors that can contribute to an overproduction of AF include maternal diabetes, syphilis, Rh isoimmunization or the presence of atypical antibodies that might lead to hemolytic disease of the newborn, certain fetal or placental (chorioangioma) abnormalities, and a recent history of maternal infection. In the presence of gestational or adult-onset diabetes, increased fetal urination can account a diagnosis of polyhydramnios, as well as a macrosomia (Dubil & Magann, 2015).
- Idiopathic causes account for 50% to 60% of the cases of polyhydramnios. Only 1% to 2% of all pregnancies are complicated by polyhydramnios. Muscular dystrophies, fetal akinesia, and skeletal dysplasias may also be present when polyhydramnios is diagnosed (Dubil & Magann, 2015, p. 351).
- In anatomically normal fetuses with otherwise unexplained polyhydramnios, diabetes should be suspected, particularly if there is fetal macrosomia or asymmetrically larger fetal abdominal circumference. These patients should be evaluated with a glucose tolerance test and treated accordingly. Polyhydramnios in diabetes is associated with increased perinatal morbidity and mortality beyond that of the diabetes itself (Dubil & Magann, 2015, p. 351).
- Uterine overdistention, however, may stimulate preterm uterine contractions and labor may ensue. These patients are at a significantly high risk for premature ROM (PROM) and cord prolapse (Dubil & Magann, 2015, p. 351)

FETAL/NEONATAL COMPLICATIONS

- Prolapsed umbilical cord at ROM is a concern, as well as an increased incidence of malpresentations.

Table 2.2 summarizes the comparisons between oligohydramnios and polyhydramnios

TABLE 2.2 Comparisons of Etiologies for Oligohydramnios and Polyhydramnios

Fluid Level	Etiologies

Oligohydramnios	PROM—most common (50%)
	Congenital genitourinary defect (14%):
	  Renal agenesis, polycystic or multicystic dysplastic kidneys, ureteral or urethral obstruction, including posterior urethral valve syndrome
	Maternal medications:
	  Prostaglandin synthetase inhibitors (e.g., indomethacin, ibuprofen, sulindac) reduce the fetal glomerular filtration rate
	  ACE inhibitors contraindicated in pregnancy can cause:
	    Twin-to-twin transfusion
	    Multiple gestation resulting in placental crowding

Polyhydramnios	Congenital anomalies • Gastrointestinal (duodenal or esophageal atresia, tracheoesophageal fistula, gastroschisis, omphalocele, diaphragmatic hernia) • Craniofacial (anencephaly, holoprosencephaly, hydrocephaly, micrognathia, cleft palate) • Pulmonary (cystic adenomatoid malformation, chylothorax) • Cardiac (malformations, arrhythmias) • Skeletal dysplasias • Fetal hydrops (immune or nonimmune) • Anemia (fetomaternal hemorrhage, parvovirus infection, isoimmunization, thalassemia) • Neuromuscular disorders (myotonic dystrophy, Pena–Shokeir) and NTDs • Neoplasias (teratomas, hemangiomas)

ACE, angiotensin-converting enzyme; NTD, neural tubular defects; PROM, premature rupture of membranes.

Sources: Data from Dubil, E. A., & Magann, E. F. (2015). Amniotic fluid volume. In R. Martin, A. Fanaroff, & M. Walsh (Eds.), *Fanaroff and Martin's neonatal-perinatal medicine: Diseases of the fetus and infant* (10th ed., pp. 340–354). Philadelphia, PA: Elsevier; Rezaee, R. L., Lappen, J. R., & Gecsi, K. S. (2013). Antenatal and intrapartum care of the high-risk infant. In A. A. Fanaroff & J. M. Fanaroff (Eds.), *Klaus and Fanaroff's care of the high-risk neonate* (6th ed., pp. 10–53). Philadelphia, PA: Elsevier.

RUPTURE OF MEMBRANES

Identifying ROM

- Pooling of fluid in vaginal vault
- Positive nitrazine testing
- Positive ferning
- Decreased AFI on ultrasound

Premature Rupture of Membranes

- ROM prior to the onset of labor, regardless of gestational age. Is the single most common diagnosis with preterm delivery.
- Preterm premature rupture of membranes is defined as ROM before 37 weeks' gestation and can be written as PPROM. See Figure 2.2 for causes of pathologic mechanisms for preterm labor.

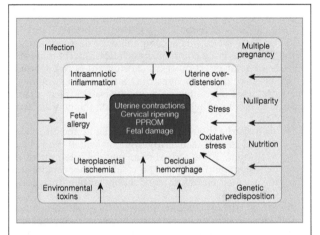

FIGURE 2.2 Pathologic mechanisms for preterm labor

Source: Reproduced with permission from Buhimsch, C. S., Mesiano, S. J., & Muglia, L. J. (2019). Pathogenesis of spontaneous preterm birth. In R. Resnik, C. J. Lockwood, T. R. Moore, M. F. Greene, J. A. Copel, & R. M. Silver (Eds.), *Creasy & Resnik's maternal-fetal medicine: Principles & practice* (9th ed., pp. 92–126e17, p. 98). Philadelphia, PA: Elsevier.

Etiology

- Smoking
- Incompetent cervix
- Multiple gestations
- Sexually transmitted diseases (STDs)/sexually transmitted infections (STIs) and other infections

Prolonged ROM

- ROM exceeding 18 hours
- Associated with prolonged labors
- Labor dystocia or "failure to progress" is a leading cause of cesarean section deliveries.

Etiology

- Pregnancies of older women
- Women with increased body mass index (BMI)
- Mothers who receive oxytocin induction and epidurals (Mercer & Chien, 2019; Simpson & O'Brien-Abel, 2014).

Diagnosis of Chorioamnionitis

- An intra-amniotic infection, better known as chorioamnionitis, can profoundly impact the morbidity and mortality of a fetus, a neonate, and/or a mother. The choriodecidual

space, fetal membranes, placenta, AF, and umbilical cord all are sites for potential microbial (usually polymicrobial) invasion (Polin & Randis, 2020, p. 404).
- The most common organisms contributing to chorioamnionitis are outlined in Table 2.3.
- During the first trimester, the presence of abnormal cervicovaginal flora (e.g., bacterial vaginosis, aerobic vaginitis) is associated with adverse pregnancy outcomes, including early preterm birth and miscarriage and microbial invasion of the amniotic cavity (Markham & Fanaroff, 2015; MIAC; Polin & Randis, 2020, p. 405).

TABLE 2.3 Organisms Associated With Chorioamnionitis

Acute Chorioamnionitis	Subclinical Chorioamnionitis
Symptomatic mother	Preterm labor or completely asymptomatic
↓	↓
Group B *Streptococcus*	*Ureaplasma urealyticum–Mycoplasma hominis*
Escherichia coli	
Streptococcus viridans	*Gardnerella vaginalis*
↓	↓
Fulminant sepsis at birth	Variable symptoms at birth
Respiratory distress	Brain injury
Cardiovascular instability	Chronic lung disease

Source: Data from Martin, R., Fanaroff, A., & Walsh, M. (Eds.). *Fanaroff and Martin's neonatal-perinatal medicine: Diseases of the fetus and infant* (11th ed., pp. 404–414). Philadelphia, PA: Elsevier.

FETAL HEART RATE MONITORING

- The ability to monitor the fetus during labor has revolutionized the care of the pregnant woman and the fetus, leading to decreases in maternal, fetal, and neonatal morbidity and mortality. Fetal status is assessed by determining fetal heart rate (FHR) at a baseline and the variability of the heart rate, as well as any accelerations or decelerations and the pattern of the heart rate over time (Nageotte, 2019; Simpson & O'Brien-Abel, 2014).
- FHR patterns are the standard language for communicating fetal status and fetal response to labor. The following terminology is recommended:
  - ○ Continuous electronic fetal monitoring (EFM) is the preferred method to assess fetal well-being during labor. Generally, EFM requires the use of an external Doppler ultrasound belted around the maternal abdomen and a second pressure transducer.
    - ■ The Doppler ultrasound plots the FHR and the pressure transducer plots the frequency and duration of uterine contractions.
    - ■ Rarely, a fetal scalp electrode is placed when there are decelerations in the FHR or the overall rate is difficult to interpret.
  - ○ FHR is reported as either reassuring or nonreassuring in order to guide clinical management (Rezaee et al., 2013, p. 27).

Categories of FHR Interpretation

CATEGORY I
- Defined as the following: baseline heart rate 110 to 160 bpm, moderate baseline variability, accelerations and/or early decelerations are present or absent, there are no late or variable decelerations.
- Interpreted to indicate that all findings are normal; predictive of normal fetal acid–base balance at the time of observation (Hackney, 2015, p. 192).

CATEGORY II
- Defined as tracings that do not meet criteria for category I or category III.
- Indeterminate interpretation, not predictive of abnormal fetal acid–base status but cannot be classified as category I or category III (Hackney, 2015, p. 192).

CATEGORY III
- Defined by absent baseline variability in the presence of recurrent late or variable decelerations or bradycardia or sinusoidal pattern.
- Interpreted to indicate abnormal fetal acid–base balance (Simpson & O'Brien-Abel, 2014, p. 448).

Normal (Reassuring) FHR

- The baseline features of the FHR are predominant characteristics that can be recognized between uterine contractions. These are the baseline rate and variability of the FHR:
  - The normal baseline FHR is between 110 and 160 bpm. Rates slower than 110 bpm are called *bradycardia*, and rates faster than 160 bpm are called *tachycardia*.
  - EFM produces an irregular line that represents the slight difference in the time interval and from beat to beat. This demonstrates the FHR variability (Hackney, 2015, p. 188; Nageotte, 2019, p. 573).

Baseline Changes

- Accelerations are a visually apparent abrupt increase in FHR above baseline. These are associated with normal FHR variability (Nageotte, 2019, p. 573).
- Decelerations are characterized as early, variable, and late:
  - Early decelerations occur when the FHR decreases concurrently with contractions.
  - Variable decelerations demonstrate an abrupt decrease from the FHR baseline lasting not more than 2 minutes. They may or may not be associated with contractions.
  - Late decelerations are identified when the FHR slows significantly and does not return to baseline until after the completion of the contraction. These are an ominous sign associated with decreases in uterine blood flow and fetal hypoxia (Nageotte, 2019, pp. 574–575).

Nonreassuring FHR

- *Bradycardia* is a baseline FHR of <110 bpm. Some fetuses have a baseline FHR of <110 bpm and are cardiovascularly normal. Others with an FHR <110 bpm may have congenital heart block.
  - Decreases in FHR may be caused by a sudden decrease in oxygenation, such as occurs with placental abruption, maternal apnea, or AF embolus; a decrease or cessation in umbilical blood flow, such as occurs with a prolapsed cord or uterine rupture; and/or a decrease in uterine blood flow, such as occurs with severe maternal hypotension (Nageotte, 2019, p. 574).
- *Tachycardia* is a baseline FHR >160 bpm. With tachycardia, loss of FHR variability is common. Although fetal tachycardia is potentially associated with fetal hypoxia, particularly when it is accompanied by decelerations of the FHR, the more common association is with maternal fever or fetal infection (e.g., chorioamnionitis). Certain drugs also cause tachycardia, such as beta-mimetic agents used for attempted tocolysis, or illicit drugs such as methamphetamine and cocaine (Nageotte, 2019, p. 574).
  - Tachycardia should not be confused with the rare event of fetal cardiac tachyarrhythmia, in which the FHR is >240 bpm. These arrhythmias may be intermittent or persistent, and they are the result of abnormalities of the cardiac electronic conduction system (Nageotte, 2019, p. 574).
- *Absent or minimal baseline variability* may be seen when the fetus experiences progressive hypoxia in cerebral and myocardial tissues. Nonhypoxic causes may be anencephaly, presence of opioids in the maternal system, or a defective cardiac conduction system (Nageotte, 2019, p. 575).
- *Sinusoidal patterns* are extremely regular and smooth with no beat-to-beat or short-term variability. This is commonly seen in Rh-sensitized infants with critical anemia, possibly leading to hydrops. It can also be seen in cases of severe fetal acidemia and as a result of maternal–fetal bleeding (Nageotte, 2019, pp. 578–579).

Maternal Interventions and the Effects on Fetus
Labor Tocolytics

- No matter which tocolytic agent the clinician chooses, the evidence supports the use of short-term tocolytic drugs to prolong pregnancy for at least 48 hours to allow for administration of antenatal steroids. This may also allow for transport of the mother to a tertiary care facility and for administration of magnesium sulfate to reduce the risk of cerebral palsy.
- Beta-mimetics:
  - Terbutaline is the β_2-adrenergic agonist that has been most commonly used in obstetrics in the United States, but its use is decreasing.
- Calcium channel blockers:
  - Dihydropyridine calcium channel blockers—or example, nifedipine and nicardipine—act on L-type calcium channels to inhibit calcium influx into myometrial cells. Reduced intracellular calcium concentrations prevent activation of myosin light chain kinase, and thereby myometrium contraction. Adverse events associated with nifedipine are usually mild and related to peripheral vasodilation, for example, flushing. In normotensive women with no underlying heart disease, there

is typically minimal effect on blood pressure due to a compensatory rise in heart rate and stroke volume.
- Magnesium sulfate:
  - Because of its familiarity and presumed safety, magnesium sulfate has been a mainstay of tocolytic therapy since 1971. Proposed mechanisms of action include competition with calcium at motor end plates and/or at plasma membrane voltage-gated channels. Maternal side effects with magnesium sulfate therapy can range from mild (e.g., flushing and somnolence) to severe (e.g., respiratory depression and cardiac arrhythmias).

Labor Induction

- Labor induction involves the stimulation of the uterus to contract before contractions begin on their own. New research suggests that induction for healthy women at 39 weeks in their first full-term pregnancies may reduce the risk of cesarean birth.
- There are several methods to start labor, which include ripening the cervix, stripping the membranes, the use of oxytocin, and rupturing the amniotic sac:
  - Ripening of the cervix uses medications that contain prostaglandins. These drugs can be inserted into the vagina or taken by mouth. The cervix can also be expanded by inserting a thin tube that has an inflatable balloon on the end into the cervix and expanded to widen the cervix.
  - Stripping of the membranes involves a healthcare professional sweeping a gloved finger over the thin membranes that connect the amniotic sac to the wall of your uterus. This action is done when the cervix is partially dilated. It may cause the body to release natural prostaglandins, which soften the cervix further and may cause contractions.
  - Oxytocin is a hormone that causes contractions of the uterus. It can be used to start labor or to speed up labor that began on its own. Contractions usually start about 30 minutes after oxytocin is given.
  - An amniotomy may be done to rupture the amniotic sac. A small hole is made in the membranes with a special tool. This procedure may be done after a woman has been given oxytocin. Amniotomy is done to start labor when the cervix is dilated and thinned and the fetus's head has moved down into the pelvis. Most women go into labor within hours after the amniotic sac breaks (their "water breaks").

See Box 2.1 for endogenous and exogenous factors affecting myometrial contractility during labor.

Maternal Analgesia

- During labor, a mother's metabolic demand increases. As the metabolic demand increases, so does the increased use of oxygen. When anxiety and pain are added, there is an increased production of catecholamines (epinephrine and norepinephrine), as well as cortisol and glucagon. If placental gas exchange is compromised, the fetus may become hypoxic and acidotic. Hence the need to address maternal analgesia.
- The goal of analgesia is pain relief while having the patient remaining conscious. This is accomplished by providing

BOX 2.1 Factors affecting myometrial contractility during labor

Uterine Stimulants
Endogenous
  Oxytocin
  Prostaglandins
  Endothelin
  Epidermal growth factor

Exogenous
  Oxytocin
  Prostaglandins

Uterine Relaxants
Endogenous
  Relaxin
  Nitric oxide
  L-Arginine
  Magnesium
  Corticotropin-releasing hormone
  Parathyroid hormone–related protein
  Calcitonin gene–related peptide
  Adrenomedullin
  Progesterone

Exogenous
  Beta-adrenergic agonists (ritodrine hydrochloride, terbutaline sulfate, salbutamol, fenoterol)
  Oxytocin receptor antagonist (atosiban)
  Magnesium sulfate
  Calcium channel blockers (nifedipine, nitrendipine, diltiazem, verapamil)
  Prostaglandin inhibitors (indomethacin)
  Phosphodiesterase inhibitor (aminophylline)
  Nitric oxide donor (nitroglycerin, sodium nitroprusside)

Source: Reproduced with permission from Norwitz, E. R., Mahendroo, M., & Lye, S. J. (2019). Physiology of parturition. In R. Resnik, C. J. Lockwood, T. R. Moore, M. F. Greene, J. A. Copel, & R. M. Silver (Eds.), *Creasy & Resnik's maternal-fetal medicine: Principles & practice* (9th ed., pp. 81–95e6, p. 92). Philadelphia, PA: Elsevier.

partial sensory receptor blockage and not full motor receptor blockage.
- Sedatives and narcotic analgesics are frequently administered alone or in combination in the first stage of labor. There is increasing evidence that opioids given systemically do not relieve the pain of labor, but do reduce anxiety and result in sedation. All drugs of this type rapidly appear in the fetal circulation when administered to the mother; therefore, predictably, there will be some sedation of the infant depending on the specific drug given, the amount, the time, and the route of administration (Thorp & Grantz, 2019, p. 755).

Neuraxial Techniques

EPIDURAL BLOCK
- Epidural labor analgesia is a catheter-based technique that provides continuous analgesia during labor through the administration of medication into the epidural space. Although it is the most difficult form of anesthesia to administer, it has the advantage of providing excellent pain relief for the first and second stages of labor and for

delivery without altering the consciousness of the mother. Analgesia is achieved by administration of local anesthetics, opioids, or both. Drug mixtures of local anesthetics and analgesics result in less motor block; this allows women who have epidural anesthesia to be more mobile during labor, and they are less likely to be confined to the supine position (Rollins & Rosen, 2018, p. 174; Thorp & Grantz, 2019, p. 756;).

- It provides significant relief from the pain of contractions and pressure on the perineum, and can be used for a vaginal delivery as well as a cesarean section delivery.
  - For patients undergoing cesarean delivery, opioids can be injected into the epidural space to provide prolonged postoperative analgesia. The rare occurrence of serious respiratory depression is the only major complication, although women may experience transient nausea, urinary retention, and pruritus (Thorp & Grantz, 2019, p. 756).
- Both retrospective- and prospective-controlled trials have demonstrated that epidural analgesia results in longer labors and a higher incidence of operative vaginal delivery and cesarean delivery than intravenous analgesia (Thorp & Grantz, 2019, p. 756).

SPINAL BLOCK
- In women without epidural analgesia, spinal analgesia can be administered in the second stage of labor near the time of anticipated delivery. A small dose of a local anesthetic, opioid, or both are injected into the subarachnoid space, and has minimal effects on motor nerve function (Rollins & Rosen, 2018, p. 175).
- Spinal anesthesia is associated with the highest incidence of maternal hypotension, and the time from onset of anesthesia to delivery of the infant is directly related to the degree of fetal metabolic acidosis resulting from uteroplacental hypoperfusion (Thorp & Grantz, 2019, p. 751).
- Contractions can be felt, but there is no pain associated with the contraction. The mother is able to ambulate has no hypotension and can have rapid pain relief.

COMBINED SPINAL-EPIDURAL ANALGESIA
- This variation of neuraxial analgesia combines the lumbar epidural technique and spinal analgesia, using an intrathecal dose to initiate analgesia. After placement of the epidural needle, but before insertion of the epidural catheter, a spinal needle is passed through the indwelling epidural needle puncturing the dura, and a small dose of local anesthetic or opioid is administered. This results in a more rapid analgesia than with an epidural. Early studies indicate it to be safe and effective (Rollins & Rosen, 2018, p. 175).

Regional Techniques

PARACERVICAL BLOCK
- A paracervical block is infrequently used to provide pain relief during the first stage of labor. The technique consists of submucosal administration of local anesthetics immediately lateral and posterior to the uterocervical junction, which blocks transmission of pain impulses at the paracervical ganglion. Complications from systemic absorption or transfer of local anesthetic can occur and there is a rare occurrence of direct fetal trauma or injection (Rollins & Rosen, 2018, p. 176). Although not advocated with enthusiasm by most authorities, this form of anesthesia is still used, especially in hospitals in which epidural anesthesia is not available (Thorp & Grantz, 2019, p. 755).

PUDENDAL BLOCK
- Pudendal block is a common form of anesthesia used for vaginal delivery. When successful, it provides adequate pain relief for episiotomy, spontaneous delivery, forceps or vacuum extraction delivery from a low pelvic station, and repair of perineal, vaginal, or cervical lacerations (Thorp & Grantz, 2019, p. 755).
  - A sheathed needle is guided to the vaginal mucosa and sacrospinous ligament just medial and posterior to the ischial spine. Injection of local anesthetic blocks sensation of the lower vagina and perineum (Rollins & Rosen, 2018, p. 176). Because the local anesthetic agent is injected well away from the parauterine vasculature, uteroplacental blood flow and FHR are not affected (Thorp & Grantz, 2019, p. 755).

General Anesthesia

- Use of general anesthesia for cesarean delivery is typically reserved for situations where neuraxial anesthesia is contraindicated or emergent delivery is needed. After denitrogenation of the lungs (i.e., preoxygenation), general anesthesia is induced by rapid-sequence administration of an intravenous (IV) induction agent, followed by a rapidly acting muscle relaxant. The trachea is intubated with a cuffed endotracheal tube, and a surgical incision is made after confirmation of tracheal intubation and adequate ventilation (Rollins & Rosen, 2018, p. 177).
  - General anesthesia is characterized by loss of consciousness, analgesia, amnesia, and skeletal muscle relaxation (Rollins & Rosen, 2018, p. 172).
  - Benefits of general anesthesia include the establishment of a secure airway and ability to control ventilation. The process is rapid and reliable onset, and there is the potential for less hemodynamic instability (Rollins & Rosen, 2018, p. 176).
- General anesthesia administration requires prompt delivery of the infant. Delivery of the infant within 90 seconds after making the uterine incision reduces the risk of fetal hypoxemia from altered uteroplacental and umbilical blood flow (Thorp & Gtrantz, 2019, p. 751).

POTENTIAL COMPLICATIONS OF THE INTRAPARTUM PERIOD

Postterm (Postdates): > 42 weeks' gestation

- The problem in defining the end of pregnancy is that the beginning of a pregnancy is seldom known; therefore, estimating dates of a spontaneous pregnancy is associated with educated guessing, resulting in accuracies of about plus or minus 2 to 3 weeks. As the end of gestation, the functioning of the placenta may take one of two paths:

- ○ If the placenta continues to function well, infants can develop macrosomia.
- ○ More commonly, the placenta functioning diminishes, resulting in an environment of placenta insufficiency. The placental insufficiency generally results in decreased nutrition and decreased oxygen exchange to the fetus, leading not only to a wide range of perinatal morbidities, but also to increased rates of perinatal mortality (Blickstein & Rimon, 2015, p. 321).

- The benefit of reducing potential fetal risks with induction of labor must be balanced against the morbidity associated with this procedure. Management of an otherwise uncomplicated pregnancy prolonged beyond the estimated date of confinement, when the woman presents with unfavorable cervical conditions, has been the subject of extensive research. (Blickstein & Rimon, 2015, p. 324).

Multiple Gestations

- With multiple gestations, there is an increased risk for preterm birth and a decreased gestational age at birth as the number of fetuses increase. PROM is a significant contribution leading to preterm birth (Rezaee et al., 2013, p. 20). In about 50% of cases, the timing of delivery of a multiple gestation will be dictated by obvious clinical concerns, such as preterm labor, preeclampsia, or poor fetal growth (Malone & D'Alton, 2019, p. 663).
  - ○ Despite these results, the American College of Obstetricians and Gynecologists suggests
  - ○ Elective delivery at 38 0/7 to 38 6/7 weeks because rates of neonatal morbidity, including respiratory distress syndrome, septicemia, and neonatal intensive care unit admission, were all lower at later gestational ages (Malone & D'Alton, 2019, p. 663).

Special Considerations

- Disparity in AF volume is a significant finding in twin oligohydramnios-polyhydramnios sequence (TOPS), of which twin-twin transfusion syndrome (TTTS) is the most severe end point. A three- to fivefold increase in morbidity and mortality is associated with TTTS. Discordant fetal weights and AF volumes as detected with ultrasound assessment can be found in monochorionic/diamniotic twins, although it has been documented in monochorionic/monoamniotic pregnancies (Dubil & Magann, 2015, p. 344).
- *Monoamniotic twinning* results in a single amniotic sac containing both twins. This setup carries a higher risk for perinatal morbidity and mortality than diamniotic twins (Malone & D'Alton, 2019, p. 670).
- Twin reversed arterial perfusion (TRAP) sequence, or acardiac twinning, is a unique abnormality of monochorionic multiple gestations in which one twin has an absent, rudimentary, or nonfunctioning heart. A bizarre range of anomalies can be seen in the acardiac twin, including anencephaly, holoprosencephaly, absent limbs, absent lungs or heart, intestinal atresias, abdominal wall defects, and absent liver, spleen, or kidneys (Malone & D'Alton, 2019, p. 670).

- *Asynchronous delivery*, or delayed-interval delivery, refers to delivery of one fetus in a multiple gestation that is not followed promptly by birth of the remaining fetus or fetuses. This an extremely rare event and usually is acceptable as the management of extreme prematurity (Malone & D'Alton, 2019, p. 666).
- *Intrauterine demise* of one fetus in a multiple gestation during the first trimester is common and is termed "vanishing twin." Original thought that the remaining twin was unaffected has now changed as data show the intrauterine demise of one fetus in a monochorionic twin pregnancy at as early as 12 weeks' gestation can result in profound neurologic injury to the surviving fetus. The risk for significant neurologic morbidity is not increased in a dichorionic gestation (Malone & D'Alton, 2019, p. 672). Intrauterine demise of one fetus in the second or third trimester is rarer.

Meconium-Stained Amniotic Fluid/Meconium Aspiration Syndrome

- Meconium aspiration syndrome (MAS) is associated with inhalation of meconium and AF during fetal life or at delivery, and is often complicated by significant pulmonary hypertension. It is among the most common causes of hypoxemic respiratory failure in term newborns who require intensive care (Parker & Kinsella, 2019, p. 672).
- Prevention of MAS has focused on decreasing exposure of the fetal and newborn lung to the noxious effects of inhaled meconium. Infusion of saline into the amniotic cavity (i.e., amnioinfusion) during labor has been studied as a means of both diluting meconium and relieving pressure on the umbilical cord, a potential cause of fetal acidemia.
  - ○ Fetal acidemia is believed to cause increased intestinal peristaltic activity that results in passage of meconium and fetal gasping, which draws meconium-contaminated AF deep into the lungs (Parker & Kinsella, 2019, p. 672)
  - ○ The presence of meconium-stained fluid may be related to fetal stress as a consequence of chorioamnionitis (Polin & Randis, 2020)

Preeclampsia

- Preeclampsia is a disorder unique to pregnancy that is characterized by poor perfusion of many vital organs (including the fetoplacental unit) that is completely reversible with the termination of pregnancy. Mothers with preeclampsia may present with a variety of signs and symptoms that range from mild to life threatening; likewise, the fetus may be minimally to severely affected (Harper, Tita, & Karumanchi, 2019, p. 812).
  - ○ Preeclampsia is distinguished between two modes: preeclampsia without severe features and preeclampsia with severe features:
    - Preeclampsia without severe features can progress to preeclampsia with severe features over the course of days; therefore, women should be monitored frequently to assess for severe features and deterioration of fetal well-being.

- Routine administration of parenteral magnesium sulfate for seizure prophylaxis is recommended in women with preeclampsia with severe features. Most seizures occur during the intrapartum and postpartum periods, when the preeclamptic process is most likely to accelerate (Harper et al. 2019, p. 824)
  - ○ The presence of a seizure changes the diagnosis of preeclampsia to eclampsia. Several additional criteria are used to differentiate mild from severe preeclampsia:
    - Elevated blood pressure (160 mmHg or higher systolic and 110 mmHg or higher diastolic on two occasions during a 6-hour window while the patient is on bed rest)
    - Proteinuria and/or oliguria (<500 mL in 24 hours)
    - Cerebral or visual disturbances
    - Respiratory distress and/or cyanosis
    - Thrombocytopenia
    - Fetal growth restriction (Rezaee et al., 2013, p. 32)

CONCLUSION

The NNP is dependent on the skill and expertise of the labor and delivery healthcare providers overseeing the care of the fetus prior to delivery. When called to attend a delivery, the NNP needs to ask or seek out the most critical and appropriate information to prepare for a successful resuscitation and stabilization. Most of the maternal history can be reviewed and provide answers to the condition of the neonate after the initial transition period. Having a broad knowledge of the events of intrapartum and the most common complications involved in labor and delivery will situate you well for certification. Remember always, the neonate's history *is* the maternal history.

REVIEW QUESTIONS

1. With a maternal diagnosis of polyhydramnios, the NNP prepares for a neonate with a possible diagnosis of neonatal:
   A. Duodenal atresia
   B. Hypoplastic lungs
   C. Liver disease

2. A velamentous insertion of the umbilical cord is associated with:
   A. Placenta previa
   B. Uterine abruptio
   C. Vasa previa

3. The main contributor to fluid dynamics in early pregnancy is the fetal:
   A. Pulmonary system
   B. Integumentary system
   C. Gastrointestinal system

4. The etiology of increased amniotic fluid may be due to decreased absorption, to overproduction, or is
   A. Idiopathic and unknown
   B. Impaired by physiology
   C. Issuing from fetal anomaly

5. The NNP is called to attend the delivery of a mother who is 30 weeks +4 days gestation and reported to have oligohydramnios since 18 weeks of gestation. The NNP know to prepare for an infant who will likely be in:
   A. Cardiopulmonary arrest
   B. Hemolytic shock
   C. Respiratory distress

REFERENCES

Blickstein, I., & Rimon, O. F. (2015). Post-term pregnancy. In R. Martin, A. Fanaroff, & M. Walsh (Eds.), *Fanaroff and Martin's neonatal-perinatal medicine: Diseases of the fetus and infant* (10th ed., pp. 10–326). Philadelphia, PA: Elsevier.

Blickstein, I., & Shinwell, E. S. (2015). Obstetric management of multiple gestation and birth. In R. Martin, A. Fanaroff, & M. Walsh (Eds.), *Fanaroff and Martin's neonatal-perinatal medicine: Diseases of the fetus and infant* (10th ed., pp. 10–320). Philadelphia, PA: Elsevier.

Buhimsch, C. S., Mesiano, S. J., & Muglia, L. J. (2019). Pathogenesis of spontaneous preterm birth. In R. Resnik, C. J. Lockwood, T. R. Moore, M. F. Greene, J. A. Copel, & R. M. Silver (Eds.), *Creasy & Resnik's maternal-fetal medicine: Principles & practice* (9th ed., pp. 92–126e17). Philadelphia, PA: Elsevier.

Dubil, E. A., & Magann, E. F. (2015). Amniotic fluid volume. In R. Martin, A. Fanaroff, & M. Walsh (Eds.), *Fanaroff and Martin's neonatal-perinatal medicine: Diseases of the fetus and infant* (10th ed., pp. 10–354). Philadelphia, PA: Elsevier.

Harper, L., Tita, A., & Karumanchi, S. (2019). Pregnancy-related hypertension. In R. Resnik, C. J. Lockwood, M. Greene, J. Copel, & R. Silver (Eds.), *Creasy and Resnik's maternal-fetal medicine: Principles and practice* (8th ed., pp 810–8738.e9) Philadelphia, PA: Elsevier, Inc.

Hoyt, M. R., & Pages-Arroyo, E. M. (2015). Anesthesia for labor and delivery. In R. Martin, A. Fanaroff, & M. Walsh (Eds.), *Fanaroff and Martin's neonatal-perinatal medicine: Diseases of the fetus and infant* (10th ed., pp. 10–390). Philadelphia, PA: Elsevier.

Hull, A.D., Resnik, R., & Silver, R. M. (2019). Placenta previa and accretea, vasa previa, subchorionic hemorrhage, and abruptio placentae. In R. Resnik, C. J. Lockwood, T. R. Moore, M. F. Greene, J. A. Copel, & R. M. Silver (Eds.), *Creasy & Resnik's maternal-fetal medicine: Principles & practice* (9th ed., pp. 786–797e4.). Philadelphia, PA: Elsevier.

Malone, F., & D'Alton, M. (2019). Multiple gestation: Clinical characteristics and management. In R. Resnik, C. Lockwood, T. Moore, M. Greene, J. Copel, & R. Silver (Eds.), *Creasy and Resnik's maternal-fetal medicine: Principles and practice* (8th ed., pp. 654–675.e5.) Philadelphia, PA: Elsevier.

Markham, K. B., & Fanaroff, A. A. (2015). Obstetric management of prematurity. In R. Martin, A. Fanaroff, & M. Walsh (Eds.), *Fanaroff and Martin's neonatal-perinatal medicine: Diseases of the fetus and infant* (10th ed., pp. 10–303). Philadelphia, PA: Elsevier.

Mercer, B M., & Chien E.K.S. (2019). Premature rupture of membranes. In R. Resnik, C. Lockwood, T. Moore, M. Greene, J. Copel, & R. Silver (Eds.). *Creasy and Resnik's maternal-fetal medicine: Principles and practice* (8th ed., pp. 712-722 e5). Philadelphia, PA: Elsevier.

Nageotte, M. (2019). Intrapartum fetal surveillance. In R. Resnik, C. Lockwood, T. Moore, M. Greene, J. Copel, & R. Silver (Eds.), *Creasy and Resnik's maternal-fetal medicine: Principles and practice* (8th ed., pp. 564–582.e2). Philadelphia, PA: Elsevier.

Norwitz, E. R., Mahendroo, M., & Lye, S. J. (2019). Physiology of parturition. In R. Resnik, C. J. Lockwood, T. R. Moore, M. F. Greene, J. A. Copel, & R. M. Silver (Eds.), *Creasy & Resnik's maternal-fetal medicine: Principles & practice* (9th ed., pp. 81–95e6). Philadelphia, PA: Elsevier.

Parker, T., & Kinsella, J. (2019). Respiratory disorders in the term infant. In C. Gleason, & S. Juul (Eds.), *Avery's diseases of the newborn* (10th ed., pp. 668–677.e3). Philadelphia, PA: Elsevier.

Polin, R., & Randis, T. M. (2019). Perinatal infections and chorioamnionitis. In R. Martin, A. Fanaroff, & M. Walsh (Eds.), *Fanaroff and Martin's neonatal-perinatal medicine: Diseases of the fetus and infant* (11th ed., pp. 11–414). Philadelphia, PA: Elsevier.

Rezaee, R. L., Lappen, J. R., & Gecsi, K. S. (2013). Antenatal and intrapartum care of the high-risk infant. In A. A. Fanaroff &

J. M. Fanaroff (Eds.), *Klaus and Fanaroff's care of the high-risk neonate* (6th ed., pp. 6–53). Philadelphia, PA: Elsevier, Inc.

Rollins, M. D., & Rosen, M. A. (2018). Obstetric analgesia and anesthesia. In C. A. Gleason & S. E. Juul (Eds.), *Avery's diseases of the newborn* (10th ed., pp. 70–179 e.2). Philadelphia, PA: Elsevier.

Ross, M. G., & Beall, M. H. (2019). Amniotic fluid dynamics. In R. Resnik, C. J. Lockwood, T. R. Moore, M. F. Greene, J. A. Copel, & R. M. Silver (Eds.), *Creasy & Resnik's maternal-fetal medicine: Principles & practice* (9th ed., pp. 62–67 e.3). Philadelphia, PA: Elsevier.

Simpson, K. R., & O'Brien-Abel, N. (2014). Labor and birth. In K. Simpson & P. Creehan (Eds.), *Perinatal nursing* (4th ed., pp. 4–444). St. Louis, MO: Lippincott Williams & Wilkins.

Thorp, J., & Grantz, K. (2019). Clinical aspects of normal and abnormal labor. In R. Resnik, C. Lockwood, T. Moore, M. Greene, J. Copel, & R. Silver (Eds.), *Creasy and Resnik's maternal-fetal medicine: Principles and practice* (8th ed., pp. 723–757.e7). Philadelphia, PA: Elsevier.

3 THE NEONATAL PHYSICAL EXAM

Vivian Lopez
Pauline D. Graziano

INTRODUCTION

The physical examination of a newborn is a comprehensive evaluation. It encompasses a review of maternal and familial health histories; antepartum, intrapartum, and delivery histories; and an assessment of gestational age (GA) and fetal growth, as well as a complete and detailed physical examination of the newborn. It is an essential tool in the assessment of the infant's transition to extrauterine life and in identifying potential risks or signs of disease processes that may threaten their well-being.

GA ASSESSMENT

GA assessment can be accomplished using several different tools. The accuracy of these varies according to when they are performed. The obstetrical estimate should be considered the most accurate and be used if the infant's physical assessment estimates GA within 2 weeks of it (Benjamin & Furdon, 2015, p. 116; Lissauer & Steer, 2013, pp. 108–109).

Prenatal GA Assessment Tools

- Last menstrual period dating (clinical estimate)
- Nagele's Rule to determine estimated date of confinement (EDC): Add 7 days to first day of last normal menstrual period and count back 3 months.
  - Accuracy dependent on regular menstrual cycles, with ovulation on day 14 of cycle, as well as accurate maternal memory of last normal cycle (Trotter, 2016, p. 25; Wilkins-Haug & Heffner, 2017, p. 1).
- First trimester:
  - GA determined using Crown–Rump length
  - Most accurate at 7 to 9 weeks' gestation
  - Accuracy within 7 days (Trotter, 2016, p. 25; Wilkins-Haug & Heffner, 2017, p. 1)
- Second trimester:
  - GA determined using biparietal diameter, head circumference, abdominal circumference, and femur length.
  - Most accurate at 18 to 20 weeks' gestation:
    - 14 to 20 weeks' gestation accuracy +/−11 days
    - 20 to 28 weeks' gestation accuracy +/−14 days
    - 29 to 40 weeks' gestation accuracy +/−21 days (Trotter, 2016, p. 25; Wilkins-Haug & Heffner, 2017, p. 1)

Postnatal GA Assessment

- Postnatal assessment of GA is based on the premise that fetal physical and neurological maturation progresses in an organized, predictable manner. This allows for a reasonably accurate estimate of GA, which is critical in determining infant risks for morbidity and proper counseling to families based on the GA of the infant (Benjamin & Furdon, 2015, p. 113).
- Postdelivery, the newborn experiences rapidly changing physiologic, biologic, and physical characteristics. GA instruments have best accuracy if used within the first 48 hours of life, before these changes are occurring. Neurologic and physical findings may also be altered due to disease processes or extreme prematurity (Benjamin & Furdon, 2015, pp. 113–117; Smith, 2017, p. 76; Trotter, 2016, pp. 26–27).

Common Newborn GA Tools

- Dubowitz:
  - 10 neurologic and 10 physical criteria
  - Combined score accuracy +/−2 weeks
  - Overestimates GA in premature infants (Benjamin & Furdon, 2015, p. 113; Trotter, 2016, pp. 26–27)
- Ballard:
  - Six neurologic and six physical criteria
  - Revised to New Ballard Tool 1991 (Benjamin & Furdon, 2015, p. 113; Fraser, 2014, p. 598; Trotter, 2016, pp. 26–27)
- New Ballard:
  - Able to assess GA between 20 and 44 weeks
  - Accuracy +/−2 weeks for well or sick infant
  - For infants with estimated GA of 20 to 28 weeks, the best timing of exam is within first 12 hours of life.
    - Limitations: Quiet, alert state required, infants affected by maternal medications, positional deformities (breech), neurological disorders, or birth asphyxia (Benjamin & Furdon, 2015, p. 113; Fraser, 2014, p. 598; Trotter, 2016, pp. 23–27)
    - See Figure 3.1 and Table 3.1

Evaluation of Anterior Vascular Lens Capsule Optic Examination

- Assesses stage of normal embryonic lens vessel development and atrophy (appear and atrophy between 27- and 34-weeks GA)
- Limitations:
  - Requires ophthalmoscope to evaluate
  - Cannot be performed before 27 weeks GA
  - Must be done within first 48 hours of life (Benjamin & Furdon, 2015, p. 114; Trotter, 2016, p. 29)
  - See Figure 3.2

Maturational Assessment of Gestational Age (New Ballard Score)

Name_____ Date/time of birth_____ Sex _____

Hospital no._____ Date/time of exam _____ Birth w eight _____

Race_____ Age when examined _____ Length_____

Apgar score: 1 minute _____ 5 minutes _____ 10 minutes_____ Head circ. _____

Neuromuscular Maturity   Examiner_____

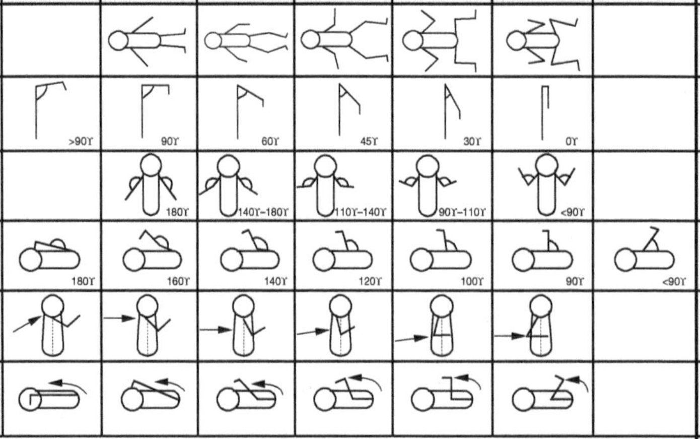

Neuromuscular Maturity Sign	Score							Record Score Here
	−1 0 1 2 3 4 5							
Posture								
Square Window (Wrist)	>90Υ	90Υ	60Υ	45Υ	30Υ	0Υ		
Arm Recoil		180Υ	140Υ–180Υ	110Υ–140Υ	90Υ–110Υ	<90Υ		
Popliteal Angle	180Υ	160Υ	140Υ	120Υ	100Υ	90Υ	<90Υ	
Scarf Sign								
Heel to Ear								

Total Neuromuscular Maturity Score

Physical Maturity

Physical Maturity Sign	Score							Record Score Here
	−1 0 1 2 3 4 5							
Skin	sticky friable transparent	gelatinous red translucent	smooth pink visible veins	superficial peeling and/or rash, few veins	cracking pale area srare veins	parchment deep cracking no vessels	leathery cracked wrinkled	
Lanugo	none	sparse	abundant	thinning	bald areas	mostly bald		
Plantar Surface	heel-toe 40–50 mm:-1 <40 mm:-2	>50 mm no crease	faint red marks	anterior transverse crease only	creases anterior 2/3	creases over entire sole		
Breast	imperceptible	barely perceptible	flat areola no bud	stippled areola 1–2 mm bud	raised areola 3–4 mm bud	full areola 5–10 mm bud		
Eye/Ear	lids fused loosely:- tightly: -21	lids open pinna flat stays folded	sl. curved pinna; soft; slow recoil	well-curved pinna; soft but ready recoil	formed and firm; instant recoil	thick cartilage ear stiff		
Genitals (Male)	scrotum flat, smooth	scrotum empty faint rugae	testes in upper canal rare rugae	testes descending few rugae	testes downgood rugae	testes pendulous deep rugae		
Genitals (Female)	clitoris prominent & labia flat	prominent clitoris & small labia minora	prominent clitoris & enlarging minora	majora & minora equally prominent	majora large minora small	majora cover clitoris and minora		

Total Physical Maturity Score

Score

Neuromuscular_____
Physical_____
Total_____

Maturity Rating

Score	Weeks
−10	20
−5	22
0	24
5	26
10	28
15	30
20	32
25	34
30	36
35	38
40	40
45	42
50	44

Gestational Age (weeks)

By dates_____
By ultrasound_____
By exam_____

FIGURE 3.1 Ballard exam

Source: From Ballard, J. L., Khoury, J. C., Wedig, K., Wang, L., Eilers-Walsman, B. L., & Lipp, R. (1991). New Ballard score, expanded to include extremely premature infants. *Journal of Pediatrics, 119*(3), 418. Reprinted by permission.

TABLE 3.1 Summary of New Ballard Criteria

Neurologic Criteria	Physical Criteria
Posture: Hip adduction and flexion increase with increasing GA	**Skin:** Transparency decreases with increasing GA Beyond 38 weeks subcutaneous tissue decreases, causing wrinkling and desquamation
Square window: Angle decreases with increasing GA Does not change after birth	**Lanugo:** Present at 20–28 weeks GA Decreases with increasing GA
Arm recoil: Recoil increases with increasing GA	**Plantar creases:** First appear on anterior sole (28–30 weeks) and increase to heel with increasing GA Not an accurate criterion after 12 hours due to drying of skin May be accelerated with oligohydramnios Absence may indicate extreme prematurity or underlying neuromuscular condition
Popliteal angle: Angle decreases with increasing GA	**Breast development:** Increases with increasing GA No difference between male and female infants
Scarf sign: Decreases with increasing GA	**Eyes and ears:** Eyes unfuse at 26–28 weeks GA Ear cartilage increases with increasing GA
Heel to ear: Decreases with increasing GA	**Genitalia:** **Female:** Clitoris becomes less visible with increasing GA Fat deposits in labia majora increase with increasing GA **Male:** Testes descend into scrotum with increasing GA Rugae of scrotum increases with increasing GA

GA, gestational age.

Sources: Benjamin, K., & Furdon, S. A. (2015). Physical assessment. In T. Verklan & M. Walden (Eds.), *Core curriculum for neonatal intensive care nursing* (5th ed., pp. 114–116). St. Louis, MO: Elsevier; Trotter, C. W. (2016). Gestational age assessment. In E. P. Tappero & M. E. Honeyfield (2014). *Physical assessment of the newborn: A comprehensive approach to the art of physical examination* (5th ed., pp. 29–36). New York, NY: Springer Publishing Company.

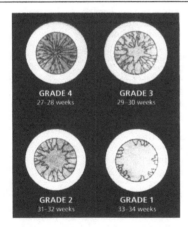

FIGURE 3.2 Anterior vascular lens gestational age assessment

Source: Reproduced with permission from Hittner, H. M., Hirsch, N. J., and Rudolph, A. J. (1977). Assessment of gestational age by examination of the anterior vascular capsule of the lens. *Journal of Pediatrics, 91*(3), 456.

EVALUATION OF GROWTH AND MATURITY

Defining Age

- GA—age from first day of last menstrual period (LMP) to day of birth
- Postmenstrual age (PMA)—age from first day of LMP to day of assessment
- Chronological age—age from day of birth to day of assessment
- Corrected age (CGA)—age from EDC to day of assessment
- See Table 3.2 (Trotter, 2016, p. 23)

GA Maturity Classifications

- Extremely Low Gestational Age Neonate (ELGAN)—24 to 28 weeks GA (Fanaroff & Klaus, 2013, p. 138)
- Preterm—Infant born before the end of 37 weeks GA
- Late preterm—Infant born between 34 0/7 and 36 6/7 weeks GA
- Term—Infant born between 38 and 42 weeks GA
- Postterm—Infant born after 42 weeks GA (Benjamin & Furdon, 2015, p. 117; Smith, 2017, p. 76)
- See Table 3.3

TABLE 3.2 Age Terminology During the Perinatal Period

Gestational age	Span of time beginning on the first day of last menstrual period and ending on the date of birth
Chronological age	Span of time beginning on the date of birth and ending on the date of assessment
Corrected age or postnatal age	Span of time beginning at the expected EDD and ending on the date of assessment
Postmenstrual age	Span of time beginning on the first day of the last menstrual period and ending on the date of assessment

EDD, date of delivery.

Growth Classifications

- Normal fetal growth requires contributions from the mother, placenta, and fetus. Intrinsic or extrinsic factors affecting any of these will ultimately affect fetal growth patterns (i.e., race, maternal overall health status, medications during pregnancy, socioeconomic factors, maternal nutrition, altitude, substance abuse, and placental function).
  - ○ A newborn's growth is assessed using birth measurements of weight, length, and head circumference. These measures should be plotted on recognized acceptable growth curves to determine infant's growth classification.
    - ■ Center for Disease Control (CDC) recommends use of World Health Organization (WHO) curves for 0 to 24 months.
    - ■ Babson and Babson fetal–infant growth graph extends intrauterine growth from 22 to 10 weeks postterm. Use CDC graphs after 50 weeks.
    - ■ Other recognized, acceptable curves also available (Benjamin & Furdon, 2015, pp. 117–119; Smith, 2017, pp. 76–77; Trotter, 2016, p. 39).
- Growth classifications are based on these growth indices regardless of GA estimation:
  - ○ Appropriate for gestational age (AGA)—growth indices between the 10th and 90th percentiles for GA
  - ○ Small for gestational age (SGA)—growth indices less than the 10th percentile for GA

TABLE 3.3 Newborn Morbidity and Mortality Risk Based on Maturity Classifications

Maturity Classification	Etiology of Risk	Possible Morbidity
Preterm	Immature systems	RDS, CLD/BPD NEC ROP Apnea IVH, neurodevelopmental risk Hypotension PDA Nutritional deficiencies, poor growth Fluid & electrolyte imbalances Temperature regulation Immunologic deficiencies, sepsis Anemia Hyperbilirubinemia Perinatal depression
Late Preterm	Immature systems	Respiratory distress Hypoglycemia Hypothermia Apnea Feeding difficulties Hyperbilirubinemia Neurodevelopmental risk Readmission
Term	Maternal health history Pre- and intrapartum medications Spontaneous vs. induction of labor Infection risk: GBS status/prophylaxis, duration of ROM, maternal fever, chorioamnionitis Fetal presentation Intrapartum risk factors: cord prolapse, precipitous delivery, prolonged labor, prolonged head to body delivery interval, signs of fetal distress Delivery mode/assistance	Affects from maternal health conditions: diabetes, thyroid disease, renal disease, iso- or alloimmunization Affects from medications: respiratory depression, hypoglycemia, NAS Immature fetal lungs, retained fetal lung fluid Infection Birth trauma: cephalohematoma, subgaleal hemorrhage, shoulder dystocia, brachial plexus injury, facial nerve injury Anemia, perinatal depression, meconium aspiration, pulmonary hypertension, HIE Transient hypoglycemia, hyperbilirubinemia

TABLE 3.3 Newborn Morbidity and Mortality Risk Based on Maturity Classifications *(cont.)*

Maturity Classification	Etiology of Risk	Possible Morbidity
Post term	• Potential placental insufficiency • Potential birth complications • Occurs in 3%–14% of all pregnancies	• Nonreassuring fetal HR tracing with labor • Meconium aspiration • Low Apgar scores • Pulmonary hypertension • HIE, birth injury • Signs of wasting • Macrosomia

BPD, bronchopulmonary dysplasia; CLD, chronic lung disease; GBS, Group B *Streptococcus*; HIE, hypoxic ischemic encephalopathy; HR, heart rate; IVH, intraventricular hemorrhage; NAS, neonatal abstinence syndrome; NEC, necrotizing enterocolitis; PDA, patent ductus arteriosus; RDS, respiratory distress syndrome; ROM, rupture of membranes; ROP, retinopathy of prematurity.

Sources: Abdulhayoglu, E. (2017). Birth trauma. In E. Eichenwald, A. Hansen, C. Martin, & A. Stark (Eds.), *Cloherty and Stark's manual of neonatal care* (8th ed., pp. 64–73). Philadelphia, PA: Wolters Kluwer; Benjamin, K., & Furdon, S. A. (2015). Physical assessment. In T. Verklan & M. Walden (Eds.), *Core curriculum for neonatal intensive care nursing* (5th ed., pp. 120–122, p. 117). St. Louis, MO: Elsevier; Smith, V. C. (2017). The high-risk newborn: Anticipation, evaluation, management, and outcome. In E. Eichenwald, A. Hansen, C. Martin, & A. Stark (Eds.), *Cloherty and Stark's manual of neonatal care* (8th ed., pp. 76–79). Philadelphia, PA: Wolters Kluwer.

- ○ Large for gestational age (LGA)—growth indices greater than the 90th percentile for GA
- ○ Occipital frontal circumference (OFC) should be plotted on growth curve as part of the determination of size—AGA, SGA, or LGA (Benjamin & Furdon, 2015, p. 126; Johnson, 2016, pp. 66–67; Vargo, 2014, p. 602).
- • Intrauterine growth restriction (IUGR)—infant, which experienced abnormal, diminished growth velocity, below expected norms for intrauterine fetal growth patterns over time. Etiology can be intrinsic or extrinsic. Additionally, classified as:
- ○ Asymmetric IUGR—also called head sparing. Disproportionate growth of weight and possibly length in comparison to relatively normal head size
- ○ Symmetric IUGR—proportional decrease in all growth indices (Benjamin & Furdon, 2015, p. 120; Lissauer & Steer, 2013, p. 105; Smith, 2017, p. 86; Trotter, 2016, p. 39; Wilkins-Haug & Heffner, 2017, pp. 4–5)
- ○ See Table 3.4

TABLE 3.4 Newborn Morbidity and Mortality Risk Based on Growth Classifications

Growth Classification	Etiology	Physical Characteristics	Associated Morbidity
AGA	• Normal growth of fetus	• Weight, length, and head circumference within established norms for GA • Weight, length, and head circumference plot between the 10th and 90th percentiles for current GA • Neuromuscular and physical maturity consistent w/ GA	• Normal newborn concerns (birth trauma, transient hypoglycemia or hypothermia, etc.) • Morbidities associated with GA (see Table 3.2)

SGA	• Nonpathologic SGA:
	  ○ Normal pattern of fetal growth
	  ○ Race
	  ○ Multiple gestation
	• Pathologic SGA (see IUGR below)
		• Nonpathologic SGA:
		  ○ Weight and/or length small for established norms for gestational age
		  ○ Weight and/or length <10th percentile for current GA
		  ○ Neuromuscular and physical maturity consistent w/ GA
		• Pathologic SGA (see IUGR below)
			• Normal newborn concerns (birth trauma, transient hypoglycemia, or hypothermia)
			• Morbidities associated with GA (see Table 3.2)

Macromia/ LGA	• Multiparity • Excessive maternal weight gain • Abnormal maternal glucose tolerance • History of previous macromic infant (incidence 22%) • Maternal diabetes (insulin-dependent, noninsulin dependent, gestational (incidence 20%–40%)	• Macrosomia (>4,000 g) • Large body with AGA head circumference	• Birth trauma • Meconium aspiration • RDS • Pulmonary hypertension • Hypocalcaemia • Hypoglycemia • Hyperinsulinemia • Polycythemia • Hyperbilirubinemia • Poor oral feeding • Infrequent—congenital heart disease or Beckwith–Wiedemann syndrome

(continued)

TABLE 3.4 Newborn Morbidity and Mortality Risk Based on Growth Classifications *(cont.)*

Growth Classification	Etiology	Physical Characteristics	Associated Morbidity
IUGR	• Maternal age • Maternal nutritional status pre- and intrapartum • Causes of placental vasoconstriction/insufficiency (maternal smoking) • Preeclampsia • Chronic hypertension • Placental concerns (size, cord anomalies, chronic abruption, choriohemangioma, placental infarction, abnormal cord implantation) • Congenital malformations or infections • Chromosomal abnormalities (incidence 22%) • Multiple gestation (physical space limitations, twin-to-twin transfusion)	• Wasted appearance of extremities • Head disproportionately large for torso • Long nails • Wizened, old-man face • Large anterior fontanel • Widened or overlapping cranial sutures • Thin umbilical with little Wharton's jelly • Scaphoid abdomen • Diminished subcutaneous fat • Dry, flaky skin • Little vernix • Possible meconium staining	• MAS • PPHN • Hypotension • ATN/renal insufficiency • Hypoglycemia • Hypothermia • Hypoxia • Polycythemia/hyperviscosity • Neutropenia • Thrombocytopenia • Sepsis • Mortality/morbidity related to underlying etiology • Congenital anomaly • Perinatal depression • Acute renal necrosis/insufficiency
Asymmetric IUGR (Head Sparing)	• Etiologic event/process occurs later in gestation during cellular hypertrophy phase and interferes with oxygen/nutrition delivery to fetus	• Weight below norm; length, and head circumference relatively normal	• See earlier • Potential for postnatal growth and development promising
Symmetric IUGR	• Etiologic event/process occurs early in gestation during cellular hyperplasia phase. • Intrinsic fetal problem (anomaly, chromosomal abnormality, congenital infection)	• Proportionate below expected growth for weight, length, and head circumference	• See earlier • Potential for growth and development likely limited due to underlying etiology

AGA, appropriate for gestational age; ATN, acute tubular necrosis; GA, gestational age; IUGR, intrauterine growth restriction; LGA, large for gestational age; MAS, meconium aspiration syndrome; PPHN, persistent pulmonary hypertension; RDS, respiratory distress syndrome; SGA, small for gestational age.

Sources: Benjamin, K., & Furdon, S. A. (2015). Physical assessment. In T. Verklan & M. Walden (Eds.), *Core curriculum for neonatal intensive care nursing* (5th ed., pp. 110–145, p. 120, 122). St. Louis, MO: Elsevier; Lissauer, T., & Steer, P. (2013). Size and physical examination of the newborn infant. In A. A. Fanaroff, J. M. Fanaroff, & M. H. Klaus (Eds.), *Klaus and Fanaroff's care of the high-risk neonate* (6th ed., pp. 109–118). Philadelphia, PA: Elsevier-Saunders; Smith, V. C. (2017). The high-risk newborn: Anticipation, evaluation, management, and outcome. In E. Eichenwald, A. Hansen, C. Martin, & A. Stark (Eds.), *Cloherty and Stark's manual of neonatal care* (8th ed., pp. 74–90, p. 87). Philadelphia, PA: Wolters Kluwer; Trotter, C. W. (2016). Gestational age assessment. In E. P. Tappero & M. E. Honeyfield (2014). *Physical assessment of the newborn: A comprehensive approach to the art of physical examination* (5th ed., pp. 39–41). New York, NY: Springer Publishing Company; Wilkins-Haug, L., & Heffner, L. J. (2017). Fetal assessment and prenatal diagnosis. In E. Eichenwald, A. Hansen, C. Martin, & A. Stark (Eds.), *Cloherty and Stark's manual of neonatal care* (8th ed., pp. 5–6). Philadelphia, PA: Wolters Kluwer.

Weight-Based Growth Classifications

• Low birth weight (LBW)—birth weight <2,500 g
• Very low birth weight (VLBW)—birth weight <1,500 g
• Extremely low birth weight (ELBW)—birth weight <1,000 g (Benjamin & Furdon, 2015, p. 117; Lissauer & Steer, 2013, p. 105; Smith, 2017, p. 76; Trotter, 2016, p. 39)

HISTORY: A KEY COMPONENT OF THE NEWBORN PHYSICAL EXAMINATION

• A comprehensive newborn assessment combines the perinatal history, GA assessment, and the neonate's physical exam. These factors assist in the identification of norms and potential risk factors for each individual infant. See Table 3.5a and b (Benjamin & Furdon, 2015, p. 122; Horns LaBronte, 2016, pp. 12–20; Johnson & Cochran, 2017, pp. 92–93; Lissauer & Steer, 2013, pp. 118–119).

NEONATAL VITAL SIGNS

• Vital signs will fluctuate based on infant state and, therefore, ideally be taken when the infant is quiet. The most accurate assessment of the infant is best achieved when the newborn is in a quiet, alert state and without signs of distress.
• Whenever possible, the complete physical examination should occur in a warm and as stress-free environment

as possible when the newborn is without signs of distress and vital signs are stable. The examination should be modified based on the response, state, and illness of the infant (Benjamin & Furdon, 2015, p. 123; Johnson & Cochran, 2017, p. 92, 94; Trotter, 2016, pp. 37–38).

Temperature

- Normal
  - Axilla temperature between 36.5°C and 37.4°C (97.7°F and 99.3°F)
- Abnormal
  - Hypothermia <36.5°C (97.7°F) for the term neonate and <36.3°C (97.3°F) in the preterm
    - Symptoms include bradycardia, apnea, decreased cardiac output, poor oral feeding, feeding intolerance, hypotension, hypoxia, irritability, respiratory distress, poor weight gain
  - Hyperthermia >37.5 °C (99.5°F) for the term neonate and >36.9°C (98.4°F) for the preterm neonate
    - Neonates are at risk because of their inability to dissipate heat. Symptoms include apnea, central nervous system (CNS) depression, hypernatremia, irritability, lethargy, weak cry, poor oral feeding, seizures, and tachycardia (Brand & Boyd, 2016, pp. 98–99).

Heart Rate

- Normal
  - Newborn HR between 95 and 160 bpm; at rest 120 to 140 bpm; with activity/crying may be ≥170; at deep sleep may decrease to 70 to 90 bpm
  - Preterm HR between 120 and 160 bpm (Johnson, 2016, p. 97; Vargo, 2016, p. 100)
- Abnormal
  - Bradycardia: HR ≤80 bpm
  - Sinus tachycardia: HR ≥160 to 180 bpm
    - Usually a physiologic response to anemia, fever, agitation, and infection (Cannon, Kovalenko, & Snyder, 2015, p. 1259; Johnson, 2016, p. 97)

Respiratory Rate

- Normal
  - Respiratory rate between 30 and 60 bpm
  - Periodic breathing (short pause in breath, between 5 and 10 seconds) common and normal
- Abnormal
  - Tachypnea: rapid, shallow breathing with rate ≥60 bpm
  - Apnea: pause in breathing of 20 seconds or longer and associated with cyanosis and/or bradycardia

TABLE 3.5A Maternal and Perinatal Histories

Maternal History	Perinatal History
• Family history: • Inherited genetic or chromosomal diseases or conditions • Chronic disorders or disabilities • Maternal history: • General health • Gravidity and parity • Infertility treatments • Prior pregnancy outcomes • Blood type and sensitizations • Chronic illnesses • Infectious disease and inherited disease screenings in pregnancy • Medications • Pregnancy complications • Age at delivery—Over 40 (chromosomal abnormalities, IUGR, microsomal), Under 16 (prematurity, IUGR) • Chronic illnesses • Surgical procedures or hospitalizations • Medications: prescribed or illicit, alcohol or tobacco use • Obstetric history: previous pregnancies, issues with infertility, previous fetal or newborn losses or problems • Social support and stressors • Education and socioeconomic status, religious or cultural considerations, language barriers or sensory deficits	• Prenatal care, LMP, EDC, ultrasound dating • Single/multiple gestation • Maternal nutrition status and weight gain • Blood type/risk for isoimmunization/Rhogam prophylaxis/positive antibody screen • Screening results: amniocentesis; ultrasounds; triple or quad screen; Group B Strep culture; congenital infections; glucose tolerance • Maternal diabetes classification and control • Maternal hypertension: chronic vs. gestational; preeclampsia or eclampsia • Fetal testing results: serum; ultrasonic; genetic testing; fetal lung maturity • Evidence of placental insufficiency • Presence of polyhydramnios, oligohydramnios, anhydramnios • Congenital TORCH infections • Abnormal fetal growth • Known anomalies (malformation vs. chromosomal)

EDC, estimated date of confinement; IUGR, intrauterine growth restriction; LMP, last menstrual period; TORCH, toxoplasmosis, other agents, rubella (also known as German measles), cytomegalovirus, and herpes simplex.

Sources: Abdulhayoglu, E. (2017). Birth trauma. In E. Eichenwald, A. Hansen, C. Martin, & A. Stark (Eds.), *Cloherty and Stark's manual of neonatal care* (8th ed., pp. 63–73, p. 63). Philadelphia, PA: Wolters Kluwer; Benjamin, K., & Furdon, S. A. (2015). Physical assessment. In T. Verklan & M. Walden (Eds.), *Core curriculum for neonatal intensive care nursing* (5th ed., pp. 110–112). St. Louis, MO: Elsevier; Fraser, D. (2014). Newborn adaptation to extrauterine life. In K. Simpson & P. Creehan (Eds.), *Perinatal nursing* (4th ed., pp. 582–583). Philadelphia, PA: Wolters Kluwer/Lippincott, Williams & Wilkins; Horns LaBronte, K. (2016). Recording and evaluating the neonatal history. In E. P. Tappero & M. E. Honeyfield (Eds.), (2014). *Physical assessment of the newborn: A comprehensive approach to the art of physical examination* (5th ed., pp. 12–20). New York, NY: Springer Publishing Company; Johnson, L., & Cochran, W. D. (2017). Assessment of the newborn history and physical examination of the newborn. In E. Eichenwald, A. Hansen, C. Martin & A. Stark (Eds.), *Cloherty and Stark's manual of neonatal care* (8th ed., pp. 92–93). Philadelphia, PA: Wolters Kluwer; Smith, V. C. (2017). The high-risk newborn: Anticipation, evaluation, management, and outcome. In E. Eichenwald, A. Hansen, C. Martin, & A. Stark (Eds.), *Cloherty and Stark's manual of neonatal care* (8th ed., pp. 74–90). Philadelphia, PA: Wolters Kluwer.

TABLE 3.5B Intrapartum and Newborn Resuscitation Histories

Intrapartum History	Newborn Birth and Resuscitation
• Preterm labor • Post dates • Bleeding: placenta previa; placental abruption • Hypertension • Reason for delivery • Labor/delivery: spontaneous labor; induction; planned; emergent • Infection risk: chorioamnionitis, GBS, PROM, fever • Infection prophylaxis • Fetal lung maturity assessment and biophysical profile • Antenatal corticosteroids • Cord prolapse • Fetal distress/fetal heart monitoring • Fetal presentation • Mode of delivery • Intrapartum drugs: magnesium sulfate; analgesia; anesthetic • Amniotic fluid stocia/appearance • Prolonged labor • Delivery difficulties: shoulder dystocia; precipitous delivery; failure to progress; nuchal cord; umbilical cord knot • Gestational age at delivery • Onset and duration of labor • Rupture of membranes: spontaneous; artificial; duration • Placental findings	Maternal/Delivery history considerations: • Known abnormal fetal growth • Previous history of SGA/LGA infants • Maternal malnutrition • History of unexpected losses • Use of tobacco or illicit drugs • Known placental insufficiency • Multiple gestation • Twin-to-twin transfusion/treatments • Placental or umbilical abnormalities • Presence of diabetes • History of congenital infection • Known congenital anomalies/malformations • Presence of polyhydramnios, oligohydramnios • Decreased fetal movement • Birth presentation • Delivery assistance: forceps; vacuum • Presence of meconium Newborn Resuscitation: • Apgar scores • Required resuscitation measures: blow by oxygen; PPV; intubation; medications; chest compressions • Presence of birth trauma

GBS, Group beta-streptococcus; LGA, large for gestational age; PPV, positive pressure ventilation; PROM, premature rupture of membranes; SGA, small for gestational age.

Sources: Abdulhayoglu, E. (2017). Birth trauma. In E. Eichenwald, A. Hansen, C. Martin, & A. Stark (Eds.), *Cloherty and Stark's manual of neonatal care* (8th ed., p. 63). Philadelphia, PA: Wolters Kluwer; Benjamin, K., & Furdon, S. A. (2015). Physical assessment. In T. Verklan & M. Walden (Eds.), *Core curriculum for neonatal intensive care nursing* (5th ed., pp. 110–112). St. Louis, MO: Elsevier; Fraser, D. (2014). Newborn adaptation to extrauterine life. In K. Simpson & P. Creehan (Eds.), *Perinatal nursing* (4th ed., pp. 583). Philadelphia, PA: Wolters Kluwer/Lippincott, Williams & Wilkins; Horns LaBronte, K. (2016). Recording and evaluating the neonatal history. In E. P. Tappero & M. E. Honeyfield (Eds.), (2014). *Physical assessment of the newborn: A comprehensive approach to the art of physical examination* (5th ed., pp. 12–20). New York, NY: Springer Publishing Company; Johnson, L., & Cochran, W. D. (2017). Assessment of the newborn history and physical examination of the newborn. In E. Eichenwald, A. Hansen, C. Martin & A. Stark (Eds.), *Cloherty and Stark's manual of neonatal care* (8th ed., pp. 92–93). Philadelphia, PA: Wolters Kluwer; Smith, V. C. (2017). The high-risk newborn: Anticipation, evaluation, management, and outcome. In E. Eichenwald, A. Hansen, C. Martin, & A. Stark (Eds.), *Cloherty and Stark's manual of neonatal care* (8th ed., pp. 74–76). Philadelphia, PA: Wolters Kluwer.

○ Apnea or bradycardia in term newborn is not normal.
  ▪ Etiologic considerations: metabolic, infectious, neurologic, or hypothermia (Boucher, Marvicsin, & Gardner, 2017, p. 107; Johnson, 2016, p. 97)

Blood Pressure

- Blood pressure (BP) values depend on GA and chronological age. It is not routinely measured in otherwise well newborns, but when indicated, the appropriate size BP cuff is critical to obtaining an accurate measure of the BP (Figure 3.3; Johnson & Cochran, 2017, p. 97).
  ○ Correct size of BP cuff is determined by measuring the circumference of the extremity. The cuff should be 40% to 50% of the circumference of the extremity (equaling 125%–155% of the diameter of the limb being measured). The cuff should be long enough to entirely encircle the extremity (Vargo, 2016, p. 105).
- Normal
  ○ Term
    ▪ Systolic: 65 to 95 mmHg
    ▪ Diastolic: 30 to 60 mmHg (Vargo, 2014, p. 612)
    ▪ Preterm

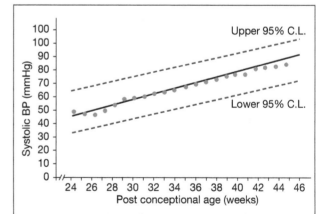

FIGURE 3.3 Linear regression of mean systolic blood pressures with 95% CIs

CIs, confidence intervals.

Source: Reproduced with permission from Gardner, S., Carter, B., Hines, M., & Hernandez, J. (Eds.), *Merenstein & Gardner's handbook of neonatal intensive care* (8th ed.). St. Louis, MO: Elsevier.

- Abnormal
  - ○ "A gradient between upper and lower extremity systolic pressure >10 mmHg should be considered suspicious for coarctation or other anomalies of the aorta" (Johnson & Cochran, 2017, p. 92)
  - ○ Hypertension: systolic >90 mmHg and diastolic >60 mmHg (Benjamin & Furdon, 2015, p. 135)

Capillary Refill (see also section "Cardiovascular")

NORMAL FINDINGS:
  - ○ Assess in central and peripheral location.
  - ○ Refill time of ≤3 seconds considered normal

ABNORMAL FINDINGS:
  - ○ Refill time of 4 or >seconds considered abnormal
  - ○ Reflection of poor perfusion/cardiac output (Benjamin & Furdon, 2015, p. 135)

Peripheral Pulses (see also section "Cardiovascular")

NORMAL FINDINGS:
  - ○ Equal intensity bilateral brachial and femoral arteries
  - ○ Graded 0 to 4 (see Chart 3.7)
    - ▪ Represent an approximate determination of cardiac output (Vargo, 2016, p. 97)

ABNORMAL FINDINGS:
  - ○ Decreased intensity of femoral compared to brachial arteries
  - ○ Unequal intensity bilaterally
  - ○ Weak pulses are noted in conditions associated with a decrease in cardiac output.
  - ○ Bounding pulses (4+) are noted when there is increased cardiac output; some conditions that are associated with this include the following:
    - ▪ Patent ductus arteriosus
    - ▪ Aortic insufficiency (Benjamin & Furdon, 2015, p. 135)

Pulse Oximetry (see also section "Cardiovascular")

- Generally not part of the initial newborn exam. Recommended universal cardiac screening for term infants between 24 and 48 hours of age.
  - ○ Abnormal results requiring additional evaluation:
  - ○ Oxygen saturation <90%
  - ○ Oxygen saturation <95% in the right hand and either foot on three measures separated by 1 hour
  - ○ >3% difference in oxygen saturation between the right hand and foot on three measures, separated by 1 hour (Johnson, 2016, p. 97; Vargo, 2016, p. 108)

HANDS-ON PHYSICAL EXAMINATION

- The physical examination is a systematic head-to-toe approach used to identify congenital anomalies, successful transition from intra- to extrauterine life, the effects of antenatal and intrapartum medications (analgesia, anesthetics) on the newborn, and signs and symptoms of life-threatening conditions requiring immediate assessment

and intervention. The infant's general appearance should be assessed prior to interacting with infant. The infant's state, alertness, movement and tone, signs of wellness or distress (color, respiratory effort, signs of nutritional status), obvious malformation, or anomaly all should be taken into consideration prior to beginning the hands-on assessment (Benjamin & Furdon, 2015, p. 122; Horns LaBronte, 2016, pp. 12–20; Johnson & Cochran, 2017, pp. 92–93; Lissauer & Steer, 2013, pp. 118–119).

Skin (Table 3.6)

TABLE 3.6 Common Dermatologic Terminology

Term	Description
Bulla	Vesicle >1 cm in diameter containing serous or seropurulent fluid
Crust	Lesion containing dried serous exudate, blood, or pus on skin surface
Cyst	Raised, palpable fluid or semifluid-filled sac
Ecchymosis	Subepidermal hemorrhage; does not blanch with pressure
Lesion	Any abnormal tissue
Macule	Discolored, flat spot <1 cm in diameter; not palpable
Nodule	Elevated lesion with indistinct border; palpable
Papule	Elevated, solid circumscribed lesion <1 cm; palpable
Petechia	Pinpoint purplish hemorrhagic spot
Plaque	Elevated lesion with circumscribed borders >1 cm or a fusion of several papules; palpable
Purpura	Elevated, cloudy, purulent fluid-filled lesion
Scale	Area of exfoliation of dead/dying skin; can be caused by excess keratin
Vesicle (blister)	Elevated, serous fluid-filled lesion <1 cm diameter
Wheal	Elevated, reddened, solid fluid-filled lesion in dermis

Original table created by Pauline D. Graziano APN, MS, NNP-BC and Vivian Lopez RN-NIC, MSN, PNP, NNP-BC 2019 using information from: Witt, C. (2015). Skin assessment. In E. P. Tappero & M. E. Honeyfield (Eds.), (2014). *Physical assessment of the newborn: A comprehensive approach to the art of physical examination* (5th ed., p. 47). New York, NY: Springer Publishing Company.

NORMAL FINDINGS
- Normal skin appearance related to GA:
  - ○ 24 to 26 weeks: Translucent—red, many visible blood vessels and scant vernix
  - ○ 35 to 40 weeks: Deep cracks—no visible blood vessels and thick vernix
  - ○ 42 to 44 weeks: Dry, peeling skin—no vernix and loss of subcutaneous fat

- Acrocyanosis bluish: Discoloration of the palms of the hands and the soles of the feet, often present at birth and may persist for up to 48 hours. Acrocyanosis longer than 48 hours should be investigated
- Plethora: Ruddy or red appearance of skin may indicate a high hemoglobin or hematocrit level
  - Polycythemia— central hematocrit >65%; places infant at risk for hypoglycemia, cyanosis, respiratory distress, or jaundice (Witt, 2015, p. 48)
- Jaundice: Yellow color of the skin and/or sclera caused by breakdown of red blood cells that then deposit the excess unconjugated bilirubin in skin
- Cutis marmorata: Bluish mottling or marbling of the skin, often in response to chilling, stress, or overstimulation caused by constriction of capillaries. Usually disappears with warming
  - Common sign in infant with trisomy 18 or trisomy 21
- Harlequin color change: Sharp, demarcated red color seen on dependent half of body when infant side lying; superior half appears pale. Seen only in newborn period; transient phenomenon, lasting as long as 30 minutes
- Erythema toxicum: Also known as "newborn rash"; it consists of small white or yellow papules or vesicles with erythematous bases and eosinophils in sterile fluid. Most often found on trunk, arms, and perineal areas (Benjamin & Furdon, 2015, p. 125; Witt, 2015, p. 49)
- Milia: Small, raised white epidermal cysts formed by an accumulation of sebaceous gland secretions. May be located on the cheeks and nose, midline palate (called Epstein Pearls) and along lingual, or buccal areas of dental ridges (called Bohn nodules; Witt, 2015, p. 49)
- Sebaceous gland hyperplasia: Occurs in 50% of newborns. Numerous tiny, <0.5 cm, white or yellow papules found on the nose, cheeks, and upper lips
- Miliaria: Result from obstruction of the sweat ducts as a result of an excessively warm, humid environment. Seen primarily over forehead, scalp, skin creases of neck, thighs, or groin area.
- Café au lait spots:
  - Flat lesion with increased melanin content; regular or irregular borders. If only 3 or fewer spots present, then there is no clinical significance
- Hyperpigmented macule (formally called 'Mongolian spot'):
  - Most common pigmented (gray to blue-green color) lesion in newborn, caused by melanocytes that infiltrate the dermis. Common locations: buttocks, flanks, and shoulders. It generally disappears over first 3 years of life.
- Pular melanosis: Benign, transient nonerythematous pustules and vesicles that occur as singular or clusters. Their rupture leaves a scaly white lesion.
- Congenital melanocytic nevus (pigmented nevus): Generally benign proliferation of melanocytes within the epithelial structures and can extend into subcutaneous fat. May include hair. Range in size from 1 to 20 cm in diameter. At risk for evolving into malignant melanoma. Treatment options include laser therapy to reduce size or surgical intervention. Repigmentation may occur post laser or surgery due to remaining nevomelanocytes in dermis.
- Capillary hemangiomas (also known as "stork bite"): Macular patches with diffuse borders that blanch with pressure; commonly located on forehead, nape of neck glabella, and eyelids

- Nevus flammeus (also known as port wine stain): Flat, sharply defined lesion commonly located on back of neck. May be abnormal if located on the face following branches of trigeminal nerve (associated with Sturge–Weber syndrome)
- Strawberry hemangioma:
  - Red, raised, circumscribed, and compressible located anywhere on body; during first 6 months of life can increase in size and then have spontaneous regression, leaving no trace. Sometimes several years before complete resolution (Witt, 2015, p. 806).
- Sucking blisters: Benign findings of skin erosion found on thumbs, index fingers, wrist, or forearm, caused by intrauterine fetal sucking

ABNORMAL FINDINGS
- Epidermolysis bullosa: Autosomal dominant or recessive genetic disorders, characterized by internal and external blistering
- Staphylococcal scalded skin syndrome: Appears in response to *Staphylococcus aureus* infection, characterized by a "scalded skin" appearance (Witt, 2015, pp. 50–51)
- Neurofibromatosis: An autosomal dominant disorder in which tumors form on peripheral nerves; cranial nerves may also be affected; characterized by presence of six or more café au lait spots (Witt, 2015, p. 52, 804, 805)

HEAD

NORMAL FINDINGS
- Anterior fontanel: Diamond shaped, from barely palpable to up to 5 cm across, flat and soft; closure at 6 to 24 months of age
- Posterior fontanel: Triangular, palpable, and small (<1 cm); closure at 2 to 3 months of age
- Sutures: Suture lines may be approximated, separated (up to 1 cm separation within normal limits) or overriding; should be mobile on palpation
- Molding: An adaptive mechanism facilitating passage of head through birth canal. Head appears elongated, asymmetrical, with cranial bones sometimes overlapping. Resolves spontaneously.
- Hair: Silky with uniform distribution and pattern of growth; can be straight or curly consistent with ethnicity; one- to two-hair whorls located in the postparietal region

ABNORMAL FINDINGS
- Findings can be normal variants or associated with syndromes or chromosomal abnormalities; 90% of all visible anomalies at birth are found in this area.
- OFC: May be affected by cranial molding, scalp edema, or hemorrhage under periosteum; most skull deformities are a result of in utero positioning, limited space, or a decrease in amniotic fluid.
- Microcephaly: OFC <10th percentile; possibly related to poor brain growth or prematurely closed/fused sutures (craniosynostosis).
  - May be an isolated finding, but may also have association with genetic syndromes and congenital infections (Benjamin & Furdon, 2015, p. 126; Johnson, 2016, p. 67).

- Macrocephaly: OFC >90th percentile on growth chart, may be an isolated finding or secondary to hydrocephalus; associated with dwarfism or osteogenesis imperfecta (OI; Benjamin & Furdon, 2015, p. 126; Johnson, 2016, p. 67).
- Fontanels (see Figure 3.4)
  - ○ Anterior fontanel (AF):
    - ▪ Very large (>5 cm across), which can be associated with hypothyroidism; may be tense and/or bulging, which can be sign of increased intracranial pressure.
  - ○ Posterior fontanel
    - ▪ Large PF (>1 cm); consider hypothyroidism, congenital infection, chromosomal abnormality, or congenital syndrome.
    - ▪ Palpable third fontanel between AF and PF along sagittal suture; possible congenital anomaly.
    - ▪ Closed fontanels (premature closure, craniosynostosis)
    - ▪ Bruit auscultated over fontanel (possible AV malformation; Benjamin & Furdon, 2015, pp. 126–127; Johnson, 2016, pp. 62–63; Vargo, 2014, pp. 603–604)

- Sutures (see Figure 3.4)
  - ○ Immobile and rigid (fused); consider craniosynostosis
  - ○ Widely separated; consider hydrocephalus or increased intracranial pressure (Benjamin & Furdon 2015, p. 126; Johnson, 2016, pp. 63–64; Vargo, 2014, p. 603)
- Shape of skull (see Figure 3.5)
  - ○ Scaphocephaly: Early closure of sagittal suture
  - ○ Plagiocephaly: Closure of suture on one side of head causing asymmetric, flattened appearance on one side of head
  - ○ Brachycephaly: Closure of coronal suture
  - ○ Dolichocephaly: Common in preterm infant. Head flattened side to side. Sutures remain unfused. Cause—positioning.
  - ○ Craniosynostosis:Early, abnormal closure of sutures
    - ▪ Significance—Primary, isolated finding, metabolic disorders, genetic abnormality, hyperthyroidism (Benjamin & Furdon, 2015, p. 126; Johnson, 2016, pp. 63–64; Vargo, 2014, pp. 602–603)
- Skull bones
  - ○ Presence of craniotabes
    - ▪ Causes: Intrauterine fundal pressure on head with breech positioning; prolonged vertex position in utero; association with hydrocephalus, or may be just an incidental finding

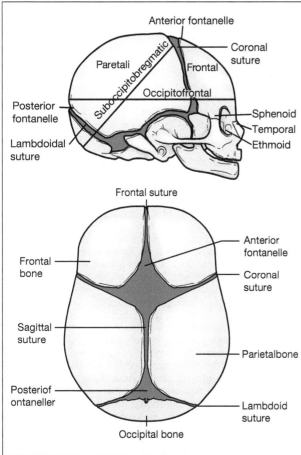

FIGURE 3.4 Neonatal skull anatomy: bones, sutures, and fontanels

Source: Reproduced from Chiocca, E. M. (2020). *Advanced pediatric assessment* (3rd ed.). New York, NY: Springer Publishing Company.

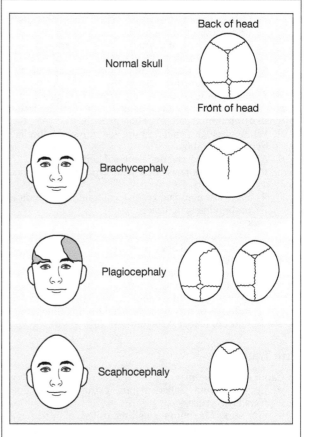

FIGURE 3.5 Newborn skulls: shapes

- Findings: Snapping sound of soft (demineralized) bones upon palpation; typically found over parietal and occipital regions along the lambdoid suture; associated with breech presentation
- Resolution: Usually spontaneous within first weeks of life (Benjamin & Furdon, 2015, p. 126; Johnson, 2016, p. 64; Vargo, 2014, p. 603)

- Skull/scalp malformation
  - Cutis aplasia
    - Cause: Most often, isolated finding can be associated with Trisomy 13.
    - Findings: An uncommon, open scalp defect. A circumscribed area that appears shiny, hairless; usual location—vertex in front of lambda
    - Resolution: Spontaneous. Area scars and remains hairless (Benjamin & Furdon, 2015, p. 128; Johnson, 2016, p. 66).
  - Encephalocele
    - Cause: Incomplete anterior neural tube closure with skull defect (cranium bifidum)
    - Findings: Protrusion of meninges and possible cerebral tissue. Covered by skin. Most commonly found in occipital region but can be found elsewhere.
    - Resolution: Severity of findings related to location and size and contents within sac (Benjamin & Furdon, 2015, p. 128; Dillon Heaberlin, 2016, pp. 184–185).
  - Anencephaly
    - Cause: Failed closure of neural tube. Results in underdeveloped cranium
    - Findings: Absent dermal covering. Exposed, hemorrhagic, fibrotic cerebral tissue
    - Resolution: Death within hours to days of birth (Dillon Heaberlin, 2016, p. 184)
- Hair abnormalities—Assess for areas of diffuse loss or abundance of hair, abnormal hair texture (brittle, fragile, twisted), abnormal pattern of hair growth.
  - White forelock (Waardenburg's syndrome)—localized hypopigmentation
  - Alopecia—abnormal deficiency of hair:
    - Diffuse loss associated with syndromic or genetic abnormality.
    - Focal loss associated with focal trauma; can indicate underlying scalp lesion
  - Whorls
    - Abnormal position or number may be associated with abnormal brain growth.
  - Hair line
    - Anterior hair line well onto forehead
    - Hirsutism—excessive hair growth may be related to metabolic disorder, genetic syndrome, drug induced, or may be an isolated finding (Benjamin & Furdon, 2015, p. 128; Johnson, 2016, p. 66).

Birth Trauma

- Caput succedaneum
  - Cause: Edema (subcutaneous, extraperiosteal fluid) from birth process
  - Findings: Maximum swelling noted at birth; may include ecchymosis, petechiae, or purpura; poorly defined edges; crosses suture lines; occurs over presenting portion of scalp; usually present with molding
  - Resolution: Spontaneous, within days (24–48 hours) of birth (Abdulhayoglu, 2017, p. 64; Benjamin & Furdon, 2015, p. 127; Johnson, 2016, p. 65; Vargo, 2014, p. 602)
- Cephalohematoma
  - Cause: Hemorrhage from rupture of superficial veins between periosteum and skull; more frequently associated with instrument-assisted deliveries; incidence about 2.5% of all live births
  - Findings: May be noted at birth or days after; well-demarcated edges; confined by suture lines; most commonly found over occipital or parietal bones; unilateral
  - Resolution: Spontaneous, within weeks to months of age; may result in palpable calcification upon resolution (Abdulhayoglu, 2017, p. 64; Benjamin & Furdon, 2015, pp. 127–128; Johnson, 2016, p. 65; Vargo, 2014, p. 602)
- Subgaleal hemorrhage–A CLINICAL EMERGENCY
  - Cause: Hemorrhage under aponeurosis. The subaponeurotic (subgaleal space) is the area between the scalp aponeurosis and pericranium. The subaponeurotic area extends from the orbital ridge to the nape of neck and laterally to the ears, which can allow for massive blood loss.
  - Findings: Fluctuant, mobile scalp mass; present at birth; crosses suture lines; poorly defined edges; can develop slowly or rapidly, resulting in shock from massive blood loss; ears may be displaced anteriorly with swelling; may have pallor and poor tone
  - Resolution: Supportive care—blood transfusion for hypovolemia; phototherapy for hyperbilirubinemia; evaluation/treatment for coagulation disorder; reabsorption occurs slowly with resolution of swelling; 14% to 22% mortality rate (Abdulhayoglu, 2017, p. 64; Benjamin & Furdon, 2015, p. 128; Johnson, 2016, pp. 65–66)
- Lacerations, Bruising, Abrasions, Subcutaneous Fat Necrosis
  - Cause: Trauma from birth process, instrumentation (fetal monitoring device, forceps, vacuum, or surgical instruments)
  - Findings: Wounds from birth process—scalp probe puncture, bruising, abrasions, lacerations, subcutaneous fat necrosis
  - Resolution: Spontaneous recovery for most; may require treatment with antibiotic ointment or sterile dressing; occasional need for plastic surgery consultation (Abdulhayoglu, 2017, p. 65; Benjamin & Furdon, 2015, p. 128; Johnson, 2016, p. 62)
- Skull Fracture Occurring During Delivery
    - Cause: Trauma from birth process/position/instrumentation
    - Findings: Palpable depression of skull; most often asymptomatic; may have neurologic depression (associated with increased intracranial hemorrhage presenting with poor tone and decreased activity) requiring neurology consultation; diagnosis confirmed with x-ray (noted fracture of skull) or head CT (if intracranial injury suspected)
  - Linear—usually of parietal bone; may be associated with dural tear; can result in herniation of brain or meninges; may result in leptomeningocele cyst development
  - Depressed—parietal or frontal bone; often associated with use of forceps

- ○ Occipital fracture—occipital bone; most often associated with breech delivery
- ○ Occipital osteodistasis—separation of basal and squamous portion of occipital bone; can result in cerebellar contusion with significant hemorrhage and possible death
  - ▪ Resolution: Uncomplicated fractures require no treatment (Abdulhayoglu, 2017, p. 65)

FACE

NORMAL FINDINGS
- Bilateral symmetry of facial shape and organs and bilateral symmetry of facial movement

ABNORMAL FINDINGS
- Asymmetry of facial shape and organs and/or asymmetry of movement; May be caused by birth trauma, prolonged intrauterine compression (multiple gestation, oligohydramnios resulting in flattened features), familial characteristic, or normal variant; or may be associated with congenital malformation, syndrome (often with distinctive facial findings), or chromosomal abnormality
- Facial nerve compression or injury: *Unilateral*
  - ○ Cause: Intrauterine position or forceps pressure
  - ○ Findings: Asymmetric facial movement or drooping of one side
  - ○ Resolution: Most recover spontaneously
- Congenital hypoplasia of depressor anguli oris (facial muscle associated with frowning)
  - ○ Cause: Unilateral hypoplasia or agenesis of depressor anguli oris muscle; may be associated with 22q11.2 deletion syndrome
  - ○ Findings: Drooping of one corner of mouth during crying; remainder of facial movement intact
  - ○ Resolution: None; cosmetic condition in infancy only
- Facial nerve compression or injury: *Symmetric*—mobius sequence
  - ○ Cause: Unknown/random occurrence; sixth (abducens) and seventh (facial) cranial nerve palsy
  - ○ Findings: Facial paralysis (unilateral or most frequently bilateral); paralysis of sideways (lateral) moving of eyes; "mask-like" face (limited facial expression during crying/laughing); may have excessive drooling, difficulty with sucking/swallowing; at risk for corneal ulceration (eyelids may remain open during sleep); other malformations/abnormalities may be present
  - ○ Resolution: Multidisciplinary follow-up required (craniofacial surgeons; ears, eyes, nose, and mouth/throat [ENT]; speech; pertussis toxin [PT]; ophthalmologist; Benjamin & Furdon, 2015, pp. 128–131; Johnson, 2016, p. 69)

EARS

NORMAL FINDINGS
- Bilateral ear shape, placement, and symmetry complete formation of both internal and external structures
- Placement of ear
  - ○ 30% of pinna located above imaginary line between inner canthus toward the occiput and tragus; helix

attached to scalp horizontal to inner eye canthus; cranial molding from birth may cause benign distortion
- Rotation of ear
  - ○ <30-degree angle from imaginary line between lobule insertion and helix
- Ear canal
  - ○ Response to auditory stimuli
  - ○ Positive startle or turn toward sound

ABNORMAL FINDINGS
- May be a normal variant/familial finding or an indication of congenital deafness. Also may be a result of intrauterine positioning or pressure, associated with renal abnormalities and/or chromosomal or syndromic disorders
- Unilateral or bilateral incomplete formation of internal or external structures
  - ○ Microtia-dysplastic ear
  - ○ Lop ear (helix folded downward)
  - ○ Cup ear (small and cupped shape): Associated with atresia of auditory meatus or conductive hearing loss
- Presence of pits, tags, or a preauricular sinus
  - ○ Often isolated finding with no other association; preauricular ear appendages (tags) can be associated with Goldenhar's syndrome or other brachial arch abnormalities (cleft lip/palate, mandible hypoplasia)
- Placement of ear
  - ○ Low set ears: >30% of pinna located below imaginary line between inner canthus and tragus; helix attached to scalp below horizontal to inner eye canthus; associated with various syndromes or chromosomal abnormalities
- Rotation of ear
  - ○ Posterior rotation: >30-degree angle from imaginary line between lobule insertion and helix
- Ear canal
  - ○ Visual absence of patent ear canal
- Response to auditory stimuli
  - ○ Lack of or diminished response to sound

Universal Hearing Screening

- Recommended for all newborns prior to discharge
- Hearing loss is one of the most common major abnormalities present at birth.

EYES

- Dysmorphisms of the eye or ocular region are most frequently cited finding of malformation syndromes.

NORMAL FINDINGS
- Distance between outer canthus can be divided equally in thirds (see Figure 3.6).
- Normal palpebral fissure length 1.5 to 2.5 cm
- No slant between inner and outer canthus; however, may be a normal racial determination.
- Eyebrows and eyelashes appear between 20 and 23 weeks GA and are located in arc above each eye. They are of equal length to the palpebral fissure.
- Eyes open spontaneously and are symmetric in size and shape.

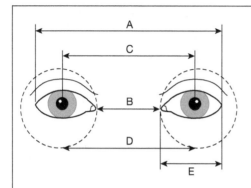

A = Outer canthal distance
B = Intracanthal distance (telecanthus)
C = Interpupilary distance
D = Intraorbital distance (hypo/hypertelorism)
E = Palpebral fissure length

FIGURE 3.6 Newborn eye

Source: Reproduced with permission from Zitelli, B. J., & Davis, H. W. (2007). *Atlas of pediatric physical diagnosis* (5th ed.). Philadelphia, PA: Mosby.

- Fused eyelids are normal up to 28 weeks GA.
- Blink reflex should be equal and symmetric.
- Pupils should be symmetric in size, shape, and reactivity to light.
- Lens clear and intact
  ○ Nearsighted at birth: By end of first week can clearly see objects 8 to 10 inches from face.
- Iris color at birth dark gray, dark blue, or brown: Permanent eye color develops near 6 months of age.
- Sclera white
- Retinal red reflex present
- Chemical conjunctivitis or edema from routine eye ointment prophylaxis may be a normal finding
- Normal eye movements
  ○ Nystagmus: Rapid involuntary eyeball movement
    ■ Normal until 3 to 4 months of age
  ○ Strabismus: Appears cross-eyed
    ■ Caused by weak musculature and muscular incoordination
    ■ Resolves spontaneously
  ○ Pseudostrabismus: Appears cross-eyed due to flattened nasal bridge and epicanthal folds

Common Birth Findings

- Birth trauma: Eyelid edema or bruising; conjunctival or subconjunctival hemorrhage; spontaneous resolution within 2 weeks of birth
- Nevus simplex: Common vascular birthmark of eyelid or glabella
- Blocked nasolacrimal duct: Causes cloudy drainage without redness or swelling; normal tear production begins at 2 to 3 months age; nasolacrimal ducts fully patent at 5 to 7 months age

ABNORMAL FINDINGS

- Distance between outer canthus cannot be divided equally in thirds (see Figure 3.6)
- Hypertelorism: Eyes spaced widely apart. Normal variant versus syndromic
- Hypertelorism: Eyes spaced closer together. Normal variant versus syndromic
- Small palpebral fissure

- Slant: Upward (outer canthus higher than inner canthus) or downward (outer canthus lower than inner) sloping of eye; may be normal variant of racial determination but may also be associated with syndromic/chromosomal abnormality
- Eyebrows that meet at the glabella (synophrys) associated with syndromes (Cornelia de Lange)
- Highly arched eyebrows
- Abnormally long-tangled eyelashes associated with syndromes (Cornelia de Lange)
- Presence of epicanthal folds: May be normal variant due to racial determination (i.e., w/up slanting palpebral fissure Asian) or a result of in utero compression from oligohydramnios (Potter's facies); prominence may be syndromic (Trisomy 21).
- Abnormal eye protrusion or enlarged eyeballs
  ○ Association hyperthyroidism or congenital glaucoma
  ○ Anophthalmos: Absent eyes
  ○ Cyclopia: Single eye
- Unable to open eyes spontaneously (after 28 weeks GA) or asymmetric opening of eyes
  ○ Ptosis: Paralytic drooping of eyelid
  ○ Sunset sign: Lid retraction with downward gaze
    ■ Associated with hydrocephaly and increased intracranial pressure
- Asymmetry or absence of blink reflex
- Coloboma: Absence or defect of ocular tissue resulting in keyhole-shaped pupil
  ○ May be sporadic finding or may be associated with Trisomy 13 or CHARGE sequence (posterior coloboma, heart defect, choanal atresia, retardation, genital and ear abnormalities)
- Infantile cataracts: Clouding of normally clear lens
  ○ Association: May be isolated finding or result of congenital rubella or CMV exposure
- Brushfield spots: White spots visualized around iris of eye
  ○ Association: May be a normal variant; however, 75% association with Trisomy 21
- Blue sclera: Blue tinted sclera; caused by thinning of sclera tissue
  ○ Association with osteogenesis imperfecta and other chromosomal abnormalities
- Absent red (retina) reflex: Possible association with congenital glaucoma, congenital cataract, retinoblastoma, or hemorrhages

- White reflex (retina) aka leukocoria: Possible association with congenital cataract, tumor, chorioretinitis
- Persistence of nystagmus after four months
- Congenital glaucoma
  ○ Cause: Abnormal development of eye's drainage system
  ○ Findings: Cornea >1 cm in diameter; excessive eye tearing; light sensitivity
  ○ Resolution: Requires immediate ophthalmology consult

NOSE

NORMAL FINDINGS

- Neonates are obligate nose breathers until 6 to 12 weeks of age
- Midline position between eyes
- Bilateral symmetry and patency of nares
- Positional deformities caused by birth process or intrauterine pressure
- Intermittent sneezing

ABNORMAL FINDINGS

- Cyanosis at rest, pink when crying (mouth breathing)
  ○ Association: Iatrogenic—excessive suctioning or choanal atresia or stenosis
- Abnormal shape or flattened, broad nasal bridge or nonmidline
  ○ May be normal variant or may be associated with syndromic abnormality
- Central proboscis with a single nare
- Nasal flaring—compensatory sign of respiratory distress
- Excessive, continuous sneezing
- Newborn abstinence syndrome

MOUTH

NORMAL FINDINGS

- Midline below philtrum, symmetrical in shape, size, and movement
- Normal reflexes present
- Suck and swallow by 32-34 weeks' GA
- Rooting and gag by 36 weeks' GA
- Hard and soft palate intact (upon inspection and palpation)
- Tongue fits within mouth, with a small singular frenulum
- Mild circumoral cyanosis during newborn period
- Epstein's Pearls: Epithelial cell masses that are benign and resolve spontaneously
- Natal teeth: Benign; often removed in newborn period due to risk of aspiration if dislodged

ABNORMAL FINDINGS

- Offset from midline, philtrum abnormalities, abnormal shape, size, or movement
  ○ Thin upper lip and flat philtrum—consider fetal alcohol syndrome
  ○ Microstomia (small mouth)—consider Trisomy 18
  ○ Macrosomia (large mouth)—consider mucopolysaccharidosis, Beckwith–Wiedemann syndrome, hypothyroidism
  ○ Micrognathia (abnormally small jaw with normal size tongue)—consider Pierre Robin, Treacher Collins, or deLange syndrome
  ○ Asymmetrical facial movement—observe at rest and crying, consider facial palsy/cranial nerve damage
- Abnormal or absent reflexes
  ○ Excessive oral secretions—consider esophageal atresia or neurologic issue associated with poor swallow or tone
- Palate
  ○ Bivid uvula
  ○ Cleft of lip, soft or hard palates—unilateral, bilateral, incomplete, or complete
  ○ Highly arched palate—caused by decreased activity or sucking in utero;—consider neuromuscular disorder
- Abnormalities of the tongue
  ○ Macroglossia (large tongue)—consider Beckwith–Wiedemann syndrome, Trisomy 21, hypothyroidism, mucopolysaccharidosis
  ○ Ankyloglossia (thick, prominent frenulum, also known as tongue-tied)
    ▪ Severe with persistence of feeding difficulties may consider frenotomy

NECK AND THROAT

NORMAL FINDINGS

- Short, thick neck with multiple skin folds. Midline trachea. Has full ROM

ABNORMAL FINDINGS

- Cystic hygroma—most common neck mass in newborn
  ○ Cause: Sequestered lymph channels that dilate into multiloculated cysts
  ○ Findings: Fluctuant mass. Most common site—lateral neck. Positive transillumination; can result in feeding difficulties or airway compromise with deviation of trachea.
  ○ Resolution: Small lesions may regress spontaneously; larger or symptomatic lesions require surgical resection.
- Redundant skin or webbed neck
  ○ Cause: Associated with Turners, Noonan's, or Down syndromes
  ○ Findings: Predominant fat pad back of neck; redundant skin back of neck. Webbed neck—excessive skinfold, usually extending from mastoid process to shoulders
  ○ Resolution: Benign symptom of syndrome; cosmetic surgical correction if desired later in life
- Thyroglossal duct cyst
  ○ Cause: Fluid-filled remnant of thyroglossal duct
  ○ Findings: Palpable nonpainful (unless infected), soft, round mass at front center of neck; moves with swallowing or tongue movement. Present at birth; most common congenital midline mass
  ○ Resolution: Normally asymptomatic until school age
- Branchial cleft cyst
  ○ Cause: Abnormal development of neck tissues leaving cystic fluid-filled pockets
  ○ Findings: Present at birth. Palpable small lump located most often near front edge of sternocleidomastoid muscle; usually unilateral, painless unless infected, may have opening on skin through which mucous drains;

if large or infected may cause difficulty in swallowing or breathing
- ○ Resolution: May require incision and drainage; antibiotics if infected: surgical removal
- Sternocleidomastoid injury or congenital muscular torticollis
  - ○ Cause: Injury to sternocleidomastoid muscle; may be congenital or caused by birth trauma; usually on right
  - ○ Findings: Contraction of neck muscle that pulls head toward affected side while chin points to opposite side; a palpable small mass at site of injury
  - ○ Resolution: PT and stretching exercises; if persists beyond 1 year may require surgical correction
- Klippel–Feil
  - ○ Defect in cervical vertebrae with decreased number of vertebrae and fusion of two or more vertebrae; neck appears shorter than normal; decreased range of motion most frequent finding; low posterior hairline additional possible finding
  - ○ X-ray of neck confirms presence of deformity
- Torticollis
  - ○ Causes: Injury sustained to the sternocleidomastoid muscle or to a cervical spine abnormality from birth trauma, intrauterine malposition, muscle fibrosis, or venous abnormality in the muscle
  - ○ Findings: Spasmodic, unilateral contraction of the neck muscles; usually appears as a firm, fibrous mass or tightness in the sternocleidomastoid muscle at approximately 2 weeks of age; head tilts laterally toward involved side with the chin rotated away from the affected shoulder.
- Brachial nerve plexus injury
  - ○ Causes: Stretching and tearing of nerve roots during birth or from pressure from maternal sacral prominence during fetal descent
  - ○ Types:
    - ■ Erb's palsy
      - • Causes: Denervation of the deltoid, supraspinatus, biceps, and brachioradialis involves cervical nerves V and VI
      - • Findings: Intact grasp ("waiter's tip"); results in upper arm paralysis and asymmetric Moro
      - • Resolution: Requires neurology and physical therapy consultations; avoid contractures of joints using passive range of motion exercises; parental education on maintaining normal joint function; reconstructive procedures if needed
    - ■ Klumpke's paralysis
      - • Cause: Involves cervical nerve VI to thoracic nerve; denervation of the intrinsic of the hand, flexors of the wrist, fingers, and sympathetics
      - • Findings: Results in lower arm paralysis, absent grasp
      - • Resolution: Requires neurology and physical therapy consultations; avoid contractures of joints using passive range of motion exercises; parental education on maintaining normal joint function; reconstructive procedures if needed

- ■ Total: Combination Erb–Duchenne paralysis and Klumpke's paralysis
  - • Causes: The denervation of entire arm from cervical nerve V to thoracic nerve
  - • Findings: In entire arm paralysis, arm remains extended and turned inward, hand flaccid ("waiter's tip")
  - • Resolution: Requires neurology and physical therapy consultations; avoid contractures of joints using passive range of motion exercises; parental education on maintaining normal joint function; reconstructive procedures if needed.

CHEST AND LUNGS

NORMAL FINDINGS
- Acrocyanosis—cyanosis of hands and feet
  - ○ Cause: Instability of peripheral circulation
  - ○ Findings: Normal in first 24 to 48 hours of life; benign in otherwise asymptomatic infant
- Symmetric chest movement, synchronous movement of abdomen
- Respiratory rate 40 to 60 bpm
- Breath sounds (see Table 3.7)—symmetrical air entry
- Pattern
  - ○ Irregular with respirations of varying depths
  - ○ Periodic breathing—5- to 20-second pause in breathing. Normal if not associated with change in color, tone, or HR
- Chest shape—symmetric, cylindrical shape
- Nipples—note placement, pigment, spacing, and amount of palpable breast tissue
  - ○ Supernumerary or accessory nipples—normal variant
  - ○ Secretions—normal variant:milky white secretions associated with breast tissue hypertrophy caused by maternal hormones
  - ○ Spacing—normal distance: less than 25% overall chest circumference

ABNORMAL FINDINGS
- Central cyanosis
  - ○ Cause: Many possible etiologies; examples include disease processes or abnormalities that result in insufficient pulmonary oxygen intake, insufficient pulmonary blood flow, or abnormal pulmonary blood flow.
  - ○ Findings: Cyanosis of mucous membranes. Always abnormal.
- Asymmetric, asynchronous movement
  - ○ Cause: Pneumothorax, phrenic nerve injury, diaphragmatic hernia, congenital heart lesion
- Abnormal breath sounds (see Table 3.7)
- Abnormal breath patterns/presence of work of breathing
  - ○ Grunting—compensatory attempt to increase intrathoracic pressure
    - ■ Allows for increased gas exchange time by trapping air within alveoli; caused by partially closed glottis
  - ○ Nasal flaring—compensatory attempt to open airways
    - ■ Widens upper airways to decrease resistance

TABLE 3.7 Abnormal Breath Sound Findings

Sound	Finding	Significance
Crackles (rales)	Fine or low pitched Heard on inspiration	Normal finding at birth as fluid clears from lungs "Wet" lungs—edema, congestion Atelectasis or inflammation
Wheeze	High pitched, "squeak" Heard loudest on expiration	Reactive airway (BPD)
Rhonchi	Loud, Low pitched, coarse	Partial obstructed airway by mucous or secretions May clear with coughing
Stridor	Rough or harsh sound Worse with inspiration	Reduced airway diameter (edema, mass, vascular ring)
Diminished	Air entry decreased	Atelectasis Effusion
Pleural friction rub	Dry, rubbing sound Inspiration or expiration	Inflammation of pleura Pleural effusion
Peristalsis in chest	Audible bowel sounds	Congenital diaphragmatic hernia

BPD, bronchopulmonary dysplasia.

Sources: Abdulhayoglu, E. (2017). Birth trauma. In E. Eichenwald, A. Hansen, C. Martin, & A. Stark (Eds.), *Cloherty and Stark's manual of neonatal care* (8th ed., pp. 70–71). Philadelphia, PA: Wolters Kluwer; Benjamin, K., & Furdon, S. A. (2015). Physical assessment. In T. Verklan & M. Walden (Eds.), *Core curriculum for neonatal intensive care nursing* (5th ed., pp. 131–133). St. Louis, MO: Elsevier; Fraser, D. (2014). Newborn adaptation to extrauterine life. In K. Simpson & P. Creehan (Eds.), *Perinatal nursing* (4th ed., pp. 81–89). Philadelphia, PA: Wolters Kluwer/Lippincott, Williams & Wilkins; Lissauer, T., & Steer, P. (2013). Size and physical examination of the newborn infant. In A. A. Fanaroff, J. M. Fanaroff, & M. H. Klaus (Eds.), *Klaus and Fanaroff's care of the high-risk neonate* (6th ed., p. 127). Philadelphia, PA: Elsevier-Saunders; Vargo, L. (2014). Newborn physical assessment. In K. Simpson & P. Creehan (Eds.), *Perinatal nursing* (4th ed., pp. 608–610, p. 599). Philadelphia, PA: Wolters Kluwer/Lippincott, Williams & Wilkins; Witt, C. (2015). Skin assessment. In E. P. Tappero & M. E. Honeyfield (Eds.), (2014). *Physical assessment of the newborn: A comprehensive approach to the art of physical examination* (5th ed., p. 48). New York, NY: Springer Publishing Company.

- ○ Retractions—substernal, subcostal, intercostal, suprasternal
  - Suprasternal retractions with gasping or stridor—possible airway obstruction
- Sneezing—normal, unless excessive or prolonged (consider neonatal abstinence syndrome)
- Coughing—always abnormal in newborn
- Apnea—pause in respiration lasting 20 seconds or longer
  - ○ Often associated with change in color, bradycardia, or decreased tone; possible causes: apnea of prematurity, infection, respiratory insufficiency, gastroesophageal reflux
- Gasping—respiratory emergency. Represents respiratory failure and acidosis.
- Chest shape
  - ○ Pectus excavation—deformity caused by excessive growth of connective tissue (cartilage) that joins the ribs to the breastbone, resulting in an inward defect of the sternum
  - ○ Depressed chest wall or funnel shaping
  - ○ Paradoxical "seesaw" movement
    - Indicates poor chest wall compliance and loss of volume; chest wall collapses with stomach bulging on inspiration
  - ○ Barrel shaped
    - Indicates air trapping or hyperinflation; may indicate cardiomegaly

- ○ Short sternum
  - Anterior chest appears short; consider Trisomy 18
- ○ Pigeon chest
  - Protrusion of sternum; consider Marfan syndrome
- Abnormal nipple discharge or placement
  - ○ Purulent discharge—mastitis. Most common organism *Staphylococcal aureus*
  - ○ Wide-spaced nipples—>25% overall chest circumference. Can be normal variant or associated with chromosomal abnormality of congenital syndrome

Birth Injury

- Fracture of the clavicles
  - ○ Cause: Most common bone injury of birth (incidence 30% of all live births), resulting from fracture of the humerus or brachial plexus palsy; 40%t undiagnosed until after hospital discharge.
  - ○ Findings: May be asymptomatic with first clinical sign a palpable callus found at 7 to 10 days of life; swelling or bone irregularity palpated over clavicle; crepitus over clavicles; may cause spasm of the sternocleidomastoid muscle or pseudoparalysis of affected extremity caused by pain on movement; asymmetric arm movement or Moro reflex; pain noted with movement of arm or shoulder; visible fracture confirmed by x-ray.
  - ○ Resolution: Supportive care; analgesia as needed; limit arm and shoulder movement: spontaneous, complete healing expected

CARDIOVASCULAR

NORMAL FINDINGS

- Color
  - Acrocyanosis—cyanosis of hands, feet, and circumoral areas
    - Cause: Instability of peripheral circulation
    - Findings: Normal in first 24 to 48 hours of life
    - Benign in otherwise asymptomatic infant
- Capillary refill—normal >3 second refill time
- Active precordium
  - Causes: Hypertrophy of ventricles; congenital heart anomaly, tachycardia; hyperthyroidism; can be present with patent ductus arteriosus (PDA)
  - Findings: Absence or presence normal finding shortly after birth of term infant; normal finding in preterm or SGA infant with decreased subcutaneous tissue; point of maximum impulse (PMI) normally located at third or fourth intercostal space, just left of midclavicular line; heartbeat seen or palpated on chest wall
- EKG
  - Nonconcerning arrhythmias—benign, requiring no treatment (see Table 3.8)
    - Sinus bradycardia (HR <80 bpm)
      - Common, transient finding in newborn
      - Cause: Parasympathetic system response to vagal stimulation
      - Normally self-resolving
  - Sinus tachycardia (HR 180–200 bpm)
    - Cause: Increased activity (crying, movement) with resultant increase demand on heart
    - Rarely requires treatment
- Auscultation examination (minimally includes assessment over aortic, pulmonic, tricuspid, and mitral valve sites)
  - Heart sounds (see Table 3.9)
  - Murmurs—note location, radiation, pitch, loudness/intensity, and timing within cycle
    - Continuous—murmur audible beyond second heart sound into diastole
    - Systolic ejection murmur—audible before first heart sound and ends at or before second heart sound; indicates flow across pulmonic valve
    - Innocent/flow murmur—normal in first 48 hours of life with transition of fetal to newborn circulation; not caused by cardiovascular disease; EKG normal; Grade I to II (see Table 3.9)
- Pulses—represent approximate estimate of cardiac output
  - Apical pulse—left ventricle during systole; normal location: fourth intracostal space, left of midclavicular line; normally the PMI
  - Peripheral pulses: Brachial (palpated at inner aspect elbow); radial (palpated at inner aspect of wrist near base of thumb); femoral (palpated in groin; midway between symphysis pubis and anterior superior iliac spine); dorsalis pedis (palpated in groove between first and second toes, slightly medial on dorsum of foot); posterior tibial (palpated below and behind ankle on inner aspect of leg)
  - Bilateral equal rate and intensity between upper and lower pulses
    - Absence or discrepancy in rate/intensity concerning for ductal dependent cardiac lesion (coarctation of the aorta)
  - Pulse grading (see Table 3.10)

ABNORMAL FINDINGS

- Color
  - Pallor or mottling
    - Compensatory peripheral vasoconstriction resulting in shunting of blood from periphery to central organs; possible causes: sepsis or cardiogenic shock

TABLE 3.8 Newborn Cardiac Arrhythmias

Arrhythmia	Cause	EKG Findings	Treatment
Sinus arrhythmia	• Normal variant	• Irregular R-R interval	• None required
Premature atrial beat	• Early beat from supraventricular focus • Normal variant in 30% of term/preterm	• P wave occurs earlier than expected in cycle • Can be inverted • Can occur on previous T-wave • PR interval normal	• Well tolerated • Usually requires no treatment • Can be seen with CHD, sepsis, hypoxia, severe RDS • If significant treat underlying cause
Premature ventricular beat	• Early beat from irritable ventricular focus causing abnormal ventricular conduction • Causes: hypoxia, irritation from invasive catheter, result of surgical procedure to treat CHD	• Wide, abnormal QRS	• Infrequent occurrence • No treatment required • Adjust tip position of invasive catheter

CHD, congenital heart disease; RDS, respiratory distress syndrome.

Sources: Benjamin, K., & Furdon, S. A. (2015). Physical assessment. In T. Verklan & M. Walden (Eds.), *Core curriculum for neonatal intensive care nursing* (5th ed., p. 133). St. Louis, MO: Elsevier; Vargo, L. (2016). Cardiovascular assessment. In E. P. Tappero & M. E. Honeyfield (2014). *Physical assessment of the newborn: A comprehensive approach to the art of physical examination* (5th ed., pp. 101–102). New York, NY: Springer Publishing Company.

TABLE 3.9 Heart Sounds in the Neonate

Sound	Represents	Location	Other
S1	• First heart sound • Closure of mitral and tricuspid valves	• Loudest at heart apex	• Intensity increases with increased cardiac output • Splitting occurs with asynchronous closure of valves • Normal variant
S2	• Second heart sound • Closure of aortic and pulmonic valves	• Loudest at base of heart	• Single sound at birth Normally split in 66% by 16 hours of age/ 80% by 48 hours • Wide split—ABNORMAL. (May be present with pulmonary stenosis, Epstein's anomaly, total anomalous venous return, tetralogy of Fallot)
S3	• Increased flow across atrioventricular valves	• Heart apex during early diastole	• Heard with PDA
S4	• Decreased compliance	• Heart apex	• Rare in neonate • Always pathologic
Ejection Click	• Normal within first 24 hours of birth	• If related to aortic valve—apex • If related to pulmonic valve—second to third intracostal space	• Abnormal finding after 24 hours of life • May be present with aortic or pulmonary stenosis, truncus arteriosus, tetralogy of fallot

PDA, patent ductus arteriosus.

Sources: Benjamin, K., & Furdon, S. A. (2015). Physical assessment. In T. Verklan & M. Walden (Eds.), *Core curriculum for neonatal intensive care nursing* (5th ed., pp. 133–134). St. Louis, MO: Elsevier; Vargo, L. (2016). Cardiovascular assessment. In E. P. Tappero & M. E. Honeyfield (2014). *Physical assessment of the newborn: A comprehensive approach to the art of physical examination* (5th ed., pp. 102–103). New York, NY: Springer Publishing Company; Vargo, L. (2014). Newborn physical assessment. In K. Simpson & P. Creehan (Eds.), *Perinatal nursing* (4th ed., p. 611). Philadelphia, PA: Wolters Kluwer/Lippincott, Williams & Wilkins.

TABLE 3.10 Peripheral Pulse Grading

0	Not palpable
+1	Very difficult to palpate. Weak, easily obliterated with pressure
+2	Difficult to palpate. Can be obliterate with pressure
+3	Easy to palpate. Normal pulse. Not easy to obliterate
+4	Strong and bounding. Not able to obliterate. Felt with PDA

PDA, patent ductus arteriosus.

Source: Benjamin, K., & Furdon, S. A. (2015). Physical assessment. In T. Verklan & M. Walden (Eds.), *Core curriculum for neonatal intensive care nursing* (5th ed., pp. 134–135). St. Louis, MO: Elsevier.

O Central cyanosis
  ▪ If no evidence of respiratory distress and/or worsens with crying, cause likely congenital heart defect (CHD). Assess by the oxygen challenge test (administration of 100% oxygen). If no improvement in saturations, etiology is likely CHD disease
O Capillary refill >3 to 4 seconds
O Precordium
  ▪ Displaced PMI—consider dextrocardia, tension pneumothorax, CHD
  ▪ Presence of heaves, taps, or thrills
    • Heave—a palpable lift; PMI that is slow and diffuse; represents ventricular dilation or volume overload
    • Tap—a palpable sharp, localized PMI; represents pressure overload and hypertrophy

    • Thrill—a palpable murmur (loud, grade IV murmur); not common in neonate
• EKG (concerning arrhythmias, see Table 3.7)
  O Bradycardia (not sinus bradycardia)
    ▪ Consider congenital heart block or cerebral defect
  O Tachycardia (not sinus tachycardia)
    ▪ Consider respiratory distress, anemia, sepsis, shock, congestive heart failure
  O Supraventricular tachycardia (HR >200 bpm)
    ▪ Medical emergency; requires immediate intervention
    ▪ Cause—abnormal extra electrical pathway. Consider Wolff–Parkinson–White syndrome or Epstein's anomaly
    ▪ Results in extreme compromise of cardiac output
    ▪ Untreated, prolonged episode can result in congestive heart failure or death within 48 hours
    ▪ Treatment includes vagal stimulation (ice to face), drug administration (adenosine), or cardioversion
• Pathologic murmurs
  O Causes: Cardiovascular disease; failed fetal circulation transition; cardiac anomaly
  O Findings: May begin or persist after 48 hours of birth; Grade II or greater (see Table 3.11)
• Pulses
  O Asymmetric or decreased in lower extremities; consider coarctation of the aorta

Universal Congenital Cardiac Heart Disease Screening

• Recommended for all newborns prior to discharge from hospital (in newborn nursery, screen should occur within 48 hours of birth)

TABLE 3.11 Heart Murmur Grading

Grade 1	Soft, barely audible
Grade 2	Soft, easily audible
Grade 3	Moderately loud, no thrill
Grade 4	Loud with thrill (palpable vibration at site)
Grade 5	Loud, audible with stethoscope lightly on chest
Grade 6	Loud, audible with stethoscope near but off chest

Sources: Benjamin, K., & Furdon, S. A. (2015). Physical assessment. In T. Verklan & M. Walden (Eds.), *Core curriculum for neonatal intensive care nursing* (5th ed., p. 134). St. Louis, MO: Elsevier; Vargo, L. (2016). Cardiovascular assessment. In E. P. Tappero & M. E. Honeyfield (2014). *Physical assessment of the newborn: A comprehensive approach to the art of physical examination* (5th ed., pp. 103–105). New York, NY: Springer Publishing Company; Vargo, L. (2014). Newborn physical assessment. In K. Simpson & P. Creehan (Eds.), *Perinatal nursing* (4th ed., p. 612). Philadelphia, PA: Wolters Kluwer/Lippincott, Williams & Wilkins.

- Screen is a comparison of pre- and postductal oximeter saturations
- Screen positive if:
  - Pre- or postductal saturation <90%
  - Pre- or postductal saturation <95% on three separate trials (at least 1 hour apart)
  - Greater than 3% difference between pre- and postductal saturations on three separate trials (at least 1 hour apart)
- Positive screen requires cardiology and NICU consultations with comprehensive evaluation of hypoxemia and echocardiogram to identify potential cardiac defect

ABDOMEN

NORMAL FINDINGS

- Appearance—soft, rounded abdomen with synchronous abdominal movement with respirations
- Umbilical cord
  - Average size 2 cm at base; normally dries and detaches within 2 weeks of birth
  - Normal color white and gelatinous
    - Yellow/green color indicates 6 to 12 hours in utero meconium staining
    - Filled with Wharton's jelly protecting one vein and two arteries
    - Absence of one artery seen in 1% of population; can be isolated finding or an association with abnormal findings of cardiovascular, gastrointestinal, or genitourinary systems
  - Cord length
    - Normal 30 to 90 cm; length determined by intrauterine space and fetal activity; decreased space or fetal activity results in short cord
    - Measure of fetal nutritional status: LGA infant—thick cord; IUGR/postdates/placental insufficiency—small, thin cord

- Audible bowel sounds—audible within first hours of life
- Patent anus
  - Appears patent; positive anal wink; passage of meconium—normally occurs within first 48 hours of birth
- Muscle tone—muscles tense with movement, crying, or upon palpation; no evidence of discomfort

ABNORMAL FINDINGS

- Appearance
  - Asynchrony of abdominal and respiratory movement associated with respiratory distress
  - Umbilical hernia—protrusion of abdominal contents at umbilicus due to weak abdominal musculature or incomplete closure of abdominal muscle wall
    - Common finding in African Americans, LBW males, and premature infants; closes spontaneously by 2 years of age
  - Diastasis recti—midline separation of rectus abdominal muscles
    - Midline, elevated ridge from sternum to umbilicus; visualized with infant crying; normal variant; resolves spontaneously
  - Sunken, scaphoid abdomen
    - Diaphragmatic hernia
  - Flaccid skinned, lumpy appearance
    - Prune belly (Eagle–Barrett syndrome)
  - Epigastric hernia—small, firm palpable fat nodule
    - Location between xyphoid and umbilicus; uncommon; surgical intervention required
  - Marked abdominal distension
    - May be iatrogenic in infant receiving positive pressure ventilation (PPV); consider bowel obstruction
- Umbilical cord
  - Omphalitis—redness encircling umbilical cord with extension onto abdomen
    - Indicative of infection; requires treatment with antibiotic
  - Patent urachus—persistence of embryonic connection between bladder and umbilicus
    - Persistent and excessive leak of clear fluid
  - Omphalomesenteric duct—persistence of embryonic tract connecting ileum to umbilicus
    - Leakage of ileal content
  - Granuloma/umbilical polyp—small, red, raw-appearing lesion
    - Located at site of separation
- Abdominal wall defects
  - Omphalocele—herniation of abdominal content into umbilical cord
    - Causes: Disruption of migration of bowel to reenter abdomen before 10th week gestation AND abdominal muscle development defect
    - Findings: Clear sac, contiguous with cord
    - Associations: 67% association with cardiac, neurologic, genitourinary, skeletal, or chromosomal abnormalities; Beckwith–Wiedemann syndrome, Trisomy 13, 18, 21

○ Gastroschisis—defect in abdominal wall allowing viscera to protrude

  ▪ Causes (theories): In utero rupture of umbilical cord hernia or possibly a vascular accident interfering with normal formation of abdominal musculature

  ▪ Findings: No sac; discrete from umbilical cord; usually to right of midline; exposed abdominal contents appear edematous, thickened, and matted as a result of in utero exposure to amniotic fluid

  ▪ Associations: Usually isolated defect; can be associated with bowel atresia and ischemic enteritis resulting from compromised mesenteric blood flow

- Perianal region
  ○ Abnormality of bowel patency/stool passage
    ▪ Not patent or no passage of meconium within first 48 hours of birth
  ○ Absence of anal wink/abnormal sphincter tone
    ▪ Consider CNS abnormality
  ○ Fistulas—anomalous connection between intestinal and genitourinary tracts
    ▪ Retrovaginal fistula—presence of meconium in vagina
    ▪ Retrourethral fistula—presence of meconium in urethral orifice
- Muscle tone
  ○ Hypertonicity—possible irritation or pain
  ○ Hypotonicity—possible neuromuscular disease, perinatal depression, neonatal depression secondary to intrapartum drug exposure

Internal Organs of the Abdomen—exam progresses from superficial to deeper structures

Liver

NORMAL FINDINGS
- 1 to 2 cm below right costal margin
- Firm, smooth, sharp edges

ABNORMAL FINDINGS
- >2 cm below right costal margin—possible associations CHD, infection, hemolytic disease, AV malformation, right-sided heart failure
- Palpated on left (sinus inversus—may be associated with cardiac defects)
- Boggy—caused by congestion/congestive heart failure
- Hard or nodular edge

Spleen

NORMAL FINDINGS
- Left side of abdomen
- If palpable felt no lower than 1 cm below left costal margin

ABNORMAL FINDINGS
- Edge palpated 1 cm below left costal margin—enlargement
- Asplenia
- Located on right—situs inversus

Kidneys

NORMAL FINDINGS
- Difficult to palpate—easiest early after birth, before feeding
- Use deep palpation—45-degree angle caudal and lateral to umbilicus
- Normal size 4.5 to 5 cm pole to pole
- Right kidney slightly lower than left

ABNORMAL FINDINGS
- Easily palpated
  ○ Enlarged— >5 cm pole to pole
    ▪ Consider hydronephrosis or cystic kidney
- Abnormal texture—not smooth or firm

Bladder

NORMAL FINDINGS
- Located 1 to 4 cm above symphysis pubis
- Can be percussed—(dull sound = urine filled)

ABNORMAL FINDINGS
- Continuous distension (consider urinary tract obstruction or CNS abnormality)
- Exstrophy of bladder
  ○ Herniation of bladder through abdominal wall
  ○ Causes: Lack of embryological development of muscle or connective tissue of abdominal wall

Abdominal Masses

- Most abdominal masses palpated at birth are of urinary tract origin (see also "Genitourinary")

NORMAL FINDINGS
- Stool palpated in colon in lower right/left quadrants
- Gaseous distension

ABNORMAL FINDINGS
- Palpated solid or cystic mass
  ○ Most common palpated masses involve urinary tract—can be cystic or solid

Groin/Femoral Region

- Observe at rest and with crying

NORMAL FINDINGS
- Flat groins
- Equal femoral pulses

ABNORMAL FINDINGS
- Weak or absent femoral pulses (consider coarctation of aorta or interrupted aortic arch)
- Full or bounding pulses—consider PDA
- Inguinal or femoral region bulges (hernia)
  ○ More common in males or very preterm
  ○ Evaluate softness and reducibility
  ○ Surgical repair required. Emergent with evidence of strangulation
- Bulge in labia majora—consider hernia or abnormal gonad position

GENITOURINARY

Male

NORMAL FINDINGS
- 2.5 to 3.5 cm in length and 1 cm wide
- Urinary meatus located distal end in the glans
- Noninflamed urethral opening
- Tight foreskin, adhered to glans (uncircumcised)
- Rugae appear near 36 weeks GA
- Testes descended into scrotum by 28 weeks GA
- Void within first 24 hours of life
- Rust color stain on diaper caused by presence of uric crystals possible
- Bruising and edema of genital and buttocks with breech presentation

Female

NORMAL FINDINGS
- Symmetric labia majora
- Term: Labia majora covers clitoris and labia minora
- Preterm: Clitoris exposed
- Presence of vaginal opening (~0.5 cm)
- Hymen tag may be observed in vagina opening
- White to pink-tinged discharge common for 2 to 4 weeks postbirth caused by maternal hormone influence

ABNORMAL FINDINGS
- Ambiguous genitalia
  - Presence of a phallic structure that is not discretely female or male
  - Abnormally located ureteral meatus
  - Inability to palpate one or both gonads in males
  - Associated with serious underlying endocrine disorders
  - Evaluation is needed with an endocrinologist, genetics, urologist, and social worker (Cavaliere, 2016, p. 134)

Male—Abnormal Findings

- Aphallia—absence of penis
- Diphallia—duplicated penis
  - Two types: bifid penis and true duplications
- Chordee—ventral bowing of penis
  - Produces a downward curvature on erection; often seen with hypospadias
- Priapism—persistent erection of penis
  - Consider spinal cord lesion
- Micropenis—abnormally small penis that is more than 2.5 standard deviations below the mean of the length and width for age using standard charts
- Displaced urethra
- Epispadias—urethral meatus located on dorsal penis
  - Less common than hypospadias
  - Three categories:
    - Balanic epispadias—meatus found at base of glans (balanus)
    - Penile epispadias—meatus on penile shaft
    - Penopubic epispadias—meatus located on symphysis, not on penis
- Hypospadias—urethral meatus located on the ventral surface of penis

- 15% associated with endocrine, chromosomal, or intersex problems
- Three categories:
  - Balanic hypospadias—meatus found at base of glans (balanus)
  - Penile hypospadias—meatus located between glans and scrotum; often associated with chordee; flattened glans and absence of ventral foreskin
  - Penoscrotal hypospadias—meatus located penoscrotal junction; associated with ambiguous genitalia, bifid scrotum, small penis, and undescended testes
- Cryptorchidism—undescended testes
  - Most common male genital abnormality; may be unilateral or bilateral
  - Occurrence: 3.7% of term; 21% to 100% preterm
  - Testes found within normal path of descent; most often below external inguinal ring
  - Usually spontaneously descends by 9 months age
- Hydrocele—large scrotal fluid–filled mass
  - Develops during normal fetal development; usually reabsorbed in utero
  - Ability to transilluminate differentiates from solid or blood-filled mass
  - Spontaneous resolution by 3 months of age
- Inguinal hernia (see section "Abdomen: Inguinal or femoral region bulges")
- Testicular torsion—twisting of testes and spermatic cord
  - Small scrotal mass
  - Scrotum appears red to bluish-red
  - Genitourinary (GU) emergency

Female—Abnormal Findings

- Periurethral cysts—most common type of mass, appearing as a whitish epithelial covering next to the unaffected urethral meatus
- Imperforate hymen
  - Suprapubic mass or mass palpated between labia majora
  - Secretions pool within vagina
- Hydrocolpos—distention of the vagina
- Hydrometrocolos—distention of the vagina and the uterus
- Clitoromegaly—an eight- to tenfold increase in clitoral index (defined as width times length)
  - Causes include endocrine abnormalities congenital adrenal hyperplasia (CAH), maternal factors such as increased androgen production, drugs, syndromes (Beckwith–Wiedemann, true hermaphroditism)

SPINE

NORMAL FINDINGS
- Spine midline and straight
- No skin disruptions or tufts of hair
- Hyperpigmented blue-gray macule (Mongolian spot)
  - Caused by concentrated melanocytes within dermis: benign
- Simple, blind ending base dimple, located midline sacrum
- Lateral curvature normal variant (in utero positioning)
- Convex curvature of lumbar and thoracic spine (best noted in sitting position)
- Extension and lateral bending of spine (noted with passive flexion)

ABNORMAL FINDINGS

- Abnormal appearing position or curve of spine
- Skin disruptions or tufts of hair
  - Isolated finding versus hidden spine defect
- Cystic masses
- Hemangioma
  - Isolated finding versus possible abnormality
- Pilonidal dimple, cyst, or sinus tract
  - Isolated finding versus hidden defect (spinal dysraphism)
  - Consider spinal lipoma, dermoid tumor, tethered cord, split cord
- Winged, elevated scapula (Sprengel's deformity)
- Asymmetric gluteal folds
  - Congenital hip dislocation
- Abnormal curvatures
  - Scoliosis—abnormal sideways curve of spine
  - Kyphosis—abnormal outward rounded curve of upper back
  - Lordosis—abnormal inward curve of lower back
  - Sacrococcygeal teratoma—most common tumor of newborn
    - Cause: Unknown; arises from fetal germ cells
    - Findings: Usual location base of coccyx, more common in females, usually benign, can be very large and result in polyhydramnios, fetal urinary obstruction (hydronephrosis), hydrops, tumor bleeding, or rupture
    - Resolution: Require surgical resection
- Spinal deformities
  - Congenital scoliosis
    - Causes: Embryonic defect—failure of vertebral formation, segmentation, or both
    - Findings: Can occur in any area of vertebral body
    - Associations: 20% to 30% incidence of associated genitourinary tract anomalies; Klippel–Feil syndrome and Sprengel's deformity
- Neural tube defects—abnormal closure of posterior neural tube
- Spina Bifida Occulta
  - Cause: Abnormal closure of posterior neural tube
  - Findings: Usually asymptomatic (no cord or meninges involvement); most common location lower lumbar or lumbosacral area; covered by skin; often an incidental finding with examination of hair tuft, dimple, sinus, or lipoma; can be associated with tethered cord
  - Resolution: Often asymptomatic requiring no treatment; surgical intervention for tethered cord if present
- Meningocele
  - Cause: Abnormal closure of posterior neural tube; meninges protrude through bony defect; usually involve several vertebrae
  - Findings: Skin covered; spinal roots and nerves normal
  - Resolution: Surgical closure of defect
- Myelomeningocele
  - Cause: Abnormal closure of posterior neural tube; bilateral broadened vertebrae or absent vertebral arches
  - Findings: Bilateral broadened vertebrae or absent vertebral arches; nerves, spinal roots, and meninges protrude into sac; spinal cord fused; neural tube exposed; most often occur in lumbar spine; >70% with associated hydrocephalus (may be associated with Arnold-Chiari malformation)
  - Resolution: Surgical intervention (neurosurgery, plastics) required as well as neurology, orthopedics, urology consultation; functional deficits of lower extremities, neurogenic bladder related to level of involvement

Birth Trauma

- Spinal cord injury
  - Causes: Hyperextension of head or neck; associated with breech vaginal delivery or severe shoulder dystocia; rate: 0.14/10,000 live births; includes spinal epidural hematoma, vertebral artery injury, traumatic cervical hematomelia, spinal arterial occlusion, transection of spinal cord
  - Findings: Depends on level of injury
    - High cervical injury or brain stem injury—stillbirth or death within hours; severe respiratory depression, shock, hypothermia
    - Upper, mid-cervical injury—central respiratory depression; lower extremity paralysis; absent deep tendon reflexes; urinary retention, and constipation
    - Below seventh cervical spine injury—may be reversible
    - Resolution: Cervical spine x-ray, CT and/or MRI; neurology, neurosurgery; focus on prevention of additional injury

EXTREMITIES: UPPER

Humerus

NORMAL FINDINGS

- Bilateral symmetry of form, length, and movement

ABNORMAL FINDINGS

- Asymmetry may indicate weakness, paralysis, injury, fracture, or infection
- Pain on palpation of movement
- Palpated mass
  - Likely hematoma formation at site of fracture
- Polydactyly
  - Causes: Congenital anomaly; isolated finding; inherited—autosomal dominant trait; more common in African Americans
  - Findings: One or more extra digits on the hands or feet; extra digit can appear as a skin tag or floppy appendage (most common)
- Macrodactyly—an enlarged finger or toe
  - Causes: Normal finding, neurofibromatosis, lymphedema, hemangioma, arterial vascular fistulas, fibrous dysplasia, lipomas
- Syndactyly—congenital webbing of the fingers and toes
  - Males twice as often as females; more common among Caucasians
  - Causes: Caused by failure of the normal necrosis of the skin that separates the fingers during sixth to eighth week of fetal gestation
  - Isolated finding versus association with other congenital anomalies, such as Apert and Streeter dysplasia; more severe the webbing the more likely of underlying bony abnormalities

Absent Bones

- Congenital absence of the radius (radial dysplasia)
  - Causes: Sporadic inheritance versus association with other congenital sequence/syndrome; VACTERL sequence (vertebral defects, anal atresia, cardiac abnormalities, tracheoesophageal abnormalities, renal, and/or limb abnormalities); Fanconi anemia; Holt–Oram syndrome
  - Findings: Hand and wrist deviated 90 degrees or more; forearm shortened with bowing of ulna; thumb usually absent or hypoplastic
- Sprengel's deformity—congenital deformity of the shoulder girdle
  - Causes: Associated with congenital spinal anomalies, Klipper–Feil syndrome and renal anomalies
  - Findings: Hypoplasia and malrotation of the scapula causing an elevated appearance; shoulder abduction and flexion are limited; most frequently unilateral but can be bilateral

Disruption Abnormalities

- Amniotic band syndrome
  - Causes: Amniotic band encircles the arms, legs, fingers, or toes; no gender or ethnic predispositions
  - Findings: Vary from mild indentation of the soft tissue to severe amputation
  - Resolution—Dependent on anatomic position and/or associated abnormalities; if vascular, lymphatic or nerve integrity compromised requires immediate surgical release of band; nonemergent may require staged surgical repairs; not life threatening unless associated with brain malformation or deep facial clefts

Elbow, Forearm, and Wrist

NORMAL FINDINGS
- Symmetry of size, shape, number of bones, and movement
- Wrist flexion increases with increasing GA

ABNORMAL FINDINGS
- See amniotic bands, neurologic birth injuries, congenital absence of radius

Hand

NORMAL FINDINGS
- Symmetry of size, shape, length, and movement
- Five digits per hand

ABNORMAL FINDINGS
- Single palm crease (Simian crease)—can be associated with Trisomy 21 (Down syndrome)
- Polydactyly, macrodactyly, syndactyly, absent bones (see above)
- Flexed fingers with index finger overlapping the third finger—consider Trisomy 18

- Puffy hands—normal finding caused by lymphedema from birth positioning; characteristic finding of some syndromes; consider Turner and Noonan syndromes
- See amniotic bands

EXTREMITIES: LOWER

Hips

NORMAL FINDINGS
- 20- to 30-degree flexion contraction normal; resolves by 4 to 6 months age
- Normal hip abduction almost 90 degrees

ABNORMAL FINDINGS
- Developmental dysplasia of the hip (DDH)
  - Positive Barlow maneuver
    - Hip is adducted while pushing thigh posteriorly
    - Palpable, sometimes audible "clunk" indicates dislocation of hip
    - Hip will be relocated by performing the Ortolani maneuver
  - Positive Ortolani maneuver
    - Thigh of the hip being tested is abducted and gently pulled anteriorly
    - Palpable, sometimes audible "clunk" will be detected as the femoral head moves over the posterior rim of the acetabulum and back into position indicating dislocation of hip
  - Treatment
    - Pavlik harness or closed reduction surgery
- Talipes equinovarus (clubfoot)
  - Causes: Positional or structural
  - Findings: Inversion of heel resulting in medial pointing of soles; forefoot curves inward; ankle in "equinus posture" (toes pointed down; heel points up).
  - Resolution: There are variations in the severity of clubfoot, and this determines treatment. Some of the treatments are conservative, such as exercises and serial casting. Some require surgical correction when nonoperative treatments are unsuccessful.
- See amniotic bands.

Legs

NORMAL FINDINGS
- Symmetry of size, shape, number of bones, and movement
- Mild bowing and internal rotation common due to intrauterine space and fetal positioning

ABNORMAL FINDINGS
- Irregularities in contour, masses, or crepitation
- Pain upon movement
- Discrepancy in knee height (Galeazzi or Allis sign)
  - Consider DDH
- Internal tibial torsion—inward twisting of tibia resulting in intoeing of foot
- Congenital absence of the tibia or fibula
  - Findings: Mild to marked shortening of the lower leg; may be partial or complete; knee is unstable with flexion contracture; absence of fibula presentation is

shortening of the involved leg with bowing of the tibia anteriorly and medially
- See amniotic bands

Ankles and Feet

NORMAL FINDINGS
- Symmetry of size, shape, length, and movement
- Five digits per foot

ABNORMAL FINDINGS
- Clubfoot (talipes equinovarus)
  - Findings: Adduction of the forefoot (points medially); pronounced varus of the heel; downward pointing of the foot and toes; lacks full range of motion, resists dorsiflexion
  - Resolution: Based on severity; exercises and serial casting; surgical correction
- Metatarsus adductus—most common congenital foot abnormality
  - Causes: Positional deformity as result of intrauterine positioning; structural deformity
  - Findings: Deformity of forefoot; metatarsal bones deviated medially
  - Resolution: Spontaneous correction with stretching exercises; casting or surgery if rigid deformity
- Rocker bottom feet—also known as congenital vertical talus
  - Findings: Prominence of calcaneus (heel bone); convex rounded bottom of foot (resembles bottom of rocking chair)
- See amniotic bands

MUSCLE MOVEMENT/TONE/REFLEXES

Evaluation of muscle tone involves resting posture, passive tone, and active tone and should be done when in an awake and alert state.

Normal Muscle Tone Findings

- Phasic: Brief, forceful contraction in response to a short duration, high-amplitude stretch; testing resistance of upper and lower extremities to movement
  - Examples of resistance are scarf sign and arm/leg recoil
  - Minimal resistance is normal at 28 weeks
  - Resistance increases with maturity
- The biceps reflex and the patellar reflex can be tested in the newborn and the patellar is the most frequently demonstrated after birth. The normal response of the patellar reflex is extension at the knee and visible contrition of the quadriceps.
- Asymmetric deep tendon reflexes may be due to central or peripheral nervous system impairment.
- Clonus: Rapid movement of a particular joint by sudden stretching of a tendon. Sustained clonus may indicate cerebral irritation (Dillon Heaberlin, 2016, p. 172).

Postural Tone

- Test the ability to resist the pull to gravity by grasping the neonate's hands and pulling slowly from the supine to a sitting position; best tested by traction response (pull-to-sit maneuver)
  - During traction, flexion occurs in the elbows, knees, and ankles
  - In term neonates, more than minimum head lag is abnormal and may indicate hypotonia
  - Neck flexion is absent in preterm infants less than 33 weeks' GA
- Strength of the lower extremities is evaluated by observing the infants stepping reflex, is noted by 37 weeks' GA (Dillon Heaberlin, 2016, p. 173)

Abnormalities of Muscle Tone

HYPOTONIA
- Focal injury to cerebellum can result in contralateral hemiparesis the face and upper extremities
- Neuromuscular diseases such as myasthenia gravis and infantile botulism can cause generalized weakness and hypotonia
- Werdnig–Hoffmann disease (disorder of lower motor neurons)
  - Flaccid weakness of the extremities
  - Continuous and rapid twitching movements of the tongue

Hypertonia

- Less common in the newborn period
- Opisthotonos (hypertonia with arching of back)—seen in bacterial meningitis, severe neonatal encephalopathy and massive intraventricular hemorrhage (IVH) and tetanus (Dillon Heaberlin, 2016, p. 174)

Developmental Reflexes

- Assessment of developmental reflexes is used to determine the overall well-being of the brain and nervous system. Reflexes are involuntary movements or actions and may be spontaneous and observed with normal newborn activity or in response to an outside action. Some reflexes are only observed during certain periods of development.
- See Table 3.12 for complete description of developmental reflexes.

BEHAVIORAL ASSESSMENT

- Behavioral assessment provides information about the infant's neurobehavioral functioning, the newborn's capability to control his or her behavior and to adapt to an environment as seen in different subsystems such as habituation, orientation, motor behavior, behavioral states, and autonomic system (Lehtonen, 2015, p. 1006).
  - The evaluation of the autonomic nervous system includes evaluation of vital sign stability, neurocutaneous stability, gastrointestinal stability, and the presence or absence or jitteriness or myoclonic jerks. See Table 3.13
  - Motor behavior is a comprehensive system that incorporates autonomic, involuntary movement, to the objective, purposeful, coordinated movement of the entire body from head to toe. It includes both physical and social activity and behavior. See Table 3.14
- State refers to the level of consciousness exhibited by the infant and is determined by the level of arousal and ability to respond to stimuli (Vittner & McGrath, 2018, p. 196).

TABLE 3.12 Developmental Reflexes in the Neonate

Reflex	Test	Response
Palmer grasp	• Stroke palm with finger	• Grasps finger • Stronger in preterm • Onset by 28 weeks' GA; well-established by 32–34 weeks • Response fades at 2–3 months • Absent reflex: CNS deficit or muscle injury
Rooting reflex	• Stroke side of cheek	• Turns head toward direction of touch • Onset by 28 weeks' GA; well-established by 32–34 weeks • Unilateral absence: facial paralysis • Bilateral absence: neurologic depression
Sucking reflex	• Finger into mouth	• Sucking • Present in utero by ~26 weeks' GA • Onset ~28 weeks' GA; well-established 32–34 weeks • Disappears by 12 months
Moro (startle) reflex	• Loud noise or gentle jolt	• Extends arms, legs, neck, then pulls back arms and legs • Onset 28–32 weeks' GA; well-established 37 weeks • Disappears at 5–6 months • Asymmetric response: brachial plexus injury or fractured clavicle • Absent: severe brain stem problem
Tonic neck (fencing position)	• Supine; turn head to one side; hold position 15 seconds	• Arm and leg extend on facial side; flex on opposite side • Onset at 35 weeks' GA; well-established 4 weeks • Disappears by 6 months • Absent: abnormal
Babinski reflex	• Stroke lateral aspect of sole from heel to ball of foot	• Hyperextension of all toes • Onset at 34–36 weeks' GA; well-established by 38 weeks • Positive response normal until 2 years of age • Persistent absence: CNS depression or spinal nerve injury
Galant reflex	• Prone; stroke down one side of spine	• Pelvis turns toward stimulated side • Present at birth • Disappears by 2 months • Asymmetric response: neurologic abnormality
Stepping reflex	• Hold upright with soles of feet touching flat surface	• Alternate stepping movements

CNS, central nervous system; GA, gestational age.

Sources: Benjamin, K., & Furdon, S. A. (2015). Physical assessment. In T. Verklan & M. Walden (Eds.), *Core curriculum for neonatal intensive care nursing* (5th ed., p. 142). St. Louis, MO: Elsevier; Boucher, N., Marvicsin, D., & Gardner, S. (2017). Physical examination, interventions, and referrals. In B. Snell & S. Gardner (Eds.), *Care of the well newborn* (pp. 130–131, p. 125). Burlington, MA: Jones and Bartlett Learning; Dillon Heaberlin, P. (2016). Neurologic assessment. In E. P. Tappero & M. E. Honeyfield (Eds.), *Physical assessment of the newborn: A comprehensive approach to the art of physical examination* (5th ed., p. 173). New York, NY: Springer Publishing Company.

TABLE 3.13 Evaluation of Autonomic System in the Neonate

System	Unstressed	Stressed	Intervention to Correct
Respiratory	• Smooth, unlabored breathing	• Tachypnea • Irregular breathing pattern • Very slow respirations • Apnea	• Reduce environmental stimulation (light, noise, activity)
Color	• Pink color	• Pale or mottled • Red • Dusky or cyanotic	• Gentle hand containment • Offer pacifier during procedures/exams • Soft voice • Slow movement transitions
Visceral	• Feeding tolerance • Smooth digestion	• Hiccups or yawns • Coughs or sneezes • Gagging or spitting up • Grunting and straining with defecation	• Pace feedings by ability and cues

TABLE 3.13 Evaluation of Autonomic System in the Neonate *(cont.)*

System	Unstressed	Stressed	Intervention to Correct
Autonomic-related motor patterns	• No tremors or twitching	• Startles • Tremors • Twitching of face or extremities	• Cluster care • Gentle repositioning while containing extremities • Use nesting or boundaries • Manage pain

Source: Data from Spruill, C. T. (2015). Developmental support. In T. Verklan & M. Walden (Eds.), *Core curriculum for neonatal intensive care nursing* (5th ed., p. 201). St. Louis, MO: Elsevier.

○ The six behavioral states of the newborn are deep sleep, light sleep, drowsiness, quiet alertness, active alertness, and crying (Boucher, Marvicsin, & Gardner, 2017, p. 105; McGrath & Vittner, 2016, pp. 195, 197).

○ The neonate's state should be noted both before and during the examination, optimally with the neonate in the quiet, alert state (Table 3.15).

• Reflects the infant's ability to integrate in the environment physiologic without disruption in state or physiologic functions (Vittner & McGrath, 2018, p. 200); see section "Autonomic and Motor Systems"). Clustering care to allow for uninterrupted sleep, arousing infant slowly, and introducing one stimulus at a time aids in organization for the infant (Table 3.16 and 3.17).

Habituation

• Infant's ability to decrease a response to a repeat stimulus. When a stimulus is repeated, the initial response will gradually disappear. Habituation provides a defense mechanism for shutting out overwhelming or uncomfortable stimuli (McGrath & Vittner, 2016, p. 203).

Testing Visual Habituation

• Shine a bright light when infant is sleeping and repeat every 5 to 10 seconds. An appropriate response is a grimace. When habituation occurs, responses will become delayed until it disappears (Vittner & McGrath, 2018, p. 204).

Testing Auditory Habituation

Use an object that makes noise and hold the object 10 to 15 inches from the baby and shake object for 1 second. Responses include startles, squirming movements, facial grimaces, and respiratory changes. When habituation occurs, infants decrease responses to stimulus (McGrath & Vittner, 2016, p. 204).

Testing Tactile Habituation

• Can be determined by stimulating the sole of the foot with a smooth object. A normal response is the infant responds by pulling foot back. When habituation occurs, the response will gradually disappear (McGrath & Vittner, 2016, p. 203).

TABLE 3.14 Evaluation of Motor Systems

System	Unstressed	Stressed	Intervention to Correct
Tone	• Consistent, normal tone for GA • Control of movement, activity, and posture	• Hypertonia or hypotonia • Limp • Hyperflexion	• Support rest periods, reduce sleep disruption • Minimize stress • Use containment and swaddling
Posture	• Improved, well-maintained posture	• Unable to maintain flexed, aligned posture	• Use boundaries, swaddling, and positioning aids to maintain flexion, containment, and alignment
Movement	• Control of movements • Midline flexion of hands/legs • Hands together or to mouth	• Stiff, extension of extremities/fingers • Neck hyperextension • Flailing movements	• Use swaddling, boundaries, nesting, or gentle hand containment • Support overall calming
Level of activity	• Activity consistent with environment and GA	• Frequent squirming • Frantic flailing activity • Lack of activity/movement	• Manage pain • Modify environment; reduce stimulation • Encourage skin to skin

Source: Data from Spruill, C. T. (2015). Developmental support. In T. Verklan & M. Walden (Eds.), *Core curriculum for neonatal intensive care nursing* (5th ed., pp. 201–202). St. Louis, MO: Elsevier.

TABLE 3.15 Assessment of Behavior and State of the Neonate

State	Behavior
Deep sleep	• Closed eyes • No spontaneous eye activity • Regular breathing
Light sleep	• Low levels of activity • Rapid eye movement possible • May startle • May make brief fussing noises • Preterm may have irregular respirations
Drowsiness	• Variable activity (mild startles, smooth movement) • Some facial movement • Eyes open and close • Breathing irregular • Response to stimuli may be delayed • May startle easily
Quiet alert	• Rarely moves • Breathing is regular • Focuses intently on individuals/objects/stimuli within focal range; widens eyes • Face bright and alert • Breathing regular
Active alert	• Moves frequently • Abundant facial movement • Appears slightly less bright and alert • Breathing irregular • Periods of fussiness • Preterm: distressed/unable to organize
Crying	• Grimacing • Eyes shut • Breathing irregular • Increased movement with color changes and marked response to internal and external stimuli

Source: Data from McGrath, J., & Vittner, D. (2016). Behavioral assessment. In E. P. Tappero & M. E. Honeyfield (Eds.), (2014). *Physical assessment of the newborn: A comprehensive approach to the art of physical examination* (5th ed., p. 198). New York, NY: Springer Publishing Company.

TABLE 3.16 The Organized Infant

General State	Behavioral Cues	Signs of Approach
• Stable vital signs • Smooth state transition with environmental interaction • Easily consoled • Able to block out overwhelming stimuli	• Quiet alert state • Focused gaze • Dilated pupils • Respirations and HR regular • Rhythmic sucking • Reaching or grasping • Hand-to-mouth movement	• Quiet alert state • Focused gaze • Dilated pupils • Respirations and HR regular • Rhythmic sucking • Reaching or grasping • Hand-to-mouth movement

HR, heart rate.

Source: Data from McGrath, J., & Vittner, D. (2016). Behavioral assessment. In E. P. Tappero & M. E. Honeyfield (Eds.), (2014). *Physical assessment of the newborn: A comprehensive approach to the art of physical examination* (5th ed., pp. 200–202). New York, NY: Springer Publishing Company.

TABLE 3.17 The Disorganized Infant

General State	Sensory Threshold Cues and Signs
• Sudden change in state • Sudden change in vital signs • Frantic, jittery movements	Overstimulated with signs of stress and fatigue: • Gaze aversion • Frowning • Sneezing, yawning, hiccupping • Vomiting • Mottling • Irregular respirations, apnea, increased oxygen needs • Changes in HR • Arching or stiffness • Finger splaying • Fussing, crying

HR, heart rate.

Source: Data from McGrath, J., & Vittner, D. (2016). Behavioral assessment. In E. P. Tappero & M. E. Honeyfield (Eds.), (2014). *Physical assessment of the newborn: A comprehensive approach to the art of physical examination* (5th ed., p. 201). New York, NY: Springer Publishing Company.

TABLE 3.18 Summary of Physical Examination of the Neonate

History	Inspection	Auscultation	Palpation	Other
SKIN • n/a	• Color, turgor, and texture • Birthmarks, lesions, petechiae, rashes, bruising • Presence of vernix • Presence of birth trauma	• n/a	• Presence of masses • Abnormal textures	• Lab work (bilirubin, hematocrit, platelet count, culture, etc.)

TABLE 3.18 Summary of Physical Examination of the Neonate *(cont.)*

History	Inspection	Auscultation	Palpation	Other
HEAD • Known fetal abnormalities	• Overall shape and size of skull • Presence of molding • Presence of birth trauma: scalp probe puncture, lacerations, bruises, abrasions, subcutaneous fat necrosis • Hair texture, quantity, distribution • Hair whorls: number and position • Hair line • Shape, integrity, movement, and symmetry of facial organs and ears • Notes abnormalities of skull of scalp: cutis aplasia, encephalocele	• n/a	• Presence and size of fontanels • Cranial sutures: approximated, separated, overriding, mobility • Presence of craniotabes • Assessment of scalp edema and bruising: caput succedaneum, cephalohematoma, subgaleal hemorrhage	• Ophthalmoscopic exam • Universal hearing screening
NECK • Known fetal abnormality	• Shape and symmetry • Presence of redundant skin or webbed neck • Presence of birth trauma • Tone, range of motion, and symmetry of movement	• n/a	• Range of motion • Reflexes • Clavicles • Masses	• Transillumination • Ultrasound
CHEST/LUNGS • Gestational age • Known fetal anomalies • Results of fetal lung maturity • Maternal steroids • Birth history	• Note landmark structures • General color, tone, activity • Assess mucous membranes • Note chest shape, movement, symmetry, and synchrony • Note respiratory rate and work of breathing • Presence of sneezing or coughing • Nipple placement, spacing, pigment, secretions	• Bilateral breath sounds. Note pitch, intensity, duration, and symmetry • Note presence of crackles, wheezes, rubs, or stridor	• Palpate clavicles for presence of crepitus or tenderness	• Transillumination • Chest x-ray
CARDIOVASCULAR • Maternal risk factors—maternal diabetes, lupus erythematosus, maternal congenital heart disease (three to four times risk of general population) • Presence of other fetal anomalies have 25% association with CHD	• General color, tone, and activity • Assess precordium: quiet, active • Capillary refill • Presence of systemic cyanosis (key indices of CHD) • Presence of edema	• Heart rate and rhythm • Heart sounds • Presence of murmurs	• Peripheral pulses: rate, rhythm, volume, character, symmetry • Location of apical pulse/PMI • Presence of heaves, taps, or thrills • Liver edge	• Universal oximetry test: CCHD screening • Oxygen challenge test • Pre- and postductal oximeter saturation comparison • Four limb blood pressure measurement • Echocardiogram

(continued)

TABLE 3.18 Summary of Physical Examination of the Neonate *(cont.)*

History	Inspection	Auscultation	Palpation	Other
ABDOMEN • Fetal ultrasound with evidence of abnormal size/shape of kidneys, distended bowel, or other masses • Presence of polyhydramnios (20%–30%) association with structural abnormalities. Most common esophageal or duodenal atresia	• Abdominal shape, movement, and skin texture • Umbilical cord characteristics: color, size, number of vessels, noted abnormalities • Presence of abdominal wall defect • Perianal region: location of organs, patency, sphincter tone, other noted abnormalities	• Perform prior to palpation • Assess four quadrants for presence and quality of bowel sounds	• Perform palpation from superficial to deep organs • Assess muscle tone • Note ability to palpate; shape and size of organs • Presence of masses	• Abdominal ultrasound • Abdominal x-ray
GENITOURINARY • Known fetal anomalies	• Evaluate external structures • Presence of urine • Presence of birth trauma	• n/a	• Palpable bladder • Presence of testes within canal or scrotum	• Abdominal ultrasound • VCUG
MUSCULOSKELETAL • Presentation • Birth history • Abnormal/decreased fetal movement	• Observe at rest and with movement • Note symmetry or abnormalities of movement • Number of digits • Presence of nails • Presence of positional deformities	• n/a	• ROM of all extremities • Evaluation for hip dysplasia/congenital hip dislocation • Positional vs. structural abnormalities	• x-rays
SPINE • Any detected fetal abnormalities	• Base of skull to coccyx • Presence of dimples, cysts, sinus tracts, tufts of hair • Skin disruption or discoloration • Symmetry of scapula and sides • Curvature of spine • Visible spinal deformities	• n/a	• Dorsal spine processes • Curvature of spine	• Spinal ultrasound
NEUROLOGIC/ BEHAVIORAL • Birth history • Abnormal/diminished fetal movement • Known fetal anomaly	• Evaluated throughout PE • Posture, muscle tone, movement, reflexes • Evaluation of cranial nerves	• n/a	• Evaluated throughout PE	• Neurology • CT/MRI • Neurodevelopmental

CCHD, critical congenital heart defect; CHD, congenital heart defect; PE, preeclampsia; ROM, rupture of membranes; VCUG, voiding cystourethrogram.

CONCLUSION

Despite the many advances in our medical technology, physical assessment remains one of the most important skills to have as a neonatal practitioner. There is no replacement for our senses in recognizing the subtle signs and symptoms that can be crucial in the timely identification of life-threatening conditions of the newborn requiring immediate intervention or transfer to a higher level of care, or in identifying potential life-altering conditions (newborn malformation/anomaly, extreme prematurity) that require timely discussion and support of the newborn's family. Expertise in the art of physical assessment should be the goal of every provider, as it remains a critical skill required to ensure good outcomes for all newborns and their families.

REVIEW QUESTIONS

1. After a prolonged labor and vaginal delivery, the nurse notes the infant has a large ecchymotic swelling over the presenting portion of the scalp that crosses suture lines, and identifies this as a:

A. Caput succedaneum
B. Cephalohematoma
C. Subgaleal hemorrhage

2. A pregnant woman is preparing to deliver vaginally an infant at 40 5/7 weeks' gestation who is large for gestational age (LGA). This infant is identified as at high risk for intrapartum:

A. Hypoextension of the neck
B. Severe shoulder dystocia
C. Umbilical cord trauma

3. Postmenstrual age (PMA) is defined as the age from first day of last menstrual period (LMP) to the day of:

A. Assessment
B. Birth
C. Confinement

4. The majority of notable, visible anomalies discovered on physical examination of a newborn infant are found in the:

A. Feet
B. Genitalia
C. Head

5. The Neonatal Nurse Practitioner (NNP) recognizes a neonatal presentation suggestive of congenital heart disease is one in which the already-present cyanosis increases with an infant's:

A. Crying
B. Dyspnea
C. Oxygen

REFERENCES

Abdulhayoglu, E. (2017). Birth trauma. In E. Eichenwald, A. Hansen, C. Martin, & A. Stark (Eds.), *Cloherty and Stark's manual of neonatal care* (8th ed., pp. 63–73). Philadelphia, PA: Wolters Kluwer.

Ballard, J. L., Khoury, J. C., Wedig, K., Wang, L., Eilers-Walsman, B. L., & Lipp, R. (1991). New Ballard score, expanded to include extremely premature infants. *Journal of Pediatrics, 119*(3), 418.

Benjamin, K., & Furdon, S. A. (2015). Physical assessment. In T. Verklan & M. Walden (Eds.), *Core curriculum for neonatal intensive care nursing* (5th ed., pp. 110–145). St. Louis, MO: Elsevier.

Boucher, N., Marvicsin, D., & Gardner, S. (2017). Physical examination, interventions, and referrals. In B. Snell & S. Gardner (Eds.), *Care of the well newborn* (pp. 101–134). Burlington, MA: Jones and Bartlett Learning.

Brand, M. C., & Boyd, H. A. (2016). Thermoregulation. In T. Verklan and M. Walden (Eds.), *Core curriculum for neonatal intensive care nursing* (5th ed., pp. 110–145). St. Louis, MO: Elsevier.

Cannon, B., Kovalenko, O., & Synder, C. (2015). Disorders of cardiac rhythm and conduction in newborns. In R. Martin, A. Faranoff, & M. Walsh. *Fanaroff and Martin's neonatal-perinatal medicine: Diseases of the fetus and infant* (10th ed., pp. 1259–1274). Philadelphia, PA: Elsevier.

Cavaliere, T. (2016). Genitourinary assessment. In E. P. Tappero & M. E. Honeyfield (Eds.), *Physical assessment of the newborn: A comprehensive approach to the art of physical examination* (6th ed., pp. 121–137). New York, NY: Springer Publishing Company.

Chiocca, E. M. (2020). *Advanced pediatric assessment* (3rd ed.). New York, NY: Springer Publishing Company.

Dillon Heaberlin, P. (2016). Neurologic assessment. In E. P. Tappero & M. E. Honeyfield (Eds.), *Physical assessment of the newborn: A comprehensive approach to the art of physical examination* (5th ed., pp. 167–192). New York, NY: Springer Publishing Company.

Fanaroff, A., & Klaus, M. (2013). The physical environment. In A. Fanaroff, & J. Fanaroff (Eds.), *Klaus and Fanaroff's care of the high-risk neonate* (6th ed., pp. 132–150). Cleveland, OH: Elsevier.

Fraser, D. (2014). Newborn adaptation to extrauterine life. In K. Simpson & P. Creehan (Eds.), *Perinatal nursing* (4th ed., pp. 581–596). Philadelphia, PA: Wolters Kluwer/Lippincott, Williams & Wilkins.

Gardner, S., Carter, B., Hines, M., & Hernandez, J. (Eds.). (2015). *Merenstein & Gardner's handbook of neonatal intensive care* (8th ed.). St. Louis, MO: Elsevier.

Goodwin, M. (2016). Abdomen assessment. In E. P. Tappero & M. E. Honeyfield (Eds.), *Physical assessment of the newborn: A comprehensive approach to the art of physical examination* (5th ed., pp. 111–120). New York, NY: Springer Publishing Company.

Horns LaBronte, K. (2016). Recording and evaluating the neonatal history. In E. P. Tappero & M. E. Honeyfield (Eds.), (2014). *Physical assessment of the newborn: A comprehensive approach to the art of physical examination* (5th ed., pp. 9–22). New York, NY: Springer Publishing Company.

Johnson, L., & Cochran, W. D. (2017). Assessment of the newborn history and physical examination of the newborn. In E. Eichenwald, A. Hansen, C. Martin & A. Stark (Eds.), *Cloherty and Stark's manual of neonatal care* (8th ed., pp. 92–102). Philadelphia, PA: Wolters Kluwer.

Johnson, P. J. (2016). Head, eyes, ears, nose, mouth, and neck assessment. In E. P. Tappero & M. E. Honeyfield (Eds.), *Physical assessment of the newborn: A comprehensive approach to the art of physical examination* (5th ed., pp. 61–78). New York, NY: Springer Publishing Company.

Lehtonen, L. (2015). Assessment and optimization of neurobehavioral development in preterm infants. In R. Martin, A. Fanaroff, & M. Walsh (Eds.), *Fanaroff and Martin's neonatal-perinatal medicine: Diseases of the fetus and infant* (10th ed., pp. 1001–1015). Philadelphia, PA: Elsevier.

Lissauer, T., & Steer, P. (2013). Size and physical examination of the newborn infant. In A. A. Fanaroff, J. M. Fanaroff, & M. H. Klaus (Eds.), *Klaus and Fanaroff's care of the high-risk neonate* (6th ed., pp. 105–132). Philadelphia, PA: Elsevier-Saunders.

McGrath, J., & Vittner, D. (2016). Behavioral assessment. In E. P. Tappero & M. E. Honeyfield (Eds.), *Physical assessment of the newborn: A comprehensive approach to the art of physical examination* (5th ed., pp. 193–219). New York, NY: Springer Publishing Company.

Smith, V. C. (2017). The high-risk newborn: Anticipation, evaluation, management, and outcome. In E. Eichenwald, A. Hansen, C. Martin, & A. Stark (Eds.), *Cloherty and stark's manual of neonatal care* (8th ed., pp. 74–90). Philadelphia, PA: Wolters Kluwer.

Spruill, C. T. (2015). Developmental support. In T. Verklan & M. Walden (Eds.), *Core curriculum for neonatal intensive care nursing* (5th ed., pp. 197–215). St Louis, MO: Elsevier.

Tappero, E. P. (2016). Musculoskeletal system assessment. In E. P. Tappero & M. E. Honeyfield (Eds.), (2014). *Physical assessment of the newborn: A comprehensive approach to the art of physical examination* (5th ed., pp. 139–166). New York, NY: Springer Publishing Company.

Trotter, C. W. (2016). Gestational age assessment. In E. P. Tappero & M. E. Honeyfield (2014). *Physical assessment of the newborn: A comprehensive approach to the art of physical examination* (5th ed., pp. 23–44). New York, NY: Springer Publishing Company.

Vargo, L. (2014). Newborn physical assessment. In K. Simpson & P. Creehan (Eds.), *Perinatal nursing* (4th ed., pp. 597–625). Philadelphia, PA: Wolters Kluwer/Lippincott, Williams & Wilkins.

Vargo, L. (2016). Cardiovascular assessment. In E. P. Tappero & M. E. Honeyfield (2014). *Physical assessment of the newborn: A comprehensive approach to the art of physical examination* (5th ed., pp. 93–110). New York, NY: Springer Publishing Company.

Wilkins-Haug, L., & Heffner, L. J. (2017). Fetal assessment and prenatal diagnosis. In E. Eichenwald, A. Hansen, C. Martin, & A. Stark (Eds.), *Cloherty and Stark's manual of neonatal care* (8th ed., pp. 1–10). Philadelphia, PA: Wolters Kluwer.

Witt, C. (2015). Skin assessment. In E. P. Tappero & M. E. Honeyfield (Eds.), (2014). *Physical assessment of the newborn: A comprehensive approach to the art of physical examination* (5th ed., pp. 45–60). New York, NY: Springer Publishing Company.

Zitelli, B. J., & Davis, H. W. (2007). *Atlas of pediatric physical diagnosis* (5th ed.). Philadelphia, PA: Mosby.

4

CLINICAL LABORATORY TEST AND DIAGNOSTIC PROCEDURES, TECHNIQUES, AND EQUIPMENT USE FOR THE NEONATE

Ke-Ni Niko Tien
Amy R. Koehn

INTRODUCTION

Infants remaining in the NICU require laboratory testing to assess their clinical status. It is important to understand physiology to properly provide integral accuracy, precision, sensitivity, specificity, and reference range of laboratory interpretation to provide a comprehensive patient care. Common laboratory tests obtained in the NICU include chemistry analysis, hematologic tests, microbiology tests, microscopy tests, blood bank tests, immunoassays, cytogenetic tests, and immunology tests (Szlachetka, 2015, pp. 235–238, 240). This chapter also covers diagnostic studies, procedures, and equipment common to patient care management in the NICU.

CLINICAL LABORATORY TESTS

Judicious Use of Laboratory Testing

- Judicious use of laboratory testing is critical in any high-acuity setting, particularly in the NICU. There are questions the neonatal nurse practitioner (NNP) should consider prior to ordering and/or obtaining a laboratory sample, which will assist in refining critical thinking skills and aid in selective use of lab work.
  - ○ Does the patient require the laboratory test?
    - ■ Are the patient examination results abnormal, whereby a laboratory test will help in diagnosis?
    - ■ Is the medical history helpful in directing which laboratory test to order?
    - ■ Does the laboratory test require too much blood volume?
    - ■ Is the laboratory test the "best" test to answer the clinical question?
  - ○ Will the laboratory test request answer the "so what" question?
    - ■ Is the laboratory result contributory to the infant's diagnosis?
    - ■ Is the laboratory result integral to the immediate clinical management of the infant?
    - ■ Does the potential benefit of the laboratory test outweigh the risk of sequelae in the patient?

  - ○ Is the laboratory test requested still applicable to current clinical status?
    - ■ Is the timing of the laboratory test appropriate?
    - ■ Has the infant's clinical status changed?
  - ○ If the laboratory sample is inadequate, faulty, or "lost," is it necessary to redraw? (Szlachetka, 2015, pp. 246–247).

Biochemical Tests

PURPOSE

- Chemical substances reflect metabolic processes and disease states in the body and measure the chemical activity or state of the body. These measurements are useful in diagnosis, planning care, monitoring of therapy, screening, and determining the severity of disease and response to treatment. Biochemical testing also provides information in the assessment of nutritional adequacy and/or toxicity (Ditzenberger, 2015, p. 192; Szlachetka, 2015, p. 237).

LABORATORY EXAMPLES

- Substances normally present with function in the circulation, such as sodium (Na^+), potassium (K^+), calcium (Ca^+), magnesium (Mg^+), phosphorus (PO4) chloride (Cl^-), and bicarbonate (HCO_3^-) (Ditzenberger, 2015, p. 192; Szlachetka, 2015, p. 237).
  - ○ *Sodium (Na+):* The normal range is between 135 and 145 mEq/L. Sodium is the major *extracellular cation* and is involved in water balance (Cadnapaphornchai, Schoenbein, Woloschuk, Soranno, & Hernández, 2016, p. 701; Halbardier, 2015, p. 152).
    - ■ Hyponatremia is a serum sodium concentration <130 mEq/L.
    - ■ Hypernatremia is a serum sodium concentration of >150 mEq/L (Wright, Posencheg, Seri, & Evans, 2018, pp. 375–376).
  - ○ *Potassium (K+):* The normal range is 3.5 to 5.5 mEq/L. Hyperkalemia can potentially be a life-threatening complication. Potassium is the major *intracellular cation* fluid and plays an essential role along with Na^+ in

regulating cell membrane potential (Cadnapaphornchai et al., 2016, p. 692; Halbardier, 2015, p. 153).

- Hypokalemia is a serum potassium concentration <3.5 mEq/L.
- Hyperkalemia is a serum potassium concentration of >6 mEq/L. A level 6.4 to 7 mEq/L can be life-threatening (Wright et al., 2018, p. 379).

○ *Calcium (Ca+)*: The normal range for serum calcium is 8.5 and 10.2 mg/dL. Serum Ca+ is transported in the forms of protein-bound Ca, inactivated Ca, and free ionized calcium (iCa, 4.4–5.3 mg/dL). Decreased level from the use of furosemide (Lasix), caffeine citrate (Cafcit), or glucocorticosteroids may negatively impact stores and result in bone demineralization (Ditzenberger, 2015, p. 192; Halbardier, 2015, p. 155).

○ *Magnesium (Mg+)*: The normal range is 1.5 to 2.5 mg/dL. Magnesium is involved with many intracellular enzyme reactions and is primarily regulated by kidneys (Halbardier, 2015, p. 158).

○ *Phosphorus (PO4−)*: The normal range is 6.5 to 7 mg/dl. A level of <4 mg/dL is an indication of decreased bone mineralization (Ditzenberger, 2015, p. 192).

○ *Bicarbonate (CO₂−)* the normal range is 22 to 26 mEq/L for neonates (Halbardier, 2015, p. 159).

- Metabolites: These are nonfunctioning waste products in the process of being cleared. Examples include bilirubin, ammonia, blood urea nitrogen (BUN), creatinine, and uric acid (Szlachetka, 2015, p. 237).

○ *Bilirubin* is a byproduct of heme breakdown. In the presence of reduced liver function, the organ is unable to excrete conjugated bilirubin into the bile ducts or biliary tract, or excessive load of unconjugated bilirubin (hemolysis) increases indirect bilirubin level (Bradshaw, 2015, p. 588).

○ *Ammonia* is a byproduct of colonic bacteria protein breakdown. When the liver is in failure, the ammonia level elevates (Bradshaw, 2015, p. 594).

○ *Blood Urea Nitrogen* (BUN) is an indirect measurement of kidney function (Sherman, 2015b, p. 726). Elevated values may indicate increased production of urea nitrogen in catabolic states (e.g., tissue breakdown). There is little to no association between BUN levels and protein intake even when changes in renal function are taken into account (Wright et al., 2018, p. 381).

○ *Creatinine (Cr)* is a valid biochemical marker for renal function for very low birth weight (VLBW) infants. In term infants, the serum creatinine level gradually decreases within the first 2 weeks of age. In preterm infants, the plasma creatinine level instead rises in the first 48 hours before falling. Each doubling of the serum creatinine level indicates an approximate 50% reduction in glomerular filtration rate (GFR; Cadnapaphornchai et al., 2016, p. 696; Ditzenberger, 2015, p. 192; Sherman, 2015b, p. 726, 729).

○ *Uric acid* may be elevated in the newborn due to the increase in nucleotide breakdown. High urinary uric acid concentrations may leave pink or red uric acid crystals in the diaper. (Cadnapaphornchai et al., 2016, p. 693).

- Substances are released from cells as a result of cell damage and abnormal permeability or cellular proliferation. Examples are alkaline phosphatase, alanine aminotransferase (ALT), aspartate aminotransferase (AST), and creatinine kinase.

○ *Alkaline phosphatase* is derived from the epithelium of the intrahepatic bile cells, and can also be found in the bone, kidney, and small intestine (Bradshaw, 2015, p. 588). The markers for management of metabolic bone disease and assessment for bone mineralization status (Ditzenberger, 2015, p. 204). Elevated alkaline phosphorus (ALP) levels indicate obstructive liver disease, hepatitis, as well as bone disease. ALP-increased serum concentration indicates decreased bone mineralization. When level is greater than 500 to 700 mg/dL, the infant is at risk for rickets (Ditzenberger, 2015, p. 102).

○ *ALT* is the formation of pyruvic acid (Bradshaw, 2015, p. 588). It will be elevated in the presence of disseminated herpes simplex virus (HSV). This lab was formerly known as serum glutamic–pyruvic transaminase (SGPT; Darras & Volpe, 2018, p. 866).

○ *AST* is the formation of oxaloacetic acid (Bradshaw, 2015, p. 588). This lab was formerly known as serum glutamic–oxaloacetic transaminase (SGOT) (Darras & Volpe, 2018, p. 866).

- ALT and AST are the most sensitive tests of hepatocyte necrosis, and the ALT-to-AST ratio can facilitate differentiating types of liver disease (Bradshaw, 2015, p. 588).

○ *Creatinine kinase* is the most useful enzyme to evaluate muscle disease and damage; however, it does not necessarily correlate with muscle weakness. Interpretation must be with the awareness that levels are usually elevated in the first several days after a vaginal delivery (Darras & Volpe, 2018, p. 866).

- Examples of drugs and toxic substances tested for in laboratory sampling are antibiotics, caffeine, digoxin, phenobarbital, and substances of abuse.

○ *Antibiotics* levels are gauged through therapeutic drug monitoring (TDM). This uses plasma medication concentrations to determine and optimize medication therapy (Domonoske, 2015, p. 217).

- There are three types of medication levels: peak, trough, and random levels (see Chapter 12 for more discussion).
  - Levels are also used to monitor therapies using caffeine citrate (Cafcit), digoxin (Lanoxin), and phenobarbital (Luminol).

○ *Substances of abuse* screening includes many forms. The sample can be obtained from urine, blood, meconium, neonatal hair, and the umbilical cord (Sherman, 2015a, pp. 48–49). Urine drug screen is the most frequently used method; however, the limitation is that it can detect only recent substance use. In contrast, meconium accumulates throughout the pregnancy, which provides higher sensitivity and detects a longer period of drug exposure (Sherman, 2015a, p. 48).

Hematologic Tests

PURPOSE

- To study the blood and blood-forming tissues of the body, such as the bone marrow and reticuloendothelial system. This area of testing also includes the study of hemoglobin (Hgb) structure, red cell membrane, and red cell enzyme activity.
  ○ Whole blood is composed of blood cells suspended in plasma fluid.
  ○ Plasma is unclotted blood that has been centrifuged to remove any cells and contains the protein fibrinogen.

LABORATORY EXAMPLES
- Blood cells: Erythrocytes (red blood cells [RBCs]), leukocytes (white blood cells [WBCs]), and thrombocytes (platelets [Plts])
  - *Hct:* The percentage of RBCs. Like Hgb, Hct levels are higher after birth and then decrease to cord values by the end of the first week of life. It should be checked along with Hgb or complete blood count (CBC) in infants at high risk, such as twins; infant of a diabetic mother (IDM); signs of plethora or hyperviscosity, hypovolemia., or hypotension; history of maternal bleeding; fetal or neonatal blood loss; suspected sepsis; or pathologic jaundice. It ranges between 48% and 60% in term infants (Diehl-Jones & Fraser, 2015, p. 664; Levy & D'Harlingue, 2013, p. 94; Manco-Johnson, McKinney, Knapp-Clevenger, & Hernández, 2016, p. 480).
  - *Hbg:* The major iron-containing component of the RBCs. It is composed of α- and β-type globin. The binding of oxygen to Hgb is influenced by temperature, pH, CO_2 pressure (PCO_2), and the concentration of RBC organic phosphates. RBCs contain 70% to 90% fetal hemoglobin (HbF) at birth and transition to adult hemoglobin (HbA) at the end of fetal life; the range is 16 to 20 g/dL in term infants. The level is higher at birth depending on gestational age or volume of placental transfusing, such as timing of cord clamping; decreases by the end of the first week of life; and reaches a physiologic nadir at 8 to 12 weeks of life (Diab & Luchtman-Jones, 2015, p. 1297; Diehl-Jones & Fraser, 2015, pp. 662–664; Manco-Johnson et al., 2016, pp. 479–480).
  - *Reticulocyte (Retic) count:* Reflects new erythroid activity, is persistently elevated with ongoing RBC destruction, is inversely proportional to gestational age at birth, and falls rapidly to less than 2% by 7 days. Persistent reticulocytosis may indicate chronic blood loss or hemolysis (Diab & Luchtman-Jones, 2015, pp. 1300–1301; Diehl-Jones & Fraser, 2015, p. 672; Manco-Johnson et al., 2016, pp. 479–480).
  - *Plt count:* Isd 150,000–400,000/mm³; thrombocytopenia (<100,000/mm³) is most likely associated with bacterial sepsis or viral infection (Diab & Luchtman-Jones, 2015, pp. 1326–1331; Diehl-Jones & Fraser, 2015, p. 666).
  - *Peripheral blood smear:* Initial evaluation of anemia to identify abnormal RBC shapes and provide clues to the etiology of the anemia (Diab & Luchtman-Jones, 2015, pp. 1300–1301; Diehl-Jones & Fraser, 2015, p. 673).
  - *Complete blood count* (CBC) is to evaluate RBCs, WBCs, and Plts.
  - *White blood cells* (WBCs) are mature in the bone marrow and lymphatic tissues. Normal range is between 9,000 and 32,000 cells per microliter at birth. It is optimal to obtain WBC after 4 hours of age, and recommended to collect the first sample at 6 to 12 hours of age (Diehl-Jones & Fraser, 2015, p. 665; Ferrieri & Wallen, 2018, pp. 558–559).
    - Leukocytosis (WBC >25,000/mm³) may be normal in a newborn infant.
    - Leukopenia (WBC <1,750/mm³) is an abnormal finding, and may indicate sepsis or pregnancy-induced hypertension.
  - WBC differential count
    - Absolute neutrophil count (ANC) = WBC × (% immature neutrophils + % mature neutrophils) × 0.01 (Diab & Luchtman-Jones, 2015, pp. 1319–1324).
      - *Neutropenia* (<1,500/mm³): is the most accurate predictor of infection. It is also associated with maternal hypertension, confirmed periventricular hemorrhage, severe asphyxia, and reticulocytosis (Letterio, Ahuja, & Petrosiute, 2013, pp. 448–452).
      - *Neutrophilia* may result from birth or other clinical conditions, such as hemolytic disease, asymptomatic hypoglycemia, trisomy 21, use of oxytocin during labor, maternal fever, stress during labor and birth, exogenous steroid administration, pneumothorax, and meconium aspiration.
    - Immature/total neutrophil (I/T) ratio = (% bands + % immature forms) ÷ (% mature + % bands + % immature forms).
      - The sensitivity is greater than 90% (Letterio et al., 2013, p. 451)
      - The value is maximum at birth and then declines to 0.12 after 72 hours of age (Ferrieri & Wallen, 2018, p. 559).
  - Eosinophils and basophils are important in allergic response.
- Plasma: Plasma proteins and coagulation factors I through XIII:
  - *Plasma proteins* interact with the endothelium, subendothelium, plts, and circulating cells to promote homeostasis (Saxonhouse, 2018, p. 1121). A drug's affinity for plasma proteins affects the medication's volume of distribution (Wilson & Tyner, 2015, p. 692). Plasma proteins also affect the plasma oncotic pressure, guiding the way fluids flow in and out of cells (Ditzenberger, 2015, p. 173).
  - *Albumin:* Synthesized in the liver, it is the most abundant protein in plasma (Bradshaw, 2015, p. 587). When hepatocellular injury occurs, the level decreases.
  - *Fibrinogen (factor I):* Soluble protein in plasma measures the circulating level of protein substrate that is required for clot formation (Diehl-Jones & Fraser, 2015, p. 667). Low level is seen in disseminated intravascular coagulation (DIC; Diehl-Jones & Fraser, 2015, p. 676).
  - *Prothrombin (factor II):* Measurement of extrinsic (triggered by tissue injury) and common portions of the coagulation cascade (Diehl-Jones & Fraser, 2015, p. 667). It measures the time needed for factor II to be converted to thrombin (Bradshaw, 2015, p. 589). Usually near normal at birth to day of life 3, and reaches adult normal values by day 5 (Manco-Johnson et al., 2016, p. 497). Decreased vitamin K-dependent clotting factors, hepatocellular injury, and biliary obstruction demonstrate a prolonged prothrombin time (PT).
  - *Activated partial thromboplastin time (aPTT) (factor III):* Is to assess intrinsic (triggered by vascular endothelial injury) and common portions of coagulation cascade (Diehl-Jones & Fraser, 2015, p. 667). Prolonged value indicates a decrease in both vitamin K-dependent factors and contact factors (XI, XII, prekallikrein). Usually, extremely prolonged without signs of excessive bleeding in a stable preterm infant with a birth weight of less than 1,000 g (Manco-Johnson et al., 2016, p. 497).

○ *International normalized ratio (INR)*: Ratio of sample PT to a normal PT (Bradshaw, 2015, p. 589)
○ *Factors IV through XIII assays:*
- Factor V—levels are low on day of life 1 and then increase to adult values within days (Saxonhouse, 2018, p. 1122t). Factor V Leiden (FVL) mutation is the most common of the serious inheritable thrombophilias (Rodger & Silver, 2019, pp. 956–959); prolonged aPTT and PT (Diab & Luchtman-Jones, 2015, p. 1334).
- Factor VII—prolonged PT with a normal aPTT (Diab & Luchtman-Jones, 2015, p. 1334).
- Factor VIII—hemophilia A, the most common inherited bleeding disorder in the neonatal period (Diab & Luchtman-Jones, 2015, pp. 1232–1233).
- Factor IX—hemophilia B; levels are reduced at birth. Repeat testing at 6 months of age for mildly affected infants is necessary to confirm the diagnosis.
- Factors X–XIII—have varying combinations of normal and abnormal PT and aPTT levels (Diab & Luchtman-Jones, 2015, p. 1334).

Microbiology Tests

PURPOSE
- Identification of infectious microorganisms causing disease. Tests include diagnostic bacteriology, mycology, virology, parasitology, and serology.

LABORATORY EXAMPLES
- Culture of body fluid:
  ○ Cultures are isolation of a pathogen, and can be obtained from blood, cerebrospinal fluid (CSF), and urine (Wilson & Tyner, 2015, p. 694). It is the most valid method to establish the diagnosis of bacterial sepsis (Pammi, Brand, & Weisman, 2016, p. 554).
    - A minimum of 1 mL of blood should be obtained to improve chances for detection of bacterial presence in the blood (Wilson & Tyner, 2015, p. 694).

Microscopy Tests

PURPOSE
- Examination of body fluids and tissues under a microscope.

LABORATORY EXAMPLES
- Blood cell counts
- Testing for fecal blood or fecal fat
- *Apt test*—is based on alkali resistance of HbF to differentiate swallowed maternal blood with neonatal blood (Manco-Johnson et al., 2016, p. 482).
- Urinalysis

Blood Bank Tests (Transfusion Medicine)

PURPOSE
- Area of blood component preparation, blood donor screening and testing, blood compatibility testing, and blood and stem cell banking.

COMMON BLOOD BANK TESTS
- *Blood typing and crossmatch.* To identify common blood group antigens, A, B, O, and Rh.

- *Direct antiglobulin test (DAT)/Coombs' test.* Positive result indicates the presence of maternal IgG antibodies in infant's RBCs (Diehl-Jones & Fraser, 2015, p. 673).
- *Indirect antiglobulin test (IAT)/indirect Coombs' test.* Positive result shows that antibodies against the infant's RBCs are present in the maternal serum (Diehl-Jones & Fraser, 2015, p. 673).
- *Erythrocyte rosette test, Kleihauer–Betke test for fetomaternal hemorrhage.* Identifies HbF in maternal blood (Diehl-Jones & Fraser, 2015, p. 673; Manco-Johnson et al., 2016, p. 481). Calculates volume of fetal–maternal hemorrhage and dose of anti-D immune globulin (Rhogam) required to prevent sensitization.

Immunoassays

PURPOSE
- Laboratory method based on antigen–antibody reactions employed in therapeutic drum monitoring (TDM), toxicology screening, detection of plasma proteins, and certain endocrine testing.
- Immunology tests evaluate immune system activity. They are used to diagnose inflammatory responses, immunodeficiency, and autoimmune disorders, (Szlachetka, 2015, p. 237).

LABORATORY EXAMPLES
- Urine and meconium toxicology test for "street drugs," latex agglutination test, and drug levels.

Cytogenetic Tests

PURPOSE
- Testing used to determine genetic composition by chromosome analysis. Laboratory examples: simple karyotype (blood, amniotic fluid, tissue, bone marrow, buccal swab), and fluorescent in-situ hybridization (FISH) (Szlachetka, 2015, p. 237).

LABORATORY EXAMPLES
- *Simple karyotype (blood, amniotic fluid, tissue, bone marrow, buccal swab)* staining techniques are used that cause dark and light bands to show up on the chromosome. Chromosomes are identified by their distance from the centromere (Schiefelbein, 2015, p. 398; Sterk, 2015, p. 771). Normal Karyotype includes 46 chromosomes, 22 pairs of autosomes, and one set of sex chromosomes.
- *FISH.* It combines the chromosome analysis with the use of the segments of fluorescence-labeled molecular markers (probes) in order to follow the hybridization of complementary pieces of DNA. FISH is powerful in diagnosing common microdeletions or microduplications and for identifying extra sets of chromosomes. (Schiefelbein, 2015, p. 398; Sterk, 2015, p. 771).
- *Comparative genomic hybridization (CGh)*: Microarray testing, it detects genetic imbalances that are too small to be picked up by routine analysis (Schiefelbein, 2015, p. 398).

Immunology Tests

PURPOSE
- Laboratory evaluation measuring immune system activity. This consists of complement activity and its cascade of activation, humoral, and cell-mediated immunity. Tests are used to diagnose inflammatory responses, immunodeficiency, and autoimmune disorders. Immunology tests including complement activity, cascade of activation, humoral, and cell-mediated immunity are used for

diagnosing inflammatory responses, immunodeficiency and autoimmune disorders (Szlachetka, 2015, p. 237).

LABORATORY EXAMPLES

- *C-reactive protein* (CRP) is a nonspecific acute-phase reactant synthesized in the liver in the first 6 to 8 hours of the infective or an inflammatory process with low sensitivity (60%). Its sensitivity, specificity, and positive predictive values improve at 24 and 48 hours.
    - It is most useful in determining effectiveness of treatment, resolution of disease, and duration of antibiotic therapy. CRP response is found to be more useful in gram-negative infections than infections with coagulase-negative *Staphylococcus* spp. Serial CRP measurements can be used to facilitate monitoring resolution of infection (Pammi et al., 2016, p. 554; Wilson & Tyner, 2015, p. 693).
- *Procalcitonin (PCT)* is induced by systemic inflammation and bacterial sepsis. Levels rise much faster than CRP. It rises at 4 hours and peaks at 6 hours with higher sensitivity and specificity than that of CRP, then plateaus 8 to 24 hours after stimulus (Ferrieri & Wallen, 2018, pp. 559–560; Pammi et al., 2016, p. 554).
- *Cytokine measurement*: Cytokines' receptors are produced by the placenta and uterine endothelial cells as well as invading macrophages. They are interferons, tumor necrosis factor-α (TNF-α), leukemia inhibitory factor, and interleukins. The balance of cytokines and proinflammatory or anti-inflammatory factors may be the key trigger for preterm labor caused by intrauterine infection or other forms of inflammation (Maltepe & Penn, 2018, p. 52; Simhan, Berghella, & Iams, 2019, pp. 686–687).
- *Complement C3 and C4*: Is part of complement system that is central to innate immune response. Concentration of C3 can be detected as early as 5 to 6 weeks' gestation (GA) and increases to 66% of adult level by 26 to 28 weeks (Weitkamp, Lewis, & Levy, 2018, pp. 454–455).
- IgG, IgM, and IgA
    - Immunoglobulin G (IgG): The predominant Ig isotype at all ages (Weitkamp et al., 2018, p. 473). It is the only immunoglobulin that freely crosses the placenta. In a disease state, they can cause hemolysis of the RBCs (Fanso, Said, & Luban, 2015, p. 1346).
    - Immunoglobulin A (IgA): Does not cross the placenta (Weitkamp et al., 2018, p. 374). Can be detected in the saliva of neonates as early as at 3 days of life. Increased umbilical cord blood (UCB) IgA concentration may suggest congenital infection such as toxoplasmosis, HIV.
    - Immunoglobulin M (IgM): The only isotype besides IgG that binds and activates complement. Postnatal IgM concentrations rise rapidly for the first month in response to antigenic stimulation. Level may elevate in the presence of bacterial and/or viral infections (Weitkamp et al., 2018, p. 474; Wilson & Tyner, 2015, p. 706).

DIAGNOSTIC STUDIES

Radiography/X-ray

- Utilizes the natural contrast between air (dark or black presentation) and fluid or tissue (white or gray) on a standard radiograph.
- It is critical to place an infant in an appropriate position to produce a high-quality and accurate image. A rotated

image may lead to a false diagnosis or abnormal central line location. The infant's arms should be extended away from the chest to prevent the scapulae from obscuring the upper lung fields (Jensen, Mong, Biko, Maschhoff, & Kirpalani, 2017, p. 67).
- Daily x-ray to evaluate the position of invasive support devices has no evidentiary support (Jensen et al., 2017, p. 70).

TERMS ASSOCIATED WITH RADIOGRAPHY
ARTIFACT

- A silhouette or shadow on the radiograph that is not part of the patient
    - Skinfold—the most common artifact seen in the neonate. It is a visible as a straight line of variable length that can travel across the diaphragm or outside the body (Ehret, 2015, pp. 253–254).
    - Artifacts present within the radiography can make interpretation difficult (see Figure 4.1).

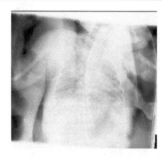

FIGURE 4.1 Artifacts within x-ray.

DENSITY

- Radiographic density varies depending on the composition of an organ or tissue. For example, a fluid-filled heart is seen as white versus black for air-filled lungs on an x-ray film (Ehret, 2015, p. 272).
- Air, fat, water (including all solid viscera: liver, spleen, kidney, pancreas, and heart), bone, and metal are the only five densities can be distinguished routinely from x-ray (Strain & Weinman, 2016, p. 159).
- Figure 4.2 demonstrates the difference in densities between the air-filled lungs and the more solid organs of the abdomen.

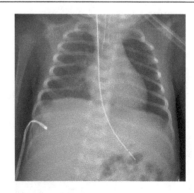

FIGURE 4.2 Radiograph showing density of lungs.

EXPOSURE
- The amount of radiation used
  - Underexposed = underpenetrated—images appear light and hazy. It is particularly difficult to view the vertebral bodies and/or any line placement due to the radiograph's brightness (Figure 4.3)
  - Overexposed = overpenetrated—images are dark and lack contrast (Ehret, 2015, p. 253, Figure 4.4)

RADIOLUCENT
- Indicates the transparency of the item being radiographed (Ehret, 2015, p. 254; Figure 4.5)

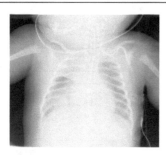

FIGURE 4.3 Example of an underexposed radiograph.

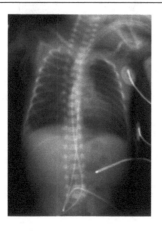

FIGURE 4.4 Example of an overexposed radiograph image.

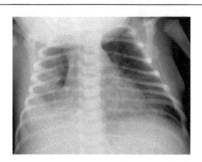

FIGURE 4.5 Rotation in a radiograph.

RADIOPAQUE
- Indicates a dense and nonpenetrable substance that cannot be radiographed (Ehret, 2015, p. 254) (Exhibit 4.1)

EXHIBIT 4.1 Radiolucent versus radiopaque

Air	Fat	Connective Tissue	Bone	Surgical Pin
Radiolucent ⟵			⟶	Radiopaque

ROTATION
- How the neonate's body is turned from the midline. This can make shadows appear larger and distorted (Ehret, 2015, p. 254)
- Figure 4.5 demonstrates rotation on an anteroposterior (AP) radiograph. Note the differences in width of the chest wall. Whichever side on which the ribs are longer is the side toward which the infant is turned.

VIEWS
- AP, cross-table lateral, and lateral decubitus views are the most commonly seen x-ray in the NICU (Jensen et al., 2017, p. 67).
- Anteroposterior view—usually shot with the infant lying on the back, chest upward (Figure 4.6).
- Cross-table lateral view—the infant lies supine and the radiograph is obtained by shooting from the infant's side through the body (Figure 4.7).

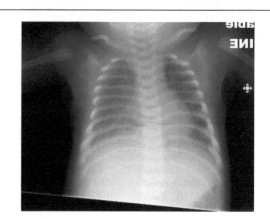

FIGURE 4.6 Anteroposterior (AP) view of an infant.

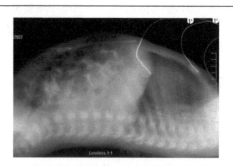

FIGURE 4.7 Cross-table lateral view of an infant.

- Lateral decubitus view is obtained with the infant lying on the side and shot back to front. A right or left lateral decubitus indicates the side on which the infant is lying. The most common example in the NICU is to obtain a left lateral decubitus (lie on left side, right side up) view to assess for free abdominal air, which will layer out over the liver (taking advantage of the contrast in densities to increase visibility; Jensen et al. 2017, p. 67, Figure 4.8).

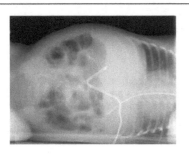

FIGURE 4.8 Lateral decubitus (left) view of an infant.

INTERPRETATION OF RADIOGRAPHS
DEVELOP A SYSTEM
- It is important to develop a systematic approach and order, as well as any anatomic and pathologic changes, when assessing a film including lung fields, mediastinum, skeletal system, and catheters (Ehret, 2015, p. 255).
- Use alphabetic approach: airway, bones, cardiac structures, diaphragm, effusions, fields and fissures, gastric fundus, and hilum and mediastinum (Jensen et al., 2017, pp. 67–68).

INDWELLING LINES AND TUBES
ENDOTRACHEAL TUBE
- Endotracheal tube (ETT) position can be confirmed on AP x-ray with midline/neutral head position and not flexed. Follow both of the main stem bronchi back to the carina and cephalad to the tip of the tube and the endotracheal tube placement should be in the mid trachea between the second and fourth thoracic vertebral bodies and at least 1 to 2 cm below the vocal cords or above the carina (Bailey, 2015, p. 289; Diblasi, & Gallagher, 2017, p. 295; Jensen et al., 2017, p. 70).

UMBILICAL ARTERY CATHETER (UAC)
- Proceeds from the umbilicus down toward the pelvis, making an acute turn into the internal iliac artery and common iliac artery advancing into the aorta. Either position is accepted practice currently.
  - ○ High position should be between the sixth and 10th thoracic vertebrae (T6–T10).
  - ○ Low position, catheter tip placed between the third and fourth lumbar vertebrae (L3–L4) (Bailey, 2015, p. 300; Ehret, 2015, p. 278; Jensen et al., 2017, p. 70).

UMBILICAL VENOUS CATHETER (UVC)
- Proceeds from the umbilicus cephalad to join the left portal vein. On lateral view, the catheter is directly distal to the abdominal wall until it passes through the ductus venosus.
  - ○ Correct placement is 0.5 to 2 cm above the diaphragm, with the catheter tip at thoracic vertebrae eight to nine. This should equate to just below the junction of the right atrium, which proceeds from the umbilicus cephalad to join the left portal vein (the junction of inferior vena cava and the right atrium; Bailey, 205, p. 302; Ehret, 2015, p. 278; Jensen et al., 2017, p. 70).

CHEST TUBE (CT)
- A lateral chest x-ray film will determine the placement. For air evacuation, anterior placement is desirable. For fluid evacuation, posterior placement is most effective (Ehret, 2015, p. 278).

PERCUTANEOUSLY INSERTED CENTRAL CATHETER (PICC) OR PERCUTANEOUS CENTRAL VENOUS CATHETER (PCVC)
- As a reference, the cavoatrial junction is located approximately two vertebral bodies below the carina on AP chest x-ray (CXR) (Jensen et al., 2017, p. 70).
- If placed in an upper extremity, the arm should be extended and at a 45-degree angle from the body for optimal evaluation, and the tip of the catheter should be in the superior vena cava (SVC). It is considered central if the tip of the catheter crosses the midclavicular line and is above the right atrium of the heart.
- If the line is placed in the lower extremities, the legs should be extended and held in place. The appropriate position should be placed in the inferior vena cava, and will be considered central once the tip of the catheter crosses to the pelvic cavity and rests below the right atrium of the heart (Ehret, 2015, p. 279).

Ultrasound (US)

- Uses an oscillating sound wave with a frequency outside the human hearing range to evaluate the density of tissues, the movement of tissue, and blood flow. It is used to evaluate internal anatomic structures and function.
- It is the most common method used for evaluation of brain parenchyma and ventricular size, myocardial function and structure, urinary tract anatomy and pathology, pelvic masses, liver anatomy, and blood flow in major vessels. Produces real-time, dynamic images using rapid, sequential images (Bailey, 2015, p. 296; Jensen et al., 2017, pp. 68–69).
- Benefits include the ease of use, ability to obtain real-time imaging, and the lack of radiation involved. Ultrasound also provides digital images that can be easily transmitted, the device is portable, and no sedation is required (Ehret, 2015, p. 279; Jensen et al., 2017, p. 68).
- Downsides to the ultrasound include the necessary skill required of the operator to obtain good images; and the mobility of the patient can make imaging challenging (Ehret, 2015, p. 279).

INDICATIONS FOR USE
BRAIN
- Ultrasonography is the ideal tool for evaluation of the newborn brain, and it is often the first step in imaging evaluations for any neurologic concern. The most common approach is through the anterior fontanel in order to obtain coronal and parasagittal views (Strain & Weinman, 2016, p. 167).
  - ○ Although ultrasonography is sensitive in noting intracranial hemorrhages and areas of increased echogenicity, it is less sensitive than a CT or MRI in defining subtle areas of anomalies (Strain & Weinman, 2016, p. 167).

HEART

- An echocardiogram (or echo) is the primary mode used to identify, size, and diagnose congenital heart disease (Scholz & Reinking, 2018, p. 809). High-frequency sound waves send vibrations through the heart, which reflect energy that is transmitted into a visual image (Ehret, 2015, p. 280).
- Two-dimensional echocardiography can define cardiac anatomy and can assess cardiac physiology by estimating pressures and gradients and evaluating cardiac function.
  - Supplemented with Doppler and color Doppler, the echocardiogram has become the primary diagnostic tool in pediatric cardiology (Swanson & Erickson, 2016, p. 654).
- A limitation to the echocardiogram is that lesions that are more distal will require other imaging modalities, such as MRI or cardiac catheterization (Scholz & Reinking, 2018, p. 810). Poor imaging technique and infant movement adversely affect echocardiogram quality (Ehret, 2015, p. 280).
- There are three types of echocardiograms: transthoracic (most common), transesophageal, and M-mode echo.
  - Noninvasive transthoracic echocardiogram is the most commonly used approach. Three-dimensional echocardiograms that offer real-time three-dimensional imaging have improved significantly and are becoming more clinically useful, especially for evaluating valve anatomy and function (Swanson & Erickson, 2016, p. 654).
  - Transesophageal echocardiography (TEE) is almost never used for infants outside of the operating room, but this imaging modality is routinely used for cardiac evaluation in the operating room immediately before and after surgical repair (Swanson & Erickson, 2016, p. 654).
  - M-mode (single dimension) echo permits evaluation of anatomic relationships of heart and vessels, and the motion of the cardiac valves; and detects pericardial fluid. Most commonly used to determine ventricular function. Two-dimensional echocardiogram has greater versatility, providing more specific information.
- Color-flow doppler echo shows patterns of blood flow, location of restrictions and/or regurgitation, and direction of motion. Continuous-wave doppler echogram shows the quantity of flow across an obstruction, and gives an estimate of pressure gradients. It is used to detect the direction of shunting, to estimate cardiac output, and to assess ventricular diastolic function (Sadowski, 2015, p. 552).
- Renal and Urinary Tract
  - Pelvic masses
- Liver anatomy
- Blood flow in major vessels
  - Doppler studies—facilitate visualization of blood flow and motion of tissue over time (Jensen et al., 2017, p. 68).
    - To locate an accessible artery or vein for vessel cannulation, such as PICC placement (Sea, 2013, p. 85)

CT

- Provides a two-dimensional visualization of anatomy and can be further enhanced by the use of a radiographic contrast agent, which can facilitate the evaluation of blood flow and assist define pathologic abnormalities. It combines a series of x-rays from various positions around an axis of rotation to generate high-quality cross-sectional images of the body (Jensen et al., 2017, p. 68; Strain & Weinman, 2016, pp. 168–172).
- Combines a series of images performed helically around an axis of rotation to generate high-quality cross-sectional images of the body. Chest CT is useful for the identification and diagnosis of space-occupying lesions such as congenital pulmonary airway malformation (CPAM), bronchopulmonary sequestration (BPS), and congenital lobar emphysema. CT and CT angiography (CTA) are also increasingly used in the diagnosis and management of severe bronchopulmonary dysplasia (BPD) and pulmonary hypertension (Jensen et al., 2017, p. 68).

MRI

- It uses radio wave to image the body and images protons and hydrogen ions within the body; and its increased sensitivity allows for more precise imaging of the smallest of structures (Strain & Weinman, 2016, pp. 172–175).
- Benefits: No ionized radiation exposure (Jensen et al, 2017, p. 70)
- Cautions: Expensive, requiring anesthesia for high-quality images, time-consuming to obtain an image (Strain & Weinman, 2016, pp. 172–175). Motion free is necessary for optimal image quality.
- Limited by its lack of availability, its expense, and the frequent need to administer anesthesia to infants to acquire high-quality images (Jensen et al., 2017, p. 70).

INDICATIONS FOR USE

- Indications for use include early diagnosis of intracranial pathologies and/or more accurate definition of tissue structures and fluid collections. May also be used as an adjuvant to clarify fetal US findings (Ehret, 2015, p.80; Strain & Weinman, 2016, p. 174).

Fluoroscopy

- Fluoroscopy produces real-time, dynamic images using rapid, sequential x-rays. Fluoroscopy is most commonly used in neonates and infants to image the gastrointestinal (GI) and genitourinary tracts. In infants with respiratory distress of unclear etiology, fluoroscopy may aid in the identification of a tracheoesophageal fistula or occult aspiration. Fluoroscopy can also assess diaphragmatic excursion and diagnose large airway disease such as tracheobronchomalacia (Jensen et al., 2017, p. 69).
- Benefits: It gives the ability to evaluate motion in real time, such as swallowing function, GI peristalsis, and diaphragmatic motion (Jensen et al., 2017, p. 69; Strain & Weinman, 2016, pp. 164–165).
- Contrast media can be given orally or per rectum, instilled into the urinary bladder, or given intravenously. Most contrast agents are compounds that use either inert barium or iodine as the material (Strain & Weinman, 2016, p. 164).
- Fluoroscopy can result in substantial radiation exposure if appropriate precautions are not used (Jensen et al., 2017, p. 69).

INDICATIONS FOR USE
RESPIRATORY SYSTEM

In infants with respiratory distress of unclear etiology, fluoroscopy may aid in the identification of a tracheoesophageal fistula or occult aspiration, fluoroscopy can also assess diaphragmatic excursion and diagnose large airway disease such as tracheobronchomalacia (Jensen et al., 2018, p. 69).

GASTROINTESTINAL SYSTEM
UPPER GI
- Upper GI series with small-bowel follow-through is used to evaluate the structure and function of the upper GI tract. A water-soluble contrast solution is swallowed and a series of x-rays are taken under fluoroscopy. A series of follow-up x-rays are obtained intermittently to evaluate emptying ability of the stomach, intestinal motility, and potential obstruction.
- Used to evaluate the structure and function of the upper GI tract. The three main areas examined are (a) the esophagus (for size, patency, reflux, and presence of fistula or swallowing abnormalities); (b) the stomach (abnormalities and motility); and (c) the small intestine (for strictures, patency, and function). A series of follow-up x-rays are obtained to evaluate the emptying ability of the stomach, intestinal motility, and potential obstruction (Ehret, 2015, p. 280; Strain & Weinman, 2016, pp. 164–165).
  - ○ If the clinical questions are malrotation and/or possible volvulus, the upper GI series is the examination of choice (Strain & Weinman, 2016, p. 165).

BARIUM ENEMA
- Barium enema is used to evaluate the structure and function of the large intestine and diagnose disorders (such as Hirschsprung's disease). A series of follow-up x-rays may be taken at timed intervals to evaluate the evacuation of the solution from the bowel. It can also be used for either diagnostic or therapeutic purposes for infants with meconium plug syndrome or meconium ileus (Ehret, 2015, p. 280; Strain & Weinman, 2016, pp. 164–165).

RENAL SYSTEM
- Voiding cystourethrogram (VCUG): It is used to evaluate the structure and function of the kidneys, bladder, and lower urinary tract.
  - ○ The infant's bladder is emptied by catheterization and then filled with a contrast solution. A series of x-rays are taken under fluoroscopy in a variety of positions during voiding. After voiding, follow-up x-rays are taken to evaluate residuals in the bladder and any reflux into the kidneys (Ehret, 2015, p. 280; Strain & Weinman, 2016, pp. 164–165).

ELECTROENCEPHALOGRAM (EEG)

- With increasing gestational age, changes in of measurable function occur, characterized principally by more refined organization of the electroencephalographic processes. Findings on an EEG are considered best in terms of the continuity of background activity, the synchrony of this activity, and the appearance and disappearance of specific waveforms and patterns (Neil & Volpe, 2018, p. 227).
  - ○ The severity of EEG abnormalities and their duration in the asphyxiated infant also are of prognostic importance.
  - ○ Depression of background activity, especially of the faster frequencies, is common after generalized insults, especially hypoxic–ischemic insults (Neil & Volpe, 2018, p. 231).

- ○ The development of continuous or intermittent discontinuity of EEG in the term infant is a very common feature of all neonatal encephalopathies. The most extreme of these discontinuous tracings is the burst-suppression pattern, which is associated with a very high likelihood of an unfavorable outcome (Neil & Volpe, 2018, p. 231).
- ○ Many neonatal electrical seizures identified by EEG are not accompanied by any motor or behavioral clinical activity, a phenomenon referred to as subclinical seizure activity or electroclinical dissociation (Parsons, Seay, & Jacobson, 2016, p. 747).
- Two common types of EEG:
  - ○ Conventional EEG is the gold standard for neonatal seizure detection, used to measure impact of neurologic insult and detect presence of seizure activity. Conventional EEG provides information about the entire cerebral cortex (Verklan, 2015, p. 763). Continuous monitoring of neonates with EEG is recommended in certain high-risk populations, including suspect neonatal seizures following acute brain injury and in neonates with clinically suspected seizures, or when neonatal epilepsy is suspected (Natarajan & Gospe, 2018, pp. 963–964).
    - ■ The procedure requires skilled technicians and experienced interpreters of the tracing (Neil & Volpe, 2018, p. 230).
  - ○ Amplitude EEG (aEEG) is a method for the continuous monitoring of cerebral electrical activity in critically ill newborns. The signal is rectified and further processed before being displayed on a modified scale. It is possible to display the corresponding, expanded raw EEG trace, which is useful for confirming possible seizure activity (Neil & Volpe, 2018, p. 235).
    - ■ Benefits include an ease of use, easy application, and bedside availability and interpretation, as well as reduced cost as compared with continuous EEG monitoring (Natarajan & Gospe, 2018, p. 964).
    - ■ Use with caution due to the fact that the device does not cover the entire brain, thereby potentially missing some focal abnormalities (Neil & Volpe, 2018, p. 235). aEEG may also be limited as it is prone to artifactual signals from movement, high-frequency oscillator ventilation, or extracorporeal membrane oxygenation (ECMO; Natarajan & Gospe, 2018, p. 964).

INDICATIONS FOR USE
- Assessment of asphyxiated term infants—the aEEG background tracings have been most useful, particularly the burst-suppression, continuous low-voltage, and flat trace patterns. Monitoring the course of aEEG changes is useful, although for identification of candidates for neuroprotective therapies, such as therapeutic hypothermia, early detection is crucial (Neil & Volpe, 2018, p. 238).
- Detection of seizures—the value of aEEG in detection of seizures has been assessed primarily in asphyxiated term infants. aEEG was not designed as a seizure monitor, although some very experienced users of the method appear skilled at seizure detection (Neil & Volpe, 2018, p. 238).
- Other uses include identifying the effect of anticonvulsant drugs, predicting postneonatal epilepsy, and predicting outcomes in premature infants with large intraventricular hemorrhages (Neil & Volpe, 2018, p. 238).

ECG/EKG

- ECG is used to measure and display the heart rate and rhythm by measuring body surface electrical potentials generated by the heart. Typically uses three electrodes: one on the upper left (LA) chest, one on the upper right (RA) chest, and one on the lower left (LL) abdomen. Typically, electrodes are color coded: LA is black, RA is white, and LL is red. (Smallwood, 2019, p. 136).
  - ○ Continuous monitoring ensures adequate heart rate and detection of life-threatening change in rate and rhythm (Smallwood, 2019, p. 136). ECG measurement also provides an alternative method of measuring heart rate in the delivery room (Owen, Weiner, & Davis, 2017, p. 277).
  - ○ Caution should be used as the technology has limits, such as inaccurate measurements caused by motion artifact (Smallwood, 2019, p. 136).

INDICATIONS FOR USE
- To identify abnormal hemodynamic burdens placed on the heart.
- It is the major tool for evaluating arrhythmias and the impact of electrolytes imbalances on electrical conductivity. Changes in ST segments or T waves may suggest myocardial ischemia. ECG can also be used to determine severity of disease by assessing the degree of atrial or ventricular hypertrophy. (Sadowski, 2015, p. 544).

TECHNIQUES/PROCEDURES IN THE NICU

There are many invasive procedures performed in NICUs every day. It is essential to have the knowledge of the indications, precautions, and potential complications associated with both the equipment and procedures.

Bag and Mask Ventilation

- Initiate when apnea or gasping respirations, heart rate is less than 100 bpm, cyanotic despite supplemental oxygen, or need for continued ventilation.
- Unresponsive apnea to stimulation or gasping respirations
- Heart rate is less than 100 beats per minute
- Persistent cyanosis despite free-flow oxygen (Niermeyer, Clarke, & Hernández, 2016, p. 63)

MASK
- It requires proper size to obtain adequate seal. Appropriate sizing should have the mask covering the chin, mouth, and nose, but not the eyes (Niermeyer et al., 2016, p. 63).

RESUSCITATION BAGS
- Including self-inflating bags, flow-inflating (anesthesia) bags, and T-piece resuscitator
- Self-inflating bags re-expand after compression, and are the only devices that can be used without a gas supply (Niermeyer et al., 2016, p. 63; Owen et al., 2017, p. 280). They do not deliver consistent tidal volumes (V_T) or inflation pressures (Niermeyer et al., 2016, p. 63).
- Flow-inflating bags require a continuous gas supply to inflate the bag (Niermeyer et al., 2016, p. 65; Owen et al., 2017, p. 280). High-peak pressures can be achieved with flow-inflating bags and deliver continuous positive airway pressure (CPAP) as well as free-flow oxygen (Niermeyer et al., 2016, p. 65).

T-PIECE
- A T-piece resuscitator is a flow-controlled and pressure-limited device and provides preset level of positive pressure and PEEP, which can achieve desired inflation pressures and respiratory times more consistently. It also requires a continuous gas supply to operate (Niermeyer et al., 2016, p. 65; Owen et al., 2017, p. 280; Verklan et al., 2015, p. 501).
- A T-piece resuscitator can be used to administer free-flow oxygen and CPAP to a spontaneously breathing infants (DiBlasi & Gallagher, 2017, p. 292).

LARYNGEAL MASK AIRWAY (LMA)
- The American Society of Anesthesiologists (ASA) Practice Guidelines for Management of the Difficult Airway include the use of supraglottic airways, of which the LMA is the most commonly used (Watters & Mancuso, 2018, p. 225). LMA does not require the visualization of the vocal cords and an instrument for insertion (Diblasi. & Gallagher, 2017, p. 298).

INDICATIONS
- Neonatal resuscitation of term and larger preterm infants with difficult airway, such as Pierre Robin sequence or micrognathia, as an aid to endotracheal intubation or in flexible endoscopy (Diblasi & Gallagher, 2017, p. 298).
- Its use in various clinical scenarios, including the following:
  - ○ In neonatal resuscitation of term and larger preterm infants
  - ○ In the difficult airway, such as in the Robin sequence, and other situations when micrognathia is profound
  - ○ As an aid to endotracheal intubation
  - ○ As an aid in flexible endoscopy
  - ○ In surgical cases in place of endotracheal intubation (Diblasi & Gallagher, 2017, p. 298)
- Limitations: Lack of small sizes, lack of ability to suction meconium from airway, leaks with high pressures, ineffective with chest compression, unable to deliver endotracheal medications (Owen et al., 2017, p. 283; Ringer, 2017, p. 1008; Verklan et al., 2015, p. 100).
- A potential complication is the aspiration of gastric contents, since the LMA does not provide an occluded airway (Watters & Mancuso, 2018, p. 225).

TECHNIQUES
- The size 1 LMA is appropriate and recommended for infants weighing 1.5 to 5 kg, although there are reports of use in infants as small as 0.8 kg (Ringer, 2017, p. 1008). An infant's neck should be slightly extended to avoid compression of soft tissues of the neck (Niermeyer et al., 2016, p. 65). The deflated mask is manually inserted into the patient's mouth and guided blindly along the hard palate, then advanced until resistance is felt. The distal tip of the LMA should rest against the upper esophageal sphincter. The balloon is inflated to form a seal in the pharynx (Watters & Mancuso, 2018, p. 228).
- An orogastric catheter should be inserted to prevent gastric distention from bag-and-mask ventilation.

Endotracheal Intubation

ORAL ENDOTRACHEAL INTUBATION
INDICATIONS
- When bag-and-mask is ineffective or undesirable to perform resuscitation, the need for mechanical ventilation, diaphragmatic hernia, or upper-airway obstruction such

as bilateral or severe unilateral choanal atresia or stenosis, pharyngeal hypotonia, and micrognathia, is present.
- Other indications include the need for administering surfactant or epinephrine (Bailey, 2015, p. 285; Niermeyer et al., 2016, p. 67; Owen et al., 2017, p. 282; Said & Rais-Bahrami, 2013d, p. 236).
- Oral intubation may be done if tracheal suction to clear the airway is needed, or a sterile culture obtained from tracheal suctioning (Bailey, 2015, p. 285).

NASAL (NASOTRACHEAL) INTUBATION
INDICATIONS
- Proponents of nasal intubation believe that fixation of the tube to the infant's face is easier and more stable because it minimizes the chance for accidental dislodgment and decreases tube movement, which can result in subglottic stenosis. Severe damage can occur from the up-and-down movement of the endotracheal tube (Diblasi & Gallagher, 2017, p. 293).
- Should be used for elective procedure when infants with copious secretions or defects of the oral anatomy are present (DiBlasi & Gallagher, 2017, p. 293; Said & Rais-Bahrami, 2013d, p. 242; Verklan et al., 2015, p. 100, 302).
- The length for correct positioning of the nasotracheal tube in the trachea is approximately 2 cm longer than the length of an orotracheal tube. The use of Magill forceps can be cumbersome in smaller infants (Said & Rais-Bahrami, 2013d, p. 243).
- Data have failed to demonstrate statistically significant differences between oral and nasal intubation with respect to tracheal injury (Diblasi & Gallagher, 2017, p. 293). Disadvantages of nasal intubation include a predisposition to sinusitis, pressure necrosis of the nares, and bleeding complications (Watters & Mancuso, 2019, p. 229).

ORAL/NASAL INTUBATION TECHNIQUE
PREMEDICATION
- Premedication should be considered for sedation of infant prior to the nonemergent intubation per institutional protocol. Medications include analgesics sedation, and followed by neuromuscular blocking agents if applicable (Bailey, 2015, p. 286).

BLADE SIZE FOR ORAL INTUBATION
- Size 00 laryngoscope blade is used for infants who weigh less than 1,000 g.
- Size 0 laryngoscope blade is used for infants who weigh 1,000 to 3,000 g.
- Size 1 laryngoscope blade is used for infants who weigh more than 4,000 g (Bailey, 2015, p. 285; Owen et al., 2017, p. 283; Said & Rais-Bahrami, 2013d, p. 236).

ENDOTRACHEAL TUBE SIZE
- Appropriate uncuffed and uniform-diameter ETT size should be selected based on an infant's weight or gestational age.
  - ETT with internal diameter (ID) of 2.5 mm is for infants who weigh less than 1,000 g or are less than 28 weeks GA.
  - ETT with ID of 3.0 mm is for infants who weigh 1,000 to 2,000 g or are between 28 and 34 weeks GA.
  - ETT with ID of 3.5 mm is for infants who weigh 2,000 to 3,000 g or are 34 to 38 weeks.
  - ETT with ID of 3.5 to 4.0 mm is for infants who weigh more than 3,000 g or are more than 38 weeks GA (Diblasi & Gallagher, 2017, p. 295; Niermeyer et al., 2016, p. 67; Owen et al., 2017, p. 282; Said & Rais-Bahrami, 2013d, p. 237; Watters & Mancuso, 2019, p. 227; Verklan et al., 2015, p. 302).

ENDOTRACHEAL TUBE—PLACEMENT
- Determine ETT insertion depth. A variety of methods have been reported for predicting insertional length, such as:
  - Nasal–tragus length (NTL)—the measurement between the infant's nasal septum and ear tragus + 1 cm
  - Using baby's weight—weight in kilograms + 6 cm. This equates to the 7–8–9 rule advocated in neonatal resuscitation program (NRP): however, this has been associated with overestimated depth insertion in infants weighing <750 g (Bailey, 2015, p. 288).
- Laryngoscope should be held between the thumb and first finger of the left hand, with the second and third fingers stabilizing the infant's chin. The blade is inserted into the vallecula and the handle of the scope raised to an angle of approximately 60 degrees relative to the bed in an upward and outward motion (Bailey, 2015, p. 288; Niermeyer et al., 2016, p. 67; Ringer, 2017, p. 1007; Said & Rais-Bahrami, 2013d, p. 240). Figure 4.9 illustrates the glottic structures as visualized through the laryngoscope.
- The ETT should be inserted to the level of vocal cord marker. If inserting a cuffed ETT, the tube is advanced until the cuff is distal to the vocal cords (Watters & Mancuso, 2019, pp. 226–227).
- Intubation attempts should be limited to 20 to 30 seconds to prevent hypoxia during the procedure.
- With the right index finger, hold the ETT against the roof of the mouth and stabilize the tube. Gently remove the laryngoscope from the mouth and stylet from the ETT (if used; Bailey, 2015, p. 288; Ringer, 2017, p. 1007).
- Use an exhaled CO_2 detector and auscultation to confirm ETT placement. The presence of vapor in the tube is not a reliable indicator.
  - Color change of the CO_2 detector may be delayed in extremely preterm infants, especially if cardiac output is low, as during bradycardia or when the neonate has little to no perfusion.
- Auscultate breath sounds bilaterally and confirm placement with a chest radiograph (Bailey, 2015, p. 286; Niermeyer et al., 2016, p. 63, 68; Ringer, 2017, p. 1007; Said & Rais-Bahrami, 2013d, p. 241; Watters & Mancuso, 2019, p. 227).

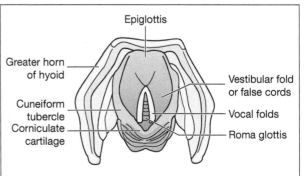

FIGURE 4.9 Anatomical illustration showing the neonatal upper airway structures.

POSSIBLE COMPLICATIONS FROM INTUBATION

- Complications of intubation may include hypoxia bradycardia, damage of the airway lining, vocal cord injury, misplacement of tube into esophagus, bronchus pain, agitation, or discomfort (Bailey, 2015, p. 288; DiBlasi & Gallagher, 2017, p. 300; Niermeyer et al., 2016, p. 68; Said & Rais-Bahrami, 2013d, p. 245).
- Observe for dislocation of endotracheal tube or unplanned extubation, for example, central cyanosis, bradycardia, decreased chest movement, breath sounds absent or diminished, lack of positive response to CO_2 detector, distended abdomen, air noises audible over stomach, or no mist or fogging in tube (Niermeyer et al., 2016, p. 63).

Thoracentesis

INDICATIONS

- The indications of thoracentesis are temporary relief of life-threatening air or fluid accumulations from the thoracic cavity. May also be used for an extrapleural drainage after surgical repair of esophageal atresia and/or tracheoesophageal fistula (Rais-Bahrami & MacDonald, 2013, pp. 255–256).

TECHNIQUE
NEEDLE ASPIRATION

- Insert an 18- to 20-gauge angiocatheter at a 45-degree angle in second, fourth, or fifth intercostal space and midclavicular line, and then decrease to a 15-degree angle once the catheter enters pleural space (Rais-Bahrami & MacDonald, 2013, p. 269).

CHEST TUBE (CT) PLACEMENT

- Types of thoracostomy tube include a polyvinyl chloride (PVC) chest tube with or without trocar, and the more commonly used pigtail catheter (Rais-Bahrami & MacDonald, 2013, p. 255).
- Elevated affected site at 60 to 75 degrees to the bed, which will allow air to rise (outer chest wall) for easy aspiration (Rais-Bahrami & MacDonald, 2013, p. 260).
- Landmarks for insertion site: Nipple and fifth intercostal spaces/midaxillary line (Rais-Bahrami & MacDonald, 2013, p. 262).
- Select appropriate insertion site and position: Anteromedial tip position for air collections and posterior tip position for fluid accumulation (Rais-Bahrami & MacDonald, 2013, p. 257).

POSSIBLE COMPLICATIONS

- Mispositioning of tube, hemorrhage, infection, needle injury to lung or adjacent structures, damage to breast tissue, pain, thoracostomy tube perforation of the lung, and nerve damage (Rais-Bahrami & MacDonald, 2013, pp. 265–266).

Umbilical Vessel Catheterization

INDICATIONS—UAC

- Frequent arterial blood sampling, continuous arterial blood gas monitoring, continuous arterial blood pressure monitoring, angiography, resuscitation (Bradshaw & Tanaka, 2016, p. 136; Said, & Rais-Bahrami, 2013b, p. 156).

INDICATIONS—UVC

- Emergency administration of drugs, fluid administration, exchange transfusion, central venous pressure monitoring, blood sampling, and central venous blood pressure monitoring and diagnosis of total anomalous pulmonary venous drainage below the diaphragm (Bradshaw & Tanaka, 2016, p. 136; Said & Rais-Bahrami, 2013c, p. 173).

CONTRAINDICATIONS FOR UAC/UVC

- Abdominal wall defects, necrotizing enterocolitis (NEC), vascular compromise below level of umbilicus, omphalitis, omphalocele, peritonitis (Said & Rais-Bahrami, 2013c, p. 173). Bleeding disorder that cannot be corrected, skin infection at the identified site, malformation or previous surgery in the desired area (Massaro & Rais-Bahrami, 2013, p. 182).

TECHNIQUE UAC/UVC

- Choice of catheter size: 3.5 Fr. in infants weighing less than 1,500 or 2,000 g and 5 Fr. in infants who are more than 1,500 or 2,000 g (Bradshaw & Tanaka, 2016, p. 137; Rabi, Kowal, & Ambalavanan, 2017, p. 85).
- Identify cord vessels:
  - The singular vein is large, thin-walled vessel, and often is situated at the 12-o'clock position (Bradshaw & Tanaka, 2016, p. 138; Said & Rais-Bahrami, 2013b, p. 160).
  - The two umbilical arteries are the continuation of the internal iliac arteries with 2 to 3 mm diameters at their origins and then become small and thickened as they approach to the umbilicus (Said & Rais-Bahrami, 2013b, p. 158).
- If the inserted catheter meets any obstruction prior to the desired distance, it may be in portal system or in an intrahepatic branch of portal vein.

PLACEMENT UAC/UVC

- High position: Several methods to estimate the distance (Rabi et al., 2017, p. 86)
  - UAC—level of thoracic vertebrae, T6 to T9 (Bradshaw & Tanaka, 2016, p. 140; Said & Rais-Bahrami, 2013b, p. 159)
- UVC—desired location is T9 to T10, just above the right diaphragm or at the junction of the inferior vena cava and the right atrium (Said & Rais-Bahrami, 2013c, p. 174).
- Never advance catheter once in place and secured, to avoid contaminated catheter into the vessel (Said & Rais-Bahrami, 2013b, p. 163).
- Low line
  - UAC—level of lumbar vertebrae, L3 to L4 (Bradshaw & Tanaka, 2016, p. 140)

POSSIBLE COMPLICATIONS

- Vessels, peritoneum or colon, false aneurysm, knot in catheter or breaking of catheter, cardiac arrhythmia, pericardial effusion, cardiac tamponade, hydrothorax, NEC, infection, hepatic necrosis, skin burns from antiseptics, hemorrhage, exsanguination, portal hypertension, or death (Bradshaw & Tanaka, 2016, p. 149; Massaro & Rais-Bahrami, 2013, p. 190; Rabi et al., 2017, p. 86; Said, & Rais-Bahrami, 2013c, p. 175).
- Microemboli or vasospasm (dusky or purple toes)
- Compromised arterial blood flow (blanching of the foot or part of the leg)

Peripheral Artery Catheterization

INDICATIONS

- When frequent blood sampling is needed and the UAC is not available, when continuous blood pressure monitoring is necessary, or when preductal measurement is needed (p. 318; Massaro & Rais-Bahrami, 2013, p. 182; Rabi et al., 2017, p. 87).

TECHNIQUE

- Allen's test to be performed to ensure ulnar artery patency, and a modified Allen test should be performed when dorsalis pedis or posterior tibial cannulation is attempted (Massaro & Rais-Bahrami, 2013, p. 183; Rabi et al., 2017, p. 87).
  - ○ The Allen's test is performed by applying pressure to both the radial and the ulnar arteries and then removing pressure from the artery that will not be cannulated. If the entire hand refills with blood, then the artery is intact and cannulation can be done (Rabi et al., 2017, p. 87)
- Cannulate the artery by inserting at a 10- to 15-degree angle to the skin with the needle bevel down, or passing needle stylet with bevel up through artery at 30- to 40-degree angle (Massaro & Rais-Bahrami, 2013, p. 184).

POSSIBLE COMPLICATIONS

- Arteriospasm, infection, extravasation of fluids, hematoma or hemorrhage, embolism or thrombus, or damage to surrounding tissues or structures are the complications.

Intravenous Line Placement (Central)

INDICATIONS

- Peripheral intravenous line—administration of IV medications, fluids, or parenteral nutrition (Said & Rais-Bahrami., 2013a, p. 142).
- PICC and midline catheter (MLC):
  - ○ Intermediate or long-term intravenous therapy, parenteral nutrition, antibiotic or other medicinal therapy, difficult venous access, irritating drug therapy, or VLBW are the indications for PICC (Bradshaw & Tanaka, 2016, p. 143).
  - ○ Repetitive blood draws—only applies to larger lumen catheters due to the risk of clotting (Rorke, Ramasethu, & Chahine, 2013, p. 194).

TECHNIQUE

- The ideal position of catheter tip should be in as large a vein as possible, such as outside the heart (not within the right atrium).
  - ○ Upper extremity—the catheter tip should be in the SVC or at the junction of the SVC and right atrium.
  - ○ Lower extremity—the catheter tip should be above the L4 to L5 or the iliac crest (Rorke et al., 2013, p. 195).
    - ■ AP and lateral radiographic views are preferred to confirm that the catheter is in a central vein, especially for the catheter placed in a lower extremity.
    - ■ Preferred insertion sites are in order as following: antecubital veins (basilic and cephalic veins), saphenous veins, scalp veins (temporal and posterior auricular veins), axillary vein, and external jugular vein (Rorke et al., 2013, p. 196).

POSSIBLE COMPLICATIONS
INSERTION SITE

- Phlebitis—the most common significant complication
- Chemical burn, nerve damage, or hematoma

CATHETER/EXTREMITY

- Infection, an air embolus, rupture of catheter
- Vascular spasm, ischemia from arteriospasm, possible necrosis
- Intravascular catheter shearing
- Embolization of catheter fragment

CATHETER TIP

- Thrombus formation, embolization of clot, infiltration
- Catheter migration

INTERNAL

- Cardiac arrhythmias
- Pericardial effusion with cardiac tamponade
- Atrial perforation with cardiac tamponade
- Infiltration/extravasation, hemorrhage, or vascular perforation (Bradshaw & Tanaka, 2016, p. 149; Jensen et al., 2017, p. 70; Ramasethu, 2013, p. 224; Rorke et al., 2013, p. 195, 208; Said & Rais-Bahrami, 2013a, p. 144)

TECHNIQUES/EQUIPMENT IN THE NICU

Cardiopulmonary Monitors

PRINCIPLES OF OPERATION

- The small alterations in voltage generated by the heart electrical impulses can be measured at the body surface with electrodes placed on the chest.
- Electrode placement is important in acquiring a signal of adequate resolution, especially in neonates with a limited surface area.
  - ○ The optimal placement to be the right mid-clavicle and the xiphoid (Fiore, 2015, pp. 522–523)
- Cardiorespiratory monitoring provides reliable and accurate data of infant's cardiac and respiratory activities, and identifies apnea/bradycardia in infants at risk as well as early warnings of potential significant changes (Fay, 2013, p. 49).
- Cardiopulmonary monitors provide a visual display of electrocardiogram with accurate heart rate and respiratory wave pattern (Bradshaw & Tanaka, 2016, p. 136).

INDICATION FOR USE

- To monitor for bradycardia (<100 beats per minute), tachycardia (>180 bpm), apnea, and tachypnea.

PRECAUTIONS

- Multiple probe applications should be avoided because this can compromise ECG signal integrity.
- Multiple applications of patches may increase the chance of skin damage (Fiore, 2015, pp. 522–523).
- Prompt patient assessment and appropriate correction should be followed immediately after monitor alarm is activated (Fay, 2013, p. 51).

Pulse Oximetry

PRINCIPLES OF OPERATION

- The most common, noninvasive, and continuous method of measuring Hgb O_2 saturation. Advantages include short response time in determining O_2 saturation and reducing the number of invasive blood gas measurements (Abubakar, 2013a, p. 65; Bradshaw & Tanaka, 2016, p. 147; Rabi et al., 2017, p. 89).
- Oxygenated Hgb (oxyhemoglobin; saturated Hgb) and reduced Hgb (deoxyhemoglobin; desaturated Hgb) absorb different light frequency, and the ratio of light absorbance is used to derive the transcutaneous oxygen saturation (Rabi et al., 2017, p. 89).

- Pulse oximetry measures the percentage of Hgb saturated with oxygen (Abubakar, 2013a, p. 65; Mathew & Lakshminrusimha, 2017, p. 97).
  - Spectrophotometry
  - Photoplethysmography

INDICATION FOR USE
- Reduce the frequency of blood gas draw.
- Titrate oxygen concentration during delivery room resuscitation and for those infants receiving supplemental oxygen
- Noninvasive continuous monitoring desaturation events in infants
- Screen critical congenital heart disease (CCHD).
- Monitor an infant's status during transport.
- Diagnose persistent pulmonary hypertension (PPHN) with ductal shunt.
- Perform car seat testing prior to discharge in infants with risk factors (Mathew & Lakshminrusimha, 2017, p. 101).

PRECAUTIONS
- It does not eliminate the need for blood gas analysis.
- Poor perfusion, ambient light and motion, shock, and severe edema will interfere with the reliability of the pulse oximeter.
- Assess the sensor site to ensure the proper circulation and skin integrity.
- Mispositioned sensor will produce falsely low readings (the penumbra effect; Abubakar, 2013a, p. 68; Mathew & Lakshminrusimha, 2017, p. 101).

Transcutaneous Carbon Dioxide Monitoring ($tcPCO_2$/P_{tcco2}/TCOM)

PRINCIPLES OF OPERATION
- Provide continuous indirect estimation of PaO_2 and $PaCO_2$ (Rabi et al., 2017, p. 90).

INDICATION FOR USE
- Trending $PaCO_2$, especially when initiating high frequency ventilation (HFV) (Rabi et al., 2017, p. 91)

PRECAUTIONS
- $TcPCO_2$ always measures greater than $PaCO_2$ due to many factors (Rabi et al., 2017, p. 90).

Transcutaneous Oxygen Monitoring ($tcPO_2$/$P_{tc}O_2$)

PRINCIPLES OF OPERATION
- Transcutaneous Po_2 ($tcPO_2$) essentially measures the PO_2 of skin. Although the PO_2 of skin is usually lower than the PaO_2, heating of the skin directly under the $tcPO_2$ electrode causes local cutaneous vasodilation resulting in the skin PO_2 approaching PaO_2. Although heating the skin causes several effects other than vasodilation, these effects on the oxygen dissociation curve, tissue oxygen consumption, and electrode oxygen consumption cancel out for most patients (Rabi et al., 2017, p. 90).

INDICATION FOR USE
- In the absence of arterial access for the effect of therapeutic ventilatory management monitoring

PRECAUTIONS
- Not reliable in older infants with chronic lung disease and infants with hyperoxemia.
- Requires frequent sensor reposition and recalibration and at the risk of thermal burns due to operating temperature.
- May underestimate PaO_2 in infants with severe acidosis, anemia, and decreased peripheral perfusion (Abubakar, 2013a, p. 70; Bradshaw & Tanaka, 2016, p. 135 & 146; Mathew & Lakshminrusimha, 2017, p. 102; Rabi et al., 2017, p. 90).

Near-Infrared Spectroscopy (NIRS)

PRINCIPLES OF OPERATION
- Relies on differential absorption of light between oxygenated and deoxygenated Hgb as well as the relatively transparent nature of tissue to infrared light to give an estimation of tissue oxygenation (Mathew & Lakshminrusimha, 2017, p. 105).

INDICATION FOR USE
- Infants who undergo cardiac surgeries
- Associate evaluations while managing of hypotension
- Monitoring of infants who have a patent ductus arteriosus (PDA)

Precautions

- True value remains unknown and venous saturation cannot be precisely determined (Mathew & Lakshminrusimha, 2017, p. 104).
- The values vary depending on the metabolic state of the tissue, following ischemic damage and during treatment with therapeutic hypothermia (Mathew & Lakshminrusimha, 2017, p. 106).

End Tidal Carbon Dioxide Monitoring (End Tidal CO_2, $Etco_2$; capnography; P_{etCO2})

PRINCIPLES OF OPERATION
- An noninvasive measurement to continuously monitor CO_2 tension through gas analysis during respiration, specifically exhaled CO_2 (Abubakar, 2013b, p. 75; Bradshaw & Tanaka, 2016, p. 135 & 146; Mathew & Lakshminrusimha, 2017, p. 102).
  - Mainstream—the sensor is in line with the ventilator circuit
  - Sidestream—the sensor is placed away from the airway
- To provide useful information on CO_2 production, pulmonary perfusion, alveolar ventilation, respiratory patterns, and the elimination of CO_2 from the lungs (Abubakar, 2013b, p. 75)

INDICATION FOR USE
- To confirm ETT placement
- To continuously monitor and evaluate exhaled CO_2 on ventilated infants and guide management (Abubakar, 2013b, p. 75; Rabi et al., 2017, p. 91).
- To monitor rate, rhythm, and effectiveness of respiration as well as systemic perfusion and metabolism (Mathew & Lakshminrusimha, 2017, p. 103).
- To provide monitoring in the operating room
- To monitor and evaluate the response to therapy in infants with severe pulmonary disease (Abubakar, 2013b, p. 75).

PRECAUTIONS

- Provides only a rough estimate of $PaCO_2$ in infants with significant lung disease (Rabi et al., 2017, p. 91)
- When the P_{etCO2} adapter is placed between the ETT and the ventilator flow sensor, tidal volume (V_T) measurements may be affected.
- Sidestream measurements tend to be less accurate when high respiratory rates occur (Mathew & Lakshminrusimha, 2017, p. 103).

Blood Gas Monitoring

- Blood gas measurement is the standard method for monitoring oxygenation, ventilation, and acid–base balance (Abubakar, 2013a, p. 65). It offers more than just basic blood gas; it also provides measurement of Hgb, electrolytes, and metabolites (Rabi et al., 2017, p. 92).

INVASIVE MONITORING

- Via arterial access (usually via umbilical artery catheter) or peripheral artery cannulation (PAC). The sample can be drawn from arterial or heel stick for capillary samples.

PRINCIPLE OF OPERATION

- Partial pressure of oxygen dissolved in whole blood detected by an electrode. The absorption of Hgb derivatives using multiple wavelengths of light (Rabi et al., 2017, p. 92)

INDICATIONS FOR USE

- The presence of an invasive, in-dwelling catheter for blood gas monitoring allows the accurate measurement of arterial blood partial pressure of oxygen (PaO_2) without disturbing the patient. Blood gas measurements performed on blood drawn from an umbilical catheter reflect post-ductal blood. It also allows direct measurement of arterial blood pressure and provides a route for obtaining other blood sample (Rabi et al., 2017, pp. 84–85).

PRECAUTIONS WITH USE

- Complications related to umbilical arterial catheters include vascular compromise and those related to malposition, infection, bleeding, and catheter-related accidents (accidental disconnection, rupture, etc.). Occasionally, catheter placement is associated with severe thrombotic complications, including frank gangrene and necrosis of the buttocks or leg (Rabi et al., 2017, p. 86).

NONINVASIVE MONITORING

- May include transcutaneous PO_2 and PCO_2, pulse oximetry, end-tidal CO_2 monitoring ,and near-infrared spectroscopy (NIRS; Mathew & Lakshminrusimha, 2017, p .105).

PRINCIPLE OF OPERATION

- Oxygen saturation monitoring is the most common, easy, and widely used method. Pulse oximetry requires no calibration or application of heat.
- Provides breath-to-breath analysis of exhaled CO_2 measured at the cutaneous capillaries (Bradshaw & Tanaka, 2016, p. 134).

INDICATIONS FOR USE

- To guide ventilator management and to ensure correct placement of endotracheal tubes

PRECAUTIONS WITH USE

- Less reliable in infants with lung disease, BPD, airway obstruction, poor perfusion, acidosis, edema, or on vasoconstrictors (Mathew & Lakshminrusimha, 2017, p. 104)
- At risk of causing skin burns
- Increase in dead space when using $TcPCO_2/TcPO_2$
- $Etco_2$ cannot be used with HFV.

Incubators/Radiant Warmers

PRINCIPLE OF OPERATION

INCUBATORS

- Controlled and enclosed environment with heated and warm air—including skin servocontrol and air servocontrol (Gardner & Hernandez, 2016, p. 120).
- Double-walled incubators have less radiant heat loss and provide a more steady temperature environment.
- Increasing the humidity within incubators can prevent evaporative heat loss and decrease the infant's metabolic rate as well as the incidence of electrolyte imbalances.

RADIANT WARMERS

- Infrared energy to heat an infant's skin
- Servocontrolled or manually controlled

INDICATIONS FOR USE

- Premature or extremely low birth weight (ELBW) infants
- Hypothermia
- Transporting infants (Rioja-Mazza, 2013, p. 26)
- Unstable infants (Rioja-Mazza, 2013, p. 25)

PRECAUTIONS

- Incubators limit the access to sick infants when extensive procedures are necessary (Gardner & Hernandez, 2016, p. 120)
- Incubators may present as a barrier to mothers and prolong feelings of fear and insecurity
- High noise levels within incubators cause negative impact on the hearing development of preterm infants.
- Malfunctions
- Weaning the incubator temperature on the air control mode should be no faster than 0.5° per 30 minutes or 1° per hour (Gardner & Hernandez, 2016, p. 124).
- Safety—keep infant 80 to 90 cm from radiant heat to avoid burns (Rioja-Mazza, 2013, p. 25).
- Insensible water loss when infants are under radiant warmers
- Manual control on a radiant warmer increases the risk of overheating or overcooling.
- Hyperthermia, dehydration (Rorke et al., 2013, p. 25)

Phototherapy

PRINCIPLE OF OPERATION

- Phototherapy uses light energy to alter the shape of bilirubin into a form that does not need conjugation. This different form is able to be excreted in the bile and urine (Kamath-Rayne, Thilo, Deacon, & Hernandez, 2016, p. 526).
- Primary uses of phototherapy are to decrease the risk of acute bilirubin encephalopathy and toxicity caused by high serum bilirubin levels and to decrease the need for exchange transfusion (Kamath-Kayne et al., 2016, p. 525).

- The most common intervention for the treatment of hyperbilirubinemia (Kamath-Rayne et al., 2016, pp. 526–530; Nassabeh-Montazami, 2013, p. 357)

INDICATIONS FOR USE
- Bilirubin rises in newborns through three mechanisms:
  - Increased production (accelerated RBC breakdown)
    - Hemolytic disease of the newborn
    - Hereditary hemolytic anemias
    - Polycythemia (a central venous Hct greater than 65%)
    - Extravascular blood (e.g., cephalohematoma, bruising from delivery)
  - Decreased excretion (liver enzyme insufficiency)
    - Decreased bilirubin conjugation or inadequate transport out of the hepatocyte
    - Biliary obstruction
  - Increased reabsorption (enterohepatic circulation)
    - Delayed passage of meconium (e.g., bowel obstruction)
    - Delayed enteral feedings (Kamath-Rayne et al., 2016, p. 514)
  - Contraindications—congenital erythropoietic porphyria or a family history of porphyria, current or history of photosensitive drug/agent use, and use of metalloporphyrin heme oxygenase inhibitors (Nassabeh-Montazami, 2013, p. 357).

MODES OF PHOTOTHERAPY
- Most effective phototherapy lights delivery output in the blue–green region, including the commercially available special blue fluorescent tubes and light-emitting diode (LED).
- Special blue fluorescent tubes provide greater irradiance than regular blue tubes because the fluorescent tubes omit light in wavelengths that penetrate the skin well and are maximally absorbed by bilirubin (Watchki, 2018, p. 1213).
  - Halogen lamps—halogen spotlight systems can provide high irradiance over a small surface area.
  - Fiberoptic systems—UV-filtered light and are frequently used as an adjunct to conventional overhead phototherapy light. Advantages include the infant can be held or nursed while receiving phototherapy and it is not necessary to cover the infant's eyes.
  - Gallium nitride LEDs—NeoBlue. It provides high spectral irradiance with minimum heat generation. It is a cost-effective device for use in phototherapy because of its long lifetime (Nassabeh-Montazami, 2013, p. 357).
- The efficacy of phototherapy depends on the irradiance (energy output) of the light (irradiance) and the amount of surface area of the infant exposed to the light (Bradshaw, 2016, p. 624; Kamath-Rayne et al., 2016, p. 527; Watchko, 2018, p. 1213).
  - The distance of the light from the infant varies among different systems to achieve the desired irradiance, 10 to 40 $\mu W/cm^2/nm$ (Nassabeh-Montazami, 2013, p. 359).
- Occlusive dressings, bandages, topical skin ointments, and plastic should not be used while the infant is receiving phototherapy to prevent burns (Nassabeh-Montazami, 2013, p. 360).

PRECAUTIONS
- Rebound—after phototherapy is discontinued, the levels should be followed for at least 24 hours to assess for rebound. A rebound of 1 to 2 mg/dL or more can occur after phototherapy is discontinued. It is most likely to occur in the late preterm infant and the infant with hemolytic disease (Kamath-Rayne et al., 2016, p. 530).
- Short-term side effects of phototherapy include increased insensible water loss and stooling, temperature instability, and rash. Eye damage may occur if coverings are not secure (Bradshaw, 2015, p. 625; Kamath-Rayne et al., 2016, p. 530; Nassabeh-Montazami, 2013, p. 360).

VENTILATORS
For discussions on invasive and noninvasive ventilator techniques and management, please see Chapter 17.

CONCLUSION

It is important to be familiar with the applications and limitations of laboratory data and diagnostic testing methods when determining appropriate care for a vulnerable neonate. This includes choosing the laboratory test which provides the most information for the necessary plan of sampling, ordering the correct diagnostic test to determine the neonate's needs, and being aware of potential side effects of all interventions performed in the NICU.

REVIEW QUESTIONS

1. Therapeutic drug monitoring (TDM) uses plasma medication concentrations to:
   A. Accumulate drugs in blood.
   B. Measure illegal substances.
   C. Optimize medication therapy.

2. Calculate the I/T ratio using the following laboratory values: WBC = 9 cells/μL, Hgb = 13 g/dL, Hct = 40%, Plts = 127,000, neutrophils = 32%, bands = 0%, lymphs = 34%, monos = 18%, esinophiles = 5%, metas = 8%, myelos = 6%, promyelos = 4
   A. 0.12
   B. 0.24
   C. 0.36

3. Calculate the absolute neutrophil count (ANC) using the following laboratory values: WBC = 3 cells/μL, Hgb = 14 g/dL, Hct = 42%, Plts = 143,000, neutrophils = 4%, bands = 2%, lymphs = 23%, monos = 18%, esinophiles = 4%, metas = 2%, myelos = 9%
   A. 120
   B. 240
   C. 360

4. When obtaining a left lateral decubitus x-ray to evaluate for free air in the abdomen, the infant should be positioned with the:
   A. Left side down.
   B. Prone position.
   C. Right side down.

5. The interpretation of an electroencephalogram (EEG) is based on three factors: the appearance and disappearance of waveforms, the synchrony of waveforms, and the:
   A. Appearance of subclinical seizures.
   B. Continuity of background activity.
   C. Electrical activity level on a standard scale.

REFERENCES

Abubakar, M. K. (2013a). Continuous blood gas monitoring. In M. G. MacDonald, J. Ramasethu, & K. Rais-Bahrami (Eds.), *Atlas of procedures in neonatology* (5th ed., pp. 65–74). Philadelphia, PA: Lippincott Williams & Wilkins.

Abubakar, M. K. (2013b). End-tidal carbon dioxide monitoring. In M. G. MacDonald, J. Ramasethu, & K. Rais-Bahrami (Eds.), *Atlas of procedures in neonatology* (5th ed., pp. 75–78). Philadelphia, PA: Lippincott Williams & Wilkins.

Bailey, T. (2015). Common invasive procedures. In T. Verklan & M. Walden (Eds.), *Core curriculum for neonatal intensive care nursing* (5th ed., pp. 282–315). St. Louis, MO: Elsevier.

Bradshaw, W. T. (2015). Gastrointestinal disorders. In M. T. Verklan & M. Walden (Eds.), *Core curriculum for neonatal intensive care nursing* (5th ed., pp. 583–631). St. Louis, MO: Saunders Elsevier.

Bradshaw, W. T., & Tanaka, D. T. (2016). Physiologic monitoring. In S. L. Gardner, B. S. Carter, M. Enzman-Hines, & J. A. Hernandez (Eds.), *Merenstein & Gardner's handbook of neonatal intensive care* (8th ed., pp. 126–144.e1). St. Louis, MO: Mosby Elsevier.

Cadnapaphornchai, M. A., Schoenbein, M. B., Woloschuk, R., Soranno, D. E., & Hernández, J. A. (2016). Neonatal nephrology. In S. L. Gardner, B. S. Carter, M. Enzman-Hines, & J. A. Hernandez (Eds.), *Merenstein & Gardner's handbook of neonatal intensive care* (8th ed., pp. 689–726). St. Louis, MO: Mosby Elsevier.

Darras, B., & Volpe, J. (2018). Evaluation, special studies. In J. Volpe, T. Inder, B. Darras, L. deVries, A. Plessis, . . . J. Perlman (Eds.), *Volpe's neurology of the newborn* (6th ed., pp. 861–873). Philadelphia, PA: Elsevier.

Diab, Y., & Luchtman-Jones, L. (2015). Hematologic and oncologic problems in the fetus and neonate. In R. J. Martin, A. A. Fanaroff, & M. C. Walsh (Eds.), *Fanaroff & Martin's neonatal-perinatal medicine: Diseases of the fetus and infant* (10th ed., pp. 1294–1343). Philadelphia, PA: Elsevier Saunders.

DiBlasi, R., & Gallagher, J. T. (2017). Respiratory care of the newborn. In J. P. Goldsmith, E. H. Karotkin, M. Keszler, & G. K. Suresh (Eds.), *Assisted ventilation of the neonate: An evidence-based approach to newborn respiratory care* (6th ed., pp. 291–309). Philadelphia, PA: Elsevier.

Diehl-Jones, W., & Fraser, D. (2015). Hematologic disorders. In M. T. Verklan & M. Walden (Eds.), *Core curriculum for neonatal intensive care nursing* (5th ed., pp. 662–688). St. Louis, MO: Elsevier Saunders.

Ditzenberger, G. R. (2015). Nutritional management. In M. T. Verklan & M. Walden (Eds.), *Core curriculum for neonatal intensive care nursing* (5th ed., pp. 172–196). St. Louis, MO: Elsevier Saunders.

Domonoske, C. D. (2015). Pharmacology. In T. Verklan & M. Walden (Eds.), *Core curriculum for neonatal intensive care nursing* (5th ed., pp. 216–234). St. Louis, MO: Elsevier Saunders.

Ehret, L. (2015). Radiologic evaluation. In T. Verklan & M. Walden (Eds.), *Core curriculum for neonatal intensive care nursing* (pp. 253–281). St. Louis, MO: Elsevier Saunders.

Fasano, R. M., Said, M., & Luban, N. L. C. (2015). Blood component therapy for the neonate. In R. Martin, A. Fanaroff, & M. Walsh (Eds.), *Fanaroff and Martin's neonatal-perinatal medicine: Diseases of the fetus and infant* (pp. 1344–1361). Philadelphia, PA: Elsevier.

Fay, R. J. (2013). Cardiorespiratory monitoring. In M. G. MacDonald, J. Ramasethu & K. Rais-Bahrami (Eds.), *Atlas of procedures in neonatology* (5th ed., pp. 49–55). Philadelphia, PA: Lippincott Williams & Wilkins.

Ferrieri, P., & Wallen, L. (2018). Newborn sepsis and meningitis. In C. Gleason & S. Juul (Eds.), *Avery's diseases of the newborn* (10th ed., pp. 553–565.e3). Philadelphia, PA: Elsevier.

Fiore, J. (2015). Biomedical engineering aspects of neonatal cardiorespiratory monitoring. In R. Martin, A. Fanaroff, & M. Walsh (Eds.), *Fanaroff and Martin's neonatal-perinatal medicine: Diseases of the fetus and infant* (pp. 522–535). Philadelphia, PA: Elsevier.

Gardner, S. L., & Hernández, J. A. (2016). Heat balance. In S. L. Gardner, B. S. Carter, M. Enzman-Hines, & J. A. Hernandez (Eds.), *Merenstein & Gardner's handbook of neonatal intensive care* (8th ed., pp. 105–121.e2). St. Louis, MO: Mosby Elsevier.

Halbardier, B. H. (2015). Fluid and electrolyte management. In M. T. Verklan & M. Walden (Eds.), *Core curriculum for neonatal intensive care nursing* (5th ed., pp. 146–161). St. Louis, MO: Saunders Elsevier.

Jensen, E. A., Mong, D. A., Biko, D. M., Maschhoff, K. L., & Kirpalani, H. (2017). Imaging: Radiography, lung ultrasound, and other imaging modalities. In J. P. Goldsmith, E. H. Karotkin, M. Keszler & G. K. Suresh (Eds.), *Assisted ventilation of the neonate: An evidence-based approach to newborn respiratory care* (6th ed., pp. 67–79). Philadelphia, PA: Elsevier.

Kamath-Rayne, B. D., Thilo, E. H., Deacon, J., & Hernández, J. A. (2016). Neonatal hyperbilirubinemia. In S. L. Gardner, B. S. Carter, M. Enzman-Hines, & J. A. Hernandez (Eds.), *Merenstein & Gardner's handbook of neonatal intensive care* (8th ed., pp. 511–536). St. Louis, MO: Mosby Elsevier.

Letterio, J., Ahuja, S. P., & Petrosiute, A. (2013). Hematologic problems. In A. A. Fanaroff & J. M. Fanaroff (Eds.), *Klaus and Fanaroff's care of the high-risk neonate* (6th ed., pp. 432–475). Philadelphia, PA: Elsevier Saunders.

Levy, J., & D'Harlingue, A. E. (2013). Recognition, stabilization, and transport of the high-risk newvorn. In A. A. Fanaroff & J. M. Fanaroff (Eds.), *Klaus and Fanaroff's care of the high-risk neonate* (6th ed., pp. 71–104). Philadelphia, PA: Elsevier Saunders.

Maltepe, E., & Penn, A. A. (2018). Development, function, and pathology of the placenta. In C. A. Gleason & S. E. Juul (Eds.), *Avery's diseases of the newborn* (10th ed., pp. 40–60.e8). Philadelphia, PA: Elsevier.

Manco-Johnson, M., McKinney, C., Knapp-Clevenger, R., & Hernández, J. A. (2016). Newborn hematology. In S. L. Gardner, B. S. Carter, M. Enzman-Hines, & J. A. Hernandez (Eds.), *Merenstein & Gardner's handbook of neonatal intensive care* (8th ed., pp. 479–510). St. Louis, MO: Mosby Elsevier.

Massaro, A. N., & Rais-Bahrami, K. (2013). Peripheral arterial cannulation. In M. G. MacDonald, J. Ramasethu, & K. Rais-Bahrami (Eds.), *Atlas of procedures in neonatology* (5th ed., pp. 182–193). Philadelphia, PA: Lippincott Williams & Wilkins.

Mathew, B., & Lakshminrusimha, S. (2017). Noninvasive monitoring of gas exchange. In J. P. Goldsmith, E. H. Karotkin, M. Keszler, & G. K. Suresh (Eds.), *Assisted ventilation of the neonate: An evidence-based approach to newborn respiratory care* (6th ed., pp. 97–107). Philadelphia, PA: Elsevier.

Nassabeh-Montazami, S. (2013). Phototherapy. In M. G. MacDonald, J. Ramasethu, & K. Rais-Bahrami (Eds.), *Atlas of procedures in neonatology* (5th ed., pp. 357–362). Philadelphia, PA: Lippincott Williams & Wilkins.

Natarajan, N., & Gospe, S. (2018). Neonatal seizures. In C. Gleason & S. Juul (Eds.), *Avery's diseases of the newborn* (10th ed., pp. 961–970.e4). Philadelphia, PA: Elsevier.

Neil, J., & Volpe, J. (2018). Specialized neurological studies. In J. Volpe, T. Inder, B. Darras, L. deVries, A. Plessis, ... J. Perlman (Eds.), *Volpe's neurology of the newborn* (6th ed., pp. 222–254.e10). Philadelphia, PA: Elsevier.

Niermeyer, S., Clarke, S. B., & Hernández, J. A. (2016). Delivery room care. In S. L. Gardner, B. S. Carter, M. Enzman-Hines, & J. A. Hernandez (Eds.), *Merenstein & Gardner's handbook of neonatal intensive care* (8th ed., pp. 47–70.e3). St. Louis, MO: Mosby Elsevier.

Owen, L. S., Weiner, G. M., & Davis, P. G. (2017). Delivery room stabilization, and respiratory support. In J. P. Goldsmith, E. H. Karotkin, M. Keszler, & G. K. Suresh (Eds.), *Assisted ventilation of the neonate: An evidence-based approach to newborn respiratory care* (6th ed., pp. 275–290). Philadelphia, PA: Elsevier.

Pammi, M., Brand, M. C., & Weisman, L. E. (2016). Infection in the neonate. In S. L. Gardner, B. S. Carter, M. Enzman-Hines, & J. A. Hernandez (Eds.), *Merenstein & Gardner's handbook of neonatal intensive care* (8th ed., pp. 537–563). St. Louis, MO: Mosby Elsevier.

Parsons, J., Seay, A., & Jacobson, M. (2016). Neurologic disorders. In S. Gardner, B. Carter, M. Hines, & J. Hernandez (Eds.), *Merenstein & Gardner's handbook of neonatal ntensive care* (8th ed., pp. 727–762). St. Louis, MO: Elsevier.

Rabi, Y., Kowal, D., & Ambalavanan, N. (2017). Blood gases: Technical aspects and interpretation. In J. P. Goldsmith, E. H. Karotkin, M. Keszler, & G. K. Suresh (Eds.), *Assisted ventilation of the neonate: An evidence-based approach to newborn respiratory care* (6th ed., pp. 80–96). Philadelphia, PA: Elsevier.

Rais-Bahrami, K., & MacDonald, M. G. (2013). Thoracostomy. In M. G. MacDonald, J. Ramasethu, & K. Rais-Bahrami (Eds.), *Atlas of procedures in neonatology* (5th ed., pp. 255–272). Philadelphia, PA: Lippincott Williams & Wilkins.

Ramasethu, J. (2013). Management of vascular spasm and thrombosis. In M. G. MacDonald, J. Ramasethu, & K. Rais-Bahrami (Eds.), *Atlas of procedures in neonatology* (5th ed., pp. 224–229). Philadelphia, PA: Lippincott Williams & Wilkins.

Ringer, S. (2017). Common neonatal procedures. In E. Eichenwald, A. Hansen, C. Martin, & A. Stark. (Eds.), *Cloherty and Stark's manual of neonatal care* (8th ed., pp. 1000–1021). Philadelphia, PA: Wolters Kluwer.

Rioja-Mazza, D. C. (2013). Maintenance of thermal homeostasis. In M. G. MacDonald, J. Ramasethu, & K. Rais-Bahrami (Eds.), *Atlas of procedures in neonatology* (5th ed., pp. 23–26). Philadelphia, PA: Lippincott Williams & Wilkins.

Rodger, M., & Silver, R. M. (2019). Coagulation disorders in pregnancy. In R. Resnik, C. J. Lockwood, T. R. Moore, M. F. Greene, J. Copel, &

R. M. Silver (Eds.), *Creasy and Resnik's maternal-fetal medicine: Principles and practice* (8th ed., pp. 949–976.e8). Philadelphia, PA: Elsevier.

Rorke, J. M., Rramasethu, J., & Chahine, A. A. (2013). Central venous catheterization. In M. G. MacDonald, J. Ramasethu, & K. Rais-Bahrami (Eds.). *Atlas of procedures in neonatology* (5th ed., pp. 23–26). Philadelphia, PA: Lippincott Williams & Wilkins.

Sadowski, S. (2015). Cardiovascular disorders. In T. Verklan & M. Walden (Eds.), *Core curriculum for neonatal intensive care nursing* (5th ed., pp. 527–582). St. Louis, MO: Elsevier.

Said, M. M., & Rais-Bahrami, K. (2013a). Peripheral intravenous line placement. In M. G. MacDonald, J. Ramasethu, & K. Rais-Bahrami (Eds.), *Atlas of procedures in neonatology* (5th ed., pp. 142–151). Philadelphia, PA: Lippincott Williams & Wilkins.

Said, M. M., & Rais-Bahrami, K. (2013b). Umbilical artery catheterization. In M. G. MacDonald, J. Ramasethu, & K. Rais-Bahrami (Eds.). *Atlas of procedures in neonatology* (5th ed., pp. 156–172). Philadelphia, PA: Lippincott Williams & Wilkins.

Said, M. M., & Rais-Bahrami, K. (2013c). Umbilical vein catheterization. In M. G. MacDonald, J. Ramasethu, & K. Rais-Bahrami (Eds.), *Atlas of procedures in neonatology* (5th ed., pp. 173–181). Philadelphia, PA: Lippincott Williams & Wilkins.

Said, M. M., & Rais-Bahrami, K. (2013d). Endotracheal intubation. In M. G. MacDonald, J. Ramasethu, & K. Rais-Bahrami (Eds.), *Atlas of procedures in neonatology* (5th ed., pp. 236–249). Philadelphia, PA: Lippincott Williams & Wilkins.

Saxonhouse, M. A. (2018). Neonatal bleeding and thrombotic disorders. In C. A. Gleason & S. E. Juul (Eds.), *Avery's diseases of the newborn* (10th ed., pp. 1121–1138.e4). Philadelphia, PA: Elsevier.

Schiefelbein, J. (2015). Genetics: From bench to bedside. In T. Verklan & M. Walden (Eds.), *Core curriculum for neonatal intensive care nursing* (5th ed., pp. 391–406). St. Louis, MO: Elsevier.

Scholz, T., & Reinking, B. (2018) Congenital heart disease. In C. Gleason & S. Juul (Eds.), *Avery's diseases of the newborn* (10th ed., pp. 801–827.e2). Philadelphia, PA: Elsevier.

Sea, S. (2013). Vessel localization. In M. G. MacDonald, J. Ramasethu, & K. Rais-Bahrami (Eds.), *Atlas of procedures in neonatology* (5th ed., pp. 85–88). Philadelphia, PA: Lippincott Williams & Wilkins.

Sherman, J. (2015a). Perinatal substance abuse. In T. Verklan & M. Walden (Eds.), *Core curriculum for neonatal intensive care nursing* (5th ed., pp. 43–57). St. Louis, MO: Elsevier.

Sherman, J. (2015b). Renal and genitourinary disorders. In T. Verklan & M. Walden (Eds.), *Core curriculum for neonatal intensive care nursing* (5th ed., pp. 719–733). St. Louis, MO: Elsevier.

Simhan, H. N., Berghella, V., & Iams, J. D. (2019). Prevention and management of preterm parturition. In R. Resnik, C. J. Lockwood, T. R. Moore, M. F. Greene, J. Copel, & R. M. Silver (Eds.), *Creasy and Resnik's maternal-fetal medicine: P les and practice* (8th ed., pp. 679–711. e10). Philadelphia, PA: Elsevier.

Smallwood, C. (2019). Noninvasive monitoring in the neonatal and pediatric care. In B. Walsh (Ed.), *Neonatal and pediatric respiratory care* (5th ed., pp. 135–148). St. Louis, MO: Elsevier.

Sterk, L. (2015). Congenital anomalies. In M. T. Verklan & M. Walden (Eds.), *Core curriculum for neonatal intensive care nursing* (5th ed., pp. 767–794). St. Louis, MO: Elsevir Saunders.

Strain, J. D., & Weinman, J. P. (2016). Diagnostic imaging in the neonate. In S. L. Gardner, B. S. Carter, M. Enzman-Hines, & J. A. Hernandez (Eds.), *Merenstein & Gardner's handbook of neonatal intensive care* (8th ed., pp. 158–180.e1). St. Louis, MO: Mosby Elsevier.

Swanson, T., & Erickson, L. (2016). Cardiovascular disease and surgical interventions. In S. Gardner, B. Carter, M. Hines, & J. Hernandez (Eds.), *Merenstein & Gardner's handbook of neonatal intensive care* (8th ed., pp. 644–688.e2). St. Louis, MO: Elsevier.

Szlachetka, D. M. (2015). Laboratory and diagnostic test interpretation. In M. T. Verklan & M. Walden (Eds.), *Core curriculum for neonatal intensive care nursing* (5th ed., pp. 235–252). St. Louis, MO: Elsevier Saunders.

Verklan, M. T. (2015). Neurologic disorders. In M. T. Verklan & M. Walden (Eds.), *Core curriculum for neonatal intensive care nursing* (5th ed., wpp. 734–766). St. Louis, MO: Elsevier.

Watchki, J. F. (2018). Neonatal indirect hyperbilirubinemia and kernicterus. In C. A. Gleason & S. E. Juul (Eds.), *Avery's diseases of the newborn* (10th ed., pp. 1198–1218.e5). Philadelphia, PA: Elsevier.

Watters, K., & Mancuso, T. (2019). Airway management. In B. Walsh (Ed.), *Neonatal and pediatric respiratory care* (5th ed., pp. 222–241). St. Louis, MO: Elsevier.

Weitkamp, J., Lewis, D. B., & Levy, O. (2018). Immunology of the fetus and newborn. In C. A. Gleason & S. E. Juul (Eds.), *Avery's diseases of the newborn* (10th ed., pp. 453–481.e7). Philadelphia, PA: Elsevier.

Wilson, D., & Tyner, C. (2015). Infectious diseases in the neonate. In T. Verklan & M. Walden (Eds.), *Core curriculum for neonatal intensive care nursing* (5th ed., pp. 689–718). St. Louis, MO: Elsevier Saunders.

Wright, C., Posencheg, M., Seri, I., & Evans, J. (2018). Fluid, electrolyte and acid-base balance. In C. Gleason & S. Juul (Eds.), *Avery's diseases of the newborn* (10th ed., pp. 368–389.e4). Philadelphia, PA: Elsevier.

5 COMMUNICATION AND PARENT/ INFANT INTERACTION

Karen Q. McDonald

INTRODUCTION

Parenting and normal parental attachment begin not at birth, but before and during pregnancy. The increase of maternal hormones during pregnancy helps with the formation of maternal bonding. After birth, the interaction between mother/father and their baby helps to build strong parental attachment and bonding.

FAMILY INTEGRATION

Normal Attachment

PREGNANCY

- The beginning of parent–infant interactions has foundation in autonomic, neurologic, and endocrinologic systems, and the emotional connection to an infant begins not at birth, but during pregnancy (Ballard, 2015, p. 634).
  - ○ Increasing levels of oxytocin throughout pregnancy encourage the formation of an emotional bond between the mother and infant by acting to reduce anxiety (Ballard, 2015, p. 632).
  - ○ Oxytocin levels in early pregnancy and the postpartum period are significantly correlated with a clearly defined set of maternal bonding behaviors, including gaze, vocalizations, positive affect, affectionate touch, attachment-related thoughts, and frequent checking of the infant (Ballard, 2015, p. 633).
- Bonding is a continuing, reciprocal process that is unique to two people and endures across time. Bonding occurs on a different timetable for mothers and fathers; mothers experience an intensifying feeling of bonding throughout the pregnancy, while the father's feelings develop and become congruent after birth (Kenner & Boykova, 2015, p. 341).
- Attachment is the quality of the bond, or affectional tie, between parents and their infant, and an individualized process that does not happen automatically. Attachment is characterized by the same qualities used to describe love. Parental love and romantic love activate the same areas of the human brain, result in brain processing of infant cues, and elevate the "bonding" hormone, oxytocin. (Gardner, Voos, & Hills, 2016, p. 821; Kenner & Boykova, 2015, p. 341).
- Table 5.1 outlines Klaus and Kennell's Nine Steps in the Process of Attachment. It is worth noting that six of the nine steps of attachment occur prior to the infant's birth.

TABLE 5.1 Klaus and Kennell's Nine Steps in the Process of Attachment

Step 1. Planning the pregnancy	This is the first step, showing investment and commitment of the parents.
Step 2. Confirming the pregnancy	Confirmation of the pregnancy begins the psychologic acceptance of the pregnancy.
Step 3. Accepting the pregnancy	Parents experience a normal feeling of ambivalence. Although the mother does not yet perceive the fetus as separate from herself, she experiences emotional changes leading toward attachment.
Step 4. Fetal movement	Feeling fetal movement leads to happy thoughts, as well as the mother starting to think of the baby as a separate person.
Step 5. Accepting the fetus	Parents begin to think of the fetus as an individual and start to imagine what the baby will be like, therefore resulting in establishing a relationship.
Step 6. Labor and birth	Parental attitudes toward the labor and delivery process may affect their reactions. Studies show that those who attend the birth are more attached to the infant than those who do not.
Step 7. Seeing	Studies have shown that immediate attachment is facilitated when the mother is able to see the baby immediately after birth.
Step 8. Touching	Nurturing maternal touch is associated with more secure attachments.
Step 9. Caregiving	Is important for psychic closure of bonding.

Source: Data from Gardner, S., Voos, K., & Hills, P. (2016). Families in crisis: Theoretical and practical considerations. In S. Gardner, B. Carter, M. Hines, & J. Hernandez (Eds.), *Merenstein & Gardner's handbook of neonatal intensive care* (8th ed., pp. 821–873). St. Louis, MO: Elsevier.

Becoming a Parent

- Becoming a parent requires a major adjustment of roles, lifestyle, and relationships. Because previous ideas and coping strategies may not be helpful, life-crisis situations challenge the individual with the potential for growth as new responses and solutions are used for problem solving (Gardner et al., 2016, p. 822).
- The ability to parent is influenced by a multitude of factors that occur before, during, and after the birth of the infant.
  - Previous life events, including degree of life stress/patterns of coping, genetic endowment, being parented, previous pregnancies, anxiety and distress about parenting role, and interpersonal relationships, affect the experience of pregnancy and parenthood. (Gardner et al., 2016, p. 822; Klaus, Kennell, & Fanaroff, 2013, p. 201).
  - Cultural differences influence (a) parental emotional responses and perceptions of their infant's illness and disability, (b) parental usage of services, and (c) parental interaction with health care providers.
    - One must be cautious in viewing parental attachment behavior through one's own cultural filter, because this may result in an incorrect assessment of parent–infant attachment (Gardner et al., 2016, pp. 822–823).
  - Infant characteristics (e.g., responsiveness/vulnerability/severity of illness), appearance, parental feelings of loyalty and hope, the behavior of health professionals, separation from the infant, an inability to protect their newborn from pain, and hospital practices may positively or negatively influence parents.
  - (Gardner et al., 2016, p. 823).

Birth and the First Days

THE INITIAL FAMILY DYNAMICS AND THE "SENSITIVE PERIOD"

- At birth, all five senses are operational and the infant is ready to cue and shape the environment, and healthy mothers are physiologically and psychologically ready for reciprocal interaction (Gardner et al., 2016, p. 821).
- The maternal cues of voice, touch and body rhythm are used to begin bonding. These cues create the response of a synchronized "dance" between the mother and infant. The sensory stimuli of touch, warmth, and odor between the mother and infant are a powerful vagal stimulant, resulting in the release of maternal oxytocin, which aids in breastfeeding and mother–infant attachment (Ballard, 2015, pp. 632, 634).
- The period of labor, birth, and the following days has been called the "sensitive period," and it is during this time that parents are most strongly influenced by the quality of care they themselves receive (Ballard, 2015, p. 634; Gardner et al., 2016, p. 822; Klaus et al., 2013, p. 207).
  - During a period referred to as "primary maternal preoccupation" of the mother, she develops a great sensitivity to and is focused on the needs of the infant. This period begins toward the end of the pregnancy and continues for a few weeks after delivery. Reciprocation of needs and responses from the infant to the mother reinforce synchronized and rewarding interactions for the dyad (Ballard, 2015, p. 634).
  - Studies have demonstrated that when fathers are given the opportunity to be alone with their newborn, they spend an amount of time equal to mothers interacting, holding, touching, and bonding with their baby (Ballard, 2015, p. 634; Klaus et al., 2013, p. 209).
- Immediately after birth, parents enter a unique period in which their attachment to their infant usually begins to blossom and in which events may have many effects on the family (Ballard, 2015, pp. 633–634).
- The birth of a newborn initiates a series of interactions with parents (particularly the mother) designed to initiate attachment and ensure survival (Gardner et al., 2016, p. 821). The high level of positive arousal that infants co-construct with their parents during their face-to-face interactions accelerates the maturation of the infant's relational skills and provides essential environmental inputs for the development of self-regulation and the process of attachment (Ballard, 2015, p. 634).
  - The first feelings of love for the infant may not be instantaneous. Many mothers express distress and disappointment when they do not experience feelings of love for their infant in the first minutes or hours after birth. Studies confirm that normal, healthy mothers may first feel love for their baby after even a week or longer (Ballard, 2015, p. 634).
- Parental attachment and appropriate caregiving behaviors are crucial for the infant's physical, psychologic, and emotional health and survival (Gardner et al., 2016, p. 821; Kenner & Boykova, 2015, p. 341).
- Early parent–infant contact facilitates parent–infant attachment and contributes to the regulation of the newborn's physiology and behavior (Gardner et al., 2016, p. 822).
- Positive effects of early and extended contact, rather than initial separation, have shown significant differences in caregiving behaviors that persist over time (Gardner et al., 2016, p. 822).
- Klaus and Klaus suggest at least 60 minutes of uninterrupted private time for parents and infants to encourage and enhance the bonding experience (Klaus et al., 2013, p. 209).

Barriers to Attachment

- Early attachment can be easily disturbed and may be permanently altered during the immediate postpartum period if a newborn requires separation from the mother for care (Ballard, 2015, p. 634).
  - Routine procedures, including weighing, measuring, bathing, blood tests, vaccines, and eye prophylaxis, should be delayed until after the first feeding is completed (Ballard, 2015, p. 633; Gardner et al., 2016, p. 821).
  - During medically necessary interventions, it is important to give parents as much interaction (or at least visual contact) with their infant as is possible (Gardner et al., 2016, pp. 822, 827; Kenner & Boykova, 2015, p. 342).

FAMILY-CENTERED CARE

- Family-centered care (FCC) principles stress that parents are the most important person in their infant's life, that they have expertise in caring for the infant, and that their values and beliefs should be central during NICU care. Adherence to these principles has been shown to have a significant positive influence on the family's ability to cope with the NICU stress. The use of FCC has been shown to enhance the likelihood of successful parent–child relationships (Gardner et al., 2016, p. 828).

1. Family-centered neonatal care should be based on open and honest communication between parents and professionals on medical and ethical issues.
2. To work with professionals in making informed treatment choices, parents must have available to them the same facts and interpretation of those facts as the professionals, including medical information presented in meaningful formats, information about uncertainties surrounding treatments, information from parents whose children have been in similar medical situations, and access to the chart and rounds discussions.
3. In medical situations involving very high mortality and morbidity, great suffering, and/or significant medical controversy, fully informed parents should have the right to make decisions about aggressive treatment for their infants.
4. Expectant parents should be offered information about adverse pregnancy outcomes and be given the opportunity to state in advance their treatment preferences if their infant is born extremely prematurely and/or critically ill.
5. Parents and professionals must work together to acknowledge and alleviate the pain of infants in the NICU.
6. Parents and professionals must work together to ensure an appropriate environment for infants in the NICU.
7. Parents and professionals must work together to ensure the safety and efficacy of neonatal treatments.
8. Parents and professionals must work together to develop nursery policies and programs that promote parenting skills and encourage maximum involvement of families with their hospitalized infants.
9. Parents and professionals must work together to promote meaningful long-term follow-up for all high-risk NICU survivors.
10. Parents and professionals must acknowledge that critically ill newborns can be harmed by overtreatment as well as undertreatment, and must insist that laws and treatment policies be based on compassion. Parents and professionals must work together to promote awareness of the needs of NICU survivors with disabilities to ensure adequate support for them and their families. Parents and professionals must work together to decrease disability through universal prenatal care.

Source: Reproduced with permission from Gardner, S., Voos, K., & Hills, P. (2016). Families in crisis: Theoretical and practical considerations. In S. Gardner, B. Carter, M. Hines, & J. Hernandez (Eds.), *Merenstein & Gardner's handbook of neonatal intensive care* (8th ed., pp. 821–873). St. Louis, MO: Elsevier.

Baby-Friendly Initiatives

- UNICEF has incorporated these evidence-based practices in its Baby-Friendly Hospital Initiative (Ballard, 2015, p. 633).
  - Among the 10 steps for a hospital to achieve Baby-Friendly designation are to *"help mother initiate breastfeeding within one hour of birth* and to *practice 'rooming in'—allow mothers and infants to remain together 24 hours a day"* (Ballard, 2015, p. 633; Klaus et al., 2013, p. 207).
- Following the introduction of the Baby-Friendly initiative in maternity units in several countries throughout the world, an unexpected observation was made: The use of "rooming in" and early contact with suckling significantly reduced the frequency of abandonment (Klaus et al., 2013, p. 208).

Skin-to-Skin Care (SSC) or Kangaroo Care

- Swedish researchers found that the infants who are placed for the first 90 minutes after birth on their mother's chest, skin to skin and covered by a blanket, cried less than babies that are dried, swaddled, and placed in a bassinet. An additional Cochrane review found that early skin-to-skin interactions between mothers and babies reduced crying, improved mother–baby interactions, kept the baby warm, and helped women to more successfully breastfeed their infant (Klaus et al., 2013, pp. 207, 209).

- Better breastfeeding
- Infant better able to maintain body temperature
- Higher initial blood glucose levels
- Lower respiratory rate
- Better heart rate stability
- Increase in affectionate maternal attachment behavior
- Lower salivary cortisol levels
- Less infant crying

Source: Data from Gardner, S., Voos, K., & Hills, P. (2016). Families in crisis: Theoretical and practical considerations. In S. Gardner, B. Carter, M. Hines, & J. Hernandez (Eds.), *Merenstein & Gardner's handbook of neonatal intensive care* (8th ed., pp. 821–873). St. Louis, MO: Elsevier.

FAMILIES IN CRISIS

- When a much-anticipated full-term baby whose mother has had an uncomplicated, problem-free pregnancy is born with any kind of problem, the parents feel an overwhelming sense of shock and disappointment. The problem or malformation of the baby can immediately cause a lowering of self-esteem and the parents may view this as a failure. Guilt is one of the overwhelming emotions that plague these parents (Gardner et al., 2016, p. 827; Kenner & Boykova, 2015, p. 331; Klaus et al., 2013, p. 201).
- Parents of infants requiring NICU care often experience high levels of stress and, as a consequence, their ability to interact optimally with their infant(s) is impaired.
- Parents of premature or sick neonates frequently experience lowered self-esteem and think of this as a failure of their capacity for reproduction and, symbolically, of their own defectiveness.
- Parental perception of support by the medical team has been shown to be inversely correlated with maternal depressive symptoms. The more support the parents feel is being given by the medical team, the fewer depressive symptoms are manifested. The perinatal health team cannot underestimate its ability to influence how the mother and family adapt (Gardner et al., 2016, p. 828).
  - Some of the care practices that can be misinterpreted by parents, leading to an increase in maternal depression, are:
    - The behavior of physicians, nurses, and hospital personnel
    - Care and support during labor, first days of life, separation of mother and infant, and rules of the hospital
    - Early comments by staff, family, and friends may have a lasting impression in the parent's minds (Gardner et al., 2016, p. 827; Kenner & Boykova, 2015, p. 332).

Influences on Parental Behavior

- A schematic diagram of the influences on paternal and maternal behavior and the hypothesized resultant disturbances are present in Figure 5.1.

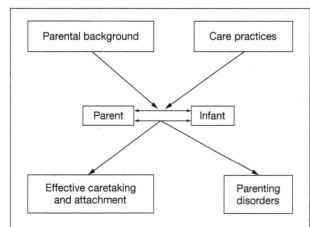

FIGURE 5.1 Schematic diagram of the major influences on paternal and maternal behavior and the resulting disturbances that we hypothesize may arise from them.

Source: Reproduced with permission from Klaus, M., Kennell., & Fanaroff, J. (2013). Care of the parents. In A. Fanaroff & J. Fanaroff (Eds.), *Klaus and Fanaroff's care of the high-risk neonate* (6th ed., pp. 201–224). Cleveland, OH: Elsevier.

- Parents' responses to stress can be determined by parenteral background and care practices.
  - Included under parental background is the parent's care by his or her own mother, practices of their culture, relationships within the family, and planning, course, and events during pregnancy.
  - Life stresses that precipitate concern for the health and survival of either her infant or herself may delay the mother's preparation for the infant and interrupt bond formation (Ballard, 2015, p. 632; Klaus et al., 2013, p. 202).
  - Some of the emotional reactions parents may exhibit when their child requires NICU care may include shock, panic, fright, anxiety, isolation, and helplessness (Gardner et al., 2016, p. 827).
    - Hospital care practices that reduce anxiety, such as avoiding unnecessary separation of an infant from parents during the "sensitive period," can contribute greatly to early attachment (Ballard, 2015, p. 632; Klaus et al., 2013, p. 202).
    - Researchers have found that parents are best able to develop a secure attachment with the premature/sick newborn when they are able to see the infant within 3 hours of delivery (Gardner et al., 2016, p. 833).
- Stresses in the NICU that affect the parent infant bond attachment are summarized in Box 5.2.
- Outcomes from altered interactions between the parent and infant result in the chance for negative (parenting disorders) and positive (effective caretaking and attachment) conclusions (Ballard, 2015, p. 632; Klaus et al., 2013, p. 202).

BOX 5.3 Six Major Sources of Parental Stress in the NICU

1. Preexisting and concurrent personal as well as family factors
2. Prenatal, perinatal, and labor and delivery experiences
3. Accepting and understanding the infant's illness and the treatment required. Also accepting the appearance of the infant during the treatment, and of those with congenital anomalies
4. Concerns for the outcome of the infant, long term and well as immediate
5. Their perceived loss of the parental role, as well as loss of personal control of the situation
6. Their trust and experience with the healthcare providers

Source: Data from Gardner, S., Voos, K., & Hills, P. (2016). Families in crisis: Theoretical and practical considerations. In S. Gardner, B. Carter, M. Hines, & J. Hernandez (Eds.), *Merenstein & Gardner's handbook of neonatal intensive care* (8th ed., pp. 821–873). St. Louis, MO: Elsevier.

- Included under parenting disorders are the vulnerable child syndrome, child abuse, failure to thrive, and some developmental and emotional problems in high-risk infants (Klaus et al., 2013, p. 2020).
- Other maladaptive parenting examples are being overprotective, or emotional disengagement and deprivation and low adherence to follow-up recommendations that may affect infant development and growth (Kenner & Boykova, 2015, p. 332).
- The most easily manipulated variables in this scheme are the separation of the infant from the mother and the practices in the hospital during the first hours and days of life. It is here, during this period, that studies have in part clarified some of the steps in parent–infant attachment (Ballard, 2015, p. 632; Klaus et al., 2013, p. 202).
  - Parents who miss out on this early interaction experience should be assured that their future relationship with their baby can still be developed. Humans do not reject their babies if they don't immediately bond. It is important that parents be given as much contact, physical or visual, as possible when medical intervention is necessary (Klaus et al., 2013, p. 209; Gardner et al., 2016, p. 822).

Facilitating Positive Parenting in the NICU

- The healthcare team can help make the NICU experience more positive in multiple ways:
  - Whenever discussing the infant with the parent make sure to refer to the baby by name and the correct gender. This helps the parents personalize this infant as theirs (Gardner et al., 2016, p. 832).
  - Facilitate opportunities for parents to be involved in their baby's care (Gardner et al., 2016, p. 832; Kenner & Boykova, 2015, p. 333).
  - Provide ongoing, positive, realistic feedback to parents (Gardner et al., 2016, p. 832).
  - Keep parents updated about their baby's medical condition and be free to answer questions (Gardner et al., 2016, p. 832).
  - Facilitate and advocate for parent/child interactions (Gardner et al., 2016, p. 832) (Kenner & Boykova, 2015, p. 333).

○ Provide opportunities for parent/child physical closeness and intimacy (Gardner et al., 2016, p. 832).
○ Allow parents to feel and/or verbalize their feelings of fear and grief, while letting them know these are normal feelings. Listening is vital for the healthcare professional at this time (Gardner et al., 2016, p. 835; Kenner & Boykova, 2015, p. 337).
○ Be consistent with the information that is given by the healthcare team (Kenner & Boykova, 2015, p. 337).

• Parents have stated that when a healthcare professional is giving information regarding their baby, they want accurate, current, and comprehensive information that is not necessarily pessimistic (Gardner et al., 2016, p. 836).
○ Many times parents may misperceive the information that they are given, so it is essential to find out their understanding of what they have been told and clarify misinformation. (Gardner et al., 2016, p. 836; Kenner & Boykova, 2015, p. 335).
○ Pictures can be very helpful when giving detailed information. Remember not to overload the parent with too much information at one time, and continually assess their understanding (Gardner et al., 2016, p. 838).

CONCLUSION

Having a sick or premature infant who requires neonatal intensive care can initiate many different emotions in parents. These include but are not limited to stress, guilt, anxiety, and fear. Healthcare professionals can help parents with these emotions by listening, giving honest, accurate, and consistent information and continually assessing parents understanding of their infant's condition.

REVIEW QUESTIONS

1. A medical problem with or malformation of an infant can lead the parents to have overwhelming feelings of:
   A. Anger.
   B. Euphoria.
   C. Guilt.

2. Parental perception of support by the medical team has been shown to be related to maternal depressive symptoms in a manner that is:
   A. Correlational.
   B. Equitable.
   C. Inverse.

3. While an infant is in an NICU, the parents should be:
   A. Allowed to visit, but not to touch or talk to the baby
   B. Given as much physical and visual contact as possible
   C. Updated routinely, but asked to stay away from the baby

4. Family-centered care has been shown to enhance parents' ability to:
   A. Cope with NICU stressors
   B. Leave the infant at night
   C. Understand the baby's care

5. Research has determined that in order to achieve maximum attachment benefit, parents and infants need to spend together a minimum of:
   A. 45 minutes
   B. 60 minutes
   C. 90 minutes

REFERENCES

Ballard, A. (2015). Normal mother-infant attachment. In R. Martin, A. Fanaroff, & M. Walsh (Eds.), *Fanaroff and Martin's neonatal-perinatal medicine: Diseases of the fetus and infant* (10th ed., pp. 632–634). Philadelphia, PA: Elsevier.
Gardner, S., Voos, K., & Hills, P. (2016). Families in crisis: Theoretical and practical considerations. In S. Gardner, B. Carter, M. Hines, & J. Hernandez (Eds.), *Merenstein & Gardner's handbook of neonatal intensive care* (8th ed., pp. 821–873). St. Louis, MO: Elsevier.
Kenner, C., & Boykova, M. (2015). Families in crisis. In T. Verklan & M. Walden (Eds.), *Core curriculum for neonatal intensive care nursing* (5th ed., pp. 331–347). St. Louis, MO: Elsevier.
Klaus, M., Kennell, J., & Fanaroff, J. (2013). Care of the parents. In A. Fanaroff & J. Fanaroff (Eds.), *Klaus and Fanaroff's care of the high-risk neonate* (6th ed., pp. 201–224). Cleveland, OH: Elsevier.

FAMILY INTEGRATION: THE GRIEVING PROCESS

Ana Arias-Oliveras

INTRODUCTION

Pregnancy, birth, and parenthood are almost universally defined as a life transition and crisis. Significant adjustments to roles, lifestyle, and relationships are required when becoming a parent. This may cause significant stress in the individual and may be heightened if the newborn is critically ill or a perinatal loss is experienced. For some parents, this may be the first time coping with a significant life challenge, creating the possibility of developing depression, impaired recall, dysfunctional parenting patterns, and poor developmental outcomes for their child (Gardner & Carter, 2016, p. 822, 827, 865; Gardner, Voos, & Hills, 2016). As highlighted in Chapter 5, the emotional connection with an infant begins during pregnancy. When a pregnancy fails to produce a live, healthy infant, it can be a life-altering event. Newborns who are born premature or with a genetic condition or congenital anomaly, or who ultimately die, are representative of the loss of the "perfect child" (Gardner & Carter, 2016, p. 868).

This chapter reviews several factors that may inhibit bonding between infant and parent(s). Such circumstances with the infant or mother as prematurity, congenital anomalies, genetic conditions, asphyxia, pregnancy or delivery complications, and mood disorders are some of many possible compounding factors that alter infant–parent bonding (Ballard, p. 632).

GRIEF

In the event of a perinatal death, the significant loss should be acknowledged and culturally appropriate rituals used, conveying compassion (Friedman, 2015, p. 640). Grief is an individualized process influenced by cultural, environmental, spiritual, and religious experiences (Gardner & Carter, 2016, p. 821, 865; Gardner et al., 2016; Klaus, Kennell, & Fanaroff, 2013, p. 215). Healing from the loss will take time, as the individual will adapt into the phase of acceptance on his or her own accord to minimize the degree of pain and suffering (Gardner & Carter, 2016, p. 865).

Stages of Grief

- Grief is the characteristic response to the loss of a valued "object"—a person or thing. For grief to occur, the individual must have valued the person or thing lost, so that the loss is perceived as significant and meaningful (Gardner & Carter, 2016, pp. 865–866; Kenner & Boykova, 2015, p. 333).
- Loss, whether real or imagined, actual or possible, is traumatic. The individual is no longer confident in himself or herself or in his or her surroundings, as both have been altered (Gardner & Carter, 2016, p. 865).
- The acceptance of the perceived "loss," the discrepancy between the idealized and the real infant, is vital for resolution of grief. When parents resolve the discrepancy between the idealized infant and the real infant (Kenner & Boykova, 2015, p. 333).
- Grief is differentiated into three categories: anticipatory grief, chronic grief, and chronic sorrow (Kenner & Boykova, 2015, p. 333). These categories are summarized in Table 6.1.

Kubler–Ross Stages of Grief

- The experience of grief is a staged process that occurs over time. Each stage of grief represents a psychologic defense mechanism used to help the individual adapt slowly to the crisis. The process of grief is dynamic and fluid rather than static and rigid.
- This process is individualized, asynchronous, and progressive at a pace manageable by the individual. Cultural and individual experiences will influence the trajectory.

TABLE 6.1 Categories of Grief

Category	Key Characteristics	Example
Anticipatory grief	Grieving prior to the loss	Parents of a preterm infant in the NICU; guarded bonding due to the potential of death or impaired neurodevelopmental outcomes
Chronic grief	Unresolved grief	Parent of an infant born at 23 weeks gestation with spastic cerebral palsy
Chronic sorrow	Cyclical, permanent grieving without resolution	A mother with multiple spontaneous abortions diagnosed with infertility

Sources: Data from Kenner, C., & Boykova, M. (2015). Families in crisis. In M. T. Verklan & M. Walden (Eds.), *Core curriculum for neonatal intensive care nursing* (5th ed., pp. 331–347). St. Louis, MO: Elsevier-Saunders.

Risk factors for pathologic grief include a history of psychiatric illness, childlessness, and poor social support.

- Knowledge of each stage is necessary to assess where an individual family member, the family as a unit, and the staff are in their grieving process (Friedman, 2015, p. 640; Gardner & Carter, 2016, p. 871).
- The stages of grief according to Kubler–Ross are summarized in Table 6.2.

Common Behaviors of Grief

- The signs and symptoms of acute grief have been well described and include both somatic and behavioral manifestations of the emotional experience of the loss. The behavior of the bereaved is characterized as ambivalent (Gardner & Carter, 2016, p. 872). These symptoms are summarized in Table 6.3.
- Men and women can have the same reactions to grief reactions but express them very differently. Women are more likely than men to express symptoms such as crying, sadness, anger, and guilt.
  - ○ This difference in symptomatology does not represent a different experience of grief, but merely a different expression of it (Gardner & Carter, 2016, p. 873).
- Maternal grief may begin with a period of shock, numbness, confusion, irritability, or anxiety, followed by intense sadness, longing, guilt, and somatic complaints (Friedman, 2015, p. 640).
- Paternal grief may be affected by the degree of investment in the pregnancy, impending parenthood, and the circumstances of birth; all affect his feelings of loss. Many men

TABLE 6.2 Kubler–Ross Stages of Grief

Stage	Key Characteristics
Denial	This stage may take a few hours to a few weeks. Characterized by feelings of disbelief after receiving bad news. The individual may compartmentalize the loss. May express anger intermittently.
Anger	Prolongation of this stage may inhibit continuation into the subsequent stages. Once the individual is aware of the significance of the loss, he or she can move onward. Social prohibition of expressing anger is prominent in some cultures and religions. This may lead to depression and a sense of guilt: "Why me?" "Is this my fault?" Anger may be expressed toward any member of the healthcare team.
	This stage may last a few months or even a few years. Can be observed concomitantly with the stage of denial. The individual may bargain with God or another spiritual/religious deity.
Depression	Significant variability in the duration of this stage. The initial acceptance of the loss may trigger depressive episodes. Social interactions with friends and family may cease or be limited.
Acceptance	Completes the grieving process.

Source: Reproduced with permission from Gardner, S., & Carter, B. (2016). Grief and perinatal loss. In S. Gardner, B. Carter, M. Hines, & J. Hernandez (Eds.), *Merenstein & Gardner's handbook of neonatal intensive care* (pp. 865–902.e5). St. Louis, MO: Elsevier.

TABLE 6.3 Common Behaviors of Grief

Somatic (physical symptoms)	GI disturbances: anorexia, diarrhea, nausea, vomiting
	Respiratory: coughing, hyperventilation, sighing
	Cardiovascular: heart palpitations, chest discomfort
	Neuromuscular: headache, syncope, vertigo, muscle weakness
Behavioral (psychologic symptoms)	Emotional changes: anger, guilt, loneliness, shame
	Dreaming, feeling of loss, nightmares
	Altered interpersonal relationships, decreased sexual drive
	Crying
	Inability to return to daily activities, fatigue
	Exhaustion, short attention span

GI: gastrointestinal.

Source: Data from Gardner, S., & Carter, B. (2016). Grief and perinatal loss. In S. Gardner, B. Carter, M. Hines, & J. Hernandez (Eds.), *Merenstein & Gardner's handbook of neonatal intensive care* (pp. 865–902.e5). St. Louis, MO: Elsevier.

have difficulty dealing with irrational behaviors, as well as with the normal ambiguity and conflict of life (Gardner & Carter, 2016, p. 873).

- Dealing with more than one grief or loss situation compounds the intensity of mourning and may prolong the grief reaction (Gardner & Carter, 2016, p. 875).

Factors Influencing the Grief Process

- Risk factors for pathologic grief include a history of psychiatric illness, childlessness, and poor social support (Friedman, 2015, p. 640). One parameter for differentiating normal from pathologic grief has been the length of time for grief to be resolved. Grief work may still be categorized as normal/uncomplicated even if it lasts longer than a year (Gardner & Carter, 2016, p. 875).
- Social prohibitions against the expression of anger, especially for women, encourage this powerful emotion to be turned inward toward the self (Gardner & Carter, 2016, p. 871). Those exhibiting maladaptive or destructive behaviors, dominant somatic symptoms, or lack of improvement over the course of months should be referred for evaluation (Friedman, 2015, p. 641).

MATERNAL POSTPARTUM MOOD DISORDERS

It is estimated that maternal mood disorders affect more than 500,000 pregnancies per year (Kelly, 2018, p. 115). Anxiety is one of the most common mental health disorders during pregnancy, followed by depression. Antepartum depression is a strong risk factor for postpartum disorders (Friedman, 2015, pp. 641–642). Depression may be affected by the cortisol levels and corticotropin-releasing hormone (CRH). Elevated levels of these hormones can lead to reduction in size of the hippocampus and other areas of the brain (Yonkers, 2018, p. 1232). Assessment and identification of a maternal mental health disorder will lead to early invention, thus inhibiting the progression of the disorder to a more severe manifestation such as postpartum psychosis (James, 2014, p. 571).

Postpartum Depression (PPD)

- The incidence of depression is variable, but can be seen up to 20% of women. Postpartum depression can be seen up to 70% in NICU mothers. Preexisting mental health conditions increase a mother's risk of developing postpartum depression. Other risk factors include familial history, lack of partner support, and low socioeconomic status.
- Symptoms of depression usually present within the first month after delivery. Symptoms include decrease in usual activities, appetite suppression, mood swings, sleep disturbance, and suicidal ideation.
- Postpartum depression is a complex, biologic, and psychologic phenomenon, which presents along a continuum. Severity of symptoms and the degree of impairment of the individual guide interventions.

Paternal Postpartum Depression

- The incidence of paternal postpartum depression is estimated at 4% to 12%. Maternal PPD is the strongest risk factor and predictor of paternal postpartum depression as the father transitions into fatherhood, while supporting his partner.
- Paternal depression usually presents after the onset of maternal depression. It may worsen 3 to 6 months after the birth of their child. Symptoms are like those of women, although subtle.
- If untreated, can impact compliance with medical care, bonding with infant and interpersonal relationships. Early treatment will minimize the potential to progress to a more severe psychiatric disorder (Gardner et al., 2016, p. 842).

Postpartum Psychosis

- Rare but serious mental health illness, occurring in 1 to 4 per 1,000 live births.
- Most often presents within the first 2 to 3 weeks postpartum, with severe clinical presentation that is an extension of those identified with depression.
  - Peak onset of symptoms is 10 to 14 days postdelivery. The following symptoms are not all-inclusive: sleep disturbances, delusions, hallucinations, and irrational behaviors. The mother is unable to discern reality from periods of delirium (Gardner et al., 2016, p. 843).
- Early identification of postpartum psychosis is extremely important to protect mother and family (Kelly, 2015, p. 117).

Assessment Tools for PPD

- Several assessment tools are available to identify women at risk for developing PPD. Current recommendation is to utilize these assessment tools at each trimester of pregnancy and intermittently in the postpartum period, because most symptoms present post discharge from the hospital.
- Various assessment tools exist; the following tools are used extensively:
  - Postpartum Depression Screening Scale (PDSS)
    - 35-item self-report Likert-type scale
    - Completed in postpartum
    - Measures depression symptomatology
    - Total score ranges 13 to 175
    - Positive screen is a score of 80 or greater
    - Most reliable tool for NICU mothers
  - Postpartum Depression Predictors Inventory–Revised (PDPI–revised)
    - Checklist that assesses 13 risk factors
    - Completed by clinician and mother
    - Completed in postpartum
    - No total score; provides detailed information on symptoms
  - Edinburgh Postnatal Depression Scale (EPDS)
    - 10-item questionnaire
    - Completed by mothers and fathers
    - Reliable and valid assessment tool for anxiety or depression disorders in fathers during antepartum period
    - Positive screen is a score of 12 or greater. Indicates likelihood of depression, not severity
    - If the woman or man has suicidal ideations, immediate intervention is necessary (Gardner et al., 2016, p. 844–851).

Intervention and Resources

- A comprehensive approach is needed, consisting of reassurance and support, nursing home visits, problem-solving education, psychoeducation, psychotherapy, and psychopharmacology.
- Paternal assistance is imperative to provide the father with guidance and reassurance to care for infant and partner. Parenting classes may be offered to enhance parenting competence, feeling confident, in control, and less frustrated.
- Monotherapy is rarely effective for major depression, but is for mild depression (Friedman, 2015, p. 639). Psychopharmacology is the most common treatment modality in conjunction with psychotherapy.
- Psychopharmacology may be necessary as the depression becomes more severe and debilitating. Classes of medication often prescribed are selective serotonin reuptake inhibitors (SSRIs), mood stabilizers, antidepressants, and antipsychotics. If the mother is breastfeeding, special considerations should be taken because all psychotropic medications enter the breast milk (Kelly, 2018, pp. 115–117).
- There is a risk for mothers to be noncompliant with prescribed medications due to concerns of fetal or neonatal exposure. Discontinuation of medication will increase the risk of relapse by more than 60% in comparison to those women who remain compliant.
- SSRIs are currently the most commonly prescribed medication to treat depression during pregnancy. Although data are inconsistent regarding fetal outcomes due to SSRI exposure, there is a suspected association with the following neonatal conditions: persistent pulmonary hypertension of the newborn (PPHN), prematurity, low birth weight, and poor neonatal adaptation syndrome (PNAS).
- Psychiatric day treatment or inpatient treatment may be necessary if it is deemed necessary based on the severity of symptoms and concern for mother to harm herself or infant (Gardner et al., 2015, p. 852).
- Support groups specific to PPD are available at the local and national level. Most often used are Depression after delivery (DAD) Inc., Postpartum Support International (PSI), and the Online PPD Support Group (Garnder, Voos, & Hills, 2015, pp. 851, 864.e7).
- Education on depression, symptoms, assessment, and interventions should be addressed with parents in the prenatal period to provide anticipatory guidance for the potential development and trajectory of postpartum depression (Gardner et al., 2016, p. 851).

PALLIATIVE CARE

- Current trends in healthcare advocate that palliative care be included with cure-oriented approaches for all patients who have a serious illness (Swaney, English, & Carter, 2016, p. 940). Curative and palliative care can be complementary and concurrent with established treatment goals of care guiding life-sustaining interventions while improving the patient's quality of life.
- The National Association of Neonatal Nurses (NANN) considers palliative and end-of-life care as integral aspects of care of the terminally ill infant. End-of-life care supports a peaceful, dignified death for the infant and the provision of support to the family and healthcare providers (NANN, 2015, p. 1).

- Treatment goals should be developed to maintain clear communication between the family, medical team, and nursing team. For parents to be involved in determining overall treatment goals and the decision-making process, they must be fully informed to consent to or refuse treatment for their child. The family's values will also affect decisions made for the infant (NANN, 2015, p. 1; Swaney et al., 2016, pp. 924, 931).
- The more complex the medical situation, the more crucial it is that parents receive consistent information, perhaps from a single designated person on the healthcare team (Swaney et al., 2016, p. 938).
- Palliative care should be considered in any of the following circumstances:
  - Life-limiting diagnosis, poor prognosis, or uncertainty of death after birth
  - Redirection of treatment goals and intense support for the family
  - Pain management during the transition period from curative to palliative care or at the end-of-life
  - Certainty of death despite life-sustaining interventions (Kenner & Boykova, 2015; Swaney et al., 2016, pp. 340, 341, 938)

Palliative Care in the NICU

- Pediatric palliative care (PPC) includes a team of pediatric providers who focus on the palliative care needs of infants and children in conjunction with cure-oriented approaches (Swaney et al., 2016, p. 940).
- Use of consistent information from all healthcare providers is important to minimize anxiety (Kenner & Boykova, 2015, p. 339). The overall goals with these conversations are to assess and develop the goals of care for their child (Fanaroff, 2015, p. 446).
- End-of-life discussions should be family-centered with an interdisciplinary team to promote clear communication, identify family goals, and assess cultural, spiritual, and religious concerns that will need to be honored.
- Create an environment that will facilitate a safe, quiet environment to have these discussions. Introduce everyone from the medical team present with their respective role. Discuss with the family their understanding of the presenting issue, then state the purpose of the meeting. Identify decision-makers if necessary. Explore options with the family. Provide moments of silence intermittently to allow the family to process the information discussed. Review relevant data, decisions (if determined by end of meeting), and options with the family and team. Offer another meeting to the family if needed (Fanaroff, 2015, pp. 31–33).

Models of Palliative Care

CONSULTATION MODEL

- Palliative care specialists are available to the NICU staff as well as all patients' families.
- Assessment of overall medical care of the patient
- Assessment of parental understanding of diagnosis and prognosis
- Assessment of parental goals and hopes for their child
- Facilitates communication between family and interdisciplinary team (Swaney et al., 2016, p. 940)

Integrative Model

- The following framework is suggested to enhance concurrent care in the NICU:
  - Admission to the NICU: Establish a care plan, review with the family, establish goals of care with the understanding that they may be modified based on the infant's medical needs.
  - Ongoing assessment and decision-making: Update family on current status, modify care plan when necessary, consult pediatric subspecialists when needed, offer a family meeting to discuss complex information, consider an ethics consult if warranted, ensure all members of the interdisciplinary team are present. During this phase of concurrent care, multiple family meetings may be necessary to allow the family time to process the change in status of their child and to make decisions regarding the medical care. Support the family during this transition. Offer services readily available to them, such as chaplain, psychosocial services, and child life services.
  - Transitional period: The family decides to either continue with curative care or withdraw life-sustaining interventions. Supportive measures remain in place with maintaining open communication with the family.
  - Bereavement: A designated team member will follow up with the family within one week of the infant's death to offer condolences. Intermittent communication within the first year after an infant's death is acceptable if the family accepts (Swaney et al., 2016, pp. 940–944).

Paradigms of Care/End-of-Life Care

- End-of-life care is an integral component of palliative care where families are supported in redirecting goals of care to ensure a holistic, dignified death for their child (NANN, 2015, p. 1).
- The transition from curative care to palliative care occurs once it had been determined that life-sustaining medical treatment is futile. Criteria for considering withholding or withdrawing life-sustaining medical treatment are:
  - Inevitability of death
  - Ineffective treatment
  - Poor quality of life (Cortezzo & Carter, 2018, p. 447; Fanaroff, 2015, p. 33)
- Unilateral decision-making is appropriate if the physician determines that medical treatment is futile with the above-mentioned criteria (Fanaroff, 2015, p. 33).
- Pregnancy milestones are very different from what was anticipated and hoped for as the focus of care shifts to pain management, grief support, preparing for the dying process, and bereavement support (Cortezzo & Carter, 2018, p. 446).

CONCLUSION

Pregnancy is most often associated with joyful emotions, expectations, wishes, and goals. At times, the pregnancy may be affected by a change in the maternal health, antenatal fetal diagnosis that may be life-limiting, or a change in the fetal well-being. Families may experience anticipatory grief while they process the information given, weigh options available, await the birth of their child, and potentially await the death of their child. Understanding the process of grief as an

individualized continuum influenced by culture, experiences, and values will enhance the support provided to families.

REVIEW QUESTIONS

1. During an intradisciplinary conference with a family in which difficult topics related to futility of care are presented, an opening to begin the conversation is to ask the family:
   A. if they want their infant to die or live with disabilities.
   B. their understanding of the infant's condition.
   C. the baby's name and if they want the child baptized.

2. Providing culturally sensitive care at the end of life includes the assessment of the family's:
   A. decision-making style
   B. preference for an autopsy
   C. religious traditions/beliefs

3. The overarching goal of family-centered care and interdisciplinary collaboration concurrent with an ongoing working relationship with the family is to establish:
   A. documentation of communication
   B. goals for care of the infant
   C. understanding of clinical terms

4. An essential component of the professional-parent relationship is:
   A. consistent, truthful communication
   B. establishing a relationship with the family
   C. providing a primary nursing team

5. One criteria for considering withholding of treatment or withdrawal of life-sustaining support is the:
   A. economics of patient care
   B. inevitability of death
   C. parents' cultural beliefs

REFERENCES

Ballard, A. R. (2015). Normal mother-infant attachment. In R. Martin, A. Fanaroff, & M. Walsh (Eds.), *Fanaroff & Martin's neonatal-perinatal medicine: Diseases of the fetus and infant* (10th ed., pp. 632–635). Philadelphia, PA: Elsevier.

Cortezzo, D. E., & Carter, B. S. (2018). Palliative care. In C. Gleason & S. Juul (Eds.), *Avery's disease of the newborn* (10th ed., pp. 446–452.e2). Philadelphia, PA: Elsevier.

Fanaroff, J. M. (2015). Medical ethics in medical care. In R. Martin, A. Fanaroff, & M. Walsh (Eds.), *Fanaroff & Martin's neonatal-perinatal medicine: Diseases of the fetus and infant* (10th ed., pp. 24–40). Philadelphia, PA: Elsevier Mosby.

Friedman, S. H. (2015). Parental mental health issues. In R. Martin, A. Fanaroff, & M. Walsh (Eds.), *Fanaroff & Martin's neonatal-perinatal medicine: Diseases of the fetus and infant* (10th ed., pp. 130–146). Philadelphia, PA: Elsevier Mosby.

Gardner, S. L., & Carter, B. S. (2016). Grief and perinatal loss. In S. Gardner, B. Carter, M. Hines, & J. Hernandez (Eds.), *Merenstein & Gardner's handbook of neonatal intensive care* (8th ed., pp. 865–902.e5). St. Louis, MO: Elsevier.

Gardner, S. L., Voos, K., & Hills, P. (2016). Families in crisis: Theoretical and practical considerations. In S. Gardner, B. Carter, M. Hines, & J. Hernandez (Eds.), *Merenstein & Gardner's handbook of neonatal intensive care* (8th ed., pp. 821–864.e7). St. Louis, MO: Elsevier.

James, D. C. (2014). Postpartum care. In K. Simpson & P. Creehan (Eds.), *Perinatal nursing* (4th ed., pp. 566–573). Philadelphia, PA: LWW.

Kelly, T. K. (2018). Maternal medical disorders of fetal significance. In C. Gleason & S. Juul (Eds.), *Avery's disease of the newborn* (10th ed., pp. 104–118e). Philadelphia, PA: Elsevier.

Kenner, C., & Boykova, M. (2015). Families in crisis. In M. T. Verklan & M. Walden (Eds.), *Core curriculum for neonatal intensive care nursing* (5th ed., pp. 331–347). St. Louis, MO: Elsevier-Saunders.

Klaus, M. H., Kennell, J. H., & Fanaroff, J. M. (2013). Care of the parents. In R. Martin, A. Fanaroff, & M. Walsh (Eds.), *Care of the high-risk neonate* (5th ed., pp. 201–224). Philadelphia, PA: Elsevier-Saunders.

National Association of Neonatal Nurses. (2015). *Palliative and end-of-life care for newborns and infants.* Position statement #3063 NANN Board of Directors. Retrieved from http://nann.org/uploads/About/PositionPDFS/1.4.5_Palliative%20and%20End%20of%20Life%20Care%20for%20Newborns%20and%20Infants.pdf

Swaney, J. R., English, N., & Carter, B. S. (2016). Ethics, values and palliative care in neonatal intensive care. In S. Gardner, B. Carter, M. Hines, & J. Hernandez (Eds.), *Merenstein & Gardner's handbook of neonatal intensive care* (8th ed., pp. 924–945.e3). Elsevier St. Louis, MO. Elsevier.

Yonkers, K. A. (2018). Management of depression and psychoses in pregnancy and in the puerperium. In R. Resnik, C. Lockwood, T. Moore, M. Greene, J. Copel, & R. Silver (Eds.), *Creasy & Resnik's maternal fetal medicine principles and practice* (8th ed., pp. 1232–1242.e3). Philadelphia, PA: Elsevier.

7 DISCHARGE PLANNING AND FOLLOW-UP

Amanda D. Bennett
Denise Kirsten

INTRODUCTION

Discharge planning should be an ongoing process between infant caregivers and the multidisciplinary team of the NICU that should facilitate a safe and seamless transition to home. The chapter reviews concepts and strategies needed for discharge planning and follow-up of the NICU patient. Standards for infants with unique and complex needs after discharge will be addressed.

THE DISCHARGE PROCESS

Basic Concepts

- Utilization of family-centered, multidisciplinary team approach to discharge planning throughout entire hospitalization will optimize transition to home and well-being of infant and caregiver.
- Families should be active participants of the care team, participating in medical rounds as well as regularly scheduled discharge planning rounds/care conferences throughout the entire hospitalization (Carter, Gratny, & Carter, 2016, p. 903; Hummel, 2014, pp. 373–374; Smith & Andrews, 2017, p. 214).

Discharge Planning

- There should be ongoing discussions between infant caregivers and NICU team, including the establishment of a clear criteria for discharge readiness.
  - Table 7.1 offers suggested criteria for discharge for both the infant and the caregiver.
- The discharge teaching plan should be tailored to meet each family's specific needs. Cultural and language needs must be assessed and incorporated in the plan.
- Families should be offered the opportunity to room in and care for their infant prior to discharge home in order to gain and demonstrate confidence and competence. Any home equipment should be delivered to the hospital prior to discharge to allow caregivers to use.

TABLE 7.1 Suggested Discharge Criteria for the Infant and Parent/Caregiver

Infant	Parent/Caregiver
Ability to maintain temperature in an open crib	Identification of at least two primary caregivers
Ability to feed without cardiopulmonary compromise	Emotional and psychosocial stability—caregivers demonstrate confidence with infant care at time of discharge • Identification of support system • Importance of self-care • Completed teaching on the dangers of shaking a baby
Demonstrates steady weight-gain pattern	Home environment acceptable to meet needs of infant after discharge from NICU
Demonstrates cardiopulmonary stability for a sufficient time frame prior to discharge	Resource availability in place (financial, utilities, transportation, etc.)
Completion of routine screening tests and immunizations for all infants • State newborn screening • Hearing screening • Congenital heart disease screening • Hepatitis B vaccination	Identification of follow-up primary care provider

(continued)

TABLE 7.1 Suggested Discharge Criteria for the Infant and Parent/Caregiver *(cont.)*

Infant	Parent/Caregiver
Completion of specialized screening tests and immunizations for infants with specialized needs • Head ultrasound • Car seat screening • Ophthalmologic examination • Palivizumab RSV prophylaxis • Routine immunizations are up to date per AAP guidelines • Scheduled appointments, or needed timing, for follow-up testing and immunizations	Caregivers have completed teaching and demonstrate competency in the following: • Provision of basic infant care • Maintain infant's thermal stability • Infant feeding (includes specialized feeding methods as well as specialized formula preparation) • Management of home feeding devices (feeding tubes, infusion pumps, stoma care, etc.) • Management of cardiopulmonary monitoring and equipment (apnea monitors, oxygen, ventilators, tracheostomy care, etc.) • Medication preparation and administration (includes knowledge of adverse effects) • Emergency plan (includes CPR training completed, emergency interventions reviewed, and contact numbers identified) • Provision of safe environment (supine positioning for sleep, car seat, smoke-free, heat, electricity, phone) • Knowledge of when to call primary care provider or seek emergency services

AAP, American Academy of Pediatrics; CPR, cardiopulmonary resuscitation; RSV, respiratory syncytial virus.

Sources: Data from Carter, A., Gratney, L., & Carter, B. S. (2016). Discharge planning and follow-up of the neonatal intensive care unit infant. In S. Gardner, B. Carter, M. Hines, & J. Hernandez (Eds.), *Merenstein & Gardner's handbook of neonatal intensive care* (8th ed., pp. 903–923). St. Louis, MO: Elsevier; Hummel, P. (2014). Discharge planning and transition to home care. In Verklan et al. (Eds.), *Core curriculum for neonatal intensive care nursing* (5th ed., pp. 373–390). St. Louis, MO: Elsevier; Smith, V. C., & Andrews, T. M. (2017). Neonatal intensive care unit discharge planning. In E. Eichenwald, A. Hansen, C. Martin, & A. Stark (Eds.), *Cloherty and Stark's manual of neonatal care* (8th ed., pp. 215–234). Philadelphia, PA: Wolters Klumer.

ANTICIPATORY GUIDANCE

- Discharge planning is a time for all neonatal health care providers to begin conversations of anticipatory guidance with the family. Anticipatory guidance describes the provision of information about what to expect from themselves and others. This term is often used involving conversations on grief after the death of an infant, but the concept may be applied to the dramatic situation of a family taking home an infant from the NICU. Knowledge of possible, likely, and unlikely encounters once at home can give the parents confidence and aid in the transition (Gardner & Carter, 2016, p. 895).
- Once transitioned to a primary care setting, anticipatory guidance should be a part of all office visits with the healthcare provider. Anticipatory guidance is crucial to the continued success of the family unit and may include topics such as:
  - Family support, family resources, maternal wellness
  - Infant behaviors, parent–child relationship, safe–sleep practices
  - Patterns of feedings, any new or recurring difficulties with oral feedings (breast or bottle), amount the infant should be feeding, and spitting versus vomiting
  - Safety issues such as car seats, smoking within the home
  - Routine infant care supplies, illness prevention, and introduction to early intervention (EI) services if appropriate (Reinhart & Gardner, 2017, pp. 345–347)

FOLLOW-UP CARE

- A comprehensive discharge summary should be completed and given to primary care providers, subspecialty providers, and the infant's caregivers. The summary should include resolved and ongoing problems, completed screening results and future screening needs (including scheduled vision and hearing follow-up), medications,

primary and specialty follow-up appointments (subspecialists, developmental follow-up, EI, etc.; Carter et al., 2016, p. 921).

Assumptions

- Each child is an individual with unique qualities, strengths, and challenges.
- Each family differs in background, social supports, finances, coping mechanisms, and expectations for their child's future.

The "High Risk" Infant

- Populations at risk for neurodevelopmental impairments include:
  - Infants with intrauterine exposure to chorioamnionitis, placental abruption, and use of tobacco or other substances regardless of gestational age
  - Preterm and late preterm infants, particularly if complicated by intrauterine growth restriction (IUGR) and/or congenital anomalies
  - Term infant who experienced persistent pulmonary hypertension requiring prolonged ventilation, nitric oxide, or extracorporeal membrane oxygenation (ECMO), or who had a history of hypoxic–ischemic injury (HII)
  - Infants of any gestational age who experienced or continue to experience:
    - Intracranial hemorrhages, seizures, periventricular leukomalacia
    - Bronchopulmonary dysplasia/chronic lung disease (BPD/CLD)
    - Feeding, growth, and/or gastrointestinal dysfunction related to necrotizing enterocolitis (NEC) or other intestinal pathology

○ Infants with complex medical conditions including dependence on technology
○ Infants with anticipated early deaths

Goals for Primary Care

- Continuum of care after discharge from the NICU
- Family education about child's development so they are empowered to optimize their child's health, growth, and development
- Prompt diagnosis and recognition of significant medical and neurodevelopmental conditions, prompting appropriate referral for community services to reduce future medical, social, and economic costs
- Anticipation of future needs to avoid or minimize secondary complications so that optimal development is promoted
  ○ Promotion of the child's integration into the family, school, and community
- Table 7.2 lists timings and expectations for post-NICU follow-up.

FOLLOW-UP SCREENINGS

Hearing

- Hearing loss is one of the most common congenital abnormalities, occurring in approximately 1.5 to 2 per 1,000 newborns (Vohr, 2018, p. 1558).
- Preterm infants are at risk for both conductive (problems with transmission of sound to cochlea) and sensorineural (damage to inner ear and auditory nerve) hearing loss, as well as auditory processing deficits.
- NICU graduates have an increased risk of developing hearing loss. When undetected, hearing loss can delay language, communication, and cognitive development. This may affect academic achievement, literacy, and social and emotional development (Carter et al., 2016, p. 907; Vohr, 2015, p. 993; Vohr, 2018, p. 1558).
  ○ Box 7.1 lists conditions associated with increased risk for hearing loss.

TABLE 7.2 Timing and Expectations for Post-NICU Follow-up Visits

Timing and Focus of Visit by Age			
Age	**Focus and/or Findings**	**Developmental Skills**	**Services**
1–3 months	• Adaptation to home • Accuracy of home medications • Oxygen administration • Formula preparation • Parental concerns	Adjusting to environment	1. Primary care coordinated services 2. Early intervention & therapies 3. NICU follow-up
4–6 months	• Inadequate catch-up growth • Identification of severe neurologic abnormality requiring intervention, occupational and/or physical therapy	• Coordination • Hearing • Vision	
8–12 months	Identification of suspected or confirmed cerebral palsy or other neurologic abnormality	• Movements • Language • Interaction	
18–24 months	• Most transient neurologic findings are resolved. • The neurologically abnormal child will show adaptation and improved functional abilities. • Potential catch-up growth should have occurred. • Administration of *Bayley Scales of Infant Development (BSID-III)* to provide assessment of cognitive functioning	• Speech • Increased physical ability	
3 years	• Administration of tests to measure cognitive function • Language may be measured.	• Language • Thinking	1. Primary care coordinated services 2. School-related services 3. Special therapy programs
4–5 years	• Measure of subtle neurologic, visuomotor, and behavioral difficulties, which may affect school performance	• Learning • Physical activity	

Sources: Data from Carter, A., Gratney, L., & Carter, B. S. (2016). Discharge planning and follow-up of the neonatal intensive care unit infant. In S. Gardner, B. Carter, M. Hines, & J. Hernandez (Eds.), *Merenstein & Gardner's handbook of neonatal intensive care* (8th ed., pp. 903–923). St. Louis, MO: Elsevier; Demauro, S. B., & Hintz, S. R. (2018). Risk assessment and neurodevelopmental outcomes. In C. Gleason & S. Juul (Eds.), *Avery's diseases of the newborn* (10th ed., pp. 971–990.e7). Philadephia, PA: Elsevier; Hack, M. (2013). The outcome of neonatal intensive care. In A. Fanaroff & J. Fanaroff (Eds.), *Klaus and Fanaroff's care of the high-risk neonate* (6th ed., pp. 525–534). Cleveland, OH: Elsevier; Wilson-Costello, D. E., & Payne, A. H. (2015). Early childhood neurodevelopmental outcomes of high-risk neonates. In R. Martin, A. Fanaroff, & M. Walsh (Eds.), *Fanaroff and Martin's neonatal-perinatal medicine: Diseases of the fetus and infant* (10th ed., pp. 1018–1031). Philadelphia, PA: Elsevier.

BOX 7.1 Conditions associated with increased risk for hearing loss

Conditions Associated With Increased Risk for Hearing Loss

1. NICU admission for > 5 days or any of the following regardless of length of stay:
   - Extracorporeal membrane oxygenation (ECMO)
   - Assisted ventilation
   - Exposure to ototoxic medications
   - Exposure to loop diuretics
   - Hyperbilirubinemia requiring exchange transfusion
2. Caregiver concern* regarding hearing, speech, language, or developmental delay**
3. Family history of permanent childhood hearing loss
4. *In utero* infections such as cytomegalovirus (CMV), herpes, rubella, syphilis, and toxoplasmosis
5. Craniofacial anomalies, including those that involve the pinna, ear canal, ear tags, ear pits, and temporal bone anomalies
6. Physical findings, such as a white forelock, that are associated with a syndrome known to include a sensorineural or permanent conductive hearing loss
7. Syndromes associated with progressive or late-onset hearing loss: neurofibromatosis, osteopetrosis, Usher syndrome, Waardenburg syndrome, Alport syndrome, Pendred syndrome, Jervell, and Lange–Neilsen syndrome
8. Neurodegenerative disorders:
   - Hunter syndrome
   - Sensory motor neuropathies (i.e., Friedreich ataxia and Charcot–Marie–Tooth syndrome)
9. Culture-positive postnatal infections associated with sensorineural hearing loss:
   - Bacterial
   - Viral (especially herpes and varicella) meningitis
10. Head trauma, especially basal skull/temporal bone fractures that require hospitalization

Sources: Data from Carter, A., Gratney, L., & Carter, B. S. (2016). Discharge planning and follow-up of the neonatal intensive care unit infant. In S. Gardner, B. Carter, M. Hines, & J. Hernandez (Eds.), *Merenstein & Gardner's handbook of neonatal intensive care* (8th ed., pp. 903–923). St. Louis, MO: Elsevier; Stewart, J. E., Bentley, J., & Knorr, A. (2017). Hearing loss in neonatal intensive care unit graduates. In E. Eichenwald, E., A. Hansen, A., C. Martin, C., & A. Stark, A. (Eds.), *Cloherty and Stark's manual of neonatal care* (8th ed., pp. 983–1068). Philadelphia, PA: Wolters Klumer; Vohr, B. (2015). Hearing loss in the newborn infant. In R. Martin, A. Fanaroff, & M. Walsh (Eds.), *Fanaroff and Martin's neonatal-perinatal medicine: Diseases of the fetus and infant* (10th ed., pp. 993–1000). Philadelphia, PA: Elsevier.

Types of Hearing Loss

- *Sensorineural hearing loss* occurs secondary to abnormal development or damage to the outer hair cells and cochlear hair cells or cranial nerve VIII that impairs neuroconduction of sound energy to the brainstem.
- *Conductive hearing loss* occurs when there is interference in the transmission of sound from the external auditory canal to the inner ear.
  - *Permanent conductive hearing loss* occurs when there is anatomic obstruction of the outer ear (atresia) or middle ear (fusion of ossicles) that blocks transmission of sound (Vohr, 2015, p. 994; Vohr, 2018, p. 1559).
  - *Transient conductive hearing loss* occurs when debris in the ear canal or fluid in the middle ear block the passage of sound waves to the inner ear.
- *Auditory dyssynchrony or auditory neuropathy* accounts for 10% of all infants diagnosed with severe permanent hearing loss. The function of the outer hair cells remains intact; however, a pathology of the inner hair cells or the myelinated fibers of cranial nerve VIII impairs neuroconduction of sound energy to the brainstem. The electric signals to the brain have responses that are dyssynchronous, so information is not relayed in a consistent manner.
  - Risk factors for dyssynchrony include extreme prematurity, severe hyperbilirubemia, hypoxia, and immune disorders. There is a genetic basis in approximately 40% of all cases.
- *Central hearing loss* occurs because of abnormal auditory processing at higher levels of the central nervous system, despite an intact auditory canal and inner ear and normal neurosensory pathways.
- *Mixed hearing loss* occurs when there is a combination of sensorineural or neural hearing loss with transient or permanent conductive hearing loss.

Screening

- The primary objective of universal newborn hearing screening during the hospital birth admission is to detect permanent hearing loss as early as possible in order to maximize language, cognitive, literacy, and social development (Carter et al., 2016, p. 907; Stewart et al., 2017, p. 996; Vohr, 2018, p. 1559).
- The two currently acceptable methods for physiologic hearing screening in newborns are the auditory brainstem response (ABR) and the evoked otoacoustic emissions (EOAEs; Stewart et al., 2017, p. 996; Vohr, 2018, p. 1560).
  - The ABR evaluates hearing via surface electrodes placed on the scalp which record neural activity in the cochlea, outer and inner hair cells, auditory nerve (VIII), and brainstem to a series of click sounds. It is reliable after 34 weeks postnatal age (Stewart et al., 2017, p. 996).
  - EOAE evaluates hearing through inserting a probe, which contains a microphone into the ear canal. It records the sound produced by outer hair cells of a normal cochlea. This method is more likely to be affected by debris or fluid in the external and middle ear, resulting in higher referral rates (Stewart et al., 2017, p. 996; Vohr, 2015, p. 994).
- Table 7.3 lists a comparison of physiologic screening methods for newborn hearing loss.

Failed Hearing Screens

- Neonatal intensive care infants have higher false-positive rates and higher failure rates than well-baby nursery infants (Vohr, 2015, pp. 993–1000).
- Infants who fail their initial screening should be rescreened before 1 month of age. If the infant is "referred" (failed the screening) after this secondary screening, the infant should have a full-scale auditory diagnostic evaluation by 3 months of age (Carter et al., 2016, p. 907; Vohr, 2015, p. 995).
  - This guideline is consistent with the Joint Committee on Infant Hearing *1-3-6 recommendation* that all infants

TABLE 7.3 Comparison of Physiologic Screening Methods for Newborn Hearing Loss

	Evoked Otoacoustic Emissions (EOAEs)	Auditory Brainstem Response (ABR)
Method of measurement	Microphone in a probe inserted into ear canal	Surface electrodes
What the test measures in response to stimulus	Records the sound produced by outer hair cells of a normal cochlea. Stimulus = sound	Record neural activity in the cochlea, outer and inner hair cells, auditory nerve (VIII), and brainstem Stimulus = click
Detects sensorineural hearing loss	Yes	Yes
Detects auditory neuropathy	No	Yes
Detects transient and permanent conductive hearing loss	Yes	Yes
Threshold for fail	30–35 dB HL	40–45 dB HL
Recommended for NICU screening	No	Yes
Recommended for well-baby screening	Yes	Yes

Sources: Data from Stewart, J. E., Bentley, J., & Knorr, A. (2017). Hearing loss in neonatal intensive care unit graduates. In E. Eichenwald, A. Hansen, C. Martin, & A. Stark (Eds.), *Cloherty and Stark's manual of neonatal care* (8th ed., pp. 983–1068). Philadelphia, PA: Wolters Klumer; Vohr, B. (2015). Hearing loss in the newborn infant. In R. Martin, A. Fanaroff, & M. Walsh (Eds.), *Fanaroff and Martin's neonatal-perinatal medicine: Diseases of the fetus and infant* (10th ed., pp. 993–1000). Philadelphia, PA: Elsevier; Vohr, B. (2018). Ear and hearing disorders. In C. Gleason & S. Juul (Eds.), *Avery's diseases of the newborn* (10th ed., pp. 1558–1566.e2). Philadelphia, PA: Elsevier.

should be screened for hearing loss no later than 1 month of age, and infants who do not pass the screen should have a comprehensive evaluation by an audiologist no later than 3 months of age for confirmation of hearing status.
- ○ Infants with confirmed hearing loss should receive appropriate intervention no later than 6 months of age from professionals with expertise in hearing loss and deafness in infants and young children (Vohr, 2018, p. 1560).
- A portion of infants who fail their initial screen are lost to follow-up. Family issues associated with poor follow-up include age of mother, insurance status, poverty level, lack of family education regarding screening, and geographical variation (Stewart et al., 2017, p. 996).

Indications for Ongoing Screening

- If a family history of hearing loss is reported for an infant who passes the initial hearing screen, ongoing surveillance is indicated with at least one follow-up audiologic assessment by 24 to 30 months of age (Vohr, 2015, p. 996).
- Any caregiver concern regarding hearing, speech, language, or developmental delay in the first 2 to 3 years of age should prompt a referral for further hearing evaluation because of the association with an increased risk for late-onset or progressive hearing loss not detected in a newborn screen (Vohr, 2015, p. 996).
- All infants should have an objective standardized screen of global development with a validated screening tool at 9, 18, and 24 to 30 months of age or at any time if the health care professional or family has concerns. Infants who do not pass the speech–language portion of a global screening or for whom there is a concern regarding hearing or

language should be referred for speech–language evaluation and audiology assessment (Vohr, 2015, p. 998).

Interventions

- All families of infants with hearing loss will benefit from a genetics consultation and counseling, as 50% of congenital hearing loss is hereditary (Vohr, 2015, p. 997).
- ○ Thirty percent of genetic hearing loss is syndromic and 70% is nonsyndromic (50% cases linked to a single gene *GJB2*). Patterns may be autosomal recessive, autosomal dominant, or X-linked.
- Every infant with confirmed hearing loss should be evaluated by an otolaryngologist with knowledge of pediatric hearing loss (Vohr, 2015, p. 997).

Audiology Devices

- Hearing aids are compact and worn either in the ear or behind the ear and can be fitted on an infant in the first month of age. They need to be replaced for growth every 6 to 8 months (Vohr, 2015, p. 997).
- Candidacy criteria for pediatric cochlear implantation currently are 18 months or older for children with severe to profound bilateral sensorineural hearing loss and 12 to 18 months for children with profound hearing loss. There are increasing reports demonstrating the beneficial effects on speech and language for infants with bilateral profound hearing loss implanted before 12 months of age.
- ○ There is a risk for bacterial meningitis with cochlear implants, with *streptococcus pneumonia* being the most common pathogen; therefore, it is essential that the patient be up-to-date on vaccinations per American Academy of Pediatrics (AAP) high-risk schedule (Vohr, 2015, p. 998).

Family Support

- There are varying degrees of stress when parents are informed that their infant has failed an initial hearing screen, with a continuum of increasing stress for families whose infants progress through the screening, diagnosis, and intervention phases of permanent hearing loss (Vohr, 2015, p. 998).
- Prompt sharing of diagnostic test results with the family and referral to EI services may facilitate the provision of needed information and support to parents to mediate stress (Vohr, 2015, p. 998).
- Half of the children identified with congenital hearing loss have been in an NICU and about 40% of children with permanent hearing loss have other disabilities, causing the potential for both financial as well as emotional stressors. It becomes important for EI case managers, and other members of the infant's care team to coordinate various support resources for the family (Vohr, 2015, pp. 998–999).

VISION

- The AAP recommends a red reflex examination prior to discharge from the hospital and all subsequent routine health supervision visits (De Alba Campomanes & Binenbaum, 2018, p. 1540).
  - Discussion regarding the implications for a present, absent, or abnormal red reflex is further discussed in Chapter 25.

Retinopathy of Prematurity (ROP)

- ROP is diagnosed by retinal examination with indirect ophthalmoscopy and should be performed by an ophthalmologist with expertise in ROP screening.
  - While direct examination is standard of care, ROP telemedicine, or retinal digital imaging, is a reasonable alternative (De Alba Campomanes & Binenbaum, 2018, p. 1553).

Screening With the First Indirect Ophthalmoscopy Exam

- All infants with a birth weight < 1,500 g or gestational age < 30 weeks should be screened for ROP.
- Infants who are born after 30 weeks gestational age or born at 1,500 to 2,000 g may be considered for screening if they have had a medically unstable course (e.g., severe respiratory distress syndrome, hypotension requiring pressor support, or surgery in the first several weeks of life).
- The first examination should occur at 31 weeks postmenstrual age (PMA) or chronologic age of 4 weeks, whichever occurs later. However, it is recommended to have the first examination before discharge from the hospital.
  - Some recommend infants who are born at < 26 weeks gestation are examined at the postnatal age of 6 to 8 weeks, those born at 27 to 28 weeks at the postnatal age of 5 weeks, those born at 29 to 30 weeks at the postnatal age of 4 weeks, and those > 30 weeks at the postnatal age of 3 weeks (Campomanes & Binenbaum, 2018, p. 1553; Carter et al., 2016, p. 907; De Alba Campomanes

& Binenbaum, 2018; Hummel, 2014, p. 376; Leeman & VanderVeen, 2017, p. 987; Martin & Crowley, 2013, p. 247; Sun, Hellstrom, & Smith, 2015, p. 1772).
- Long-term follow-up determined by the degree of ROP. Infants needing laser or cryotherapy for ROP require ongoing assessment of retina, as well as evaluations for refractive errors, strabismus, and amblyopia (Leeman & VanderVeen, 2017, p. 991; Sun et al., 2015, pp. 1772–1773).
- It is the NICU medical team's clinical and medicolegal responsibility to schedule needed ROP examinations prior to discharge from the NICU, as well as stressing to caregivers the absolute necessity of keeping these appointments postdischarge (Carter et al., 2016, p. 907; De Alba Campomanes & Binenbaum, 2018, p. 1557).

Prior to Discharge

- The following conditions place children at high risk of eye disease and should be referred for examination by a pediatric ophthalmologist for follow-up postdischarge:
  - History of prematurity, as this leads to an increased risk for ROP, amblyopia, strabismus, myopia, and astigmatism. There is also increased risk for alterations in vision function: acuity, color vision, contrast sensitivity, visual processing, visual attention, pattern discrimination, visual recognition memory, and visual–motor integration.
  - History of metabolic or genetic diseases
  - Significant developmental delay or neurologic problems, including periventricular leukomalacia (PVL) and other cerebral lesions, which can result in strabismus, nystagmus, visual field deficits, and perceptual difficulties and may not be recognized until school age or later.
  - Systemic diseases associated with eye abnormalities
  - A family history of retinoblastoma, childhood cataracts or glaucoma, inherited retinal disorders, or blindness in childhood
  - Those whose parents needed glasses at a very young age

Postdischarge

- The neonatal healthcare teams should provide ongoing eye-related education and support, especially toward reducing the risk of pediatric acute head trauma (shaken baby syndrome). This should be discussed with all parents and caregivers (De Alba Campomanes & Binenbaum, 2018, p. 1557; Hummel, 2014, pp. 383–384).
  - Viewing of educational videos on shaken baby syndrome (if available)
  - Discussion about crying and parental stress during the first few months of age
- The neonatal healthcare team may also provide support for the families of children with visual impairment, ensuring early, anticipatory referral to state commissions for the blind, EI services, and ongoing encouragement for parents to maximally utilize such resources when they are available (De Alba Campomanes & Binenbaum, 2018, p. 1557).
- Children should have an eye examination at every well-child visit. Primary care eye examinations and vision assessments continue to be vital for the detection of

conditions that may result in visual impairment or blindness, lead to problems with school or social performance, signal the presence of a serious systemic disease, or threaten the child's life (De Alba Campomanes & Binenbaum, 2018, p. 1557; Örge & Grigorian, 2015, p. 1734).

- Infants with the following findings should be referred for examination by a pediatric ophthalmologist:
  - ○ The absence of visual responsiveness by a corrected gestational age (CGA) of 2 months
  - ○ Absent, poor, or paradoxical pupillary response, nystagmus or roving eye movements after 2 to 3 months of age
  - ○ Any misalignment after 3 to 4 months of age
  - ○ Poor fixation and following after 3 months of age
  - ○ Any child with corneal opacification
  - ○ Persistence of nasolacrimal duct obstruction at 12 months of age
  - ○ Strabismus and nystagmus developing in the first 3 to 6 months of age
  - ○ Intraretinal, preretinal, or subretinal hemorrhage past 1 month of age
    - ▪ The presence of any retinal hemorrhage in an infant is highly associated with abuse

NEUROSENSORY AND DEVELOPMENTAL ASSESSMENT

Correction for Gestational Age

- Noting the age when an infant achieves milestones such as gross-motor, fine-motor, language, and adaptive skills help determine if delays are present. However, controversy exists regarding the need to correct for degrees of prematurity, that is, whether to use the child's chronological age or to use the corrected age for degree of prematurity (Carter et al., 2016, p. 911; Demauro & Hintz, 2018, p. 988).
- The best evidence supports the use of correction for prematurity. By convention, most healthcare providers correct through 2 years of age (Carter et al., 2016, p. 911; Stewart, Hernandez, & Duncan, 2017, p. 194), although reports exist describing the use of correction until 3 years of age (Hack, 2013, p. 528).
- For the extremely low gestational age newborn (ELGAN) infant, those born at 23 to 25 weeks, some literature suggests continued correction through 5 years of age (Hack, 2013, p. 528). Although no overall consensus exists, whatever standard is set should be followed consistently by all team members involved in the infant's care (Demauro & Hintz, 2018, p. 988).

Neurodevelopmental Assessment

- *Neurodevelopmental handicap* has been defined in children who have a neurologic abnormality or a developmental quotient or IQ of less than 80 (Carter et al., 2016, p. 914; Hack, 2013, p. 530). More currently, the World Health Organization (WHO) categorizes handicap/disability with emphasis placed on the interaction of functioning and disability, health condition of the individual, and environmental factors (Carter et al., 2016, p. 912).
- *Neurologic abnormality* is usually classified by neurologic diagnosis, which can include hypotonia or hypertonia, cerebral palsy (spastic diplegia or quadriplegia),

hydrocephalus, blindness, or deafness. (Demauro & Hintz, 2018, p. 984; Hack, 2013, p. 530).

- *Developmental delay* is a more recent term used to describe a deficit in any one of the five development domains: cognition, motor, language, adaptive, and social–emotional skills. (Carter et al., 2016, p. 913).
- *Global developmental delay* is used to define deficits in two or more areas of development with scores more than two deviations below the referenced standards (Carter et al., 2016, p. 913).
- Neurologic examination during infancy is best based on changes in muscle tone that occur within the first year (Hack, 2013, p. 530). A detailed, structured neurologic examination as early as full-term corrected age in high-risk infants is highly correlated with neuromotor outcomes at least until 1 year of age (Demauro & Hintz, 2018, p. 988).
- The scale developed by Claudine Amiel-Tison provides a qualitative method to assess neurologic integrity, which leads to the categorization of *normal, suspect,* or *abnormal* during the first year after term.
  - ○ Measures the decrease in passive muscle tone (head control, back support, sitting, standing, and walking) contrasted with the progressive increase in active muscle tone that occur together during infancy. It also documents visual and auditory responses and some primitive reflexes (Hack, 2013, p. 530; Wilson-Costello & Payne, 2015, p. 1024).

DEVELOPMENTAL ASSESSMENT

- The Bayley Scales of Infant Development is the most commonly used tool for monitoring early cognitive and motor development for high-risk infants.
  - ○ The 2006 (newest) version contains five scales: cognitive, language, motor, social–emotional, and adaptive behavior, the latter two in the form of parent questionnaires. This edition of the Bayley Scales does not generate a "mental developmental index," but rather separate cognitive and language scores (Wilson-Costello & Payne, 2015, p. 1024).
- Multiple tools are available to use for developmental assessment of both the infant and child. Examples are listed in Table 7.4.

Early Intervention (EI)

- Some infants may have risks to their development that are evident at discharge. Early identification of infants at high risk of poor outcomes, for example, an infant with a significant history of intraventricular hemorrhages, allows for timely referrals to EI therapies.
  - ○ EI has been shown to improve neurobehavioral development with improved cognitive outcomes and parent–child interactions (Carter et al., 2016, p. 913; Wilson-Costello & Payne, 2015, p. 1028).
- Referral can be made by the neonatal medical team, the primary care provider, follow-up clinic specialists, or the family itself.
- Each child receives a multidisciplinary assessment and service coordinator. Based on the child's assessment, various services with various focus intensities may include occupational therapy, physical therapy, speech therapy, audiology services, vision services, family education with

TABLE 7.4 Psychomotor and Cognitive Assessment Tools

Test	Age Range	Components	IQ	Most Popular

The Bayley Scales of Infant Development (BSID-III) 2006	1–42 months (first administer at 8–12 months)	1. Cognitive composite score
		2. Language composite score
		  a. Receptive
		  b. Expressive
		3. Motor composite score
		  a. Gross
		  b. Fine
		4. Social–emotional score (per parent report)
		5. Adaptive behavior score (per parent report)
			No	X

Griffiths-III 2016	2 versions: 0–2 years and 2–8 years		No	
Ages and Stages Questionnaire	3 months–5 years	Qualitative only—parents provide information about child development	No	
Wechsler Preschool and Primary Scale of Intelligence (WPPSI-IV) 2012	2 years 6 months–7 years 7 months	Verbal, performance, and full-scale scores with means of 100	Yes	X
Wechsler Intelligence Scale for Children (WISC-V) 2014	6 years 0 months–16 years 11 months	Verbal, performance, and full-scale scores with means of 100	Yes	
Wechsler Individual Achievement Test (WIAT-III) 2009	4 years 0 months–50 years 11 months	Identifies academic strengths and weaknesses Used in clinical, research, and educational settings	Yes	
Differential Ability Scales (DAS-III) 2007	2 years 6 months–17 years 11 months		Yes	
Stanford-Binet Intelligence Scale 2003	2 years–elementary school years	Measure of intelligence highly correlated with school performance	Yes	
Kaufman Assessment Battery for Children (K-ABC II) 2004	3 years–10 years	Subscales to assess various components of intelligence	Yes	

Sources: Data from Carter, A., Gratney, L., & Carter, B. S. (2016). Discharge planning and follow-up of the neonatal intensive care unit infant. In S. Gardner, B. Carter, M. Hines, & J. Hernandez (Eds.), *Merenstein & Gardner's handbook of neonatal intensive care* (8th ed., pp. 903–923). St. Louis, MO: Elsevier; Demauro, S. B., & Hintz, S. R. (2018). Risk assessment and neurodevelopmental outcomes. In C. Gleason & S. Juul (Eds.), *Avery's diseases of the newborn* (10th ed., pp. 971–990.e7). Philadelphia, PA: Elsevier; Hack, M. (2013). The outcome of neonatal intensive care. In A. Fanaroff & J. Fanaroff (Eds.), *Klaus and Fanaroff's care of the high-risk neonate* (6th ed., pp. 525–534). Cleveland, OH: Elsevier; Wilson-Costello, D. E., & Payne, A. H. (2015). Early childhood neurodevelopmental outcomes of high-risk neonates. In R. Martin, A. Fanaroff, & M. Walsh (Eds.), *Fanaroff and Martin's neonatal-perinatal medicine: Diseases of the fetus and infant* (10th ed., pp. 1018–1031). Philadelphia, PA: Elsevier.

focus on infant growth and development, family counseling, social work services, and transportation for therapies outside the home.

○ *Individuals With Disabilities Education Act*: A federal mandate that each state provides services up to 3 years of age for those children with developmental delays or conditions that lead to developmental delay. Each state establishes criteria for referral to EI and services provided within the parameters set by the government.

SPECIALIZED FOLLOW-UP

Immunizations

- The AAP recommends that all preterm infants receive routine immunizations at their chronologic age, rather than their corrected age.
- Influenza immunization is recommended yearly for child and caregivers.

- Respiratory syncytial virus (RSV) prophylaxis Palivizumab (Synagis®) is recommended for all high-risk infants and young children by the AAP.

Growth and Nutrition

- Many extremely low birth weight (ELBW), very low birth weight (VLBW), and IUGR infants experience delayed growth and require catch-up after discharge.
  - *Postnatal growth failure* or *extrauterine growth restriction* is a weight less than the 10th percentile for CGA.
- Optimal growth after discharge is a good measure of physical, neurological, and environmental well-being.
- Catch-up of head circumference occurs only during the first 6 to 12 months after the expected date of delivery.
- Specialized feedings for the first 6 to 9 months postdischarge are needed in infants with ongoing and catch-up requirements not met by term infant formulas
  - Increased calorie postdischarge formulas with increased protein, minerals, and long-chain polyunsaturated fatty acids
  - Continued fortification of breast milk or exclusive breast milk feedings with two to three bottles per day of increased calorie postdischarge formulas
- Vitamin and iron supplementation
  - Vitamin D: 400 IU per day is minimal requirement, which may be achieved by a combination of formula and/or supplement (Abrams & Tiosano, 2015, p. 1477; Poindexter & Ehrenkranz, 2015, p. 607).
  - Iron: 2 to 4 mg/kg day, which may be achieved by a combination of formula and/or supplement to start at 1 month of age and continue to 12 months.

OUTCOMES

School-Age Outcomes

- Infants who have severe cognitive, motor, or neurosensory impairments in early years (2–3 years of age) are nearly always found to have moderate or severe impairments at school age (Demauro & Hintz, 2018, p. 980).
- Few studies have compared school-age outcomes among premature infants over time. Most of the school-age outcome studies of very premature children have compared these survivors with children of normal birth weight. Findings demonstrate former preterm infants have neurologic dysfunction, lower intelligence, and poorer performance on tests of language and academic achievement (Wilson-Costello & Payne, 2015, pp. 1025–1026).
  - These lower scores may be related to difficulties with memory, visuomotor, and fine and gross motor function, and spatial concepts and executive function (Hack, 2013, p. 533).
  - Deficits include mild cognitive impairment (IQ 1–2 SD below the mean or 70–84); learning, emotional, behavior, motor coordination, and executive function disorders; and poor academic achievement. The most immature infants have the highest risk for poor cognitive outcome (Demauro & Hintz, 2018, pp. 979–980).
  - Although most children with VLBW remain in the regular school system, many have difficulty coping with the demands of classroom learning and require individualized education and remedial resources (Hack, 2013, p. 533; Wilson-Costello & Payne, 2015, pp. 1025–1026).
- Children with social advantages (two-parent household, educated parents, employed parents) demonstrate more cognitive gains through early childhood than those without social advantages (Demauro & Hintz, 2018, p. 980).

Behavioral Problems

- The most commonly reported childhood behavioral problems of prematurity are disorders of attention and hyperactivity, emotional difficulties, and socialization issues. Rates of attention deficit hyperactivity disorder (ADHD) range from 20% to 30% for preterm children versus 5% to 10% for term-born children (Wilson-Costello & Payne, 2015, p. 1025). Neurobehavioral or psychiatric problems, including autism spectrum disorders (ASDs), are reported with higher frequency in school-aged former preterm children than in the general population (Demauro & Hintz, 2018, p. 980).
- Internalizing problems, such as depression, anxiety, and poor adaptive skills, have all been associated with prematurity, resulting in socialization and peer relationship difficulties. Internalizing symptoms manifest as shyness, social maladaptation, anxiety, and withdrawn behavior (Demauro & Hintz, 2018, p. 980; Hack, 2013, p. 533; Wilson-Costello & Payne, 2015, pp. 1025–1026).
  - Furthermore, motor delays due to prematurity may compromise playground skills, causing peer victimization and rejection (Wilson-Costello & Payne, 2015, pp. 1025–1026).
- Table 7.5 identifies school-age outcomes related to prematurity.

Young Adult Outcomes

- Overall, results suggest that neurodevelopmental and growth sequelae of prematurity persist into young adulthood. Traditionally, educational attainment, employment, independent living, marriage, and parenthood have been considered as markers of successful transition to adulthood.
  - When compared with controls of normal birth weight, young adults with VLBW have poorer educational achievement. Preterm infants as adults have significantly lower income, and are less likely to get married and become parents (Demauro & Hintz, 2018 p. 981; Wilson-Costello & Payne, 2015, pp. 1025–1026).
- Even in adults without neurosensory or cognitive impairment, impairments in learning or executive function may interfere with educational and vocational achievement. Executive function refers to a collection of processes that are responsible for purposeful, goal-directed behavior, such as planning, setting goals, initiating, using problem-solving strategies, and monitoring thoughts and behavior. Executive function deficits primarily involve impairments in response inhibition and mental flexibility (Demauro & Hintz, 2018, p. 981; Hack, 2013, p. 533).
- Adolescents and young adults who were born preterm are found to show deficits in executive function on tasks of verbal fluency, inhibition, cognitive flexibility, planning and organization, and working memory, as well as

TABLE 7.5 School-Age Outcomes of Prematurity

Neurodevelopmental Impairment				
Cognitive	**Motor**	**Sensory**	**Behavioral**	**Other**
• Cognitive delay ○ Most common NDI in children born prematurely • Global developmental delay • Learning disabilities ○ Variable cognitive abilities	• CP • DCD ○ Fine-motor incoordination ○ Sensorimotor integration problems	• Hearing impairment • Visual impairment	• ADHD • ASD • Internalizing symptoms ○ Shyness ○ Depression ○ Anxiety ○ Poor adaptive skills	• Language delay ○ Receptive and expressive language ○ Visual–perceptual problems • Executive functioning problems

ADHD, attention-deficit hyperactivity disorder; ASD, Autism spectrum disorders; CP, Cerebral Palsy; DCD, developmental coordination disorder; NDI, neurodevelopmental impairment.

Sources: Data from Carter, A., Gratney, L., & Carter, B. S. (2016). Discharge planning and follow-up of the neonatal intensive care unit infant. In S. Gardner, B. Carter, M. Hines, & J. Hernandez (Eds.), *Merenstein & Gardner's handbook of neonatal intensive care* (8th ed., pp. 903–923). St. Louis, MO: Elsevier; Demauro, S. B., & Hintz, S. R. (2018). Risk assessment and neurodevelopmental outcomes. In C. Gleason & S. Juul (Eds.), *Avery's diseases of the newborn* (10th ed., pp. 971–990.e7). Philadelphia, PA: Elsevier; Hack, M. (2013). The outcome of neonatal intensive care. In A. Fanaroff & J. Fanaroff (Eds.), *Klaus and Fanaroff's care of the high-risk neonate* (6th ed., pp. 525–534). Cleveland, OH: Elsevier; Hummel, P. (2014). Discharge planning and transition to home care. In Verklan et al. (Eds.), *Core curriculum for neonatal intensive care nursing* (5th ed., pp. 373–390). St. Louis, MO: Elsevier; Stewart, J. E., Bentley, J., & Knorr, A. (2017). Hearing loss in neonatal intensive care unit graduates. In E. Eichenwald, A. Hansen, C. Martin, & A. Stark (Eds.), *Cloherty and Stark's manual of neonatal care* (8th ed., pp. 983–1068). Philadelphia, PA: Wolters Klumer; Wilson-Costello, D. E., & Payne, A. H. (2015). Early childhood neurodevelopmental outcomes of high-risk neonates. In R. Martin, A. Fanaroff, & M. Walsh (Eds.), *Fanaroff and Martin's neonatal-perinatal medicine: Diseases of the fetus and infant* (10th ed., pp. 1018–1031). Philadelphia, PA: Elsevier.

verbal and visuospatial memory. These individuals may have a lower IQ on formal testing, and fewer attend college than normal birth-weight, term-born controls (Hack, 2013, p. 534).

- Medical sequelae of prematurity more chronic illnesses such as asthma or cerebral palsy, and less physical activity, which impact on respiratory, cardiovascular, and renal function. There is a higher incidence of hypertension, visceral obesity, asthma, neurodevelopmental problems, and perturbations in glucose–insulin homeostasis. Surviving ELBW infants are far more likely to have cerebral palsy (CP), blindness, and deafness compared with term-born matched controls.
  - ○ Overall, 23 to 27 weeks' gestation-born adults are 7.5 times more likely to have a medical disability affecting the ability to work, as compared with term-born adults.
  - ○ In adulthood, preterm survivors are more likely to receive disability pensions than term-born controls (Demauro & Hintz, 2018. p. 981; Wilson-Costello & Payne, 2015, pp. 1025–1026).

CONCLUSION

A stay in the NICU is but a short time frame of a preterm or ill infant's life experience. Infants are not "healed" upon leaving the NICU; on the contrary, the effects of their initial condition and the care they received in the NICU can have lifelong implications. It is because of these implications that preparing the infant and family for discharge is important and impactful toward the successful transition to home and a stable family unit. Family involvement, planning, and coordination are all crucial to the safe transition home and the ongoing well-being of the infant and family.

REVIEW QUESTIONS

1. National recommendations state that all preterm infants receive routine immunizations at their:
   A. chronologic age
   B. corrected age
   C. restricted age

2. The type of hearing loss which accounts for a large portion of infants diagnosed with permanent hearing loss is:
   A. auditory dyssynchrony
   B. sensorineural hearing loss
   C. conductive hearing loss

3. When compared to the evoked optoacoustic emissions (EOAE) auditory test, the auditory brainstem responses (ABR):
   A. is not recommended for the NICU
   B. detects auditory neuropathy
   C. uses a microphone in the ear

4. The neonatal nurse practitioner (NNP) is arranging follow-up appointments for a patient who had a complex start to life. Born at 35 weeks, the infant had a spontaneous bowel perforation shortly after birth requiring surgery. The subsequent recovery course was uneventful, and the NNP now is preparing for discharge. With regard to the need for a screening exam for retinopathy of prematurity (ROP), the NNP recognizes an exam is necessary:
   A. as an outpatient in 3 weeks
   B. 2 days prior to discharge
   C. when the infant is 6 months of age

5. A infant born at 25 weeks' gestation is going home on a preterm formula, and the mother wants to know how long she should feed her infant the preterm formula. The NNP answers based on the knowledge that extremely low gestation age newborn (ELGAN) neonates require preterm formula for at least:
   A. 3 to 5 months
   B. 6 to 9 months
   C. 12 to 15 months

REFERENCES

Abrams, S. A. (2017). Osteopenia (metabolic bone disease) of prematurity. In E. Eichenwald, A. Hansen, C. Martin, & A. Stark (Eds.), *Cloherty and Stark's manual of neonatal care* (8th ed., pp. 853–858). Philadelphia, PA: Wolters Kluwer.

Abrams, S. A., & Tiosano, D. (2015). Disorders of calcium, phosphorus, and magnesium metabolism in the neonate. In R. Martin, A. Fanaroff, & M. Walsh (Eds.), *Fanaroff and Martin's neonatal-perinatal medicine: Diseases of the fetus and infant* (10th ed., pp. 1460–1489). Philadelphia, PA: Elsevier.

Adamkin, D. H., Radmacher, P. G., & Lewis, S. (2013). Nutrition and selected disorders of the gastrointestinal tract. Part one: Nutrition for the high-risk infant. In A. Fanaroff & J. Fanaroff (Eds.), *Klaus and Fanaroff's care of the high-risk neonate* (6th ed., pp. 151–844). Cleveland, OH: Elsevier.

Anderson, D. M., Poindexter, B. B., & Martin, C. R. (2017). Nutrition. In E. Eichenwald, A. Hansen, C. Martin, & A. Stark (Eds.), *Cloherty and Stark's manual of neonatal care* (8th ed., pp. 248–284). Philadelphia, PA: Wolters Kluwer.

Angelidou, A. I., & Christou, H. A. (2017). Anemia. In E. Eichenwald, A. Hansen, C. Martin, & A. Stark (Eds.), *Cloherty and Stark's manual of neonatal care* (8th ed., pp. 755–767). Philadelphia, PA: Wolters Kluwer.

Baley, J. E. (2015). Schedule for immunization of preterm infants. In R. Martin, A. Fanaroff, & M. Walsh (Eds.), *Fanaroff and Martin's neonatal-perinatal medicine: Diseases of the fetus and infant* (10th ed., pp. 1837–1838). Philadelphia, PA: Elsevier.

Blackburn, S. T. (2018). Neurologic, muscular, and sensory systems. In S. Blackburn (Ed.), *Maternal, fetal, & neonatal physiology* (5th ed., pp. 497–542). Maryland Heights, MO: Elsevier.

Carter, A., Gratney, L., & Carter, B. S. (2016). Discharge planning and follow-up of the neonatal intensive care unit infant. In S. Gardner, B. Carter, M. Hines, & J. Hernandez (Eds.), *Merenstein & Gardner's handbook of neonatal intensive care* (8th ed., pp. 903–923). St. Louis, MO: Elsevier.

Christensen, R. D. (2018). Neonatal erythrocyte disorders. In C. Gleason & S. Juul (Eds.), *Avery's diseases of the newborn* (10th ed., pp. 1152–1179e.4). St. Louis, MO: Elsevier.

Colaizy, T. T., Demauro, S. B., Mcnelis, K. M., & Poindexter, B. B. (2018). Enteral nutrition for the high-risk neonate. In C. Gleason & S. Juul (Eds.), *Avery's diseases of the newborn* (10th ed., pp. 1009–1022e.4). St. Loius, MO: Elsevier.

De Alba Campomanes, A. G., & Binenbaum, G. (2018). Eye and vision disorders. In C. Gleason & S. Juul (Eds.), *Avery's diseases of the newborn* (10th ed., pp.1536–1557). Philadelphia, PA: Elsevier.

Demauro, S. B., & Hintz, S. R. (2018). Risk assessment and neurodevelopmental outcomes. In C. Gleason & S. Juul (Eds.), *Avery's diseases of the newborn* (10th ed., pp. 971–990.e7). Philadelphia, PA: Elsevier.

Diab, Y., & Luchtman-Jones, L. (2015). Hematologic and oncologic problems in the fetus and neonate. In R. Martin, A. Fanaroff, & M. Walsh (Eds.), *Fanaroff and Martin's neonatal-perinatal medicine: Diseases of the fetus and infant* (10th ed., pp. 1294–1343). Philadelphia, PA: Elsevier.

Gardner, S., & Carter, B. (2016). Grief and perinatal loss. In S. Gardner, B. Carter, M. Hines, & J. Hernandez (Eds.), *Merenstein & Gardner's handbook of neonatal intensive care* (8th ed., pp. 865–902.e). St. Louis, MO: Elsevier.

Hack, M. (2013). The outcome of neonatal intensive care. In A. Fanaroff & J. Fanaroff (Eds.), *Klaus and Fanaroff's care of the high-risk neonate* (6th ed., pp. 525–534). Cleveland, OH: Elsevier.

Hummel, P. (2014). Discharge planning and transition to home care. In Verklan et al. (Eds.), *Core curriculum for neonatal intensive care nursing* (5th ed., pp. 373–390). St. Louis, MO: Elsevier.

Leeman, K. T., & VanderVeen, D. K. (2017). Retinopathy of prematurity. In E. Eichenwald, A. Hansen, C. Martin, & A. Stark (Eds.), *Cloherty and Stark's manual of neonatal care* (8th ed., pp. 986–992). Philadelphia, PA: Wolters Kluwer.

Martin, R. J., & Crowley, M. A. (2013). Respiratory problems. In A. Fanaroff & J. Fanaroff (Eds.), *Klaus and Fanaroff's care of the high-risk neonate* (6th ed., pp. 244–269). Cleveland, OH: Elsevier.

Örge, F. H., & Grigorian, F. (2015). Examination and common problems of the neonatal eye. In R. Martin, A. Fanaroff, & M. Walsh (Eds.), *Fanaroff and Martin's neonatal-perinatal medicine: Diseases of the fetus and infant* (10th ed., pp. 1734–1766). Philadelphia, PA: Elsevier.

Poindexter, B. B., & Ehrenkranz, R. A. (2015). Nutrient requirements and provision of nutritional support in the premature neonate. In R. Martin, A. Fanaroff, & M. Walsh (Eds.), *Fanaroff and Martin's neonatal-perinatal medicine: Diseases of the fetus and infant* (10th ed., pp. 592–612). Philadelphia, PA: Elsevier.

Reinhart, K., & Gardner, S. (2017). Health maintenance visits in the first month of life. In B. Snell & S. Gardner (Eds.), *Care of the well newborn* (pp. 331–354). Burlington, MA: Jones & Bartlett Learning.

Smith, V. C., & Andrews, T. M. (2017). Neonatal intensive care unit discharge planning. In E. Eichenwald, A. Hansen, C. Martin, & A. Stark (Eds.), *Cloherty and Stark's manual of neonatal care* (8th ed., pp. 215–234). Philadelphia, PA: Wolters Kluwer.

Soul, J. S. (2017). Intracranial hemorrhage and white matter injury/periventricular leukomalacia. In E. Eichenwald, A. Hansen, C. Martin, & A. Stark (Eds.), *Cloherty and Stark's manual of neonatal care* (8th ed., pp. 760–789). Philadelphia, PA: Wolters Kluwer.

Stewart, J. E., Bentley, J., & Knorr, A. (2017). Hearing loss in neonatal intensive care unit graduates. In E. Eichenwald, A. Hansen, C. Martin, & A. Stark (Eds.), *Cloherty and Stark's manual of neonatal care* (8th ed., pp. 983–1068). Philadelphia, PA: Wolters Kluwer.

Stewart, J. E., Hernandez, F., & Duncan, A. F. (2017). Follow-up care of very preterm and very low birth weight infants. In E. Eichenwald, A. Hansen, C. Martin, & A. Stark (Eds.), *Cloherty and Stark's manual of neonatal care* (8th ed., pp. 192–201). Philadelphia, PA: Wolters Kluwer.

Sun, Y., Hellstrom, A., & Smith, L. E. H. (2015). Retinopathy of prematurity. In R. Martin, A. Fanaroff, & M. Walsh (Eds.), *Fanaroff and Martin's neonatal-perinatal medicine: Diseases of the fetus and infant* (10th ed., pp. 1767–1774). Philadelphia, PA: Elsevier.

Verklan, T., & Walden, M. (2014). *Core Curriculum for Neonatal Intensive Care Nursing.* (5th ed.). St. Louis, MO: Elsevier.

Vohr, B. (2015). Hearing loss in the newborn infant. In R. Martin, A. Fanaroff, & M. Walsh (Eds.), *Fanaroff and Martin's neonatal-perinatal medicine: Diseases of the fetus and infant* (10th ed., pp. 993–1000). Philadelphia, PA: Elsevier.

Vohr, B. (2018). Ear and hearing disorders. In C. Gleason & S. Juul (Eds.), *Avery's diseases of the newborn* (10th ed., pp. 1558–1566.e2). Philadelphia, PA: Elsevier.

Wilson-Costello, D. E., & Payne, A. H. (2015). Early childhood neurodevelopmental outcomes of high-risk neonates. In R. Martin, A. Fanaroff, & M. Walsh (Eds.), *Fanaroff and Martin's neonatal-perinatal medicine: Diseases of the fetus and infant* (10th ed., pp. 1018–1031). Philadelphia, PA: Elsevier.

8 THERMOREGULATION

Amy Koehn
Tosha Harris

INTRODUCTION

Thermoregulation is the foundation of neonatal care. Neonates, specifically the very low birth weight (VLBW) infant, are challenged from birth to interact and function within in an environment that is starkly different than that of the protective womb; this is both physiologically and developmentally taxing. Years of research have culminated in a body of knowledge and advanced technology dedicated to thermoregulation. The importance of temperature regulation has been supported by the recommendations from the World Health Organization (WHO) and the Neonatal Resuscitation Program, and by the practice guidelines of the Golden Hours protocol. NICU clinicians must make use of available equipment appropriately in order to avoid or minimize thermal irregularities. Clinician interventions, or lack thereof, provided in the delivery suite and daily in the NICU can have lasting effects on neonatal development. This chapter discusses the principles, both physiological and pathophysiological, of thermoregulation and interventions to minimize heat loss, and provides a brief overview of the utilization of equipment to assist in the maintenance of a neutral thermal environment (NTE).

PRINCIPLES OF THERMOREGULATION

- Neonatal hypothermia after delivery is a worldwide issue, occuring in all climates. Thermal management of the newborn during the first few hours of life is critical to prevent detrimental effects of cold stress and hypothermia (Fraser, 2016, p. 587). Adverse consequences associated with cold stress remains an important contributor to neonatal mortality and morbidity, and the potential impact of optimal thermal care provision on infant health is huge (Agren, 2015, p. 502; Brand & Boyd, 2015, p. 95; Chatson, 2017, p. 185).
  - The cost of heat production is an important contributor to infant morbidity and mortality. Even modest long-term exposure to cold will increase thermogenesis, consume oxygen and substrate stores, and impact negatively on growth (Agren, 2015, p. 504).
- These risks have prompted organizations such as the Neonatal Resuscitation Program and the WHO to stress the importance of normal body temperatures in the delivery room and preventing early postnatal hypothermia (Fanaroff & Klaus, 2013, p. 136; Hodson, 2018, p. 364)
- The neonate is most vulnerable to heat loss during the first minutes following birth (Hodson, 2018, p. 361). The primary challenge in thermal management of newborns is the prevention of hypothermia, because the neonate is expected to transition from a warm, moist environment to a much colder, drier environment. The newborn's ability to maintain temperature control after birth is determined by external environmental factors and internal physiologic processes (Brand & Boyd, 2015, p. 102; Fraser, 2016, p. 586).
- The infant's core temperature decreases rapidly, owing mainly to evaporation from his or her moist body. These losses may result in a fall of 2°C to 3°C within the first 30 to 60 minutes after birth if the newborn is extremely premature or no wrapping, drying, or clothing is applied in a larger newborn. In addition to evaporative losses from amniotic fluid, losses to cooler room air and cooler structures in the room such as walls also result in large radiant and convective heat losses (Brand & Boyd, 2015, p. 102; Fanaroff & Klaus, 2013, p. 137; Hodson, 2018, pp. 361–362).

Physiology of Thermoregulation

- Thermoregulation is defined as the means by which the neonate's body temperature is maintained by balancing heat generation and heat loss in a changing environment and is a critical component in the physiologic adaptation to extrauterine life (Cheffer & Rannalli, 2016, p. 345).
- The exposure to cold, clamping of the umbilical cord, and the general "stress of being born" induce a thermal response. This response is part of a homeostatic system with input (detectors) and output (effectors) that is aimed at preserving body temperature (Agren, 2015, pp. 503–504). Thermal receptors in the skin affect the infant's response to cold stimuli. The most prominent and sensitive skin receptors are in the trigeminal area of the face (Brand & Boyd, 2015, p. 100).
- If environmental cooling exceeds the infant's thermoregulatory response of energy output, the core temperature will drop along with a decrease in oxygen consumption. This "Q10 effect" of decreased metabolism when the environmental temperature falls below a critical point is the basis for the use of induced hypothermia in other clinical situations. The increase in oxygen consumption and the increase in metabolic output are considered important contributors to increased morbidity and mortality especially in extremely low birth weight (ELBW) infants (Hodson, 2018, p. 363).

Assessing Temperature in the Neonate

- The neonate's temperature at birth will be reflective of the intrauterine temperature. If the mother has a fever, it is common for the neonate's temperature to be elevated. It is important to distinguish between environmental, iatrogenic, and infectious causes of elevations in neonatal temperatures (Brand & Boyd, 2015, p. 100).
- The optimal temperature for a specific infant cannot be defined by a single central temperature; rather, it is defined

by the range of measurable skin temperatures that are associated with minimal heat production. This implies an optimal central or core temperature (Hodson, 2018, p. 363). The control range refers to the range of environmental temperatures at which body temperature can be kept constant (Fanaroff & Klaus, 2013, p. 136).

- Early detection and management of hypothermia and hyperthermia are essential to the well-being of neonates. Frequent temperature measurements and observation are key to early detection until the infant's temperature is stable (Brand & Boyd, 2015, p. 99). A drop in skin temperature may be the first sign of hypothermia. The core temperature may not fall until the infant can no longer compensate (Gardner & Hernandez, 2016, p. 110).
- In critically ill infants, the skin temperature is usually routinely monitored in addition to axillary temperature readings. A skin probe is secured to the right upper quadrant of the abdomen. The temperature probe should not be placed under the axilla or any other position except as recommended by the manufacturer (Gardner & Hernandez, 2016, p. 110).
- The use of low-reading thermometers (from 29.4°C/85°F) is recommended because temperature readings <34.4°C (94.0°F) can go undetected with routine thermometers (Chatson, 2017, p. 186).
- Rectal temperatures should not be used due to the risk of intestinal perforation and because the core temperature may not decrease until the neonate has totally decompensated (Brand & Boyd, 2015, p. 99).

Goals for Environmental and Neonatal Temperatures

- The control range refers to the range of environmental temperatures at which body temperature can be kept constant by means of regulation. The environmental range of the infant is more limited than that of the adult because of less insulation. The control range for an adult is 0°C (32°F), but for the full-term infant it is 20°C to 23°C (68–73.4°F; Fanaroff & Klaus, 2013, p. 136).
- For the healthy term infant, standard thermal care guidelines include maintaining the delivery room temperature at 72°F (25°C; Chatson, 2017, p. 187).
  - ○ The chilled environment of the surgical suite poses extra challenges to the newborn for thermoregulation (Gardner & Hernandez, 2016, p. 122). Coordination between neonatal and surgical staff is necessary to prevent heat loss during transport to and while in the surgical suite.
- The WHO advocated a 10-step "warm chain," which includes the following elements: environmental modification such as warming the delivery room and examination or transport areas: skin-to-skin holding, mother–baby care, and breastfeeding; delayed bathing and weighing; immediate drying and clothing/blanketing; and adequate staff training in recognition and management of cold stress (Shaw-Battista & Gardner, 2017, p. 80).
- Axillary temperatures are commonly used as they are easy to obtain, are minimally invasive, and correlate well with core temperature. When taken properly, axillary temperatures provide readings as accurate as rectal and core temperature methods (Brand & Boyd, 2015, p. 99; Gardner & Hernandez, 2016, p. 110; Hardy, D'agata, & Mcgrath, 2016, p. 376). Recommended neonatal temperature ranges are presented in Table 8.1.

TABLE 8.1 Recommended Neonatal Temperatures

Infant	Recommended Temperature Range
Full term	36.5–37.5°C (97.7–99.5° F).
Preterm	35.6–37.3°C (96.0–99° F) OR 36.3°C and 36.9°C (97.3°F and 98.4°F)
VLBW	36.7–37.3°C (98.0–99.0° F)

Sources: Data from Brand, M., & Boyd, H. (2015). Thermoregulation. In T. Verklan, M. Walden (Eds.), *Core curriculum for neonatal intensive care nursing* (pp. 95–109). St. Louis, MO: Elsevier; Gardner, S., & Hernandez, J. (2016). Heat balance. In S. Gardner, B. Carter, E. Hines, & J. Hernandez (Eds.), *Merenstein & Gardner's handbook of neonatal intensive care* (8th ed., pp. 105–125). St. Louis, MO: Elsevier; Hodson, A. (2018). Temperatures regulation. In C. Gleason & S. Juul (Eds.), *Avery's diseases of the newborn* (10th ed., pp. 361–367). Philadelphia, PA: Elsevier.

Neonates at Risk

- The neonate born before 28 weeks' gestation presents a major challenge in the prevention of heat loss. Hypothermia is reported to occur in the most ELBW neonates on their admission to an NICU and is especially hard to prevent in neonates born at less than 25 weeks' gestation (Hodson, 2018, p. 364).
- Infants at high risk of hypothermia at delivery are listed in Box 8.1.
- Neonatal physiology plays a significant role in the rapid development of hypothermia and hyperthermia. The physiologic characteristics of the neonate that lend to thermal irregularities are listed in Box 8.2.

BOX 8.1 Infants at greatest risk of hypothermia

- Less than 28 weeks' gestation
- A birthweight less than 1,500 g
- Intrauterine growth restriction
- Affected by maternal sedation
- Neurologic complications (e.g., asphyxia)
- Abdominal wall, neural tube, or other open skin defects

Sources: Data from Brand, M., & Boyd, H. (2015). Thermoregulation. In T. Verklan, M. Walden (Eds.), *Core curriculum for neonatal intensive care nursing* (pp. 95–109). St. Louis, MO: Elsevier; Chatson, K. (2017). Temperature control. In E. Eichenwald, A. Hansen, C. Martin, & A. Stark (Eds.), *Cloherty and Stark's manual of neonatal care* (8th ed., pp. 185–191). Philadelphia, PA: Wolters Kluwer; Hodson, A. (2018). Temperatures regulation. In C. Gleason & S. Juul (Eds.), *Avery's diseases of the newborn* (10th ed., pp. 361–367). Philadelphia, PA: Elsevier.

Cold Stress

- When heat loss is greater than the infant's ability to conserve and produce heat, the newborn is no longer in thermal neutrality: in such a case, the body temperature drops, and the newborn is cold stressed and becomes hypothermic.
  - ○ Hypothermia in a newborn is defined as body temperature below 36.3–36.5°C (97.3–97.7°F) measured as an axillary temperature (Shaw-Battista & Gardner, 2017, p. 81).
- The WHO developed a classification system to underscore the importance of intervention. Three levels are defined in Table 8.2.

BOX 8.2 Physiologic reasons for hypothermia in neonates

1. The infant has a small amount or veritable absence of subcutaneous fat for insulation, along with decreased levels of brown fats and decreased glycogen stores. Thermoregulation in neonates is affected by the type and amount of accumulated fat, which in turn is affected by both gestational age and birth weight.
2. Neonates also have a large surface area-to-mass ratio compared with adults. Even healthy term newborns are at risk for heat loss due to their relatively large body surface area.
3. In term neonates, the surface area-to-body mass ratio is three times greater than that of an adult.
4. There is a lower capacity for heat storage because of the higher temperature of the body shell in relation to the environment and the larger surface-to-volume ratio.
5. Preterm infants often have poor vasoconstrictor control.
6. The hypothalamus, which regulates temperature, is immature.
7. Neonates have decreased spontaneous muscle activity and poorly developed shivering thermogenesis. Term newborns have the ability to maintain this flexed posture, whereas preterm and compromised newborns may lack the muscle tone for this posturing, making them more vulnerable to cold stress.
8. There are increased evaporative losses and transepidermal insensible water loss due to thin permeable skin, allowing water to evaporate from the skin surface. Heat lost by evaporation is known as transepidermal water loss (TEWL).

Sources: Data from Brand, M., & Boyd, H. (2015). Thermoregulation. In T. Verklan & M. Walden (Eds.), *Core curriculum for neonatal intensive care nursing* (pp. 95–109). St. Louis, MO: Elsevier; Chatson, K. (2017). Temperature control. In E. Eichenwald, A. Hansen, C. Martin, & A. Stark (Eds.), *Cloherty and Stark's manual of neonatal care* (8th ed., pp. 185–191). Philadelphia, PA: Wolters Kluwer; Fanaroff, A., & Klaus, M. (2013). The physical environment. In A. Fanaroff & J. Fanaroff (Eds.), *Klaus and Fanaroff's care of the high-risk neonate* (6th ed., pp. 132–150). Cleveland, OH: Elsevier; Fraser, D. (2016). Newborn adaptation to extrauterine life. In K. Simpson & P. Creehan (Eds.), *Perinatal nursing* (4th ed., pp. 581–596). Philadelphia, PA: Wolters Kluwer/Lippincott Williams & Wilkins; Hodson, A. (2018). Temperatures regulation. In C. Gleason & S. Juul (Eds.), *Avery's diseases of the newborn* (10th ed., pp. 361–367). Philadelphia, PA: Elsevier; Shaw-Battista, J., & Gardner, S. (2017). Newborn transition: The journey from fetal to extrauterine life. In B. J. Snell & S. Gardner (Eds.), *Care of the well newborn* (pp. 69–100). Burlington, MA: Jones & Bartlett Learning.

TABLE 8.2 The WHO Classification of Hypothermia

Cold stress or mild hypothermia	Temperature 36.0–36.4°C
Moderate hypothermia	Temperature 32.0–35.9°C
Severe hypothermia	Temperature below 32°C

Source: Data from Hodson, A. (2018). Temperatures regulation. In C. Gleason & S. Juul (Eds.), *Avery's diseases of the newborn* (10th ed., pp. 361–367). Philadelphia, PA: Elsevier.

- Consequences of cold stress include a cycle of peripheral vasoconstriction, increased oxygen and glucose consumption, depletion of glycogen, pulmonary vasoconstriction, hypoglycemia, hypoxia, anaerobic metabolism, and metabolic acidosis. (Chatson, 2017, p. 186; Shaw-Battista & Gardner, 2017, p. 81).
- VLBW infants' limited ability to produce heat, their increased evaporative water loss at birth secondary to extremely thin skin, as well as their small heat capacity (the result of their large surface-to-volume ratio) make them unusually susceptible to cold stress (Fanaroff & Klaus, 2013, p. 138).
- After the immediate newborn period, the more common and chronic problem facing premature infants than actual hypothermia is caloric loss from unrecognized chronic cold stress that results in excess oxygen consumption and slow weight gain (Chatson, 2017, p. 186).

Neonatal Cold Injury

- This is a rare, extreme form of hypothermia that may be seen in low birth weight (LBW) infants and term infants with central nervous system (CNS) disorders. Core temperature can fall below 32.2°C (90° F) and infants may have a bright red color because of the failure of oxyhemoglobin to dissociate at low temperature. They may also have central pallor or cyanosis. The skin may show edema and sclerema, and occasionally there is generalized bleeding, including pulmonary hemorrhage (Chatson, 2017, p. 186).

Rewarming Techniques

- It is controversial whether warming should be rapid or slow, but it is established that rewarming too rapidly may further compromise the already cold-stressed infant and result in apnea. Setting the abdominal skin temperature to 1°C higher than the core temperature or setting it to 36.5°C on a radiant warmer will produce slow rewarming (Chatson, 2017, p. 186). Another practice is to set the difference between the skin and the ambient air temperature at less than 1.5°C (2.7°F), which results in minimal oxygen consumption (Gardner & Hernandez, 2016, p. 123).
  - ○ Efforts to block heat loss by convection, radiation, evaporation, and conduction should be initiated (Gardner & Hernandez, 2016, p. 124).
- If hypothermia is mild, slow rewarming is preferred. External heat sources should be slightly warmer than the skin temperature and gradually increased until the neutral thermal environmental temperature range is attained (Gardner & Hernandez, 2016, p. 123).
- For more extreme hypothermia (i.e., core temperatures less than 35°C [95°F]), a more rapid rewarming with radiant heaters (servo control 37°C [98.6°F]) or heated water mattresses prevents prolonged metabolic acidosis or hypoglycemia and decreases mortality risk (Gardner & Hernandez, 2016, p. 123).
  - ○ The infant may benefit from a normal saline bolus, supplemental oxygen, and from correction of metabolic acidosis (Chatson, 2017, p. 186). Volume expanders may be needed to maintain an adequate blood pressure. Apnea and seizures may occur as a result of hypoxia or decreased cerebral blood flow after vasodilation (Gardner & Hernandez, 2016, p. 124).
- Skin, axillary, and environmental temperatures should be measured and recorded every 30 minutes during the rewarming period. During the rewarming process, the hypothermic infant should be observed for hypotension as vasodilation occurs (Gardner & Hernandez, 2016, p. 124).

MECHANISMS OF HEAT PRODUCTION

- After birth, newborns must adapt to their relatively cold environment through the metabolic production of heat because they are not able to generate an adequate shivering response (Chatson, 2017, p. 185).
- Oxidative glucose, fat, and protein metabolism, nonshivering thermogenesis (NST) of brown fat, and muscle activity are all mechanisms to generate heat in the term newborn. Peripheral vasoconstriction helps prevent heat loss, as does normal newborn flexion (decreased body surface area exposed to air) (Shaw-Battista & Gardner, 2017, p. 80).
- Temperature receptors sensing a low temperature stimulate increased sympathetic output from the CNS, resulting in norepinephrine release, which in turn stimulates β-adrenergic receptors in brown fat, increasing cyclic adenosine monophosphate (AMP) production (Hodson, 2018, p. 363). Thus, the thermoregulatory system of the homeothermic infant adjusts and balances heat production, skin blood flow, sweating, and respiration in such a way that the body temperature remains constant within a control range of environmental temperatures (Fanaroff & Klaus, 2013, p. 135).
    ○ Different thresholds of the effector response for nonshivering and shivering thermogenesis explain the differences observed between hypothermic adults and neonates. In the range of normal to near-normal body temperature (≥36°C), shivering thermogenesis will be nonoperative in the neonate, and chemical thermogenesis dominates (Agren, 2015, p. 506).
- When exposed to cold stress, thermal receptors in skin transmit messages to the CNS, activating the sympathetic nervous system and triggering metabolism of brown fat, a process that utilizes glucose and oxygen and produces acids as a by product. Once utilized, brown fat stores are not replaced (Fraser, 2016, p. 586).

Brown Adipose Tissue (BAT)

- A cold-exposed infant depends primarily on chemical thermogenesis to avoid hypothermia. Exposure to cold induces a sympathetic surge that acts on receptors in brown fat stores. BAT, also known as brown adipose tissue, is highly vascularized and innervated by sympathetic neurons (Chatson, 2017, p. 185) and generates more energy than any other tissue in the body; hence its importance in thermoregulation (Brand & Boyd, 2015, p. 100). Brown fat comprises most of the fat content of the newborn.
    ○ The metabolic rate of a newborn has been observed to increase up to threefold when maximally stimulated by cold. However, in the preterm infant fat stores are scarce and nutritional provision often suboptimal, limiting their thermogenic capacity (Agren, 2015, p. 504).
- NST produces energy output and hence heat production through the oxidation of fatty acids. The presence of the protein thermogen in brown fat uncouples β-oxidation, resulting in metabolic production of heat. Glucose or glycerol appears to be an alternative fuel utilized for this purpose.
- Although all metabolically active tissues can generate heat (Brand & Boyd, 2015, p. 101):
    ○ Norephinephrine acts in the brown fat tissue to stimulate lipolysis. Most of the free fatty acids are re-esterified or oxidized; both reactions produce heat (Chatson, 2017, p. 185).
    ○ A heavy concentration of blood vessels gives BAT its characteristic brown color and serves to conduct heat into the circulation (Brand & Boyd, 2015, p. 101). BAT is located in the interscapular, paraspinal spaces (Agren, 2015, p. 504) as well as around the kidneys and adrenal glands; at the nape of the neck, the scapula, and axilla; in the mediastinum, and around the trachea, heart, lungs, liver, and abdominal aorta kidneys and adrenal glands (Fraser, 2016, p. 586).
- The amount of available BAT is dependent on gestational age. It begins to appear at 25 to 26 weeks in the fetus but is probably not an efficient participant in thermogenesis at this stage of development. (Hodson, 2018, p. 363), so only a minimal amount is available in VLBW infants. Production of brown fat begins around 26 to 28 weeks' gestation and continues for 3 to 5 weeks after birth (Fraser, 2016, p. 586).

Nonshivering Thermogenesis (NST)

- Shivering is an involuntary method of heat production that is rarely seen in the neonatal population. Physical activity can generate heat, but only late preterm and term infants have enough muscle tone to produce heat by this method and this may only be effective for a short time. The neonate only shivers after prolonged cold stress that leads to decreased spinal cord temperature (Brand & Boyd, 2015, p. 101).
- NST is the major method of heat production in the neonate. NST is triggered when skin temperature decreases to less than 35°C to 36°C (95–96.8°F). NST produces energy output and hence heat production through the oxidation of fatty acids, largely from brown fat (Hodson, 2018, p. 363).
    ○ The initiation of NST at birth depends on cutaneous cooling, separation from the placenta, and the euthyroid state (Fanaroff & Klaus, 2013, p. 133).
    ○ NST relies on the availability of BAT and therefore is limited in ELBW infants (Brand & Boyd, 2015, p. 101).
- Infants less than 32 weeks of gestation do not have enough BAT to produce significant amounts of heat by NST (Brand & Boyd, 2015, p. 101).

Mechanisms of and Interventions to Minimize Heat Transfer

- The term "golden hour" is used in reference to strategies implemented in the delivery room to improve the outcome of neonates. A major focus during the "golden hour" is prevention of heat loss (Brand & Boyd, 2015, p. 95).
- The mechanisms of heat transfers are complex, and the contribution of each component involves four means of loss: (a) by radiation; (b) by conduction; (c) by convection; and (d) by evaporation (Chatson, 2017, p. 187; Cheffer & Rannalli, 2016, p. 345; Fanaroff & Klaus, 2013, p. 134; Gardner & Hernandez, 2016, p. 122).
    ○ All modes of heat transfer influence thermal balance, and the relative contribution of each mode changes with maturity, postnatal age, disease state, and care environment (Agren, 2015, p. 502).
    ○ The physiologic control mechanisms of the infant may alter the internal gradient (i.e., vasomotor) to change skin blood flow. The external gradient is of a purely physical nature. The large surface-to-volume ratio of the infant (especially those weighing less than 2 kg) in

relation to the adult and the thin layer of subcutaneous fat increase the heat transfer in the internal gradient (Fanaroff & Klaus, 2013, p. 134).

Radiant Heat Loss

- Radiation is the transfer of heat through infrared energy transfer from a warm object to a cooler object that is not in direct contact. Heat transfer is affected by the temperature gradient and the distance and angle between the heat source and the skin surface (Brand & Boyd, 2015, p. 96). This mechanism of heat loss is influenced by the mean temperature of the skin and the mean temperatures of the surrounding walls, as well as the temperature gradient to nearby objects of lesser temperature (the newborn loses heat by radiation to nearby cooler surfaces such as crib, isolette, windows, or other objects (Fraser, 2016, p. 587; Hodson, 2018, p. 362; Shaw-Battista & Gardner, 2017, p. 80).
  - Radiation can be responsible for 40% or more of heat loss, so it has been the focus of most research studies (Hodson, 2018, p. 362).
  - Radiant heat loss is related to the temperature of the surrounding surfaces, not air temperature (Fanaroff & Klaus, 2013, p. 134). Many variables can influence the degree of heat loss, including body surface area, environmental temperature, the type of external heat source, clothing, blankets, caps, heat shields, and swaddling (Hodson, 2018, p. 362).

Interventions to Minimize

- Standard thermal care guidelines include maintaining the delivery room at an ambient air temperature at 72°F/25°C. A radiant warmer should be used during resuscitation and stabilization (Chatson, 2017, p. 190).
  - Preterm newborns need additional protection from heat losses, including higher ambient temperature and the use of plastic wraps (without drying; Hodson, 2018, p. 364).
    - To avoid hypothermia, it is recommended that low birth weight infants be placed directly in a sterile food or medical grade plastic bag or wrapped with occlusive wrap after delivery (Fraser, 2016, p. 586).
  - Heat loss from the head is clinically important and can be significantly reduced with a three-layered hat, and the neonate's head should remain covered (Chatson, 2017, p. 187; Fanaroff & Klaus, 2013, p. 143; Hardy et al., 2016, p. 377).

Evaporative Heat Loss

- Evaporation is heat transfer due to water vaporizing from the large surface area of wet skin and to the duration of exposure into the drier surrounding air as when a newborn wet with amniotic fluid is subjected to dry and cooler surroundings air (Shaw-Battista & Gardner, 2017, p. 80). In the case of premature infants with thin permeable skin, evaporative heat loss occurs through TEWL. The more immature the newborn, the larger the relative surface area (Hodson, 2018, p. 362).
  - Evaporative heat losses are inversely related to ambient humidity, and measures to increase the vapor pressure close to the skin simplify fluid and thermal management of extremely preterm infants (Agren, 2015, p. 502).

- The amount of insensible water loss from the skin is inversely related to gestational age. At 25 weeks of gestation, premature infants can lose 15 times more water through their skin than term neonates. This water loss is inversely proportional to gestational age until about 33 weeks of gestation, when TEWL is similar to that of a term infant (Brand & Boyd, 2015, p. 100).
- The magnitude of water loss through the skin is related to maturity at birth, when the tiniest infants have evaporative heat losses that are many times higher than those of a term infant when cared for under similar environmental conditions (Agren, 2015, p. 502; Fraser, 2016, p. 586).
  - In very small infants (<1,500 g), high total body water, very thin skin that is unusually permeable because the keratin layer of the skin has not matured, and relatively large body surface area result in increased evaporative losses in premature infants. This is even more significant in VLBW and especially in ELBW infants (Brand & Boyd, 2015, p. 97; Fanaroff & Klaus, 2013, p. 134; Fraser, 2016, p. 586).

Interventions to Minimize

- Drying the infant immediately after birth in the delivery room reduces evaporative heat loss (Agren, 2015, p. 507)
  - Do not bathe the neonate without first evaluating the consequences of cold stress on the neonate's clinical condition (Hardy et al., 2016, p. 377).
- Ideally, a preheated gel mattress, with a warm bassinette, warm blankets, and a radiant heat source should be in place. Immediate drying, swaddling (once stabilized), and placement of a cap will reduce evaporative heat loss (Hodson, 2018, p. 364).
- Insensible water loss through the skin continues to contribute to evaporative heat loss and decreases over the first few days after birth. The rate of evaporative water loss depends on the ambient humidity and increases at humidity levels below 50% (Hodson, 2018, p. 362).
  - Because evaporative loss is related to ambient relative humidity, incubator humidification will decrease heat loss; the higher the humidity, the lower the evaporation. However, in most situations, a higher evaporative loss can be compensated for by a higher air temperature (convective gain; Agren, 2015, p. 507).

Convection Heat Loss

- Convection is heat transfer due to air currents or drafts the transfer of heat from a solid object to surrounding air (Brand & Boyd, 2015, p. 96; Fraser, 2016, p. 587). Heat loss due to convection is determined by the airflow around the infant, the mean temperature of the ambient air, the mean temperature of the skin, and the exposed surface area of the infant (the amount of exposed) skin surface and amount of air turbulence created by drafts (Chatson, 2017, p. 187; Fraser, 2016, p. 587; Hodson, 2018, p. 362; Shaw-Battista & Gardner, 2017, p. 80).

Interventions to Minimize

- Remain vigilant to the presence of radiant heat loss to cold walls or windows and convection heat loss in the path of air-conditioning vents (Hardy et al., 2016, p. 377).
- The relatively larger brain of the newborn is a major heat source, the largest surface area of the body. The brain of the infant is 12% of body weight compared with 2% in

the adult, and heat loss from the head is clinically important and can be significantly reduced with a three-layered hat made of wool and gauze when not under the radiant warmer greatly conserves heat (Fanaroff & Klaus, 2013, p. 143; Fraser, 2016, p. 586).

Conductive Heat Loss

- Conduction is the transfer of heat via direct contact when two solid objects of different temperatures come in contact (Fraser, 2016, p. 587), such as from the infant's warm body to a cold table or cold blankets (Chatson, 2017, p. 187; Shaw-Battista & Gardner, 2017, p. 80).
- The rate of heat transfer varies with the temperature gradient and the amount of skin in contact with the surface. Heat is transferred more readily from the skin to a metal object than from the skin to a cloth surface (Brand & Boyd, 2015, p. 95).
  - ○ Conductive heat losses contribute minimally to energy expenditure and depend on the thermal conductivity of the mattress, which is low in incubators and under radiant warmers (Hodson, 2018, p. 362).

Interventions to Minimize

- Mechanisms for preventing conductive heat loss immediately after birth include using a preheated radiant warmer, warm blankets for drying, and covering scales and x-ray plates with warm blankets (Fraser, 2016, p. 587).
  - ○ External heat sources, including skin-to-skin care (SSC) and transwarmer mattresses, have demonstrated a reduction in the risk of hypothermia (Chatson, 2017, p. 190).
  - ○ Prewarm linens and equipment that will come into contact with the neonate (Hardy et al., 2016, p. 377).
  - ○ The term and near-term vigorous infant may preferably be placed skin-to-skin on the mother's chest and covered by dry blankets, enabling conductive transfer of maternal heat to the infant and minimizing any ongoing heat loss. Alternatively, the infant may be dried and wrapped with dry blankets (Agren, 2015, p. 507).
  - ○ Figures 8.1 summarizes methods of heat loss and interventions to minimize.

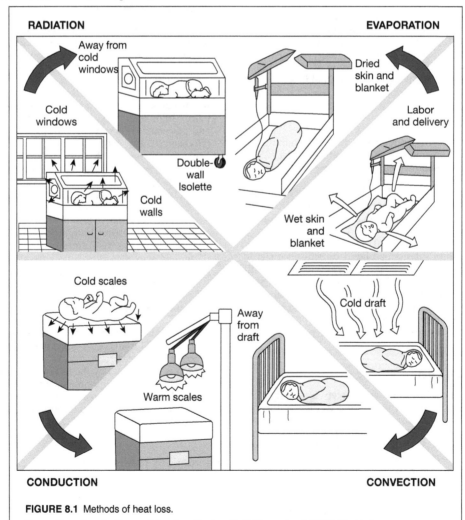

FIGURE 8.1 Methods of heat loss.

Source: Reproduced with permission from Gardner, S., & Hernandez, J. (2016). Heat balance. In S. Gardner, B. Carter, E. Hines, & J. Hernandez (Eds.), *Merenstein & Gardner's handbook of neonatal intensive care* (8th ed., pp. 105–125). St. Louis, MO: Elsevier.

NEUTRAL THERMAL ENVIRONMENTS (NTEs)

- Minimizing heat loss and maintaining the newborn in a thermally neutral environment are important steps in facilitating a normal neonatal transition (Shaw-Battista & Gardner, 2017, p. 80).
- The concept of an optimum thermal environment for newborn infants evolved during the 1960s. This "thermoneutral zone" or thermal neutral environment (TNE) refers to the range of temperature within which the infant can maintain a normal body temperature at minimal metabolic rate (as measured by oxygen consumption) with use of nonevaporative processes (vasoconstriction, vasodilation, and/or changes in posture) only (Agren, 2015, p. 505; Cheffer & Rannalli, 2016, p. 345; Hodson, 2018, p. 363).
- In the NICU, infants require a thermoneutral environment to minimize energy expenditure and optimize growth (Chatson, 2017, p. 190). Caregivers strive to maintain the infant in a warm environment (the NTE, or the so-called "zone of thermal comfort"; Fanaroff & Klaus, 2013, p. 135).
  - ○ Thermoneutral conditions exist when heat production measured by oxygen consumption is minimal and core temperature is within the normal range (Chatson, 2017, p. 186).
  - ○ A number of factors affect the temperature needed to maintain thermal stability, including gestational age, birth weight, chronologic age, humidity, proximity to outside walls and windows, and the use of positioning devices, clothing, or swaddling (Brand & Boyd, 2015, p. 105).
- Thermal management relies on simple principles and requires frequent individual evaluation and adjustment.
  - ○ Thermal care benefits from a protocol-driven approach based on guidelines that minimize variation in practice.
  - ○ Such guidelines should specify ranges for normal body and skin temperatures and thermal environment recommendations specifying in which situations incubators, radiant warmers, heated mattresses, and SSC are applicable, and when to use continuous temperature measurement (peripheral/central) and infant servo or air control (Agren, 2015, p. 509).
- There are three options to achieve a stable and desirable skin temperature of 36.0–36.5°C:
  - ○ Manual control of incubator temperature (Hodson, 2018, p. 364)
  - ○ Servo control of incubator air temperature
  - ○ Servo control of abdominal skin temperature (using an abdominal skin probe)
    - ■ Whether a heat panel or incubator is used, a probe is placed on the infant's abdomen to measure skin temperature. If the infant's skin temperature decreases, the warming device increases its heat output (Fanaroff & Klaus, 2013, p. 143).
      - • An anterior abdominal temperature of 37.0°C is generally recommended for servo control of radiant heat output, at least as a starting point (Agren, 2015, p. 508).
- Both incubators and radiant warmers have been in use in NICUs for several decades and remain the focus of heat management. Each of these warming devices has undergone sophisticated evolution and remains effective in providing a TNE for infants of differing sizes and with differing illnesses (Hodson, 2018, p. 364).

- ○ Comparisons of the superiority of the incubator over the radiant warmer have shown no differences in outcome. Both methods are effective and safe and appropriate for the care of the ELBW newborn, with recognition of small differences in insensible water loss (Hodson, 2018, p. 365).
- After stabilization, the preterm infant may either be nursed in an incubator or under a radiant warmer. For extremely preterm infants, measures to reduce insensible water and heat loss through the skin are recommended at least during the first week of life. In the incubator, this is accomplished by use of high ambient relative humidity, and under the radiant warmer, by use of a plastic wrap (Agren, 2015, p. 510).

Environmental Temperatures

- Because of the relationship between metabolic rate and body temperature, both fluid and nutritional requirements for growth are intimately linked with temperature regulation. This is especially important to the small premature infant maintained in a slightly cool environment (Fanaroff & Klaus, 2013, p. 138).
  - ○ Fewer calories would be required for maintenance of body temperature if the infant was in a warmer environment; thus, in the NTE, caloric intake can be more effectively used for growth (Fanaroff & Klaus, 2013, p. 138).
- The home environment should be kept at a temperature that prevents cold stress. A room temperature that is comfortable for the parent usually is suitable for the infant. The infant should be in clothing appropriate for the room temperature. For example, if the parent requires a sweater to be comfortable, the infant probably also requires a sweater.
  - ○ Parents often overdress the infant or overheat the home, and this may cause hyperthermia. Parents should be given written instructions before discharge on how and when to take an axillary temperature, when to call the physician, and how to maintain a comfortable environment for their infant (Gardner & Hernandez, 2016, p. 125).

Servo-Control Radiant Warmers

- This device and the primitive delivery room heaters led to the development of the current radiant warmers now in common use in NICUs. They produce overhead heat in the infrared range distributed in a uniform fashion to the infant and controlled by an abdominal skin thermistor. The high-power output of the device explains the effectiveness and speed with which a hypothermic infant can be warmed. Radiant warmers provide excellent accessibility and visibility for the care of the newborn infant assessment and management of the seriously ill infant on admission and have, therefore, become widely used in neonatal intensive care (Agren, 2015, p. 508).
  - ○ The temperature probe itself, not the skin temperature, controls heat output (Hodson, 2018, pp. 364–365). Radiant warmers should always be used with a servo control to prevent overheating (Brand & Boyd, 2015, p. 102).
- The radiant warmer provides radiant heat to maintain temperature while providing improved access to the infant for assessment and procedures when compared to an incubator (Brand & Boyd, 2015, p. 106). Infant skin temperature servo control has the advantage of providing a more

stable body temperature under changing care conditions, different ventilation modes, opening of port holes, and so on (Agren, 2015, p. 507).

- ○ An increase in insensible water loss occurs when infants are cared for in radiant warmers. This increased fluid loss poses a risk for fluid and electrolyte imbalance. Careful documentation of intake, output, and weight are essential in managing infants cared for in radiant warmers. Convective losses are also increased in a radiant warmer. Care should be taken to minimize drafts (Brand & Boyd, 2015, p. 106).
- The desired skin temperature used for skin servo control is generally 36.0°C to 36.5°C (96.8–97.7°F; Gardner & Hernandez, 2016, p. 114).
- Overheating can occur if the probe becomes detached or covered with a blanket (Hodson, 2018, p. 364) may lead to overwarming, although usually this is not severe (Agren, 2015, p. 507). Both the infant and the incubator temperatures must be compared together, so the infant's true condition is not masked (Fanaroff & Klaus, 2013, p. 143). On the other hand, harmful overheating can rapidly occur unless careful monitoring (preferably continuous) of infant temperature is instituted (Agren, 2015, p. 508).
- Conductive thermal support may also be provided by the use of a heated mattress. The mattress should always be prewarmed and the temperature never set lower than the desired body temperature, because this will lead to significant conductive heat loss and impact negatively on body temperature and weight gain (Agren, 2015, pp. 508–509).
  - ○ A transparent heat shield positioned over the infant may influence the heat exchange (occurring through convection, evaporation, and radiation) and result in reduced losses of heat. However, such a shield positioned between the infant and radiant heat source will also disrupt the servo-control mechanism and reduce direct radiant heat delivery to the infant, which may interfere with thermal control (Agren, 2015, p. 508).

Servo-Control Incubators

- Incubators are designed to decrease all four forms of heat loss, namely evaporation, conduction, radiation, and convection. Double-walled incubators further decrease heat loss primarily, due to radiation and, to a lesser degree, conduction (Chatson, 2017, p. 191).
  - ○ Incubator covers can be used to decrease radiant heat loss from incubator walls, to decrease radiant loss in cold climates, and to decrease radiant gain in hot climates, especially on sunny days.
- Skin mode or servo control can be set so that the incubator's internal thermostat responds to changes in the infant's skin temperature to ensure a normal temperature despite any environmental fluctuations (Chatson, 2017, p. 190).
  - ○ Safety features to prevent overheating include the setting of upper limits of air temperature and alarms to alert the nurse to a detached probe.
  - ○ In this mode, the nurse must document the neonate's axillary temperature, the incubator set point, the skin temperature, and the air temperature (Brand & Boyd, 2015, p. 103).
  - ○ When incubators are in cool surroundings (e.g., during transfer), the inner surface temperature of the single-walled incubator declines to well below that

of the air temperature in the incubator (Fanaroff & Klaus, 2013, p. 134).

- The incubator is controlled either thermostatically by air or infant temperature. Both modes are capable of providing a stable thermoneutral environment. However, their respective advantages and disadvantages need to be understood to properly conduct incubator care (Agren, 2015, p. 507).
  - ○ Air temperature servo control usually provides a more stable environment, but makes it necessary to frequently determine infant temperature, thus adding further to the load of procedures disturbing the infants.
  - ○ For both modes, it is essential that procedures such as intravenous (IV) line insertion and intubation are performed through the portholes, and not through the large access panel at the front of the incubator (Agren, 2015, p. 507).
- An anterior abdominal skin temperature of 36.5°C has been widely used for servo control of incubator air temperature, but may be too low to ensure thermoneutrality. An abdominal skin (or back to mattress) temperature setting of 37.0°C may be preferable (Agren, 2015, p. 507).
- Humidity should be used with VLBW infants to reduce evaporative heat loss through TEWL. Evaporative heat loss is the major source of thermal instability in the first few weeks of life due to increased body surface area, increased skin permeability, and increased extracellular fluid (Brand & Boyd, 2015, p. 105).
- Because evaporative loss is related to ambient relative humidity, incubator humidification will decrease heat loss; the higher the humidity, the lower the evaporation. However, in most situations a higher evaporative loss can be compensated for by a higher air temperature (convective gain) and a too low incubator humidity will only increase metabolic demand if the infant is nursed below thermoneutral temperature.
- There is less need for humidity after the first week of life due to maturation of the infant's skin and decreased insensible water loss from TEWL. Barrier maturation usually develops in 2 to 4 weeks. This may take longer in extremely premature infants. Continuing high humidity beyond the first week may slow skin maturation (Brand & Boyd, 2015, p. 106).
  - ○ High incubator ambient humidity (70%–90%) is only vital in situations wherein high insensible water loss per se complicates fluid management, i.e., in extremely preterm infants during the first postnatal week(s).
  - ○ An increased risk of Pseudomonas infections has been demonstrated with the use of incubator humidification when condensation of vapor on the inner incubator walls occurs, which, therefore, should be avoided (Agren, 2015, p. 507).

Weaning From Servo Control

- Premature infants in relatively stable condition can be dressed in clothes and caps and covered with a blanket. The intervention offers a broader range of safe environmental temperatures. Heart rate and respiration should be continuously monitored because the clothing may limit observation (Chatson, 2017, p. 191).
- Weaning from the incubator can typically be started when the infant is physiologically stable, at least 32 weeks' corrected gestational age, weighs at least 1,500 g and takes 100

kcals/kg/day, and provided there is no medical indication for continuing incubator/warmer care, such as the need for close observation (Fanaroff & Klaus, 2013, p. 143).
  ○ Body weight attainment serves as a useful indicator as the infant approaches a weight of at least 1,500 g and takes 100 kcals/kg/day (Fanaroff & Klaus, 2013, p. 143).
- Crib nursing of full-term infants requires a room temperature of at least 24°C (75°F), while infants of 1,500 g should be in an environment of 26°C to 28°C (79–82°F). The smaller infants should be fully dressed, including a head covering, and may require a room temperature of 30°C (86°F) (Hodson, 2018, p. 365).

Skin-to-Skin Practices

- SSC has been practiced long before the concept of "kangaroo mother care" for preterm infants was introduced (Agren, 2015, p. 508). "Kangaroo mother care" was originally used as an effective way for mothers to keep their full-term babies warm while breastfeeding, and subsequently as an alternative method of caring for LBW babies in resource-limited countries.
  ○ In these original versions, the infant is placed skin-to-skin in a vertical position between the mother's breasts and under her clothes and is exclusively (or almost exclusively) breastfed (Hodson, 2018, p. 365).
- Skin-to-skin contact conserves infant heath through tucked positioning and covering, and positively contributes to thermal gain from continuous adult body heat, and has been shown to be more effective for the prevention and treatment of newborn hypothermia than either an incubator or radiant warmer (Shaw-Battista & Gardner, 2017, p. 80).
- During kangaroo care, the patents' clothing around the sides and back of the infant forms a "pouch" that provides insulation and reduces nonevaporative losses (and possibly evaporation losses). ELBW infants in particular require careful temperature monitoring during kangaroo care to avoid both heat stress and cooling (Blackburn, 2013, p. 672).
- Skin-to-skin (kangaroo) is appropriate-for-gestational age (AGA) and SGA infants experience a beneficial warming effect and a stable skin and core temperature when held skin to skin.
  ○ Mothers exhibit thermal synchrony with the infants so that their body temperature increases or decreases to maintain the infant's thermal neutrality.
  ○ Skin-to-skin contact between mother and infant reduces conductive and radiant heat loss and is an excellent way to maintain a neutral thermal condition for the healthy newborn.
- SSC has been proven to enhance physiological stability and is recommended. In SSC, the kangaroo position reduces infant heat loss by minimizing the skin surface exposed to the environment, and enables conductive heat gain through the skin-to-skin contact between infant and parent.
  ○ Studies in more immature infants have shown that SSC can be safely applied, and without an increase in metabolic rate, as early as during the first week after birth in stable 28- to 30-week infants, and from the second week in infants born at a gestational age of 25 to 27 weeks (Agren, 2015, p. 508).

  ○ During SSC, extremely preterm infants were able to both maintain and increase their body temperature after the drop that occurred during transfer from the incubator (Gardner & Hernandez, 2016, p. 122; Hodson, 2018, p. 365).
- SSC, provided by the mother or father, has been introduced for babies requiring neonatal intensive care—even extremely premature infants and those on ventilators (Hodson, 2018, p. 365). The infants were studied early (first week) after birth and during intensive care, including mechanical ventilation. The study shows that ambient air temperature and humidity are lower during SSC compared with incubator care (Agren, 2015, p. 508).
  ○ Enhanced parental bonding, facilitation of breastfeeding, better sleep patterns, and procedural pain relief are some of SSC's purported benefits (Hodson, 2018, p. 365).
- Several guidelines regarding SSC in the NICU have been published, but since it requires intensive staffing support, resources, and parent participation, development of individualized unit guidelines has been recommended (Hodson, 2018, p. 365)
- Studies have been performed mainly in countries with limited availability to neonatal intensive care, with increasingly known effects and benefits in the moderately preterm and LBW infant.
- At birth, term infants placed skin to skin against their mother or who experience skin-to-skin contact later maintain their temperature as well as infants cared for in standard heating units (Blackburn, 2013, p. 671).
- Studies of skin-to-skin (kangaroo) care with stable preterm infants demonstrate that most infants maintain adequate thermal control during this type of holding.

Hyperthermia

- The fetus is incapable of independent thermoregulation; heat production and heat loss are controlled by the maternal–fetal thermal gradient (Blackburn, 2013, p. 661).
  ○ Maternal hyperthermia results in fetal hyperthermia and can lead to compromised fetal oxygen uptake, lower Apgar scores, hypotonia, and increased incidence for advanced resuscitation and oxygen support following delivery (Blackburn, 2012, p. 661).
  ○ Maternal fever related to infection early in pregnancy been associated with increased risk for anencephaly, neural tube defects, microcephaly, cleft lip, facial dysmorphosis, and altered growth patterns (Blackburn, 2012, p. 659).
- Neonatal hyperthermia (37.5–38.0°C or 99.5–100.4°F), may be caused by maternal fever secondary to epidural anesthesia or infection, environmental factors, cardiac defects, drug withdrawal, infection, dehydration, CNS dysfunction related to birth trauma or malformations, or medications (Blackburn, 2012, p. 673; Brand & Boyd, 2015, p. 97; Fanaroff & Klaus, 2013, p. 145).
- The most common causes for neonatal hyperthermia are iatrogenic and environmental in nature (Gardner & Hernandez, 2016, p. 124; Gardner & Snell, p. 297). High room temperatures, improperly set heating controls (i.e., radiant warmer left in manual-control mode or excessive servo-control temperature setting), malpositioned temperature probes, excessive swaddling, and conditions that alter heat control, such as phototherapy use and incubator sun exposure, have been linked to neonatal hyperthermia

(Chatson, 2017, p. 191; Fanaroff & Klaus, 2013, p. 145; Gardner & Hernandez, 2016, p. 124).

- The neonate is more susceptible to heat stress due to its larger surface-to-volume ratio, lower heat storage capacity, and narrower temperature control range (Blackburn, 2012, p. 675).

Presentation

- Hyperthermia causes an increase in metabolic demands, resulting in an increase in oxygen consumption (Blackburn, 2012, p. 673).
- While environmental conditions may the primary causation of neonatal hyperthermia, it is important to also assess for signs of infection. Servo-controlled incubators will have decreased heater output in response to increasing infant skin temperatures, thus keeping the infant's temperature within a normal range (Garder & Hernandez, 2016, p. 112).
  - ○ Clinicians should closely monitor infants requiring decreased incubator heat support (Gardner & Hernandez, 2016, p. 112)
  - ○ Sepsis in infants may present with hypothermia or hyperthermia (Gardner & Hernandez, 2016, p. 112). Hypothermia is more likely to occur in premature infants with bacterial sepsis. Term infants are more likely to present with hyperthermia as a sign of infection (Wilson & Tyner, 2015, p. 699).

TABLE 8.3 Neonatal Hyperthermia—Environmental Versus Infection Presentation

Environmental	Infection
Generally warm to touch, with trunk and extremities the same temperature	Cool to touch, with extremities significantly cooler than trunk
Skin appears flushed or ruddy in color	Skin appears pale-blue, hypoperfused
Vasodilation	Vasoconstricted

Sources: Data from Agren, J. (2015). The thermal environment of the intensive care nursery. In R. Martin, A. Fanaroff, & M. Walsh (Eds.), *Fanaroff and Martin's neonatal-perinatal medicine: Diseases of the fetus and infant* (10th ed., pp. 502–512). Philadelphia, PA: Elsevier; Chatson, K. (2017). Temperature control. In E. Eichenwald, A. Hansen, C. Martin, & A. Stark (Eds.). *Cloherty and Stark's manual of neonatal care* (8th ed., pp. 185–191). Philadelphia, PA: Wolters Kluwer; Fanaroff, A., & Klaus, M. (2013). The physical environment. In A. Fanaroff & J. Fanaroff (Eds.), *Klaus and Fanaroff's care of the high-risk neonate* (6th ed., pp. 132–150). Cleveland, OH: Elsevier; Gardner, S., & Hernandez, J. (2016). Heat balance. In S. Gardner, B. Carter, E. Hines, & J. Hernandez (Eds.), *Merenstein & Gardner's handbook of neonatal intensive care* (8th ed., pp. 105–125). St. Louis, MO: Elsevier.

- Sweating is usually not present in infants <36 weeks, but may occur in term infants (Gardner & Hernandez, 2016, p. 124).
- Hyperthermic infants may be irritable, restless, lethargic, hypotonic, apneic, tachypneic, tachycardic, or have a weak or absent cry. Vasodilation to increase heat loss may cause hypotension and dehydration as a result of increased insensible water losses (IWL). Seizures and apnea may also occur as a result of high internal temperatures (Blackburn, 2012, p. 675; Gardner & Hernandez, 2016, p. 124; Hodson, 2018, p. 366).

- Infants with temperature irregularities should be monitored closely for any changes in their behavioral, feeding, and respiratory patterns. Axillary temperatures should be evaluated frequently in any infant exhibiting these changes or who feel cool or warm to touch (Gardner & Hernandez, 2016, p. 124).

Treatment

- The primary approach to treating hyperthermia is to remove any external sources of heat and to promote heat loss (i.e., removing extra blankets or clothes; Gardner & Hernandez, 2016, p. 112). Environmental temperature should be lowered approximately every 30 minutes by 0.5°C (Hodson, 2018, p. 366).
- Fluid status should be monitored by assessing the infant's intake and output, serum electrolyte assays, serum and urine osmolality, skin turgor, and mucous membranes. Total intake volume should be adjusted as needed to replace IWL. Blood pressure measurements should be assessed frequently to monitor for hypotension; volume resuscitation should be provided as needed. Assisted ventilation should be provided for persistent apnea or apnea that does not respond to stimulation. Infants with significant hyperthermia should be assessed for subtle seizure signs such as facial grimacing, horizontal eye deviation, nystagmus, eye blinking or fluttering, or staring; tremors, apnea, decorticate posturing, rowing, stepping, or pedaling movements; and tongue thrusting, nonnutritive sucking, lip smacking, or drooling (Gardner & Hernandez, 2016, p. 125; Verklan, 2015, p. 759).
- Discharge education related to thermal regulation should focus on proper axillary temperature-taking technique, newborn care, and signs and symptoms of illness (Box 8.3).

BOX 8.3 Parent teaching and temperature regulation

- Teach parents how to take an axillary temperature on their newborn and maintain the axillary temperature 36.5°C and 37.4°C (97.7° and 99.3°F).[5]
- Teach parents how to dress their infant with clothes and blankets and use an appropriate environmental temperature to maintain the baby's temperature in the above range.
- Teach parents appropriate safety precautions, which include verbal and written information about recognizing signs and symptoms of a sick infant, as well as how the infant acts, including temperatures either higher than or, more commonly, lower than the range of 36.5–37.4°C (97.7–99.3°F).
- Teach parents to notify their infant's primary health care provider immediately or to take the infant to the nearest emergency department for temperatures out of the above range, especially if the baby's feeding pattern changes.

Source: Reproduced with permission from Gardner, S., & Hernandez, J. (2016). Heat balance. In S. Gardner, B. Carter, E. Hines, & J. Hernandez (Eds.), *Merenstein & Gardner's handbook of neonatal intensive care* (8th ed., pp. 105–125). St. Louis, MO: Elsevier.

CONCLUSION

The significance of thermal regulation in the neonatal population cannot be overstated. An understanding of the physiology and mechanics of thermoregulation is a basic requirement of neonatal care. Beginning at delivery and continuing throughout the neonatal period, infants require a thermally neutral environment to facilitate transition to the extrauterine life, to lower energy expenditure in order to utilize caloric intake to optimize growth, and to lower oxygen consumption. Evidence-based practice guidelines and protocols focusing on thermal management minimize practice variations and promote an environment in which the infant can grow and thrive.

REVIEW QUESTIONS

1. Additional humidity within an isolette is needed for the very low birthweight infant to minimize heat loss from:
   A. convection
   B. evaporation
   C. radiation

2. Brown fat production in the fetus begins during gestation at approximately:
   A. 23–25 weeks
   B. 26–28 weeks
   C. 29–31 weeks

3. A former 26-week, now 9-days-old infant is requiring increased isolette heat support despite corrective measures and is now tachycardic and hypotensive. The neonatal nurse practitioner (NNP) recognizes the correct response is to be concerned for a/an:
   A. disseminated septicemia
   B. overstimulation of receptors
   C. patent ductus arteriosus (PDA)

4. The NNP examines a 65-day-old, 1.74 kg, former 33 weeks and finds the infant dressed and swaddled with several blankets in his crib and with recorded axillary temperatures of 98.0–98.4°F (36.7–37°C). Additionally, the growth curve reveals stagnate growth for the past two weeks. The NNP suspects the infant is experiencing:
   A. cold stress resulting in poor overall weight gain
   B. normal premature infant 2-month growth lag
   C. poor growth due to nonfortification of feedings

5. A newly born neonate at 24 3/7 weeks' gestation is placed in an isolette and provided with 85% humidity. The NNP instructs the bedside nurse to keep the isolette walls as dry as possible due to concerns for the infant developing:
   A. hyperthermia
   B. polyuria
   C. septicemia

REFERENCES

Agren, J. (2015). The thermal environment of the intensive care nursery. In R. Martin, A. Fanaroff, & M. Walsh (Eds.), *Fanaroff and Martin's neonatal-perinatal medicine: Diseases of the fetus and infant* (10th ed., pp. 502–512). Philadelphia, PA: Elsevier.

Blackburn, S. (2013). Thermoregulation. In S. Blackburn (Ed.), *Maternal, fetal, & neonatal physiology: A clinical perspective* (4th ed., pp. 657–679). Maryland Heights, MO: Elsevier.

Brand, M., & Boyd, H. (2015). Thermoregulation. In T. Verklan, M. Walden (Eds.), *Core curriculum for neonatal intensive care nursing* (pp. 95–109). St. Louis, MO: Elsevier.

Chatson, K. (2017). Temperature control. In E. Eichenwald, A. Hansen, C. Martin, & A. Stark (Eds.), *Cloherty and Stark's manual of neonatal care* (8th ed., pp. 185–191). Philadelphia, PA: Wolters Kluwer.

Cheffer, N., & Rannalli, D. (2016). Transitional care of the newborn. In S. Mattson & J. Smith (Eds.), *Core curriculum for maternal-newborn nursing* (5th ed.). St. Louis, MO: Elsevier.

Fanaroff, A., & Klaus, M. (2013). The physical environment. In A. Fanaroff & J. Fanaroff (Eds.), *Klaus and Fanaroff's care of the high-risk neonate* (6th ed., pp. 132–150). Cleveland, OH: Elsevier.

Fraser, D. (2016). Newborn adaptation to extrauterine life. In K. Simpson & P. Creehan (Eds.), *Perinatal nursing* (4th ed., pp. 581–596). Philadelphia, PA: Wolters Kluwer/Lippincott Williams & Wilkins.

Gardner, S., & Hernandez, J. (2016). Heat balance. In S. Gardner, B. Carter, E. Hines, & J. Hernandez (Eds.), *Merenstein & Gardner's handbook of neonatal intensive care* (8th ed., pp. 105–125). St. Louis, MO: Elsevier.

Hardy, W., D'agata, A., & Mcgrath, J. (2016). The infant at risk. In S. Mattson & J. Smith (Eds.), *Core curriculum for maternal-newborn nursing* (5th ed.). St. Louis, MO: Elsevier.

Hodson, A. (2018). Temperatures regulation. In C. Gleason & S. Juul (Eds.), *Avery's diseases of the newborn* (10th ed., pp. 361–367). Philadelphia, PA: Elsevier.

Shaw-Battista, J., & Gardner, S. (2017). Newborn transition: The journey from fetal to extrauterine life. In B. J. Snell & S. Gardner (Eds.), *Care of the well newborn* (pp. 69–100). Burlington, MA: Jones & Bartlett Learning.

Verklan, M. (2015). Neurologic disorders. In T. Verklan & M. Walden (Eds.), *Core curriculum for neonatal intensive care nursing* (5th ed., pp. 734–766). St. Louis, MO: Elsevier.

Wilson, D., & Tyner, C. (2015). Infectious diseases in the neonate. In T. Verklan & M. Walden (Eds.), *Core curriculum for neonatal intensive care nursing* (5th ed., pp. 689–718). St. Louis, MO: Elsevier.

9 RESUSCITATION AND DELIVERY ROOM STABILIZATION

Jodi M. Beachy
Barbara Snapp

INTRODUCTION

A successful resuscitation and stabilization require good communication, teamwork, and a thorough understanding of neonatal transitional physiology. This chapter discusses transition, resuscitation, and preparation for transport to another healthcare facility if needed.

The American Academy of Pediatrics (AAP) provides the Neonatal Resuscitation Program (NRP), which is considered the gold standard for neonatal resuscitation and issues a completion certificate which many hospitals require for all the nursing staff in women's and children's services (AAP/NRP, 2019). Although there is an NRP algorithm on the specific steps of resuscitation, this chapter outlines the key components that contribute to understanding normal and abnormal transitional physiology and the science behind proper neonatal resuscitation.

TRANSITION TO EXTRAUTERINE LIFE

General Assessment of Transition

- Transition from a fetus to neonate requires significant physiological adaptation.
- Approximately 10% of newborns will need assistance after delivery in order to transition successfully (Cheffer & Rannalli, 2016, p. 345).
- Immediately after birth, the infant should cry vigorously.
- The need for intervention is determined by the heart rate (HR) and respiratory effort.
- Auscultation of the heart is preferred over digital palpation of the cord (Leon & Finer, 2013, p. 57).
- The Apgar score is not a reliable indicator of the need for resuscitation.
- Low HR and poor respiratory effort are the primary indicators for resuscitation.
- Cardiac monitoring provides the most accurate HR assessment.
- Pulse oximetry is more reliable than a visual assessment of the infant's color (Leon & Finer, 2013, p. 57).
- The newborn may have bradycardia or HR averaging less than 100 beats per minute (bpm) in the first minute post-delivery, but should rise to 140 to 160 bpm by 3 minutes.
- The infant may also experience tachycardia (HR greater than 160 bpm) for the first few minutes after delivery (Leon & Finer, 2013, p. 57; Owen, Weiner, & Davis, 2017, p. 275).
- After birth it is normal for respirations to be somewhat irregular, with mild grunting and nasal flaring (Levy & D'Harlingue, 2015, p. 80).
- Fine rales are normal and may be heard throughout lungs as the lung fluid is cleared (Verklan, 2015, p. 62).

- Successful transition includes the ability to maintain temperature, sustain respiratory effort, and support systemic perfusion throughout the body (Katheria & Finer, 2018, p. 272).

Physiology of Adaptations After Delivery

PULMONARY

- To adapt to extrauterine life, the infant's lungs must fill with air and begin to exchange gases without the placenta.
- Pulmonary vascular resistance (PVR) decreases as blood flows to the lungs.
- Several days prior to delivery, there is a biochemical dehydration of the lungs as fluid is actively moved to the interstitium and then drained through pulmonary and lymphatic systems (Goldsmith, 2015, p. 462).
- The infant's normal opening breath generates 20 to 70 cm water (H_2O) pressure, the amount required to replace lung fluid with air.
- Changes in arterial oxygenation (PaO_2) and carbon dioxide ($PaCO_2$) during delivery affect chemoreceptors, which control depth and rhythm of respirations (Niermeyer, Clarke, & Hernandez, 2016, p. 47).
- The change in the environment from in utero temperature to external environmental temperature, plus touch and noise, can stimulate initial respirations (Verklan, 2015, p. 62).
- A vigorous newborn can generate an adequate functional residual capacity (FRC) with the initial breath. Naturally occurring surfactant reduces surface tension maintaining FRC (Katheria & Finer, 2018, p. 274).
- Lung compliance improves with the help of catecholamines, especially circulating epinephrine (Verklan, 2015, pp. 62–63).

CARDIOVASCULAR

- After birth, the PVR falls drastically while systemic blood pressure increases.
- When the umbilical cord is clamped, the low-pressure placenta is removed and systemic vascular resistance increases.
- The end-of-fetal circulation involves closure of three shunts:
  - Ductus venosus: A right-to-left shunt that closes within minutes of birth due to a cessation of blood flow. Normally gone by 1 week of age in the majority of full-term infants, some will remain open longer in premature infants.
  - Foramen ovale: An opening separating the two atria, allowing for left-to-right blood flow. The foramen ovale usually closes anatomically with the rising left-sided blood pressure, but may remain for up to 30 months.

○ Ductus arteriosus: Closes within days after birth, but may remain patent for several days. By 96 hours, the ductus should be functionally closed in full-term infants; it may occur later in premature infants. Anatomic closure normally occurs by 3 months of age (Blackburn, 2013, pp. 297–299; Owens, Weiner, & Davis, 2017, p. 275).

Hematologic

- The transition from Hg F (fetal hemoglobin [HgF] with a high affinity for oxygen) to Hg A (adult hemoglobin [HgA] with a lower affinity for oxygen) is associated with a rightward shift of the oxyhemoglobin dissociation curve (Martin & Crowley, 2013, pp. 244–269; Verklan, 2015, p. 60).
- The infant transitions from the production of HgF to the production of HgA via increased interaction with 2,3-diphosphoglycerate, which decreases the red cell affinity for oxygen by 3 to 6 months of age.
- Hemoglobin levels increase after birth and then decrease by the seventh day of life (Blackburn, 2013, p. 249).

Metabolic

- Glycogen is a polysaccharide that produces glucose to provide energy to the newborn during transition (Verklan, 2015, p. 60).
- The fetal glucose level is approximately 70% to 80% of maternal glucose level.

NEONATAL RESUSCITATION

Education

- Follow current NRP guidelines.
- Offer mock codes and simulations for knowledge, practice, and quality improvement.
- Review NRP at least annually.
- Review and discuss (debrief) all neonatal codes for quality improvement (Lyndon, O'Brien-Abe, & Rice Simpson, 2014, p. 663; Pappas & Robey, 2015, p. 80).

Preparation

- Develop a system of effective teamwork. Effective teams have clear communication and good leadership. Poor communication and lack of teamwork lead to poor outcomes.
- Have a checklist to evaluate and update equipment as needed.
- Test team-alert system for an appropriate response time (Lyndon, O'Brien-Abe, & Rice Simpson, 2014, p. 663; Pappas & Robey, 2015, p. 80).

Preparation in the Delivery Room

- Preparation is one of the most important factors for successful neonatal resuscitation (Katheria, & Finer, 2018, p. 276).
- Anticipate the needs of the neonate by gestational age, number of fetuses, and other fetal/maternal risk factors.
- Formulate a plan for the correct endotracheal tube size, medications, fluids, and equipment (see Table 9.1).
- Assemble the team and have clear role assignment.

TABLE 9.1 Equipment List for Neonatal Resuscitations

Thermal regulation	Radiant warmer Temperature sensor Blankets Warming mattress/plastic bag <32 wks
Suction equipment	Bulb syringe Mechanical suction device with tubing Suction catheters (8, 10, 12, Fr) Shoulder roll
Ventilation	Self-inflating bag with reservoir (cannot give free-flow oxygen or CPAP) Flow inflating bag (needs gas source, can give blended oxygen 21%–100% oxygen and CPAP) T-piece (needs gas source, PIP/PEEP can be set, can delivery 21%–100% oxygen) Appropriate neonatal-sized mask (covers mouth and nose but not eyes). Oxygen Compressed air, oxygen blender, flow meter 8 Fr feeding tube and syringe Stethoscope
Intubation	Laryngoscope with blades (00, 0, 1) Batteries, bulbs Endotracheal tubes (2.5, 3.0, 3.5) Tube securing device/tape/scissors Colorimetric end-tidal CO_2 detectors Laryngeal mask Pulse oximeter Oral airway
Medications	Epinephrine (0.1 mg/mL concentration) 0.5–1 mL/kg via ETT 0.1–0.03 mL/kg via UVC Normal saline/lactated ringers 10 mL/kg UVC insertion supplies
Monitors	Pulse oximeter/sensor Place on right hand/wrist ECG monitor/leads

CO_2, carbon dioxide; CPAP, continuous positive airway pressure; ECG, electrocardiogram; ETT, endotracheal tube; Fr., French; PEEP, positive end-expiratory pressure; PIP, peak inspiratory pressure; UVC, umbilical venous catheter.

Sources: Data from Goldsmith, J. P. (2015). Overview and initial management of delivery room resuscitation. In R. J. Martin & A. A. Fanaroff (Eds.), *Fanaroff and Martin's neonatal-perinatal medicine* (10th ed., pp. 460–470). Philadelphia, PA: Saunders; Katheria A., & Finer, N. (2018). Newborn resuscitation. In C. Gleason & S. Juul (Eds.), *Avery's diseases of the newborn* (10th ed., pp. 24, 273–288). St. Louis, MO: Elsevier Saunders.

- Pre-warm the room to prevent hypothermia. Obtain plastic wrap and chemically activated warming pad as needed for gestational age of 32 weeks or less. Avoid drafts.
- Gather equipment and ensure proper function.
- Use all resources available for anticipated resuscitation.
- Have the current NRP algorithm available and visible.
- Communicate clearly with the family as to the expected resuscitation and possible outcomes (Pappas & Robey, 2015, pp. 79–81).

Behavioral Skills for Effective Teamwork

- Know your environment.
- Anticipate and make a plan.

- Assume leadership role as assigned.
- Use effective and open communication.
- Delegate the workload.
- Use all available information to plan the resuscitation.
- Recruit more help as needed.
- Remain professional (Pappas & Robey, 2015, p. 81).

Physiology of Resuscitation

- The goal of resuscitation is to prevent morbidity and mortality.
- The most important task is to provide effective ventilation.
- Effective ventilation leads to reduced PVR, which increases blood flow to the lungs and pumps oxygenated blood through the coronary arteries, thus perfusing the heart and increasing the HR (Owen, Davis, & TePas, 2015, p. 276).

Resuscitation Goals

- A neutral thermal environment as hypothermia increases the risk of hypoglycemia, acidosis, and respiratory distress, which may contribute to greater morbidity/mortality
- Good lung expansion and normal breathing to increase oxygen levels to the targeted range
- Adequate cardiac output (Owen, Weiner, & Davis, 2017, p. 278; Ringer, 2017, p. 34)

Initial Resuscitation Steps

- Dry infant with dry, warm blankets and remove wet blankets.
- Infants less than 32 weeks require plastic wrap and a thermal mattress (Niermeyer, Clarke, & Hernandez, 2016, p. 55).
- Stimulate term infants by gently rubbing the back, trunk, extremities, or head.
- Quick assessment after delivery includes:
  - Is the baby term?
  - Is the baby breathing and crying?
  - Is there good tone?
  - If "no" to any of these questions, move the infant to a preheated warmer for further evaluation (Niermeyer, Clarke, & Hernandez, 2016, p. 50).
- Position and clear airway (if needed).
- Place infant on back, head in midline with neck slightly extended; a shoulder pad (towel or blanket) may be needed for infants with large occiput.
- Clear airway as gently as possible with the least invasive method possible. Wipe the nose and mouth with dry towel.
- Suction mouth, then nose, to prevent aspiration.
- Use bulb syringe (preferable) or wall suction catheter.
- Set the suction pressure to 80 to 100 mm mercury (mmHg).
- Avoid deep suction that is prolonged or vigorous, especially during first few minutes, due to risk of trauma, edema, bradycardia, and desaturations, which will cause a delay in PaO_2 rise.
- Prolonged suctioning may cause apnea from vagal stimulation of posterior pharynx and vagus nerve (Niermeyer Clarke, & Hernandez, 2016, pp. 55–56; Pappas & Robey, 2015, p. 85).
- Clearing of the airway is not necessary for every newborn. Suction if secretions are present and obstructing the airway, if there are breathing issues, or if the infant needs bag and mask ventilation (Owen, Weiner, & Davis, 2017, p. 279).

Evaluate Respirations, Oxygenation, and HR

PULSE OXIMETRY

- Use pulse oximetry whenever resuscitation and/or oxygen is needed (Leone & Finer, 2013, p. 57).
- Pulse oximetry is a device that uses a light source (red and infrared) and transmits it to a light receiver. Hemoglobin absorbs the infrared light and deoxyhemoglobin absorbs the red light. The ratio is calculated as a percent of oxygen saturation (SPO_2). The percent of oxygen displayed does not equal partial pressure of oxygen (PaO_2; Carlo & Ambalavana, 2015, pp. 270–288).
- Place the pulse oximeter probe on the preductal right upper extremity. Preductal readings are preferred immediately after birth, as the readings are more reliable than post-ductal saturation readings, which are prone to shunting discrepancies (Ringer, 2017, p. 38).
- Preductal oxygen levels generally should be above 85% to 95% after 10 minutes (Pappas & Robey, 2015, p. 86). Avoid hyperoxia by using the targeted SPO_2 range (Niermeyer, Clarke, & Hernandez, 2016, p. 56). See Table 9.2.

TABLE 9.2 Target Preductal Saturation Goals after Birth (by Minutes of Age)

1 minute	60%–65%
2 minutes	65%–70%
3 minutes	70%–75%
4 minutes	75%–80%
5 minutes	80%–85%
10 minutes	85%–95%

Source: Data from Pappas, B. E., & Robey, D. L. (2015). Neonatal delivery room resuscitation. In M. T. Verklan & M. Walden (Eds.), *Core curriculum of neonatal intensive care nursing* (pp. 77–94). St. Louis, MO: Saunders.

- Pulse oximeters do not always give reliable readings in the first few minutes after delivery.
- Pulse oximetry does not detect changes in carbon dioxide (CO_2).

CARDIAC MONITORING

- Cardiac monitoring is more accurate than pulse oximetry for determining the infant's response to resuscitation. Pulse oximetry relies on circulation, which may be poor; and the cardiac monitor measures the heart's electrical activity.
- EKG leads should be placed when compressions are anticipated/begun (Katheria & Finer, 2018, p. 279).

Oxygen Delivery

BLOW-BY OXYGEN

- Begin oxygen blow-by at flow rate of 5 L per minute and adjust the fraction of inspired oxygen (FiO_2) to meet the preductal saturations per minute-of-life target range.
- Begin blow-by as needed when the HR is above 100 bpm and respiratory rate is adequate but saturations remain below NRP guidelines. Slowly withdraw oxygen as infant's saturations reach the target range (Niermeyer, Clarke, & Hernandez, 2016, pp. 56–58; Pappas & Robey, 2015, p. 89).

POSITIVE PRESSURE VENTILATION (BAG AND MASK)

- Effective assisted ventilation is the single most important intervention in newborn resuscitation (Katharina & Finer, 2018, p. 281; Wyckoff & Goldsmith, 2015, p. 489).
- Delaying effective ventilation negatively impacts an infant's respiratory efforts (Niermeyer, Clarke, & Hernandez, 2016, p. 49).

Indications for Positive Pressure Ventilation (PPV)

- Begin PPV, after initial steps, if the infant is without respiratory effort or has gasping respirations. The lack of respiratory effort increases the partial pressure of carbon dioxide ($PaCO_2$), lowering blood pH and causing metabolic acidosis.
- Start PPV if the HR is below 100 bpm even if breathing.
- If saturations are out of target range with 100% blow-by, start PPV (Niermeyer, Clarke, & Hernandez, 2016, pp. 56–59).

Function and Physiology of PPV

- With adequate lung inflation, FRC is created and oxygenation maintained (Levy & D'Harlingue, 2015, p. 57).
- Surfactant deficiency inhibits the development of adequate FRC and causes alveolar collapse and bradycardia.

Steps in Giving PPV

- Turn on the air and oxygen blend to the bag and mask (Niermeyer, Clarke, & Hernandez, 2016, p. 52).
- Begin at 21% for full-term infants and 21% to 30% for infants under 35 weeks (Katheria & Finer, 2018, p. 489).
- Start with an initial positive end-expiratory pressure (PEEP) setting of 5 cm of water (H_2O) and a peak inspiratory pressure (PIP) setting of 20 cm H_2O.
- Prepare appropriate mask size. Mask should cover chin, mouth and nose, but not eyes (Niermeyer, Clarke, & Hernandez, 2016, p. 59).
- Position infant and make sure that airway is clear.
- Apply mask and apply proper seal with the fingers in "C" shape around the mask. Apply gentle pressure to the neonate's face. There should be no leaks between mask and face (Niermeyer, Clarke, & Hernandez, 2016, p. 59).
- Provide PPV at a rate of 40 to 60 breaths per minute.
- Use an initial PIP of 20 cm H_2O and increase to 30 cm H_2O or more as needed for chest movement. PIP should be limited to the lowest pressure required to create adequate chest rise and aeration of the lungs.
- Continue to observe frequently for good chest expansion, improved HR, and targeted saturations.
- Spontaneous breathing is a sign of effective ventilation and overall improvement (Niermeyer, Clarke, & Hernandez, 2016, pp. 59–60).
- Delivering PEEP with PPV will improve FRC, inflate alveoli, and reduce work of breathing (Owen, Davis, & TePas, 2015, pp. 471–481).
- Place orogastric tube through mouth (to maximize ventilation through nose) after several minutes of ventilation to prevent air distention elevating the diaphragm and reducing lung volume (Pappas & Robey, 2015, p. 87).

Continuous Positive Airway Pressure (CPAP)

- Once respirations and HR are established, CPAP will:
  - Minimize lung injury caused by pressure ventilation.
  - Improve gas exchange.
  - Increase lung compliance by stabilizing the chest wall FRC (Niermeyer, Clarke, & Hernandez, 2016, p. 59).
- It is preferable to use a T-piece resuscitator with an appropriately sized mask.
- The PEEP may need to be increased for effective ventilation.
- Mask must have a secure seal to deliver PEEP and oxygen (Katheria & Finer, 2018; Niemeyer, Clark, & Hernandez, 2016).

Endotracheal Intubation (ETT)

INDICATIONS

- Used for prolonged PPV or failure to respond to initial resuscitation measures
- Appropriate in the presence of a diaphragmatic hernia or other congenital anomalies
- Needed for surfactant administration
- Suction of trachea is needed.

Confirmation of Endotracheal Tube (ETT) Placement

- Bilateral breath sounds are heard near axilla, condensation in tube, chest rise, HR increase, and color change of colorimetric carbon dioxide detector.
- The longer it takes to achieve effective PPV, the longer it takes for the infant's respiratory effort to become effective.
- Risks: Intubation can cause trauma to the trachea, mouth, pharynx, and vocal cords. Hypoxia and bradycardia may occur if procedure takes more than 30 seconds per attempt (Leone & Finer, 2013, p. 61; Niermeyer, Clarke, & Hernandez, 2016 pp. 61–62).

Laryngeal Mask Airway (LMA)

INDICATIONS

- Unable to intubate, Trisomy 21, Pierre Robin, other airway anomalies

LIMITATIONS

- Medications cannot be given through an LMA, nor can the infant be suctioned through the LMA. Generally, it is not used for infants under 1.5 kg or under 31 weeks' gestation (Katheria & Finer, 2018, p. 283; Owen, Weiner, & Davis, 2015, p. 283).

Use of Acronym MRSOPA

- Acronym is used to help remember resuscitation steps in proper order. See Box 9.1.

Chest Compressions

- Chest compressions are a rare occurrence in neonatal resuscitation (Leon & Finer, 2013, p. 61).
- Primary goal is to perfuse the heart and brain.

BOX 9.1 MRSOPA Mnemonic

> **Ma**sk repositioned on the face and check seal
> **Re**position of airway, avoiding hyperextension or flexion of the neck
> **S**uction mouth and nose
> **O**pen mouth slightly with jaw lifted forward
> **P**ressure increase gradually
> **A**irway alternative with intubation or laryngeal mask airway

Source: Data from Pappas, B. E., & Robey, D. L. (2015). Neonatal delivery room resuscitation. In M. T. Verklan & M. Walden (Eds.), *Core curriculum of neonatal intensive care nursing* (pp. 77–94). St. Louis, MO: Saunders.

- Begin chest compressions per NRP guidelines.
  - If HR less than 60 bpm despite 30 seconds of effective bag and mask (with time given for MRSOPA) in tandem with PPV. Plan to intubate.
  - Increase FiO$_2$ to 100% once chest compressions begin.
- Beginning chest compression too early may interfere with proper ventilation.
- Thumb technique is preferred and should be used whenever possible.
- Two thumbs are preferred as it improves the depth of compressions, is more accurate than the hand around chest method and is less fatiguing for the provider (Katheria & Finer, 2018, pp. 489–491).

PHYSIOLOGY OF CHEST COMPRESSIONS
- Chest compressions squeeze the heart and pushes it against the spine, increasing intrathoracic pressure creating blood circulation (Wyckoff & Goldsmith, 2015, pp. 489–490).

Method
- Placement of thumbs should be on the lower one-third of the sternum between the nipples. A compression is straight down (to minimize lung or rib damage) to one-third of anterior–posterior chest diameter while hands encircle chest.
- Compressions deeper than one-third of the chest diameter do not improve hemodynamics and increase the risk of injury (Wyckoff & Goldsmith, 2015, pp. 489–491).
- Use a 3:1 ratio with 90 compressions to 30 breaths.
- Fingers or thumbs should remain on the chest to prevent complications from incorrect placement and unproductive time reestablishing correct placement (Katheria & Finer, 2018, pp. 489–491).
- The two-thumb technique is preferred as it more effective in increasing blood pressure during asphyxial asystole (Wyckoff & Goldsmith, 2015, pp. 489–499).

COMPLICATIONS AND RISKS OF CHEST COMPRESSIONS
- Liver laceration due to dislocation of xiphoid process may occur if compressions are performed too low on the sternum.
- Rib fractures, flail chest when the rib breaks and becomes detached, and pneumothorax may occur if compressions are performed off to the side of sternum (Niermeyer, Clarke, & Hernandez, 2016, p. 64).

Medications Used in Resuscitation

EPINEPHRINE
Indications
- HR less than 60 beats a minute despite 60 seconds of adequate coordinated ventilation and compressions. The heart is now without energy (adenosine triphosphate or ATP) and will no longer beat adequately.

Effect
- Epinephrine increases the HR and improves contractility through the action of beta receptor agonists restricting blood vessels and relaxing lung airways (Wyckoff & Goldsmith, 2015, pp. 491–492), counteracting the vasodilation caused by acidosis.

Route
- Umbilical venous catheter (UVC) placement has better effectiveness and absorption and is more reliable than through endotracheal tube
- Pulmonary fluid retention may dilute an endotracheal dose and a right-to-left shunt may bypass the pulmonary circulation (Katheria & Finer, 2018, pp. 284–286).

Dose
- Calculate dose (0.1–0.3 mL/kg intravenous (IV) push or ETT 0.5 to 1 mL/kg, followed with 1 mL normal saline (NS) neonatal concentration (0.1 mg/mL). May be repeated every 3 to 5 minutes.

RISKS
- Extravasations
- Hepatic injury (seen with low-lying UVC)
- Adverse drug effects
- Hypertension
- Hyperadrenergic effect (Katheria & Finer, pp. 284, 491–492; Niermeyer, Clarke, & Hernandez, 2016, pp. 64–66).
- High epinephrine dose risks: hypertension, hyperadrenergic state, germinal matrix hemorrhage, and cardiac damage.

Volume Expanders

Indications
- To improve a poor response to resuscitation after adequate ventilation and oxygenation or evidence of acute blood loss, suspected shock, or hypovolemia
- Increases circulating blood volume

Use
- Given after adequate resuscitation and the administration of epinephrine (Pappas, & Robey, 2017, p. 89; Ringer, 2017, p. 47).

Types of Volume Expanders

- Normal saline NS (preferred), Ringer's lactate, and O-negative blood (Pappas & Robey, 2015, p. 89)
- O-negative blood has the benefit of volume and oxygen-carrying capacity (Katheria & Finer, 2018, pp. 492–493).

Effect
- Fluids increase circulating blood volume to improve hypovolemia, and for effective closure of right-to-left circulatory shunts (Ringer, 2017, p. 33) and improved tissue perfusion (Pappas & Robey, 2015, p. 89).

Route
- IV infusion

Dose
- 10 mL/kg over 5 to 10 minutes via peripheral IV or UVC
- May repeat if no improvement after assessed for adverse effects and results.

Risks

- Volume overload and intraventricular hemorrhage (Niermeyer, Clarke, & Hernandez, 2016, p. 66)

Post-Resuscitation Care

- After significant resuscitation, close assessment of the infant is crucial. Any or all of the following may need to be assessed:
  ○ Vital signs, including temperature
  ○ Neurological status
  ○ Breath sounds, work of breathing (look for grunting, nasal flaring, and retractions, symmetry of chest movement)
  ○ Ventilation and oxygenation through arterial (preferable) or capillary blood gases
  ○ Blood glucose and electrolytes
  ○ Anemia, hypovolemia or polycythemia, hyperviscosity
- Perfusion and cap refill (Katheria & Finer, 2018, p. 288; Pappas & Robey, 2015, pp. 92–94; Owen, Weiner, & Davis, 2017, p. 290)

Complicated Resuscitation Situations

- Pneumothorax:
  ○ Unequal breath sounds
  ○ Sudden deterioration
  ○ Shifted or distant heart sounds
  ○ Uneven chest (Wyckoff & Goldsmith, 2015, p. 495)
- Choanal atresia:
  ○ Signs include:
    ▪ Cyanosis when not crying and pink when crying
    ▪ Obstruction of nares (Pappas & Robey, 2015, p. 90)
- Pulmonary hypoplasia may be indicated by difficult ventilation due to small lungs.
- Congenital diaphragmatic hernia
  ○ Cardinal signs include:
    ▪ Scaphoid abdomen
    ▪ Bowel sounds in chest
    ▪ One-sided decreased breath sounds
    ▪ 85% of the defects are found on the left side, as the right side is blocked by the liver (Pappas & Robey, 2015, pp. 90–91; Wyckoff & Goldsmith, 2015, p. 495).
- Maternal anesthesia or narcotic use affecting the infant may present as persistent respiratory depression (Pappas & Robey, 2015, p. 90).

DELAYED CORD CLAMPING (DCC)

Definition

- Blood flow to infant from the placenta will continue for 1 to 2 minutes after birth (Niermeyer, Clarke, & Hernandez, 2016, p. 50).
- Delayed umbilical cord clamping is defined as a 30- to 60-second pause before clamping the cord in order to allow for placental transfusion of blood to the infant (Katheria & Finer, 2018, pp. 277–279).

Benefits

- DCC is especially beneficial to premature infants, but is also recommended for full-term infants.
  ○ Decreases the need for transfusions
  ○ Increases hemoglobin and iron stores in early infancy
  ○ Reduces anemia during first 6 months of life
  ○ Increases cardiac output
  ○ Increases circulatory stability

- Increases blood volume by 15% to 20% with an additional of 30-150 ml of blood from the placenta
- Improves physiologic stability
- Increases lung-fluid absorption
- Increases oxygen-carrying capacity to tissues
- Decreases intraventricular hemorrhage for all grades
- Decreases necrotizing enterocolitis (NEC)
- Has shown no increased morbidities, but is shown to decrease mortality (Katheria & Finer, 2018, pp. 277–279; Niermeyer, Clarke, & Hernandez, 2016, p. 50).

Risks of Delay Cord Clamping

- Transient tachypnea
- Polycythemia and/or hyperbilirubinemia (Katheria & Finer, 2018, p. 277)

CORD BLOOD GAS

- Cord blood gases have a broader range of normal than postnatal blood gas values (Barry, Deacon, Hernandez, & Jones, 2016, pp. 154–155).
- Cord blood gases provide information on how the fetus's condition is immediately prior to delivery (Lyndon, O'Brien, & Rice Simpson, 2014, p 481). See Table 9.3.

TABLE 9.3 Cord Blood Gas Ranges

Measure	Venous	Arterial
Ph	7.25–7.45	7.18–7.38
pCO_2 (mmHg)	26.8–49.2	32.2–65.8
PaO_2 (mmHg)	17.2–40.8	5.6–30.8
HCO_3 (mmol/L)	15.8–24.2	17–27
Base deficit (mmol/L)	0–8	0–8

Source: Data from Barry, J., Deason, J., Hernandez, C., & Jones, M. D. (2016). Acid-base homeostasis and oxygenation. In Gardner et al. (Eds.), *Handbook of neonatal intensive care.* St Louis, MO: Elsevier.

Occasions for Cord Blood Sampling

- Cord blood samples are performed when events of pregnancy or labor are connected to adverse outcomes in the neonate.
- These may include:
  ○ Severe intrauterine growth restriction (IUGR)
  ○ Abnormal fetal HR tracings
  ○ Cesarean section for fetal compromise
  ○ A low five-minute Apgar score (Barry, Deacon, Hernandez, & Jones, 2016, pp. 154–155)
  ○ Preterm and postterm infants
  ○ Multiparous gestations
  ○ Thick meconium stained amniotic fluid
  ○ Maternal thyroid disease (Lyndon, O'Brien-Abel, & Rice, Simpson, 2014, p. 481)

Sample Collection

- The cord can be saved, but must be drawn by 1 hour after birth if at room temperature and by 6 hours if refrigerated (Barry, Deacon, Hernandez, & Jones, 2016, pp. 154–155).

Principles of Cord Gas Interpretation

- In utero, the umbilical cord vein transports oxygenated blood from the placenta to the fetus and the umbilical arteries transport blood back to the placenta (Barry, Deacon, Hernandez, & Jones, 2016, pp. 154–155).
- The umbilical cord arterial blood gas is more valuable than the umbilical cord venous blood gas for determining neonatal acid base status because it represents both the fetal and uteroplacental states (Lyndon, O'Brien-Abel, & Rice SImpson, 2014, p. 481).
- Umbilical venous blood reflects the uteroplacental state only.
  - Metabolic acidosis occurs when decreased oxygenation leads to increased lactic acid, decreased bicarbonate, and increased base deficit (BD; Lyndon, O'Brien, & Rice Simpson, 2013, p. 481).

PREDICTIVE VALUE

- Asphyxia is caused by an interruption in exchange of gases and metabolic acidosis (Niermeyer Clarke, & Hernandez, 2016, pp. 48–49).
- The pH as a solo indicator is a poor predictor of long-term outcomes.
- pH less than 7.00 with abnormal neurologic assessment is associated with poor outcomes.
- Encephalopathy is seen in 10% of infants with base deficit (BD) of 12 to 16 mmol/L and in 40% of those infants with a BD over 16 mmol/L (Lyndon, O'Brien-Abel, & Rice Simpson, 2014, p. 481).

NEONATAL TRANSPORT

Levels of Care

The AAP and the American College of Obstetricians and Gynecologists in their *Guidelines for Perinatal Care* established classifications of perinatal resources according to different levels of care. These include:

Level I: Well Newborn Nursery
- Provide NRP and S.T.A.B.L.E (Sugar, Airway, Blood Pressure, Lab Work, and Emotional Support), postnatal care for stable full-term infants, stabilize and care for infants 35 to 37 weeks if stable, and stabilize ill infants and those less than 35 weeks to prepare for transfer.

Level II: Special Care Nursery
- Care for infants 32 weeks and above, infants after intensive care, some assisted ventilation; stabilize infants less than 32 weeks for transport.

Level III: Neonatal Intensive Care
- Care for infants less than 32 weeks. Provide full respiratory support and appropriate support services, and perform MRI and echocardiology.

Level IV: Regional NICU
- Provide level III care plus provide surgery and facilitate outreach (Rojas, Furlong Craven, & Rush, 2016, pp. 33–34).

Regionalization

- Data show that the transfer of high-risk pregnant women has better outcomes than transfer of the infant after delivery. When this is not possible, neonatal transport to the appropriate level care offers a second option that will also improve outcomes (Insoft, 2017, pp. 425–426).
- The regionalization of neonatal care has led to the development of specialized teams to transfer infants from outlying hospitals to a higher level of care.
- The composition of the team is less significant than the experience and skill level of the team members. Transport teams often bring a level of care that may not be available at the referral center and require a high level of competency (Insoft, pp. 425–426).

Education and Skills

- Minimal education requirements are standardized by the AAP Section on Transport Medicine (SOTM, 2019). At minimum, the teams need to be educated by participating in the NRP and the American Heart Association basic life support (BLS) training.
- The team members need to be well versed on neonatal physiology (Insoft, pp. 425–426) and able to anticipate the possibility of deterioration during transport and respond (O'Mahony & Woodward, 2018, p. 350).
- A minimum of two years' experience in level III NICU is recommended (Rojas, Furlong Craven, & Rush, 2016, pp. 33–34).
- Team members should have comprehensive education, maintain continuing education, and maintain skills with skills labs (Insoft, pp. 425–426).
- Stabilization may include intubation for control of the airway and/or the placement of central lines for access (O'Mahony & Woodward, 2018, p. 350).
- Other skills include treatment of pneumothorax, treatment of shock, ability to treat cyanotic heart disease with medication (Levy & D'Harlinque, 2015, p. 99), bag and mask ventilation, venous and arterial access, intubation, and placement of LMA (Bowen, 2015, p. 413).

Unique Physiological Impact of Air and Ground Transportation

- During air transportation, there is a greater risk of hypoxia with the increase in altitude as the alveolar partial pressure of oxygen falls.
- Ground transportation can be jarring to the neonates.
- Both transports can incur high noise levels, and some teams will use ear protection on the neonate to reduce the high noise levels.
- Thermoregulation can be a challenge when dealing with outside temperatures and altitude (Insoft, pp. 426–427).

Legal Issues

- The liability and level of responsibility between receiving and referring personnel is a shared responsibility and is open to legal interpretation.
- The responsibilities of the receiving institution increase from time of accepting the patient to the arrival at receiving hospital (Bowen, 2015, p. 424; O'Mahony & Woodward, 2018, p. 353).
- Parents must be told of risks and benefits of transportation (Bowen, 2015, p. 424).

CONCLUSION

The transition from intrauterine to extrauterine existence is a critical time with multiple, important, and necessary physiological changes occurring simultaneously. Any disruption in these processes can threaten the life of the infant and/or create lifelong morbidities. Although the steps in neonatal resuscitation are clearly outlined by the AAP NRP, the NNP must have a thorough understanding of underlying physiological principles to not only comprehend the "how to," but, perhaps, more importantly, the "why." A basic tenet of neonatology is providing care appropriate for gestational age, and resuscitation measures must be correctly tailored and adjusted to each and every delivery in order to achieve the desired outcomes.

Key Points

1. Thoroughly plan and prepare for a resuscitation.
2. Ensure excellent communication with obstetrical colleagues, parents, and team members.
3. Understand underlying physiological transition principles.
4. Follow the NRP algorithm.
5. Recognize that *effective* ventilation is the most important resuscitation step.
6. Debrief in order to improve outcomes.

REVIEW QUESTIONS

1. An appropriate situation in which to consider obtaining cord blood gases is when an infant is:
   A. assigned a 5-minute Apgar of less than 3
   B. compromised by a one-time tight nuchal cord
   C. designated as large for gestational age

2. Benefits of delayed cord clamping include increased:
   A. cardiac output
   B. fluid retention
   C. bilirubin levels

3. An appropriate indication for the use of epinephrine (Adrenalin) during a neonatal resuscitation event is when the heart rate remains low despite adequate ventilation and compressions for a duration of:
   A. 40 seconds
   B. 60 seconds
   C. 90 seconds

4. The correct statement regarding ECG cardiac monitoring during a newborn resuscitation is that ECG leads:
   A. are not as accurate as the use of a stethoscope
   B. depend on adequate circulation for accuracy
   C. should be placed when compressions are initiated

5. The most appropriate location for a mother to deliver an infant who is at 31 weeks' gestation and has known congenital anomalies is at a hospital with a NICU designated Level:
   A. II
   B. III
   C. IV

REFERENCES

AAP/NRP. (2019). *Neonatal resuscitation.* Retrieved from https://www.aap.org/en-us/continuing-medical-education/life-support/NRP/Pages/NRP.aspx

AAP/SOTM. (2019). *Section on transport medicine.* Retrieved from https://www.aap.org/en-us/about-the-aap/Sections/Section-on-Transport-Medicine/Pages/SOTM.aspx

Barry, J., Deason, J., Hernandez, C., & Jones, M. D. (2016). Acid-base homeostasis and oxygenation. In S. L. Gardner, B. S. Carter, M. E. Hires & J. A. Hernandez (Eds.), *Handbook of neonatal intensive care.* (8th ed. pp. 145-157.e1). St. Louis, MO. Elsevier, Inc.

Blackburn, S. (2013). *Maternal, fetal & neonatal physiology, a clinical perspective* (pp. 247–150, 295–300, 337–341). St. Louis, MO: Saunders.

Bowen, S. L. (2015). Intrafacility and interfacility neonatal transport. In M. T. Verklan & M. Walden (Eds.), *Core curriculum of neonatal intensive care nursing* (pp. 407–425). St. Louis, MO: Saunder.

Carlo, W. A., & Ambalavana, N. (2015). Assisted ventilation. In A. A. Fanaroff (Ed.), *Klaus & Fanaroff's care of the high risk neonate* (6th ed., pp. 270–288). St. Louis, MO: Elsevier-Saunders.

Cheffer, N., & Rannalli, D. (2016). Transitional care of the newborn. In S. Mattson & J. Smith (Eds.), *Core curriculum maternal-newborn nursing* (pp. 345–362). Philadelphia, PA. Elsevier, Inc.

Goldsmith, J. P. (2015). Overview and initial management of delivery room resuscitation. In R. J. Martin & A. A. Fanaroff (Eds.), *Fanaroff and Martin's neonatal-perinatal medicine* (10th ed., pp. 460–470). Philadelphia, PA: Saunders.

Insoft, R. (2017). Transport of the intubated neonate. In J. Goldsmith, E. Karotkin, G. Suresh, & M. Keszler (Eds.), *Assisted ventilation of the neonate, an evidence-based approach to newborn respiratory care* (6th ed., pp. 425–430). St. Louis, MO: Saunders Elsevier.

Katheria A., & Finer, N. (2018). Newborn resuscitation. In C. Gleason & S. Juul (Eds.), *Avery's diseases of the newborn* (10th ed., pp. 24, 273–288). St. Louis, MO: Elsevier Saunders.

Leon, T. A., & Finer, N. (2013). Resuscitation at birth. In M. H. Klaus, & A. A. Fanaroff (Eds.), *Klaus and Fanaroff's care of the high risk neonate* (6th ed., pp. 54–70). St. Louis, MO: Elsevier Saunders.

Levy, J., & D'Harlingue, A. (2015). Recognition, stabilization, and transport of the high-risk newborn. In M. H. Klaus & A. A. Fanaroff (Eds.), *Klaus and Fanaroff's care of the high risk neonate* (6th ed., pp. 71–104). St. Louis, MO: Elsevier-Saunders.

Lyndon, A., O'Brien-Abel, N., & Rice Simpson, K. (2014). Fetal assessment during labor. In K. R. Simpson & P. A. Creenhan (Eds.), *AWHONN's perinatal nursing* (pp. 480–482). Philadelphia, PA: LWW.

Manco-Johnson, M., McKinney, C., Knapp-Clevenger, R., & Hernandez, J. A. (2017). Newborn heatology. In S. L. Gardner, B. S. Carter, M. E. Hines, & I. A. Hernandez (Eds.), *Handbook of neonatal intensive care* (pp. 479–510). St Louis, MO: Elsevier.

Martin, R. J., & Crowley, M. A. (2013). Respiratory problems. In A. Fanaroff & J. Fanaroff (Eds.), *Klaus and Fanaroff's care of the high risk neonate* (6th ed., pp. 244–269). St. Louis, MO: Elsevier-Saunder.

Niermeyer, S., Clarke, S., & Hernandez, J. (2016). Delivery room care. S. L. Gardner, B. S. Carter, M. E. Hines, & J. A. Hernandez (Eds.), *Handbook of neonatal intensive care* (pp. 47–70). St. Louis, MO: Elsevier.

O'Mahony, L., & Woodward, G. (2018). Neonatal transport. In C. A. Gleason, & S. E. Juul (Eds.), *Avery's diseases of the newborn* (10th ed., pp. 347–353). St. Louis, MO: Elsevier Saunders.

Owen, L., Davis, P., & TePas, A. B. (2015). Role of positive pressure ventilation in neonatal resuscitation. In R. J. Martin, A. A. Fanaroff, & M. C. Walsh (Eds.), *Fanaroff & Martin's neonatal-perinatal medicine: Disease of the fetus and infant* (10th ed., pp. 471–281). St. Louis, MO: Elsevier Mosby.

Owen, L. S., Weiner, G. M., & Davis, P. G. (2017). Delivery room stabilization and respiratory support. In J. Goldsmith, E. Karotkin, G. Suresh, & M. Keszler (Eds.), *Assisted ventilation of the neonate, an evidence-based approach to newborn respiratory care* (6th ed., pp. 275–290). St. Louis, MO: Saunders Elsevier.

Pappas, B. E., & Robey, D. L. (2015). Neonatal delivery room resuscitation. In M. T. Verklan & M. Walden (Eds.), *Core curriculum of neonatal intensive care nursing* (pp. 77–94). St. Louis, MO: Saunders.

Ringer, S. A. (2017). Resuscitation in the delivery room. In E. Eichenwald, A. Hansen, C. Martin, & A. Stark (Eds.), *Cloherty and Stark's manual of neonatal care* (8th ed., p. 33). Philadelphia, PA: Lippincott, Williams & Wilkins.

Rojas, M., Furlong Craven, H., & Rush, T. (2016). Perinatal transport and level of care. In S. Gardner, B. Carter, M. Hines, & J. Hernandez (Eds.), *Handbook of neonatal intensive care* (pp. 33–34). St. Louis, MO: Elsevier.

Verklan, T. M. (2015). Adaptation to extrauterine life. In T. M. Verklan & M. Walden (Eds.), *Core curriculum of neonatal intensive care nursing* (pp. 58–63). St. Louis, MO: Saunders.

Wyckoff, M., & Goldsmith, J. (2015). Chest compression, medications and special problems in neonatal resuscitation. In R. J. Martin, & A. A. Fanaroff (Eds.), *Fanaroff & Martin's neonatal-perinatal medicine* (10th ed., pp. 489–493). St. Louis, MO: Elsevier Mosby.

10 NEONATAL NUTRITION

Julie E. Williams
Hope Mckendree
Karen Stadd

INTRODUCTION

Proper nutrition is imperative to ensure optimal neonatal growth and development. Term infants are often able to successfully transition to extrauterine life as they have received the appropriate amount of nutrient accretion. Preterm infants have a limited amount of nutrient accretion and, therefore, a lower reserve than term infants. The success of the preterm infant's postnatal growth and development is dependent on the management of the infant's medical conditions and nutritional demands. As medical technology continues to improve preterm survival rates, it is crucial to maximize nutritional requirements for optimal growth and development.

PHYSIOLOGY OF DIGESTION AND ABSORPTION

Principles of Gastrointestinal (GI) Development and Function

- Morphogenesis and cellular differentiation affect the embryologic formation of the GI tract. However, functional digestive development continues following birth (Dimmitt, Sellers, & Sibley, 2018, p. 1032).
- Postnatal GI function and development are influenced by genetic endowment, gut trophic factors, and hormonal regulatory mechanisms involved with enteral feeding initiation and feeding type (Blackburn, 2013, p. 418).
- Maintenance of GI development and function requires interaction with the intrauterine environment, followed with postnatal exogenous environmental exposures (McElroy, Frey, Torres, & Maheshwari, 2018, p. 1054).

Embryology of the GI Tract

- A series of folding, lengthening, and luminal dilation during the fourth week of gestation results in formation of the:
  - foregut (esophagus, stomach, duodenum, liver, and pancreas)
  - midgut (jejunum, ileum, ascending colon, and transverse colon)
  - hindgut (descending colon, sigmoid colon, and rectum; Dimmitt al., 2018, p. 1032)
- During the sixth week of gestation, the small intestines and colon herniate into the umbilical cord due to the rapid growth of the liver, permitting direct communication between the fetal GI tract and the in utero environment (Dimmitt et al., 2018, p. 1032; Parry, 2015, p. 1365).

Therefore, the fetal intestinal tract is bathed in amniotic fluid during the early second trimester (McElroy et al., 2018, p. 1054).
- Intestinal villi appear during 8 to 11 weeks' gestation, acquiring finger-like shape by 14 weeks' gestation (Parry, 2015, p. 1365).
- By 20 weeks' gestation, the abdominal cavity migrates into the umbilical cord by rotating counterclockwise around the superior mesenteric artery, resulting in the colon being located anterior to the small intestines, with the cecum located in the right lower quadrant (Dimmitt et al., 2018, p. 1032). During this 270-degree rotation, the duodenum becomes fixed in the retroperitoneal position from the pylorus to the ligament of Treitz. Any failure of rotation and fixation can cause twisting of the bowel on its mesentery, with subsequent interruption of blood flow to the intestines (Parry, 2015, p. 1365).
  - The basic morphogenesis of the fetal GI tract is completed by the second trimester, but additional in utero and postnatal functional maturation is still necessary (Dimmitt et al., 2018, p. 1032).

Role of Amniotic Fluid

- Amniotic fluid is considered the first environmental exposure required for GI development, which varies in volume and composition over the gestational period. This dynamic fluid initially consists of water and solute from maternal plasma, which is delivered to the fetus via the placenta. By the second half of pregnancy, the fetus actively contributes to the volume and composition of amniotic fluid via swallowing and urination (McElroy et al., 2018, p. 1054).
- Amniotic fluid is enriched with hormones, cytokines, growth factors, nutrients, and other plasma proteins to facilitate GI development and the associated immune system (McElroy et al., 2018, p. 1054).
- Fetal swallowing of amniotic fluid occurs by 8 to 11 weeks' gestation, progressively reaching 500 mL/day in the third trimester (McElroy et al., 2018, p. 1054).
- By the end of the third trimester, amniotic fluid provides approximately 25% of the enteral protein intake of a term breastfed infant (Poindexter & Ehrenkranz, 2015, p. 597).

Meconium Production

- Meconium consists of material and secretions such as ingested amniotic fluid, lanugo, intestinal cells, bile salts, and pancreatic enzymes that are created by or swallowed by the fetus in utero (Blackburn, 2013, p. 420).

GI Development

- Phases of GI development span from early embryogenesis until the introduction of solid foods in late infancy to early childhood (McElroy et al., 2018, p. 1054).
  - ○ Phase I: Embryonic organogenesis and primitive gut formation
  - ○ Phase II: The GI tract becomes a tubular structure with the formation of villi, initiating the functional role of the intestinal epithelium.
  - ○ Phase III: Rapid linear intestinal growth and cellular differentiation for specific physiologic functions
  - ○ Phase IV: The intestinal microbiome is established immediately after birth from environmental exposures, including response to dietary factors present in human milk or formula.
  - ○ Phase V: Refinement and maturation of structural intestinal development and mucosal immunity occur after weaning from breast milk or formula while introducing solid food (McElroy et al., 2018, p. 1054).

Functional Development

- GI organs develop and acquire different digestive capacities during embryogenesis (Dimmitt et al., 2018, p. 1037).
- Intestinal transport of amino acids (AAs) is seen by 14 weeks of gestation, followed by intestinal transport of glucose by 18 weeks' gestation and fatty acid by 24 weeks' gestation (Ditzenberger, 2015, p. 172).
- Major gut-regulating polypeptides (gastrin, motilin, cholecystokinin, pancreatic polypeptide, and somatostatin) act locally to regulate gut growth and development. They are present in limited amounts by the end of the first trimester and reach adult distribution by term (Blackburn, 2013, p. 418).
- Gastric gland secretion activity is seen by 20 weeks of gestation, and salivary amylase and mucosal glucoamylase are functionally active after 27 weeks' gestation (Ditzenberger, 2015, p. 172).
- Lingual and gastric lipase are present by 26 weeks' gestation in limited volume and function (Dimmitt et al., 2018, p. 1037).

Functions of the GI Tract

- The primary function of the GI tract is digestion and absorption of ingested nutrients from food. The small intestine is responsible for digestion and absorption of nutrients, where the colon absorbs more than 80% of water left after passage through the small intestine (Parry, 2015, p. 1365).
- The GI tract serves as the largest defense barrier and immune organ in the body by protecting against dietary and environmental antigens (McElroy et al., 2018, p. 1054).

Immunity

- Physical and chemical barriers within the GI tract prevent epithelial adherence and translocation of pathogens between paracellular spaces. The first layer of immune defenses includes the acidic stomach environment, compounded with numerous digestive enzymes and bile salts along the entire GI tract (McElroy et al., 2018, p. 1054). Gastric acid, bile salts, and pancreatic secretions inhibit potential pathogenic bacterial growth (Dimmitt et al., 2018, p. 1036).
- Healthy intestinal microbiomes are necessary to compete with pathogenic organisms for cell surface binding sites. Consequently, protective gut flora regulates intestinal inflammation by increasing the production of anti-inflammatory cytokines and decreasing proinflammatory cytokines (McElroy et al., 2018, p. 1054).
- Preterm infants are at increased risk for altered mucosal immunity and intestinal bacterial colonization due to an underdeveloped immune system, hospital environmental exposures, and medical interventions (McElroy et al., 2018, p. 1054).
- Delayed or absent enteral nutrition leads to a lack of luminal nutrients, resulting in decreased intestinal mass, mucosal enzyme activity, and gut permeability (Poindexter & Ehrenkranz, 2015, p. 597).

Digestion

- Digestion consists of breaking down carbohydrates, proteins, and fats into smaller molecules (monosaccharides, oligopeptides, AAs, free fatty acids, and monoglycerides), which are transported into absorptive intestinal epithelial cells, followed by the portal circulation (Dimmitt et al., 2018, p. 1037).
- Biochemical and physiologic capacities for limited digestion and absorption are present by 28 weeks' gestation (Blackburn, 2013, p. 415; Ditzenberger, 2015, p. 172).
- Enteroglucagon promotes intestinal mucosal growth. Gastrin stimulates gastric mucosa and exocrine pancreas growth. Motilin and neurotensin stimulate the development of gut motility (Blackburn, 2013, p. 418).
- Preterm infants are born with an underdeveloped GI tract, with immature function such as limited production of gut digestive enzymes and growth factors and decreased gut absorption of lipids due to low levels of pancreatic lipase, bile acids, and lingual lipase (Blackburn, 2013, p. 418; Ditzenberger, 2015, p. 172).
- Enteral feeding is a major stimulus for hormonal regulatory mechanisms needed to mediate gut development after birth in both preterm and term infants. Gastric inhibitory peptide promotes glucose tolerance (Blackburn, 2013, pp. 418–419).

GI Motility

- GI motility refers to the coordinated movement of food from ingestion to elimination, including suck–swallow, esophageal, stomach, and intestinal peristalsis.
- Immature gut motility and gastric emptying are a major limitation to enteral digestion, which progressively improves after 30 to 32 weeks' gestation until term (Blackburn, 2013, p. 420; Ditzenberger, 2015, p. 172).
- Passage of meconium is an essential step in the initiation of intestinal function. Most full-term infants pass meconium within 48 hours of birth (Blackburn, 2013, pp. 420–422).
- Delayed passage of stool and constipation are common complications among preterm infants. Only 37% of preterm infant pass meconium by 24 hours of life, 69% by 48 hours of life, and 99% by 9 days of life (Blackburn, 2013, p. 420).

ASSESSMENT OF NEONATAL GROWTH

- Accretion of most nutrients occurs during the latter portion of the second trimester and throughout the third trimester in preparation for a term delivery.
- Term infants have adequate minerals, glycogen, and fat stores to meet the demands of the first few days of relative starvation experienced immediately after birth (Anderson, Poindexter, & Martin, 2017, p. 248).
- Preterm infants miss out on in utero accretion of fat, glycogen, iron, calcium, and phosphorus stores. Therefore, early and appropriate nutrition is essential for the growth and neurodevelopmental outcomes of the preterm infant (Adamkin, Radmacher, & Lewis, 2013, p. 151).

Growth and Nutritional Assessment

- Postnatal growth begins with a period of weight loss, primarily due to extracellular water loss. Consequently, it is recommended to use the birth weight for nutritional calculations until birth weight is regained (Adamkin et al., 2013, p. 152).
  - The total body water of the term infant represents 75% of total body weight; 40% is distributed in the extracellular compartment and 35% within the intracellular compartment (Adamkin et al., 2013, p. 153).
  - Postnatal weight loss in the term infant can range from 5% to 10% of birth weight and usually occurs within the first week (Anderson et al., 2017, p. 248).
- Early nutrition in the preterm infant is essential for the attenuation of weight loss and a faster return to birth weight. Preterm infants quickly experience hypoglycemia and catabolism if not provided with early nutrition therapy, and early nutritional deficits can take weeks to months to replenish (Anderson et al., 2017, p. 248; Brown et al., 2016, p. 380).
- Preterm infants are at high risk for postnatal growth failure for many reasons:
  - The gap between the nutritional needs and the nutrition provided
    - Infants often receive less protein and fewer calories than necessary for protein accretion and growth. Less-than-ideal protein and caloric intake is the primary reason for postnatal growth failure.
  - Increased energy expenditure
    - Preterm infants have increased energy expenditure due to environmental factors, such as losses from low humidity and convection.
  - Increased energy consumption
    - Daily physiologic demands, such as maintenance of a normal temperature, breathing, nutrient digestion, and absorption, require constant energy usage.
  - Stress-induced hormones
    - Stress-induced hormones, such as corticosteroids and catecholamines, are catabolic and limit the production and action of anabolic growth factors (Brown et al., 2016, p. 380).
- Goals for the postnatal growth of preterm infants are based on the intrauterine growth of a fetus of the same gestational age (Anderson et al., 2017, p. 248; Brown et al., 2016, p. 382; Olsen, Leick-Rude, Dusin, & Rosterman, 2016, p. 365). See Table 10.1 for the goals of postnatal anthropometric growth in the preterm infant.

TABLE 10.1 Goals for Postnatal Anthropometric Growth in the Preterm Infant

Gestational Age	Weight Gain
24–32 weeks	15 to 20 g/kg/day
33–36 weeks	14 to 15 g/kg/day
37–40 weeks	7 to 9 g/kg/day
Corrected/Adjusted Age	
40 weeks–3 months	30 g/day
3–6 months	12 g/day
6–9 months	15 g/day
9–12 months	10 g/day
Other Anthropometric Measures	
Length	1 cm/week
Head circumference	1 cm/week

Sources: Data from Adamkin, D., Radmacher, P., & Lewis, S. (2013). Nutrition and selected disorders of the gastrointestinal tract. In A. Fanaroff & J. Fanaroff (Eds.), *Klaus and Fanaroff's care of the high-risk neonate* (6th ed., pp. 151–200). Cleveland, OH: Elsevier; Anderson, D., Poindexter, B., & Martin, C. (2017). Nutrition. In E. Eichenwald, A. Hansen, C. Martin, & A. Stark (Eds.), *Cloherty and Stark's manual of neonatal care* (8th ed., pp. 248–284). Philadelphia, PA: Wolters Kluwer; Blackburn, S. (2013). Gastrointestinal and hepatic systems and perinatal nutrition. In S. Blackburn (Ed.), *Maternal, fetal, & neonatal physiology: A clinical perspective* (pp. 393–442). Maryland Heights, MO: Elsevier/Saunders.

- At a minimum, infant growth monitoring should consist of a daily weight. The extremely preterm infant may require a weight check more frequently in the first few days of life. Additionally, each infant's weight gain should be evaluated every week and plotted on a growth chart (Olsen et al., 2016, p. 365).
  - Linear growth and head circumference represent lean mass growth and can potentially predict neurodevelopmental outcomes (Brown et al., 2016, p. 380).
- Length and head circumference should be monitored weekly and plotted on a growth chart (Olsen et al., 2016, p. 365).
- Utilization of a length board should be encouraged and can improve the validity of the measurements. The accuracy of the measurement can be increased by utilizing the tonic–neck reflex to straighten the hip and the knee (Brown et al., 2016, p. 380).

Postnatal Growth Velocity

- Extremely preterm infants with a suboptimal growth trajectory while hospitalized are more likely to have a weight, length, and head circumference below the 10th percentile at 18 months corrected age (Colaizy, Demauro, Mcnelis, & Poindexter, 2018, p. 1019).
- Optimal nutrition is essential for the attainment of appropriate growth and development. Therefore, it is important for the clinician to continuously assess the infant's nutritional status.

○ The nutritional assessment should include the infant's gestational age, intrauterine growth, and nutrition; and an assessment of the current nutritional status, as well as an evaluation over time.

○ Non-nutritional status, including illness, medications, and stress (surgery and infection), should also be assessed (Adamkin et al., 2013, p. 181).

○ It may be difficult to assess growth measurement in preterm infants during the first week of life due to calorie and fluid restriction as a result of illness (Olsen et al., 2016, p. 365).

WEIGHT
- It is important to obtain weights on the same scale and at the same time daily. The addition or subtraction of equipment should be noted, and an assessment of whether weight gain is reflective of true growth (new tissue deposition), excess fat deposition, or water retention should be completed (Adamkin et al., 2013, pp. 181–182).
- Weight gain should be expressed as grams/kg/day in preterm infants (Adamkin et al., 2013, p. 181).
  To calculate: (change in weight in kilograms ÷ current weight in kilograms) ÷ number of days = g/kg/day
  ○ Example: A preterm infant weighs 1,500 g today. Seven days ago, the infant weighed 1,300 g. What is the daily weight gain in g/kg/day over the last 7 days?
  1,500 g − 1,300 g = 200 g in weight gain over 7 days
  200 g ÷ 1.5 kg = 133.33 g/kg
  133.33 g/kg ÷ 7 days = 19 g/kg/day
- The average goal for preterm infant's weight gain is approximately 15 to 20 g/kg/day (Brown et al., 2016, p. 382).
- Inadequate weight gain or weight loss is a sign of inadequate caloric intake (Olsen et al., 2016, p. 365).

LENGTH
- Growth in length reflects lean mass growth. After long periods of insufficient nutrition, linear growth can be affected (Brown et al., 2016, p. 380; Olsen et al., 2016, p. 365).

HEAD CIRCUMFERENCE (HC)
- In normal infants, HC growth correlates with brain development.
- During periods of acute illness, head growth is slower than that of the normal fetus. Normal head growth does not

occur until the infant has recovered despite high caloric intake. The longer the infant has a suboptimal head size, the higher the neurodevelopment risk.

- HC growth is the least affected with poor nutrition (Olsen et al., 2016, p. 365).
- See Table 10.2 for the growth velocity of preterm infants from term to 24 months.

PONDERAL INDEX
- Also known as the weight–length index, it is used to assess the quality of an infant's growth. Tissue accretion and organ growth are seen along with increases in both weight and length, and can be seen on the Ponderal Index (Brown et al., 2016, p. 382).

Growth Charts

- Growth charts provide a method of tracking serial weights, length, and HC measurements. Several charts are available; however, Fenton and Olsen are used for preterm infants. The Fenton chart allows the infant to be monitored from 22 to 50 weeks postmenstrual age (Anderson et al., 2017, p. 249).
- Term-infant growth charts also include incremental growth curves for weight, length, and HC and are developed by the National Center for Health Statistics and the National Center for Chronic Disease Prevention and Health Promotion (Ditzenberger, 2015, p. 193).
- See Figures 10.1 Fenton Preterm Growth Chart for Boys and 10.2 Fenton Preterm Growth Chart for Girls (Anderson et al., 2017, pp. 250–251).

Laboratory Assessment

- Electrolytes: sodium, potassium, chloride, and bicarbonate are used to assess renal function and fluid status (Ditzenberger, 2015, p. 192).
- Blood urea nitrogen (BUN) and creatinine (Cr) (Ditzenberger, 2015, p. 192):
  ○ In the first weeks of life, BUN is not a good marker of protein intake or tolerance in the preterm infant, but represents fluid status (Ditzenberger, 2015, p. 192). Cr and Cr clearance are good indicators for renal function for the preterm infant (Ditzenberger, 2015, p. 192).

TABLE 10.2 Growth Velocity of Preterm Infants From Term to 24 Months (Range includes ±1 SD)

Age From Term (month)	Weight (g/day^{-1})	Length (cm/month^{-1})	Head Circumference (cm/month^{-1})
1	26–40	3–4.5	1.6–2.5
4	15–25	2.3–3.6	0.8–1.4
8	12–17	1–2	0.3–0.8
12	9–12	0.8–1.5	0.2–0.4
18	4–10	0.7–1.3	0.1–0.4

Source: Reproduced with permission from Adamkin, D., Radmacher, P., & Lewis, S. (2013). Nutrition and selected disorders of the gastrointestinal tract. In A. Fanaroff & J. Fanaroff (Eds.), *Klaus and Fanaroff's care of the high-risk neonate* (6th ed., pp. 151–200). Cleveland, OH: Elsevier.

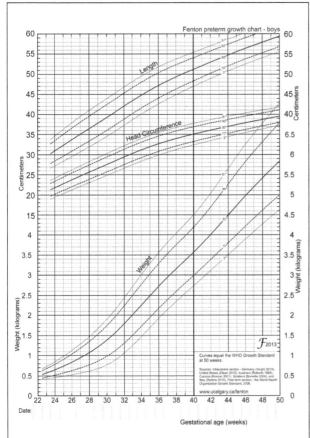

FIGURE 10.1 Reproduced with permission from Fenton, T. Fenton Preterm Growth Chart for Boys.

Source: Fenton Preterm Growth Chart Site, University of Calgary. Retrieved from https://www.ucalgary.ca/fenton/2013chart

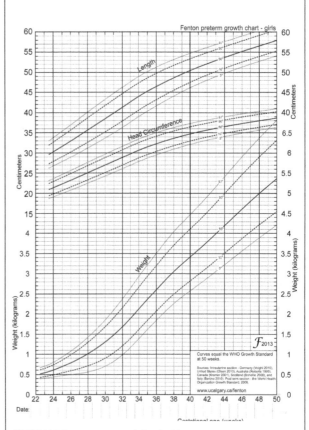

FIGURE 10.2 Fenton preterm growth chart for girls

Source: Reproduced with permission from Fenton T. Fenton Preterm Growth Chart Site, University of Calgary. Retrieved from https://www.ucalgary.ca/fenton/2013chart

- ■ The BUN level does not usually correlate with AA intake during the first postnatal weeks, even with changes in renal function. Studies have demonstrated safety with early protein administration without abnormal elevations of ammonia or BUN levels (Denne, 2018, p. 1024).
- In the critically ill extremely preterm infant, serum glucose, electrolytes, BUN, and Cr should be monitored 2 to 3 times per day during the first 2 days at least and then daily as needed (Adamkin et al., 2013, p. 154).
- Plasma triglyceride levels
  - ○ Monitor plasma triglycerides after each increase in the dose of intravenous (IV) fat. A serum triglyceride level below 200 mg/dL indicates lipid tolerance (Adamkin et al., 2013, p. 164).
- Calcium, magnesium, phosphorus, and alkaline phosphatase:
  - ○ Calcium, phosphorus, and alkaline phosphatase are used to assess for metabolic bone disease and bone mineralization status.
  - ○ Decreased calcium and phosphorus levels or increased alkaline phosphatase levels (levels greater than 500 mg/dL) are indicators of bone demineralization.

- ○ Magnesium is important to plasma membrane excitability, energy storage, transfer and production. It is also important to calcium and bone homeostasis. (Ditzenberger, 2015, p. 192)
  - ■ Elevated alkaline phosphatase levels generally precede radiographic changes by approximately 2 to 4 weeks.
- ○ Serum phosphorus levels of <4 mg/dL may be early signs of decreased bone mineralization.
- ○ Calcium levels may remain normal despite depletion of calcium bone stores (Adamkin et al., 2013, p. 172, 182; Ditzenberger, 2015, p. 192).
- Vitamin D
  - ○ Vitamin D levels are important to assess when evaluating for rickets. 25-hydroxycholecalciferol (25-OH vitamin D) levels are usually normal, while 1, 25 dihydroxycholecalciferol (1, 25-OH vitamin D) levels may be elevated due to increased parathyroid hormone levels and low serum phosphorus levels (Adamkin et al., 2013, p. 172).
- Total serum protein, albumin, transferrin, retinol-binding protein, and prealbumin
  - ○ These biochemical markers can be used to assess for protein malnutrition, especially albumin levels, which

may serve as an indicator of insufficient energy and protein intake (Adamkin et al., 2013, p. 182; Olsen et al., 2016, p. 365).

NUTRITIONAL REQUIREMENTS FOR TERM INFANTS

Parenteral Energy (Calorie) Requirements

- Term infants require 100 to 120 mL/kg/day of parenteral nutrition (PN), and a caloric intake of 80 to 90 kcal/kg/day (Ditzenberger, 2015, pp. 175–176).
  - ○ Parenteral nutrition promotes optimal postnatal growth and neurodevelopment similar to the rate of a fetus at the same gestational age, or along a growth curve consistent with the birth weight.
  - ○ The caloric requirements for the parenterally fed infant are less than that of the enterally fed infant due to lower fecal losses, activity levels (Blackburn, 2013, p. 427), and the absence of calories necessary for absorption and digestion of food (Denne, 2018, p. 1030).

Protein (AA) Requirements

- Protein makes up lean body mass and is essential for optimal growth. Early protein solutions preserve endogenous protein stores by limiting catabolism to ensure a positive nitrogen balance and promote insulin secretion (Adamkin et al., 2013, p. 159; Denne, 2018, p. 1025; Olsen et al., 2016, pp. 356, 378; Poindexter & Ehrenkranz, 2015, p. 598).
- Term infants need between 1.5 and 2.5 g/kg/day of protein (Blackburn, 2013, p. 427; Brown et al., 2016, p. 385).
  - ○ 1 gram of protein equals 4 kcals/g (Anderson et al., 2017, p. 260).
- Calculation of protein for PN solution
  - ■ Determine total gram/kg/day of protein needed
  - ■ gram/kg/day × weight (kg) = gram/day
  - ■ (gram/day ÷ mL/day) × 100 = % AAs
  - ○ Calculation example: A 3-kg infant starting total parenteral nutrition (TPN) at 1.5 g AAs/kg/day is receiving 80 mL TPN fluid/kg/day. The infusion rate is 10 mL/h, to give a total of 240 mL in 24 hours.
    - ■ Calculate grams of AA to add to TPN
      - • g/kg/day × weight (kg) = g/day
      - • 1.5 g/kg/day × 3 kg = 4.5 g/day
      - • Calculate the grams per mL
      - • 4.5 g/day ÷ 240 mL = 0.1875 g/mL
      - • Calculate grams of AA per 100 mL base solution or the % AA.
      - • 0.1875 g/mL × 100 mL = 1.875 g of AA added to every 100 mL of base solution or 1.875% AA in the solution
    - ■ Calculate kcal per kg delivered from protein:
      - • 1 g of protein = 4 kcal
      - • 4.5 g/day × 4 kcal/g = 18 kcal or
      - • 1.5 g/kg/day of AA × 4 kcal/g = 6 kcal/kg/day from protein or a total of 18 kcals (Carlson & Shirland, 2010, pp. 7–8).
- It is not necessary to provide increased protein for the term infant unless required due to illness (Brown et al., 2016, p. 387). However, term infants experiencing sepsis, surgical stress, and steroids can have increased protein catabolism, resulting in decreased accretion of protein (Poindexter & Ehrenkranz, 2015, p. 599).

Lipid (Fat) Requirements

- Standard 20% lipid emulsions containing long-chain triglycerides (LCTs) and phospholipids serve as a concentrated source of nonprotein calories (NPC), which promotes nitrogen retention (Denne, 2018, p. 1026; Olsen et al., 2016, p. 363).
  - ○ Twenty percent IV lipid is preferred to 10% due to fewer phospholipids per gram of fat which are associated with high triglyceride levels, increased cholesterol, and low-density lipoprotein levels (Ditzenberger, 2015, p. 176).
    - ■ Omegaven is a fish–oil-based 10% fat emulsion and is used in the United States only under compassionate use protocols for treatment of PN-associated liver disease (Denne, 2018, p. 1023; Poindexter & Ehrenkranz, 2015, p. 608).
  - ○ The composition of IV lipid solutions is shown in Table 10.3.

TABLE 10.3 Oil Composition of Parenteral Lipid Emulsions

	Intralipid 20%	Liposyn II 20%	Omegaven	SMOF
Oil composition				
Soybean	x	x		x
Safflower		x		
Fish			x	x
Medium-chain triglycerides				x
Olive oil				x

SMOF, soybean oil, MCT oil, olive oil, fish oil.

Sources: Data from Denne, S. (2018). Parenteral nutrition for the high-risk neonate. In C. Gleason & S. Juul (Eds.), *Avery's diseases of the newborn* (10th ed., pp. 1023–1031e2). Philadelphia, PA: Elsevier; Poindexter, B., & Ehrenkranz, R. (2015). Nutrient requirements and provision of nutritional support in the premature neonate. In R. Martin, A. Fanaroff, & M. Walsh (Eds.), *Fanaroff and Martin's neonatal-perinatal medicine: Diseases of the fetus and infant* (10th ed., pp. 592–612). Philadelphia, PA: Elsevier.

- Term infants require 2 to 4 g/kg/day of parenteral, IV lipid emulsion.
  - ○ Intravenous 20% lipid emulsion is 2 kcal/mL or approximately 10 kcal/g (Anderson et al., 2017, p. 260).
    - ■ Calculation to determine the intralipids for PN:
      - Determine gram/kg/day.
      - Calculate gram/day.
      - Convert gram/day into ml/day.
      - Calculate mL/kg/day and hourly rate of administration (Carlson & Shirland, 2010, pp. 5–6).
    - ■ Calculation example: A 3-kg infant needs to receive 0.5 g/kg/day of 20% IV lipids solution. Calculate the fluid rate and calories.
      - Determine gram/kg/day of IV lipids needed— 0.5 g/kg/day
      - Calculate grams/day of IV lipids.
      - Weight of infant × desired gram/kg/day = g/day
      - 3 kg × 0.5 g/kg/day = 1.5 g/day
      - Convert gram/day into mL/day.
      - 1.5 g/day ÷ 0.2 (20% IV lipids solution) = 7.5 mL/day
      - Calculate mL/hr of IV lipids.
      - ml/day ÷ 24 hr/day = mL/hr
      - 7.5 ÷ 24 = 0.3125 mL/hr
- Two methods to calculate calories from intralipids:
  - ○ #1 – g/kg/day of lipids × weight in kg × 10 kcals/g
    - ■ Example—A 3-kg term infant receives 0.5 g/kg of IV 20% lipid emulsion. How many kcal/kg is delivered?
      - 0.5 g/kg of IV 20% lipid emulsion × 10 kcals/g = 5 kcals/kg.
  - ○ #2 – mL/day × 2 kcal/mL of lipid
    - ■ Example: A 3-kg term infant is received 7.5 mL of IV 20% lipid emulsion per day. How many kcals/kg/day is delivered?
      - 7.5 mL/day × 2 kcal/mL ÷ 3 kg = 5 kcal/kg
- IV lipids should be infused over 24 hours (Poindexter & Ehrenkranz, 2017, p. 601).

Carbohydrate (Glucose) Requirements

- Glucose is considered the IV source of carbohydrate, and the main energy substrate for nothing by mouth (NPO) infants receiving PN (Adamkin et al., 2013, p. 159; Poindexter & Ehrenkranz, 2015, p. 594).
  - ○ A dextrose solution of less than 12.5% can be used peripherally. A solution of 15% to 30% can be used centrally (Olsen et al., 2016, p. 367).
- Glucose is the primary energy substrate for the brain (Poindexter & Ehrenkranz, 2015, p. 594).
- With long-term PN, at least 50% of total calories should be provided as carbohydrates (Olsen et al., 2016, p. 362).

GLUCOSE INFUSION RATE

- The glucose infusion rate (GIR) maintains normal plasma glucose concentrations to meet energy requirement demands (Denne, 2018, p. 1025).
  - ○ Endogenous glucose production is estimated at 4 mg/kg/min (Olsen et al., 2016, p. 367).
- An appropriate GIR for a full-term infant is approximately 4 to 5 mg/kg/min; however, a preterm infant often requires

a GIR of approximately 6 to 10 mg/kg/min (Poindexter & Ehrenkranz, 2015, p. 601).
  - ○ Maximize nutrition delivery by advancing GIRs by 1 to 2 mg/kg/min as able by increasing dextrose concentration and/or infusion rate to maximize caloric delivery without causing iatrogenic hyperglycemia (Anderson et al., 2017, p. 261).
- 1 gram of dextrose equals 3.4 kcal.
- Glucose calculations for PN:
  - ○ Calculate the percentage of dextrose from the desired GIR.
    - ■ mg/kg/min (desired) × kg = mg glucose/min
    - ■ mg/min ÷ 1,000 mg/g = gram/min
    - ■ gram/min × 1,440 min/day = gram/day
    - ■ gram/day ÷ total ml/day × 100 = % dextrose
  - ○ Example: A 3-kg term infant is going to receive 80 mL/kg/day. The nurse practitioner would like to administer a GIR of 6 mg/kg/min. What percent dextrose should the practitioner order?
    - ■ Calculate mL/kg/day
      - 80 mL/kg/day × 3 kg = 240 mL/day of IV fluids
    - ■ Calculation of percentage of dextrose needed from desired mg/kg/min (6 mg/kg/min)
      - mg/kg/min (desired) × kg = mg of glucose/min
      - 6 mg/kg/min × 3 kg = 18 mg of glucose/min
      - mg/min ÷1,000 mg/g = gram of glucose/min
      - 18 mg/min ÷ 1,000 mg/g = 0.018 g of glucose/min
      - gram of glucose/min × 1,440 min/day = gram of glucose/day
      - 0.018 g of glucose/min × 1,440 min/day = 25.92 g/day
      - gram/day ÷ mL/day (80 mL/kg/day) × 100 = % dextrose needed
      - 25.92 g/day ÷ 240 mL/day × 100 = 10.8% dextrose needed
    - ■ Calculate GIR from known dextrose concentration (%).
      - % dextrose ÷ 100 × mL/day = gram/day
      - gram/day ÷ 1,440 min/day = gram/min
      - gram/min × 1,000 mg/g = mg/min
      - mg/min ÷ kg = mg/kg/min
  - ○ Example: A term infant weighs 3 kg and is receiving 100 mL/kg/day of dextrose 15% solution.
    - ■ Calculation:
      - ml/kg/day × weight in kg = mL/day
      - 100 × 3 = 300 mL/day of dextrose 15% IV fluids
      - % dextrose ÷ 100 × mL/day = gram/day
      - 15 ÷ 100 × 300 mL/day = 45 g/day
      - gram/day ÷ 1,440 min/day = gram/min
      - 45 g/day ÷ 1,440 min/day = 0.03125 g/min
      - gram/min × 1,000 mg/g = mg/min
      - 0.03125 × 1,000 mg/g = 31.3 mg/min
      - mg/min ÷ kg = mg/kg/min
      - 31.3 mg/min ÷ 3 kg = 10.4 mg/kg/min (GIR; Carlson & Shirland, 2010, pp. 6–7).

Enteral Energy (Calorie) Requirements

- The enteral caloric intake requirement for term and near-term infants is 100–120 kcal/kg/day (Ditzenberger, 2015, p. 176).
- Breastfed term newborns require slightly less caloric intake than the formula-fed term newborn for maintenance and

growth due to the amount of energy required to metabolize formula (Blackburn, 2013, p. 427).

Protein (AA) Requirements

- Term infants need between 2 and 2.5 g/kg/day of enteral protein (Ditzenberger, 2015, p. 177).
- Protein intake can be calculated based on the feeding regimen of the infant, due to varying protein content of formula versus breast milk.
  - Calculation of enteral protein
    - Calculate the total volume of feeds per day.
    - Determine how many grams of protein per 100 mL are in the current feed.
    - Total mL of feed × protein content of feed = total protein per day
    - Total grams per day ÷ weight in kg = g/kg of protein
  - A 3.5-kg term infant is receiving 50 mL of unfortified human milk every 3 hours. How many grams of protein is the infant receiving?
    - Calculate the total volume of feeds per day
    - 50 mL × 8 feeds (infant feeds every 3 hours) = 400 mL
    - Determine how many grams of protein per 100 mL are in breast milk.
    - Mature human milk has 0.9 g of protein per 100 mL
    - Total mL of feed × protein content of feed = total protein per day
    - 400 mls × 0.9 g/100 mL = 3.6 g of protein per day
    - Total grams of protein per day ÷ weight in kg = gram/kg of protein
    - 3.6 g ÷ 3.5 kg = 1.03 g/kg of protein

Lipid (Fat) Requirements

- Term infants require 3 to 4 g/kg/day of fat enterally (Ditzenberger, 2015, p. 177).
  - Calculation of enteral fat:
    - Calculate the total volume of feeds per day.
    - Determine how many grams of fat per 100 mL are in the current feed.
    - Total mL of feed × fat content of feed = total fat per day
    - Total grams of fat per day ÷ weight in kg = grams/kg of fat
  - A 3.5-kg term infant is receiving 50 mL of unfortified human milk every 3 hours. How many grams of fat is the infant receiving?
    - Calculate the total volume of feeds per day.
    - 50 mL × 8 feeds (infant feeds every 3 hours) = 400 mL per day
    - Determine how many grams of fat per 100 mL are in the current feed.
    - Mature human milk has 3.5 g of fat per 100 mL
    - Total mL of feed × fat content of feed = total fat per day
    - 400 mL × 3.5 g fat/100 mL = 14 g of fat per day
    - Total grams of fat per day ÷ weight in kg = grams/kg of fat
    - 14 g ÷ 3.5 kg = 4 g/kg of fat

Carbohydrate (Lactose/Oligosaccharides) Requirements

- Term infants require approximately 40% of daily carbohydrate intake, or 8 to 12 g/kg/day enterally (Ditzenberger, 2015, p. 176).

- To calculate enteral kcal/kg/day:
  - Multiply grams/kg/day × 3.4 kcal/g of carbohydrates = kcal/kg/day.
  - Multiply kcals × weight in kg = total kcal/day.
  - Or
  - Determine total enteral intake per day.
  - [Multiply the total volume of feeds in mL × (kcal of feed ÷ 30)] ÷ weight in kg.
  - A term 3.5-kg infant is receiving 8 g/kg/day of carbohydrates from his enteral nutrition. How many kcal/kg/day is the infant receiving?
    - Multiply grams/kg/day × 3.4 kcal/g of carbohydrates = kcal/kg/day.
    - 8 g/kg/day × 3.4 kcal/g of carbohydrates = 27.2 kcal/kg/day.
    - Multiply kcals × weight in kg = total kcal/day.
    - 27.2 kcal × 3.5 kg = 95.2 total kcals from carbohydrates.
  - A term 3.5-kg infant is receiving human milk fortified to 22 kcal/oz. He eats 60 mL every 3 hours. How many kcal/kg/day is the infant receiving?
    - Determine total enteral intake per day.
    - 60 mL × 8 meals a day = 480 mL a day.
    - [Multiply the total volume of feeds in mL × (kcal of feed ÷ 30)] ÷ weight in kg
    - [480 mL × (22 kcal/oz ÷ 30)] ÷ 3.5 kg = 100 kcal/kg/day.
- For the term infant, human milk can be fortified with powdered infant formula, medium-chain triglycerides (MCT) or corn oil, and/or SolCarb, also known as maltodextrin. Fortification should occur in 2 to 3 kcal/oz increments with a max of 30 kcal/oz (Anderson et al., 2017, p. 275).

NUTRITIONAL REQUIREMENTS OF PRETERM INFANTS

General Considerations

- The goal of nutritional support for the high-risk infant is to provide postnatal support that will mimic in utero growth.
  - Nutritional intake should account for tissue losses while permitting tissue accretion.
  - Maximal nutritional support for the preterm infant is limited by the functional immaturity of the renal, GI, and metabolic system as well as any acute illnesses.
  - Infants delivered preterm miss out on the fat, glycogen, iron, calcium, and phosphorus stores that accrue during the third trimester of pregnancy (Adamkin et al., 2013, p. 151).
- Nutritional requirements for the preterm infant are estimated based on body composition and fetal protein accretion at varying gestational ages (Blackburn, 2013, p. 427).

Fluid Requirements

- Preterm infants have higher nutritional needs than term infants, including water and caloric requirements, due to more substantial insensible water losses (IWL; Blackburn, 2013, p. 427).
  - Daily fluid requirements are influenced by IWLs from the respiratory and GI tract, skin, urinary losses, and drainage tube losses. The use of humidified isolettes can minimize IWLs (Adamkin et al., 2013, p. 153).

- Total body water (TBW) is inversely proportionate to gestational age. The 24-weeks' gestation infant has a TBW of more than 90% of her total body weight. Sixty-five percent of the TBW is extracellular, 25% is intracellular, and 1% is in fat stores. The initial diuresis of the preterm infant is considered physiologic and due to the state of relative extracellular fluid volume with an excess of (Adamkin et al., 2013, pp. 151–152).
    - In the preterm infant, postnatal weight loss can range from 10% to 15% of birth weight during the first week, with a return to birth weight by 14 to 21 days (Anderson et al., 2017, p. 248).
- Preterm infants require 120 to 150 mL/kg/day of fluid parenterally and 150 to 200 mL/kg/day enterally (Ditzenberger, 2015, p. 177).
    - The use of larger volumes of fluid (160–180 mL/kg/day) to prevent weight loss can increase the risk of developing a patent ductus arteriosus (PDA), cerebral IVH, bronchopulmonary dysplasia (BPD), and necrotizing enterocolitis (NEC) (Adamkin et al., 2013, p. 152).
- Fluid within the first few days of life should result in urine output of 1 to 3 mL/kg/hr, a urine-specific gravity of 1.008 to 1.012 (Adamkin et al., 2013, p. 152).

Energy (Calorie) Requirements

- Preterm infant energy requirements are determined by total energy expenditure, energy excretion, and energy stored in new tissue for growth. See Table 10.4 for the estimated daily energy requirements for preterm infants.
- Total energy expenditure is comprised of basal metabolic rate, thermoregulation, activity, digestion, and metabolism.
- Energy excretion encompasses heat loss by radiation and evaporation, as well as fecal and urinary losses (Brown et al., 2016, p. 384).
- Extremely preterm infants require approximately 50 to 70 kcal/kg/day for weight maintenance and an additional 45 to 70 kcal/kg/day above maintenance for growth.
    - The European Society for Paediatric Gastroenterology and Nutrition (ESPGHAN) recommends an energy intake of 110 to 135 kcal/kg/day for preterm infants.

- Small for gestational age (SGA) infants and infants with increased metabolic needs, such as intrauterine growth restriction (IUGR) infants who have a higher basal metabolic rate per kilogram body weight may require higher energy intake to attain adequate growth (Adamkin et al., 2013, p. 157; Blackburn, 2013, p. 427; Poindexter & Ehrenkranz, 2015, p. 595).

Parenteral Energy (Calorie) Requirements

- Caloric needs for infants receiving PN are lower than infants enterally fed due to lower activity levels and fecal losses, averaging 80 to 110 kcal/kg/day (Blackburn, 2013, p. 427).
- Goal calories for full PN in the extremely preterm infants are 90 to 100 kcal/kg/day (Denne, 2018, p. 1023).
    - An increase in caloric intake above 120 kcal/kg/day through the addition of calories does not result in proportionate increases in weight gain. The higher the caloric intake, the higher the energy consumed through excretion, tissue synthesis, and diet-induced thermogenesis (Adamkin et al., 2013, p. 158).
    - An increase in the enteral protein-to-energy ratio is necessary to increase lean body mass and decrease fat deposition (Adamkin et al., 2013, p. 158). ⟶ non-protein cal.
- In the parenterally fed preterm infant, NPCs are derived from glucose and lipids. An NPC intake of greater than 70 NPC/kg/day and a protein intake of 2.7 to 3.5 g/kg/day will allow the infant to exhibit nitrogen accretion and growth rates similar to in utero levels (Adamkin et al., 2013, p. 158).
    - Providing a balanced carbohydrate and lipid approach (60:40) to NPCs improves protein accretion and minimizes overall energy expenditure (Denne, 2018, p. 1026).
    - Excess energy expenditure occurs if a disproportionate amount of NPCs is given as glucose. Even at a higher protein intake, a parenterally fed extremely preterm infant may require 80 to 90 kcal/kg of nonprotein energy supplies for growth (Poindexter & Ehrenkranz, 2015, p. 601).

TABLE 10.4 Estimated Daily Energy Requirements for Preterm Infants

Factor	Enterally Fed (kcal/kg/day)	Parenterally Fed (kcal/kg/day)
Energy expenditure		
Basal metabolic rate	40–50	40 – 50
Activity	0–5	less
Thermoregulation	0–5	0–5
Synthesis (energy cost of growth)	15	15
Energy stored	20–30	20 - 30
Energy excreted	15	less
Total requirements	90–120	80–110

Sources: Data from Blackburn, S. (2013). Gastrointestinal and hepatic systems and perinatal nutrition. In S. Blackburn (Ed.), *Maternal, fetal, & neonatal physiology: A clinical perspective* (pp. 393–442). Maryland Heights, MO: Elsevier/Saunders; Brown, L., Hendrickson, K., Evans, R., Davis, J., Sollosy Anderson, M., & Hay, W. W., Jr. (2016). Enteral nutrition. In S. Gardner, B. Carter, M. Enzman-Hines, & J. Hernandez (Eds.), *Merestein & Gardner's handbook of neonatal intensive care* (8th ed., pp. 377–418). St. Louis, MO: Elsevier.

Protein (AA) Requirements

- The goal of providing AAs is to mimic in utero protein accretion. Fetal protein accretion is 3 to 4 g/kg/day (Blackburn, 2013, p. 427; Poindexter & Ehrenkranz, 2015, p. 592). Infants receiving no AAs after birth lose more than 1.5% of their daily body protein when they should be accumulating 2% per day. By 3 days, a 10% protein deficiency occurs (Denne, 2018, p. 1023).
  - ○ Starter or stock PN (premade AA solution with dextrose) is recommended for preterm infants within the first 24 hours of postnatal life to compensate for high protein losses, even if providing a lower caloric intake (Poindexter & Ehrenkranz, 2015, p. 597).
- Extremely preterm infants experience higher protein losses than the term infant in the absence of IV AA (Poindexter & Ehrenkranz, 2015, p. 593).
  - ○ Inadequate protein intake can increase the risk of postnatal growth restrictions in preterm infants through the alteration of growth factors, including serum insulin-like growth factor (IGF)-I (Blackburn, 2013, p. 427).
  - ○ Preterm infants who develop postnatal growth failure have a higher neurodevelopmental risk.
- Preterm infants who are fed diets fortified with protein have shown improved neurodevelopment test scores into adolescent years (Brown et al., 2016, p. 385).
- Protein requirements are inversely related to body weight (Poindexter & Ehrenkranz, 2015, p. 593).
  - ○ An average protein intake of 3.5 g/kg/day is recommended for most preterm infants less than 30 weeks (Brown et al., 2016, p. 386; Poindexter & Ehrenkranz, 2015, p. 593).
  - ○ Extremely preterm infants may require a protein intake of approximately 4 g/kg/day (Brown et al., 2016, p. 386; Poindexter & Ehrenkranz, 2015, p. 593).
  - ○ A protein intake as high as 4.5 g/kg/day may be required to compensate for protein deficits (Brown et al., 2016, p. 387).

- ○ See Table 10.5 for estimated daily nutrition for the term and preterm infant.
- The quality of protein or AA composition in PN is important for nitrogen utilization. There are certain AAs that neonates are unable to produce (essential) or produce in limited quantities (semi-essential). Therefore, it is recommended to provide these AAs exogenously (Adamkin et al., 2013, pp. 161–162). Essential AAs include cysteine, tyrosine, and taurine (Poindexter & Ehrenkranz, 2015, p. 600).
- Two main types of AA solutions are commercially available; adult AA solutions and neonatal/pediatric solutions:
  - ○ The standard adult AA solution is not ideal for infants because it contains little to no tyrosine, cysteine, or taurine and relatively high concentrations of glycine, methionine, and phenylalanine.
  - ○ Neonatal/pediatric crystalline AA solutions have a larger amount of nonessential AAs, more branched chain AAs, less methionine and phenylalanine, and more tyrosine, cysteine, and taurine than adult AA solutions. Neonatal/pediatric AA solutions also have a lower pH; this allows for the addition of greater concentrations of calcium and phosphorus (Adamkin et al., 2013, p. 162).
    - The addition of cysteine can produce metabolic acidosis if the PN solution is not appropriately buffered with acetate (Poindexter & Ehrenkranz, 2015, p. 600).
- Metabolic overload can occur with protein intakes greater than 5 g/kg/ per day. Infants can experience irritability, late metabolic acidosis, azotemia, edema, fever, lethargy, diarrhea, elevated BUN, and poor developmental outcomes (Blackburn, 2013, p. 427).

Lipid (Fat) Requirements

- Fat provides the major source of nonprotein energy for growing preterm infants (Olsen et al., 2016, p. 595; Poindexter & Ehrenkranz, 2015, p. 595).

TABLE 10.5 Estimated Daily Nutrition for the Term and Preterm Infant

Nutritional Content	Term Infant	Preterm Infant
Fluid requirements		
Parenteral	100–120 mL/kg/day	120–150 mL/kg/day
Enteral	120–150 mL/kg/day	150–200 mL/kg/day
Calories/energy		
Parenteral	80–90 kcal/kg/day	80–110 kcal/kg/day
Enteral	100–120 kcal/kg/day	110–135 kcal/kg/day
Protein		
Parenteral	1.5–2.5 g/kg/day	3.5–4.5 g/kg/day
Enteral	1.5–2.5 g/kg/day	3.5–4.5 g/kg/day
Fats/Lipid		
Parenteral	2–4 g/kg/day	2–3.5 g/kg/day
Enteral	3–4 g/kg/day	3–4 g/kg/day

(continued)

TABLE 10.5 Estimated Daily Nutrition for the Term and Preterm Infant *(cont.)*

Nutritional Content	Term Infant	Preterm Infant
Carbohydrates		
Parenteral	10–15 g/kg/day	10–15 g/kg/day
Enteral	8–12 g/kg/day	8–12 g/kg/day

Sources: Data from Blackburn, S. (2013). Gastrointestinal and hepatic systems and perinatal nutrition. In S. Blackburn (Ed.), *Maternal, fetal, & neonatal physiology: A clinical perspective* (pp. 393–442). Maryland Heights, MO: Elsevier/Saunders; Ditzenberger, G. (2015). Nutritional management. In M. T. Verklan & M. Walden (Eds.), *Core curriculum for neonatal intensive care nursing* (5th ed., pp. 172–196). St. Louis, MO: Elsevier; Poindexter, B., & Ehrenkranz, R. (2015). Nutrient requirements and provision of nutritional support in the prematrure neonate. In R. Martin, A. Fanaroff, & M. Walsh (Eds.), *Fanaroff and Martin's neonatal-perinatal medicine: Diseases of the fetus and infant* (10th ed., pp. 592–612). Philadelphia, PA: Elsevier.

- Long-chain polyunsaturated fatty acids (PUFAs) like arachidonic acid and docosahexaenoic acid (DHA) are sources of omega-6 fatty acids and essential to neurologic and vision development (Blackburn, 2013, p. 429).
- Initiate IV lipids cautiously per recommendations, starting with 0.5 to 1 g/kg/day and advance by 0.5 g/kg every 1 to 2 days as tolerated, to a maximum of 3 g/kg/day (Olsen et al., 2016, p. 367).
- Preterm infants require 2 to 3.0 g/kg/day of parenteral lipids (Ditzenberger, 2015, p. 179).
- Lipids are necessary to provide infants with energy in the form of essential fatty acids (EFAs) and to prevent EFA deficiency (Adamkin et al., 2013, p. 163).
  - EFA deficiency can develop within 72 hours in the preterm infant. The provision of 0.5 g to 1.0 g/kg/day of IV lipid can prevent the development of fatty acid deficiency (Poindexter & Ehrenkranz, 2015, p. 595).
  - Linoleic acid is an EFA necessary for the formation of arachidonic acid and docosahexaenoic. Linoleic acid is associated with cognition and vision and should account for about 3% of total calories (Ditzenberger, 2015, p. 179).

Carnitine

- Added to PN increases tolerance of IV lipids. Although the addition of carnitine results in increased tolerance to IV lipids, there is contradicting data on increase weight gain and nitrogen retention. Therefore, carnitine is recommended only for low birth weight infants requiring PN for over 2 to 3 weeks. Carnitine dosages of 8 to 10 mg/kg/day have been used without side effects (Adamkin et al., 2013, p. 165).

Carbohydrate (Dextrose) Requirements

- Carbohydrates are the principal energy substrate for preterm infants in PN (Adamkin et al., 2013, p. 160).
  - Preterm infants require parenteral carbohydrates administration at 10 to 15 g/kg/day (Adamkin et al., 2013, p.158; Ditzenberger, 2015, p. 178).
  - Carbohydrates should provide 40% of postnatal caloric intake (Anderson et al., 2017, p. 260).
- Infants weighing above 1,000 g initially tolerate 10% glucose solution (Olsen et al., 2016, p. 326; Poindexter & Ehrenkranz, 2015, p. 601).

- Extreme preterm infants have a predisposition toward hyperglycemia, but may initially require a 5% glucose solution due to higher fluid needs from increased insensible losses (Denne, 2018, p. 1025; Poindexter & Ehrenkranz, 2105, p. 601).
- Extreme preterm infants should start with a GIR of at least 4 to 6 mg/kg/min. Many small infants will initially be unable to tolerate a certain glucose load but will eventually develop tolerance if they are presented with just enough glucose to keep their glucose levels high yet not enough to cause glycosuria (Burris, 2017, p. 323).

Anions

- Anions are provided as either acetate or chloride (Poindexter & Ehrenkranz, 2015, p. 605).
  - The immature kidneys contribute to acidosis by failing to reabsorb HCO_3 and to excrete hydrogen. The addition of acetate aids with correction of hyperchloremic metabolic acidosis (Halbardier, 2015, p. 161).
  - The addition of chloride aids with correction of metabolic alkalosis due to increased renal losses from diuretic therapy (Halbardier, 2015, p. 161).

Vitamins, Mineral, and Trace Elements

- Trace elements should be added to PN as infants have very little endogenous stores (Adamkin et al., 2013, p. 166).
- The peak fetal accretion of minerals occurs during the third trimester, placing preterm infants at increased risk for osteopenia (Poindexter & Ehrenkranz, 2015, p. 606).
  - The limited solubility of current PN solutions does not supply enough calcium and phosphorus to support optimal bone mineralization. However, adding cysteine to PN improves the calcium and phosphorus solubility by lowering the pH (Denne, 2018, p. 1025; Olsen et al., 2016, p. 369; Poindexter & Ehrenkranz, 2015, p. 606).
- Preterm infants need:
  - 60 to 90 mg/kg/day of parenteral calcium
  - A ratio of calcium to phosphorus of 1.7 to 2.0:1 should be the goal (Adamkin et al., 2013, p. 172; Poindexter & Ehrenkranz, 2015, p. 606).
  - 45 to 60 mg/kg/day of phosphorus
  - 4 to 7 mg/kg/day of magnesium
  - 120 to 160 IU/day vitamin D (Adamkin et al., 2013, p. 166; Ditzenberger, 2015, p. 178)

- Preterm infants are born with low stores of trace elements because in utero accumulation occurs during the last trimester of pregnancy (Poindexter & Ehrenkranz, 2015, p. 606).
    - Dosing of trace elements in PN contributes less than 0.01% of total body weight. Requirements for preterm infants are not well defined.
        - Recommendations include adding zinc and selenium early in PN administration, where other trace elements are probably not needed until the first 2 weeks of life (Poindexter & Ehrenkranz, 2015, p. 606). Supplementing very preterm infants with selenium has been associated with reduced sepsis (Olsen et al., 2016, p. 369).
    - Iron is not recommended unless an infant is receiving PN for longer than 2 months (Denne, 2018, p. 1028).
    - It is recommended to reduce or omit copper and manganese from PN in patients with impaired biliary excretion and/or liver disease because they are excreted in the bile (Anderson et al., 2017, p. 263).
    - The recommended intakes of vitamins for the term and preterm infants on PN are shown in Table 10.6.
    - The recommended intake of trace elements in PN for the term and preterm infants are shown in Table 10.7.

Delivery of Parenteral Nutrition

- Both peripheral and central venous catheters are used to deliver PN and IV fat (Poindexter & Ehrenkranz, 2015, p. 608).
    - Central venous delivery is recommended for patients who require PN for a duration greater than 1 week (Anderson et al., 2017, p. 260).
    - Central venous delivery allows for more concentrated formulations and caloric density (Olsen et al., 2016, p. 356; Poindexter & Ehrenkranz, 2015, p. 608).
- Peripherally infused PN should not exceed an osmolality of 900 mOsm/L.
    - The osmolality limitation can result in limited carbohydrate and AA delivery.
    - Noncentral PN solutions do not allow dextrose concentrations above 12.5% (Anderson et al., 2017, p. 260; Olsen et al., 2016, p. 364).

Complications of Parenteral Nutrition Delivery

- Electrolyte imbalance/glucose instability—This common, preventable complication of electrolyte imbalance and glucose instability can be corrected by manipulating the constituents of the infusate (Poindexter & Ehrenkranz, 2015, p. 608).

TABLE 10.6 Parenteral Vitamin Intake for Term and Preterm Infants

Vitamin	Term (daily dose)	Preterm (dose/kg per day)
Fat soluble		
Vitamin A (IU)	2,300	700–1,500
Vitamin D (IU)	400	40–260
Vitamin E (IU)	7	2.8–3.5
Vitamin K (µg)	200	10 -80
Water Soluble		
Vitamin B$_6$ (µg)	1,000	150–200
Vitamin B$_{12}$ (µg)	1	0.3–0.7
Vitamin C (mg)	80	15–32
Biotin (µg)	20	5–8
Folic acid (µg)	140	40–90
Niacin (mg)	17	4.0–6.8
Pantothenate (mg)	5	1–2
Riboflavin (µg)	1,400	150–200
Thiamin (µg)	1,200	200–350

Sources: Data from Anderson, D., Poindexter, B., & Martin, C. (2017). Nutrition. In E. Eichenwald, A. Hansen, C. Martin, & A. Stark (Eds.), *Cloherty and Stark's manual of neonatal care* (8th ed., pp. 248–284). Philadelphia, PA: Wolters Kluwer; Denne, S. (2018). Parenteral nutrition for the high-risk neonate. In C. Gleason & S. Juul (Eds.), *Avery's diseases of the newborn* (10th ed., pp. 1023–1031e2). Philadelphia, PA: Elsevier; Ditzenberger, G. (2015). Nutritional management. In M. T. Verklan & M. Walden (Eds.), *Core curriculum for neonatal intensive care nursing* (5th ed., pp. 172–196). St. Louis, MO: Elsevier.

TABLE 10.7 Parenteral Intake of Trace Elements for Term and Preterm Infants

Trace Element	Term (µg/kg per day)	Preterm (µg/kg per day)
Chromium	0.20	0.05–0.30
Copper	20	20–29
Iodide	1	1
Manganese	1	1
Molybdenum	0.25	0.25
Selenium	2	1.5–4.5
Zinc	250	400

Sources: Data from Denne, S. (2018). Parenteral nutrition for the high-risk neonate. In C. Gleason & S. Juul (Eds.), *Avery's diseases of the newborn* (10th ed., pp. 1023–1031e2). Philadelphia, PA: Elsevier; Ditzenberger, G. (2015). Nutritional management. In M. T. Verklan & M. Walden (Eds.), *Core curriculum for neonatal intensive care nursing* (5th ed., pp. 172–196). St. Louis, MO: Elsevier.

- Hepatic dysfunction—Infants who receive PN for greater than 2 weeks are at risk for cholestatic jaundice. The risk further increases with prematurity and the duration of PN without enteral feedings (Olsen et al., 2016, p. 375; Poindexter & Ehrenkranz, 2015, p. 608).
  - The primary complication of PN arises from hepatic dysfunction with a noted direct bilirubin level greater than 2 mg/dL (Poindexter & Ehrenkranz, 2015, p. 608).
- Bacteremia/fungemia—Sepsis is a potentially lethal complication of PN delivery from central line-associated bloodstream infections, which increases with prematurity and prolonged duration of PN (Olsen et al., 2016, p. 378).
  - IV lipids provide a rich growth medium for skin flora that has colonized indwelling catheters (Poindexter & Ehrenkranz, 2015, p. 608).
  - There have been numerous reports *of Malassezia furfur* fungemia in infants receiving IV lipids (Poindexter & Ehrenkranz, 2015, p. 608).
- Negative oxidant effects—Photoprotection of bags, syringes, and tubing are recommended for PN delivery, as exposure of PN to light may generate peroxides with negative oxidant effects. These can induce vasoconstriction, decrease mesenteric blood flow, and increase oxidant stress associated with higher occurrences of BPD (Olsen et al., 2016, p. 371).
- Adverse effects from IV lipids—Lipid infusion rates in excess of 0.25 g/kg per hour can be associated with decreased oxygenation (Adamkin et al., 2013, p. 163; Poindexter & Ehrenkranz, 2015, p. 601).
  - IV fat can displace indirect bilirubin from binding sites on serum albumin, even with adequate lipid metabolism; therefore, use with caution in infants with significant hyperbilirubinemia (Adamkin et al., 2013, p. 163).

Enteral Energy (Calorie) Requirements

- An enterally fed, stable preterm can achieve reasonable growth about 120 kcal/kg/day (Blackburn, 2013, p. 427).

Protein and AA Requirements

- Preterm infants have a higher protein fractional protein accretion rate than term infants. Therefore, they require 3.5 to 4 g/kg/day of enteral protein (Brown et al., 2016, p. 385).
- Enteral protein sources include whey and casein (Brown et al., 2016, p. 386).

Lipid (Fat) Requirements

- Preterm infants require 3 to 4 g/kg/day of fat enterally (Ditzenberger, 2015, p. 179).
- Preterm infants have a limited ability enterally to absorb and digest certain fats because of low levels of pancreatic lipase, bile acids, and lingual lipase (Adamkin et al., 2013, p. 170; Brown et al., 2016, p. 387; Poindexter & Ehrenkranz, 2015, pp. 595–596).
- MCTs do not require bile for emulsification and are absorbed by passive diffusion. MCTs are better absorbed than LCTs; however, long-chain fatty acids are essential for brain development (Adamkin et al., 2013, p. 170; Olsen et al., 2016, p. 378).

Carbohydrate Requirements

- The preterm infant's enteral carbohydrate requirement is approximately 8 to 12 g/kg/day. Most preterm infant formulas include glucose polymers as a major source of carbohydrates. Glucose polymers provide increased caloric density without increasing osmolality (Poindexter & Ehrenkranz, 2015, p. 595).

Vitamins, Minerals, and Trace Elements

- Preterm infants can sustain normal vitamin D levels with 400 IU of vitamin D.
- In addition, they should receive:
  - 185 to 210 mg/kg/day of calcium
  - 123 to 140 mg/kg/day of phosphorus
  - 8.5 to 10 mg/kg/day of magnesium (Adamkin et al., 2013, p. 172)

ENTERAL FEEDINGS

Feeding Methods

- Enteral feeding is the preferred method for nourishing all infants. However, high-risk neonates require the gradual introduction of enteral feedings in conjunction with supplemental PN (Anderson et al., 2017, p. 278).
- Most high-risk infants start feeding via nasogastric/orogastric (NG/OG) tubes; these tube feedings are commonly used for bolus or continuous feeding methods in the preterm or sick infant until it is safe to introduce oral feedings (Anderson et al., 2017, p. 278).
  - Neonatal feeding tubes consist of radio-opaque material for radiographic visualization. Polyurethane or silicone-based feeding tubes are recommended for indwelling use up to 30 days. Polyvinylchloride-based feeding tubes are intended for nonindwelling intermittent use (Anderson et al., 2017, p. 278).
  - Optimal feeding tube size is determined by weight.
    - A 5 French feeding tube is used for infants less than 1,000 g.
    - Infants weighing 1,000 g or greater require a 6 to 8 French gastric tube (Ditzenberger, 2015, p. 189).
- Transpyloric (nasoduodenal and nasojejunal) feedings should be considered for lung protection secondary to the risk of aspiration in infants with severe chronic lung disease (CLD) and/or gastroesophageal reflux. Transpyloric feedings are routinely placed under guided fluoroscopy and should always be infused continuously due to the intestines limited capacity for expansion (Anderson et al., 2017, p. 278).
  - Lingual and gastric lipase secretions are bypassed when infants are receiving transpyloric feeding, resulting in increased risk for fat malabsorption (Anderson et al., 2017, p. 278).
- Gastrostomy tubes may be considered for infants who are unable to take sufficient oral feeding volumes for adequate growth/hydration (Anderson et al., 2017, p. 278).

Standardized Feeding Guidelines

- Enteral feeding practices vary from center to center, despite recommended evidence-based feeding guidelines for preterm infants. Standardized feeding guidelines have shown improved nutritional outcomes with optimized growth, reduced duration of PN, and decreased incidence of NEC (Poindexter & Ehrenkranz, 2015, p. 598).

Gut Priming

- Gut priming can be administered as a fixed dose regardless of gestational age. Alternatively, a low volume per kilogram may be delivered, divided into aliquots.
  - Optimal timing to start gut priming is by the first or second day of life as the absence of any enteral feeding leads to villous atrophy in the preterm infant (Anderson et al., 2017, p. 268; Poindexter & Ehrenkranz, 2015, p. 597).
- Trophic/minimal enteral feedings are usually low-volume and hypocaloric to promote intestinal maturation, with a volume of < 24 mL/kg/day.

- Trophic feedings improve feeding tolerance, maturation of the preterm intestine (both structurally and functionally), and reduce liver dysfunction. They do not contain sufficient calories to sustain somatic growth (Poindexter & Ehrenkranz, 2015, p. 597).
- Use full-strength colostrum/preterm human milk or pasteurized donor human milk (PDHM) to start gut priming (Anderson et al., 2017, p. 268).
  - Full-strength 20 kcal/oz preterm formula is preferred over not feeding when human milk supply is insufficient or donor breast milk has been declined. Contraindications for gut priming include, but are not limited to, severe hemodynamic instability, medical treatment for patent ductus arteriosus, indications of ileus or clinical signs of intestinal pathology, or suspected or confirmed NEC (Anderson et al., 2017, p. 268).

Rate of Advancement of Enteral Feeds

- Feeding practices vary among institutions since there is limited information regarding the most appropriate way to advance feedings in preterm infants.
- Use 20 kcal/oz human milk or preterm formula (full strength) and advance feeding volume in the following suggested manner:
  - Enteral feedings should cautiously be advanced by 20 to 30 mL/kg per day in preterm infants.
  - Extremely preterm infants may need a slower advancement 15 to 25 mL/kg/day.
  - As enteral volumes are increased, the PN or IV fluid volume should be decreased to balance the total fluid volume (Poindexter & Ehrenkranz, 2015, p. 598).
- The caloric density can be advanced from 20 to 24 kcal/oz in preterm infants when the feeding volume has reached 100 mL/kg/day.
  - It is the recommendation not to increase feeding volume further until the new caloric density has been tolerated for approximately 24 hours (Poindexter & Ehrenkranz, 2015, p. 598).

Gastric Residuals

- In many institutions, the measurement of gastric residuals is a common practice to evaluate feeding tolerance. However, there is little data supporting the utility of gastric residuals in the diagnosis of feeding intolerance or NEC (Poindexter & Ehrenkranz, 2015, p. 598).
  - Gastric residuals of the milk given at the previous feeding with a volume greater than 30% may warrant further evaluation. Additionally, residuals greater than 10–15 mL is considered excessive (Ditzenberger, 2015, p. 189).
- Antiperistalsis may cause bile-stained residuals secondary to immature gut motility, which is not enough information to withhold feedings (Ditzenberger, 2015, p. 189).
- It is not recommended to stop enteral feedings based on residuals without other symptoms of feeding intolerance (Poindexter & Ehrenkranz, 2015, p. 598).
  - Clinical manifestations in conjunction with concerning residuals that provide reasons for further investigation include:
    - Abdominal distention with visible bowel loops, erythema, abdominal tenderness

- Bloody stools
- Apnea and bradycardia
- Emesis (evaluate color and consistency; Ditzenberger, 2015, p. 189).

HUMAN MILK, COMPOSITION AND USES

- Human milk remains the gold standard for healthy term infants and most high-risk preterm infants. Human milk provides many nutritional and non-nutritional advantages for the term and preterm infants (Poindexter & Ehrenkranz, 2015, p. 602).
- Human milk has a low renal solute load, the ideal AA composition for newborns, an easily digestible and absorbable form of lipid, and contains human milk bile salts (Blackburn, 2013, p. 429).
- Milk obtained from mothers of preterm infants differs from that of mothers of term infants. The initial milk composition of the preterm mother reflects what is believed to be the nutritional needs of the preterm infant. However, the composition of the milk changes over the first month after birth and resembles term milk by 1 month (Blackburn, 2013, p. 429).
- The nutritional content of human milk can vary based on:
  - ○ Gestational age at the time of delivery
    - Preterm human milk is higher in cholesterol, phospholipids, and very long chain PUFAs than term milk. Preterm milk also has a higher sodium and chloride levels than that of mothers of term infants. As lactation progresses, the total fat content increases and cholesterol and phospholipid content decreases (Anderson et al., 2017, p. 268; Ditzenberger, 2015, p. 180; Poindexter & Ehrenkranz, 2015, p. 596).
  - ○ Expression and storage
    - Freezing human milk can change its composition by reducing the antioxidant properties, rupturing the fat globules, altering the casein component of the protein, and decreasing the fat and caloric content (Hurst & Puopolo, 2017, p. 290; Snell & Gardner, 2017, p.165).
  - ○ Hindmilk versus foremilk
    - Foremilk is lower in fat than hindmilk (Snell & Gardner, 2017, p.145)
  - ○ Use of feeding tube
    - Human milk fat and MCT additives adhere to the feeding tube, altering the nutritional content of the milk (Ditzenberger 2015, p. 192).
- During the first few postpartum days, mothers produce colostrum. Colostrum has less carbohydrates, fats, and calories than mature milk. However, it is higher in sodium, chloride, potassium, and protein than mature milk because of increased concentrations of globulins and lactoferrin. Colostrum has protective and anti-infective properties (Blackburn, 2012, p. 155).
- Changes occur as maternal milk transitions to mature milk:
  - ○ The concentration of immunoglobulins, protein, lactoferrin, sodium, chloride, and carotenoids decrease. For example, the protein content and composition decrease from 2 g/dL at birth to 1 g/dL in mature milk. The whey:casein ratio changes from 80:20 at the start of lactation to 55:45 in mature milk (Poindexter & Ehrenkranz, 2015, p. 593).
  - ○ The concentration of lactose, fat, and caloric density increases (Blackburn 2012, p. 155).

Nutrient Components of Human Milk

PROTEIN

- The leading whey protein in human milk is α–lactalbumin, which is high in AAs. Other human milk proteins include lactoferrin, serum albumin, lysozyme, secretory immunoglobulin A, IgA, IgG, IgM, and casein (Blackburn, 2013, p. 155, 428).
- Human milk contains less protein than cow's milk. The higher levels of nonprotein nitrogen and the AA composition of human milk are easier for digestion (Blackburn, 2013, p. 428).
- Human milk provides more than 45 enzymes, growth factors, and bioactive substances to promote growth and development, enhance gut maturation, and protect the infant from infection. It is ideal nutrition for the term and most preterm infants (Blackburn, 2013, p. 429).

FAT

- Fats are the primary source of energy in human milk and many formulas; it provides high calories without increasing the osmotic load (Blackburn, 2013, p. 429).
- Triglycerides are the primary component of human milk fat. Infants require both saturated and unsaturated fatty acids for neurologic and vision development (Blackburn, 2013, p. 429).
- Fats make up about 30% to 52% of the total caloric density of human milk and formulas (Adamkin et al., 2013, p. 170; Blackburn, 2013, p. 428; Brown et al., 2016, p. 380).
- At 3 days' lactation, the total fat content of human milk is about 2 g/dL. Mature milk has a fat content of 4 to 5 g/dL (Poindexter & Ehrenkranz, 2015, p. 596).
  - ○ Human fat globules contain fatty acids like linoleic, linolenic, oleic, palmitic, arachidonic, and DHAs. Arachidonic and DHAs are long-chain PUFAs (Blackburn, 2013, p. 429).
  - ○ Preterm human milk is higher in cholesterol, phospholipids, and very long-chain PUFAs. As lactation progresses, the total fat content increases and cholesterol and phospholipid content decreases (Poindexter & Ehrenkranz, 2015, p. 596).
- The fat content of human milk varies with circumstance:
  - ○ Mothers of preterm infants have higher PUFA.
  - ○ Phospholipids and cholesterol are higher in early lactation.
  - ○ Higher volumes of human milk production are associated with lower fat content.
  - ○ Mothers on low-fat diets are associated with milk production with a lower fat content.
  - ○ Milk fat content increases the longer a breastfeeding session continues (Blackburn, 2013, p. 429).
- Due to a limited bile salt pool and decreased pancreatic lipase levels, preterm infants poorly absorb LCTs (chain lengths of 14–20 carbons). MCT–carbon chain lengths of 8 to 12 carbons do not require bile for emulsification and are a good alternative to LCTs (Adamkin et al., 2013, p. 170).
  - ○ Shorter chain fatty acids can be absorbed intact across the intestinal and gastric mucosa. Medium-chain fatty acids (MCFAs) enhance calcium and magnesium absorption and are associated with rapid gastric emptying (Blackburn, 2013, p. 429).
  - ○ Excessive fat intake from MCFAs is associated with a risk of EFA deficiency (Blackburn, 2013, p. 429).

○ Human milk contains between 8% and 12% of MCTs as fat (Poindexter & Ehrenkranz, 2015, p. 596).

○ Between 10% and 50% of the fat in preterm formulas is MCFAs (Blackburn, 2013, p. 429).

○ Inadequate fat or a lack of EFA can result in metabolic problems, skin disorders, and poor growth. Excessive fats can result in ketosis (Blackburn, 2013, p. 428).

CARBOHYDRATES

- Carbohydrates comprise 40% to 50% of the caloric content of human milk and most formulas. Inadequate carbohydrates result in hypoglycemia. Excessive carbohydrates result in diarrhea (Adamkin et al., 2013, p. 168; Blackburn, 2013, p. 428).
- The primary carbohydrate in human milk is lactose. Lactose is an essential source of energy for the developing brain. Other carbohydrates include glucose, nucleotides, sugars, glycolipids, glycoproteins, and oligosaccharides (Adamkin et al., 2013, p. 168; Blackburn 2012, p. 155).
- Preterm infants have little difficulty digesting lactose-based formulas despite an immaturity of lactase (Adamkin et al., 2013, p. 168). Feedings containing lactose stimulate lactase activity and lactose utilization (Blackburn, 2013, p. 428).
- Alternative carbohydrates can be used for infants who are unable to tolerate lactose or when greater carbohydrate absorption is needed. It is important to note that infants require some lactose for calcium and magnesium absorption.

  ○ Oligosaccharides are glucose polymers that function as prebiotics by promoting the development of intestinal bacterial flora and inhibiting bacterial adhesion, which minimizes the risk of GI infections. Oligosaccharides are a major element in human milk (Blackburn, 2013, pp. 155, 429). See Box 10.1 for Advantages of Glucose Polymers.

BOX 10.1 Advantages of glucose polymers

1. Readily available from natural resources like corn syrup solids
2. Provide a high caloric density without considerably increasing the renal solute load
3. Do not significantly increase osmotic load or risk of diarrhea and water loss
4. Faster gastric emptying than lactose or glucose
5. Digestion is independent of lactase and amylase
6. Glucose polymers are digested by glucoamylase, which is present in adequate supply in the preterm infant.

Sources: Data from Blackburn, S. (2013). Gastrointestinal and hepatic systems and perinatal nutrition. In S. Blackburn (Ed.), *Maternal, fetal, & neonatal physiology: A clinical perspective* (pp. 393–442). Maryland Heights, MO: Elsevier/Saunders.

Vitamins and Minerals

- Human milk has a calcium and phosphorus concentrations appropriate for the full-term infant. Preterm infants receiving human milk must receive additional calcium, phosphorus, and vitamin D. Insufficient consumption of calcium, phosphorus, and vitamin D can result in rickets of prematurity (Adamkin et al., 2013, p. 172).

Human Milk Fortification

- Preterm human milk, when compared to the preterm infant's nutritional requirement, is lower in protein, calcium, phosphorus, iron, vitamins, and sodium (Blackburn, 2013, p. 431). Fortification of human milk can help minimize nutrient deficiencies for the preterm infant (Anderson et al., 2017, p. 269).

  ○ The preterm infant would require large volumes—180 mL/kg/day to 200 mL/kg/day—of unfortified human milk to mimic in utero weight gain of approximately 15 g/kg/day (Adamkin et al., 2013, p. 175).

- Human milk fortifiers contain protein, carbohydrates, calcium, phosphate, vitamins, sodium, and other substances. Fortification can lead to increases in weight gain, length, and HC in the short term. However, some preterm infants may experience slower weight gain when compared to formula due to the variable protein content of human milk (Blackburn, 2013, p. 431).

  ○ Absorption and nutrient retention of fortified human milk are similar to that of infants fed preterm formula (Adamkin et al., 2013, p. 169).

- The osmolarity of formulas and human milk mixtures increase by roughly the same percentage as the caloric increase. The renal solute load and osmolarity must be considered when concentrating formulas/human milk beyond 24 cal/oz (Ditzenberger, 2015, p. 186).
- Preterm infants less than 1,500 g should receive fortified human milk or fortified PDHM when available (Brown et al., 2016, p. 396).

  ○ Human milk-fed infants weighing < 1,500 g may be fortified with bovine milk-based HMF when receiving approximately 100 mL/kg of feeding volume.

  ○ Larger infants may be considered for the addition of HMF once they reach full volume (Anderson et al., 2017, p. 274).

Pasteurized Donor Human Milk

- Donor human milk is pasteurized human milk obtained from an accredited milk bank and utilized in the preterm infant when maternal human milk supply is unavailable. The composition of donor milk may vary based on the gestational age at the time of donation. Additionally, donor milk changes throughout lactation (Brown et al., 2016, p. 398).

  ○ Very low birth weight (VLBW) infants and those born < 32 weeks qualify for PDHM in most institutions because of their increased risk factors. PDHM is used as supplementation until the mother can provide 100% human milk or as a replacement for formula if the mother chooses not to provide human milk (Anderson et al., 2017, p. 269).

Breast Milk Storage and Handling

- It is important to collect, handle, and store breast milk appropriately to ensure nutritional quality and most importantly microbiological safety.

  ○ Appropriate hand hygiene is required before beginning the human milk collection process (Furman & Schanler, 2018, p. 1007; Hurst & Puopolo, 2017, p. 290).

  ○ Human milk collection kits should be rinsed, cleaned with hot soapy water, and air-dried (Ditzenberger,

2015, p. 187; Furman & Schanler, 2018, p. 1007; Hurst & Puopolo, 2017, p. 290).
- ○ Milk storage containers should be hard plastic or glass (Hurst & Puopolo, 2017, p. 290).
- ○ Each storage container should contain milk from one expression. The container should be labeled with a name, date, and time of pumping (Furman & Schanler, 2018, p. 1007; Hurst & Puopolo, 2017, p. 290).
- ○ Human milk should not be stored in plastic bags for preterm infants (Hurst & Puopolo, 2017, p. 290).
- Human milk must be frozen if not used within 24 hours after collection (Hurst & Puopolo, 2017, p. 290).
  - ○ Recent evidence suggests that human milk may be stored at 4°C in the refrigerator for up to 96 hours without increased bacterial count, and minimal changes in macronutrients, total fat, protein IgA, and lactoferrin (Ditzenberger, 2015, p. 188).
  - ○ Human milk can be stored safely from 3 to 6 months in the rear of the freezer compartment or in a deep freezer for 6 to 12 months (Ditzenberger, 2015, p. 187; Hurst & Puopolo, 2017, p. 290).
  - ○ It may be safe to freeze human milk for longer than recommended under appropriate conditions; however, the nutritional quality may decrease secondary to lipid degradation (Hurst & Puopolo, 2017, p. 290).
  - ○ Freezing human milk preserves many of the immunologic and nutritional benefits (Ditzenberger, 2015, p. 187; Furman & Schanler, 2018, p. 1007).
- Human milk must be thawed completely, using tepid running water or a commercial human milk thawing machine. Never use hot water or warm in the microwave oven (Ditzenberger, 2015, p. 188; Furman & Schanler, 2018, p. 1007).
  - ○ Thawed human milk must be stored in a refrigerator at 4°C and used within 24 hours (Ditzenberger, 2015, p. 188).
  - ○ Do not refreeze human milk after it has been thawed (Ditzenberger, 2015, p. 188; Furman & Schanler, 2018, p. 1007).

Lactation Support for Mothers

- The benefits of providing human milk to preterm infants begin with early encouragement and education to mothers about expressing and storing human milk (Ditzenberger, 2015, p. 187; Hurst & Puopolo, 2017, p. 288).
- Early discussions about the importance of human milk increase the incidence of lactation initiation without causing maternal stress and/or anxiety (Ditzenberger, 2015, p. 187).
- Pumping should begin soon after delivery in order to establish a generous milk supply.
  - ○ The first 24 to 48 hours postpartum may only yield a small amount of colostrum before sizable milk production begins. Maternal milk increases from approximately 50 mL/day to 500 to 600 mL/day by 36 hours postpartum (Ditzenberger, 2015, p. 187).
  - ○ Mothers require encouragement to pump a minimum of eight times per day in order to establish an adequate milk supply. A break in frequency can cause a significant decrease in milk supply (Ditzenberger, 2015, p. 187).
    - ■ By day 10 to 14, the milk production goal should be approximately 600 to 750 mL/day. Milk production will typically plateau by 14 days postpartum (Ditzenberger, 2015, p. 187).

- ○ Once milk production is established, milk supply is maintained by pumping six or more times per day with a minimum of 45 pumping times per week (Ditzenberger, 2015, p. 187).
- ○ Providing a supportive environment for mothers in addition to regular breast massage with proper technique can facilitate optimal milk expression. For example, it is essential to have a properly fitted milk expression shield and to simultaneously pump both breasts with a high-quality breast pump (Ditzenberger, 2015, p. 187).

Contraindications for Human Milk

- Illicit drugs concentrated in mother's human milk can cause neonatal intoxication and death (Snell & Gardner, 2017, p. 146). See Chapter 26 for a discussion of breastfeeding in the presence of specific drugs.
- Some prescription or over-the-counter medication, including cytotoxic drugs, are contraindications to breastfeeding (Ditzenberger, 2015, p. 185).
- Mothers with active type 1 and 2 human T-lymphotrophic virus infection should not breastfeed (Furman & Schanler, 2018, p. 1001).
- Varicella lesions must be crusted over before direct breastfeeding. Although pumped milk may be provided, the infant should be separated from the mother during an active varicella infection (Furman & Schanler, 2018, p. 1001; Snell & Gardner, 2017, p. 146).
- In developed countries, breastfeeding is contraindicated in mothers with HIV because of safer available alternatives (Snell & Gardner, 2017, p. 146).
- Infants with galactosemia are unable to receive maternal human milk or donated human milk (Furman & Schanler, 2018, p. 1001; Hurst & Puopolo, 2017, p. 291).

INFANT FORMULAS

Preparation of Formulas

- Most standard formulas have a ready-to-feed, powder, and liquid concentrate form allowing the option of fortification.
  - ○ Formulas should not be concentrated to more than 30 kcal/oz due to the resulting high renal solute load (Adamkin et al., 2013, p. 178).
  - ○ The use of powder infant formulas for fortification should be avoided in hospitalized newborns unless there is no other option, due to the risk of Cronobacter sakazakii infection (Brown et al., 2016, p. 402).
- Caloric density of formula can be increased through the addition of powder and/or liquid concentrate, glucose polymers, or fat (e.g., vegetable or MCT oil; Adamkin et al., 2013, p. 179; Brown et al., 2016, p. 402).
- When increasing the caloric density of a feeding, careful attention must be paid to the calorie distribution of carbohydrates, proteins, and fats. Total calories should be distributed as 35% to 65% from carbohydrates, 30% to 55% from fat, and 8% to 16% from protein (Adamkin et al., 2013, p. 179).

Preterm Infant Formulas

- Preterm infant formulas are whey predominant, with a whey:casein ratio of 60:40 (Adamkin et al., 2013, p. 170, 178; Brown et al., 2016, p. 401).

○ These formulas have a higher protein concentration, of 3.6 to 4.2 g protein/kg/day (Adamkin et al., 2013, p. 178).

○ Compared to human milk, whey-predominant formulas have higher levels of methionine, threonine, lysine, and branched AAs (Poindexter & Ehrenkranz, 2015, p. 594).

○ High protein infant formulas are indicated:

■ For infants who are volume restricted; to promote wound healing; for infants with inadequate growth in length and/or HC; and for infants weighing less than 1,500 g (Brown et al., 2016, p. 390).

● Preterm infant formulas are comprised of approximately 50% LCTs and up to 50% MCTs (Adamkin et al., 2013, p. 178; Poindexter & Ehrenkranz, 2017, p. 604).

○ Due to differences in metabolism, formulas with MCTs improve nitrogen, calcium, and magnesium absorption. Approximately half of the fat in preterm infant formula is in the form of MCTs (Adamkin et al., 2013, p. 171).

● The iron content of preterm formulas varies from the low content 3 mg elemental iron/L to fortified with an iron content of 15 mg elemental iron/L (Adamkin et al., 2013, p. 178).

Standard Infant Formulas

● Most standard formulas are whey predominant with a whey-to-casein protein ratio of 60% to 40%. Casein-predominant cow milk formulas have a whey:casein ratio of 18:82 (Poindexter & Ehrenkranz, 2015, p. 594).

○ Casein protein requires more energy to digest and is more likely to be incompletely digested due to its tougher curds. The curds of whey are softer (Blackburn, 2013, p. 428).

● The fat content of standard formulas includes all LCTs from vegetable oils, including soy and coconut (Adamkin et al., 2013, p. 178).

● Standard formulas are available as iron-fortified or non-fortified/low iron forms. Iron-fortified formulas contain 12 mg/L of elemental iron, or 2 mg/kg/day for infants receiving 108 kcal/kg/day. Low-iron formulas contain 1.5 mg/L of elemental iron, or 0.2 mg/kg/day (Adamkin et al., 2013, p. 178).

Soy Formulas

● Soy formulas are lactose-free and recommended for infants with galactosemia, with primary lactase deficiency, or for

infants recovering from secondary lactose intolerance, vegan families, or infants with IgE-mediated cow's milk protein allergy (Adamkin et al., 2013, p. 179; Brown et al., 2016, p. 402).

● LCTs in the form of vegetable oils, usually coconut and soy oil, make up the fat content in soy formulas (Adamkin et al., 2013, p. 179).

● Soy protein formulas are not recommended for the preterm infant due to their low calcium and phosphorus content, poorer quality of protein, lower digestibility, and bioavailability. Preterm infants fed soy protein formulas are at increased risk of developing osteopenia and experience slower weight gain and lower protein and albumin concentrations despite supplementation (Adamkin et al., 2013, p. 179; Brown et al., 2016, p. 402).

Protein Hydrolysate Formulas

● Protein hydrolysate formulas are designed for infants with allergies to cow's milk or soy protein and are sometimes used in the management of infants with bowel resections or intractable diarrhea. Elemental formulas have also been used in infants with severe liver disease and fat malabsorption, infants with short bowel syndrome, and dysmotility syndromes (Brown et al., 2016, p. 402).

● The protein source in these elemental formulas are derived from free AAs, and many are lactose free (Adamkin et al., 2013, p. 179; Brown et al., 2016, p. 402).

● Fat content is comprised of both medium chain and LCTs (Adamkin et al., 2013, p. 179).

● Some of these formulas are elemental with easily absorbable carbohydrates (e.g., monosaccharides or glucose polymers (Adamkin et al., 2013, p. 179).

Post-Discharge Transitional Formulas

● Post-discharge formulas have increased concentrations of calcium, phosphorus, zinc, vitamins, and trace elements to promote and support linear growth (Adamkin et al., 2013, p. 180).

● Post-discharge transitional formula or fortified human milk should be provided to the preterm infants who remain below normal weight at discharge (Brown et al., 2016, p. 417).

● Preterm infants with normal weight for postmenstrual age at the time of discharge may be fed similar to term infants of the same gestational age (Brown et al., 2016, p. 417).

● See Table 10.8 for the indication for use of different formulas.

TABLE 10.8 Indication for Use of Infant Formulas

Clinical Condition	Suggested Type of Infant Formula	Rationale
Allergy to cow's milk protein or soy protein	Extensively hydrolyzed protein or free amino acids	Impaired digestion/utilization of intact protein
Bronchopulmonary dysplasia	High energy, nutrient dense	Increased energy requirement, fluid restriction
Biliary atresia	Semi elemental, containing reduced LCT (~45%), with supplemented MCT (~55%)	Impaired intraluminal digestion and absorption of long-chain fats
Chylothorax (persistent)	High-energy formula	Lower fluid and sodium intake; increased energy requirement

(continued)

TABLE 10.8 Indication for Use of Infant Formulas *(cont.)*

Clinical Condition	Suggested Type of Infant Formula	Rationale
Cystic fibrosis	Semi-elemental formula, containing reduced LCT (~45%), with supplemented MCT (~55%) or standard formula with pancreatic enzyme supplementation	Impaired intraluminal digestion and absorption of long-chain fats
Galactosemia	Soy protein-based formula	Lactose free
Gastroesophageal reflux	Standard formula, Enfamil A.R.	Consider small, frequent feedings
Hepatic insufficiency	Semi-elemental formula, containing reduced LCT (~45%), with supplemented MCT (~55%)	Impaired intraluminal digestion and absorption of long-chain fats
Lactose intolerance	Low-lactose formula	Impaired digestion or utilization of lactose
Lymphatic anomalies	Significantly reduced LCT (—15%), with supplemented MCT (~84%)	Impaired absorption of long-chain fats
Necrotizing enterocolitis	Preterm formula or semi-elemental formula, if indicated	Impaired digestion
Renal insufficiency	Standard formula	
	Similac PM 60/40	Low phosphate content, low renal solute load

LCT, long-chain triglyceride; MCT, medium-chain triglyceride.

Source: Reproduced with permission from Anderson, D., Poindexter, B., & Martin, C. (2017). Nutrition. In E. Eichenwald, A. Hansen, C. Martin, & A. Stark (Eds.), *Cloherty and Stark's manual of neonatal care* (8th ed., pp. 248–284). Philadelphia, PA: Wolters Kluwer.

ENTERAL SUPPLEMENTS

Oral Dietary Supplements

FATS
- MCTs offers 8.3 kcal/g or 7.7 kcal/mL.
- LCTs offers 4.5 kcal/mL.

CARBOHYDRATES
- Maltodextrin (for use with term infants only) offers 3.8 kcal/g or 8 kcal/teaspoon (powder).

PROTEIN
- Extensively hydrolyzed casein protein offers 3.6 kcal/g or 4 kcal/ 6 mL.

Enteral Electrolyte Requirements

- Sodium, potassium, and chloride are necessary for growth and play an important role in the water, acid/base balance (Ditzenberger, 2015, p. 180).
  - Many preterm infants, especially VLBW infants, may require sodium supplements until renal tubular function matures (Ditzenberger, 2015, p. 180).
- Preterm human milk has higher sodium and chloride levels than that of mothers of term infants; however, these infants may still need additional supplementation until the renal tubular function matures (Anderson et al., 2017, p. 268; Ditzenberger, 2015, p. 180).
- Preterm infant formulas contain higher amounts of sodium, potassium, and chloride than do term infant formulas (Ditzenberger, 2015, p. 180).

Enteral Vitamins and Mineral Requirements

- Vitamins are organic substances that are essential to normal metabolism; however, they are not synthesized by the body (Poindexter & Ehrenkranz, 2015, p. 607).
- Infants of undernourished mothers as well as preterm infants have lower blood levels of water-soluble vitamins at birth (Poindexter & Ehrenkranz, 2015, p. 607).
- Freezing or pasteurization may decrease the vitamins and minerals in human milk (Poindexter & Ehrenkranz, 2015, p. 607).
- Vitamins are categorized by their solubility:
  - Fat-soluble vitamins include vitamins A, D, E, and K (Poindexter & Ehrenkranz, 2015, p. 607).
  - Water-soluble vitamins include vitamin B complex and vitamin C. Folic acid is not included in liquid multivitamins because there is a lack of stability; they can be given separately as indicated (Poindexter & Ehrenkranz, 2015, p. 607–608).

Vitamin A

- Colostrum contains the highest amounts of vitamin A. Vitamin A content in preterm and term human milk are comparable, then decline as the human milk matures (Colaizy et al., 2018, p. 1013).
- Improving vitamin A levels in the preterm infant is associated with decreased incidence of CLD, also known as BPD (Colaizy et al., 2018, p. 1013).
- Vitamin A supplementation in extremely preterm infants during the first month after birth affects survival without neurodevelopmental impairment (Picciano, McGuire, & Coates, 2011, p. 830).

Vitamin K (Phytonadione)

- Vitamin K is the only vitamin routinely given immediately after birth (Colaizy et al., 2018, p. 1013). Human milk does not provide adequate amounts of vitamin K; therefore, a dose is given after birth to protect infants from hemorrhage (Picciano et al., 2011, p. 836). There is also an association with human milk and the development of an intestinal microflora that makes less vitamin K (Furman & Schanler, 2018, p. 996).
  - ○ Recommended vitamin K dosing at the time of birth is 1 mg intramuscular (IM) injection in both term and preterm neonates more than 1,000 g birth weight.
  - ○ Dosing for preterm infants less than 1,000 g is 0.3 mg (Poindexter & Ehrenkranz, 2015, p. 607).

Vitamin D

- Vitamin D supplementation is recommended for breastfed or formula-fed infants unless taking at least 1,000 mL/day of vitamin D–fortified formula (Anderson et al., 2017, p. 282).
  - ○ Vitamin D plays a vital role in skeletal growth and maturation. Four hundred international units per day of vitamin D is recommended to prevent osteopenia, otherwise known as vitamin D deficiency rickets, in preterm infants (Abrams, 2017, p. 857; Picciano et al., 2011, p. 832; Poindexter & Ehrenkranz, 2015, p. 607).
  - ○ Vitamin D in human milk is dependent on maternal vitamin D levels (Furman & Schanler, 2018, p. 996).
- Vitamin D supplementation is recommended in the exclusively breastfed infant secondary to the inadequate amounts of vitamin D in human milk (Anderson et al., 2017, p. 282).

Vitamin E

- Vitamin E supplementation in preterm infants has been debated by many experts.
  - ○ The American Academy of Pediatrics (AAP) does not recommend pharmacological doses of vitamin E for the prevention or treatment of retinopathy of prematurity, BPD, and/or IVH. However; 6 to 12 IU/kg/d of vitamin E enterally has been recommended for extremely preterm infants for optimal nutritional support (Picciano et al., 2011, p. 835).
- Term and preterm human milk provide adequate amounts of vitamin E (Picciano et al., 2011, p. 835).

Iron

- Preterm infants are more likely to develop iron deficiency, which can have a negative impact on brain development (Poindexter & Ehrenkranz, 2015, p. 607). Delayed cord clamping may increase iron stores for both term and preterm infants (Colaizy et al., 2018, p. 1012).
- Preterm infants that receive human milk are more likely to have iron deficiency secondary to the decrease in iron concentration during the progression of lactation (Colaizy et al., 2018, p. 1012).
- The iron content of many preterm formulas and HMFs is not sufficient; therefore, additional iron supplementation is necessary (Poindexter & Ehrenkranz, 2015, p. 607).
- Infants receiving an erythrocyte-stimulating agent such as erythropoietin may need a higher dose of iron (Poindexter & Ehrenkranz, 2015, p. 607).
  - ○ Preterm infants require iron supplementation to be started between 2 and 4 weeks of age with a recommended dose of 2 to 4 mg/kg/day (Anderson et al., 2017, p. 278; Poindexter & Ehrenkranz, 2015, p. 607).

Calcium/Phosphorous

- The nutritional goal for preterm infants is to obtain a bone mineralization pattern similar to that of the fetus in an effort to prevent osteopenia and fractures (Colaizy et al., 2018, p. 1011), as calcium and phosphorus are the primary components of the skeleton (Poindexter & Ehrenkranz, 2015, p. 606).
- The recommended daily requirement for enteral calcium is 120 to 200 mg/kg (Poindexter & Ehrenkranz, 2015, p. 606).
- Recommended daily requirements for phosphorus are 60 to 140 mg/kg (Poindexter & Ehrenkranz, 2015, p. 606).
  - ○ Preterm infants require sufficient amounts of calcium and phosphorus early in hospitalization prior to exclusive breastfeeding (Poindexter & Ehrenkranz, 2015, p. 606).
  - ○ Calcium and phosphorus exist in ionized and complex forms that are easily absorbed in human milk (Colaizy et al., 2018, p. 1011).
  - ○ Preterm human milk contains approximately 250 mg of calcium in addition to 140 mg of phosphorus per liter (Colaizy et al., 2018, p. 1011). The calcium:phosphorus (Ca:P) ratio should be approximately 2:1, which is similar to the ratio in human milk (Poindexter & Ehrenkranz, 2015, p. 606).
- *Magnesium*
- An estimated 60% of the body's magnesium is found in the bones (Poindexter & Ehrenkranz, 2015, p. 606).
  - ○ Daily requirements for magnesium are 8 to 12 mg/kg (Poindexter & Ehrenkranz, 2015, p. 606).
  - ○ Preterm human milk contains approximately 30 mg of magnesium per liter (Poindexter & Ehrenkranz, 2015, p. 606).
- Infants born to diabetic mothers often present with transient hypomagnesemia (Poindexter & Ehrenkranz, 2015, p. 606).

Omega-3 Fatty Acids

- Omega-3 fatty acids play an important role in visual and neurological development, in addition to immune function, protecting the body from inflammation, and decreasing the risk for many chronic degenerative diseases. Supplementing infants with longer chain polyunsaturated fatty acid (LCPUFA) has been shown to improve neural development, especially, when infants are fed formula.
- Omega-3 fatty acids supplementation includes alpha-linolenic acid (ALA), LCPUFA metabolites, eicosapentaenoic acid (EPA), and DHA. Human milk contains a variety of omega-3 fatty acids and is greatly dependent on the mother's diet (Picciano et al., 2011, p. 845).
- Infant formulas are made with corn, coconut, safflower, and soy oils unless they are fortified with LCPUFAs (Picciano et al., 2011, p. 845).

Zinc

- Zinc is highly bioavailable in human milk; however, the quantity declines over the course of lactation (Picciano et al., 2011, p. 841).

- Preterm recommendations for zinc intake are 1 to 3 mg/kg/d, and can be achieved through the use of term or preterm formulas as well as HMFs (Picciano et al., 2011, p. 841).
- Most formulas are supplemented with zinc to contain 5 to 7 mg/L with preterm formulas containing roughly 5 to 10 mg/L (Picciano et al., 2011, p. 841).

Fluoride

- Fluoride intake by infants can vary widely depending on whether the infant is fed human milk or formula. There is a difference in fluoride content in ready-to-feed formulas versus powder formulas that require reconstitution with water. Fluoride intake by formula-fed infants can be as high as 1.0 mg per day. However, there is variability based on the water source (Picciano et al., 2011, p. 844).
- Fluoride concentration in human milk is 4 to 15 mg/L, which results in intakes of 3 to 12 mg/kg/day (Picciano et al., 2011, p. 844).
- Fluoride supplements are not recommended in infants under 6 months of age (Picciano et al., 2011, p. 844).

Iodine

- Iodine is found in the developing brain, muscle, heart, pituitary, and kidney. However, it is concentrated in the thyroid gland (Picciano et al., 2011, p. 842).
- Iodine is the most common nutrient deficiency worldwide, causing transient hypothyroidism. However, iodine deficiency is not as common in the United States (Wassner & Belfort, 2017, p. 902).
  - Iodine deficiency disorders include mental retardation, hypothyroidism, goiter, cretinism, and growth and developmental abnormalities (Picciano et al., 2011, p. 843).
- Iodine content in human milk is contingent on maternal intake. Human milk and bovine milk-based infant formulas are typically a good source of this mineral (Picciano et al., 2011, p. 842).

INFANTS WITH SPECIAL NUTRITIONAL REQUIREMENTS

Bronchopulmonary Dysplasia

- Infants with BPD often require a balance between proper nutrition and a required fluid restriction as BPD can cause an increase in metabolic demand and energy requirements by 20% to 40% (Ditzenberger, 2015, p. 186). Monitor ongoing growth parameters to ensure continued growth is not compromised (Anderson et al., 2017, p. 281).
- When fluid restrictions are implemented, it is important to monitor adequate caloric and micronutrient intake as higher caloric needs may be required in order to promote healing and tissue growth (Ditzenberger, 2015, p. 186). Infants with BPD often require a caloric density of 30 kcal/oz to achieve desired growth targets (Anderson et al., 2017, p. 268).
- Transitioning from gavage to oral feedings may require different approaches in the duration and feeding volume based on the infant's energy status and respiratory demands (Ditzenberger, 2015, p. 186).

Inborn Errors of Metabolism

- An individualized diet must be established based on the metabolic defect. Modified formula preparation containing all but the aberrant AAs should be used. For example, an infant with galactosemia should be fed a lactose-free formula (Anderson et al., 2017, p. 868).
- It is important to withhold enteral feedings for infants with inborn errors of metabolism (IEM) until the infant is neurologically stable. The infant may have difficulty establishing oral feedings until the acute phase is over. An OG (oral gastric) or NG (nasogastric) tube should be considered if there is a significant neurological compromise.

Cardiac Defects

- Infants with cardiac defects have increased metabolic demand and tend to have poor growth. Higher metabolic rate and oxygen consumption secondary to increased cardiac and respiratory workload may cause fatigue, resulting in tachypnea and poor feeding. Infants with cardiac defects often display poor feeding with fewer cues and are less responsive to the caregiver during periods of feeding.
- Fortification of human milk/formula at an increased caloric density is imperative to ensure higher caloric needs are met in efforts to restrict total fluid intake (Ditzenberger, 2015, p. 186).

Short Bowel Syndrome

- Infants with short bowel syndrome have reduced intestinal length because of surgical resection resulting from a congenital anomaly or NEC. Also, intestinal hypoxia from NEC can cause atrophy of essential villi as a result of the reduced intestinal length; there is a reduction in the intestinal absorptive surface areas
- Enteral feedings may potentially be achieved with a minimum of 25 cm of small bowel with an intact ileocecal valve, or with 40 cm of small bowel without an ileocecal valve (Ditzenberger, 2015, pp. 186–187). However, these numbers are not absolute. Intestinal failure occurs anytime the intestines no longer have the ability to meet energy, fluid, and electrolyte requirements, regardless of remaining length (Javid, Riggle, & Smith, 2018, p. 1096)
- Long-term PN may be required to promote linear growth, depending on the length of the remaining bowel and nutritional status (Ditzenberger, 2015, pp. 186–187). The goal of intestinal rehabilitation is to slowly advance enteral feeds and wean PN as the remaining bowel undergoes the process of intestinal adaptation (Javid et al., 2018, p. 1096).

Gastroesophageal Reflux

- Intestinal dysmotility secondary to prematurity is most commonly the root cause of emesis during the initiation and advancement of enteral feeds in the preterm infant. If these episodes do not compromise the infant's respiratory status or growth, only continued close monitoring is required (Anderson et al., 2017, p. 280).
- There is no clear evidence linking gastroesophageal reflux (GER) and apnea episodes, therefore, it is not recommended to use promotility agents with uncomplicated apnea of prematurity (Anderson et al., 2017, p. 280).

- Modifications of the feeding regimen can improve emesis in the preterm infant, including:
  - ○ Lengthening the duration of the feeding (sometimes to the point of using continuous feeding)
  - ○ Reduction in feeding volume
  - ○ The removal of nutritional additives
  - ○ Use of specialized formulas (Anderson et al., 2017, pp. 279–280)
- Therapeutic maneuvers to help decrease emesis include:
  - ○ Reposition the infant to elevate the head and upper body.
  - ○ Position either prone or right side down (Anderson et al., 2017, p. 280).
- Infants may require an evaluation of their anatomy if the achievement of full-volume feeds is prevented by recurrent episodes of symptomatic emesis.

Intrauterine Growth Restriction

- IUGR infants have increased energy requirements secondary to low stores of energy, nutrients, and minerals (Brown et al., 2016, p. 415).
- An individualized management plan is essential for IUGR infants because they may not tolerate enteral feeding advancement as well as normally grown infants. Additionally, they do not always respond to the increased nutrient intake with adequate rates of growth (Brown et al., 2016, p. 415).
  - ○ The IUGR population is at risk for NEC (Brown et al., 2016, p. 415). Providers tend to proceed with caution when initiating early feedings in this population. However, there is no evidence correlating early feedings with NEC (Calkin & Devaskar, 2015, p. 232).

Necrotizing Enterocolitis

- NEC is the most commonly acquired GI emergency in the NICU and predominantly affects preterm infants (Weinert and Martinez-Rios, 2015, p. 547).
  - ○ Hypoxic-ischemic events and/or asphyxia episodes may place term infants at a higher risk of developing NEC (Brown et al., 2016, p. 416).
- There are multiple bioactive factors in human milk that influence host immunity, inflammation, and mucosal protection (Caplan, 2015, p. 1426); therefore, preterm infants exclusively fed with expressed human milk are at decreased risk for developing NEC (Weitkamp, Premkumar, & Martin, 2017, p. 364).
  - ○ Preterm infants can be given minimal enteral feedings with mother's colostrum/human milk, which has the potential to improve gut development after injury. Human milk can potentially colonize the gut with a more favorable microbiome (Brown et al., 2016, p. 416).
- Infants with NEC are at higher risk for malnutrition secondary to increased nutrient losses and malabsorption; therefore, it is imperative to support the infants' nutritional needs with PN, specifically through the acute phase (Brown et al., 2016, p. 416).
- In the case of surgical NEC, neonates are at increased risk for nutritional deficiencies caused from the stress of illness and surgery. Therefore, human milk feedings are preferred because they are safe while preserving the integrity of the intestinal mucosa. Additionally, enteral feedings promote the continued development of the GI tract (Brown et al., 2016, p. 416).

CONCLUSION

The development and function of the GI system are vital to human growth and long-term survival. A thorough understanding of fluid, electrolytes, GI development, physiology, and disease process are crucial to ensure adequate growth and nutrition in the critically ill neonate. This chapter highlights GI embryology, physiology, parenteral, and enteral nutrition. The effects of nutrition on the neonate with multisystem disease processes were further discussed.

REVIEW QUESTIONS

1. A 36-week infant born 1 month ago currently weighs 3.62 kilograms. The previous weight 7 days ago was 3.5 kg. What is the 7-day weight gain in grams (gm) per kilogram (kg) per day (d)?
   A. 1.2 gm/kg/d
   B. 3.3 gm/kg/d
   C. 4.7 gm/kg/d

2. An infant is eating 75 mL every 3 hours of human milk at 20 kcal/oz. The current weight is 3.62 kg. What is the intake in kilocalories (Kcal) per kilogram (kg) per day (d)?
   A. 106 kcal/kg/day
   B. 111 kcal/kg/day
   C. 115 kcal/kg/day

3. Infants with necrotizing enterocolitis (NEC) are at high risk for malnutrition; therefore, it is imperative to support the infants' nutritional needs with:
   A. parenteral nutrition
   B. oral omega acids
   C. corticosteroids

4. An infant has been NPO for an extended period of time due to impaired biliary excretion. Regarding the delivery of parenteral nutrition, the nutritionist recommends the reduction or omission of
   A. chromium
   B. manganese
   C. selenium

5. One contraindication for breastfeeding includes an infant's diagnosis of:
   A. cytomegalovirus
   B. galactosemia
   C. microcephaly

REFERENCES

Abrams, S. (2017). Osteopenia (metabolic bone disease) of prematurity. In E. Eichenwald, A. Hansen, C. Martin, & A. Stark (Eds.), *Cloherty and Stark's manual of neonatal care* (8th ed., pp. 853–857). Philadelphia, PA: Wolters Kluwer.

Adamkin, D., Radmacher, P., & Lewis, S. (2013). Nutrition and selected disorders of the gastrointestinal tract. In A. Fanaroff & J. Fanaroff (Eds.), *Klaus and Fanaroff's care of the high-risk neonate* (6th ed., pp. 151–200). Cleveland, OH: Elsevier.

Anderson, D., Poindexter, B., & Martin, C. (2017). Nutrition. In E. Eichenwald, A. Hansen, C. Martin, & A. Stark (Eds.), *Cloherty and Stark's manual of neonatal care* (8th ed., pp. 248–284). Philadelphia, PA: Wolters Kluwer.

Blackburn, S. (2013). Gastrointestinal and hepatic systems and perinatal nutrition. In S. Blackburn (Ed.), *Maternal, fetal, & neonatal physiology: A clinical perspective* (pp. 393–442). Maryland Heights, MO: Elsevier/ Saunders.

Brown, L., Hendrickson, K., Evans, R., Davis, J., Sollosy Anderson, M., & Hay, W. W., Jr. (2016). Enteral nutrition. In S. Gardner, B. Carter, M. Enzman-Hines, & J. Hernandez (Eds.), *Merestein & Gardner's handbook of neonatal intensive care* (8th ed., pp. 377–418). St. Louis, MO: Elsevier.

Burris, H. (2017). Hypoglycemia and hyperglycemia. In E. Eichenwald, A. Hansen, C. Martin, & A. Stark (Eds.), *Cloherty and Stark's manual of neonatal care* (8th ed., pp. 312–334). Philadelphia, PA: Wolters Kluwer.

Calkin, K., & Devaskar, S. (2015). Interuterine growth restriction. In R. Martin, A. Fanaroff, & M. Walsh (Eds.), *Fanaroff and Martin's neonatal-perinatal medicine: Diseases of the fetus and infant* (10th ed., pp. 227–235). Philadelphia, PA: Elsevier.

Caplan, M. (2015). Neonatal necrotizing enterocolitis. In R. Martin, A. Fanaroff, & M. Walsh (Eds.), *Fanaroff and Martin's neonatal-perinatal medicine: Diseases of the fetus and infant* (10th ed., pp. 1423–1432). Philadelphia, PA: Elsevier.

Carlson, C. A., & Shirland, L. (2010). *Neonatal parenteral and enteral nutrition: A resource guide for the student and novice neonatal nurse practitioner.* Retrieved from http://nann.org/uploads/Membership/MembersOnllyPDFS/Neonatal_Parenteral_and_Enteral_Nutrition.pdf

Colaizy, T., Demauro, S., Mcnelis, K., & Poindexter, B. (2018). Enteral nutrition of the high risk neonate. In C. Gleason & S. Juul (Eds.), *Avery's diseases of the newborn* (10th ed., pp. 1009–1022). Philadelphia, PA: Elsevier.

Denne, S. (2018). Parenteral nutrition for the high-risk neonate. In C. Gleason & S. Juul (Eds.), *Avery's diseases of the newborn* (10th ed., pp. 1023–1031e2). Philadelphia, PA: Elsevier.

Dimmitt, R., Sellers, Z., & Sibley, E. (2018). Gastrointestinal tract development. In C. Gleason & S. Juul (Eds.), *Avery's diseases of the newborn* (10th ed., pp. 1032–1038). Philadelphia, PA: Elsevier.

Ditzenberger, G. (2015). Nutritional management. In M. T. Verklan & M. Walden (Eds.), *Core curriculum for neonatal intensive care nursing* (5th ed., pp. 172–196). St. Louis, MO: Elsevier.

Furman, L., & Schanler, R. J. (2018). Breastfeeding. In C. Gleason & S. Juul (Eds.), *Avery's diseases of the newborn* (10th ed., pp. 991–1008). Philadelphia, PA: Elsevier.

Halbardier, B. (2015). Fluid and electrolyte management. In M. T. Verklan & M. Walden (Eds.), *Core curriculum for neonatal intensive care nursing* (5th ed., pp. 146–161). St. Louis, MO: Elsevier.

Hurst, N., & Puopolo, K. (2017). Breastfeeding and maternal medications. In E. Eichenwald, A. Hansen, C. Martin, & A. Stark (Eds.), *Cloherty and Stark's manual of neonatal care* (8th ed., pp. 285–295). Philadelphia, PA: Wolters Kluwer.

Javid, P., Riggle, K., & Smith, C. (2018). Necrotizing enterocolitis and short bowel syndrome. In C. Gleason & S. Juul (Eds.), *Avery's diseases of the newborn* (10th ed., pp. 1090–1097e.2). Philadelphia, PA: Elsevier.

McElroy, S., Frey, M., Torres, B., & Maheshwari, A. (2018). Innate and mucosal immunity in the developing gastrointestinal tract. In C. Gleason & S. Juul (Eds.), *Avery's diseases of the newborn* (10th ed., pp. 1054–1067). Philadelphia, PA: Elsevier.

Olsen, S., Leick-Rude, M. K., Dusin, J., & Rosterman, J. (2016). Total parenteral nutrition. In S. Gardner, B. Carter, M. E. Hines, & H. Jacinto (Eds.), *Merestein & Gardner's handbook of neonatal intensive care* (8th ed., pp. 360–376). St. Louis, MO: Elsevier.

Parry, R. (2015). Development of the neonatal gastrointestinal tract. In R. Martin, A. Fanaroff, & M. Walsh (Eds.), *Fanaroff and Martin's neonatal-perinatal* (10th ed., pp. 1364–1370). Philadelphia, PA: Elselvier/Saunders.

Picciano, M., McGuire, M., & Coates, P. (2011). Nutrient supplements. In S. Yaffe & J. Aranda (Eds.), *Neonatal and pediatric pharmacology: Therapeutic principles in practice* (4th ed., pp. 827–846). Philadelphia, PA: Lippincott Williams & Wilkins.

Poindexter, B., & Ehrenkranz, R. (2015). Nutrient requirements and provision of nutritional support in the prematrure neonate. In R. Martin, A. Fanaroff, & M. Walsh (Eds.), *Fanaroff and Martin's neonatal-perinatal medicine: Diseases of the fetus and infant* (10th ed., pp. 592–612). Philadelphia, PA: Elsevier.

Snell, B., & Gardner, S. (2017). Newborn and neonatal nutrition. In B. Snell & S. Gardner (Eds.), *Care of the well newborn* (pp. 135–190). Burlington, MA: Jones & Bartlett Learning.

Wassner, A. J., & Belfort, M. B. (2017). Thyroid disorders. In E. Eichenwald, A. Hansen, C. Martin, & A. Stark (Eds.), *Cloherty and Stark's manual of neonatal care* (8th ed., pp.892–909). Philadelphia, PA: Wolters Kluwer.

Weinert, D., & Martinez-Rios, C. (2015). Diagnostic imaging of the neonate. In R. Martin, A. Fanaroff, & M. Walsh (Eds.), *Fanaroff and Martin's neonatal-perinatal medicine: Diseases of the fetus and infant* (10th ed., pp. 536–558). Philadelphia, PA: Elsevier.

Weitkamp, J., Premkumar, M., & Martin, C. (2017). Necrotizing enterocolitis. In E. Eichenwald, A. Hansen, C. Martin, & A. Stark (Eds.), *Cloherty and Stark's manual of neonatal care* (8th ed., pp. 353–365). Philadelphia, PA: Wolters Kluwer.

11 FLUIDS AND ELECTROLYTES

Carolyn J. Herrington
Leanne M. Nantais-Smith

INTRODUCTION

Fluid and electrolyte management, acid–base homeostasis, and parenteral and enteral nutritional therapies are central in the management of the sick newborn. Management approaches have changed significantly over time, moving from restrictive fluid-management approaches in the 1950s to the current, more liberalized approach. Those early restrictive approaches resulted in hyperosmolarity, exaggerated hyperbilirubinemia, and hypoglycemia, all of which further complicated management and outcomes in these infants. The current approach recommends a more liberal approach to initial fluid management, but ideal approaches continue to remain somewhat uncertain. The principles of fluid and electrolyte management also vary based on the gestational age (GA) and the disease process of the infant (Nyp, Brunkhorst, Reavy, & Pallotto, 2016, pp. 315–318).

PRINCIPLES OF FLUID AND ELECTROLYTE MANAGEMENT

- Physiologically, infants are different from children and adults in several ways. Basic metabolic rates are significantly higher in newborns, which creates a need for increased delivery per kilogram of body weight.
- Sodium excretion is 10% of that of older children and adults because the glomerular filtration rate (GFR) is five to 10 times lower and sodium reabsorption in the proximal and distal renal tubules is decreased (Doherty, 2017, p. 296), which makes them more vulnerable to sodium overload (Nyp et al., 2016, p. 315).
- Total body water (TBW) distributions are also significantly different from those of older children and adults and vary significantly across GAs as well (Nyp et al., 2016, p. 315).

Total Body Water

- The TBW varies from 85% to 90% in the extremely low birth weight (ELBW) infant to 75% in the term newborn infant (Halbardier, 2015, p. 146).
  - Prior to birth, the major factor controlling TBW is maternal status.
  - After birth, the infant assumes the homeostatic control of TBW content as well as fluid and electrolyte balance (Doherty, 2017, p. 296).
- The TBW is composed of both the intracellular and extracellular fluid compartments (ICF and ECF respectively). The ECF is further broken down into the intravascular space (IVS) and the interstitial space (IS; Doherty, 2016, p. 296).

Intracellular

- Water and biomolecules are contained within the cells surrounded by a cell membrane. The cell membrane allows movement of water and electrolytes inside and outside the cell via transport mechanisms, such as diffusion and sodium or potassium transport carriers.
  - Protein transporters in the cell membrane require energy to transport ions—for example, sodium, potassium, and chloride—back and forth between the ICF to ECF.
  - The major intracellular solutes are proteins that support cell function, organic phosphates that participate in energy production and storage, and charged ions.
  - Potassium is the major cation of the ICF (Wright, Posencheg, Seri, & Evans, 2018, p. 369).
  - Any disorder or disease that disrupts maintenance of normal pH can affect fluid and electrolyte balance by interfering with normal cell function, such as limiting the production of protein cell membrane transport carriers or disabling oxygen-requiring active ion transport mechanisms (Wright et al., 2018, p. 383).

Extracellular

- The extracellular compartment is comprised of water and biomolecules contained outside the cell. The major cation of the ECF is sodium and the major anion is chloride. The ECF is divided into two compartments:
  - The intravascular space (IVS) contains the fluid component of the blood, which circulates in the blood vessels.
  - The interstitial space (IS) is comprised of fluid within the tissues that surround all cells not contained in the IVS.
- A capillary membrane divides the intravascular and interstitial compartments. The major differences in the composition between the IVS and IS are proteins. Proteins in the IVS exert an osmotic pressure.
  - Movement of fluid between the IVS and IS is determined by filtration and reabsorption.
  - When capillary hydrostatic pressure (blood pressure) exceeds blood oncotic pressure, fluid moves from the IVS into the tissue (filtration).
  - When capillary oncotic pressure (from circulating albumin) exceeds capillary hydrostatic pressure, fluid moves into the IVS (reabsorption).
    - Excess fluid not reabsorbed is drained by the lymphatic system and returns to the IVS via the subclavian veins (Wright et al., 2018, p. 370).
- The composition of the ICF and ECF differs in the concentration of each solute—for example, higher potassium concentration in the ICF, higher sodium concentration in the ECF—but the osmolality of the spaces must remain

equal. This is maintained by selective permeability of the cell membrane to solutes and energy-dependent protein transport carriers.

- Derailment in maintenance of normal fluid and electrolyte balance, caused by critical illness, asphyxia, cardiovascular compromise, loss of capillary wall integrity, can lead to hypovolemia, cell damage from fluid overload shifts via osmosis, loss of oncotic pressure in the IVS from protein leakage and edema, or failure of electrolyte transport pumps due to hypoxia (Wright et al., 2018, pp. 369–373).
  - Edema results when there is an abnormal accumulation of fluid in the IS. Etiology of edema can include decreased capillary oncotic pressure from inadequate protein intake or kidney glomerular disease, increased capillary hydrostatic pressure, increased capillary wall permeability from infection affecting the integrity of the capillary wall, or hypertension from venous obstruction (Wright et al., 2018, pp. 370–371).
  - The kidneys play a major role in maintaining normal fluid and electrolyte balance in the ECF via sodium and water reabsorption. This control is compromised in the preterm infant, leading to sodium and bicarbonate losses in the urine and the inability to handle large fluid volumes or sodium boluses (Wright et al., 2018, pp. 371–371).
  - Management of fluid and electrolytes in the sick newborn and preterm infant is a careful balance between excesses or deficits in fluid or electrolytes, anticipated losses and growth needs, and challenges to normal function resulting from developmental compromise or critical illness (Wright et al., 2018, p. 374).

Transitional Changes at Birth

- Both GA and chronologic age affect relationships between ICF and ECF compartments. These changes are primarily the result of maturation in the heart, kidney, and endocrine systems (Wright et al., 2018, p. 373).
- After birth, the infant enters a physiologic transitional phase as the body shifts from the intrauterine to extrauterine life (Doherty, 2017, p. 296). The degree of TBW loss and intracompartmental shifts is related primarily to GA.
  - These shifts are also influenced by the fat content of the infant (less fat content in the small for gestational infant, for instance, and greater fat content in the infant of the diabetic mother) as well as any disease processes in the infant (asphyxia, respiratory distress syndrome, and pneumonia; Nyp et al., 2016, p. 319).

- After birth, the first shift in fluid balance occurs as the ECF compartment contracts and the infant loses interstitial fluid through diuresis (Nyp et al., 2016, p. 319). This shift ideally occurs over the first 3 to 5 days of life (Nyp et al., 2016, p. 319).
  - The preterm infant may lose 10% to 15% of the TBW, while the healthy term infant loses 5% to 10% of the TBW (Nyp et al., 2016, p. 319). Weight loss is generally regained over the first 7 to 10 days of life as muscle growth occurs and fat stores increase (Nyp et al., 2016, p. 319).
- Diuresis is secondary to change in the glomerular filtration, which begins to increase after birth due to the increase in cardiac output, renal blood flow, and increasing glomerular permeability following clamping of the cord (Nyp et al., 2016, p. 320).
  - Diuresis is accompanied by natriuresis, which results in increased loss of sodium in the urine. This increased sodium loss produces an initial negative sodium balance, but is not generally associated with a need for sodium supplementation in the first 24 to 48 hours of life (Nyp et al., 2016, p. 319).
- The goal of fluid and electrolyte management during this period is to provide sufficient fluid intake to allow the physiologic ECF losses to occur gradually over the first 3 to 5 days of life, while maintaining normal electrolyte balances and circulating IVS volumes to support cardiovascular function (Doherty, 2017, p. 299).
- Subsequently, the goal of fluid and electrolyte balance is to provide the appropriate supplementation to maintain homeostasis and support growth (Doherty, 2017, p. 299).

Insensible Loss/Gain

- Another important factor that must be taken into consideration is the expected insensible water losses (IWLs) that occur in the newborn period through the pulmonary and cutaneous systems (Nyp et al., 2016, p. 232).
  - Insensible losses cannot be directly measured, but are calculated as the provider assesses intake, output, and weight change in the infant. The external environment also influences the degree of insensible loss. Table 11.1 shows the estimated IWL, which can guide the practitioner.
  - IWL can be calculated using this formula (Doherty, 2017, p. 296):
    IWL = fluid intake – urine output + weight change
  - Average IWLs for infant in incubators during the first 7 days of life are estimated at:

TABLE 11.1 Factors That Affect IWL

Decrease IWL	Increase IWL
Heat shield or double-walled incubators	Inversely related to gestational age and weight
Plastic blankets	Respiratory distress
Clothes	Ambient temperature above thermoneutral
High relative humidity (ambient ventilator gas)	Fever
Emollient use	Radiant warmer
	Phototherapy
	Activity

Source: Reproduced with permission from Nyp, M., Brunkhorst, J. L., Reavy, D., & Pallotto, E. K. (2016). Fluid and electrolyte management. In S. L. Gardner, B. S. Carter, M. E. Hines, & J. A. Hernandez (Eds.), *Merenstein & Gardner's handbook of neonatal intensive care* (pp. 315–336). St. Louis, MO: Elsevier.

- BW (birthweight) 750–1,000 g = ~80 mL/kg/day
- BW 1001–1250 g = ~50 mL/kg/day
- BW 1,251–1,500 g = ~45 mL/kg/day
- BW >1,501 g = ~25 mL/kg/day

Assessing Fluid and Electrolyte Balance

MATERNAL, FETAL, AND PERINATAL INFLUENCE

- Several factors must be evaluated in the assessment of fluid and electrolyte balance. An initial review of maternal history is critical since the newborn's status is a reflection of the maternal status at birth, gradually reflecting the extrauterine transition over the first 24 hours of life (Doherty, 2017, p 298).
  - Oxytocin, maternal diuretic use, and infusion of hypotonic intravenous (IV) fluid may result in maternal and fetal hyponatremia (Doherty, 2017, p. 298).
  - Use of antenatal steroids can enhance lung maturation in the preterm infant and may also enhance skin maturation, which will decrease IWL and, in turn, reduce the risk of hyperkalemia (Doherty, 2017, p. 298).
- Fetal and perinatal factors such as oligohydramnios may be associated with congenital renal abnormalities such as renal agenesis, polycystic kidney disease, or posterior urethral valves. Severe hypoxia or asphyxia at birth can lead to renal tubular necrosis (Doherty, 2017, p. 398), which will require a decrease in total fluid goals in these infants.

Physical Assessment

- The importance of a thorough assessment of the infant's status is critical to management of fluid and electrolyte balance.
- Daily weights are essential in helping to determine fluid losses and planning fluid goals. Acute changes in weight are reflective of the TBW (Doherty, 2017, p. 298). Weight is the most sensitive indicator of IWL (Nyp et al., 2016, p. 327).
  - Increases in weight may be indicative of fluid compartment shifts from IVS into the interstitial compartment, as seen in the infant with acute sepsis or peritonitis, or with long-term use of paralytics (Doherty, 2017, p. 298).
- The skin and mucosal membranes are less helpful in evaluating overall hydrational status (Doherty, 2017, p. 298) unless dehydration is significant. Decreased skin turgor, sunken anterior fontanelle, and dry mucous membranes are often very late signs (Nyp et al., 2016, p. 327).
- Tachycardia can be seen in ECF excess (e.g., heart failure) as well as in hypovolemia (e.g., acute blood loss, intravascular fluid shifts; Doherty, 2017, p. 298).
- Capillary refill should be less than 3 seconds and is best assessed over the forehead or sternum (Nyp et al., 2016, p. 327).
  - Delayed capillary refill indicates decreased perfusion, but is not a specific indicator of hydration.
  - Decreases in blood pressure are a late sign of hypovolemia (Doherty, 2017, p. 298).
- All fluids administered must be accurately measured, including flushes for medications, especially in the most critically ill infants (Wright et al., 2018, p. 381).

- Strict and accurate measurement of intake and output are critical. Diapers must be weighed. Any source of measurable fluid loss must be measured and included in fluid evaluation.
  - Normal urine output after the first 24 hours should be 1 to 3 mL/kg/h; however, the ELBW infant may not have decreased urine output in response to ECF depletion early on, as a result of marked renal immaturity (Doherty, 2017, p. 299).
  - Although stool output is not calculated separately, normal fluid loss in the stool is calculated at 5 to 10 mL/kg/day. See Table 11.2.

Laboratory Assessment

- Serum electrolytes, blood urea nitrogen (BUN), creatinine (Cr), glucose, and acid–base status are central in managing fluids and electrolytes, and should be measured in the ELBW infant every 4 to 6 hours in the first few days of life due to their increased rates of IWL (Doherty, 2017, p. 299; Nyp et al., 2016, p. 327).
- Urine electrolytes and specific gravity (SG) reflect renal concentration/dilutional capabilities and the quantity of sodium (Na^+) reabsorbed or excreted, but are altered when the infant is on diuretics (Doherty, 2017, p. 299).
- Fractional excretion of Na^+ (FENa) reflects the balance between GFR and tubular reabsorption of Na^+ and can be calculated:
  - FENa = (urine Na^+ × plasma Cr)/ (plasma Na^+ × urine Cr) × 100.
  - Levels of <1% are indicative of prerenal failure secondary to decreased renal blood flow; levels of 2.5% are associated with acute kidney injury (AKI), however, levels of >2.5% are often found in infants <32 weeks GA due to renal immaturity, which results in increased Na^+ excretion (Doherty, 2017, p. 299).
- Acid–base balance measured as arterial pH, carbon dioxide tension ($PaCO_2$), and Na^+ bicarbonate provide indirect evidence of intravascular volume depletion related to the effect of decreased tissue perfusion and the development of lactic acidosis (Doherty, 2017, p. 299).

Fluid

FLUID REQUIREMENTS

- The goal of fluid and electrolyte management is to allow appropriate initial losses during the first 5 to 6 days of life, while maintaining normal serum osmolality and intravascular volume.
- Initial fluid goals will vary depending upon the GA of the infant, taking into account the IWL, weight change, serum electrolytes, urine output, and cardiovascular stability.
- Recommended initial fluid-goal volumes vary significantly. Ongoing fluid adjustments must be guided by weight change, intake, measurable output, IWL, and electrolyte balance, to maintain the gradual decrease in ECF to 5% to 10% for the term infant and 10% to 15% for the preterm infant in the first 5 to 6 days of life (Doherty, 2017, p. 299).
  - At less than 24 hours of age:
    - Birth Weight (BW) <1,000 g require ~100 to 150 mL/kg/day
    - BW 1,000–1,500 g require ~80–100 mL/kg/day
    - BW >1,500 g require ~60–80 mL/kg/day

TABLE 11.2 Ranges of Estimated Water Loss

Weight (G)	Ranges of Water Loss (mL/kg/day)		Day 1[a]	Days 2–3[a]	Days 4–7[a]
Less than 1,250	IWL[b]	40–170			
	Urine	50–100			
	Stool	5–10			
	TOTAL	95–280	120	140	150–175
1,250–1,750	IWL[b]	20–50			
	Urine	50–100			
	Stool	5–10			
	TOTAL	75–160	90	110	130–140
More than 1,750	IWL[b]	15–40			
	Urine	50–100			
	Stool	5–10			
	TOTAL	70–150	80	90	100–200

IWL, Insensible water loss; VLBW, very low birth weight.

Increment for phototherapy: 20 to 30 mL/kg/day if patient is in open warmer and has radiant phototherapy. No adjustment if baby is in humidified environment and/or has fiberoptic phototherapy source.

Increment for radiant warmer: 20–30 mL/kg/day

Maintenance solutes: glucose: 7–12 g/kg/day (4–8 g/kg in VLBW infants)

Na: 1–4 mEq/kg/day (2–8 mEq/kg/day in VLBW infants)

K: 1–4 mEq/kg/day

Cl: 1–4 mEq/kg/day

Ca: 1 mEq/kg/day

[a]Adjustment based on a urine flow rate of 2 to 5 ml/kg/hr and a stable weight.

[b]May be reduced by 30% if the infant is on a ventilator.

Source: Reproduced with permission from Nyp, M., Brunkhorst, J. L., Reavy, D., & Pallotto, E. K. (2016). *Fluid and electrolyte management.* In S. L. Gardner, B. S. Carter, M. E. Hines, & J. A. Hernandez (Eds.), *Merenstein & Gardner's handbook of neonatal intensive care* (pp. 315–336). St. Louis, MO: Elsevier.

○ At 24 to 48 hours of life
  ■ BW <1,000 g require ~120–150 mL/kg/day
  ■ BW 1,000–1,500 g require ~100–120 mL/kg/day
  ■ BW >1,500 g require ~ 80–120 mL/kg/day
○ At more than 48 hours of life
  ■ BW <1,000 g require ~140–190 mL/kg/day
  ■ BW 1,000–1,500 g require ~120–160 mL/kg/day
  ■ BW >1,500 g require ~120–160 mL/kg/day

MAINTENANCE FLUID REQUIREMENTS
- Maintenance fluid volumes are calculated using anticipated IWL, urine and stool output, and any other measurable losses (GI output, chest tubes, etc.; Nyp et al., 2016, p. 324).
- Maintenance fluid generally increases 20 to 40 mL/kg/day per day over the first few days of life (Nyp et al., 2016, p. 326). The actual fluid goal (ml/kg/day) must be guided by the latest evidence that shows that fluid maintenance must provide adequate hydration without increasing the risks for patent ductus arteriosus (PDA), necrotizing enterocolitis (NEC), and intraventricular hemorrhage (IVH; Nyp et al., 2016, p. 326).

DEFICIT FLUID REQUIREMENTS
- Initially there are no deficit fluid losses in the newborn infant. However, in conditions that cause fluid shifts to the interstitial compartment (NEC, acute sepsis, long-term paralytics), fluid goals may need to be increased to maintain appropriate intravascular fluid volumes (Nyp et al., 2016, p. 324).

Electrolyte Requirements

MAINTENANCE ELECTROLYTE REQUIREMENTS
- Initially Na[+] and K[+] supplementation are not required in the first 24 hours in newborn infants, but supplementation may be required after 24 to 48 hours of life based on fluid balance and electrolyte levels (Doherty, 2017, p. 299; Nyp et al., 2016, p. 325).
- Sodium is supplemented as chloride, acetate, or phosphate in amounts of 2 to 3 mEq/kg/day (Nyp et al., 2016, p. 326). Infants with mild metabolic acidosis may benefit from sodium acetate supplementation rather than chloride (Nyp et al., 2016, p. 325).

- Potassium is not provided until adequate urine output has been established (Nyp et al., 2016, p. 325). Once urine output has been established, K$^+$ supplementation is added in 1 to 2 mEq/kg/day but may increase to 3 to 4 mEq/kg/day (Olsen, Leick-Rude, Dusin, & Rosterman, 2016, p. 363).
- Elemental calcium should be provided in the first day of life for most newborns (20–60 mg/kg/day) as elemental calcium (Ca^{+2}) increasing over the course of the first few days of life to 60 to 80 mg/kg/day (Denne, 2018, p. 1024).

DISORDERS OF FLUID AND ELECTROLYTE IMBALANCE

Dehydration

- Dehydration may occur when appropriate fluid management is not achieved. This may be the result of losses through uncommon routes (chest tubes, gastric tubes, ventriculostomy drainage) that were neglected in the intake and output. Third space losses due to NEC, sepsis, gastroschisis, or omphalocele (Doherty, 2017, p. 300) can be difficult to measure.
- Diagnosis: Signs of dehydration include weight loss greater than the anticipated physiologic losses, decreased urine output, and increased urine specific gravity (SG).
  - Other signs of dehydration include tachycardia and hypotension, metabolic acidosis, and increases in BUN (Doherty, 2017, p. 300).
  - The <32-week infant may not present with decreased urine output despite having a fluid deficit, due to the inability of the immature renal tubules to concentrate urine (Nyp et al., 2016, p. 320).
- Management: Fluids must be administered to correct the fluid deficit and maintenance fluid requirements will need to be adjusted to reflect the intake and output (Doherty, 2017, p. 300).
  - Acute symptomatic dehydration with normal serum sodium can be treated with bolus(es) of normal saline (NS) at 10 mL/kg to improve cardiac function (Doherty, 2017, p. 300).

Edema

- Excessive intake of isotonic fluids will precipitate edema and signs of fluid overload. Development of edema can also occur under conditions such as heart failure, sepsis, and long-term use of paralytics (Doherty, 2017, p. 300).
- Diagnosis: Signs of edema often include exaggerated weight gain and may also include periorbital edema, edema of the extremities, and hepatomegaly (Doherty, 2017, p. 301).
- Management: The goal of therapy in edema is Na$^+$ restriction (to decrease total body Na$^+$) and/or fluid restriction (in the case of low serum Na$^+$). Again, the overall fluid balance must be carefully assessed to ensure that the IVS is adequate.

Sodium

- Sodium is the primary extracellular cation and is intricately involved in water balance. Na$^+$ is the major electrolyte controlling tonicity of the fluid compartments.
  - Normal serum Na$^+$ levels range from 135 to 145 mEq/L. Normal body Na$^+$ requirements are generally 2 to 4 mEq/kg/day, although, in the case of the preterm infant, higher Na$^+$ intake may be required due to greater renal Na$^+$ losses due to renal immaturity (Wright et al., 2018, p. 375).
  - Elevated serum Na$^+$ creates a hyperosmolar situation where water shifts from intracellular to extracellular spaces, resulting in cellular dehydration.
  - Low serum Na$^+$ creates a hypoosmolar situation where water shifts from the extracellular space to the intracellular spaces, resulting in cellular edema (Halbardier, 2015, p. 152).

Hyponatremia

- Evaluation of hyponatremia begins with determining whether the etiology is due to factitious hyponatremia due to hyperlipidemia, hypoosmolar hyponatremia due to osmotic changes, excess free water, or increased sodium losses (Doherty, 2017, p. 301).
- Hyponatremia is defined as serum Na$^+$ less than 130 mEq/L (Nyp et al., 2017, p. 330). Serum Na$^+$ <120 mEq/L may cause seizures or coma (Doherty, 2017, p. 301).
  - Hyperlipidemia can create a factitiously low serum Na$^+$ because the elevated lipids remain in a solid phase in the serum after sample preparation and displace the water content in the serum, creating a lower Na$^+$ concentration per liter in the plasma (Nyp et al., 2016, p. 322).
- *Hyponatremia due to ECF volume depletion.* This condition can result from diuretic therapy, osmotic diuresis (secondary to significant hyperglycemia), renal losses related to immaturity of the preterm kidney, adrenal salt-losing disorders (e.g., congenital adrenal hyperplasia), excessive losses in gastrointestinal (GI) secretions/diarrhea, and conditions that cause third spacing (e.g., NEC, tissue sloughing; Doherty, 2017, p. 301; Nyp et al., 2016, p. 330).
  - Diagnosis: Signs of volume depletion include decreased weight, poor skin turgor, tachycardia, rising BUN, and metabolic acidosis (Doherty, 2017, p. 301). Decreased urine output may be seen in infants with relatively mature kidneys (>32 weeks' GA) as well as increased SG (due to renal urinary concentration) and low FENa (Doherty, 2017, p. 301).
  - Management: The goal of therapy is to decrease ongoing Na$^+$ loss, provide Na$^+$ supplementation as well as fluid deficit replacement, and adjust maintenance Na$^+$ and fluid supplementation (Doherty, 2017, p. 301). Serum Na$^+$ deficit can be calculated with the following formula:
    Sodium deficit = (sodium desired – actual serum sodium) × 0.6 × weight (kg).
  - For example, a 1.5 kg infant has a serum Na$^+$ of 130 mEq/L. The target goal is 140 mEq/L. Substitute these values in the above equation:
    Sodium deficit = (140–130) × 0.6 × 1.5 kg.
    Or:
    Sodium deficit = 10 × 0.6 × 1.5
  - The sodium deficit for this infant is 9 mEq. Generally, only one-half of this deficit is replaced, slowly over several hours, and the serum Na$^+$ level is checked again (Nyp et al., 2016, p. 330).
- *Hyponatremia with normal ECF volume.* This condition can result from excess fluid administration, and in

syndrome of inappropriate antidiuretic hormone (SIADH). Etiologies for SIADH include pain, opiate administration, IVH, asphyxia, meningitis, pneumothorax, and positive pressure ventilation (Doherty, 2017, p. 301; Nyp et al., 2016, p. 330).

- ○ Diagnosis: Signs of SIADH include weight gain without apparent edema, decreased urine output, and increased SG. Signs of excessive fluid administration include high urine output and low SG (Doherty, 2017, p. 301).
- ○ Management: The goal of therapy is to restrict fluids unless the serum Na⁺ is <120 mEq/L, or there are neurologic symptoms such as seizure or coma. In mild hyponatremia the goal of therapy is reduction in total fluids. When the serum Na⁺ is <120 mEq/L, furosemide therapy may be initiated while decreasing fluid goals and replacing the urinary output with hypertonic NaCL (3%). (Doherty, 2017, p. 301.)

- • *Hyponatremia due to ECF volume excess.* This condition can result from conditions associated with fluid shifts from the IVS to the interstitial compartment (third spacing), such as overwhelming sepsis, heart failure, abnormal lymphatic drainage, and the use of neuromuscular paralytics (Doherty, 2017, p. 298).
  - ○ Diagnosis: Signs of third spacing include increase in weight with edema, low urine output, rising BUN, rising SG, and low FENa (in infants with mature renal function, for example, >32 weeks GA; Doherty, 2017, p. 302).
  - ○ Management: The goal of therapy is to treat the underlying etiology and restrict free water to normalize serum osmolality (Doherty, 2017, p. 302). Restricting Na⁺ and improving cardiac output may be beneficial (Doherty, 2017, p. 302).

Hypernatremia

- • Evaluation of hypernatremia begins with determining whether the condition results from increased Na⁺ supplementation, decreased ECF volume, excessive urine output, or excessive administration of isotonic or hypertonic fluids. Hypernatremia is defined as a serum Na⁺ >150 mEq/L (Halbardier, 2015, p. 153).
- • *Hypernatremia with normal or deficient ECF volume.* This condition can result from increased renal losses (urine) and IWL in the very low birth weight (VLBW) infant (Doherty, 2017, p. 303). IWL may be increased due to skin sloughing, antidiuretic hormone (ADH) deficiency subsequent to IVH, and increased renal (urine) losses (Doherty, 2017, p. 303).
  - ○ Diagnosis: Signs include weight loss, tachycardia, hypotension, metabolic acidosis, decreasing urine output, and increasing SG (Doherty, 2017, p. 303). SG may also be low in the infant with diabetes insipidus (DI), whether central or nephrogenic (Doherty, 2017, p. 303).
  - ○ Management: The goal of therapy is to increase free water administration to reduce the serum Na⁺ while avoiding ECF excess. Serum Na⁺ reduction should be achieved slowly, no greater than 1 mEq/kg/h to avoid too rapid a change in the serum osmolality (Doherty, 2017, p. 303). Hypernatremia is not always indicative of excess body Na⁺; the VLBW infant may present with hypernatremia in the first 24 hours of life due to

free water deficits related to ECF contraction and IWL (Doherty, 2017, p. 303).

- • *Hypernatremia with ECF volume excess.* This condition can result from excessive administration of isotonic or hypertonic fluids, particularly in conditions resulting in decreased cardiac output (Doherty, 2017, p. 303).
  - ○ Diagnosis: Signs of hypernatremia with ECF include weight gain accompanied by edema. Vital signs such as heart rate, blood pressure, urine output, and SG are often normal, but the FENa will be elevated (Doherty, 2017, p. 303).
  - ○ Management: The goal of therapy is to restrict Na⁺ administration (Doherty, 2017, p. 303).

Potassium

- • Potassium is the primary intracellular cation and is measured indirectly in the serum (Wright et al., 2018, p. 369). K⁺ shifts between the ICF and ECF based on pH of the serum. An increase of 0.1 pH units in the serum will result in a decrease of 0.6 mEq/L in serum K⁺ concentration (Doherty, 2017, p. 307). Normal total body K⁺ is a product of normal intake (1–2 mEq/kg/day) and excretion through the GI tract and renal system. Normal serum K⁺ levels range from 3.5 to 5.5 mEq/l (Doherty, 2017, p. 307).

Hypokalemia

- • Evaluation of hypokalemia requires a determination of whether the primary etiology is increased loss of K⁺ or inadequate intake. Hypokalemia can result in arrhythmias, ileus, renal concentrating defects, and coma in the infant (Doherty, 2017, p. 307).
  - ○ Diagnosis: Signs of hypokalemia include generalized muscle weakness, decreased T waves, and ST depression.
  - ○ Management: The goal of therapy is to decrease losses and gradually increase K⁺ supplementation. Hypokalemia related to the use of loop diuretics (e.g., furosemide) can be treated with K⁺ supplementation. Changing to K⁺-sparing diuretics (e.g. spironolactone) as early as possible when long-term diuretic therapy is indicated will reduce renal losses (Nyp et al., 2016, p. 335).

Hyperkalemia

- • Evaluation of hyperkalemia begins with determining the underlying etiology. The source of the sample must be central to confirm diagnosis, since capillary samples may be elevated by squeezing causing cell lysis and release of intracellular K⁺ (Halbardier, 2015, p. 154).
  - ○ Initial therapy for hyperkalemia is often initiated emergently, but all therapies provide only temporary reduction in the serum K⁺.
  - ○ Conditions commonly associated with hyperkalemia include acidosis (with or without tissue damage), cephalohematoma, hemolysis, hypothermia, asphyxia, ischemia, acute kidney injury (AKI), adrenal insufficiency, and IVH, or can be iatrogenic due to excess K⁺ administration (Doherty, 2017, p. 307; Nyp et al., 2016, p. 331).
  - ○ Non-oliguric hyperkalemia often occurs in the ELBW infant in the first few days of life even without K⁺ administration, due to relatively low GFR and intra- to

extracellular K^+ shifts due to decreased activity of the Na–K–ATPase system (Doherty, 2017, p. 311; Nyp et al., 2016, p. 331).
- ○ Symptomatic hyperkalemia may be seen at levels >6 mEq/L (Doherty, 2017, p. 307).
- Diagnosis: Signs of hyperkalemia may include cardiovascular instability as bradyarrhythmias or tachyarrhythmias, or cardiovascular collapse, but the infant may also be asymptomatic in the early stages (Doherty, 2017, p. 308).
  - ○ ECG changes are often the first sign of hyperkalemia. Electrocardiographic findings are altered as the serum K^+ rises, presenting with varying levels of peaked T waves (secondary to increased repolarization of the cardiac tissue), flattened P waves, and increased PR intervals (secondary to suppression of atrial conductivity). These changes are followed by widening and slurring of the QRS complex (secondary to delay in ventricular conduction as well as delays in myocardial conduction), with eventual development of supraventricular tachycardia, ventricular tachycardia, bradycardia, or ventricular fibrillation (Doherty, 2017, p. 308).
- Management: The goal of therapy is to remove all sources of exogenous K^+ (IV solutions, medications, enteral feedings if they contain K^+), rehydrate if indicated, and evaluate serum and total ionized calcium levels.
  - ○ There are three stages in pharmacologic therapy: stabilization of the conductive tissue, dilution and intracellular shifting of K^+, and facilitating K^+ excretion.
  - ○ If calcium levels are low, calcium supplementation is indicated to protect cardiac function (Doherty, 2017, p. 308; Nyp et al., 2016, p. 331).
- Stabilization of the conductive tissue can be accomplished by Na^+ or Ca^{+2} administration. Ca^{+2} is generally the first step, infusing 1 to 2 mL/kg IV of calcium gluconate over 15 to 30 minutes (Doherty, 2017, p. 308; Nyp et al., 2016, p. 331). In cases where the infant is also hyponatremic, normal saline bolus may be beneficial in adjusting the Na^+ level and adding a dilutional factor (Doherty, 2017, p. 308).
- Antiarrhythmic agents (lidocaine or bretylium) may be added to treat refractory ventricular tachycardia (Doherty, 2017, p. 308).
- Dilution is accomplished be evaluating overall hydration and correcting fluid administration to promote adequate circulating volumes (Doherty, 2017, p. 308). Fluid administration must always be evaluated in the face of renal functionality; the infant with AKI will often not be able to accommodate additional fluid loads (Nyp et al., 2016, p. 331).
- Sodium bicarbonate ($NaHCO_3$) may be used to shift the pH slowly.
- Insulin will enhance intracellular K^+ uptake by stimulating the membrane-bound NA-K ATPase (Doherty, 2017, p. 308; Nyp et al., 2016, p. 331).
  - ○ Glucose infusion must always accompany insulin to maintain normal serum glucose. Insulin therapy may start with a bolus dose of insulin and glucose, followed by continuous infusion of D10W with human regular insulin. Many institutions have their own glucose/insulin cocktails that can be ordered from the pharmacy.
  - ○ Insulin binds to the plastic IV tubing so the tubing must be flushed well in attempt to saturate the binding sites prior to administration (Doherty, 2017, p. 308; Nyp et al., 2016, p. 331). Significant hypoglycemia

and seizures may occur, which mandates frequent evaluation of blood glucose (Nyp et al., 2016, p. 331).
- The use of β2-adrenergic agents (such as albuterol) will enhance K^+ uptake as well, although they are not commonly used in the neonatal population; the mechanism for this is thought to be stimulation of the Na–K ATPase activity (Doherty, 2017, p. 309).
- K^+ excretion can be facilitated with diuretic therapy by increasing renal blood flow and improving Na^+ delivery in the distal tubules (Doherty, 2017, p. 309).
- In the infant with oliguria and reversible AKI, peritoneal dialysis and double-volume exchange transfusions may be considered as potentially life-saving measures (Doherty, 2017, p. 309).
  - ○ Peritoneal dialysis can be successful in the infants <1 kg and should be considered in situations where the newborn's overall clinical status is appropriate and there is a reasonable chance for recovery with good long-term outcome (Doherty, 2017, p. 309). Other sources suggest that peritoneal dialysis in the VLBW infant may be technically difficult to impossible, particularly in infants with accompanying NEC (Nyp et al., 2016, p. 331).
  - ○ Double volume exchange transfusions should be conducted with fresh blood <24 hours old, or deglycerized red blood cells that have been reconstituted with fresh frozen plasma (Doherty, 2017, p. 309).
- Cation exchange resin solutions may also enhance K^+ excretion by exchanging Na^+ or Ca^{+2} ions for K^+ (Na^+ or Ca^{+2} polystyrene sulfonate). These resins may be given orally or rectally, although the literature remains inconclusive relative to risk/benefit ratios in neonates (Doherty, 2017, p. 309; Nyp et al., 2016, p. 331).

Calcium

- Calcium is essential for several biochemical processes, including coagulation, neuromuscular excitability, cell membrane integrity and function, and cellular enzymatic and secretory activity (Doherty, 2017, p. 326). Serum calcium levels are regulated by parathyroid levels and 1,25-dihydroxyvitamin D (calcitriol); (Doherty, 2017, p. 327). Calcium can be measured as total serum calcium or as ionized calcium. Normal ranges for calcium are 8.5 to 10.2 mg/dL for total serum calcium and 4.4 to 5.3 mg/dL for ionized calcium (Halbardier, 2015, p. 155).

Hypocalcemia

- Hypocalcemia is a common finding in critically ill infants due to the interrelationship between calcium levels, parathyroid hormone, and calcitriol (Nyp et al., 2016, p. 329). At birth the infant's calcium supply across the placenta ceases abruptly and parathyroid hormone responds by rising, which causes release of Ca^{+2} from the bone, increasing Ca^{+2} resorption in the renal tubule, and stimulating the renal production of calcitonin resulting in a rise in serum Ca^{+2} (Doherty, 2017, p. 327). This response is gradual over the first 48 hours of life and is more diminished in the preterm and sick newborn. Normal Ca^{+2} nadir occurs at approximately 48 hours of life and is well tolerated in the healthy term newborn (Nyp et al., 2016, p. 329). Early Ca^{+2} supplementation may be required in the preterm infant, the critically ill newborn, and the ill infant of the diabetic mother.

- Conditions that are associated with low calcium due to hypoparathyroidism are DiGeorge sequence (hypoplasia or absence of the parathyroid, and Kenny–Caffey syndrome), pseudohypoparathyroidism secondary to maternal hyperparathyroidism, hypomagnesemia, vitamin D deficiency, alkalosis and bicarbonate use, shock, sepsis, and phototherapy (Doherty, 2017, p. 327). The mechanism for phototherapy-induced hypocalcemia is thought to be secondary to decreased melatonin secretion, which increases bone absorption of Ca^{+2}. Late-onset hypocalcemia may be related to high phosphate intake, which decreases serum Ca^{+2} (Doherty, 2017, p. 327).
- Diagnosis: Signs of hypocalcemia may include jitteriness, irritability, or twitching, increased extensor tone, clonus, hyperreflexia, and stridor secondary to laryngospasm (Doherty, 2017, p. 327; Nyp et al., 2016, p. 329).
  - Hypocalcemia is defined as total serum Ca^{+2} less than 7 mg/dL or ionized Ca^{+2} less than 4 mg/dL (0.8–1 mmol/L). Calcium is present as total serum Ca^{+2} (free serum Ca^{+2} plus albumin bound Ca^{+2}) and ionized Ca^{+2} (Doherty, 2017, p. 327; Nyp et al., 2016, p. 329). It is critical to measure ionized Ca^{+2} when assessing for hypocalcemia since hypoalbuminemia will decrease the level of total circulating serum Ca^{+2} (Nyp et al., 2016, p. 329.
- Management: The goal of therapy is to provide calcium supplementation. Serum magnesium levels should be obtained prior to calcium supplementation to make certain that the serum magnesium is normal, since calcium and magnesium absorption are interrelated (Koves, Ness, Nip, & Salehi, 2018, p. 1343).
  - Calcium gluconate 10% solution is preferred for IV supplementation (Nyp et al., 2016, p. 329) and may be given over 10 to 15 minutes for management of seizures or cardiac failure (Doherty, 2017, p. 330).
  - In circumstances where hypocalcemia occurs in the infant who is taking enteral nutrition, calcium glubionate syrup may be used orally; however, this will increase osmolarity and may cause GI irritation or diarrhea (Doherty, 2017, p. 329).
  - The best approach is to prevent hypoglycemia by providing IV Ca^{+2} supplementation in the first day of life for infants at greatest risk for hypocalcemia (Nyp et al., 2016, p. 329).

SPECIAL CONCERNS WITH IV CA^{+2} SUPPLEMENTATION

- Rapid infusion of Ca^{+2} may cause bradyarrhythmias.
- Calcium can cause hepatic necrosis if given through an umbilical venous catheter (UVC) that is improperly positioned in the hepatic portal veins.
- Rapid infusion of calcium into an umbilical arterial catheter (UAC) can cause arterial spasm which may result in intestinal necrosis.
- Calcium and bicarbonate are incompatible and cannot be infused together.
- Extravasation of Ca^{+2} into the subcutaneous tissue can cause severe necrosis and calcifications (Doherty, 2017, p. 329).

Hypercalcemia

- Hypercalcemia is defined as total serum Ca^{+2} >11 mg/dL, or ionized Ca^{+2} >1.45 mmol/L. Infants with calcium levels in this range are often asymptomatic; however, infants presenting with total serum Ca^{+2} >16 mg/dL (ionized Ca^{+2} >1.8 mmol/L) may require immediate treatment (Doherty, 2017, p. 330).
  - Conditions associated with hypercalcemia may be iatrogenic due to excessive vitamin D intake, excessive Ca^{+2} supplementation, or inadequate phosphorus supplementation in infants receiving parenteral nutrition (PN) (Nyp et al., 2016, p. 330).
  - Other conditions that may be associated with hypercalcemia include hyperparathyroidism, hyperthyroidism, Williams syndrome, and hypophosphatasia, or due to thiazide diuretics (Doherty, 2017, p. 332; Nyp et al., 2016, p. 330).
- Diagnosis: Signs of hypercalcemia may include history of poor feeding, emesis, lethargy, irritability, constipation, and polyuria (Nyp et al., 2016, p. 330). Infants with hypercalcemia secondary to hyperthyroidism may present with hypotonia, encephalopathy, hepatosplenomegaly, anemia, and extra skeletal calcifications (Doherty, 2017, p. 331).
- Management: The goal of therapy for infants with significant hypercalcemia is dependent upon the etiology.
  - Emergent medical treatment for symptomatic infants, or infants with total serum Ca^{+2} >16 mg/dL (ionized Ca^{+2} >1.8 mmol/L is volume expansion (to provide dilution) with 0.9% NaCl to promote renal excretion of calcium (Doherty, 2017, p. 332; Nyp et al., 2016, p. 330).
  - Furosemide can be given to promote renal excretion of calcium (Doherty, 2016, p. 332; Nyp et al., 2016, p. 330).
    - Inorganic phosphate may lower serum Ca^{+2} if the infant is hypophosphatemic, by inhibiting Ca^{+2} mobilization from the bone and promoting mineral accretion in the bone (Doherty, 2017, p. 332; Nyp et al., 2016, p. 330).
    - Glucocorticoids are effective in treating hypervitaminosis A and D and can also facilitate reduction of serum Ca^{+2} secondary to fat necrosis by inhibiting bone mobilization and intestinal absorption (Doherty, 2017, p. 333; Nyp et al., 2016, p. 330).
  - If hypercalcemia is iatrogenic secondary to inadequately balanced Ca^{+2}/Phos supplementation in PN, adjusting the supplementation will correct serum Ca^{+2}.
  - Iatrogenic hypercalcemia related to PN is often associated with the removal of phosphorous in an effort to decrease the Na or K supplementation (Doherty, 2017, p. 331).
  - Hypercalcemia may also be seen in the ELBW infant as a result of an inability to utilize the amount of Ca^{+2} being provided in the PN (Doherty, 2017, p. 331).

Magnesium

- Magnesium is required for optimal function of intracellular enzyme systems. Magnesium should be provided as 0.25 to 0.5 mEq/kg/day (Olsen et al., 2016, p. 363).

Hypomagnesemia

- Hypomagnesemia is defined as serum levels <1.6 mg/dl. Hypomagnesemia is uncommon in the infant, but when present is most often seen in conjunction with hypocalcemia (Doherty, 2017, p. 333).

- Diagnosis: Signs of hypomagnesemia may include apnea and poor motor tone (Doherty, 2017, p. 333).
- Management: The goal of therapy for symptomatic hypomagnesemia is to provide magnesium supplementation with magnesium sulfate (Doherty, 2017, p. 333). Serum calcium levels must also be measured, and if hypocalcemia is present, it must be treated concurrently.

Hypermagnesemia

- Hypermagnesemia is defined as serum magnesium > 3 mg/dL. The most common etiology for newborn hypermagnesemia is secondary to maternal therapy for preterm labor or preeclampsia (Doherty, 2017, p. 333).
- Diagnosis: Signs of symptomatic hypermagnesemia include apnea, respiratory depression, lethargy, hypotonia, hyporeflexia, poor suck, decreased peristalsis, and delayed passage of meconium. Newborns are often asymptomatic until levels exceed 6 mg/dL (Doherty, 2017, p. 333).
- Management: The goal of therapy for hypermagnesemia is generally the removal of exogenous magnesium. Enteral feedings are delayed until the infant demonstrates good suck and has adequate intestinal motility (Doherty, 2017, p. 334).
- Table 11.3 summarizes ranges for serum electrolytes at the low (hypo-) normal, and high (hyper-) values.

ACID–BASE BALANCE

- Cells function at their maximal metabolic function in a stable, homeostatic environment. Normal pH range is approximately 7.35 to 7.45 (Halbardier, 2015, p. 158; Wright et al., 2016, p. 383).
  - ○ The Henderson–Hasselebalch equation calculates plasma pH (Barry, Deacon, Hernandez, & Jones, 2016, p. 145). The pH is a negative logarithm that measures the level of hydrogen ions (H+), which means that there is an inverse relationship between the pH and H+. The pH decreases with a rise in H+ and increases with a fall in H+. The pH remains normal when there is a balance in changes of carbon dioxide (CO_2) and bicarbonate (HCO_3).
- Regulation of pH is determined by chemical buffers in body fluids, elimination of PCO_2 (H+ and water) by the lungs, and reabsorption or elimination of H+ or HCO_3 by the kidneys (Wright et al., 2016, p. 383). The classification of acidosis and alkalosis is determined by the system causing the pH derangement (Halbardier, 2015, p. 159).
  - ○ *Respiratory acidosis* results from inadequate alveolar ventilation, leading to an excess of CO_2 and a decrease in pH. Inadequate alveolar ventilation can result from prematurity, neurologic compromise, or medications (Dell, 2015, p. 625).
  - ○ *Respiratory alkalosis* results from alveolar hyperventilation, leading to a decrease in CO_2 and an increase in pH. Excessive alveolar ventilation can result from mechanical overventilation, tachypnea, or anxiety (Dell, 2015, p. 625).
  - ○ *Metabolic acidosis* results either from an excess of acid in the ECF or a loss of buffer, leading to a decrease in pH. Conditions such as hypoxia, immature renal tubular function, or diarrhea can result in metabolic acidosis (Dell, 2015, pp. 624–625; Doherty, 2017, p. 306; Halbardier, 2015, pp. 159–160).
    - The anion gap helps distinguish metabolic acidosis from a pathologic condition, such as asphyxia, or a physiologic condition, such as an increased threshold for bicarbonate excretion in the neonate (Doherty, 2017, pp. 277–278; Halbardier, 2015, pp. 159–160; Nyp et al., 2016, p. 321).
    - Metabolic acidosis in the presence of an increased anion gap (>15 mEq/L) may be caused by a/an
      - acute renal failure
      - inborn error of metabolism
      - lactic acidosis
      - toxins (e.g., benzyl alcohol)
  - ○ *Metabolic alkalosis* results from a loss of acids or an increase in bases. Vomiting or diuretics can induce metabolic alkalosis. Treatment depends on the underlying cause and can be guided by urine chloride levels. For example, a low urinary chloride is suggestive of vomiting or continuous nasogastric suction, whereas high urinary chloride may be associated with hypokalemia or early diuretic therapy (Dell, 2015, p. 625; Doherty, 2017, p. 307; Halbardier, 2015, pp. 159–160).
    - Metabolic alkalosis in the presence of a *low urinary chloride* (<10 mEq/L) may be caused by GI losses

TABLE 11.3 Normally Accepted Ranges for Serum Electrolytes

	Hypo-	Normal	Hyper-
Na+	<130 mEq/L	135–145 mEq/L	>150 mEq/L
K+	<3.5 mEq/L	3.5–5.5 mEq/L	> 6.5 mEq/L
Ca+2	<7 mg/dL	8.5–10.2 mg/dL	> 11 mg/dL
iCa+2	<1.1 mmol/L <4.4 mg/dL	1–1.4 mmol/L 4.4–5.3 mg/dL	> 1.45 mmol/L > 5.8 mg/dL
Mg+2	<1.5 mg/dL	1.5–2.5 mg/dL	>3 mg/dL

Sources: Data from Abrams, S. A., & Tiosano, D. (2015). Disorders of calcium, phosphorous, and magnesium metabolism in the neonate. In R. J. Martin, A. A. Fanaroff, & M. C. Walsh (Eds.), *Fanaroff & Martin's neonatal-perinatal medicine: Diseases of the fetus and infant* (pp. 1474–1479). Philadelphia, PA: Elsevier; Halbardier, B. H. (2015). Fluid and electrolyte management. In M. T. Verklan & M. Walden (Eds.), *Core curriculum for neonatal intensive care nursing* (pp. 146–161). St. Louis, MO: Elsevier.

(e.g., vomiting, gastric suction, diarrhea, or the use of diuretic therapies.

■ Metabolic alkalosis in the presence of a *high urinary chloride* (>20 mEq/L) may be caused by alkali administration, massive transfusion of blood products, diuretic therapy, or Bartter syndrome associated with mineralocorticoid excess.

- Correction of a pH imbalance results from manipulation the body system causing the problem; that is, correction of respiratory acidosis via manipulation of ventilator rate to control the level of carbon dioxide (acid); (Dell, 2015, p. 621).
- Compensation of a pH imbalance results from a response from the system not directly causing the pH imbalance; for example, kidney reabsorption of HCO_3 (buffer) as compensation for chronic respiratory acidosis (Dell, 2015, p. 621).
- *Management of respiratory and metabolic acidosis and alkalosis* is centered around treatment of the underlying cause. Normalization of respiratory acidosis or alkalosis may involve manipulation of ventilator rate (correction) acutely or involve kidney response by increasing bicarbonate

reabsorption (compensation) in chronic permissive hypercapnia accompanying bronchopulmonary dysplasia (BPD); (Dell, 2015, pp. 385–389).

○ Management of metabolic acidosis usually involves corrective action by treating the underlying circulatory problem while providing volume and/or sodium bicarbonate treatment (Doherty, 2017, pp. 305–306). In critically ill infants with metabolic acidosis, K^+ levels must be closely monitored due to the intricate shifts of K^+ and H^+ ions during metabolic acidosis and treatment with sodium bicarbonate (Wright et al., 2018, p. 387)

- Using these normal blood gas ranges (Table 11.4), blood gases can be assessed for acid–base status; however, GA, disease, and clinical status must be considered when evaluating blood gases and acid–base status.
- Table 11.5 demonstrates four examples of blood gases reflective of acid-base imbalances, possible causes, and possible corrective interventions to normalize acid–base balance.

TABLE 11.4 Established Blood Gas Ranges for Neonates

Normal Blood Gas Values			
pH	$PaCO_2$	PaO_2	HCO_3-
7.35–7.45	35–45 mmHg	50–80- mmHg	22–26 mEq/L

Source: Data from Fraser, D., & Diehl-Jones, W. (2015). Assisted ventilation. In M. T. Verklan & M. Walden (Eds.), *Core curriculum for neonatal intensive care nursing* (pp. 487–511). St. Louis, MO: Elsevier.

TABLE 11.5 Acid Base Imbalances (Four Examples)

Arterial Blood Gas		Acid Base Imbalance	Cause/Mechanism	Possible Intervention	Expected Outcome
pH/$PaCO_2$(mm/Hg)/PaO_2(mm/Hg)/HCO_3(mEq/L)			One possible cause	Correction	Repeat ABG
7.25/60/50/22	→	Respiratory acidosis pH < 7.35, $PaCO_2$ > 45	CNS depression with hypoventilation	Mechanical ventilation with IMV	7.30/45/65/24
7.50/28/70/24	→	Respiratory alkalosis	RDS with mechanical hyperventilation	Decrease IMV	7.43/38/70/24
7.25/40/55/15	→	Metabolic acidosis pH < 7.35, HCO_3 < 22	Decreased tissue perfusion with lactic acid production	Reestablish perfusion. Consider bicarb administration	7.30/45/62/20
7.49/38/72/28	→	Metabolic alkalosis pH < 7.45, HCO_3 < 26	Excessive base (acetate) in TPN	Change TPN additives (acetate to chloride)	7.43/40/70/24

Source: Data from Fraser, D., & Diehl-Jones, W. (2015). Assisted ventilation. In M. T. Verklan & M. Walden (Eds.), *Core curriculum for neonatal intensive care nursing* (pp. 487–511). St. Louis, MO: Elsevier.

IMV, intermittent mandatory ventilation; RDS, respiratory distress syndrome; TPN, total parenteral nutrition.

Factors Affecting Acid/Base Balance

- Renal tubular acidosis (RTA) is most commonly associated with tubular damage in the kidney and should be considered in infants with a metabolic acidosis with a normal anion gap and a urine pH less than 6.5. There are three types of RTA, and treatment varies depending on the type (Dell, 2015, pp. 625–627).
- Dehydration has an impact on fluid and electrolyte and acid-base balance. The severity of the imbalance depends on the precipitating factors for dehydration, the etiology of the associated sodium balance (depleted, normal, or excess ECF water content), and the response to treatment (Doherty, 2017, pp. 300–302).
- GI losses/surgery—Intestinal decompression and postoperative metabolic response impact both fluid and electrolyte balance and acid–base homeostasis (Nyp et al., 2016, pp. 382–383; Wright et al., 2016, p. 334).
- NEC is characterized by tissue edema and increased IS fluid, alteration in electrolytes due to GI decompression, and circulatory compromise affecting fluid/electrolyte and acid–base balance (Nyp et al., 2016, pp. 382–383; Wright et al., 2018, pp. 332–333).
- Diarrhea is a precipitating factor in metabolic acidosis with a normal anion gap. Treatment of the underlying cause and supportive treatment with fluid and electrolyte replacement is often necessary in severe diarrhea (Doherty, 2017, p. 306).
- Vomiting places the infant at risk for metabolic alkalosis with low urinary chloride. Severe vomiting in the infant may require fluid and electrolyte replacement (Doherty, 2017, pp. 306–307).

Common Problems Associated With Fluid and Electrolyte Imbalance

- SIADH occurs when the body is unable to excrete water due to an excessive amount of ADH.
  - ○ The resulting water retention leads to a dilutional hyponatremia. Serum and urine chemistry and osmolality can assist in determining if SIADH is the etiology of hyponatremia. Infants with oliguria, water retention, serum hyponatremia, low serum osmolality, increased urine osmolality, and no acid–base disturbance is suggestive of SIADH (Wright et al., 2018, p. 382).
- DI is an uncommon disorder in the newborn and is characterized by a decrease in ADH (vasopressin) secretion from the posterior pituitary (central DI), or lack of response to ADH by the renal tubules (nephrogenic DI), resulting in polyuria and hypernatremia. Serum and urine chemistry and osmolality show elevated serum sodium and osmolality, low urine osmolality, and low serum ADH levels (Wright et al., 2018, p. 382).
- Early versus late-onset hyponatremia is determined by the timing of occurrence. Early-onset hyponatremia occurs in the first few days of life, whereas late-onset hyponatremia occurs after the first week of life (Halbardier, 2015, p. 152).
  - ○ Determination of late-onset hyponatremia due to ECF volume depletion, normal ECF volume, or ECF volume excess will determine management (Doherty, 2017, pp. 300–301, Wright et al., 2018, pp. 375–376).
- Oliguria is defined as urine output less than 1 mL/kg/hr. Investigation into the etiology of oliguria (prerenal, parenchymal, and post-renal) will determine the management (Doherty, 2017, pp. 303–304).
  - ○ AKI has a significant effect on fluid and electrolyte and acid–base balance. AKI can occur with or without oliguria.
- PDA can be affected by fluid and acid-base imbalance (overhydration and metabolic acidosis) and may also affect fluid and electrolyte status.
  - ○ Choice of pharmacologic management for closure of PDA (indomethacin vs. ibuprofen) will impact the severity of the fluid and electrolyte imbalance (Wright et al., 2018, p. 382).
- Asphyxia secondary to insufficient oxygen delivery to the cells often results from decreased perfusion (ischemia) or inadequate ventilation (hypoxia/hypercarbia) and can damage renal tubules, resulting in decreased urine output. SIADH often develops after perinatal depression, exacerbating fluid and electrolyte imbalance by increasing fluid retention and risk for hyponatremia.
  - ○ Management focuses on restriction of fluid delivery to basal needs plus insensible losses, strict output measurement of urine volume and sodium, and diligent fluid and electrolyte replacement during the oliguric and ensuing polyuric (tubule recovery) phases (Nyp et al., 2016, p. 333).
- Bronchopulmonary dysplasia (BPD) may result from the fluid and electrolyte management of the neonate, especially the necessary high fluid and sodium needs of the neonate in the first days after birth, accompanied by sluggish contraction of the ECF and expected loss of fluid in the first week of life (Wright et al., 2018, pp. 381).
  - ○ Infants with BPD, who require increased caloric support in the presence of high metabolic needs are at increased risk for fluid and electrolyte imbalances.
  - ○ High nutrition and caloric needs often require higher daily fluid goals that lead to volume overload and fluid retention, resulting in exacerbation of pulmonary disease.
  - ○ Diuretics are often used to manage fluid retention; however, this results in electrolyte abnormalities due to urine electrolyte losses (Nyp et al., 2016, p. 332). Diuretics have significant impact on both fluid and electrolyte and acid/base balance. The extent of the imbalances depends on the type of diuretic used in treatment (Nyp et al., 2016, pp. 334–335).
  - ○ Table 11.6 provides a brief description of action and outcomes of common diuretics used in the NICU.

GLUCOSE HOMEOSTASIS

Fetal Physiology

- Throughout pregnancy, the mother supplies most of the glucose for the fetus via facilitated diffusion across the placenta. Fetal glucose levels are approximately 70% of maternal values (Rozance, McGowan, Price-Douglas, & Hay, 2016, p. 337).
- During the fetal period the fetus produces very little glucose, although the enzymes to facilitate gluconeogenesis are present in the third month of gestation (Rozance et al., 2016, p. 337). In periods of extreme stress where maternal glucose levels fall, the fetus can utilize ketone bodies for energy (Rozance et al., 2016, p. 337).

TABLE 11.6 Action and Outcomes of Common Diuretics Used in the NICU

	Mechanism of Action	Effects	Monitor for
Thiazide Diuretics			
Chlorothiazide	Inhibits Cl reabsorption in the distal tubule	Increased Na⁺ loss, decreases Ca⁺ losses	May increase renal calcium reabsorption
Hydrochlorothiazide	Inhibits Na⁺ reabsorption in distal convoluted tubule, collecting tubule, and early collecting duct	Increased reabsorption of NaCl	Hyponatremia, Hypokalemia
Sprionolactone	Inhibits effect of aldosterone on the collecting tubules	Increased Na⁺ loss, spares K⁺ losses	Hyperkalemia
Loop diuretics			
Furosemide	Blocks chloride transport in the thick ascending loop of Henle	Increased loss of Cl⁻, Na⁺, K⁺, Ca⁺² Subsequent water loss	Hypocalcemia Hypercalciuria, Nephrocalcinosis Hypomagnesemia, Hyponatremia, Hypokalemia, Hypovolemia Bone demineralization

Sources: Data from Fraser, D., & Diehl-Jones, W. (2015). Assisted ventilation. In M. T. Verklan & M. Walden (Eds.), *Core curriculum for neonatal intensive care nursing* (pp. 487–511). St. Louis, MO: Elsevier; Nyp, M., Brunkhorst, J. L., Reavy, D., & Pallotto, E. K. (2016). Fluid and electrolyte management. In S. L. Gardner, B. S. Carter, M. E. Hines, & J. A. Hernandez (Eds.), *Merenstein & Gardner's handbook of neonatal intensive care* (pp. 315–336). St. Louis, MO: Elsevier.

- The fetus begins to produce glycogen as early as the ninth week of gestation and continues to increase production throughout gestation, with the majority of glycogen production and storage occurring in the last trimester (Rozance et al., 2016, p. 337).
- The fetus also stores energy as fat, with most of the fat storage occurring in the last trimester as well (Rozance et al., 2016, p. 337).

Neonatal Physiology

- At birth, the maternal glucose supply abruptly ceases with the separation from the placenta, and the infant assumes responsibility glucose homeostasis (Rozance et al., 2016, p. 339). Several processes are required for successful adaptation.
  - Initially, catecholamine levels rise sharply as a result of delivery into a cooler, extrauterine environment and the physical separation of the placenta (Rozance et al., 2016, p. 339).
  - Glucagon levels rise, receptor sensitivity increases, and fetal glucagon/insulin ratios shift as catecholamine levels rise (Rozance et al., 2016, p. 339).
  - Rising glucagon and norepinephrine levels activate hepatic glycogen phosphorylase, and the rapidly decreasing glucose levels stimulate cortisol secretion, which stimulates hepatic glucose-6-phophatase activity (Rozance et al., 2016, p. 339).
- The newborn's ability to achieve glucose homeostasis is dependent upon the balance between hepatic glucose output and glucose utilization in the brain and peripheral tissues (Rozance et al., 2016, p. 339).
- Increased metabolic demands (e.g., prematurity, respiratory distress, and cold stress) will increase demand for glucose that may exceed hepatic rates of glycogenolysis and gluconeogenesis (Rozance et al., 2016, p. 339).
- Box 11.1. lists indications for routine blood glucose monitoring in the neonate.

BOX 11.1 Indications for Routine Blood Glucose in the Neonate

Maternal Conditions
- Presence of diabetes or abnormal result of glucose tolerance test
- Preeclampsia and pregnancy-induced or essential hypertension
- Previous macrosomic infants
- Substance abuse
- Treatment with beta-agonist tocolytics
- Treatment with oral hypoglycemic agents
- Late antepartum to intrapartum administration of intravenous glucose

Neonatal conditions
- Prematurity
- Intrauterine growth restriction
- Perinatal hypoxia–ischemia
- Sepsis
- Hypothermia
- Polycythemia–hyperviscosity
- Erythroblastosis fetalis
- Iatrogenic administration of insulin
- Congenital cardiac malformations
- Persistent hyperinsulinemia
- Endocrine disorders
- Inborn errors of metabolism

Source: Reproduced with permission from Rozance, P. J., McGowan, J. E., Price-Douglas, W., & Hay, W. W., Jr. (2016). Glucose homeostasis. In S. L. Gardner, B. S. Carter, M. E. Hines, & J. A. Hernandez (Eds.), *Merenstein & Gardner's handbook of neonatal intensive care* (pp. 337–359). St. Louis, MO: Elsevier.

Assessing Glucose Homeostasis in the Newborn

- Glucose concentrations in the newborn can be measured at the bedside (point of care [POC]) or in the laboratory. POC measurements rely on reagent strips and measure whole blood glucose (Burris, 2017, p. 312).

- Reagent strips are subject to false positives and false negatives, and thus, laboratory analysis must be performed to accurately determine hypoglycemia.
- POC glucose levels generally run 15% below plasma blood glucose samples run in the laboratory (Burris, 2017, p. 318).
- Glucose concentrations calculated in the laboratory are completed on plasma and must be run quickly after the sample is drawn to limit the uptake of glucose by the red blood cells in the sample (Burris, 2017, p. 316).

Hypoglycemia

- Agreement on absolute blood or plasma glucose concentrations that define hypoglycemia continues to vary, ranging from 20 mg/dL in premature infants (30 mg/dL in term infants) to plasma concentrations less than 45 mg/dL regardless of gestation in the first day of life (Rozance et al., 2016, p. 339). Beyond the first 48 hours of life, any infant with plasma glucose levels <60 mg/dL should be evaluated for hypoglycemia (Burris, 2017, p. 313).
- Signs of hypoglycemia may include tremors, jitteriness, exaggerated Moro, high-pitched or weak cry, apnea, tachypnea, irregular respirations, cyanosis, lethargy, hypotonia, poor feeding, hypothermia, or seizures (Armentrout, 2015, p. 163; Burris, 2017, p. 316)

MANAGEMENT OF THE ASYMPTOMATIC NEWBORN AT RISK

- Initial screens for infants at risk for hypoglycemia (e.g., small for gestational age [SGA], infants of diabetic mothers [IDM] large for gestational age [LGA], and late preterm infants) should be completed in the first hour of life.
- If the infant is otherwise stable and asymptomatic, the infant may be fed, and the glucose rechecked 1 hour later (Burris, 2017, p. 313).
  - ○ If the repeat glucose remains <25 mg/dL, the infant should be treated with IV glucose.
  - ○ If the second blood glucose is 25 to 40 mg/dL, feeding may be considered rather than treating with IV glucose in the otherwise healthy infant (Burris, 2017, p. 313).
- An alternative therapy that may be helpful for healthy breastfed infants is 40% dextrose gel placed in the buccal mucosa (Burris, 2017, p. 318; Rozance et al., 2016, p. 337) in addition to putting the infant to breast. Studies have shown that the use of 40% dextrose gel may reduce the need for NICU admissions due to hypoglycemia and decrease the use of formula supplementation for these infants in the first 2 weeks of life (Burris, 2017, p. 318).

MANAGEMENT OF THE SYMPTOMATIC INFANT

- When the newborn is symptomatic, IV therapy should be initiated with a bolus of IV D10W. The bolus should be followed with maintenance IVF D10W to provide a glucose infusion rate (GIR) of 6 to 8 mg/kg/min (Burris, 2017, p. 318).
- Refractive hypoglycemia, or hypoglycemia with onset beyond the first day of life, requires an endocrinology consult for further evaluation (Armentrout, 2015, p. 167). Adjunct therapies for persistent hypoglycemia include:
  - ○ Corticosteroids may be used to decrease peripheral glucose utilization and enhance gluconeogenesis.
  - ○ Glucagon may be used in the term infant to stimulate glycogenolysis and release glycogen stores form hepatic stores when insulin concentrations are normal.

If hyperinsulinism is present, the dose must be adjusted significantly.
  - ○ Diazoxide may be used to inhibit insulin secretion.
  - ○ Somatostatin may be used to inhibit insulin and growth hormone release.
  - ○ Pancreatectomy may be necessary to decrease insulin production and secretion (Rozance et al., 2016, p. 354).

Hyperglycemia

- Hyperglycemia is defined as point of care (POC) >120–125 mg/dL or plasma glucose >150 mg/dL. Onset of hyperglycemia may be seen within the first day of life and usually begins within the first 3 days of life.
- Signs of hyperglycemia may include glycosuria, dehydration, weight loss, fever, ketosis, metabolic acidosis, and failure to thrive (Armentrout, 2015, p. 169).
- The primary concern with hyperglycemia is related to hyperosmolarity and osmotic diuresis. An osmolarity of >300 mOsm/L is associated with osmotic diuresis and each 18 mg/dL increase in blood glucose concentration will increase serum osmolarity by 1 mOsmL (Burris, 2017, p. 321).
- When blood glucose reaches 450 to 720 mg/dL (hyperosmolar) ICF can shift to the extracellular compartment. It is postulated that the resultant decrease in the ICF may result in IVH (Burris, 2017, p. 321).
- Management: The primary goal of therapy is prevention and early detection of hyperglycemia.
  - ○ The initial GIR for all infants is 4 to 6 mg/kg/min (Burris, 2017, p. 323). Blood glucose should be checked regularly and adjustments to GIR made appropriately.
  - ○ Care should be taken to calculate GIR with changes in total fluid goals to prevent significant increases in GIR (Burris, 2017, p. 323).
  - ○ If the newborn develops hyperglycemia significant enough to warrant treatment (>250 mg/dL) despite efforts to decrease GIR and subsequently decrease blood glucose, insulin therapy may be required (Burris, 2017, p. 323). However, studies have reported that routine prophylactic use of insulin to prevent development of hyperglycemia in the VLBW infant is associated with a significant increase in morbidity, including increases in hypoglycemic episodes, and that there was no improvement in long-term outcomes of infants treated with insulin (Burris, 2017, p. 324; Rozance et al., 2016, p. 357).

PARENTERAL THERAPY

- The goal of PN therapy is to provide adequate nutrients to prevent energy deficiency and negative nitrogen balance (Anderson, Poindexter, & Martin, 2017, p. 260). In addition to prevention of negative balances, the goal is to promote appropriate weight gain and growth in the newborn until adequate enteral calories can be achieved (Anderson et al., 2017, p. 260).
- Indications for PN in newborns include VLBW and ELBW infants, infants with congenital and/or surgical disorders (e.g., gastroschisis, tracheal esophageal fistula, malrotation, obstruction, NEC, intestinal perforation, short bowel syndrome) and infants with renal failure. (Ditzenberger, 2015, p. 180). The sick term infant may also require PN.

PN should be initiated in the first day of life for these infants (Olsen et al., 2016, p. 361).

- Other factors to be considered in evaluating the newborn for PN are the type of IV access that is optimal. For infants with relatively short-term requirements (<7 days), where nutritional requirements can be met with dextrose solutions no greater than 12.5%, peripheral access may be sufficient (Anderson et al., 2017, p. 260). However, in infants who are anticipated to require longer term PN, or whose nutritional needs will require dextrose >12.5%, central access will be required.
- Central access can be obtained with UVCs, or peripherally inserted central catheters. Maximum osmolarity for solutions to be delivered through peripheral catheters must not exceed 900 mOsm/L (Anderson et al., 2017, p. 260).
- Central access must be obtained if the osmolarity of the PN will exceed 900 mOsm/L. PN solutions exposed to light generate peroxides, which may induce vasoconstriction and oxidant stress affecting the pulmonary and mesenteric perfusion.
- Lipid oxidation also occurs with exposure to light. Covering PN and intralipid (IL) solutions, including tubing, may reduce these oxidant effects, enhance IL metabolism, and lower circulating triglyceride levels (Olsen et al., 2016, p. 371).

Caloric Requirements

- Caloric goals for PN are lower than those for enteral nutrition and will vary based on the GA of the infant and the type of illness. These goals range from 80 to 100 kcal/kg/day (Ditzenberger, 2015, p. 181; Olsen et al., 2016, p. 360).

Water Requirements

- Fluid goals also vary initially based on GA with the goal of 100 to 150 mL/kg/day by 5 to 6 days of life (Ditzenberger, 2015, p. 181; Olsen et al., 2016, p. 361).

Carbohydrate Requirements

- Dextrose provides the carbohydrate source for the newborn. Initial GIR is 4 to 6 mg/kg/min. and is advanced by 1 to 2 mg/kg/day as the newborn tolerates to a goal of 11 to 12 mg/kg/min (Anderson et al., 2017, p. 261) or 13 to 17 mg/kg/min (Ditzenberger, 2015, p. 181).
- Dextrose concentrations available are 5% to 10% solutions. Every 1% of dextrose is equal to 1 g of dextrose per dL (Ditzenberger, 2015, p. 181).
- The caloric density of dextrose is 3.4 kcal/g (Anderson et al., 2017, p. 260). GIR can be calculated using the following formulas:
  - GIR in mg/kg/minute = (dextrose % concentration × mL/kg/day) divided by 144.
    Or:
  - GIR = (D × rate)/(6 × weight) (Burris, 2017, p. 319)

Protein Requirements

- Recommended protein requirements range from 2.25 to 4 g/kg/day. Higher protein requirements are needed in the most preterm infants (Ditzenberger, 2015, p. 182), with recommendations for protein of 2–3 g/kg/day beginning the first day of life for the VLBW and ELBW infant (Anderson et al., 2017, p. 262).

- Protein should be increased daily to a maximum of 3 g/kg/day for the term infant and 4 g/kg/day for the most preterm infant (Ditzenberger, 2015, p. 183).

Fat Requirements

- Recommended fat requirements vary depending upon the source, but the most recent recommendations are to initiate 2 g/kg of lipid in the first day of life for infants <1,500 g, advancing to 3 g/kg in the second day of life (Anderson et al., 2017, p. 262).
- The ELBW infant often has a lower tolerance for IL, which may require initiating IL at a lower rate and/or advancing the dose more gradually (Anderson et al., 2017, p. 262).
- Lipids are infused over 24 hours to promote optimal clearance (Anderson et al., 2017, p. 262). Essential fatty acid deficiency can be eliminated by providing 0.5 to 1 mL of IL/kg/day (Ditzenberger, 2015, p. 182). Twenty percent lipid emulsion is the most commonly supplied formulation, and the most common lipid solutions used in the United States were soy-based or a combination of soy/safflower. Twenty percent solutions of IL provide 2.2 kcal/mL (or approximately 10 kcal/g) (Anderson et al., 2017, p. 262; Ditzenberger, 2015, p. 182).
- Omegaven is a lipid emulsion made only from fish oil, which is high in anti-inflammatory ω-3 fatty acids. The use of fish oil emulsion is recommended in management of parenteral nutrition-associated cholestasis (PNAC) or parenteral nutrition-associated liver disease (PNALD), but has not been demonstrated to prevent PNALD in infants (Denne, 2018, p. 1026). Omegaven was Food and Drug Administration (FDA) approved in the United States in 2018 and is available by prescription (Anderson et al., 2017, p. 266).
- SMOF lipids are a combination of **S**oybean oil, **M**edium chain triglycerides, **O**live oil, and **F**ish oil. SMOF lipids are also higher in anti-inflammatory ω-3 fatty acids and have been introduced for management of PNALD (Kaplan et al., 2015, p. 1667). SMOF lipids are also FDA approved for use in the United States.
- Table 11.7 summarizes the metabolic requirements for the low birth weight infant.

TABLE 11.7 Metabolic Requirements for the Low Birth Weight Infant

Physiologic Activity	Kcal/kg/day
Energy expended	40–60
Resting metabolic rate	40–50
Activity	0–5
Thermoregulation	0–5
Synthesis	15
Energy stored	20–30
Energy excreted	15
Total energy intake	90–120

Source: Reproduced with permission from Ditzenberger, G. R. (2015). Nutritional management. In M. T. Verklan & M. Walden (Eds.), *Core curriculum for neonatal intensive care nursing* (pp. 172–196). St. Louis, MO: Elsevier.

Electrolyte and Mineral Requirements

- Initial sodium, potassium, and calcium requirements for the infant requiring PN were reviewed earlier in the chapter.
- Na^+ and K^+ supplementations are not required in the first 24 hours in newborn infants, but supplementation may be required after 24 to 48 hours of life based on fluid balance and electrolyte levels (Doherty, 2017, p. 299; Nyp et al., 2016, p. 325).
  - ○ Sodium is supplemented as chloride, acetate, or phosphate in amounts of 2 to 3 mEq/kg/day (Nyp et al., 2016, p. 326; Olsen et al., 2016, p. 361). Infants with mild metabolic acidosis may benefit from sodium acetate supplementation rather than chloride (Nyp et al., 2016, p. 325).
- Potassium is not provided until adequate urine output has been established (Nyp et al., 2016, p. 325). Once urine output has been established, K^+ supplementation is added in 1 to 2 mEq/kg/day but may increase to 3 to 4 mEq/kg/day (Olsen et al., 2016, p. 361).
- Elemental calcium should be provided in the first day of life for most newborns (20–60 mg/kg/day) as elemental Ca^+, increasing over the course of the first few days of life to 60 to 80 mg/kg/day (Denne, 2018, p. 1024).
- Phosphorous must be provided to promote calcium absorption and should be initiated on the second day of life. 45 to 60 mg/kg/day will provide adequate substrate; however, calcium and phosphorous may precipitate in solution if not carefully balanced. Calcium:phosphorous ratios of 1.7:1 by weight, or 1.3:1 by molar ratio, are optimal. The addition of cysteine lowers the pH, which improves solubility (Denne, 2018, p. 1027).
- Magnesium is required for optimal function of intracellular enzyme systems. Magnesium should be provided as 0.25 to 0.5 mEq/kg/day (Olsen et al., 2016, p. 363).
- Adjustments to electrolyte supplementation are made daily initially, guided by serum lab values and overall fluid management requirements.

Vitamins and Trace Elements

- Vitamins are essential in many metabolic processes (Brown et al., 2016, p. 391). There are currently no parenteral vitamin sources designed exclusively for preterm infants, however, M.V.I. Pediatric is the solution currently used for infants. The dose will vary from 2.5 mL/day for infants <2.5 kg, and 5 mL/day for infants >2.5 kg/day (Anderson et al., 2017, p. 263).
- Trace elements are provided in the first few days of life and provide selenium, copper, chromium, iron, fluoride, manganese, molybdenum, and zinc (Denne, 2018, p. 1028).

Other Additives

- Carnitine facilitates the transfer of long-chain fatty acids into the mitochondria. Prenatal stores are quickly depleted leaving the preterm infant who requires prolonged PN at risk. Carnitine can be added at 10 mg/kg/day; however, not all NICUs currently add carnitine (Anderson et al., 2017, p. 267).
- Cysteine is synthesized from methionine and provides a substrate for taurine production. Preterm infants are low in enzyme hepatic cystathionine required to convert methionine to cysteine and thus, cysteine is commonly added to infant PN. Cysteine also lowers the pH the solution and reduces the risk for calcium/phosphorous precipitation (Anderson et al., 2017, p. 267).
- Table 11.8 identifies the suggested goals for PN components

TABLE 11.8 Suggested Goals for PN Components

Component	Daily Amount
Calories	
Dextrose 3.4 kcal/g	10–15 g/kg
Lipids 2.0 kcal/ml (20%) solution	1–3 g/kg
Protein (6.25 g protein = 1 g N_2)	3.5-4 g/kg
Electrolytes	
Sodium	3 mEq/kg
Potassium	2–3 mEq/kg
Chloride	3–4 mEq/kg
Acetate	3 mEq/kg
Phosphate	2 mM/kg
Calcium	3 mEq/kg
Magnesium	0.3 mEq (range 0.25–0.5 mEq/kg) or 20 mg/kg (range 10–40 mg/kg) of elemental magnesium
Vitamins	
MVI-Ped	1 vial*
Vitamin A	0.7 mg
Thiamine (B_1)	1.2 mg
Riboflavin (B_2)	1.4 mg
Niacin	17 mg
Pyridoxine (B_6)	1 mg
Ascorbic acid (C)	80 mg
Ergocalciferol (D)	10 mcg
Vitamin E	7 mg
Pantothenic acid	5 mg
Cyanocobalamin	1 mcg
Folate	140 mcg
Vitamin K	200 mcg
Trace elements	
Zinc (zinc sulfate)†	300 mcg/kg
Copper (cupric sulfate)†	20 mcg/kg
Manganese sulfate†	5 mcg/kg
Chromium chloride†	0.2 mcg/kg
Selenium	2 mcg/kg

*MVI Pediatric (Astra Pharmaceuticals), reduced amount provided for very low birth weight infants (see text)

Source: Reproduced with permission from Olsen, S. L., Leick-Rude, M. K., Dusin, J., & Rosterman, J. (2016). Parenteral nutrition. In S. L. Gardner, B. S. Carter, M. E. Hines, & J. A. Hernandez (Eds.), *Merenstein & Gardner's handbook of neonatal intensive care* (pp. 360–376). St. Louis, MO: Elsevier.

Risks Associated With PN Use

- Delivery of PN often includes placement of central lines. Mechanical risks for central line use include pneumothorax, hemithorax, air embolism, cardiac perforation, and cardiac tamponade. Risks may also include malposition, catheter occlusion, thrombosis, catheter migration, and phlebitis (Olsen et al., 2016, p. 372).
  - Line position must be verified by x-ray when the line is inserted, and lines must be evaluated daily for evidence that the line remains secure.
  - All x-rays are obtained after insertion of a central line should be reviewed to verify that the line remains in optimal position (Olsen et al., 2016, p. 372).
  - Infection is always a risk with central line use. The use of dedicated line insertion teams, as well as insertion and maintenance bundles, are associated with decreased incidence of central-line related sepsis infections (CLABSIs); (Olsen et al., 2016, p. 373).
- Cholestasis and osteopenia may develop in the newborn with prolonged duration of PN (Anderson et al., 2017, p. 265; Ditzenberger, 2015, p. 182; Olsen et al., 2016, p. 373).

CONCLUSION

Best practices in diagnosis and management of fluid and electrolyte abnormalities in the sick newborn require more than knowledge of physiological principles. Astute clinical knowledge of disease processes and impact on the newborn, careful attention to changes in fluid and electrolyte levels, and timely adjustments in fluid and electrolyte supplementation to maintain homeostasis are equally critical in the safe and appropriate management of the sick newborn with fluid and electrolyte imbalances.

REVIEW QUESTIONS

1. The total body water (TBW) content in the extremely low birth weight (ELBW) infant is inversely related to gestational age, which means that as:
   A. gestational age decreases, TBW increases.
   B. postnatal age increases, TBW increases.
   C. TBW increases, gestational age increases.

2. An abnormal accumulation of fluid in the interstitial space (IS) caused by increased capillary hydrostatic pressure and increased capillary wall permeability is termed:
   A. edema
   B. oncotic
   C. solute

3. Calculate the insensible water loss (IWL) for a 1.5 kg infant with a total fluid intake of 150 mL/kg/day, a urine output of 3 mL/kg/hr., and a weight loss of 200 g.
   A. −56 mL
   B. −70 mL
   C. −83 mL

4. The NNP orders dextrose fluids for a 4-hours-old preterm infant and knows supplementation with which electrolytes is not necessary?
   A. calcium (Ca^{+2})
   B. bicarbonate (HCO_3^-)
   C. sodium (Na^+)

5. Hyponatremia in the newborn may result from which of the following?
   A. delayed administration of isotonic solutions.
   B. excessive administration of hypertonic solutions.
   C. excessive administration of isotonic solutions.

REFERENCES

Anderson, D. M., Poindexter, B. B., & Martin, C. R. (2017). Nutrition. In E. C. Eichenwald, A. R. Hansen, C. R. Marin, & A. R. Stark (Eds.), *Cloherty and Stark's manual of neonatal care* (pp. 248–284). Philadelphia, PA: Wolters Kluwer.

Armentrout, D. (2015). Glucose management. In M. T. Verklan, & M. Walden (Eds.), *Core curriculum for neonatal intensive care nursing* (pp. 162–171). St. Louis, MO: Elsevier.

Barry, J. S., Deacon, J., Hernandez, C., & Jones, M. D. (2016). Acid-base homeostasis and oxygenation. In S. L. Gardner, B. S. Carter, M. E. Hines, & J. A. Hernandez (Eds.), *Merenstein & Gardner's handbook of neonatal intensive care* (pp. 145–157). St. Louis, MO: Elsevier.

Brown, L. D., Hendrickson, K., Evans, R., Davis, J., Anderson, M. S., & Hay, W. A. (2016). Enteral nutrition. In S. L. Gardner, B. S. Carter, M. E. Hines, & J. A. Hernandez (Eds.), *Merenstein & Gardner's handbook of neonatal intensive care* (pp. 377–418). St. Louis, MO: Elsevier.

Burris, H. H. (2017). Hypoglycemia and hyperglycemia. In E. C. Eichenwald, A. R. Hansen, C. R. Marin, & A. R. Stark (Eds.), *Cloherty and Stark's manual of neonatal care* (pp. 312–325). Philadelphia, PA: Wolters Kluwer.

Dell, K. M. (2015). Fluid, electrolyte, and acid-base homeostasis. In R. J. Martin, A. A. Fanaroff, & M. C. Walsh (Eds.), *Fanaroff and Martin's neonatal-perinatal medicine: Diseases of the fetus and infant* (pp. 613–629). Philadelphia, PA: Elsevier.

Denne, S. C. (2018). Parenteral nutrition for the high-risk neonate (pp 1023–1031). In C. A. Gleason & S. E. Juul (Eds.), *Avery's diseases of the newborn* (pp. 368–389). Philadelphia, PA: Elsevier

Ditzenberger, G. R. (2015). Nutritional management. In M. T. Verklan & M. Walden (Eds.), *Core curriculum for neonatal intensive care nursing* (pp. 172–196). St. Louis, MO: Elsevier.

Doherty, E. G. (2017). Fluid and electrolyte management. In E. C. Eichenwald, A. R. Hansen, C. R. Marin, & A. R. Stark (Eds.), *Cloherty and Stark's manual of neonatal care* (pp. 296–311). Philadelphia, PA: Wolters Kluwer.

Halbardier, B. H. (2015). Fluid and electrolyte management. In M. T. Verklan & M. Walden (Eds.), *Core curriculum for neonatal intensive care nursing* (pp. 146–161). St. Louis, MO: Elsevier

Koves, I. H., Ness, K. D., Nip, A. S., & Salehi, P. (2018). Disorders of calcium and phosphorous metabolism. In C. A. Gleason & S. E. Juul (Eds.), *Avery's diseases of the newborn* (pp. 1333–1350). Philadelphia, PA: Elsevier

Nyp, M., Brunkhorst, J. L., Reavy, D., & Pallotto, E. K. (2016). Fluid and electrolyte management. In S. L. Gardner, B. S. Carter, M. E. Hines, & J. A. Hernandez (Eds.), *Merenstein & Gardner's handbook of neonatal intensive care* (pp. 315–336). St. Louis, MO: Elsevier.

Olsen, S. L., Leick-Rude, M. K., Dusin, J., & Rosterman, J. (2016). Total parenteral nutrition. In S. L. Gardner, B. S. Carter, M. E. Hines, & J. A. Hernandez (Eds.), *Merenstein & Gardner's handbook of neonatal intensive care* (pp. 360–376). St. Louis, MO: Elsevier.

Rozance, P. J., McGowan, J. E., Price-Douglas, W., & Hay, W. W., Jr. (2016). Glucose homeostasis. In S. L. Gardner, B. S. Carter, M. E. Hines, & J. A. Hernandez (Eds.), *Merenstein & Gardner's handbook of neonatal intensive care* (pp. 337–359). St. Louis, MO: Elsevier.

Wright, C. J., Posencheg, M. A., Seri, I., & Evans, J. R. (2018). Fluid, electrolyte, and acid-base balance. In C. A. Gleason & S. E. Juul (Eds.), *Avery's Diseases of the newborn* (pp. 368–389). Philadelphia, PA: Elsevier.

12 PRINCIPLES OF NEONATAL PHARMACOLOGY

Sandra L. Smith

INTRODUCTION

Pharmacotherapeutics, or the use of medications to treat disease, is one of the most common responsibilities of the NNP and requires knowledge of pharmacokinetics and pharmacodynamics during the perinatal period. This includes (a) neonatal/infant pharmacokinetics and pharmacodynamics and the effects of drug therapy on the neonate and (b) neonatal effects of drugs used by mothers who are breastfeeding. There is great variability in pharmacokinetics and pharmacodynamics in the neonate and infant due to rapid changes in physiology and the effect of various disease states on the neonate (Allegaert, Ward, & Van Den Anker, 2018, p. 419; Blackburn, 2018, p. 196).

Aspects of pharmacokinetics and pharmacodynamics applied to the neonate are presented to assist the NNP in understanding various drug therapies. Rationales for dose adjustment and management of the neonate as they relate to drug therapy are covered, as well as changes in drug metabolism during infancy. The effects of maternal drug use on infants who are fed human milk are discussed. Drug tolerance and withdrawal are described. Specific drug treatments are presented in subsequent chapters.

NEONATAL PHARMACOKINETICS

- Pharmacokinetics is the mathematical relationship between drug dose and blood levels over time. Pharmacokinetic processes include absorption, distribution, metabolism (biotransformation), and excretion (Allegaert et al., 2018, pp. 419–421; Blackburn, 2018, pp. 180–181; Wade, 2015, p. 665).

Absorption

- Absorption is the process of drug movement from the administration site (gastrointestinal, intravenous (IV), intramuscular, intrapulmonary/inhaled, and subcutaneous) across membranes and into the systemic circulation (Allegaert et al., 2018, p. 419; Domonoske, 2015, pp. 220–221; Wade, 2015, p. 665).

Distribution

- Drug distribution is the movement of drug to various tissues or the site of action and/or extravascular space (Wade, 2015, p. 666).
  - Properties of drugs affecting distribution include lipid solubility, size (molecular weight), and degree of ionization. Only free, unbound drug crosses membranes and can exert a pharmacologic action and be metabolized and excreted (Allegaert et al., 2018, p. 420; Katzung, 2018, pp. 3–10; Wade, 2015, p. 666).
    - Drugs diffuse across membranes passively along a concentration gradient by facilitated carrier-mediated transport, endocytosis, and exocytosis (Katzung, 2018, pp. 7–9).
  - Infant properties that influence drug distribution include organ blood flow, pH, body fat content, extracellular fluid space, amount of total body water (TBW), and plasma protein-binding capacity (Allegaert et al., 2018, p. 420; Blackburn, 2018, pp. 198–199; Wade, 2015, p. 666).
    - Physiologic differences among preterm infants, term infants, children, and adults that affect distribution include (a) TBW content, (b) body fat content, (c) protein (primarily albumin) content, (d) protein binding affinity, and (e) competition for protein binding with other substances, primarily bilirubin (Allegaert et al., 2018, p. 420; Blackburn, 2018, pp. 198–199).
    - TBW is higher in preterm infants (~85%) compared to term infants (~75%) and adults (~50%–65%), thus affecting the distribution of water-soluble drugs (Allegaert et al., 2018, p. 420; McClary, 2015b, p. 65520).
    - Body fat content is lower in the newborn and increases during the first 5 months of infancy as TBW decreases, thereby affecting the distribution of lipophilic drugs (Allegaert et al., 2018, p. 420; Blackburn, 2018, p. 199; McClary, 2015b, p. 655).
    - Protein binding is lower in the infant due to lower circulating proteins, and the circulating protein available has a lower binding affinity in the infant, thus more free drug is available for distribution to tissues (Allegaert et al., 2018, p. 420; Blackburn, 2018, p. 199; McClary, 2015b, p. 655).
    - Bilirubin freely binds with protein and competes with drugs for protein binding sites, thus the amount of unbound drug varies with bilirubin levels (Allegaert et al., 2018, p. 420; McClary, 2015b, p. 655).
  - Measurements of serum drug concentrations include free and protein-bound drug; however, in the infant, the amount of free drug may be higher than in the adult due to the protein-binding differences between infants and adults (Allegaert et al., 2018, p. 420; Wade, 2015, p. 666).
  - Volume of Distribution (Vd): the hypothetical amount of volume needed to dissolve a given amount of drug, also called apparent Vd (Allegaert et al., 2018, p. 422;

Blackburn, 2018, p. 198; Domonoske, 2015, p. 222; Herbert, 2013, p. 33; Holford, 2018, pp. 42–45).

- Drugs with high Vd are found extensively in the tissues rather than plasma and are not homogeneously distributed, whereas drugs found mostly in plasma have a smaller Vd (Holford, 2018, p. 42; Wade, 2015, p. 666).
- Vd is influenced by gestational age due to the rapid changes in TBW and fluid shifts (Allegaert et al., 2018, p. 428; Wade, 2015, p. 666).
- Infants with large extracellular fluid volumes have increased Vd for water-soluble drugs and may reduce peak drug values and affect drug excretion (Blackburn, 2018, p. 198).
- Decreased body fat in preterm and intrauterine growth-restricted infants decreases the Vd for lipophilic drugs (Blackburn, 2018, p. 199).

Bioavailability

- Bioavailability is defined as the amount of drug administered that reaches the circulation or as the amount of drug delivered to the site of action (Domonoske, 2015, p. 216; Wade, 2015, p. 665).
- Intravenously administered drugs are considered 100% bioavailable and are the standard by which the bioavailability of orally and intramuscularly administered drugs is determined (Wade, 2015, p 665).
- Bioavailability of orally administered drugs may be limited by drug formulation, solubility, dissolution, or stability in an acidic environment, or be reabsorbed by enterocytes back into the gut lumen (Wade, 2015, p. 665).

Metabolism

- Drug metabolism is the biotransformation of drug into inactive and active metabolites; occurs in the liver, kidney, intestinal mucosa, and lungs; and is generally classified as Phase I or Phase II metabolism (Allegaert et al., 2018, p. 420; Blackburn, 2018, p. 201; Domonoske, 2015, p. 224; McClary, 2015b, pp. 655–657; Wade, 2015, p. 666).
  - ○ Phase I metabolism: enzymatic drug conversion to metabolites via oxidation, reduction, and hydrolysis (Blackburn, 2018, p. 181; Domonoske, 2015, p. 224).
    - Cytochrome P450 (CYP450) enzymes mediate Phase I metabolism and are present in many tissues, but they are most highly concentrated in hepatic tissues (Allegaert et al., 2018, pp. 655–657; McClary, 2015b, pp. 420–421).
      - CYP450 enzymes have variable expression and maturation across the life span, thus the enzyme responsible for metabolism of a given drug may be more or less active in the infant depending on gestational and postnatal age (Allegaert et al., 2018, p. 421; Blackburn, 2018, p. 200; McClary, 2015b, pp. 656–657).
      - Examples of drugs metabolized via Phase I reactions: phenytoin, phenobarbital, ibuprofen, diazepam, indomethacin (Blackburn, 2018, p. 181).
  - ○ Phase II metabolism: enzymatic drug biotransformation via the addition (conjugation) of a substance to the drug metabolite (Domonoske, 2015, p. 224; McClary, 2015b, p. 657).

- Phase II reactions are glucuronidation (glucuronide conjugation), acetylation, methylation, glycine conjugation, glutathione conjugation, and sulfate conjugation (Blackburn, 2018, p. 181; McClary, 2015b, p. 657).
  - Primary enzymes in Phase II metabolism include uridine 5′-diphosphoglucuronosyltransferases (UGTs), glutathione S-transferase, and sulfotransferase (McClary, 2015b, p. 657).
  - Phase II enzyme activity is variable in infants, with glucuronidation activity typically low at birth and sulfate conjugation activity more active at birth (McClary, 2015b, p. 657).
  - Examples of drugs metabolized via Phase II reactions include:
    - ○ Morphine and acetaminophen via glucuronidation (Allegaert et al., 2018, p. 421; Blackburn, 2018, p. 181).
    - ○ Dopamine and epinephrine via methylation (Blackburn, 2018, p. 181).
- Factors affecting metabolism that may result in prolonged or unpredictable drug half-life and decreased drug clearance include age-related enzyme maturation, nutrition, illness, drug interactions, hepatic blood flow, drug transport, protein synthesis, protein binding, biliary secretion, and genetic variation (pharmacogenomics; Allegaert et al., 2018, pp. 420–421; Blackburn, 2018, pp. 200–201; Wade, 2015, pp. 666–667).
  - ○ The rate of drug metabolism is low at birth in term infants and even lower in premature infants regardless of the route of metabolism. The development of individual drug-metabolizing enzymes varies widely among neonates and may be delayed in premature neonates (Blackburn, 2018, pp. 200–201; McClary, 2015b, p. 657).
  - ○ Many enzymes responsible for metabolism of drugs have significant development during the first month of life; therefore, dosing regimens at birth may not be appropriate at 3 to 4 weeks of life, necessitating dose and dose–interval adjustments (Blackburn, 2018, p. 200; McClary, 2015b, p. 657).
  - ○ Predicting clearance is difficult and dosing regimens must be individualized based on patient response, tolerance, and drug levels. Decreased clearance and prolonged half-life often require drug administration with longer dosing intervals (Blackburn, 2018, pp. 200–201; McClary, 2015b, p. 657).

Excretion

- The excretion or elimination of unchanged drug or drug metabolites from the body occurs via the renal, biliary, cutaneous, and pulmonary systems. Renal excretion is an important excretory pathway for unchanged drugs or drug metabolites in neonates and infants (Allegaert et al., 2018, p. 421; Blackburn, 2018, pp. 201; Domonoske, 2015, p. 225; Wade, 2015, pp. 666–667).
  - ○ Renal mechanisms of drug elimination include glomerular filtration, active secretion at the proximal tubule, and reabsorption at the distal tubule (Allegaert et al., 2018, p. 421; McClary, 2015b, p. 657; Wade, 2015, pp. 666–667).
    - Altered renal elimination occurs in the neonate due to reduced renal function, glomerular filtration rate, and creatinine clearance (Allegaert et al., 2018,

p. 421; Blackburn, 2018, pp. 201; McClary, 2015b, p. 657; Wade, 2015, p. 667).

- ◾ Factors affecting renal drug clearance include pathologic processes such as hypoxemia, poor perfusion, hypothermia, concurrent renal disease, and exposure to nephrotoxic drugs (Allegaert et al., 2018, p. 421; Blackburn, 2018, pp. 201; McClary, 2015b, p. 657; Wade, 2015, p. 667).
- ○ Hepatic mechanisms of drug elimination include metabolism, bile excretion, fecal elimination, and enterohepatic recirculation (Allegaert et al., 2018, p. 421; Wade, 2015, pp. 666–667).
  - ◾ Liver blood flow and hepatic enzyme activity affect hepatic excretion (Allegaert et al., 2018, p. 421; Wade, 2015, pp. 666–667).
  - ◾ Drug elimination is decreased in patients with decreased albumin levels, altered protein binding, poor liver blood flow, and liver enzyme alterations (Allegaert et al., 2018, p. 421; Wade, 2015, p. 667).

Pharmacokinetic Models of Drug Elimination

- • Pharmacokinetic models of drug elimination are zero-order, first-order, or multicompartment first order. These models entail mathematical calculations of the relationships between the dose selected (mg/kg) and the desired serum concentrations (peak and trough) influenced by the body's ability to clear the drug, the volume of distribution (Vd), half-life ($T_{1/2}$), and elimination rate constant (Kel; Allegaert et al., 2018, p. 428; Wade, 2015, p. 669).

ZERO-ORDER OR SATURATION PHARMACOKINETICS

- • A constant amount of drug is eliminated per unit of time regardless of serum concentration (Allegaert et al., 2018, p. 424; Wade, 2015, p. 668). Concepts relative to zero-order pharmacokinetics include enzyme/transport systems and drug dose.
  - ○ Enzymes or transport system receptors are saturated with drug, thereby preventing proportional drug elimination (Allegaert et al., 2018, p. 424).
  - ○ Small dose increases result in large serum concentration changes until receptors are free from drug (Allegaert et al., 2018, p. 424).
  - ○ Examples of drugs with zero-order kinetics: caffeine, diazepam, furosemide, indomethacin, phenytoin (Allegaert et al., 2018, p. 424; Wade, 2015, p. 668).

FIRST-ORDER PHARMACOKINETICS

- • Mathematically described as the equation of a straight line, first-order pharmacokinetics is also called single-compartment first-order kinetics (Allegaert et al., 2018, p. 423).
  - ○ A constant *percentage* of drug is eliminated over time; it is a *proportional rate* of elimination (Allegaert et al., 2018, p. 423; Wade, 2015, pp. 667–668).
  - ○ The compartment is the fluid and tissue where drugs penetrate. These spaces include vascular, interstitial, spinal fluid, and tissues (Domonoske, 2015, p. 222).
    - ◾ Central compartment: the vascular space where hydrophilic drugs accumulate, typically the blood volume (Allegaert et al., 2018, p. 422).
    - ◾ Peripheral compartment: tissues and other fluid spaces where lipophilic drugs accumulate (Allegaert et al., 2018, p. 422).

- ◾ Diffusion between the central compartment and peripheral compartments is influenced by molecular size of drug, polarity of drug, and protein binding of drug (Allegaert et al., 2018, p. 422).
- ○ Circulating/plasma drug concentration is the mathematical relationship between drug dose and Vd (Allegaert et al., 2018, p. 422) expressed as follows: Plasma Drug Concentration (mg/L) = Dose (mg/kg)/Vd (L/kg) (Allegaert et al., 2018, p. 422).
- ○ Half-life: the time needed for the concentration of drug in plasma to decrease by 50% due to elimination (Figure 12.1; Allegaert et al., 2018, p. 423; Wade, 2015, p. 667).

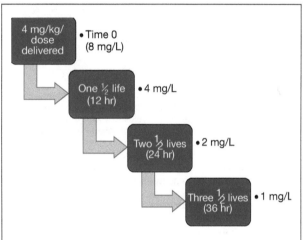

FIGURE 12.1 Example of a drug with a half-life of 12 hours. The drug plasma concentration decreases by one-half every 12 hours; thus the half-life is equal to 12 hours.

MULTICOMPARTMENT FIRST-ORDER PHARMACOKINETICS

- • The biphasic elimination of drugs from the circulation id divided into two phases: alpha phase and beta phase (Figure 12.2; Allegaert et al., 2018, pp. 423–424; Wade, 2015, pp. 668–669).
  - ○ *Alpha phase:* the distribution and elimination of a drug in serum. This phase is typically rapid; however, the length of time varies as the alpha phase is drug dependent. For example, the alpha phase for gentamicin is 60 minutes: 30 minutes to infuse, 30 minutes to complete the alpha phase. (Wade, 2015, p. 673).
  - ○ *Beta phase:* the elimination phase, which is slower and longer than the alpha phase due to the elimination rate constant, the clearance, and volume of distribution unique to each infant (see Pharmacokinetic Calculations section; Allegaert et al., 2018, p. 423).

Pharmacokinetic Calculations

- • Clinicians at the bedside use pharmacokinetic calculations for therapeutic drug monitoring (TDM) to guide dosing for individual patients, achieve effective serum concentrations, and avoid toxic drug concentrations (Allegaert et al., 2018, p. 425; Wade, 2015, pp. 669–670).
- • The calculations require a knowledge of exponential and logarithmic functions and a step-by-step approach considering the infusion time, alpha phase, and serum peak and

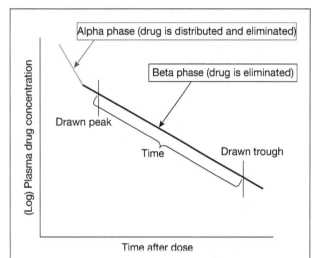

FIGURE 12.2 Multicompartment first-order pharmacokinetics is the basis for pharmacokinetic calculations. The length of the alpha phase is drug dependent. Peak and trough drug levels are drawn during the beta phase of elimination when calculating drug kinetics. The drug peak is drawn at the beginning of the beta phase of elimination. The drug trough is ideally drawn at the time the next dose is due to be administered.

Source: Data from Allegaert, K., Ward, R. M., & Van Den Anker, J. N. (2018). Neonatal pharmacology. In C. A. Gleason & S. E. Juul (Eds.), *Avery's diseases of the newborn* (10th ed., pp. 419–431). Philadelphia, PA: Elsevier.

trough concentrations (Allegaert et al., 2018, pp. 425–428; Wade, 2015, pp. 669–670).

- Measured peaks and troughs are used in these equations, but estimated peaks and troughs can be calculated using exponential equations. Key aspects of the calculations include the following and are detailed with examples by Wade (2015, p. 673) and Allegaert et al. (2018, pp. 422–428):
  - The elimination rate constant (Kel): the natural logarithm (ln) of the measured peak (Cp_0) divided by the measured trough (Cp) drug levels divided by the time (t) elapsed between when the peak and trough were drawn (Wade, 2015, p. 673).
    - $(\ln[Cp_0/Cp]/t)$
  - Half-life: the natural logarithm of 2 (ln2) divided by the Kel, where ln2 = 0.693 (Wade, 2015, p. 673).
    - $(0.693/Kel)$
  - Vd (L/kg) = Dose (mg/kg)/(Serum Peak [mg/L]-Serum Trough [mg/L]) where the serum peak minus the serum trough is the change in concentration (ΔC) (Allegaert et al., 2018, p. 428).
    - $Vd \ (L/kg) = Dose \ (mg/kg)/\Delta C$
- The true peak and trough can be calculated prior to calculating the Vd for a more accurate Vd, but the measure peak and trough may be used.
  - True peak equation: $Cp_0 = Cp/e^{-kt}$ where Cp_0 = true peak, Cp = measured peak, e = exponential function, k = Kel, t = length of time in hours between the time the peak was drawn and the time the true peak would occur.
  - True peak occurs at the end of the alpha phase and beginning of the beta phase.

- Gentamicin alpha phase is 60 minutes (30 minutes for infusion plus 30 minutes for alpha phase to complete), and the peak may be drawn 60 minutes after the infusion ends to ensure that the drawn peak is within the beta phase of elimination by 0.5 hours. Peaks may be drawn 30 minutes after the infusion ends, assuming that the beta phase begins 30 minutes after the infusion is complete (Allegaert et al., 2018, p. 428).
  - If the time between the drawn peak and the beginning of the beta phase is equal to 0, the drawn peak and true peak will be the same.
- True trough equation: $Cp = CP_0(e^{-kt})$ where Cp = true trough, Cp_0 = drawn trough, e = exponential function, k = Kel, t = length of time in hours between the time the drawn trough and true trough would occur.
  - The true trough occurs at the time the dose is to be given.
  - If t = 0 (the drawn trough was obtained at the time the dose was due) the drawn trough and true trough will be the same.
- Clearance (Cl): the rate of drug removal from the blood over time.
  - $Cl \ (L/hr/kg) = Vd \ (L/kg) \times Kel(hr^{-1})$ (Allegaert et al., 2018, p. 424; Wade, 2015, pp. 669–673).
- Clinical examples see Allegaert et al. (2018, p. 428) and Wade (2015, pp. 673–674).

Steady-State Concentration

- Occurs with repetitive drug dosing due to drug accumulation. The amount of drug administered equals the amount of drug eliminated and occurs after the fourth dose of drug given; however, the time it takes to reach steady-state concentration is mostly dependent upon drug half-life and can be reached sooner if the dosing interval is shorter than the drug half-life (Allegaert et al., 2018, p. 426; Holford, 2018, pp. 49–54). When steady state is reached:
  - Peak levels will be the same after each dose and trough levels will be the same before each dose (Allegaert et al., 2018, p. 426).
- The practitioner can use pharmacokinetic data when adjusting drug doses based upon changes in volume of distribution, elimination, and Cl, and knowledge of pharmacokinetics assists the practitioner in predicting drug concentrations over time. Pharmacokinetics describes mathematical relationships but does not provide the practitioner with knowledge about drug effects (Allegaert et al., 2018, p. 419; Wade, 2015, p. 665, 670–671).
- In contrast, *pharmacodynamics* are drug properties the practitioner uses when selecting specific drug therapies to achieve a desired effect.

PHARMACODYNAMICS

Pharmacodynamics is the relationship between drug concentrations in the serum and the effects of the drug on the body. These effects include therapeutic and toxic effects (Domonoske, 2015, pp. 217–218; Holford, 2018, p. 52; Wade, 2015, pp. 670–671).

- Pharmacodynamic properties are drug specific and reflect the (a) mechanism of action, (b) potency, (c) toxicity characteristics, (d) efficacy, and (e) desired outcome (Wade, 2015, p. 671).

- Many drugs bind to receptors and the pharmacodynamics of these receptor-binding drugs are altered in the neonate due to changes in receptor binding, receptor density (number of receptors available), downstream signal transduction, disease states, maturity, and concomitant use of other drugs (Wade, 2015, p. 671).
- Pharmacodynamic properties of antimicrobials are a unique application for use by practitioners and include elimination of the pathogenic microbe, avoiding toxicity of drug, and minimizing the development of antimicrobial resistance (Wade, 2015, pp. 666, 671).
- Pharmacodynamics is used to determine antibiotic killing concentrations needed to eradicate infection based on the minimum inhibitory concentration (MIC), area under the concentration curve (AUC), post-antibiotic effect (PAE) and serum drug level, specifically the drug peak or maximum concentration (Cp_{max}; Wade, 2015, p. 671).
  - MIC: the lowest antimicrobial concentration that prevents visible growth of an organism after 24 hours of incubation, which varies by organism being treated (Domonoske, 2015, p. 226).
  - AUC: the measure of total drug exposure from time of administration to time of complete elimination. AUC remains above zero with repeated drug dosing (Wade, 2015, p. 671).
  - PAE: continued killing or suppression of an organism for a period of time after the drug is removed (Wade, 2015, p. 672).

PHARMACOKINETIC AND PHARMACODYNAMICS SPECIFIC TO ANTIBIOTIC THERAPY

- Concentration-dependent killing of microbes is killing dependent on the Cp_{max} to MIC ratio (Cp_{max}/MIC; Wade, 2015, p. 672).
  - Goal: to increase the peak concentration with the dose to achieve more bacterial killing, for example with gentamicin (Wade, 2015 p. 671).
- Time-dependent killing: killing is dependent on the percent of time the drug concentration is above the MIC of the organism being treated (Wade, 2015, p. 672).
  - Goal: improve extent of drug exposure with short dosing intervals; for example, with beta-lactam antibiotics (e.g., ampicillin; Wade, 2015, pp. 671–672).
- Time-dependent killing with PAE: killing is related to the AUC/MIC ratio or the amount of total drug exposure relative to the organism's MIC (Wade, 2015, p. 672).
  - Goal: augment the drug exposure using both dose and interval adjustments; for example, with vancomycin (Wade, 2015, p. 672).
- Drug efficacy is influenced by how the drug is administered to the neonate. Pharmacodynamics is therapeutic and toxicity profiles of drugs that are influenced by the drug mechanism of action, potency, toxicity characteristics, and desired outcome (Wade, 2015, p. 671).

PRINCIPLES OF ADMINISTRATION

- Concepts of significance to drug administration include the (a) selected route of administration, (b) drug dosage, and (c) interval between doses (Allegaert et al., 2018, pp. 419–420; McClary, 2015a, p. 654).

- Tolerance and weaning from drug therapy must also be considered when determining the administration of specific drugs (Allegaert et al., 2018, p. 427; Domonoske, 2015, p. 230).
- Withdrawal from drug therapy has implications for administration choices. Pharmacokinetic and pharmacodynamic principles previously described affect drug administration choices (Allegaert et al., 2018, p. 419).

Routes of Administration

- Common routes of administration and their challenges in the neonate include the following (Allegaert et al., 2018, p. 419):

IV ADMINISTRATION

- Slow IV infusion rates, small volumes of drugs, dead space in IV tubing, and limits to volumes used to flush IV lines are limitations seen in neonates. Therefore, IV-infused drugs need to be infused as close to the neonate as possible (Allegaert et al., 2018, p. 419).

INTRAMUSCULAR AND SUBCUTANEOUS ADMINISTRATION

- Poor perfusion to the muscle limits absorption with these routes; drug may deposit and remain at the injection site for a prolonged period and neonates are at risk for sclerosis at the injection site or abscess development (Allegaert et al., 2018, p. 420).
  - Muscle and subcutaneous tissues are limited in the preterm and low birth weight infant, limiting the use of these sites for drug therapy (Blackburn, 2018, pp. 198; Domonoske, 2015, p. 221).
  - Gestational age and health status of the neonate may result in delayed or erratic absorption from the muscle (Blackburn, 2018, pp. 198).

ORAL ADMINISTRATION

- Oral drug absorption is dependent on gastric emptying time, gastric pH, intestinal enzyme activity, intestinal bacteria colonization, hepatic metabolism, and enterohepatic recirculation, which are altered in the preterm and ill neonate (Allegaert et al., 2018, p. 420; Blackburn, 2018, pp. 197–198; Domonoske, 2015, pp. 219–220).
  - Oral drug absorption is altered in the neonate due to decreased bile salts and pancreatic enzymes, slower gut transit time, delayed gastric emptying and motility, mucus in the stomach, gastric and duodenal pH differences, high levels of beta-glucuronidase, gut metabolic enzymes and drug transporters, intestinal flora, and intestinal surface area (Blackburn, 2018, p. 197).
  - Oral drug absorption matures by 4 to 5 months of life (Blackburn, 2018, p. 197).

OTHER ADMINISTRATION ROUTES

- Buccal, lingual, rectal, and topical administration are associated with variable absorption (Allegaert et al., 2018, p. 420).
  - Rectal absorption may be greater in neonates due to the well-vascularized rectum (Blackburn, 2018, p. 198).
  - Neonates have increased skin permeability and surface area to body weight, resulting in increased risk for toxic reactions from topically applied substances (Blackburn, 2018, p. 198).

Dosage/Interval

- Dosing and interval regimens are determined based on individual drug pharmacokinetic and pharmacodynamic properties. TDM assumes that total plasma drug concentrations correlate with drug dose and with circulating unbound drug concentrations and unbound drug concentration at the site of action (Allegaert et al., 2018, p. 425).
  - TDM: laboratory measurements of a drug's serum level that may directly influence the prescriber's dosing choice. Useful when (a) there is a high correlation between therapeutic effect and serum level rather than dose, (b) the drug has a narrow therapeutic range, and (c) maintaining the drug level within the range reduces toxicity and improves efficacy, thereby improving outcomes (Allegaert et al., 2018, p. 425; Domonoske, 2015, pp. 216–217).
    - Therapeutic range: the drug concentration range that is highly efficacious with a low risk of toxicity in most patients (Domonoske, 2015, pp. 216–217).
    - Patient response is the ultimate goal of therapy, not whether the drug level is in a specified range (Allegaert et al., 2018, p. 425).
  - Dose and interval determinations and changes in the neonate must take into consideration the following:
    - Drug metabolism is reduced in the neonate and improves over time as enzyme systems mature (Allegaert et al., 2018, pp. 420–421; McClary, 2015b, pp. 655–657; Wade, 2015, pp. 666–668).
    - Clearance of drugs is reduced in neonates and improves as renal function improves (Allegaert et al., 2018, p. 421; Wade, 2015, p. 667).
    - Volume of distribution is higher in neonates due to fluid shifts that change over the first week of life (Allegaert et al., 2018, p. 420; Wade, 2015, p. 666).
    - Half-life of drugs is prolonged in the neonate and increases as drug metabolic processes mature during the first month to year of life (McClary, 2015b, p. 657).
    - Dosages and intervals must be individualized in the neonate based on therapeutic response and monitoring of selected plasma drug concentrations (McClary, 2015b, pp. 655–657).

Withdrawal

- Drug dependence is the physiologic condition whereby the neonate requires regular drug administration for physiologic well-being (Domonoske, 2015, p. 230). Abrupt discontinuation of a drug on which a neonate or infant has developed dependence may result in withdrawal symptoms (Domonoske, 2015, p. 230).
  - Drug withdrawal in the neonate is primarily related to antenatal fetal exposure to drugs or secondarily to long-term opioid treatment during the infant's hospitalization; however, other drugs may result in withdrawal-type signs and symptoms (Hudak, 2015, p. 683).
  - Among the maternal effects of opioid use that may affect the fetus are premature rupture of membranes and preterm birth, fetal death, and low birth weight (Hudak, 2015, p. 683; Wallen & Gleason, 2018, p. 126).
    - Fetal effects of maternal opioid use may include exposure to infectious agents and fluctuating opioid concentrations resulting in intermittent withdrawal in utero (Hudak, 2015, pp. 683–685).
    - Neonatal withdrawal occurs in 55% to 94% of neonates with antenatal exposure to opioids (Hudak, 2015, p. 685).
    - The onset of signs of withdrawal are variable depending on the opioid used by the mother, type of opioid used, and the gestational age of the infant (Hudak, 2015, p. 686).
  - Infants who develop dependence may benefit from a tapered-dose regime when discontinuing a drug in order to prevent withdrawal symptoms (Domonoske, 2015, p. 230).
- Other drugs associated with signs of drug withdrawal that are not necessarily the same as opioid signs include nicotine, marijuana, benzodiazepines, cocaine, methamphetamine, and selective serotonin reuptake inhibitors (SSRIs); however, the neonatal signs seen in neonates whose mothers took SSRIs is believed to be due to the hyper-serotonergic state resolving rather than drug withdrawal (Hudak, 2015, p. 690; Wallen & Gleason, 2018, p. 128, 131–137).

Tolerance and Weaning

- Tolerance is the diminished response to a drug during a course of drug therapy, usually occurring over a long-term course; therefore, higher drug doses may be needed to achieve the same therapeutic effect (Domonoske, 2015, pp. 218–230; Zastrow, 2018, p. 28).
- Tolerance develops due to receptor-drug interactions and the characteristic of the drug as either an agonist or antagonist when bound to receptor sites (Correia, 2018, pp. 70–71; Domonoske, 2015, pp. 218–230; Zastrow, 2018, pp. 21–25).
  - Receptors interact with a drug, initiating events leading to drug effects, with drug–receptor complexes determined by the number of receptors available, the affinity of the receptor for the drug, and the agonist or antagonist action of the drug–receptor complex (Zastrow, 2018, pp. 20–25).
  - Agonists are drugs that activate when bound with the receptor (Zastrow, 2018, pp. 21–23).
  - Antagonists are drugs that interfere with the receptor–agonist interaction (Zastrow, 2018, pp. 23–25).
- The full action of some drugs may occur even if some receptors are not complexed with drug (Zastrow, 2018, pp. 23–25).
- The persistence of drug effects post discontinuation of the drug, while not tolerance per se, may occur due to the slow metabolism of drug, or the slow dissolution of protein-drug complexes, or when drugs have a high volume of distribution due to lipophilic attributes and are slowly released to the central compartment after discontinuation (Allegaert et al., 2018, p. 427; McClary, 2015b, p. 657; Zastrow, 2018, p. 49).
- Downregulation of receptors at a rate faster than the genesis of new receptors may limit the strength and duration of drug effects, another type of tolerance (Trevor, 2018, p. 389; Zastrow, 2018, p. 38).
- Opioids are a class of drugs where infants may develop tolerance when the drug is used long term, and dose adjustments should be made for the desired effect (Allegaert et al., 2018, p. 427; Schumacher, Basbaum, & Naidu, 2018, pp. 559, 564–565; Wallen & Gleason, 2018, pp. 133–134).

DRUGS AND BREASTFEEDING

- Transfer of drugs into breast milk is determined by drug molecular weight, protein binding, lipid solubility, and ionization (Berlin, 2015, p. 42; McClary, 2015a, p. 660).
- The amount of drug excreted in breast milk is markedly less than the maternal dose (Berlin, 2015, p. 42; Blackburn, 2018, p. 209; McClary, 2015a, p. 660).
  - The relative infant dose (RID) is an estimate of the infant's drug exposure via breast milk and can be calculated using a known milk concentration compared to an infant therapeutic dose or the weight-adjusted maternal dose when an infant dose is not well established (Taketomo, Hodding, & Kraus, 2017, p. 2179).
  - When calculating the RID, the milk concentration is used to estimate the amount of drug ingested by the infant (Taketomo et al., 2017, p. 2179).
    - Estimated daily infant dose via breast milk (mg/kg/day) = drug concentration in breast milk (mg/mL) × volume of breast milk ingested (mL/kg/day; Taketomo et al., 2017, p. 2179).
    - The daily dose received by the infant is then compared to either the dose used therapeutically in infants or the weight-adjusted maternal dose (Taketomo et al., 2017, p. 2179).
  - Generally, an RID of 10% or less is considered acceptable, but individual drugs must be evaluated for infant effects (McClary, 2015a, pp. 660–661; Taketomo et al., 2017, p. 2179).
    - Other considerations include gestational and postnatal age of the infant, amount of milk ingested, properties of maternal medications, medical conditions of the infant, and medications the infant is receiving (Taketomo et al., 2017).
- Providing human milk and breastfeeding are rarely contraindicated due to maternal pharmacotherapy, as most drugs are considered safe with few exceptions (Berlin, 2015, p. 49; Blackburn, 2018, p. 209; McClary, 2015a, p. 660).
  - Drugs contraindicated during breastfeeding include drugs of abuse (heroin, cocaine, etc.), lithium, beta-blocking agents (atenolol, satalol), and amiodarone (Berlin, 2015, p. 49; McClary, 2015a, pp. 662–663).
  - Mothers in a methadone program are encouraged to breastfeed, as the RID is ~3% and may theoretically alleviate some withdrawal symptoms in the infant (McClary, 2015a, p. 663).
- Oral contraceptives may be used by breastfeeding mothers, but the recommendations include using the lowest dose possible and to begin taking oral contraceptives after breastfeeding has been well established in order to minimize lactation suppression (Berlin, 2013, pp. 49–50; Blackburn, 2018, p. 210; McClary, 2015a, p. 662).
- Monitoring infant growth, sleep, activity, and behavioral responses is recommended if the mother is taking medication for which there are infant concerns. Correlate infant signs with maternal drug ingestion (Berlin, 2013, p. 50; Blackburn, 2018, p. 211; McClary, 2015a, p. 663).

CONCLUSION

Drug therapy is one of the many responsibilities of the NNP. Safe drug prescribing depends on the NNP applying basic principles of pharmacokinetics and pharmacodynamics to the neonate and infant (Allegaert et al., 2018, p. 430). Pharmacokinetic parameters (Vd, half-life, Cl) may be used in developing individualized dosing and drug dose intervals to achieve desired drug exposure levels; however, more pharmacokinetic study in neonates is needed to ensure that effective dose and pharmacodynamic targets are achieved in the neonate and infant (Wade, 2015, p. 672).

Neonates and infants fed breast milk or those who are breastfeeding may be exposed to maternal drugs. Providing human milk and breastfeeding is rarely contraindicated due to maternal pharmacotherapy, as most drugs are considered safe with few exceptions (Berlin, 2015, p. 49; Blackburn, 2018, p. 209; McClary, 2015a, p. 660). The RID may be calculated if the neonate or infant is exposed to maternal medications via breast milk (Taketomo et al., 2017, p. 2179). Monitoring infant growth, sleep, activity, and behavioral responses is recommended if the mother is taking medication for which there are infant concerns (Berlin, 2013, p. 50; Blackburn, 2018, p. 211; McClary, 2015a, p. 663).

REVIEW QUESTIONS

1. The NNP is considering the dose and dose interval for gentamicin and recognizes that steady-state concentration is primarily dependent on a drug's:
   A. clearance
   B. half-life
   C. interval

2. First-order kinetics with regard to drug removal means that the amount of drug removed over time is:
   A. biphasic
   B. constant
   C. a percentage

3. A neonate is receiving caffeine and is reported to have tachycardia with a heart rate of 206 beats per minute during sleep. The NNP recognizes a possible etiology as altered metabolism of caffeine and understands that the:
   A. clearance of caffeine is impaired
   B. first-order kinetics have been met
   C. zero-order kinetics have been reached

4. When the NNP orders an oral medication, there is understanding that the amount of bioavailable drug for that infant will be affected by first-pass metabolism through the:
   A. kidney
   B. liver
   C. lung

5. The most erratic drug absorption in the neonate occurs with drugs given via the:
   A. intramuscular route
   B. intrarectal route
   C. intravenous route

REFERENCES

Allegaert, K., Ward, R. M., & Van Den Anker, J. N. (2018). Neonatal pharmacology. In C. A. Gleason & S. E. Juul (Eds.), *Avery's diseases of the newborn* (10th ed., pp. 419–431). Philadelphia, PA: Elsevier.

Berlin, C. M. (2013). Medications and the breastfeeding mother. In D. R. Mattison (Ed.), *Clinical pharmacology during pregnancy* (pp. 41–53). Waltham, MA: Elsevier.

Blackburn, S. T. (2018). Pharmacology and pharmacokinetics during the perinatal period. In S. T. Blackburn (Ed.), *Maternal, fetal, and neonatal physiology* (5th ed., pp. 180–214). Philadelphia, PA: Elsevier.

Domonoske, C. D. (2015). Pharmacology. In M. T. Verklan, M. Walden, NANN, & AACN (Eds.), *Core curriculum for neonatal intensive care nursing* (5th ed., pp. 216–234). Philadelphia, PA: Elsevier.

Herbert, M. F. (2013). Impact of pregnancy on maternal pharmacokinetics of medications. In D. R. Mattison (Ed.), *Clinical pharmacology during pregnancy* (pp. 17–39). Waltham, MA: Elsevier.

Holford, N. H. G. (2018). Pharmacokinetics and pharmacodynamics: Rational dosing and the time course of drug action. In B. G. Katzung (Ed.), *Basic and clinical pharmacology* (14th ed., pp. 41–55). New York, NY: McGraw-Hill Education.

Hudak, M. L. (2015). Infants with antenatal exposure to drugs. In R. J. Martin, A. A. Fanaroff, & M. C. Walsh (Eds.), *Fanaroff and Martin's neonatal perinatal medicine: Diseases of the fetus and infant* (10th ed., pp. 682–695). Philadelphia, PA: Elsevier.

Katzung, B. G. (2018). Introduction: The nature of drugs and drug development and regulation. In B. G. Katzung (Ed.), *Basic and clinical pharmacology* (13th ed., pp. 1–19). New York, NY: McGraw-Hill Education.

McClary, J. D. (2015a). Principles of drug use during lactation. In R. J. Martin, A. A. Fanaroff, & M. C. Walsh (Eds.), *Fanaroff and Martin's neonatal perinatal medicine: Diseases of the fetus and infant* (10th ed., pp. 660–664). Philadelphia, PA: Elsevier.

McClary, J. D. (2015b). Principles of drug use in the fetus and neonate. In R. J. Martin, A. A. Fanaroff, & M. C. Walsh (Eds.), *Fanaroff and Martin's neonatal perinatal medicine: Diseases of the fetus and infant* (10th ed., pp. 648–659). Philadelphia, PA: Elsevier.

Schumacher, M. A., Basbaum, A. I., & Naidu, R. K. (2018). Opioid agonists and antagonists. In B. G. Katzung (Ed.), *Basic and clinical pharmacology* (14th ed., pp. 553–574). New York, NY: McGraw-Hill Education.

Taketomo, C. K., Hodding, J. H., & Kraus, D. M. (2017). *Pediatric and neonatal dosage handbook* (24th ed.). Hudson, OH: Wolters Kluwer.

Trevor, A. J. (2018). Sedative-hypnotic drugs. In B. G. Katzung (Ed.), *Basic and clinical pharmacology* (14th ed., pp. 381–395). New York, NY: McGraw-Hill Education.

Wade, K. C. (2015). Pharmacokinetics in neonatal medicine. In R. J. Martin, A. A. Fanaroff, & M. C. Walsh (Eds.), *Fanaroff and Martin's neonatal perinatal medicine: Diseases of the fetus and infant* (10th ed., pp. 665–675). Philadelphia, PA: Elsevier.

Wallen, L. D., & Gleason, C. A. (2018). Prenatal drug exposure. In C. A. Gleason & S. E. Juul (Eds.), *Avery's diseases of the newborn* (10th ed., pp. 126–144). Philadelphia, PA: Elsevier.

Zastrow, M. V. (2018). Drug receptors and pharmacodynamics. In B. G. Katzung (Ed.), *Basic and clinical pharmacology* (14th ed., pp. 20–40). New York, NY: McGraw-Hill Education.

13 PHARMACOLOGY: COMMON DRUG THERAPIES

Shawn Sullivan

INTRODUCTION

This chapter serves to review medications routinely used in the care of the neonate. It is not intended to be an exhaustive list of all drug therapies and is not intended as an in-depth source on pharmacotherapeutics. Drug dosage and timing of onset and/or duration are not included as these will likely differ between institutions and neonates; the reader is directed to resources such as *Lexicomp Pediatric & Neonatal Dosage Handbook* or the *Red Book: 2018 Report of the Committee on Infectious Diseases* for dosing and therapeutic monitoring guidelines. The focus of this chapter is on understanding the mechanisms of action of drugs, available routes, and things to consider when ordering and/or managing an infant receiving the therapy.

ANALGESIA/NARCOTICS ANESTHETICS AGENTS

25% Sucrose Solution (Sweet-Ease)

- Use: Used to calm or soothe in times of stress and for short-term analgesia during minor procedures such as heel sticks, orogastric (OG)/nasogastric (NG) tube placement, and venipunctures.
- Mechanism of action: Exact mechanism is unknown; it has been proposed that sucrose induces endogenous opioid release.
- Route: Oral (PO)
- Considerations: Give 2 minutes prior to painful procedure; may be repeated. Place sucrose on tip of the tongue; this is where taste buds for sweet taste are located. May be more effective when used with nonnutritive sucking. *Not effective if given NG.* No long-term data are available. Some do not support use in extremely premature or critically ill infants.

Acetaminophen (Tylenol)

- Use: Analgesia, antipyretic
- Mechanism of action: Activation of descending serotonergic inhibitory pathways in the central nervous system (CNS)
- Clearance: Hepatic metabolism, renal excretion
- Route: PO, per rectum (PR), intravenous (IV)
- Considerations: Potentiates opioid therapy; is not effective alone for surgical pain. No effect on pain from heel sticks. Use with caution in hepatic failure; half-life may increase twofold or more. Do not use in infant with G6PD. Prophylactic administration prior to vaccination may decrease the immune response of some vaccines.

Ibuprofen (Motrin)

- Use: Antipyretic, mild analgesic; *not recommended for analgesia in infants <6 months of age.*
- Mechanism of action: Inhibits COX-1 and 2 enzymes, which results in decreased formation of prostaglandin precursors
- Clearance: Hepatic metabolism, renal excretion
- Route: PO, IV
- Considerations: If given IV, ensure infant is well hydrated. Use with caution in infants with hepatic and renal failure (Taketomo, Hodding, & Kraus, 2018, pp. 1034–1039).

Fentanyl (duragesic)

- Use: Relief of pain; preoperative medication; adjunct to general or regional anesthesia; has also been used for sedation and intranasally for analgesia
- Mechanism of action: Binds with stereospecific receptors at many sites within CNS, increases pain threshold, alters pain reception, inhibits ascending pathways. Is highly lipophilic, redistributed into muscle and fat
- Clearance: Hepatic metabolism
- Route: IV or subcutaneous (Sub-Q)
- Considerations:
  - Give intermittent IV doses slowly; rapid infusion may cause chest wall rigidity.
  - Monitor for CNS and respiratory depression, hypotension, decreased gastric/intestinal motility, urinary retention.
  - Renal and/or hepatic dysfunction may alter kinetics.

Morphine (Duramorph)

- Use: Management of moderate-to-severe acute and chronic pain, neonatal abstinence and iatrogenic drug withdrawal, and palliative care management of dyspnea
- Mechanism of action: Binds to opioid receptors in CNS, causing inhibition of ascending pain pathways, altering the perception of and response to pain
- Clearance: Hepatic metabolism, renal and fecal excretion
- Route: PO, intramuscular (IM), IV, Sub-Q
- Considerations: Monitor for CNS and respiratory depression, hypotension, decreased gastric/intestinal motility,

urinary retention, risk for necrotizing enterocolitis (NEC), increased intracranial pressure (ICP). Slower onset but longer duration than fentanyl. IV is the preferred route. Oral doses are half as effective as parenteral dose. Start with lower dose in the opioid-naive infant; infant with previous or prolonged exposure may need higher dosing.

○ For discussion regarding morphine use in the treatment of neonatal abstinence syndrome (NAS), please see Chapter 26, on Intrauterine Drug Exposure.

Opioid Agonists

NALOXONE (NARCAN)

- Use: Complete or partial reversal of opioid drug effects
- Mechanism of action: Pure opioid antagonist that competes and displaces opioids at opioid receptor sites
- Clearance: Hepatic metabolism, renal excretion
- Route: IM, IV, endotracheal tube (ET), Sub-Q
- Considerations: Because naloxone's duration is shorter than most opioids, repeat dosing may be necessary. Not recommended as part of initial resuscitative measures in the delivery room for neonates with respiratory depression; support ventilation to improve oxygenation and heart rate.

General Anesthesia

PROPOFOL (DIPRIVAN)

- Use: Induction and maintenance of general anesthesia.
- Mechanism of action: Short-acting lipophilic IV anesthetic. Causes global CNS depression.
- Clearance: Hepatic metabolism, renal and fecal excretion
- Route: IV
- Considerations: May cause hypotension to monitor blood pressure; ensure cardiac/respiratory and oxygen saturation monitoring.

KETAMINE (KETTLER)

- Use: Preanesthetic sedation, induction, and maintenance of anesthesia
- Mechanism of action: Produces a cataleptic-like state in which the patient is dissociated from the surrounding environment by direct action on the cortex and the limbic system. Low doses produce analgesia and modulate central sensitization, hyperalgesia, and opioid tolerance. Reduces polysynaptic spinal reflexes.
- Clearance: Hepatic metabolism, renal excretion
- Route: IV, IM
- Considerations: Risk of airway obstruction, laryngospasm, and apnea. Monitor cardiovascular effects, heart rate, blood pressure, respiratory rate, oxygen saturation.

Topical/Local Anesthetics

LIDOCAINE-PRILOCAINE (EMLA)

- Use: Topical anesthetic for intact skin to provide minor analgesia for minor procedures
- Mechanism of action: Stabilization of neuronal membranes and inhibiting ionic fluxes required for the initiation and conduction of neuronal impulses.
- Route: Topical
- Considerations: Maximum application time 1 hour

ANTIBACTERIAL DRUGS

Agents That Target Bacterial Cell Wall Synthesis

BETA-LACTAM COMPOUNDS – PENICILLINS

- Uses: Treatment of infections caused by susceptible organisms; active against some gram-positive organisms, some gram-negative organisms such as *Neisseria gonorrhoeae*, and some anaerobes and spirochetes
- Mechanism of action: Penicillins, like all β-lactam antibiotics, inhibit bacterial growth by interfering with the transpeptidation reaction of bacterial cell wall synthesis. The exact mechanism of cell death is not completely understood, but autolysins are involved in addition to the disruption of cross-linking of the cell wall (Deck & Winston, 2015a, p. 771).
- Clearance: Excreted mostly unchanged by kidneys
  ○ Natural penicillins—penicillin G (Pfizerpen)
    ▪ These have the greatest activity against Gram-positive organisms, Gram-negative cocci, and non-β-lactamase-producing anaerobes
  ○ Penicillinase-resistant penicillins—methicillin, nafcillin (Nallpen), oxacillin (Bactocill)
    ▪ These penicillins are resistant to staphylococcal β-lactamases. They are active against staphylococci and streptococci spp.
  ○ Aminopenicillins—ampicillin (generic), amoxicillin (Amoxil)
  ○ β-lactam-β-lactamase inhibitor combinations—amoxicillin–clavulanic acid (Augmentin), ampicillin–sulbactam (Unasyn), and piperacillin–tazobactam (Zosyn)
    ▪ These drugs retain the antibacterial spectrum of penicillin and have improved activity against Gram-negative rods (Deck & Winston, 2015a, pp. 774–775).

BETA-LACTAM COMPOUNDS—CEPHALOSPORINS

- Uses: Cephalosporins are used parenterally for the treatment of lower respiratory tract, skin, and skin structure, urinary tract, and bone and joint infections caused by susceptible Gram-positive or Gram-negative bacteria, and also are used parenterally for the treatment of meningitis and septicemia/bacteremia caused by susceptible Gram-positive or Gram-negative bacteria.
- Mechanism of action: Cephalosporins are like penicillin but are more stable to many bacterial β-lactamases and, therefore, have a broader spectrum of activity.
- Clearance: Excreted mostly unchanged by kidneys
- First generation: First-generation cephalosporins are very active against Gram-positive cocci, such as streptococci and staphylococci. *Escherichia coli*, *Klebsiella pneumoniae*, and *Proteus mirabilis* are often sensitive to first-generation cephalosporins.
  ○ Cefazolin (Ancef)
  ○ Cephalexin (Keflex; Deck & Winston, 2015a, p. 776)
- Second generation: Second-generation cephalosporins are relatively active against organisms inhibited by first-generation drugs, but in addition they have extended Gram-negative coverage. *Klebsiella* spp. (including those resistant to first-generation cephalosporins) are usually sensitive. As with first-generation agents, no member of this group is active against enterococci or *Pseudomonas aeruginosa*.
  ○ Cefoxitin (generic)
  ○ Cefuroxime (Ceftin)

- Third generation: Compared with second-generation agents, third-generation cephalosporins have expanded Gram-negative coverage, and some are able to cross the blood–brain barrier. Third-generation drugs may be active against *Citrobacter, Serratia marcescens*, and *Providencia* and against β-lactamase-producing strains of *Haemophilus* and *Neisseria*.
  - Cefotaxime (Claforan)
  - Ceftazidime (Fortaz)
  - Ceftriaxone (Rocephin)
- Fourth generation: Fourth-generation cephalosporins are more resistant to hydrolysis by chromosomal β-lactamases (e.g., those produced by Enterobacter). However, like the third-generation compounds, it is hydrolyzed by extended spectrum β-lactamases. Cefepime has good activity against *P. aeruginosa*, Enterobacteriaceae, methicillin-susceptible *Staphylococcus aureus*, and *Streptococcus pneumoniae*. It is highly active against *Haemophilus* and *Neisseria sp*. It penetrates well into cerebrospinal fluid.
  - Cefepime (Maxipime)
- Fifth generation: Beta-lactam antibiotics with activity against methicillin-resistant staphylococci are currently under development. Ceftaroline is the first such drug to be approved for clinical use in the United States. Ceftaroline has increased binding to penicillin-binding protein 2a, which mediates methicillin resistance in *staphylococci*, resulting in bactericidal activity against these strains.
  - Ceftaroline fosamil (Teflaro; Deck & Winston, 2015a, pp. 778–779)

BETA-LACTAM COMPOUNDS—CARBAPENEMS
- Mechanism of action: The carbapenems are structurally related to other β-lactam antibiotics and have a wide spectrum with good activity against most Gram-negative rods, including *P. aeruginosa*, Gram-positive organisms, and anaerobes. Carbapenems penetrate body tissues and fluids well, including the cerebrospinal fluid.
- Clearance: Hepatic metabolism, renal excretion
  - Imipenem (Primaxin)
  - Meropenem (Merrem; Deck & Winston, 2015a, p. 781)

GLYCOPEPTIDES
- Mechanism of action: Inhibits cell-wall synthesis by binding firmly to the end of a developing peptidoglycan cell-wall matrix. This inhibits the transglycosylase, preventing further elongation of peptidoglycan and cross-linking. The peptidoglycan is thus weakened, and the cell becomes susceptible to lysis. The cell membrane is also damaged, which contributes to the antibacterial effect.
- Clearance: No apparent metabolism; renal excretion primarily through glomerular filtration
  - Vancomycin (Vancocin)

Agents That Target Protein Synthesis

AMINOGLYCOSIDES
- Aminoglycosides exhibit concentration-dependent killing; that is, higher concentrations kill a larger proportion of bacteria and kill at a more rapid rate. They also have a significant post-antibiotic effect, such that the antibacterial activity persists beyond the time during which the drug is measurable. When administered with a cell-wall active antibiotic (a β-lactam or vancomycin), aminoglycosides may exhibit synergistic killing against certain bacteria (Deck & Winston, 2015b, p. 801).

- Mechanism of action: Aminoglycosides are irreversible inhibitors of protein synthesis, but the precise mechanism for bactericidal activity is unclear. Protein synthesis is inhibited by aminoglycosides in at least three ways: (1) interference with the initiation complex of peptide formation; (2) misreading of mRNA, which causes incorporation of incorrect amino acids into the peptide and results in a nonfunctional protein; and (3) breakup of polysomes into nonfunctional monosomes (Deck & Winston, 2015b, pp. 799–800).
- Clearance: Mostly unchanged renal excretion
  - Amikacin (Amikin)
    - Is slightly more active against *P. aeruginosa; Enterococcus faecalis* is susceptible to both gentamicin and tobramycin, but *E. faecium* is resistant to tobramycin. Gentamicin and tobramycin are otherwise interchangeable clinically (Deck & Winston, 2015b, p. 804).
  - Gentamicin (Garamycin)
    - It is effective against both Gram-positive and Gram-negative organisms, and many of its properties resemble those of other aminoglycosides (Deck & Winston, 2015b, p. 803).
  - Neomycin (Mycitracin)
    - Drugs of the neomycin group are active against Gram-positive and Gram-negative bacteria and some mycobacteria (Deck & Winston, 2015b, p. 804).
  - Tobramycin (Tobradex)
    - Tobramycin has almost the same antibacterial spectrum as gentamicin with a few exceptions. Gentamicin is slightly more active against *S. marcescens*

MACROLIDES
- The macrolides are a group of closely related compounds characterized by a macrocyclic lactone ring to which deoxy sugars are attached. The antibacterial action of macrolides may be inhibitory or bactericidal. Inhibition of protein synthesis occurs via binding to ribosomal RNA, and peptide chain elongation is prevented. As a result, peptidyl-tRNA is dissociated from the ribosome (Deck & Winston, 2015c, p. 792).
- Clearance: Hepatic metabolism, excretion through feces
  - Erythromycin (Erythrocin)
    - Erythromycin is active against susceptible strains of Gram-positive organisms, especially pneumococci, streptococci, staphylococci, and corynebacteria. Gram-negative organisms such as *Neisseria* sp, *Treponema Pallidum*, and *Campylobacter* species are susceptible.
  - Azithromycin (Zithromax)
    - It is resistant to many enzymes that inactivate gentamicin and tobramycin and, therefore, can be used against some microorganisms resistant to the latter drugs. Many Gram-negative bacteria, including many strains of *Proteus, Pseudomonas, Enterobacter,* and *Serratia,* are inhibited by amikacin (Deck & Winston, 2015b, p. 804).
- Miscellaneous class
  - Clindamycin (Cleocin)
    - Is a chlorine-substituted derivative of lincomycin. Clindamycin is very similar to erythromycin, as it inhibits protein synthesis by interfering with the formation of initiation complexes with aminoacyl translocation reactions. The binding site is identical with that for erythromycin.

- *Bacteroides* spp and other anaerobes, both Gram positive and Gram negative, are usually susceptible. *Enterococci* and gram-negative aerobic organism are generally resistant (Deck Winston, 2015c, p. 794).

Agents That Target Nucleic Acid

FLUOROQUINOLONES

- Quinolones block bacterial DNA synthesis and prevent the relaxation of positively supercoiled DNA required for normal transcription and replication.
- Clearance: Mostly hepatic metabolism, excreted mostly unchanged in both urine and feces
  - Ciprofloxacin (Cipro) and levofloxacin (Levaquin) possesses excellent Gram-negative activity and moderate-to-good activity against Gram-positive bacteria.
  - Moxifloxacin (Avelox) has improved activity against Gram-positive organisms, particularly *S. pneumoniae* and some staphylococci.

SULFONAMIDES

- Sulfonamides with varying physical, chemical, pharmacologic, and antibacterial properties are produced by attaching substituents to the amino group of the sulfanilamide.
- Sulfonamides inhibit both Gram-positive bacteria, such as Staphylococcus sp and Gram-negative enteric bacteria such as *E. coli, K. pneumoniae, Salmonella, Shigella*, and *Enterobacter* sp, as well as *Nocardia* sp, *Chlamydia trachomatis*, and some protozoa.
- Clearance: Metabolized via colonic flora, excreted primarily in urine
  - Trimethoprim–sulfamethoxazole (Bactrim)
    - TMP-SMZ is active against most *S. aureus* strains, both methicillin-susceptible and methicillin-resistant, and against respiratory tract pathogens such as *Haemophilus* sp, *Moraxella catarrhalis*, and *K pneumoniae* (Beauduy & Winston, 2015, pp. 810–812).

Miscellaneous Agents

METRONIDAZOLE

- Indicated for treatment of anaerobic or mixed intra-abdominal infections (in combination with other agents with activity against aerobic organisms), *Clostridium difficile* infection, and brain abscess.
- Metronidazole is selectively absorbed by anaerobic bacteria and sensitive protozoa. Once taken up, it is nonenzymatically reduced by reacting with reduced ferredoxin. This reduction results in products that accumulate in and are toxic to anaerobic cells.
- Clearance: Heptic metabolism, urine, and fecal excretion (Deck & Winston, 2015d, p. 865)

ANTIFUNGAL AGENTS

Amphotericin B (Fungizone)

- Use: Treatment of progressive, potentially life-threatening susceptible fungal infections; owing to its broad spectrum of activity and fungicidal action, amphotericin B remains a useful agent for nearly all life-threatening mycotic infections.
- Mechanism of action: Exploits the difference in lipid composition of fungal and mammalian cell membranes (ergosterol is found in the cell membrane of fungi, whereas the predominant sterol of bacteria and human cells is cholesterol). Amphotericin B alters the cell membrane permeability in susceptible fungi, causing leakage of cell components and resultant cell death. Some binding to human membrane sterols does occur, probably accounting for the drug's prominent toxicity.
- Clearance: Renal excretion, eliminated over 7 days, and may be detected in urine for up to 7 weeks after being discontinued.
- Route: IV
- Considerations:
  - Therapy with amphotericin B is often limited by toxicity, especially drug-induced renal impairment. Monitor renal function frequently during therapy.
  - Monitor liver function tests; abnormalities are occasionally seen, as is a varying degree of anemia due to reduced erythropoietin production by damaged renal tubular cells.

Amphotericin B (liposomal formulation) (AmBisome)

- Use: Treatment of systemic fungal infection
- Mechanism of action: Alters cell membrane permeability in susceptible fungi, causing leakage of cell components resulting in cell death
- Clearance: Exhibits nonlinear kinetics, excreted through kidneys over 24 hours
- Route: IV
- Considerations: *Not preferred in neonates due to poor penetration into the CNS, kidney, urinary tract and eye.* Monitor blood urea nitrogen (BUN), serum creatinine liver function tests, serum electrolytes—especially potassium and magnesium, I/O, monitor for s/s hypokalemia.

Fluconazole (Diflucan)

- Use: Treatment of suspected or proven candidiasis
- Mechanism of action: Interferes with fungal cytochrome P450 activity, decreasing ergosterol synthesis and inhibiting cell-wall synthesis.
- Clearance: Excreted mostly unchanged in urine
- Route: PO, IV
- Considerations: Monitor liver and renal function, serum potassium, complete blood count (CBC) with differential and platelet count. Should not be used until speciation has been completed because *Candida krusei* and *Candida glabrata* are resistant.

Miconazole (Lotrimin)

- Use: Treatment of superficial cutaneous infections with *Candida albicans*
- Mechanism of action: Inhibits biosynthesis of ergosterol damaging the fungal cell-wall membrane, which increases permeability causing leakage of nutrients.
- Route: Topical cream, ointment, powder
- Considerations: Monitor for worsening symptoms

Nystatin (Bio-Statin [Oral]/Nyamyc [Topical])

- Use: Treatment of cutaneous and mucocutaneous fungal infections caused by susceptible *Candida* species
- Mechanism of action: Binds to sterols in fungal cell membrane, changing the cell-wall permeability, allowing for leakage of cellular contents.
- Route: PO, Topical, cream, ointment
- Considerations: The oral suspension should be retained in the mouth for as long as possible. Paint nystatin into the recesses of the mouth and avoid feeding for 5 to 10 minutes.

ANTIVIRAL AGENTS

Acyclovir (Zovirax)

- Use: Treatment and prophylaxis of herpes simplex virus (HSV-1, HSV-2) infections, herpes simplex encephalitis, herpes zoster infection, and varicella–zoster infections
- Mechanism of action: A competitive inhibitor of HSV DNA polymerase and terminates DNA chain elongation. Because it requires certain conditions for activation, the active metabolite accumulates only in infected cells.
- Clearance: Glomerular filtration and tubular secretion
- Route: PO, IV
- Considerations: Monitor urinalysis, BUN, serum creatinine, CBC, liver function, neuro and nephrotoxicity, and neutrophil count twice weekly.

Ganciclovir (Cytovene)

- Use: Treatment of congenital cytomegalovirus; activity is up to 100 times greater than that of acyclovir.
- Mechanism of action: The activated compound inhibits viral DNA polymerase and causes termination of viral DNA elongation.
- Clearance: Renal excretion is linearly related to creatinine clearance.
- Route: IV
- Considerations:
  ○ Neutropenia, anemia, thrombocytopenia, and pancytopenia may occur. Monitor CBC with differential and platelet count, urine output (UOP), serum creatinine, ophthalmologic exams, liver enzymes, B/P urinalysis.
  ○ Treatment with ganciclovir is improving neurologic outcomes; however, there is potential for future reproductive system effects.

Valganciclovir (Valcyte)

- Use: Long-term treatment of CMV with the goal of reduced hearing loss and developmental delay. Chronic suppression therapy has reduced transmission rates. Also effective in preventing CMV infection following transplantation.
- Mechanism of action: Rapidly converts to ganciclovir in the body and inhibits viral DNA synthesis.
- Clearance: Metabolized by intestinal mucosal cells and excreted through kidneys
- Route: PO
- Considerations: Monitor CBC with differential and platelet count, serum creatinine at baseline, and periodically during therapy. Also used for the prevention of CMV disease in high-risk patients undergoing heart transplant 1 month of age and greater: Begin within

10 days of transplant; continue therapy until 100 days posttransplant.

Zidovudine (Retrovir; AZT)

- Use: Decrease the rate of clinical disease progression and prolong survival in HIV-infected individuals. Use during pregnancy shows significant reductions in the rate of vertical transmission.
- Mechanism of action: Interferes with the HIV viral RNA-dependent DNA polymerase, resulting in inhibition of viral replication
- Clearance: Renal excretion
- Route: PO, IV
- Considerations:
  ○ Routinely monitor CD cell counts for status of immune status.
  ○ Concurrent use of phenytoin, methadone may result in elevated zidovudine levels. In contrast, the use of zidovudine may decrease phenytoin levels.
  ○ Hazardous drug—use appropriate precautions for receiving, handling, administration, and disposal. Gloves should be worn during any handling (Baley & Leonard, 2013, p. 359; Safrin, 2015, pp. 836, 839, 840, 849; Taketomo et al., 2018, pp. 53, 939, 2024, 2083–2084).

CARDIOVASCULAR DRUGS

Antiarrhymic Drugs

ADENOSINE (ADENOCARD)
- Use: Treatment of supraventricular tachycardia
- Mechanism of action: Slows conduction time through the atrioventricular (AV) node, interrupting the reentry pathway through the AV node restoring normal sinus rhythm.
- Clearance: Removed from circulation by vascular endothelial cells and erythrocytes, metabolized intracellularly, excreted by kidneys
- Route: Rapid IV
- Considerations: EKG monitoring required during use. Equipment for resuscitation and trained personnel should be immediately available. Adenosine decreases conduction through AV node and may produce first-, second-, and third-degree heart block.

AMIODARONE (CORDARONE)
- Use: Management of ventricular arrhythmias
- Mechanism of action: Inhibits adrenergic stimulation; effects sodium, potassium, and calcium channels; and prolongs the action potential and refractory period in myocardial tissue, decreases AV conduction and sinus node function.
- Clearance: Hepatic metabolism, excreted in urine and feces
- Route: PO, IV
- Considerations: Monitor cardiac and respiratory status, thyroid function, electrolytes, serum glucose.

FLECAINIDE (TAMBOCOR)
- Use: Prevention and treatment of ventricular arrhythmia, prevention of supraventricular tachycardia
- Mechanism of action: Slows conduction of electrical impulses within the heart
- Clearance: Excreted primarily as unchanged drug in urine
- Route: PO

- Considerations: EKG, heart rate, blood pressure, periodic serum concentrations after fifth dose and after dose changes. Therapeutic trough 0.2 to 1 mcg/mL

LIDOCAINE (XYLOCAINE)
- Use: Treatment of ventricular arrhythmias
- Mechanism of action: Suppresses automaticity of conduction tissue by increasing electrical stimulation threshold of ventricle, blocks both the initiation and conduction of nerve impulses by decreasing the neuronal membrane's permeability to sodium ions.
- Clearance: Hepatic metabolism, renal excretion
- Route: IV, IO, ET
- Considerations: Continuous EKG monitoring. Monitor serum concentrations with continuous infusions. Do not exceed 20 mcg/kg/min in patients with shock, hepatic disease cardiac arrest, or congestive heart failure (CHF).

MEXILETINE (MEXITIL)
- Use: Management of life-threatening ventricular arrhythmias
- Mechanism of action: Class 1B antiarrhythmic, structurally related to lidocaine, which inhibits inward sodium current, decreases rate of rise of phase 0, increases effective refractory period/action potential duration ratio.
- Clearance: Hepatic metabolism, renal excretion altered by urinary acidification or alkalinization
- Route: PO
- Considerations: Monitor serum concentrations, liver enzymes, CBC, EKG, heart rate.

ANTIHYPERTENSIVE DRUGS

α or β Receptor Antagonist

LABETALOL (TRANDATE)
- Use: PO—treatment of hypertension alone or in combination particularly with thiazide or loop diuretics IV—treatment of severe hypertension
- Mechanism of action: Limited use in neonates. These drugs have both beta-blocking and vasodilating effects. Blood pressure is lowered by reduction of systemic vascular resistance.
- Clearance: Hepatic metabolism, renal excretion
- Route: PO, IV
- Dose: PO 0.5 to 1 mg/kg/dose, maximum 10 mg/kg/day, IV 0.2 to 1 mg/kg/dose: 0.25 to 3 mg/kg/hour
- Onset/duration: PO 20 minutes to 1 hour, IV within 5 minutes. Duration is dose-dependent; PO 8 to 12 hours, IV 16 to 18 hours.
- Considerations: Contraindicated in heart failure and borderline personality disorder (BPD). Monitor blood pressure, heart rate, EKG. When monitoring IV dosing, monitor for length of infusion and for several hours after infusion is stopped due to prolonged duration of action.

Angiotensin-Converting Enzyme (ACE) Inhibitors

CAPTOPRIL (CAPOTEN)
- Use: Treatment of hypertension, CHF, reduction of after load
- Mechanism of action: Angiotensin-converting enzyme inhibitors block the production of angiotensin II, leading to a decrease in release of aldosterone and norepinephrine. ACE inhibitors also increase the production of bradykinin. The result is a decrease in peripheral vascular resistance.
- Clearance: Cleared >95% unchanged via renal system
- Route: PO
- Considerations: Monitor for hypotension; some experience significant drop in blood pressure, start with lower dosing; may cause oliguria, hyperkalemia, and renal failure; monitor BUN, serum creatinine, serum potassium, CBC with differential; try to give on empty stomach; food decreases absorption.

ENALAPRIL (VASOTEC)
- Use: Management of hypertension, symptomatic heart failure, and symptomatic left ventricular dysfunction
- Mechanism of action: Angiotensin-converting enzyme inhibitors block the production of angiotensin II, leading to a decrease in release of aldosterone and norepinephrine. ACE inhibitors also increase the production of bradykinin. The result is a decrease in peripheral vascular resistance.
- Clearance: Hepatic metabolism, renal excretion; renal dysfunction will increase peak and trough levels.
- Route: PO; IV form used primarily for hypertensive crisis
- Considerations: May cause prolonged hypotension. Use lower initial dose in patients with hyponatremia, hypovolemia, severe CHF, decreased renal function, or in those receiving diuretics. May cause oliguria, hyperkalemia, renal failure. May cause dry, hacking cough. Monitor blood pressure, renal function, white blood cell (WBC), serum potassium, and serum glucose. Monitor for angioedema and anaphylactoid reaction.

α-Receptor Antagonist

PROPRANOLOL (INDERAL)
- Use: Management of hypertension, supraventricular arrhythmias, tetralogy of Fallot cyanotic spells
- Mechanism of action: Decreases hypertension primarily by decreasing cardiac output. Inhibits the stimulation of renin production by catecholamines.
- Clearance: Hepatic metabolism, metabolites excreted in urine
- Route: PO, IV
- Considerations: PO route—monitor heart rate/blood pressure; a resting bradycardia may indicate need or dose change. IV route—monitor EKG, blood pressure, heart rate.

Calcium-Channel Blockers

AMLODIPINE (NORVASC)
- Use: Treatment of hypertension
- Mechanism of action: Decreases peripheral resistance and blood pressure by the inhibiting calcium influx into arterial smooth muscle cells
- Clearance: Hepatic (dysfunction will slow metabolism), renal excretion
- Route: PO
- Considerations: May cause an increase in heart rate within 10 hours of administration secondary to vasodilating

activity. Monitor blood pressure, heart rate, and liver function.

NICARDIPINE (CARDENE)
- Use: Short-term treatment of hypertension when PO not feasible
- Mechanism of action: Decreases peripheral resistance and blood pressure by inhibiting calcium influx into arterial smooth muscle cells.
- Clearance: Hepatic metabolism, renal excretion. Will be altered with hepatic and/or renal dysfunction.
- Route: IV—continuous infusion
- Considerations: Blood pressure, heart rate, hepatic, and renal function. Monitor blood pressure carefully with the initiation of therapy and dose changes.

NIFEDIPINE (PROCARDIA)
- Use: Severe hypertension
- Mechanism of action: Calcium channel blocker
- Clearance: Hepatic metabolism, renal excretion
- Route: PO, sublingual
- Considerations: *Current pediatric blood pressure guidelines do not recommend use because other safe and effective alternatives are available.* Monitor blood pressure, CBC, platelets, periodic liver enzymes, heart rate, s/s of CHF, and peripheral edema.

Vasodilators

DIAZOXIDE (PROGLYCEM)
- Use: Management of hypoglycemia related to hyperinsulinemia
- Mechanism of action: Opens ATP-dependent potassium channels on pancreatic beta cells in the presence of ATP and Mg, resulting in hyperpolarization of the cell and inhibition of insulin release.
- Clearance: Urine excretion
- Route: PO
- Considerations: Use the least amount of drug that produces the desired effect. Monitor blood glucose, serum uric acid, electrolytes, BUN, renal function, aspartate aminotransferase (AST), CBC with differential and platelets, urine glucose and ketones, blood pressure, and heart rate.

HYDRALAZINE (APRESOLINE)
- Use: PO—treatment of essential hypertension. IV—management of severe hypertension when oral therapy is not possible or when urgent reduction in blood pressure is necessary.
- Mechanism of action: Vasodilator relaxes smooth muscle of arterioles, decreasing systemic vascular resistance
- Clearance: Hepatic metabolism, renal excretion
- Route: PO, IV
- Considerations: May cause tachycardia. Give PO with food. Monitor blood pressure and heart rate.

SODIUM NITROPRUSSIDE (NIPRIDE)
- Use: Management of hypertensive crisis
- Mechanism of action: Dilates both arterial and venous vessels. Reduces preload and afterload
- Clearance: Nitroprusside combines with hemoglobin to produce metabolites, renal excretion
- Route: IV continuous infusion

- Considerations: Heart rate and blood pressure, renal and hepatic function, measure cyanide and thiocyanate blood levels.

Management of Congestive Heart Failure

DIGOXIN (LANOXIN)
- Use: Treatment of mild-to-moderate heart failure, to slow ventricular rate in supraventricular tachyarrhythmias
- Mechanism of action: Inhibition of sodium/potassium pump in myocardial cells, results in increase in intracellular sodium, which promotes calcium influx via the sodium–calcium exchange pump, leading to increased contractility.
- Clearance: Metabolism via sugar hydrolysis in the stomach or by reduction by intestinal bacteria, renal excretion
- Route: PO, IV
- Considerations: Narrow therapeutic window. Dosage must be individualized. Consider renal function. When transitioning from IV to oral, decrease dose by 20% to 25%. Monitor heart rate and rhythm, periodic EKG, electrolytes, renal function; sinus bradycardia is a sign of toxicity. Trough concentrations should be followed 3 to 5 days after start of therapy and after dose changes. Therapeutic levels 0.5 to 2 ng/mL

Management of Patent Ductus Arteriosus (PDA)

IBUPROFEN (NEOPROFEN)
- Use: PDA closure
- Mechanism of action: Inhibits COX-1 and 2 enzymes, which results in decreased formation of prostaglandin precursors.
- Clearance: Hepatic metabolism, renal excretion
- Route: PO, IV
- Considerations: Monitor vital signs, CBC, serum electrolytes, BUN, Cr, glucose, bilirubin, calcium, monitor for bleeding, heart murmur, echocardiogram.

INDOMETHACIN (INDOCIN)
- Use: Closure of hemodynamically significant PDA, prophylaxis of PDA, and prevention of intraventricular hemorrhage
- Mechanism of action: Inhibits COX-1 and 2 enzymes, which results in decreased formation of prostaglandin precursors.
- Clearance: Hepatic metabolism, renal excretion
- Route: IV
- Considerations: In general, may give at 12-hour intervals if UOP is ≥1 mL/kg/hr after first dose; use 24-hour interval if <1 mL/kg/hr after first dose. *Dose should be held if UOP <0.6 mL/kg/hr or anuria is noted.* Monitor BMP, platelet count, UOP, heart murmur, echocardiogram.

Vasopressors

DOBUTAMINE (DOBUTREX)
- Use: Short-term management of patients with cardiac decompensation
- Mechanism of action: Stimulates beta-1 receptors, resulting in increased myocardial contractility and cardiac output.

Also has mild beta-2 agonist activity, which makes it useful for mild vasodilatation.
- Clearance: Hepatic metabolism, renal excretion
- Route: IV, IO
- Considerations: Infuse in a large vein. Monitor blood pressure, EKG, heart rate, UOP.
  - ○ To calculate rate of infusion: (mL/hour) = dose(mcg/kg/min) × weight × 60 minutes divided by the concentration (mcg/mL)

DOPAMINE (INTROPIN)
- Use: Increase cardiac output, blood pressure, and urine flow as an adjunct in the treatment of shock and hypotension which persists after adequate fluid volume replacement; also used in low doses to increase renal perfusion.
- Mechanism of action: Stimulates both adrenergic and dopaminergic receptors; lower doses are mainly dopaminergic-stimulating and produce renal mesenteric vasodilatation; higher doses are both dopaminergic- and beta-1 adrenergic-stimulating and produce cardiac stimulation and renal vasodilatation; large doses stimulate alpha-adrenergic receptors.
- Clearance: Renal, hepatic metabolism, renal excretion
- Route: Continuous IV
- Considerations: Monitor blood pressure, EKG, heart rate, UOP; monitor skin for temperature and color changes. Ensure proper IV placement. If extravasation occurs, do not flush line; stop infusion and attempt to aspirate the extravasated solution, then remove catheter.

EPINEPHRINE (ADRENALIN)
- Use: Treatment of bradycardia, cardiac arrest, cardiogenic shock
- Mechanism of action: Stimulates alpha, beta, and beta2-adrenergic receptors, resulting in relaxation of smooth muscle of the bronchial tree, cardiac stimulation (increasing myocardial oxygen consumption), and dilatation of skeletal muscle vasculature. Small doses can cause vasodilatation via beta2-vascular receptors; large doses may produce constriction of skeletal and vascular smooth muscle.
- Clearance: Taken up by the adrenergic neuron and metabolized by monoamine oxidase (MAO), renal excretion
- Route: IV, IO, ET
- Considerations: Titrate by 0.01 mcg/kg/min as needed to stabilize mean blood pressure. Monitor EKG, heart rate, blood pressure, site of infusion for excessive blanching/extravasation; cardiac and blood pressure monitoring required during infusion.

NOREPINEPHRINE (LEVOPHED)
- Use: Treatment of shock that persists after adequate fluid volume replacement, severe hypotension, septic shock, and in neonates with persistent pulmonary hypertension-induced circulatory failure.
- Mechanism of action: Stimulates beta 1-adrenergic receptors and alpha-adrenergic receptors, causing increased contractility and heart rate as well as vasoconstriction, thereby increasing systemic blood pressure and coronary blood flow clinically; alpha effects (vasoconstriction) are greater than beta effects (inotropic and chronotropic effects).

- Clearance: Metabolized by catechol-o-methyltransferase (COMT) and MAO, renal excretion
- Route: IV
- Considerations: Blood pressure, heart rate, intravascular volume, UOP, peripheral perfusion. Ensure proper IV placement. If extravasation occurs, do not flush line; stop infusion and attempt to aspirate the extravasated solution, then remove catheter.

Anticoagulant Therapy

UNFRACTIONATED HEPARIN (HEPARIN)
- Use: Systemic—prophylaxis and treatment of thromboembolic disorders and anticoagulant for ECMO and dialysis procedures. Local—heparin lock solution to maintain patency of IV sites.
- Mechanism of action: Potentiates the action of antithrombin III and thereby inactivates thrombin and prevents conversion of fibrinogen to fibrin.
- Clearance: Metabolism in the liver and spleen, renal excretion
- Route: IV
- Considerations: Prior to start of systemic therapy, ensure imaging has been completed, obtain baseline CBC with diff, pertussis toxin (PT), partial thromboplastin time (PTT); then monitor serially.
- Adjustment of dose is based on clinical response, serial evaluation of thrombus, and lab values. Monitor PTT 4 hours after initial bolus, change in dose, and then every 24 hours once therapeutic dose is achieved. Rare occurrence of heparin-induced thrombocytopenia

ENOXAPARIN (LOVENOX)/LOW-MOLECULAR WEIGHT HEPARIN (LMWH)
- Use: Inpatient treatment of or prophylaxis thromboembolic disorders and anticoagulant for extracorporeal and dialysis procedures.
- Mechanism of action: Small effect on the activated PTT and strongly inhibits anti-Xa
- Clearance: Hepatic metabolism, renal excretion
- Route: Sub-Q
- Considerations: Monitor CBC with diff, stool for occult blood, serum creatinine and potassium anti-Xa 4 to 6 hours after Sub-Q injection; after levels are therapeutic for 24 to 48 hours, monitor weekly. Do not rub injection site as bruising may occur.

Reversal of Anticoagulation

PROTAMINE (PROTAMINES)
- Use: Treatment of heparin overdose
- Mechanism of action: A highly alkaline protein molecule with a large positive charge, has weak anticoagulant activity when administered alone. When given in the presence of heparin (strongly acidic and negatively charged) a stable salt is formed, and the anticoagulant activity of both drugs is nullified. In the presence of LMWH, protamine completely reverses the antifactory Xa activity of LMWH.
- Clearance: Renal excretion
- Route: IV
- Considerations—administer slow IV push not more than 5 mg/min; rapid IV infusion causes hypotension. Monitor coagulation tests and cardiac status during administration.

GASTROINTESTINAL DRUGS

Histamine H₂ Antagonist

RANITIDINE (ZANTAC)
- Use: Short-term and maintenance treatment of duodenal ulcers, gastric ulcers, gastroesophageal (GE) reflux, and erosive esophagitis
- Mechanism of action: Competitive inhibition of histamine at H2-receptors of the gastric parietal cells, which inhibits gastric acid secretion; gastric volume and hydrogen ion concentrations are reduced.
- Clearance: Hepatic metabolism, renal excretion
- Route: PO, IV
- Considerations: Sixfold increased risk of NEC, infection, and mortality in very low birth weight (VLBW) infants. Monitor AST/alanine aminotransferase (ALT) serum creatinine, occult blood with gastrointestinal (GI) bleeding; when used to prevent GI bleeding, measure intragastric pH and try to maintain >4.

FAMOTIDINE (PEPCID)
- Use: Short-term treatment for GE reflux
- Mechanism of action: Competitive inhibition of histamine at H2 receptors of the gastric parietal cells, which inhibits gastric secretion.
- Clearance: Hepatic metabolism, renal excretion
- Route: PO, IV
- Considerations: Monitor CBC, gastric pH, occult blood with GI bleeding, renal function.

Prokinetics

METOCLOPRAMIDE (REGLAN)
- Use: Symptomatic treatment of GE reflux
- Mechanism of action: Blocks dopamine receptors and, when given in higher doses, also blocks serotonin receptors in chemoreceptor trigger zone of the CNS; enhances the response to acetylcholine of tissues in the upper GI tract, causing enhanced motility and increased gastric emptying without stimulating gastric, biliary, or pancreatic secretions: increases lower esophageal sphincter tone.
- Clearance: Hepatic metabolism, renal excretion
- Route: PO, IM, IV
- Considerations: Monitor blood pressure and heart rate when rapid IV administration is used, monitor for dystonic reactions.

Proton Pump Inhibitors (PPIs)

LANSOPRAZOLE (PREVACID)
- Use: Short-term treatment of GE reflux, erosive esophagitis
- Mechanism of action: Decreases acid secretion in gastric parietal cells through inhibition of an enzyme system, blocking the final step in gastric acid production.
- Clearance: Hepatic metabolism, excretion through feces
- Route: PO
- Considerations: Monitor CBC, liver function, renal function, serum gastrin levels. Best if given 30 mins prior to meals.

OMEPRAZOLE (PRILOSEC)
- Use: Short-term treatment of GE reflux, erosive esophagitis

- Mechanism of action: Suppresses gastric basal and stimulated acid secretion by inhibiting the parietal cell H+/K+ ATP pump
- Clearance: Hepatic metabolism, renal excretion
- Route: PO
- Considerations: Use of PPIs may increase the rate of GI infections; increased frequency of osteoporosis and fractures. Use the lowest effective dose. Consider supplementation of vitamin D and calcium.

PANTOPRAZOLE (PROTONIX)
- Use: Treatment of GE reflux, erosive esophagitis, gastritis
- Mechanism of action: Suppresses gastric basal and stimulated acid secretion by inhibiting the parietal cell H+/K+ ATP pump
- Clearance: Hepatic metabolism, excreted in urine and feces
- Route: PO, IV
- Considerations: Thrombocytopenia, ascites, pulmonary deterioration, and renal and hepatic failure have been reported. Use of PPIs may increase the rate of GI infections; increased frequency of osteoporosis and fractures. Use the lowest effective dose. Consider supplementation of Vitamin D and calcium.

ERYTHROMYCIN (EES)
- Use: Prokinetic GI motility agent
- Mechanism of action: Inhibits RNA-dependent protein synthesis during elongation; blocks the transpeptidation binding to the 50S ribosomal subunit.
- Clearance: Hepatic metabolism, excreted in feces
- Route: PO
- Considerations: Therapy started after the start of enteral feedings. Efficacy has not been demonstrated in the majority of trials; use in neonates with PNA <14 days of age has been associated with a 10-fold increase in pyloric stenosis.

NEUROLOGIC DRUGS

Anticonvulsants

PHENOBARBITAL (LUMINAL)
- Use: Management of generalized tonic–clonic seizures, status epilepticus, and cortical focal seizures
- Mechanism of action: Acts on gamma-aminobutyric acid (GABA) receptors. Decreases excitability of the postsynaptic neuron status epilepticus.
- Clearance: Hepatic metabolism, renal excretion
- Route: PO, IV
- Consideration: *Drug of choice for neonatal seizures.* Therapeutic level 20 to 40 μg/mL. May need additional respiratory support at higher doses.

FOSPHENYTOIN (CEREBYX)
- Use: Management of generalized tonic–clonic status epilepticus
- Mechanism of action: Diphosphate ester salt that acts as a water-soluble prodrug of phenytoin. Phenytoin acts by stabilizing neuronal membranes and decreasing seizure activity by increasing efflux or decreasing influx of sodium ions across cell membranes in the motor cortex during generation of nerve impulses.

- Clearance: Fosphenytoin is converted by hydrolysis to phenytoin, phenytoin undergoes hepatic metabolism and renal excretion
- Route: PO, IM, IV
- Dose: *Use the neonatal IV phenytoin dosing guidelines to dose fosphenytoin using doses in phenytoin equivalents (PEs) equal to the phenytoin dose. Phenytoin 1 mg = fosphenytoin 1 PE. Do not change the doses when changing between fosphenytoin for phenytoin as they are not equivalent on an mg-to-mg basis.*
- Consideration: Monitor CBC with differential and platelet count, serum glucose, therapeutic levels of total phenytoin 8 to 15 mcg/mL.
    - ○ Added if seizures are not controlled by phenobarbital alone. *Measure trough serum phenytoin, not fosphenytoin.* Obtain trough 48 hours after IV loading dose.

PHENYTOIN (DILANTIN)
- Use: PO—management of generalized tonic–clonic and complex partial seizure including grand mal
- Mechanism of action: Decreases neuron excitability
- Clearance: Hepatic metabolism, renal excretion
- Route: PO, IV
- Consideration: *Administer slowly at a maximum 0.5 to 1 mg/kg/min to avoid cardiac arrhythmia.* Monitor CBC with differential, liver function monitor trough. Following IV infusion flush with normal saline (NS) to avoid irritation.
    - ○ Phenytoin is a vesicant, and there is conflicting information regarding use of hyaluronidase with infiltration.

LEVETIRACETAM (KEPPRA)
- Use: Adjunctive therapy in the treatment of partial onset seizures, myoclonic seizures, and primary generalized tonic–clonic seizures.
- Mechanism of action: The precise mechanism by which it exerts its antiepileptic effect is unknown; however, studies suggest one or more of the following effects: inhibition of calcium channels; displacement of negative modulators; reduction of potassium current; and/or binding to synaptic proteins.
- Clearance: Metabolized by enzymatic hydrolysis, renal excretion
- Route: PO, IV
- Considerations: Few prospective studies; monitor seizure frequency, severity, and duration; CNS depression, diastolic blood pressure, renal function, CBC.

PYRIDOXINE (VITAMIN B6)
- Use: Employed for the treatment of pyridoxine-dependent seizures or treatment of drug-induced deficiency
- Mechanism of action: Precursor to pyridoxal, which functions in the metabolism of proteins, carbohydrates, and fats; also aids in the release of liver- and muscle-released glycogen and the synthesis of GABA in the CNS and heme.
- Clearance: Hepatic metabolism, renal excretion
- Route: PO, IM, IV
- Considerations: Neonates with intractable seizures not responsive to antiepileptic drug therapy may receive an empiric trial of pyridoxine. Monitor EEG while giving dose-diagnostic when seizures cease within minutes

and the EEG normalizes within minutes to hours. Protect from light.

Sedatives

DIAZEPAM (VALIUM)
- Use: Management of general anxiety, relief of skeletal muscle spasms and muscle spasticity, adjunct therapy in convulsive disorders
- Mechanism of action: Binds to stereospecific benzodiazepine receptors on the postsynaptic GABA neuron at several sites in the CNS.
- Clearance: Hepatic metabolism, renal excretion
- Route: IV
- Consideration: Not recommended as a first-line agent. Use only after multiple agents have failed.

LORAZEPAM (ATIVAN)
- Use: Management of anxiety (anxiolytic) and amnestic often used for preprocedure sedation
- Mechanism of action: Binds to stereospecific benzodiazepine receptors on the postsynaptic GABA neuron at several sites in the CNS.
- Clearance: Hepatic metabolism, renal excretion
- Route: IV—Limited data available
- Considerations: may cause respiratory depression, hypotension, use lowest effective dose. Dependence develops with prolonged use. Monitor respiratory status, blood pressure, heart rate, CBC with diff and liver function with long-term use. Use with caution, there is concern regarding neurotoxicity.
- Antidote: Flumazenil
    - ○ For benzodiazepine reversal, 10 mcg/kg over 15 seconds, may repeat after 45 seconds and then every minute until maximum cumulative dose of 50 mcg/kg.

MIDAZOLAM (VERSED)
- Use: Preprocedural sedation, anxiolysis, amnesia for diagnostic or radiographic procedures. Continuous infusions maybe used in sedation of intubated and mechanically ventilated patients.
- Mechanism of action: Binds to specific GABA receptor subunits at CNS neuronal synapses, facilitating GABA-mediated chloride ion channel opening frequency-enhance membrane hyperpolarization
- Clearance: Hepatic metabolism, renal excretion
- Route: IM, IV, intranasal
- Considerations: May cause hypotension with rapid administration; give over 2 to 5 minutes. Use lowest effective dose. Dependence develops with prolonged use. Use with caution. There is concern regarding neurotoxicity. Several studies report significant adverse effects and no clinical benefit. Several cases of myoclonus have been reported.
    - ○ Antidote: Flumazenil
        - For benzodiazepine reversal, 10 mcg/kg over 15 seconds, may repeat after 45 seconds and then every minute until maximum cumulative dose of 50 mcg/kg.

RENAL DRUGS

Loop Diuretics

FUROSEMIDE (LASIX)
- Use: Management of edema associated with heart failure, hepatic or renal disease, used alone or in combination with antihypertensives to treat hypertension
- Mechanism of action: Inhibits reabsorption of sodium and chloride in the ascending loop of Henle and proximal and distal renal tubules, causing increased excretion of water, sodium, chloride magnesium, and calcium.
- Clearance: Hepatic metabolism, excretion through urine and feces
- Route PO, IM, IV—oral and IM/IV doses are not interchangeable
- Considerations: Monitor electrolytes, renal function, blood pressure, I/O, hearing; risk for hypokalemia and renal calcifications with chronic use. Risk for ototoxicity increased in the premature infant due to prolonged half-life and with concomitant use of an aminoglycoside.

BUMETANIDE (BUMEX)
- Use: Management of edema associated with heart failure, hepatic or renal disease, including nephrotic syndrome; has been used to reverse oliguria in preterm neonates and used alone or in combination with antihypertensives to treat hypertension.
- Mechanism of action: Inhibits chloride and sodium reabsorption in ascending loop of Henle and proximal renal tubule causing increased excretion of water and electrolytes. It does not appear to act in the distal tubule.
- Clearance: Hepatic metabolism, renal excretion
- Route: PO, IM, IV
- Considerations: Higher end of dosing may be needed for patients in heart failure. Has been used to reverse oliguria in preterm infants. Monitor electrolytes, renal function, blood pressure, UOP. May displace bilirubin.

Thiazide Diuretics

CHLOROTHIAZIDE (DIURIL)
- Use: Treatment of edema due to heart, renal failure, management of hypertension alone or in combination with antihypertensive, treatment of BPD, treatment of central diabetes insipidus
- Mechanism of action: Inhibits sodium and chloride reabsorption in the distal tubules causing increased excretion of sodium chloride and water resulting in diuresis. Loss of potassium, hydrogen ions, magnesium phosphate, and bicarbonate also occur. Thiazide diuretics decrease calcium excretion.
- Clearance: Not metabolized, renal excretion as unchanged drug
- Route: PO, IV
- Considerations: Electrolytes, BUN, creatinine, hyperglycemia, blood pressure, I/O, weight

HYDROCHLOROTHIAZIDE (HCTZ) (MICROZIDE)
- Use: Management of edema related to heart failure, hepatic cirrhosis or corticosteroid therapy, renal dysfunction, management of hypertension alone, or in combination with

other antihypertensives, has also been used for BPD, central diabetes insipidus (DI), idiopathic hypercalciuria
- Mechanism of action: Inhibits sodium and chloride reabsorption in the distal tubules causing increased excretion of sodium chloride and water resulting in diuresis. Loss of potassium, hydrogen ions, magnesium phosphate, and bicarbonate also occur. Thiazide diuretics decrease calcium excretion.
- Clearance: Not metabolized, renal excretion as unchanged drug
- Route: PO
- Considerations: Monitor electrolytes, BUN, creatinine, hyperglycemia, blood pressure, I/O, weight.

Potassium-Sparing Diuretics

SPIRONOLACTONE (ALDACTONE)
- Use: Management of edema and sodium retention, prophylaxis against hypokalemia patients on digoxin
- Mechanism of action: Competes with aldosterone for receptor sites in the distal renal tubule increasing sodium chloride and water losses while conserving potassium and hydrogen ions.
- Clearance: Hepatic metabolism, renal excretion
- Route: PO
- Considerations: Generally used in combination with a thiazide diuretic. Use with caution in infants with renal impairment. Monitor electrolytes—primarily hyperkalemia, renal function, I/O, weight.

Combination Diuretic Therapy

HYDROCHLOROTHIAZIDE AND SPIRONOLACTONE (ALDACTAZIDE)
- Use: Treatment of edema, hypertension, BPD
- Mechanism of action: The product is a fixed combination of equal mg proportions of components.
- Route: PO
- Considerations: Monitor serum electrolytes, BUN, creatinine, blood pressure, fluid balance, body weight, heart rate.

Inhibitors of Carbonic Anhydrase Diuretics

ACETAZOLAMIDE (DIAMOX)
- Use: Mild diuretic, correction of metabolic alkalosis
- Mechanism of action: Reversible inhibition of the enzyme carbonic anhydrase resulting in reduction of hydrogen ion secretion at renal tubule and an increased renal excretion of sodium, bicarbonate, and water.
- Clearance: Renal excretion
- Route: PO, IV
- Considerations: Monitor serum electrolytes, CBC, and platelet count.

RESPIRATORY DRUGS

Bronchodilators

ALBUTEROL (VENTOLIN)
- Use: Treatment of bronchospasm, adjunct therapy for hyperkalemia
- Mechanism of action: Relaxes bronchial smooth muscle by action on beta2-receptors with little effect on heart rate.

- Route: Oral inhalation, nebulization
- Considerations: Monitor serum potassium, oxygen saturation, heart rate, pulmonary function respiratory rate, use of accessory muscles during respiration suprasternal retractions, blood gases. May cause insomnia, excitability.

IPRATROMIUM (ATROVENT)
- Use: Treatment of bronchospasm associated with asthma and as a bronchodilating agent in bronchopulmonary dysplasia and neonatal respiratory distress.
- Mechanism of action: Blocks the action of acetylcholine at parasympathetic sites in bronchial smooth muscle causing bronchodilatation
- Route: Oral inhalation, nebulization
- Considerations: Nimited data optimal dosing not established

BOSENTAN (TRACLEER)
- Use: Treatment of pulmonary arterial hypertension
- Mechanism of action: Endothelin receptor antagonist that blocks endothelin receptors on endothelium and vascular smooth muscle (stimulation of these receptors is associated with vasoconstriction).
- Clearance: Hepatic metabolism, excreted through feces
- Route: PO
- Considerations:
  - Serum transaminase levels (AST and ALT) and bilirubin should be determined prior to start of therapy and monitored at monthly intervals thereafter. There have been reported cases of hepatic failure. Discontinue therapy in patients who develop elevated transaminase levels either in combination with symptoms of hepatic injury or increased bilirubin.
  - Bosentan is a hazardous agent—wear gloves when handling tablets/capsules. The National Institute of Occupational Safety and Health recommends double gloving, gown and eye protection when administering an oral liquid/tube feeding administration if there is a risk for vomiting or spitting.

Inhalants

NITRIC OXIDE (INO) (INOMAX)
- Use: Treatment of hypoxic respiratory failure associated with clinical or echocardiographic evidence of pulmonary hypertension, used in conjunction with ventilator support.
- Mechanism of action: In neonates with persistent pulmonary hypertension, nitric oxide improves oxygenation. Nitric oxide relaxes vascular smooth muscle. When inhaled, pulmonary vasodilatation occurs and an increase in the partial pressure of arterial oxygen results.
- Route: Oral inhalation
- Considerations: Monitor respiratory status including arterial blood gases (ABGs) with close attention to PaO_2, methemoglobin measured within 4 to 8 hours after start and then periodically during treatment, vital signs. Contraindicated in infants depending on right to left hunting of blood. Avoid abrupt discontinuation; may lead to worsening hypotension, oxygenation. Elevations of methemoglobin and nitrogen dioxide may be signs of overdose. Use in infants <34 weeks is not recommended. May only be delivered by an INOmax DSIR nitric oxide delivery system.

Inhaled Steroids, Corticosteroids.

BECLOMETHASONE (QVAR)
- Use: Treatment of bronchial asthma
- Mechanism of action: Controls the rate of protein synthesis; depresses the migration of polymorphonuclear leukocytes, fibroblasts; reverses capillary permeability and lysosomal stabilization at the cellular level to control inflammation
- Route: Oral inhalation
- Considerations: Check mucous membranes for signs of fungal infection, monitor growth, monitor symptoms of asthma.

BUDESONIDE (PULMICORT)
- Use: Maintenance therapy and prophylaxis of bronchial asthma
- Mechanism of action: Controls the rate of protein synthesis, depresses the migration of polymorphonuclear leukocytes, fibroblasts; reverses capillary permeability and lysosomal stabilization. Has potent glucocorticoid activity and weak mineralocorticoid activity.
- Route: Oral inhalation, nebulization
- Considerations: Orally inhaled corticosteroids may cause a reduction in growth velocity titrate to lowest effective dose. Monitor mucous membranes for signs of fungal infection, monitor for asthma, regular eye exams, monitor blood pressure, signs and symptoms hypercorticism or adrenal suppression. Prolonged use may increase the risk for secondary infection, may mask acute infection or prolong/exacerbate viral infections, and limit response to vaccines.

Inhaled Steroids, Mineralocorticoid

FLUTICASONE (FLOVENT)
- Use: Anti-inflammatory agent, anti-asthmatic, treatment of bronchopulmonary dysplasia
- Mechanism of action: Fluticasone belongs to a group of corticosteroids which utilizes a fluorcarbothioate ester linkage at the 17-carbon position; extremely potent vasoconstriction and anti-inflammatory activity. The effectiveness of inhaled fluticasone is due to its direct effect.
- Route: Oral inhalation
- Considerations: Monitor growth, mucous membranes for signs of fungal infection, ocular effects such as cataracts, increased ocular pressure, glaucoma, bone mineral density, hepatic impairment, possible eosinophilic conditions. Monitor for signs of asthma. Monitor for HPA axis suppression.

Respiratory Stimulants

CAFFEINE CITRATE (CAFCIT)
- Use: Treatment of apnea of prematurity
- Mechanism of action: CNS stimulant that increases medullary respiratory center sensitivity to carbon dioxide, stimulates central inspiratory drive, and improves diaphragmatic contractility.
- Clearance: Hepatic metabolism, renal excretion
- Route: IV, PO
- Considerations: Monitor for tachycardia, number and severity of apnea spells, serum caffeine levels—therapeutic

8 to 20 mcg/mL, potentially toxic >20 mcg/mL, toxicity >50 mcg/mL. Administer with caution in patients with gastric esophageal reflux, impaired renal or hepatic function, seizure disorders, or cardiovascular disease. May be associated with risk for necrotizing enterocolitis.

Systemic Steroids, Cortiosteroids

BETAMETHASONE (CELESTONE)
- Use: Prevention of respiratory distress syndrome (RDS), treatment of infantile hemangioma
- Mechanism of action: Anti-inflammatory. Controls the rate of protein synthesis; depresses the migration of polymorphonuclear leukocytes, fibroblasts; reverses capillary permeability and lysosomal stabilization at the cellular level to prevent or control inflammation.
- Clearance: Hepatic metabolism, renal excretion
- Route: IM, IV
- Considerations: No contraindications exist to antenatal treatment; benefits of treatment may diminish if preterm labor stops and pregnancy continues more than a week. Adrenal suppression with failure to thrive has been reported in infants receiving intralesional corticosteroid injections. May cause osteoporosis or inhibition of bone growth. Risk of bone fracture increased with >four courses of therapy. Monitor blood pressure, serum glucose, serum potassium, calcium, hemoglobin, occult blood loss. May cause hypercortisolism or suppression of hypothalamic–pituitary–adrenal (HPA) axis. HPA axis suppression may lead to adrenal crisis. Withdrawal and discontinuation of corticosteroids should be done slowly and carefully. Prolonged use may increase the risk for secondary infection, may mask acute infection or prolong/exacerbate viral infections.

DEXAMETHASONE (DECADRON)
- Use: Prevention of RDS, anti-inflammatory
- Mechanism of action: A *long-acting* corticosteroid with minimal sodium-retaining potential. Decreases inflammation by suppression of neutrophil migration, decreased production of inflammatory mediators, and reversal of increased capillary permeability.
- Clearance: Hepatic metabolism, renal excretion
- Route: PO, IM, IV
- Considerations: In premature neonates, the use of high-dose dexamethasone approximately >0.5 mg/kg/day for the prevention or treatment of BPD has been associated with adverse neurodevelopmental outcomes, including higher rates of cerebral palsy, without additional clinical benefits of lower doses. Dexamethasone may increase the effects/toxicity of loop and thiazide diuretics. Monitor hemoglobin, occult blood loss, blood pressure, serum glucose, serum potassium; monitor for osteopenia with long/multiple courses of therapy.

HYDROCORTISONE (SOLU-CORTEF)
- Use: Anti-inflammatory, treatment of primary or secondary adrenocorticoid deficiency, management of septic shock, hypoglycemia, hypotension, and treatment of bronchopulmonary dysplasia
- Mechanism of action: A *short-acting* corticosteroid with minimal sodium-retaining potential. Decreases inflammation by suppression of neutrophil migration, decreased

production of inflammatory mediators, and reversal of increased capillary permeability.
- Clearance: Hepatic metabolism, renal excretion
- Route: PO, IV
- Considerations: Monitor electrolytes, serum glucose, blood pressure; monitor growth/weight; monitor for suppression of HPA suppression, associated with GI perforation in low birth weight infants.

PREDNISOLONE (PEDIAPRED)
- Use: Anti-inflammatory used in treating bronchopulmonary dysplasia
- Mechanism of action: Decreases inflammation by suppression of migration of polymorphonuclear leukocytes and reversal of increased capillary permeability, suppresses the immune system by reducing activity and volume of the lymphatic system
- Clearance: Hepatic metabolism, renal excretion
- Route: PO
- Considerations: Dose depends on the condition being treated and response of patient, dosage for infants should be based on disease severity and patient response rather than rigid adherence to dosing guidelines. Consider alternate day therapy for long-term therapy. Monitor blood pressure, weight, electrolytes, serum glucose, bone mineral density with long-term therapy, risk for fractures increased with >four courses of corticosteroids.

Surfactant Therapy

BERACTANT (SURVANTA)
- Use: Treatment of RDS in premature infants with birth weight <1,250 g or evidence of surfactant deficiency, treatment of RDS with x-ray confirmation of RDS and requiring mechanical ventilation, has also been used for treatment of meconium aspiration syndrome in term and near-term infants.
- Mechanism of action: replaces deficient or ineffective endogenous lung surfactant in neonates with RDS or in neonates at risk of developing RDS. Surfactant prevents the alveoli from collapsing during expiration by lowering surface tension between air and alveolar surfaces.
- Route: ET
- Considerations: Continuous heart rate and oxygen saturation should be monitored during administration; bradycardia and oxygen desaturation are frequently noted during dosing, pause dosing to initiate corrective measures then resume. Produces rapid improvements in lung oxygenation and compliance may require frequent adjustments to oxygen and ventilator settings. Monitor frequent ABG sampling to prevent post-dosing hyperoxia and hypocarbia. Pulmonary hemorrhage has been reported. Do not suction airway for 1 hour after instillation unless significant airway obstruction occurs.

PORACTANT ALFA (CUROSURF)
- Use: Treatment of RDS in preterm infants
- Mechanism of action: endogenous pulmonary surfactant reduces surface tension at the air–liquid interface of the alveoli during ventilation and stabilizes the alveoli against collapse at resting transpulmonary pressures.
- Route: ET

- Considerations: Continuous heart rate and oxygen saturation should be monitored during administration. Produces rapid improvements in lung oxygenation and compliance may require frequent adjustments to oxygen and ventilator settings. Monitor frequent ABG sampling to prevent post-dosing hyperoxia and hypocarbia. Pulmonary hemorrhage has been reported. Do not suction airway for 1 hour after instillation unless significant airway obstruction occurs.

IMMUNIZATIONS/VACCINES, IMMUNE GLOBULIN, AND OTHER BIOLOGICS

Passive Immunization

HEPATITIS B VACCINATION (ENERGIX; RECOMBIVAX HB)

- Use: Immunization against all known subspecies of Hepatitis B virus. HepB vaccine is used for pre-exposure and post-exposure protection and provides long-term protection. Pre-exposure immunization with HepB vaccine is the most effective means to prevent HBV transmission. Accordingly, HepB immunization is recommended for all infants, children, and adolescents through 18 years of age. Infants should receive HepB vaccine as part of the routine childhood immunization schedule.
- Mechanism of action: HepB vaccines stimulate immunity through the production of specific antibodies. Vaccines licensed in the United States have a 90% to 95% efficacy for preventing HBV infection and clinical HBV disease among susceptible children and adults.
- Route: IM
- Dose: 0.5 mL
- Schedule:
  - ○ Mother is HBsAg-negative:
    - ▪ One dose within 24 hours of birth for all medically stable infants ≥2,000 g.
      - • Infants ≤2,000 g: Administer one dose at chronological age 1 month or hospital discharge.
  - ○ Mother is HBsAg-positive:
    - ▪ Administer HepB vaccine and 0.5 mL of hHpatitis B immune globulin (HBIG; at separate anatomic sites) within 12 hours of birth, regardless of birth weight.
    - ▪ For infants ≤2,000 g, administer three additional doses of vaccine (total of four doses) beginning at age 1 month. Test for HBsAg and anti-HBs at age 9 to 12 months. If HepB series is delayed, test 1 to 2 months after final dose.
  - ○ Mother's HBsAg status is unknown:
    - ▪ Administer HepB vaccine within 12 hours of birth, regardless of birth weight.
      - • For infants ≤2,000 g, administer 0.5 mL of HBIG in addition to HepB vaccine within 12 hours of birth.
      - • Administer three additional doses of vaccine (total of four doses) beginning at age 1 month. Determine mother's HBsAg status as soon as possible. If mother is HBsAg-positive, administer 0.5 mL of HBIG to infants ≥2,000 g as soon as possible, but no later than 7 days of age.
  - ○ Routine series: Three-dose series at 0, 1 to 2, 6 to 18 months (use monovalent HepB vaccine for doses administered before age 6 weeks). Infants who did not

receive a birth dose should begin the series as soon as feasible.
    - ▪ Minimum age for the final (third or fourth) dose: 24 weeks.
    - ▪ Minimum intervals: Dose 1 to dose 2: 4 weeks/dose 2 to dose 3: 8 weeks/dose 1 to dose 3: 16 weeks. (When four doses are administered, substitute "dose 4" for "dose 3" in these calculations.)
- Considerations: Hepatitis B vaccine preparations differ by concentration; when dosed by volume, the equivalent dose is the same between products.

DIPHTHERIA, TETANUS, AND ACELLULAR PERTUSSIS (DTAP; DAPTACEL, INFANRIX)

- Use: Diphtheria and tetanus toxoids and pertussis vaccine (DTaP) consists of a mixture of the detoxified toxins (toxoids) of diphtheria and tetanus and inactivated *Bordetella pertussis* that have been adsorbed onto an aluminum salt. Diphtheria and tetanus toxoids and acellular pertussis vaccines contain PT.
- Mechanism of action: Promotes active immunity to diphtheria, tetanus, and pertussis by inducing production of specific antibodies.
- Route: IM
- Dose: 0.5 mL schedule: Five-dose series at 2, 4, 6, 15 to 18 months, 4 to 6 years
- Considerations: Same product should be used for entire series, shake vial well prior to withdrawing (Taketomo et al., 2018, pp. 665–667).

HAEMOPHILUS INFLUENZAE TYPE B (HIB)

- Use: Protection against H influenza. The Hib conjugate vaccine consists of the Hib capsular polysaccharide (polyribosylribotol phosphate [PRP]) covalently linked to a carrier protein. Protective antibodies are directed against PRP.
- Mechanism of action: Stimulates production of anticapsular antibodies and provides active immunity to Hib. Vaccination provides protective antibodies to 95% of infants who are vaccinated with a 2- or 3-dose series.
- Route: IM injection
- Dose: 0.5 mL. Schedule: Four-dose series at 2, 4, 6, 12 to 15 months
- Considerations: Minimum age for first dose is 6 weeks. Do not restart if doses have been missed; refer to current immunization guidelines for schedule and timing of dose based on patient age and previous number of doses.

INFLUENZA VIRUS VACCINE, INACTIVATED (FLUZONE)

- Use: Promotes immunity to seasonal influenza virus. Strains selected for inclusion in the seasonal vaccine may change yearly in anticipation of the predominant influenza strains expected to circulate in the United States. The American Academy of Pediatrics (AAP) recommends annual use of inactivated influenza vaccines (IIVs) in all people 6 months and older.
- Mechanism of action: Promotes immunity by inducing specific antibody production
- Route: IM
- Dose: 0.25 mL. Schedule: One to two doses separated by 4 weeks; ≥6 months of age number of doses are dependent on flu vaccination history.
- Considerations:

- ○ Flu seasons vary in their timing and duration from year to year; vaccination should occur as soon as vaccine is available and, if possible, by the end of October.
- ○ The effectiveness of influenza vaccines depends primarily on the age and immune competence of vaccine recipients, the degree of similarity between the viruses in the vaccine and those in circulation, and the outcome being measured.

PNEUMOCOCCAL CONJUGATE (PREVNAR 13)
- Use: Immunization against *S. pneumoniae* infections
- Mechanism of action: PCV13 is composed of purified capsular polysaccharide serotypes which are all individually conjugated to a nontoxic variant of diphtheria toxin carrier protein.
- Route: IM
- Dose: 0.5 mL given in a four-dose series at 2, 4, 6, 12 to 15 months
- Considerations: Do not restart if doses have been missed; refer to current immunization guidelines for schedule and timing of dose based on patient age and previous number of doses.

INACTIVATED POLIO VACCINE (IPV)
- Use: Provides active immunity against poliovirus
- Mechanism of action: As an inactivated virus vaccine, polio vaccine induces active immunity against the three serotypes, which are grown in Vero cells or human diploid cells and then inactivated. Administration of IPV results in seroconversion in 95% or more of vaccine recipients to each of the three serotypes after two doses and results in seroconversion in 99% to 100% of recipients after three doses.
- Route: IM
- Dose: 0.5 mL. Four doses of IPV are recommended for routine immunization of all infants and children in the United States.
- Considerations: Do not restart if doses have been missed; refer to current immunization guidelines for schedule and timing of dose based on patient age and previous number of doses.

Active Immunization

ROTAVIRUS VACCINE (ROTARIX, ROTATEQ)
- Use: Routine immunization to prevent rotovirus gastroenteritis
- Mechanism of action: A live vaccine; replicates in the small intestine and promotes active immunity to rotavirus gastroenteritis. Virus from live vaccines may be transferred to nonvaccinated persons by physical contacts. Viral shedding occurs within the first weeks of administration.
- Route: PO
- Dose:
  - ○ Rotarix: 1 mL; schedule: Two-dose series at 2 and 4 months
  - ○ RotaTeq: 2 mL; schedule: Three-dose series at 2, 4, and 6 months
    - Administer to inner cheek if infant spits out portion of dose; do not administer replacement dose.
    - Series should not be restarted if a dose is missed. If doses have been given, restart with the applicable dose number and separate doses by 4 weeks; total three doses.

- Considerations:
  - ○ Not routinely administered in NICU
  - ○ Immunocompromised patients should not receive live vaccines.
  - ○ Contraindicated in infants with a history of intussusception or severe combined immunodeficiency syndromes (SCIDS). The series should not be started after 15 weeks 0 days of age and should be completed by 8 months of age.

Biologicals

HEPATITIS B IMMUNE GLOBULIN (HUMAN) HBIG
- Use: Provide prophylactic postexposure passive immunity for infants born to HBsAg positive mothers. HBIG provides short-term protection (3–6 months) and is indicated in specific postexposure circumstances. Transmission of perinatal HBV infection can be prevented in approximately 95% of infants born to HBsAg-positive mothers by early active and passive immunoprophylaxis of the infant.
- Mechanism of action: HBIG is a nonpyrogenic sterile solution containing immunoglobin G (IgG) specific to Hepatitis B surface antigen (HBsAg). Standard immune globulin is not effective for post-exposure prophylaxis against HBV infection, because concentrations of anti-HBs are too low.
- Route: IM injection
- Dose:
  - ○ Neonates born to HBsAg positive mothers: 0.5 mL within 12 hours after birth
  - ○ Neonates born to mothers with unknown status at birth:
    - BW <2 kg: 0.5 mL within 12 hours of birth
    - BW >2 kg: 0.5 mL within 7 days of birth.
- Consideration: May give at the same time as Hepatitis B vaccine—use different site. Do not mix in same syringe; vaccine will be neutralized. Do not shake vial, avoid causing foaming of content.

IMMUNE GLOBULIN INTRAVENOUS (IGIV) (BIVIGAM)
- Use: Treatment of primary humoral immunodeficiency syndromes, SCIDS, acute and chronic thrombocytopenia
- Mechanism of action: Replacement therapy for primary and secondary immunodeficiencies, and IgG antibodies against bacteria, viral, parasitic, and mycoplasma antigens, provides passive immunity by increasing the antibody titer and antigen–antibody reaction potential
- Route: IV
- Dose: Varies based on goal of treatment
- Considerations: Consider osmolarity and concentration when selecting product. Infuse as slowly as indication and stability of patient allow. Monitor renal function, UOP, hematocrit and hemoglobin levels, platelet count in patients with idiopathic thombocytopenia (ITP), infusion reactions, anaphylaxis, volume status, pulmonary adverse reactions, clinical response as defined by disease state.

Varicella–Zoster Immune Globulin (VariZig)
- Use:
  - ○ Routine immunization against varicella virus
  - ○ Post-exposure prophylaxis of varicella
    - Newborn of mother who had onset of chickenpox within 5 days before delivery or within 48 hours after delivery

- Hospitalized premature infants >28 weeks' gestation who were exposed during the neonatal period and whose mother has no history of chicken pox
- Hospitalized premature infant (<28 weeks' gestation or <1,000 g) regardless of maternal history and who were exposed during the neonatal period
- Mechanism of action: Varicella vaccine is a live attenuated preparation of the serially propagated and attenuated viral strain. Antibodies obtained from pooled human plasma of individuals with high titers of varicella–zoster provide passive immunity. Infection occurs when the virus comes in contact with the mucosa of the upper respiratory tract or the conjunctiva of a susceptible person. Person-to-person transmission occurs either from direct contact with varicella zoster virus (VZV) lesions from varicella or herpes zoster or from airborne spread. Varicella is much more contagious than is herpes zoster. Skin lesions appear to be the major source of transmissible VZV. The incubation period usually is 14 to 16 days, with a range of 10 to 21 days after exposure to rash. Patients are contagious from 1 to 2 days before onset of the rash until all lesions have crusted.
- Route: IM injection
- Dose: The recommended dose of vaccine is 0.5 mL, administered subcutaneously.
- Considerations: There is no evidence varicella zoster immune globulin (VZIG) modifies established varicella–zoster infections. Administration should begin as soon as possible (ideally within 96 hours) and within 10 days of exposure. High-risk, susceptible patients who are re-exposed >3 weeks after a prior dose of VZIG should receive another full dose. Monitor for signs and symptoms of varicella infection for 28 days after VZIG administration.

CONCLUSION

Making decisions surrounding medication therapy for a neonate is a complex task deserving careful thought and consideration. Benefits of treatment weighed against risks of exposure to drugs should be balanced and discussed within the healthcare team and a pharmacist specializing in neonatal medicines if available. Drug therapy decisions should also take into account the particular medications available within a healthcare system, rules governing their use, and individualized abilities to administer and monitor their usage.

REVIEW QUESTIONS

1. The NNP is notified by a RN of a 3-weeks-old term infant with a heart rate of 70 bpm. The infant has a known ventricular septal defect (VSD) and is receiving digoxin (Lanoxin) for pulmonary over circulation. The NNP recognizes the sinus bradycardia is a sign of a/an:
   A. acute toxicity
   B. momentary finding
   C. therapeutic level

2. The steroid medication dosed based on disease severity, condition being treated, and the response of patient rather than standardized dosing guideline is:
   A. betamethasone (Celestone)
   B. hydrocortisone (Solu-Cortef)
   C. prednisolone (Pediapred)

3. Following administration of surfactant to an infant who is 36 weeks' gestational age with respiratory distress syndrome (RDS), the NNP realizes the need to:
   A. Decrease the mechanical pressures as compliance improves.
   B. Monitor the infant closely for respiratory acidosis due to hypercarbia.
   C. Repeat the dosing in 2 to 4 hours to maximize the therapeutic effect.

4. The NNP is providing medical management of an infant with a hemodynamically significant patent ductus arteriosus (PDA) by ordering indomethacin (Indocin) every 12 hours. The 0.73 kg infant has a urine output of 8 mL in 24 hours. The correct action to take regarding the medication therapy is to:
   A. Continue the current dosing.
   B. Discontinue subsequent doses.
   C. Increase the interval to every 24 hours.

5. Rapid intravenous administration of fentanyl (Duragesic) may lead to:
   A. chest wall rigidity and the inability to ventilate the infant
   B. hypotension resulting in the need for vasopressor support
   C. urinary retention leading to inability of the infant to void

REFERENCES

Baley, J., & Leonard, E. (2013). Infections in the neonate. In A. Fanaroff & J. Fanaroff (Eds.), *Klaus and Fanaroff's care of the high-risk neonate* (6th ed., pp. 346–367). Cleveland, OH: Elsevier.

Beauduy, C., & Winston, L. (2015). Sulfonamides, trimethoprim, & quinolones. In B. Katzung & A. Trevor (Eds.), *Basic & clinical pharmacology* (13th ed., pp. 807–814). New York, NY: McGraw-Hill Education.

Benowitz, N. (2018). Antihypertensive agents. In B. Katzung & A. Trevor (Eds.), *Basic & clinical pharmacology* (13th ed., pp. 169–190). New York, NY: McGraw-Hill Education.

Cadnapaphornchai, M., Schoenbein, M. B., Woloschuk, R., Soranno, D., & Hernandez, J. (2016). Neonatal nephrology. In S. Gardner, B. Carter, M. Hines, & J. Hernandez (Eds.), *Merenstein & Gardner's handbook of neonatal intensive care* (8th ed., pp. 689–726.e4). St. Louis, MO: Elsevier.

Deck, D., & Winston, L. (2015a). Beta-lactam & other cell wall- & membrane-active antibiotics. In B. Katzung & A. Trevor (Eds.), *Basic & clinical pharmacology* (13th ed., pp. 769–787). New York, NY: McGraw-Hill Education.

Deck, D., & Winston, L. (2015b). Aminoglycosides & spectinomycin. In B. Katzung & A. Trevor (Eds.), *Basic & clinical pharmacology* (13th ed., pp. 799–806). New York, NY: McGraw-Hill Education.

Deck, D., & Winston, L. (2015c). Tetracyclines, macrolides, clindamycin, chloramphenicol, streptogramins, & oxazolidinones. In B. Katzung & A. Trevor (Eds.), *Basic & clinical pharmacology* (13th ed., pp. 788–798). New York, NY: McGraw-Hill Education.

Deck, D., & Winston, L. (2015d). Miscellaneous antimicrobial agents; disinfectants, antiseptics & sterilants. In B. Katzung & A. Trevor (Eds.), *Basic & clinical pharmacology* (13th ed., pp. 865–872). New York, NY: McGraw-Hill Education.

Eilers, H., & Yost, S. (2015). General anesthetics. In B. Katzung & A. Trevor (Eds.), *Basic & clinical pharmacology* (13th ed., pp. 421–439). New York, NY: McGraw-Hill Education.

Gardner, S., Hines, M., & Agarwal, R. (2016). Pain and pain relief. In S. Gardner, B. Carter, M. Hines, & J. Hernandez. (Eds.), *Merenstein & Gardner's handbook of neonatal intensive care* (8th ed., pp. 218–261.e8). St. Louis, MO: Elsevier.

Guttentag, S. (2017). Respiratory distress syndrome. In E. Eichenwald, A. Hansen, C. Martin, & A. Stark (Eds.), *Cloherty and Stark's manual of neonatal care* (8th ed., pp. 436–460). Philadelphia, PA: Wolters Kluwer.

Kenagy, D., & Vogt, B. (2013). The kidney. In A. Fanaroff & J. Fanaroff (Eds.), *Klaus and Fanaroff's care of the high-risk neonate* (6th ed., pp. 410–431). Cleveland, OH: Elsevier.

Kimberlin, D. W., Brady, M. T., Jackson, M. A., & Long, S. S. (2018). *Red book 2018 : Report of the committee on infectious diseases* (31st ed.). Elk Grove Village, IL: American Academy of Pediatrics.

McClary, J. (2013). Drug dosing table. In A. Fanaroff & J. Fanaroff (Eds.), *Klaus and Fanaroff's care of the high-risk neonate* (6th ed., pp. 546–562). Cleveland, OH: Elsevier.

McQuaid, K. (2018). Drugs used in the treatment of gastrointestinal disease. In B. Katzung, M. Weitz, & P. Boyle (Eds.), *Basic & clinical pharmacology* (13th ed., pp. 1052–1083). New York, NY: McGraw-Hill Education.

Parsons, J., Seay, A., & Jacobs, M. (2016). Neurologic disorders. In S. Gardner, B. Carter, M. Hines, & J. Hernandez (Eds.), *Merenstein & Gardner's handbook of neonatal intensive care* (8th ed., pp. 727–762.e3). St. Louis, MO: Elsevier.

Safrin, S. (2015). Antiviral agents. In B. Katzung, M. Weitz, & P. Boyle (Eds.), *Basic & clinical pharmacology* (13th ed., pp. 835–864). New York, NY: McGraw-Hill Education.

Samuels, J., Munoz, H., & Swinford, R. (2017). Neonatal kidney conditions. In E. Eichenwald, A. Hansen, C. Martin, & A. Stark (Eds.), *Cloherty and Stark's manual of neonatal care* (8th ed., pp. 366–400). Philadelphia, PA: Wolters Kluwer.

Scher, M. (2013). Brain disorders of the fetus and neonate. In A. Fanaroff & J. Fanaroff (Eds.), *Klaus and Fanaroff's care of the high-risk neonate* (6th ed., pp. 476–524). Cleveland, OH: Elsevier.

Sheppard, D., & Lampiris, H. (2015). Antifungal agents. In B. Katzung & A. Trevor (Eds.), *Basic & clinical pharmacology* (13th ed., pp. 825–834). New York, NY: McGraw-Hill Education.

Spruill, C., & LaBrecque, M. (2017). Preventing and treating pain and stress among infants in the newborn intensive care unit. In E. Eichenwald, A. Hansen, C. Martin, & A. Stark (Eds.), *Cloherty and Stark's manual of neonatal care* (8th ed., pp. 1022–1042). Philadelphia, PA: Wolters Kluwer.

Taketomo, C., Hodding, J., & Kraus, D. (2018). *Lexicomp pediatric & neonatal dosage handbook* (25th ed.). Hudson, OH: Wolters Kluwer.

14 GENETICS

Tami Wallace
Terri Schneider-Biehl
Ana Arias-Oliveras
Amy Koehn

INTRODUCTION

When a neonate is born with a congenital anomaly, chromosomal abnormality, or an inborn error of metabolism, they require assessment and management by a team of neonatal and multidisciplinary experts. Advances in medical technology have provided clinicians with the ability to diagnose many genetic abnormalities and diseases antenatally, but many may still not be evident until after delivery. A genetic evaluation can be multifaceted and quite complex. This evaluation includes a physical examination to identify dysmorphic features, a family history identifying lineage etiology, and skill in evaluating laboratory results. This evaluation must use a logical and disciplined methodologic process to ensure accurate diagnosis (Mathews & Robin, 2016). Early evaluation may enhance the appropriate treatment, provide a timely diagnosis, and optimize outcomes and prognosis for some infants and their families. This chapter provides a broad overview of genetic processes, diagnostic options, and treatments that are currently widely available.

GENETIC BASICS

Terminology

- *Chromosome*: This is a structure in a cell nucleus that has genes and transports genetic information. It is composed of complex, linear DNA molecules with structural proteins. Chromosomes are located in the nuclei of a cell. The expected total number of chromosomes in humans is 46 (diploid number). Of these, 44 are autosomes and two are sex chromosomes (Bajaj & Gross, 2015, p. 130; Matthews & Robin, 2016, pp. 763–766; Schiefelbein, 2015, p. 391).
  - A normal human karyotype has 46 chromosomes, 22 sets of autosomes, and one set of sex chromosomes. Genetic material is stained, and chromosomes are arranged by size and banding patterns. Each chromosome has a long arm, referred to as the q arm, and a short, or p arm; these are joined by a centromere (Bajaj & Gross, 2015, p. 144; Haldeman-Englert, Saitta, & Zackai, 2018).
- *Gene*: A gene is the functional unit of heredity (Matthews & Robin, 2016, p. 764). The small unit is responsible for inherited single characteristics, such as biochemical, physical, or physiologic traits. It is aligned in a linear sequence along with other genes along a chromosome.
- *DNA*: Deoxyribonucleic acid is a molecule that stores, processes, and duplicates vital hereditary information. It has two long strands, which form a double helix. Each DNA strand is composed of four nucleotides: guanine (G), adenine (A), thymine (T), and cytosine (C).
- The term *diploid* indicates the presence of the normal two copies (46) of all chromosomes (Matthews & Robin, 2016, p. 764).
  - *Haploid* indicates only one copy of all chromosomes (23) is present (Matthews & Robin, 2016, p. 764).
  - *Triploidy* indicates three sets, for a total of 69 chromosomes (Bajaj & Gross, 2015, p. 130).
  - *Tetraploidy* indicates four sets for a total of 96 chromosomes (Bajaj & Gross, 2015, p. 130).
  - The term *aneuploid* is used to describe any genotype in which the total chromosome number is not a multiple of 23. This indicates a net loss or gain of genetic material (Bajaj & Gross, 2015, p. 130; Matthews & Robin, 2016, p. 764).
- A person's *genotype* is the actual genetic makeup of an individual (Matthews & Robin, 2016, p. 764). This cannot be known without in-depth genetic analysis (Parikh & Mitchell, 2015, p. 436).
- *Phenotype* is a term used to describe the identifiable features and possible dysmorphisms of an individual. In clinical practice, phenotype refers to a collection of specific traits and physical findings, and the results of medical tests, such as laboratory, pathologic, and radiologic studies (Matthews & Robin, 2016, p. 764; Parikh & Mitchell, 2015, p. 436).
- A *congenital anomaly* is an internal or external structural defect that is present at birth. It may or may not be immediately visible (Matthews & Robin, 2016, p. 764).
  - It is important to distinguish the concepts of *congenital* and *genetic*, terms that are often confused. Congenital merely indicates that the feature is present at birth, and congenital features can have genetic or nongenetic causes (Parikh & Mitchell, 2015, p. 436).

Genetic Testing

KARYOTYPE

- To analyze chromosomes, a karyotype is produced (Figure 14.1). A karotype is the standard pictorial arrangement of chromosome pairs (Matthews & Robin, 2016, p. 764). The pairs are organized according to size and the evaluated for overall structure and banding pattern. Standardized reporting is guided by the International System for Cytogenetic Nomenclature

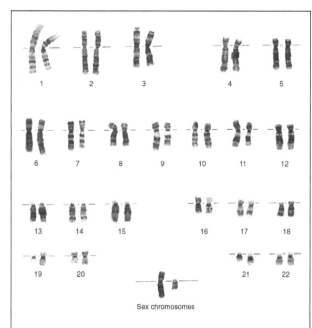

FIGURE 14.1 Karoytpe of a normal male

Source: Reproduced with permission from Bajaj, K., & Gross, S. J. (2015). Genetic aspects of perinatal disease and prenatal diagnosis. In R. Martin, A. Fanaroff, & M. Walsh (Eds.), *Fanaroff and Martin's neonatal-perinatal medicine: Diseases of the fetus and infant* (10th ed., pp. 130–146). Philadelphia, PA: Elsevier.

○ Chromosome report format: total chromosomal number, sex chromosomes, abnormalities. Example: The report may read 47, XX, + 21; this should be interpreted as 47 total chromosomes, XX (girl), extra 21st chromosome (trisomy 21; Bajaj & Gross, 2015, p. 130).

CHROMOSOMAL MICROARRAY (CMA)
● CMA is considered the first-line genetic test in neonates with multiple anomalies. It allows for the detection of deletions and duplications too small to be seen in a high-resolution chromosome analysis, and is able to identify an additional 5% to 10% of cases with genomic imbalance compared with routine karyotyping (Parikh & Mitchell, 2015, p. 454; Sterk, 2015, p. 771).
　○ CMA can also identify deletions or duplications, known as *copy number variants,* that may or may not be associated with the phenotype of the neonate. Thus, care must be taken when interpreting the CMA results (Parikh & Mitchell, 2015, p. 454).

FLUORESCENCE IN SITU HYBRIDIZATION (FISH)
● FISH testing can be ordered if there is a high level of suspicion for a known microdeletion syndrome not detectable by routine cytogenetic analysis. An example is testing for 22q11 deletion/velocardiofacial/DiGeorge syndrome or Williams syndrome.
　○ Testing with FISH has shown that a significant number of neonates with conotruncal heart defects have a 22q11 microdeletion, so this testing is indicated in all patients with truncus arteriosus, interrupted aortic arch, and tetralogy of Fallot (Parikh & Mitchell, 2015, p. 454).

○ A DNA probe is labeled with a fluorochrome, and the fluorescent signal is visible with microscopy. The number of signals can be counted (one signal = a specific genetic sequence). It is relatively rapid, but some chromosomal structural abnormalities may be missed as "the test detects genetic sequence, not its location" (Bajaj & Gross, 2015, p. 144; Haldeman-Englert et al., 2018; Sterk, 2015, p. 771).
○ A full karyotype should still be performed (Haldeman-Englert et al., 2018).

COMPARATIVE GENOMIC HYBRIDIZATION (ARRAY-CGH)
● This technology blends molecular techniques with cytogenetics and allows the genome to be scanned at a higher resolution than conventional techniques. It can measure the difference between two different DNA samples in copy number (dosage) of a particular segment of DNA. Thus, microscopic gains and losses from a patient sample can be quantified (Matthews & Robin, 2016, p. 768).

CHROMOSOMAL STRUCTURE ABNORMALITIES
● A *deletion* denotes a loss of a chromosomal segment (Schiefelbein, 2015, p. 394). This mechanism is responsible for a partial monosomy in the affected chromosome (Matthews & Robin, 2016, p. 767).
　○ Loss of material from the end of a chromosome is known as a *terminal deletion.*
　○ An *interstitial deletion* involves loss of chromosomal maternal that does not include the ends (Matthews & Robin, 2016, p. 767).
● *Duplication* of the DNA region that contains a gene results in a new mutation (Schiefelbein, 2015, p. 394). It is considered as a partial trisomy of a chromosome (Matthews & Robin, 2016, p. 767).
● *Nondisjunction* occurs when paired chromosomes fail to separate during cell division (Schiefelbein, 2015, p. 394). It is the most common mechanism for aneuploidy.
● *Translocation* occurs when a chromosomal agent attaches at an abnormal site, either in the wrong position on the same chromosome or attached on another chromosome (Schiefelbein, 2015, p. 394).
　○ *Unbalanced translocation* results in partial trisomy or monosomy (Matthews & Robin, 2016, p. 767).
Figure 14.2 summarized these structural anomalies.

Etiologies of Dysmorphology
● Anomalous external physical features are called *dysmorphisms* and can be clues to the underlying cause or developmental defect. A useful approach to determining the etiology of a congenital anomaly is to consider whether it represents a malformation, deformation, or disruption of normal development (Parikh & Mitchell, 2015, p. 436).

MALFORMATION/DISRUPTION/DEFORMATION
● A *malformation* implies an abnormal morphogenesis of the underlying tissue owing to a genetic or teratogenic factor. Malformations are a primary structural defect that results from a localized error of morphogenesis and that results in abnormal development (Matthews & Robin, 2016, p. 764). The effects are primary structural defects in

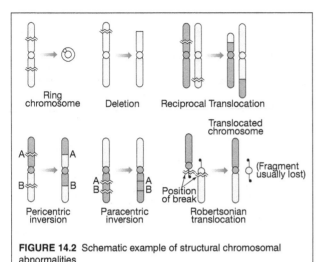

FIGURE 14.2 Schematic example of structural chromosomal abnormalities

Ring chromosome

Deletion

Reciprocal Translocation

Translocated chromosome

(Fragment usually lost)

Pericentric inversion

Paracentric inversion

Position of break

Robertsonian translocation

tissue formation, such as a neural tube defect or a congenital heart defect (Parikh & Mitchell, 2015, p. 436; Sterk, 2015, p. 768).

- A *deformation* results from abnormal mechanical forces, such as intrauterine constraint, acting on otherwise normal tissues (e.g., club foot). A variety of maternal factors can cause fetal constraint, and common examples include breech or other abnormal positioning in utero, oligohydramnios, and uterine anomalies (Parikh & Mitchell, 2015, p. 436; Sterk, 2015, p. 768).

- A *disruption* represents the destruction or interruption of intrinsically normal tissue. Disruptions usually affect a body part, not a specific organ (e.g., amniotic bands). Monozygotic twinning and prenatal cocaine exposure are common predisposing factors for disruptions on the basis of vascular interruption (Parikh & Mitchell, 2015, p. 436; Sterk, 2015, p. 768).

ASSOCIATION/SYNDROME/SEQUENCE

- An *association* refers to a nonrandom occurrence of multiple malformations for which no specific or common etiology has been identified (Parikh & Mitchell, 2015, p. 437).
  - Example: VATER/VACTERL Association, **V**ertebral, **A**nal, **C**ardiac, **T**racheal, **E**sophageal, **R**enal, **L**imb (radial).
    - Although the VACTERL association has been associated with certain conditions such as maternal diabetes, a genetic cause for the spectrum of malformations has not (Parikh & Mitchell, 2015, p. 467).

- A *syndrome* is a pattern of anomalies with a single specific cause (usually genetic). Previously known as an association, it is now known that CHARGE is a syndrome that originates from mutations in the CHD7 gene. These mutations have been discovered as causative in over half of affected children, although the exact mechanism for the multiple malformations is not clear at this time.
  - CHARGE: **C**oloboma, **H**eart anomalies, choanal **A**tresia, **R**estriction of growth and development, **G**enital and **E**ar (Parikh & Mitchell, 2015, p. 437; Sterk, 2025, p. 768).

- *Sequence* refers to a pattern of multiple anomalies derived from a single known or presumed cause.

- An example is the oligohydramnios sequence, often referred to as Potter syndrome. Potter syndrome demonstrates a constellation of features, which are primarily due to a lack of amniotic fluid during gestation (Parikh & Mitchell, 2015, p. 436; Sterk, 2015, p. 768).
- Another example is Pierre Robin sequence, in which features are altered due to a malformed mandible, which causes the tongue to move backward and upward in the oral cavity (Parikh & Mitchell, 2015, p. 437).

PRINCIPLES OF INHERITANCE

Mendelian Inheritance

AUTOSOMAL DISORDERS

- Single-gene traits for which mutations cause predictable disease are described as exhibiting Mendelian inheritance because they follow the rules that he originally described.
- Variants of a gene are called *alleles*. Some versions of the gene are *mutations*, not all of which cause disease. Mutations to genetic traits can either be inherited from parents or develop de novo, meaning the mutation occurred as a random error (Bajaj & Gross, 2015, p. 132).
- Autosomal dominant
  - The phenotype of one allele will express itself over a recessive allele.
  - Approximately half of Mendelian disorders are inherited in an autosomal dominant fashion. This indicates that the phenotype usually appears in every generation, with each affected person having an affected parent. For each offspring of an affected parent, the risk of inheriting the mutated allele is 50% (Bajaj & Gross, 2015, p. 132; Sterk, 2015, p. 769).
- Autosomal recessive
  - An autosomal recessive condition occurs when an individual possesses two mutant alleles that were inherited from heterozygous parents (Bajaj & Gross, 2015, p. 133).
  - An individual with one normal allele does not manifest the disease because the normal gene copy is able to compensate (Bajaj & Gross, 2015, p. 134). The phenotype of the recessive allele will not be expressed in the presence of a dominant allele. The phenotype of the recessive allele will be expressed only when two of the recessive alleles are present.
  - If both parents are carriers of a mutated allele, 25% of offspring have the autosomal recessive disease.
    - Consanguineous parents (individuals who are second cousins or closer) present an increased risk for passing an autosomal recessive disorder to an offspring because there is a higher likelihood that both parents carry the same recessive mutation (Bajaj & Gross, 2015, p. 134; Sterk, 2015, p. 769).
- Sex linked
  - Disorders caused by abnormalities on one of the sex chromosomes. They may be dominant or recessive. Disorders of genes located on the X chromosome have a characteristic pattern of inheritance that is affected by gender.
    - Males with an X-linked mutant allele are described as being hemizygous for that allele. Males have a 50% chance of inheriting a mutant allele if the mother is a carrier.

- Females can be homozygous dominate-type allele, homozygous mutant allele, or a heterozygote (Bajaj & Gross, 2015, p. 134).
  - X-linked recessive disorders are generally seen in males and rarely seen in females who are homozygous for the mutation. An X-linked recessive mutation is phenotypically expressed in all males (Bajaj & Gross, 2015, p. 134).

Non-Mendelian Patterns

- Multifactorial or complex
  - *Multifactorial* or *complex* inheritance disorders have a greater incidence than disorders secondary to chromosomal or single-gene mutations. These disorders affect certain families more than others, but do not follow Mendelian patterns of inheritance or fit into the non-Mendelian inheritance phenomenon (Bajaj & Gross, 2015, p. 136). These occur when one or more genetic susceptibility factors combine with environmental factors and random developmental events (Parikh & Mitchell, 2015, p. 437).
- Mitochondrial inheritance (mtDNA)
  - Mitochondrial DNA is located only in the mitochondria of a cell and inherited entirely from maternal side. More than 100 different mutations in mtDNA have been identified to cause disease in humans. Most of these involve the central nervous system or musculoskeletal system.
    - Mitochondrial disease typically manifests as dysfunction in high energy-consuming organs such as the brain, muscle, heart, and kidneys. Poor growth, muscle weakness, loss of coordination, or developmental delay are common (Bajaj & Gross, 2015, p. 135).
- Epigenetics
  - Epigenetics refers to modification of genes that determines whether a gene is expressed or not.
    - Imprinting refers to a phenomenon in which genetic material is differentially expressed depending on whether it was inherited from the father or the mother. Classic examples of disorders related to genomic imprinting are Prader–Willi and Angelman syndromes. Both these syndromes involve the long arm of chromosome 15 (Bajaj & Gross, 2015, p. 135).

GENETIC (CHROMOSOMAL) DISORDERS

Trisomy

TRISOMY 21 AKA DOWN SYNDROME
Incidence and Etiology

- Affected individuals have three copies of chromosome 21, for a total of 47 chromosomes (Sterk, 2015, p. 772).
- More than 90% Trisomy 21 syndromes occur secondary to meiotic nondisjunction, but 3% to 5% of cases are caused by a translocation that could be either de novo or inherited from a balanced translocation–carrier parent that subsequently becomes unbalanced and trisomic in the baby (Haldeman-Englert et al., 2018, p. 213; Sterk, 2015, p. 771).
  - Of these infants, 25% receive the extra chromosome from their father. Familial transmission is autosomal dominate (Schiefelbein, 2015, p. 403).
- The more common occurrence of Down syndrome in babies of older mothers led to the recommendation for

prenatal karyotyping in the presence of advanced maternal age (>35 years) at the time of conception (Haldeman-Englert et al., 2018, p. 213).
  - Incidences are reported at one in 270 pregnancies in mothers aged 35 to 39 years and one in 100 for mothers aged 40 to 44 years. By ages 45 to 50 mothers have a one in 50 chance of conceiving an infant who will be affected with Trisomy 21 (Schiefelbein, 2015, p. 403; Sterk, 2015, p. 773).

CLINICAL FEATURES AND ASSOCIATED ANOMALIES

- Most patients with Down syndrome, if it is not diagnosed prenatally, are usually recognized at birth because of the typical phenotypic features (Haldeman-Englert et al., 2018, p. 213).
- Physical features may include brachycephaly, up-slanted palpebral fissures, epicanthal folds, Brushfield spots in irises, a flattened nasal bridge, small posteriorly rotated ears, a prominent tongue, and short neck with excessive nuchal folds. The hand may have single palmar creases and fifth finger clinodactyly; the foot may have an exaggerated gap between the first and second toes. Hypotonia is also often noted (Haldeman-Englert et al., 2018; Sterk, 2015, p. 773).
  - Cardiac defects occur in 50% of infants with Trisomy 21. The most frequent defects are atrioventricular canal defects, but also ventricular septal defect (VSD), ASD, TOF, and patent ductus arterioles (PDA) (Haldeman-Englert et al., 2018, p. 214; Sterk, 2015, p. 773).
  - Gastrointestinal anomalies may include duodenal atresia and Hirschsprung disease. Rarer findings are esophageal atresia, fistulas, and webs (Schiefelbein, 2015, p. 404).

COMPLICATIONS AND OUTCOMES

- Patients with Down syndrome demonstrate a wide range of developmental abilities, with highly variable personalities. Central hypotonia with concomitant motor delay is most pronounced in the first 3 years of life, as are language delays. Early intervention and developmental therapy are necessary for maximizing the developmental outcome (Haldeman-Englert et al., 2018, p. 214).
- Significantly decreased postnatal growth velocity is encountered in these patients. Separate growth curves have been devised for patients with Down syndrome (Haldeman-Englert et al., 2018, p. 214).
- An initial ophthalmologic evaluation is also indicated in the first few months of life, and then annually, because strabismus, cataracts, myopia, and glaucoma have been shown to be more common in children with Down syndrome (Haldeman-Englert et al., 2018, p. 214).
- Bone marrow dyscrasias, such as neonatal thrombocytopenia, and transient self-resolving myeloproliferative disorders, such as leukemoid reaction, have been observed during the first year of life. An elevated rate of leukemia with a relative risk 10 to 18 times greater than normal up to age 16 years has been identified (Haldeman-Englert et al., 2018, p. 214; Sterk, 2015, p. 773).
- The most common causes of death in patients with Down syndrome are related to congenital heart disease, to infection (e.g., pneumonia) that is thought to be associated with defects in T-cell maturation and function, and to malignancy. Once medical and surgical interventions for the correction of associated congenital malformations are complete and successful, the long-term survival rate is good. However, less than half of patients survive to 60 years, and

less than 15% survive past 68 years (Haldeman-Englert et al., 2018, p. 214; Sterk, 2015, p. 774).

Trisomy 18 aka Edwards Syndrome

INCIDENCE AND ETIOLOGY

- Affected individuals have three copies of chromosomes 18 for a total of 47 chromosomes (Sterk, 2015, p. 774).
- Occurs most frequently due to nondisjunction (80%), but also may be caused by a partial trisomy, translocation, or mosaicism (5%; Schiefelbein, 2015, p. 404; Sterk, 2015, p. 774).
  - ○ Severe pattern: Handicaps are severe with short life expectancy.
  - ○ Mosaic pattern: Some cells have the normal complement of genetic material; the remaining have the trisomy 18 pattern. Infants are less severely affected and have a longer life expectancy.
  - ○ Partial pattern: Dependent on the portion of the chromosome affected, affects range from minimal handicaps and few abnormalities to partial syndrome with less profound developmental delays and longer survival (Sterk, 2015, p. 774).
- Trisomy 18 is associated with a high rate of intrauterine demise. It is estimated that only 5% of conceptuses with trisomy 18 survive to birth and that 30% of fetuses in whom trisomy 18 is diagnosed by second-trimester amniocentesis die before the end of the pregnancy (Haldeman-Englert et al., 2018, p. 215; Sterk, 2015, p. 774).

CLINICAL FEATURES AND ASSOCIATED ANOMALIES

- Phenotypic features that are notable at birth include intrauterine growth restriction (IUGR) with a small narrow cranium with prominent occiput, open metopic suture, low-set and posteriorly rotated ears, and micrognathia. Characteristic are clenched hands with overlapping fingers, hypoplastic nails, and rocker bottom feet (Haldeman-Englert et al., 2018, p. 215; Schiefelbein, 2015, p. 404; Sterk, 2015, p. 774).
- Additional malformations include heart defects (ASD, VSD, PDA, pulmonic stenosis, aortic coarctation), cleft palate, club foot deformity, renal malformations (horseshoe, ectopic kidneys), brain anomalies, choanal atresia, eye malformations, vertebral anomalies, hypospadias, cryptorchidism, and limb defects (Haldeman-Englert et al., 2018, p. 215; Sterk, 2015, p. 776).

COMPLICATIONS AND OUTCOMES

- There is a high rate of intrauterine demise. Death after delivery is usually from central apnea or congestive heart failure (Bajaj & Gross, 2015; Haldeman-Englert et al., 2018).
- The prognosis in this disorder is extremely poor, with more than 90% of babies succumbing in the first 6 months of life and only 5% alive at 1 year old. Causes of death include central apnea, infection, and congestive heart failure (Haldeman-Englert et al., 2018, p. 215; Schiefelbein, 2015, p. 405).
- Infants will full trisomy are usually fragile, and prognosis for survival is poor. Those who survive the first year deal with feeding, growth, and developmental issues. They are generally are unable to walk unsupported and are capable of only limited verbal communication (Sterk, 2015, p. 776).

Trisomy 13 aka Patau Syndrome

INCIDENCE AND ETIOLOGY

- Affected individuals have three copies of the chromosome 13 for a total of 47 chromosomes. It is the fourth most common autosomal dominate disorder resulting from chromosomal nondisjunction (Sterk, 2015, p. 776).
- Approximately 2% to 3% of fetuses with trisomy 13 survive to birth, with a frequency of one in 12,500 to one in 21,000 live births (Haldeman-Englert et al., 2018, p. 216).
- Abnormal noninvasive screening, such as ultrasound or maternal screens, identifies risk and prompt genetic testing. There is a high rate of intrauterine demise. It is unusual for infants to survive out of the newborn period (Bajaj & Gross, 2015).

CLINICAL FEATURES AND ASSOCIATED ANOMALIES

- Infants with Trisomy 13 are known to have multiple midline malformations, which may include congenital heart disease, cleft palate, holoprosencephaly, renal anomalies, and postaxial polydactyly. Eye anomalies and scalp defects can suggest the diagnosis. Brain malformations such as microcephaly and holoprosencephaly are found in more than half of patients with concomitant seizure disorders (Haldeman-Englert et al., 2018, p. 216; Schiefelbein, 2015, p. 405; Sterk, 2015, p. 777).
  - ○ Aplasia cutis congenita is a congenital absence of skin involving the scalp. Lesions have sharp margins and may present as ulcers, bullae, or scars. Most defects are small and superficial (Sterk, 2015, p. 777).
- Congenital heart disease is present in approximately 80% of patients, usually VSD, ASD, PDA, or dextrocardia. Limb anomalies, such as postaxial polydactyly, single palmar creases, and hyperconvex narrow fingernails, are also seen (Haldeman-Englert et al., 2018, p. 216).

COMPLICATIONS AND OUTCOMES

- The presence of holoprosencephaly is the single most important factor predicting survival (Sterk, 2015, p. 777).
- Prognosis is extremely poor, with 80% mortality in the neonatal period and less than 5% of patients surviving to 6 months old. Developmental delays are profound, and many patients are blind and deaf. Feeding difficulties are typical (Haldeman-Englert et al., 2018, p. 216; Schiefelbein, 2015, p. 405).

MONOSOMY

Turner Syndrome (45, X)

INCIDENCE AND ETIOLOGY

- Turner syndrome described a phenotype associated with loss of all or part of one copy of the X chromosome in approximately one in 2,500 female infants. Studies indicate that approximately 80% of cases, it is the paternally derived X chromosome that is lost.
  - ○ The 45, X karyotype or loss of one entire X chromosome accounts for approximately half of the cases.
  - ○ A variety of X chromosome anomalies, including deletions and translocations, account for the remainder of the causes (Haldeman-Englert et al., 2018, p. 216; Sterk, 2015, p. 778).

CLINICAL FEATURES AND ASSOCIATED ANOMALIES

- Turner syndrome exhibits a wide variety of presentations. At birth, notable findings are short stature, webbed neck, low posterior hairline, broad nasal bridge, low set ears with anomalous auricles, ptosis of eyelids, shield chest, and lymph edema of hands and feet. The syndrome is associated with congenital heart disease, which may include bicuspid aortic valve, coarctation of the aorta, valvular aortic stenosis, and mitral valve prolapse (Haldeman-Englert et al., 2018, p. 216; Sterk, 2015, p. 778).

COMPLICATIONS AND OUTCOMES

- Growth issues, especially short stature, are the predominant concern in childhood and adolescence; growth hormone therapy has been shown to increase final adult height, but the age of initiation of therapy not yet established.
- Primary ovarian failure caused by gonadal dysplasia (streak gonads) can result in delay of secondary sexual characteristics and primary amenorrhea (Haldeman-Englert et al., 2018, p. 216; Sterk, 2015, p. 779).

DELETION SYNDROME

DiGeorge Syndrome—22q11.2 Deletion

INCIDENCE AND ETIOLOGY

- Patients with classically termed conditions DiGeorge, velocardiofacial, and conotruncal anomaly face syndromes all reflect features of the same genomic disorder, a deletion of 22q11.2, which is the most commonly occurring microdeletion syndrome in humans. Estimates indicate that 22q11.2 microdeletion syndrome occurs in approximately one in 1,000 fetuses.
- Most 22q11 deletions occur as de novo events, with less than 10% of them being inherited from an affected parent (Haldeman-Englert et al., 2018, p. 218). Both parents must be tested to determine carrier status (Sterk, 2015, p. 777).

CLINICAL FEATURES AND ASSOCIATED ANOMALIES

- Clinical features include facial dysmorphia, which may include hooded eyelids, hypertelorism, overfolded ears, bulbous nasal tip, a small mouth, and micrognathia.
- Most patients with a deletion receive the diagnosis following identification of significant cardiovascular malformations, conotruncal cardiac anomaly including interrupted aortic arch type B, truncus arteriosus, or tetralogy of Fallot.
- With further evaluation, often aplasia or hypoplasia of the thymus and parathyroid glands are noted, along with functional T-cell abnormalities and hypocalcemia (Haldeman-Englert et al., 2018, p. 218).
  - Hypocalcemia occurs in 60% of neonates; severe cases will cause seizures (Sterk, 2015, p. 778).

COMPLICATIONS AND OUTCOMES

- Developmental delays or learning disabilities have been reported in most patients with 22q11.2 deletion syndrome, and a wide range of developmental and behavioral findings have been observed in young children.
  - In the preschool years, affected children were most commonly found to be hypotonic and developmentally

delayed, with language and speech difficulties; however, one-third of patients functioned within the average range (Haldeman-Englert et al., 2018, p. 218; Sterk, 2015, p. 778).
- Death is primarily related to severity of cardiac defects (Sterk, 2015, p. 778).

SINGLE-GENE DISORDER

Cystic Fibrosis

INCIDENCE AND ETIOLOGY

- Cystic fibrosis (CF), the most common autosomal recessive disease in live-born infants, is the result of mutations of a large gene on chromosome 7 that encodes the cystic fibrosis transmembrane conductance regulator (CFTR) protein (Bajaj & Gross, 2015, p. 141; Gross & Gheorghe, 2018, p. 166).
- The carrier rate differs based on ethnic origin; individuals of Asian descent have the lowest carrier rates and Ashkenazi Jewish and non-Hispanic White individuals have the highest (Gross & Gheorghe, 2018, p. 167).

CLINICAL FEATURES AND ASSOCIATED ANOMALIES

- Multiorgan disorder impacts the pulmonary, pancreatic, and gastrointestinal systems, but does not affect intelligence.
- This disorder can present very early in life with meconium ileus, which is an obstruction of the ileum as a result of thick meconium plugs. On abdominal x-rays, the small bowel loops may have a ground-glass appearance (Neuhauser sign) resulting from dilated loops of bowel with bubbles of gas and meconium without air–fluid levels.
  - Half of the infants presenting with meconium ileus develop complications, including peritonitis, volvulus, atresia, and necrosis.
  - The presence of meconium plug syndrome, which is a temporary obstruction of the distal colon, should also raise concerns for the possibility of cystic fibrosis (CF) (Larson-Nath, Gurram, & Chelimsky, 2015, p. 1382).
- Another common presentation of CF is chronic diarrhea secondary to pancreatic fat malabsorption (Larson-Nath et al., 2015, p. 1383).
- Infants can present less commonly with extrahepatic biliary duct obstruction as a result of thick inspissated bile. Therefore, CF should be included in the differential diagnosis of any neonate with prolonged conjugated hyperbilirubinemia (Larson-Nath et al., 2015, p. 1383).

COMPLICATIONS AND OUTCOMES

- The screening program is less accurate in children with less common alleles; therefore, a normal newborn screen does not rule out the presence of CF. The diagnosis is confirmed by a sweat chloride test showing a chloride greater than 60 mEq/L, which is present in 99% of patients with CF (Larson-Nath et al., 2015, p. 1383).
- Early and presymptomatic diagnosis through screening leads to early nutritional therapy, pancreatic enzyme replacement, and antibiotic prophylaxis for pulmonary infection (Sahai & Levy, 2018, p. 343).

○ Median survival is approximately 37 years, with respiratory failure as the most common cause of death (Bajaj & Gross, 2015, p. 142).

• It is important for providers to discuss with their patients that a negative screen decreases the risk of being a carrier, but does not eliminate it completely because screening does not test for all possible mutations (Gross & Gheorghe, 2018, p. 167).

• Cell-based therapies, advances in bone marrow transplantation, direct treatment of metabolic disorders, and mutation-specific interventions for cystic fibrosis and have all provided hope to families with a child in whom diagnosis, but not curative therapy. Now a new technology, clustered regularly interspaced short palindromic repeats (CRISPR)/CRISPR-associated protein-9 nuclease (Cas9) holds out a new promise that targeted gene editing may be possible to apply on an individual basis (Cotton & Murray, 2018, p. 189).

IMPRINTING DISORDER

Beckwith–Wiedemann syndrome

INCIDENCE AND ETIOLOGY

• Beckwith–Wiedemann syndrome affects approximately 1 in 14,000 newborns and manifests itself as an overgrowth syndrome in the neonatal period (Haldeman-Englert et al., 2018, p. 222).

• Genetic studies in patients with Beckwith–Wiedemann syndrome have identified three major subgroups of patients: familial, sporadic, and chromosomally abnormal. Sporadic causes 85% of cases, with the remaining being due to inherited autosomal dominant 11p15, methylation of H19/IGF2, and mutation of CDK1C gene (Devaskar & Garg, 2015, p. 1449; Haldeman-Englert et al., 2018, p. 223).

○ Mutations causing overexpression of the paternal allele or underexpression of the maternal allele can result in an imbalance of expression, leading to the overgrowth and tumor formation encountered in these patients (Haldeman-Englert et al., 2018, p. 223).

○ It has been observed that pregnancies that are the result of assisted reproductive therapy (ART) are at an increased risk for rare imprinting disorders, such as Beckwith–Wiedemann syndrome, suggesting that epigenetic changes may occur as a result of ART (Bajaj & Gross, 2015, p. 145).

CLINICAL FEATURES AND ASSOCIATED ANOMALIES

• The characteristic findings are macrosomia, abdominal wall defect, and macroglossia. Often called congenital overgrowth syndrome (Devaskar & Garg, 2015, p. 1448). Hemihypertrophy caused by asymmetric growth is common, as is visceromegaly of various organs, including the spleen, kidneys, liver, pancreas, and adrenal gland (Haldeman-Englert et al., 2018, p. 222).

○ Other common features are being large for gestational age (somatic overgrowth), macroglossia, transverse ear lobe crease, renal abnormalities, visceromegaly, hemihypertrophy, abdominal wall defects.

• Hypoglycemia is present in at least half the cases, and may be manifested soon after birth. Endocrine evaluation of the few reported cases has not been consistent. However, based on the clinical features of hypoglycemia with low free fatty acids (FFAs) and ketones and autopsy findings of islet cell hyperplasia, it is believed that hypoglycemia is caused by hyperinsulinism in this syndrome (Devaskar & Garg, 2015, p. 1449).

COMPLICATIONS AND OUTCOMES

• Treatment of hypoglycemia may require high caloric intake and therapy to inhibit insulin secretion. May require central line for increase in glucose infusion rates. Medication therapy can include diazoxide and octreotide.

• Infants with this disorder are predisposed to certain malignancies (adrenal carcinoma, nephroblastoma) and appear to have an increased risk for malignancies associated with hemihypertrophy (Devaskar & Garg, 2015, p. 1449).

○ Routine ultrasonograms from the neonatal time through the school-age years (approximately 8 years old) are necessary because the increased risk of malignant tumors, especially Wilms tumor. The estimated risk is as high as 8% for patients with hemihypertrophy (Haldeman-Englert et al., 2018, p. 222).

NONCHROMOSOMAL DISORDERS

Malformation Disorders

OSTEOGENESIS IMPERFECTA (OI)

Incidence and Etiology

• Disorder is caused by mutations of COL1Al and COL1A2 genes on chromosomes 17q21 and 17q22.l. The result of the mutation is an abnormality of type I collagen. Overall incidence is three to four per 100,000 (Sterk, 2015, p. 780). The more severe forms of OI are the result of abnormal collagen synthesis rather than decreased production (Tiller & Bellus, 2018, p. 1454).

• Type II and III are generally spontaneous dominant acting gene mutation with approximately a 6% reoccurrence risk. Other types are mostly autosomal dominate and rate recessive forms (Haldeman-Englert et al., 2018).

CLINICAL FEATURES AND ASSOCIATED ANOMALIES

• Clinical features: Six clinical types (in decreasing order of severity) have been identified; types I, II, and III are considered severe (Sterk, 2015, p. 780).

• All clinical types share common findings of low birthweight, short stature, macrocephaly, triangular-appearing facies (with a bossed, broad forehead and a tapered, pointed chin), blue sclerae, and short-limbed extremities (Sterk, 2015, p. 781; Tiller & Bellus, 2018, p. 1454).

○ Associated findings are hearing loss, platelet dysfunction, and scoliosis (Sterk, 2015, p. 781)

COMPLICATIONS AND OUTCOMES

• Depending on the type of osteogenesis, treatment will vary extensively (Sterk, 2015, p. 781).

• Sixty percent of affected babies are stillborn or die during the first day of life, and 80% die by 1 month. Those severely affected with OI type II are not expected to survive the neonatal period (Tiller & Bellus, 2018, pp. 1454, 1456).

INBORN ERRORS OF METABOLISM (IEM)

Incidence and Etiology

- The term *inborn errors of metabolism* was coined in the early 20th century to describe diseases caused by errors and variations in chemical pathways (Cotton & Murray, 2018, p. 183).
- IEM are genetic biochemical disorders in which the function of a protein is compromised, resulting in alteration of the structure or amount of the protein synthesized.
    - These gene mutations produce deficiencies in enzymes, cofactors, transport proteins, and cellular processes. Interruptions of any of the steps in the formation of the coenzyme can lead to disease (Sterk, 2015, p. 789).
- IEM is most often due to an autosomal recessive inheritance. Other mechanisms of inheritance are autosomal dominant and sex-linked. The majority of mutations are of no consequence; however, others produce disease states ranging from mild to severe (Sterk, 2015, p. 789).
- IEM can be classified into three groups:
    - Defects involving complex molecules result from defective function of enzymes responsible for breaking down complex glycosaminoglycans and sphingolipids. Symptoms are not generally evident at birth as pathologic metabolites accumulate slowly.
    - Disorders of fatty acid metabolism are defects concerning the intermediary metabolism of small molecules-glucose, lactate, amino acids, organic acids, and ammonia.
    - Metabolic disorders in which there is insufficient generation of energy by the mitochondria are complex processes involving problems in either the manufacture, the failure of delivery, the inability to break down, or the deficient function of mitochondrial substrates and energy-generating systems (Sterk, 2015, p. 789).

Clinical Presentation and Associated Anomalies

- An infant may or may not present with an IEM in the newborn period. Consider IEM as a differential diagnosis in any an otherwise healthy infant with an acute decompensation of unknown etiology. Early recognition of the symptoms can lead to appropriate medical interventions, and a delay in treatment may have severe consequences, such as impaired neurodevelopmental outcomes or death.
- Symptoms of possible IEMs include:
    - Neurologic changes in activity and/or muscle tone, new onset of seizures
    - Cataracts, glaucoma, dislocated lenses of the eyes
    - Respiratory changes ranging from tachypnea to apnea
    - Cardiomyopathies
    - Onset of vomiting, long-term failure to gain weight
    - Jaundice, hepatomeglay, refractory hypoglycemia
    - Unusual body or uninary odor (Sterk, 2015, p. 790)
- An initial laboratory workup when IEM is suspected includes:
    - Blood gas analysis and lactate level, serum electrolytes, glucose, and ammonia level, urinalysis (urine pH, ketones)

- Newborn Screening
    - Newborn screening is a practice to test all newborns for specific disorders that can cause serious health issues. The goal is to identify IEM that will lead to early treatment and prevention of major sequelae (Sterk, 2015, p. 790).
    - With the introduction of mass spectrometry, a single blood spot can detect greater than 50 disorders. Each state can choose which tests are collected; however, all states are required to screen for phenylketonuria (PKU), hypothyroidism, and glactosemia (Sahai & Levy, 2018, p. 333; Sterk, 2015, p. 790).
- Second-line workup includes:
    - Serum and urine amino acids and urine organic acids (Cederbaum, 2018, pp. 215–220; Matthews & Robin, 2016, pp. 776–777)

Complications and Outcomes

- Specific genetic biomarkers may be obtained later in the clinical course once a full family history is completed by the genetic or metabolic pediatric specialist, in addition to a full assessment of laboratory results and a full physical examination. Some IEM may need to be supplemented with radiographic testing, such as an MRI of the brain.
- Genetic testing of the biological parents of the infant/child will be beneficial for future pregnancies.

DISORDERS OF METABOLISM

- Disorders of metabolism are classified as carbohydrate disorders, urea cycle disorders, amino acid metabolism disorders, organic acidemias, fatty acid oxidation disorders, ketone metabolism disorders, primary lactic acidosis, lysosomal storage disorders, and congenital disorders of glycosylation. See Table 14.1 for a summary of IEMs by classification.

Carbohydrate Disorders

- The most common disorder is galactosemia, a defect in one of three enzymes in the galactose metabolic pathway.
- Most often presents in the newborn period.
- Identified on newborn screen (Merritt & Gallagher, 2018)

Further details on carbohydrate disorders are summarized in Table 14.2.

Urea Cycle Disorders

- Defective process, caused by an inhibited synthesis of urea from ammonia
- Two common pathways: proximal and distal urea cycle disorders
- Most often presents within the first 24 hours of life.
- Most common clinical presentation is poor feeding, lethargy.
- Hyperammonemia present (Merritt & Gallagher, 2018, pp. 236–238)

Further details on urea cycle disorders are summarized in Table 14.3.

TABLE 14.1 Summary of Inborn Errors of Metabolism Classification

Amino Acid/Urea Cycle Disorders	Organic Acid Disorders	Fatty Acid Oxidation Disorders	Others
Phenylketonuria	Maple syrup urine disease	Medium chain Acyl-CoA Dehydrogenase deficiency	Congenital adrenal hyperplasia
Homocystinuria	Isovaleric acidemia	Short-chain Acyl-CoA Dehydrogenase deficiency	Galactosemia
Hypermethionemia	Propionic acidemia	Very long chain Acyl-CoA Dehydrogenase deficiency	Sickle cell disease
Argininosuccinic acidemia	Glutaric acidemia type I	Glutaric acidemia type II	Hemoglobinopathies
Citrullinemia	Isolbutyrul—CoA dehydrogenase deficiency	Carnitine palmityl transferase deficiency	Congenital hypothyriodism
Argininemia	3-Hydroxy-3 methylglutaryl-CoA lyase deficiency	Carnitine/acylcarnitine translocase deficiency	
Tyrosinemia types I and II	2-Mehylbutyryl-CoA dehydrogenase deficiency	Multiple CoA carboxylase deficiency	
	3-Methylcrotonyl-CoA carboxylase deficiency	Trifunctional protein deficiency	

Sources: Data from Matthews, A. L., & Robin, N. H. (2016). Genetic disorders, malformations, and inborn errors of metabolism. In S. Gardner, B. Carter, M. Hines, & J. Hernandez (Eds.), *Merenstein & Gardner's handbook of neonatal intensive care* (8th ed., pp. 763–785). St. Louis, MO: Elsevier; Sahai, I., & Levy, H. (2018). Newborn screening. In C. Gleason & S. Juul (Eds.), *Avery's diseases of the newborn* (10th ed., pp. 332–346.e3). Philadelphia, PA: Elsevier.

TABLE 14.2 Carbohydrate Metabolism Disorder

Disorder	Defective Process	Characteristics
Galactosemia Galactose-1-phosphate uridyltransferase deficiency (GALT) Galactokinase (GALK) Uridine diphosphate Galactose-4-epimerase(GALE)	A defect in one of three enzymes in the galactose metabolic pathway	GALT – Clinical jaundice – Coagulopathy – Most common in newborn period – Identified on the newborn screen (NBS) – Cataracts – *Escherichia coli* sepsis if untreated – Liver failure if untreated GALE – May be identified on NBS – Deficient enzyme activity in red blood cell (RBC) – Liver failure if untreated GALK – Cataracts
Glycogen storage diseases (GSDs) Hepatic glycogen storage diseases Muscular glycogen storage diseases	– defective glycogen synthesis – abnormal utilization for energy production – categorized by how they affect liver	Hypoglycemia Infantile cardiomyopathy Muscular glycogen storage diseases—most common form of GSD in the neonatal period. Also a lysosomal storage disease
Fructose metabolism hereditary fructose intolerance (HFI)	Abnormal enzyme activity in liver tissue and/or sequencing of ALDOB	– Most often later infancy – Hypoglycemia, pallor, GI disturbances

GI, gastrointestinal.

Source: Data from Merritt, J. L., & Gallagher, R. (2018). Inborn errors of carbohydrate, ammonia, amino acid, and organic acid metabolism. In C. Gleason & S. Juul (Eds.), *Avery's diseases of the newborn* (10th ed., pp. 230–252.e4). Philadelphia, PA: Elsevier.

Amino Acid Metabolism Disorders

- Most common disorder is maple syrup urine disease, which is caused by a branched-chain α-ketoacid dehydrogenase (BCKAD) complex deficiency.
- Presents within the first 48 hours of life
- Clinical presentation is poor feeding, lethargy, and having an odor of maple syrup (Merritt & Gallagher, 2018, pp. 238–241).

Further details on amino acid metabolism disorders are summarized in Table 14.4.

Organic Acidemias

- Defects in pathways of catabolism of more than one of the following: leucine, isoleucine, valine
- Clinical presentation consistent with those of hyperammonemia

- Most disorders in this category present within the newborn period except for glutaric aciduria type 1 (Merritt & Gallagher, 2018, pp. 242–245).

Further details on organic acidemias are summarized in Table 14.5.

Fatty Acid Oxidation Disorders

- Defective pathway: Failure of β-oxidation within, or transport of fatty acids into, the mitochondria
- Most common disorder: medium-chain acyl-CoA dehydrogenase deficiency.
- Presents in the newborn period (Merritt & Gallagher, 2018, pp. 245–248)

Further details on fatty acid oxidation disorders are summarized in Table 14.6.

TABLE 14.3 Urea Cycle Disorder (UCD)

Disorder	Defective Process	Characteristics
Proximal UCD N-acetylglutamate synthase deficiency (NAGS) Carbamyl phosphate synthetase I (CPSI) deficiency Ornithine transcarbamylase deficiency (OTCD) Distal UCD Argininosuccinate synthetase deficiency Argininosuccinate lyase deficiency Arginase 1 deficiency	Inhibited synthesis of urea from ammonia	– Onset ~24 hours of life – Poor feeding – Emesis – Hyperventilation – Altered level of consciousness; lethargy – Symptoms secondary to hyperammonemia – Encephalopathy – Seizures - Hallmark sign: hyperammonemia Delayed treatment fatal

Source: Data from Merritt, J. L., & Gallagher, R. (2018). Inborn errors of carbohydrate, ammonia, amino acid, and organic acid metabolism. In C. Gleason & S. Juul (Eds.), *Avery's diseases of the newborn* (10th ed., pp. 230–252.e4). Philadelphia, PA: Elsevier.

TABLE 14.4 Amino Acid Metabolism Disorder

Disorder	Defective Process	Characteristics
Maple syrup urine disease	Branched-chain α-ketoacid dehydrogenase (BCKAD) complex deficiency	– Onset within 48 hours of life – Poor feeding – Irritability – Lethargy – Seizure-like activity – Apnea – High-pitched cry – Maple syrup odor
Nonketotic hyperglycinemia (NKH)	Defective synthesis of glycine	– Onset ~ first week of life – Apnea – Seizures Milder forms of NKH present later in infancy
Hyperhomocystinemias and remethylation disorders	Deficiency of the cystathionine β-synthase enzyme	Does not present in the newborn period
Phenylketonuria	Deficiency of phenylalanine hydroxylase resulting in decreased levels of tyrosine	– Most common IEM – Severe phenotype if presents in newborn period – Developmental delays – Intellectual delays – Eczema – Hypopigmented skin and hair

Source: Data from Merritt, J. L., & Gallagher, R. (2018). Inborn errors of carbohydrate, ammonia, amino acid, and organic acid metabolism. In C. Gleason & S. Juul (Eds.), *Avery's diseases of the newborn* (10th ed., pp. 230–252.e4). Philadelphia, PA: Elsevier.

TABLE 14.5 Organic Acidemias

Disorder	Defective Process	Characteristics
Methylmalonic acidemia	Elevation of methylmalonic acid	– Onset day of life 2–3 – GI disturbances – Lethargy – Seizures – Identified with urine organic acids subsequent to an abnormal NBS
Propionic acidemia	Deficiency of propionyl–CoA carboxylase	Symptoms consistent with hyperammonemia Identified with urine organic acids and DNA testing
Multiple carboxylase deficiency	Defects in holocarboxylase Synthetase deficiency And biotinidase deficiency	– Metabolic acidosis – Lactic acidosis – Encephalopathy
Glutaric aciduria type 1	Deficiency of glutaryl–CoA dehydrogenase	– Delayed onset ~ 6–18 months

Source: Data from Merritt, J. L., & Gallagher, R. (2018). Inborn errors of carbohydrate, ammonia, amino acid, and organic acid metabolism. In C. Gleason & S. Juul (Eds.), *Avery's diseases of the newborn* (10th ed., pp. 230–252.e4). Philadelphia, PA: Elsevier.

Ketone Metabolism Disorders

- Defective process: Inability to use ketone bodies, 3-hydroxybutyric acid, and acetoacetic acid, for energy generation
- Severe phenotype is HMG-CoA lyase deficiency, which is an autosomal recessive disease. Presents in the newborn period, around day 3 of life, with symptoms such as vomiting, lethargy, hyperketotoic hypoglycemia, metabolic acidosis, and metabolic acidosis. HMG-CoA lyase deficiency is confirmed by the mutation analysis of the HMGCL gene.
- Succinyl-CoA 3-ketoacid-CoA transferase deficiency presents within the first week of life with severe ketosis, lactic acidosis, hypoglycemia, and coma. Most patients do not survive.
- Clinical presentation is consistent with hyperammonemia (Merritt & Gallagher, 2018, p. 248).

Primary Lactic Acidosis

- Defective process: Abnormal energy metabolism-multifactorial. Primary defect in the mitochondrial electron transport chain (ETC) or the tricarboxylic acid (TCA) cycle.

- Presents with profound metabolic acidosis.
- Moderate hyperammonemia (Merritt & Gallagher, 2018, pp. 248–251)

Further details on primary lactic acidosis disorders are summarized in Table 14.7.

Lysosomal Storage Disorders (LSDs)

- Defective process: Deficiency in a specific lysosomal enzyme/transport
- 20 LSDs will appear in the newborn period (Thomas, Lam, & Berry, 2018, pp. 253–272).

Further details on lysosomal storage disorders are summarized in Table 14.8.

Congenital Disorders of Glycosylation

- Defective process: Defects in the process of modifying proteins, lipids, or sugar molecules/chains
- Onset variable based on phenotype (Thomas et al., 2018, pp. 264–267)

Further details on congenital disorders of glycosylation are summarized in Table 14.9.

TABLE 14.6 Fatty Acid Oxidation Disorders (FAOD)

Disorder	Defective Process	Characteristics
	Failure of β-oxidation within, or transport of fatty acids into, the mitochondria	Severe phenotypes present within 24–48 hours of life Hypoglycemia Liver disease/failure Cardiomyopathy
Medium-chain Acyl-CoA dehydrogenase deficiency (MCADD)		Most common FAOD Most common etiology of sudden infant death syndrome (SIDS) Severe phenotypes present in the newborn period

Source: Data from Merritt, J. L., & Gallagher, R. (2018). Inborn errors of carbohydrate, ammonia, amino acid, and organic acid metabolism. In C. Gleason & S. Juul (Eds.), *Avery's diseases of the newborn* (10th ed., pp. 230–252.e4). Philadelphia, PA: Elsevier.

TABLE 14.7 Primary Lactic Acidosis

Disorder	Defective process	Characteristics
Pyruvate dehydrogenase complex deficiency		Profound lactic acidosis Low to normal lactate-to-pyruvate ratio Moderate hyperammonemia
Pyruvate carboxylase deficiency		Lactic acidosis in the newborn period Developmental delays
Electron transport chain defects		Presents ~ 3 months of age
Benign infantile mitochondrial myopathy, cardiomyopathy, or both		Congenital hypotonia at birth
Barth syndrome		Anemia Ringed sideroblasts Exocrine pancreatic dysfunction
Early lethal lactic acidosis		Onset with first 72 hours of life Poor prognosis

Source: Data from Merritt, J. L., & Gallagher, R. (2018). Inborn errors of carbohydrate, ammonia, amino acid, and organic acid metabolism. In C. Gleason & S. Juul (Eds.), *Avery's diseases of the newborn* (10th ed., pp. 230–252.e4). Philadelphia, PA: Elsevier.

TABLE 14.8 Lysosomal Storage Disorders

Disorder	Defective Process	Characteristics
Niemann–Pick C Disease	Defective transport of lipoprotein	Variable onset Conjugated hyperbilirubinemia in newborn period
Gaucher disease type 2 (acute neuropathic)	Deficiency of lysosomal glucocerebrosidase	Infantile onset of severe central nervous system (CNS) involvement
GM1 gangliosidosis	Deficiency in lysosomal β-galactosidase	Coarse, thick skin Hirtuism on forehead and neck Dysmorphic facial features
Farber lipogranulomatosis	Deficiency of lysosomal acid ceramidase	Onset 2 weeks to 4 months of age Aphonia Poor weight gain Intermittent fever
Galactosialidosis	Deficiency of two lysosomal enzymes, neuraminidase, and β-galactosidase	Onset birth to 3 months of age Ascites Edema Coarse facial features Inguinal hernias Hypotonia
Wolman disease	Deficiency of lysosomal acid lipase	Onset birth to first few weeks of life GI disturbances Failure to thrive Abdominal distention
Infantile sialic acid storage disease	Defective lysosomal sialic acid transporter	Hepatosplenomegaly Ascites Hypopigmentation, Hypotonia
I-Cell disease (mucolipidosis type II)		Corneal clouding Organomegaly Hypotonia Gingival hyperplasia Low birthweight (BW)

Source: Data from Thomas, J. A., Lam, C., & Berry, G. (2018). Lysosomal storage, peroxisomal, and glycosylation disorders and Smith–Lemli–Opitz syndrome presenting in the neonate. In C. Gleason & S. Juul (Eds.), *Avery's diseases of the newborn* (10th ed., pp. 253–272.e3). Philadelphia, PA: Elsevier.

TABLE 14.9 Congenital Disorders of Glycosylation

Disorder	Defective Process	Characteristics
Combined glycosylation defects	Defective glycosylation	Microcephaly Seizures Hypotonia Cutis laxa Hepatic involvement

Source: Data from Thomas, J. A., Lam, C., & Berry, G. (2018). Lysosomal storage, peroxisomal, and glycosylation disorders and Smith–Lemli–Opitz syndrome presenting in the neonate. In C. Gleason & S. Juul (Eds.), *Avery's diseases of the newborn* (10th ed., pp. 253–272.e3). Philadelphia, PA: Elsevier.

Perixomal Disorders

- Defective process: Absence or dysfunction a peroxisomal enzyme. May involve more than one enzyme.
- Clinical presentation variable; may include dysmorphic craniofacial features, glaucoma, cataracts.
- Onset variable (Thomas et al., 2018, pp. 267–269)

Further details on perixomal disorders are summarized in Table 14.10.

TABLE 14.10 Perixomal Disorders

Disorder	Defective Process	Characteristics
Zellweger syndrome	Fails to import newly synthesized peroxisomal proteins into the peroxisome	Cataracts Glaucoma Seizures Dysmorphic facial features Hepatomegaly Generalized weakness Hypotonia

Source: Data from Thomas, J. A., Lam, C., & Berry, G. (2018). Lysosomal storage, peroxisomal, and glycosylation disorders and Smith–Lemli–Opitz syndrome presenting in the neonate. In C. Gleason & S. Juul (Eds.), *Avery's diseases of the newborn* (10th ed., pp. 253–272.e3). Philadelphia, PA: Elsevier.

CONCLUSION

Although individual conditions may be rare, the cumulative number of infants admitted to the NICU with a potentially genetic condition is significant. Recent advances in knowledge and technology have made the need for collaborative practice increasingly important. The neonatal provider requires multiple skills to be able to care for these infants and their families. The provider must have advanced physical assessment skills, the ability to identify dysmorphology, and a working knowledge of how to start a basic genetic evaluation. Any evaluation of this scale should be tailored to the infant's medical status, be mindful of infant blood volume, be fiscally responsible, and minimize infant pain and discomfort. These infants may require extensive multidisciplinary care and coordination of this becomes an important role of the NNP. The NNP must act as an advocate for these infants and their families. The NNP's knowledge infant physiology, testing, infant pain, and family stress, and their role as coordinators of care, make them uniquely qualified to act as advocates. The NNP must also possess skills not covered in this chapter, including the ability to compassionately deliver unexpected news, provide family support, and knowledge of local, regional, national, and online resources.

REVIEW QUESTIONS

1. The term *dysmorphism* indicates:
   A. anomalous external physical features
   B. malformed morphogenesis of tissue
   C. nonstandard forces pulling on tissues

2. The NNP is called to attend the delivery of a premature infant. The infant has respiratory distress after birth and requires intubation. The intubation is difficult due to the size of the mouth, but the procedure is successful. On brief exam after resuscitation the NNP noted the infant has clenched hands and rocker-bottom feet, and becomes concerned the infant has:
   A. Trisomy 13
   B. Trisomy 18
   C. Trisomy 21

3. The finding of aplasia cutis congenita on the admission exam of a newborn leads the NNP to further evaluate the infant for:
   A. DiGeorge syndrome
   B. Trisomy 13 pattern
   C. Urea cycle disorder

4. The NNP is caring for a 4-day-old infant who was admitted to the NICU for hypocalcemia. The infant required multiple boluses and a daily supplement to maintain low normal serum levels. On exam of the fifth day, the infant exhibits some cyanosis, requires, oxygen, and has a new murmur. The NNP considers evaluating the infant for:
   A. 11p15 methylation association
   B. 17q21.1 COL1A1 mutations
   C. 22q11.2 deletion syndrome

5. Inborn errors of metabolism are genetic, biochemical disorders in which the function, structure, or volume is altered in a key pathway of:
   A. carbohydrate synthesis
   B. fatty acid synthesis
   C. protein synthesis

REFERENCES

Bajaj, K., & Gross, S. J. (2015). Genetic aspects of perinatal disease and prenatal diagnosis. In R. Martin, A. Fanaroff, & M. Walsh (Eds.), *Fanaroff and Martin's neonatal-perinatal medicine: Diseases of the fetus and infant* (10th ed., pp. 130–146). Philadelphia, PA: Elsevier.

Cederbaum, S. (2018). Introduction to metabolic and biochemical genetic diseases. In C. Gleason & S. Juul (Eds.), *Avery's diseases of the newborn* (10th ed., pp. 224–229). Philadelphia, PA: Elsevier.

Cotton, M., & Murray, J. (2018). The human genome and neonatal care. In C. Gleason & S. Juul (Eds.), *Avery's diseases of the newborn* (10th ed., pp. 180–189.e2). Philadelphia, PA: Elsevier.

Devaskar, S. U., & Garg, M. (2015). Disorders of carbohydrate metabolism. In R. Martin, A. Fanaroff, & M. Walsh (Eds.), *Fanaroff and Martin's neonatal-perinatal medicine: Diseases of the fetus and infant* (10th ed., pp. 1434–1459). Philadelphia, PA: Elsevier.

Gross, S., & Gheorghe, C. (2018). Genetic aspects of perinatal diseases and prenatal diagnosis. In C. Gleason & S. Juul (Eds.), *Avery's diseases of the newborn* (10th ed., pp. 154–173). Philadelphia, PA: Elsevier.

Haldeman-Englert, C. R., Saitta, S. C., & Zackai, E. H. (2018). Chromosome disorders. In C. Gleason & S. Juul (Eds.), *Avery's diseases of the newborn* (10th ed., pp. 211–223.e2). Philadelphia, PA: Elsevier.

Larson-Nath, C., Gurram, B., & Chelimsky, G. (2015). Disorders of digestion in the neonate. In R. Martin, A. Fanaroff, & M. Walsh (Eds.), *Fanaroff and Martin's neonatal-perinatal medicine: Diseases of the fetus and infant* (10th ed., pp. 1379–1394). Philadelphia, PA: Elsevier.

Matthews, A. L., & Robin, N. H. (2016). Genetic disorders, malformations, and inborn errors of metabolism. In S. Gardner, B. Carter, M. Hines, & J. Hernandez (Eds.), *Merenstein & Gardner's handbook of neonatal intensive care* (8th ed., pp. 763–785). St. Louis, MO: Elsevier.

Merritt, J. L., & Gallagher, R. (2018). Inborn errors of carbohydrate, ammonia, amino acid, and organic acid metabolism. In C. Gleason & S. Juul (Eds.), *Avery's diseases of the newborn* (10th ed., pp. 230–252.e4). Philadelphia, PA: Elsevier.

Parikh, A. S., & Mitchell, A. L. (2015). Congenital anomalies. In R. Martin, A. Fanaroff, & M. Walsh (Eds.), *Fanaroff and Martin's neonatal-perinatal medicine: Diseases of the fetus and infant* (10th ed., pp. 436–457). Philadelphia, PA: Elsevier.

Sahai, I., & Levy, H. (2018). Newborn screening. In C. Gleason & S. Juul (Eds.), *Avery's diseases of the newborn* (10th ed., pp. 332–346.e3). Philadelphia, PA: Elsevier.

Schiefelbein, J. (2015). Genetics: From bench to bedside. In T. Verklan & M. Walden (Eds.), *Core curriculum for neonatal intensive care nursing* (5th ed., pp. 391–406). St. Louis, MO: Elsevier.

Sterk, L. (2015). Congenital anomalies. In T. Verklan & M. Walden (Eds.), *Core curriculum for neonatal intensive care nursing* (5th ed., pp. 747–794). St. Louis, MO: Elsevier.

Thomas, J. A., Lam, C., & Berry, G. (2018). Lysosomal storage, peroxisomal, and glycosylation disorders and Smith–Lemli–Opitz syndrome presenting in the neonate. In C. Gleason & S. Juul (Eds.), *Avery's diseases of the newborn* (10th ed., pp. 253–272.e3). Philadelphia, PA: Elsevier.

Tiller, G., & Bellus, G. (2018). Skeletal dysplasias and heritable connective tissue disorders. In C. Gleason & S. Juul (Eds.), *Avery's diseases of the newborn* (10th ed., pp. 1450–1657.e2). Philadelphia, PA: Elsevier.

15 THE NEUROLOGIC SYSTEM

Carrie Lewis
Antonette Hurst
Amy R. Koehn

INTRODUCTION

The nervous system is one of the first organ systems to evolve following conception. Through intricate and complex interactions between biochemicals, vessels, circuits, and pathways, the brain and nervous system link to and communicate with other body systems to maintain physiologic homeostasis. Maternal health, genetics, pharmaceuticals and pharmacological therapies, infection, and the environment can all influence and alter fetal development and postnatal neurological function. Sequala associated with compromised neurodevelopment can range from treatable conditions to severe neurological devastation. This chapter provides a review of fetal neurological development and the most commonly encountered neuromal formations and neurological disorders.

Embryology and Growth and Development of the Neurologic System

- Neural crest/neural tube
  - Normal development of the central nervous system (CNS) involves several steps. Different steps of brain development and maturation are controlled by the individual genes and the environment in which these genes are exposed (Gressens & Hüppi, 2015, p. 836). Neurulation is the process in which neuroectodermal cells transform into the neural tube. The neural tube will transform into the brain and spinal cord. Three stages of neurulation are:
    - Neural plate formation/modeling: in the fetus, this appears during the third week after conception.
    - Neural groove formation also develops in the third week after conception.
    - Closure of the neural groove starts at the fourth week of postconception beginning with formation of the neural crests. Closure begins in the lower medulla and moves both rostrally and caudally to form the neural tube (Gressens & Hüppi, 2015, p. 836).
- Neuronal development and migration (Du Plessis & Volpe, 2018, p. 34)
  - Neuronal proliferation occurs during weeks 10 to 20 of gestation.
  - Neuronal migration occurs during weeks 12 to 24 of gestation.
- Porencephalic development
  - During weeks 5 to 10 of gestation (Gressens & Hüppi, 2015, p. 837)
  - Bifurcation of neural tube forming left and right forebrain
  - Forebrain—telencephalon and diencephalon (thalamus, hypothalamus) create the cerebral hemispheres (Du Plessis & Volpe, 2018, p. 34).
  - Midbrain—mesencephalon
  - Hindbrain–rhombencephalon
  - Thalamus and hypothalamus (Huang & Doherty, 2018, p. 857)
- Anatomy of the brain
  - Cerebellum—complexity of neurons that influence coordination, muscle tone, posture, and equilibrium (Darras & Volpe, 2018, p. 861). Contains vermis and hemispheres and growth continues into the second year of life, hence the vulnerability of the preterm infant (Huang & Doherty, 2018, p. 857).
  - Cerebrum
    - Cortical lobes consist of frontal, parietal, temporal, and occipital.
    - Corpus callosum—largest bundle of nerve fibers connecting the hemispheres. Completion of corpus callosum takes ~11 weeks and the developing connections synthesize throughout adolescences (Huang & Doherty, 2018, p. 860).
    - Lateral ventricles
  - Brainstem development of the following structures occurs after the neural tube is completed:
    - Midbrain—vision, hearing, sleep/wake, motor control, temperature regulation
    - Pons carries sensory messages to the thalamus, conducts signals to brain down to cerebellum.
    - Medulla control center for involuntary functions

Congenital Malformations of the Central Nervous System

- Disorders from the prosencephalon
  - Agenesis of the corpus callosum (ACC)
    - **Incidence and Etiology**
      - The corpus callosum is the largest commissure-composed of bundles of nerve fibers that connect the two hemispheres. When absent, the fiber bundles run parallel to the ventricle in an anterior to posterior direction rather than connecting. These fibers are Probst bundles and are a useful distinguishing feature (Huang & Doherty, 2018, pg. 861).
      - ACC is a common malformation and represents ~50% of midline defects. (Gressens, & Hüppi, 2015, pgs. 856). It can be partial or complete and often times involving loss of posterior segments. (Huang & Doherty, 2018, p. 861) Prevalence in the general population is 0.5 in 10,000 where as in children with neurodevelopmental disabilities it is 600 in 10,000.
      - Callosal formation is affected by genetic and environmental factors. Has been shown to

be inherited by all modalities of transference (Huang & Doherty, 2018, pg. 860–861).

- Alcohol exposure has the highest incidence where 7% of children with fetal alcohol syndrome are affected. (Huang & Doherty, 2018, p. 860).
- Prenatal infections can cause ACC but it is rare. It more commonly causes a thinning of the corpus callosum (Huang & Doherty, 2018, p. 860).

■ **Clinical Presentation and Associated Findings**
- ACC is often associated with other neuronal migration abnormalities including craniofacial anomalies, midline ocular/nasal clefts or other defects, holoprosencephaly and Dandy–Walker malformation (Gressens & Hüppi, 2015, pp. 856–857). Metopic synostosis is also associated (Cohen & Robinson, 2015, p. 983; Huang & Doherty, 2018, p. 861).
- Seventeen percent of the time, ACC is associated with chromosomal aneuploidy (chromosomes 13, 18, and 21). ACC in the presence of associated disorders is considered to have a poor prognosis (Cohen & Robinson, 2015, p. 983; Huang & Doherty, 2018, p. 861).
- When isolated, ACC can go unnoticed. (Gressens & Hüppi, 2015, p. 856; Huang & Doherty, 2018, p. 860).

■ **Diagnosis**
- A fetal MRI at 20 to 22 weeks' gestation may be helpful in identifying ACC and/or other cerebral findings (Huang & Doherty, 2018, p. 861).
- Postnatal: Metabolic testing will help determine the presence or absence of ACC and any other associated chromosomal anomalies (Huang & Doherty, 2018, p. 861).

■ **Treatment and Outcomes**
- Long-term developmental follow-up is dependent on severity (Gressens & Hüppi, 2015, p. 856) and may involve subspecialty consultations such as neurology, ophthalmology, genetics, audiology, and developmental pediatrics (Huang & Doherty, 2018, p. 861).
- Patients with known ACC have been shown to have specific impairment in abstract reasoning, problem solving, category fluency, and difficulty with higher-level language comprehension (Huang & Doherty, 2018, p. 861).

○ Holoprosencephaly
■ **Incidence and Etiology**
- Holoprosencephaly refers to an entire spectrum of cleavage disorders sharing a common embryologic origin. The essential abnormality is the incomplete separation of the prosencephalon along one or more of its three major planes: horizontal, transverse, and sagittal occurring no later than the fifth and sixth weeks of gestation (Du Plessis & Volpe, 2018, p. 37–38; Gressens & Hüppi, 2015, p. 855).
- Holoprosencephaly is the most common brain malformation, with its frequency estimated to be approximately one in 10,000 to one in 20,000 live births (Du Plessis & Volpe, 2018, p. 38; Gressens & Hüppi, 2015, p. 855; Huang & Doherty, 2018, p. 860).
- Up to 45% of holoprosencephaly is caused by chromosomal abnormalities detectable by standard karyotyping. The most common chromosome abnormalities are trisomies 13 and 18 (Huang & Doherty, 2018, p. 860). Holoprosencephaly is also observed in several syndromes, including the Smith–Lemli–Opitz syndrome. Causes of holoprosencephaly are variable, with genetic, chromosomal, syndromic, and environmental etiologies. Some familial cases have been reported (Gressens & Hüppi, 2015, p. 856).
- The incidence is more than 60-fold greater (i.e., 1/250) in studies of miscarried or aborted human embryos and fetuses, suggesting that holoprosencephaly is often accompanied by early embryonic loss (Gressens & Hüppi, 2015, p. 855).

■ **Clinical Presentation and Associated Findings**
- Holoprosencephaly is characterized by a single midline lateral ventricle, incomplete or absent interhemispheric fissure, absent olfactory system, midfacial clefts, and hypotelorism (Parsons, Seay, & Jacobson, 2016, p. 730).
- Disorders of prosencephalic development often have concurrent facial anomalies and forebrain alterations (Blackburn, 2013, p. 529; Verklan, 2015, p. 734).
- Facial anomalies are present in up to 80% to 90% of holoprosencephaly cases. The findings may range from cyclopia (a single central eye) with a nose-like structure (proboscis) above the eye, or even no eye at all and a rudimentary nasal structure, the proboscis, often located above the midline to cebocephaly (a flattened single nostril situated centrally between the eyes; Huang & Doherty, 2018, p. 860). Less severe facial deformities include marked ocular hypotelorism with or without a proboscis (ethmocephaly) and ocular hypoelorism (Du Plessis & Volpe, 2018, pp. 38, 40; Parsons et al., 2016, p. 730).
- Neurological features in the most severe cases are obvious from the neonatal period. Infants exhibit frequent apneic spells, stimulus-sensitive tonic spasms (Du Plessis & Volpe, 2018, pp. 38, 40). May also present with low tone and microcephaly Only about 40% of children have epilepsy, but one-third of these will have intractable epilepsy (Huang & Doherty, 2018, p. 860). Seizures occur in a minority (Du Plessis & Volpe, 2018, p. 40).
- Endocrinological abnormalities are very common. Various abnormalities of hypothalamic function (e.g., poikilothermia, diabetes insipidus, or inappropriate antidiuretic hormone secretion; Du Plessis & Volpe, 2018, pp. 38, 40).
- Diabetes insipidus occurs in up to 70% of patients, with hypothyroidism,

hypoadrenocorticism, and growth hormone deficiency being less common (Huang & Doherty, 2018, p. 860).

■ **Diagnosis**
  – Prenatal ultrasonography is adept at identifying a fetus with holoprosencephaly. A fetal MRI may then clarify the diagnosis and severity of the malformation. If a variant of holoprosencephaly is discovered, an amniocentesis for chromosome array and possibly DNA sequencing is indicated (Huang & Doherty, 2018, pp. 859–860).
  – Holoprosencephaly can be divided into three variants based principally on the severity of the cleavage abnormality in the cerebral hemispheres and deep nuclear structures. The DeMyer classification scheme includes alobar, semilobar, and lobar divisions.
    • Alobar holoprosencephaly is the most severe disturbance and includes a single anterior ventricle contained within a holosphere with complete lack of separation of the prosencephalon. There may be a fusion of thalami and an absence of any or all of the interhemispheric fissure, corpus callosum, and third ventricle.
    • Semi-lobar holoprosencephaly occurs when there is a failure of separation of the anterior hemispheres with presence of a posterior portion of the inter-hemispheric fissure and less severe fusion of deep nuclear structures. This somewhat milder form will still have distinct hemispheres and the presence of a portion of the posterior corpus callosum.
    • Lobar holoprosencephaly is identified when the cerebral hemispheres are nearly fully separated, and the fissure along almost the entire midline and separation or near separation of the thalami. Deep nuclear structures are nearly or totally separated and the posterior callosum is well developed, although the anterior callosum may be some- what underdeveloped. The third ventricle is present and frontal horns are partially formed and the corpus callosum is present; however, the frontal lobes may still be hypoplastic according to the severity of the malformation (Du Plessis & Volpe, 2018, pp. 37–38; Gressens & Hüppi, 2015, p. 855; Huang & Doherty, 2018, p. 859).

■ **Treatment**
  – Prognosis is related to the severity of the defect, involvement of other organ systems, and the genetic cause (Huang & Doherty, 2018, p. 860). The most severe forms of holoprosencephaly result in death in the first year. Subsequent neurological deficits relate to the nature of the neuropathological features (Du Plessis & Volpe, 2018, p. 40).

• Cortical defects in migration
  ○ Lissencephaly
    ■ **Incidence and Etiology**
      – A neuronal migrations disorder that results in a smooth appearance of the cortical surface of the brain caused by absent or reduced gyri (Huang & Doherty, 2018, p. 865; Verklan, 2015, p. 735).
        • An important distinguishing development is the normal fetal brain is smooth early in gestation with convolutions forming throughout gestation. Lissencephaly is a cortical migrational disorder resulting in agyria, pachygyria, and other issues in term infants (Parsons, Seay, & Jacobson, 2017, p. 730).
      – Estimated to occur 1.2/100,000 births with Type 1 Isolated lissencephaly or LIS1. LIS1 accounts for 40% of cases. This comes from deletions and mutations or a particular gene that gives way for absent or decreased gyri. Depending on which particular genes are affected determine the degree of cell motility and degree of mutations. Lissencephalies may be X-linked (Gressens & Hüppi, 2015, pp. 859, 865).
        • Dominant and recessive mutations are also found and are related to different mutations of genes, creating sex-linked differences in severities of disorders (Gressens & Hüppi, 2015, p. 859; Huang & Doherty, 2018, p. 865).
        • Neuronal migrations disorders can be linked to several environmental factors, such as cocaine and alcohol exposure and TORCH infections (Gressens & Hüppi, 2015, p. 861).
      – Miller–Dieker syndrome combines LIS1 with dysmorphic features (Gressens & Hüppi, 2015, p. 859).

    ■ **Clinical Presentation**
      – Seizures may be the first clinical manifestation in the early postnatal period (Verklan, 2015, p. 735).
      – Clinical features of lissencephaly include hypotonia, feeding problems, and decreased movement sometimes presenting with arthrogryposis in the newborn (Parsons, Seay, & Jacobson, 2017, p. 730). Infants with LIS1 often have hypotonia, spastic quadriparesis, and seizures. Ambiguous genitalia, may also be noted (Huang & Doherty, 2018, p. 865).
      – Miller–Dieker syndrome will demonstrate additional findings of dysmorphic facial features such as malrotated and positioned ears, large, narrow forehead, micrognathia long philtrum, short/turned-up nose, flat nasal bridge, and thin upper lip (Gressens & Hüppi, 2015, p. 859). Other possible characteristics are, retrognathia, retinal hypervascularization, and digital abnormalities (Parsons, Seay, & Jacobson, 2017, p. 730).

    ■ **Diagnosis**
      – Prenatal ultrasounds are adept at intrauterine diagnosis. In cases when mother has no to limited prenatal care, individual clinical presentation and testing are key (Huang & Doherty, 2018, p. 865).

- Postnatally, an electroencephalography (EEG), computerized tomography (CT) cranial ultrasound, (US) and magnetic resonance imaging (MRI) of the brain are all helpful in establishing a diagnosis (Verklan, 2015, p. 760).

■ **Treatment and Outcome**

- Microcephaly and myoclonic epilepsy are commonly noted to occur over the first year of life. Poor head growth resulting in microcephaly usually occurs within the first year in type I lissencephaly. Neonatal seizures may also occur, but seizures are more commonly present at 6 to 12 months of age (Huang & Doherty, 2018, p. 865; Parsons, Seay, & Jacobson, 2017, p. 730).
- Like most disorders causing long-term neurodevelopmental delays, early interventions and identification of support are crucial. Prognosis of lissencephalies is very poor. Typically, seizures and spastic quadriparesis limit long-term achievements (Huang & Doherty, 2018, p. 865).

- Congenital cerebellar anomalies
  ○ Hydrocephalus
    ■ **Incidence and Etiology**
      - A category of ventriculomegaly that results in ventricular dilation by an accumulation of cerebral spinal fluid (CSF) due to CSF production exceeding CSF absorption. Can result from abnormalities anywhere in the CSF pathway; however, the majority of cases are caused by decreased absorption due to an obstruction.
        • Impaired CSF flow distal to the fourth ventricle foramina results in communicating hydrocephalus.
        • Enlargement of any or all ventricles due to an obstruction of CSF flow upstream or at the fourth ventricle foramina is called noncommunicating hydrocephalus.
      - The majority of cases of fetal hydrocephalus is due to decreased CSF absorption which is essentially obstructive in nature (duPlessis, Robinson, & Volpe, 2018, p. 61)
      - Etiology is typically heterogenous, but most cases result from developmental disorders of the brain and its CSF circulatory system. Major causes have been identified as Dandy–Walker malformation, Chiari type malformation, and aqueductal stenosis.
        • Dandy–Walker malformation is the result of abnormal development of the rhombencephalon at weeks 7 to 10 in gestation (Gressens & Hüppi, 2015, p. 857). Exact etiology is unnkown (Gressens & Hüppi, 2015, p. 857; Huang & Doherty, 2018, p. 861). Consists of three major abnormalities (1) Enlargement of the posterior fossa (occipital cranial prominence) with upward displacement of the tentorium, (2) Cystic dilation of the fourth ventricle, and (3) Partial or complete ACC (Gressens & Hüppi, 2015, p. 857; Huang & Doherty, 2018, p. 869). Dandy–Walker malfor-

mation accounts for 5% to 10% of congenital hydrocephalus. 75% of infants with Dandy–Walker malformation will have hydrocephalus. (Gressens & Hüppi, 2015, p. 857).
        • Arnold–Chiari malformation (Chiari malformation Type-II) is a primary neurulation defect which occurs during weeks 3 to 4 in gestation and presents in the second trimester (Robinson & Cohen, 2015, p. 973; Volpe et al., 2018, pp. 3, 15). There is displacement of the medulla, cerebellum, and fourth ventricle into the cervical canal, blocking adequate CSF drainage. It is almost always exclusively seen with open neural tube defects (Gressens & Hüppi, 2015, p. 855; Huang & Doherty, 2018, p. 873; duPlessis & Volpe, 2018, p. 15).
        • Aqueductal stenosis is an obstructive noncommunicating hydrocephalus occurring when CSF is unable to drain from the third ventricle into the fourth ventricle due to a congenital obstruction in the aqueduct of Slyvius connecting the third and fourth ventricle. CSF collects into the cranial cavity and leads to lateral and third ventricular dilation, causing compression of blood flow and brain growth. This develops between 15 and 17 weeks' gestation, the time of rapid elongation of the mesencephalon and evolution of the normal constriction of the aqueduct (duPlessis et al., 2018, p. 62; Robinson & Cohen, 2015, p. 973).
    ■ **Clinical Presentation and Associated Findings**
      - Neonatal presentation is a markedly enlarging head, full anterior fontanelle, and separated cranial sutures, full (bulging) and tense fontanelles, increased frontal-occipital circumference (FOC), "Setting-sun" eyes, and visible scalp veins (duPlessis et al., 2018, p. 64; Verklan, 2015, p. 745)
      - Sequelae of this hydrocephalus may include apnea, respiratory distress with inspiratory stridor, depressed gag, weak cry, quadriparesis, or dysphagia. These are typically the result of brainstem or cranial nerve dysfunction. Hindbrain dysfunction can be the result of compression or ischemic factors. Also can be caused by the abnormal development of the cranial nerve nuclei in the brainstem. Highest mortality is seen when stridor, apnea, cyanotic spells, and dysphagia are all present (Huang & Doherty, 2018, p. 876; du Plessis & Volpe, 2018, pp. 15–16).
      - A widening of the squamosal suture, the suture that runs horizontally above the ear between the temporal and parietal bones, is a useful sign for indicating increased intracranial pressure (ICP). Ventricular dilation occurs before rapid head growth or increased ICP is seen (Robinson & Cohen, 2015, p. 973; Volpe et al., 2018, p. 15).
      - Careful neonatal assessment should be made for signs of specific etiological types of congenital

hydrocephalus, such as the flexion deformity of the thumbs (which can often be detected by fetal US) characteristic of approximately 50% of cases of X-linked aquductal stenosis, the occipital cranial prominence of the Dandy-Walker formation, and the chorioretinitis of intrauterine infection by toxoplasmosis or cytomegalovirus (duPlessis et al., 2018, p. 64).

■ **Diagnosis**
– Ventriculomegaly is usually readily recognized by experienced ultrasonographers on prenatal ultrasounds, but may on occasion be mistaken for other fluid-filled supratentorial lesions, such as hydranencephaly or holoprosencephaly. These issues are readily resolved by fetal MRI (duPlessis et al., 2018, p. 61).

■ **Treatment and Outcomes**
– The options for postnatal treatment of symptomatic hydrocephalus are individualized to the needs of each infant, and require consideration of the comorbidities, overall prognosis, and parental preferences (duPlessis et al., 2018, p. 65).
– Hydrocephalus, regardless of etiology, can be managed with temporary procedures such as a ventricular access device (VAD), or ventriculo-subgaleal shunt (VSGS), or permanent ventriculoperitoneal (VP) shunt insertion.
  • The main complications for shunts include infections and malfunction. The risk of early shunt infection has been reduced by implementation of specific protocols and typically averages 5%–7.5% (duPlessis et al., 2018, p. 66).
– The prognosis of congenital hydrocephalus is dependent on the underlying cause, the extent of secondary parenchymal brain injury, the treatment options, and the complications of intervention. Overall, the incidence of serious associated brain anomalies in fetal hydrocephalus is generally approximately 60% to 70% (duPlessis et al., 2018, p. 67).
  • Shunting soon after birth often produces a far better outcome than would be assumed with minimal motor deficit and only a mild to moderate deficit in intellect (OParsons, Seay, & Jacobson, 2017, p. 735).
○ Abnormality of the Cranium
○ Craniosynostosis
  ■ **Incidence and Etiology**
  – Craniosynostosis is premature fusion of one or more of the sutures of the skull which then prevent appropriate growth of the brain and, occasionally, facial dysmorphisms (Robinson & Cohen, 2015, pp. 980–983; Johnson, 2018, p. 63; Evans, Hing, & Cunningham, 2018, p. 1424).
    • Sagittal craniosynostosis is the most common type, occurring 1/1,000 births, fourfold occurrence in males compared to females. Commonly known as scaphocephaly (one or more sagittal sutures are fused, creating an elongated appearance of the skull).

• Unilateral coronal craniosynostosis is present when one of the coronal sutures is prematurely fused, creating some asymmetry in the eyes, forehead, and nose, causing a flattening of the forehead on the same side of suture fused. This is commonly known as plagiocephaly.
• Bilateral coronal craniosynostosis results when both coronal sutures are prematurely closed, causing flattening and widening of the skull structure.
• Metopic craniosynostosis is identified by the triangular-shaped head with point at the forehead (trigonocephaly) (Robinson & Cohen, 2015, pp. 980–983).

■ **Clinical Presentation and Associated Findings**
– Primary findings are a misshapen head, facial asymmetry, syndactyly, bossing of forehead, hydrocephalus (Cohen & Robinson, 2015, pp. 980–985). Viewing the head from above may facilitate assessment of skull shape (Johnson, 2018, p. 63).
– The most significant concerns for the newborn with craniosynostosis are airway compromise (specifically, upper airway obstruction) and intracranial hypertension. Obstructive sleep apnea is common in Apert, Pfeiffer, and Crouzon syndromes (Evans et al., 2018, p. 1428).
– Conductive and mixed hearing loss, most commonly due to middle ear disease, ossicular abnormalities, and external auditory canal stenosis or atresia, can be present in syndromic craniosynostosis (Evans et al., 2018, p. 1429).
– Syndromic associations include:
  • Crouzon syndrome's common feature are brachycephaly, exophthalmos, and small maxillary bone (Cohen & Robinson, 2015, p. 984).
  • Apert syndrome is a triad of dysmorphic noted at birth. Craniosynostosis, small maxillary bone, and syndactyly of hands and feet (Cohen & Robinson, 2015, p. 984).
  • Pfeiffer syndrome is similar to features of Crouzon and Apert syndrome with additions of other dysmorphias. Three types exist, with third type being the most severe and presenting with clover leaf scalp shape (Cohen & Robinson, 2015, pp. 984–985).

■ **Diagnosis**
– The diagnosis of craniosynostosis is usually made on clinical criteria. Cases of single suture involvement may be identified by skull radiographs demonstrating sclerosis along all or part of the fused suture and compensatory changes. For complex cases, CT or three-dimensional CT scanning can help to delineate the pathologic process (Robinson & Cohen, 2015, p. 980)

■ **Treatment and Outcomes**
– A craniofacial team made up of the appropriate specialties allows proper planning and coordination so that the patient may receive the best possible care. Recommend involvement of a craniofacial team, including members specializing

in pediatrics, neurosurgery, ophthalmology, oral surgery, orthodontics, otolaryngology, nursing, nutrition, plastic surgery, and social work (Evans et al., 2018 pp. 1429–1430).
- Multiple operative options are available, ranging from minimally invasive to traditional surgery. bone grafting and excising (Cohen & Robinson, 2015, p. 983). Although the specific timing of the surgical treatment may differ between teams, it is generally accepted that individuals with synostosis should undergo cranial surgery in the first year of life. Cranioplasty involves release of fused sutures and repositioning and reconstruction of the calvaria, so as to prevent increased ICP and progressive abnormal craniofacial development (Evans et al., 2018, p. 1430).

Neural Tube Defects

- Neural tube defects occur when there is failure of the folds to fuse and form the neural tube. There is a secondary malformation of the skeletal structure and skin covering. These abnormalities cover a wide spectrum of defects (Bauer & Doherty, 2018, p. 873).
- Anencephaly
  - **Incidence and Etiology**
    - Anencephaly represents nearly one-half of all open NTDs, about 0.28/1,000 births (du Plessis & Volpe, 2018, p. 7)
    - Typically occurs within the first 4 weeks of gestation and is a complete failure of the rostral neuropore to close, leaving the remainder of the brain atrophied (Huang & Doherty, 2018, p. 875).
    - This affects more females then males, and geographic locations are a factor (Bauer & Doherty, 2018, p. 875).
  - **Clinical Presentation**
    - Three-fourths of these infants are stillborn. If born alive, most die within 24 hours of life. Some have been reported to survive up to 2 months of age (Bauer & Doherty, 2018, p. 874–875; Gressens & Hüppi, 2015, p. 854).
    - Due to the lack of normal cranial structures, the eyes appear to be large and protruding on ultrasound, giving a distinct facies noted on ultrasound (Bauer & Doherty, 2018, p. 877).
    - Seen in congruency with polyhydramnios (Bauer & Doherty, 2018, p. 873)
  - **Diagnosis**
    - Fetal ultrasound (Bauer & Doherty, 2018, p. 875)
  - **Treatment and Outcomes**
    - Palliative care for infants born alive.
    - Prenatal detection rate is high; in turn, individuals choose termination (duPlessis & Volpe et al., 2018, p. 8).
- Encephalocele
  - **Incidence and Etiology**
    - Occurs before 26 days post conception.
    - Cranial skull defects that contain brain tissue in the pocket that protrudes from the skull.
    - An encephalocele typically forms in the occipital region and affects the meninges; therefore, severity depends on the locations and amount of brain tissue involved (Bauer & Doherty, 2018, p. 876; Gressens & Hüppi, 2015, p. 854).
  - **Clinical Presentation**
    - Large mass noted around infants skull or face
    - Wide bridge nose and wide-spaced eyes can be a sign of internal encephaloceles (Bauer & Doherty, 2018, pp. 876–877).
    - May present with hydrocephalus due to the high relationship with other CNS defects such as ACC, anomalous venous drainage, and Chiari malformations (Bauer & Doherty, 2018, pp. 876–877).
    - Also associated with a large variety of chromosomal disorders, such as Dandy–Walker, Goldenhar, Walker–Warburg, and several trisomies, such as 13 and 18 (Gressens & Hüppi, 2015, pp. 854).
  - **Diagnosis**
    - Can be seen on fetal ultrasounds
    - Postnatal transillumination can be used; x-rays, ultrasounds, CT, MRI with angiography, and venography is preferred (Huang & Doherty, 2018, pp. 876–877).
  - **Treatment and Outcomes**
    - Surgery is indicated soon after birth in some cases.
    - Other cases require palliative care due to the severity of the lesion (Huang & Doherty, 2018, pp. 876–877).
- Meningocele
  - **Incidence and Etiology**
    - Has a dermal covered protruding sac that contains the meninges and is associated with spina bifida. The spinal cord is typically intact and unaffected; however, there are rare cases where there can be cord anomalies (Cohen & Robinson, 2015, p. 990).
    - Occurs during gestational weeks 4 to 7 or during secondary neurulation (Volpe et al., 2018, p. 6)
    - Most commonly noted to be located in the thoracic spine (Volpe et al., 2018, p. 27). Fluid-filled skin covered protrusion is noted along spine (Volpe et al., 2018, p. 27).
  - **Clinical Presentation and Associated Findings**
    - In the neonatal period, infants do not tend to have neurologic deficits.
    - Later deficits can include incontinence and disturbances in gait, all associated with tethered cord (Volpe et al., 2018, p. 28).
  - **Diagnosis**
    - Often seen on prenatal ultrasounds
    - Postnatal diagnosis consists of clinical assessments, spinal ultrasounds, and MRI (Huang & Doherty, 2018, p. 877).
  - **Treatment and Outcomes**
    - Surgical correction shortly after birth
    - Folic acid supplementation has not been noted to decrease the incidence (Volpe et al., 2018, p. 26). However, other sources discuss that 70% of NTD have been prevented due to the practice of preconception supplementation (Cohen & Robinson, 2015, p. 990).
- Myelomeningocele (MMC)
  - **Incidence and Etiology**
    - Affects the posterior neural tube closure and contains meninges and neural tissues. It affects all layers of the spinal cord, vertebrae, nerves, and skin (Gressens & Hüppi, 2015, p. 854).

- Three-fourths of these defects are located in the lumbar regions.
- Occurs during gestational weeks 3 to 4 or during primary neurulation (Volpe et al., 2018, p. 3).
- The higher the location of defect, the poorer the prognosis. (Cohen & Robinson, 2015, p. 990).
○ **Clinical Presentation**
- Varying sizes of openings along the spine, open without sac or with fluid-filled transparent sac intact.
- Neurologic impairments are noted below the lesion.
- May present as part of findings associated with Trisomy 18 or Chiari Type II malformation.
  - Associated hydrocephalus may lead to clinical signs or symptoms of increased intracranial pressure. (Cohen & Robinson, 2015, p. 991; Huang & Doherty, 2018, p. 876).
○ **Diagnosis**
- Usually prenatally diagnosed through the use of ultrasonography. Increased alpha fetoprotein (AFP) levels may also be indicative of MMC.
○ **Treatment and Outcomes**
- Surgical closure is the primary treatment, occurring approximately 48 to 72 hours after birth. Early intervention typically enhances cognitive outcomes and decreased incontinence problems (Huang & Doherty, 2018, p. 876).
  - Remains at risk for chronic urinary tract infections
- For significant hydrocephalus involvement, a ventricular peritoneal (VP) shunt may be indicated.
- Long-term care of kids with MMC includes a multiple-disciplinary approach including urology, physical therapy, neurosurgery, OT, PT, and developmental care (Huang & Doherty, 2018, p. 876)

Congenital Neuromuscular Disorders

- Myotonic dystrophy
  ○ **Incidence and Etiology**
  - Myotonic dystrophy is the most common disorder affecting musculature.
  - It is an autosomal dominant disorder passed on by the mother. This heredity pattern makes the disease more severe as generations pass it along to their kin due to the excessive amounts of cytosine thymine guanine (CTG) which repeat and repeat, worsening the disease (Darras & Volpe, 2018, p. 927–928).
  ○ **Clinical Presentation**
  - The most striking clinical features are respiratory and feeding difficulties, arthrogryposis (especially of the lower extremities), symmetrical facial paralysis, and hypotonia.
    - The respiratory impairment may be so severe that the newborn infant fails to establish adequate ventilation and requires intubation and mechanical ventilation in the absence of lung disease (Darras & Volpe, 2018, pp. 922–923).
  - A head circumference within the upper half of the normal range is more common than overt macrocephaly, although approximately 70% of infant will present with macrocephaly, with or without accompanying ventricular dilatation when examined on CT or MRI (Darras & Volpe, 2018, p. 925).

○ **Diagnosis**
- The diagnosis is suspected if the mother has clinical or EMG features of myotonic dystrophy or if she has a confirmed genetic diagnosis; the diagnosis is made in the neonate by identifying the abnormally expanded CTG repeat in the DMPK gene.
  - The diagnosis is supported particularly by demonstrating myotonic discharges on the electromyogram (EMG) elicited by direct muscular percussion of the neonate.
- Additional information can be discovered by evaluating the serum creatine kinase (CK) levels and CSF for elevated protein levels (Darras & Volpe, 2018, pp. 924–925; Gressens & Hüppi, p. 880; Neil & Volpe, 2018, p. 438).
○ **Treatment and Outcomes**
- The clinical course relates clearly to the severity of the disease. Neonatal mortality can be as high as 40% in extreme cases, but typically ranges from 15% to 20%. For those that survive into young adulthood, gastrointestinal problems are common
- For optimal development, adequate nutrition and ventilation must be ensured, and respiratory support and tube feedings may be needed for extended periods of time (Darras & Volpe, 2018, p. 923–928; Wilson-Costello & Payne, 2015, pp. 1018–1021).
- Spinal muscular atrophy (SMA)
  ○ **Incidence and Etiology**
  - The SMAs are predominantly autosomal recessive disorders characterized by degeneration of the anterior horn cells in the spinal cord and motor nuclei in the lower brainstem. (Bass, Lotze, & Miller, 2015, p. 951; Darras & Volpe, 2018, p. 889).
  - Approximately 95% of individuals with SMA are homozygous for a deletion of exon 7 of the survival motor neuron (SMN) gene (SMN1) on chromosome 5q13. (Bass, Lotze, & Miller, 2015, p. 951).
    - SMA type 1 is often referred to as Werdnig-Hoffmann disease. This severe form of SMA (i.e., type 1) is defined by onset before 6 months of age, failure to develop the ability to sit unsupported, and death usually by less than 2 years of age (Darras & Volpe, 2018, p. 889; Bass, Lotze, & Miller, 2015, p. 951).
  ○ **Clinical Presentation**
  - Severe hypotonia related to a combination of atrophic and hypertrophic muscle fibers (Bass, Lotze, & Miller, 2015, p. 951)
    - Most infants exhibit generalized weakness, but when it is possible to make a distinction between proximal and distal muscles, a proximal more than distal distribution is discernible. (Darras & Volpe, 2018, p. 891).
  - The pattern of weakness of limbs leads to a characteristic posture, characterized particularly by a frog-leg posture with the upper extremities abducted and either externally rotated or internally rotated (jug handle) at the shoulders (Darras & Volpe, 2018, p. 891).
  - Respiratory distress with most symptoms noted with weak intercostal musculature. There is associated distention of the abdomen and intercostal recession during inspiration known as paradoxical breathing. This gives rise to the characteristic

Bell-shaped chest deformity (Bass, Lotze, & Miller, 2015, p. 951; Darras & Volpe, 2018, p. 891–892)

- Poor suck/swallow reflex, weak cry, excess oral secretions with inability to self-clear secondary to weak bulbar muscles (Bass et al., 2015, pp. 951–952)
- Particularly noteworthy differential diagnostic features in the neurological examination include the presence of normal sphincter and sensory functions
  - The infant will have an alert expression with a furrowed brown and normal eye movements due to the sparing of the upper cranial nerves (Bass, Lotze, & Miller, 2015, p. 951; Darras & Volpe, 2018, p. 892).

○ **Diagnosis**
- Decreased or lost fetal movement often noted by the mother in the late stages of pregnancy (Bass, Lotze, & Miller, 2015, p. 951; Darras & Volpe, 2018, p. 892)
- The muscle biopsy of a patient with Werdnig-Hoffmann disease, with clinically apparent findings at birth or in the first month, usually exhibits advanced changes of denervation (Darras & Volpe, 2018, p. 893)
  - With the advances made in the genetic diagnosis of this disorder, biopsies are rarely needed. (Bass et al.,2015, pp. 951–952)

○ **Treatment and Outcomes**
- Serious disturbances of sucking and swallowing early in infancy may lead to frequent aspiration of the oropharynx, and usually institution of tube feeding are required to ensure adequate nutrition
- Tracheostomy and mechanical ventilation are often necessary, and surveillance for respiratory infection must be diligent
- Quality of life discussion are important at various events throughout the infant's growth and development. (Darras & Volpe, 2018, p. 895–896).

Cranial Hemorrhages

- Subdural hemorrhage
  - ○ **Incidence and Etiology**
    - Most likely to occur under circumstances where the infant is subjected to unusual or rapid deforming stresses such as compression, molding, or stresses on extraction during delivery (Inder et al., 2018, p. 600).
      - Large head and small birth canal
      - Unusually compliant skull
      - Unusually rigid pelvic structures
      - Short duration of labor not allowing pelvis structures to dilate or an unusually long labor in which the head is subjected to prolonged compression and molding
      - Atypical presentation (breech, face, or brow)
      - Difficult vacuum extraction, challenging forceps, or rotational maneuvers (Inder et al., 2018, p. 600).
    - Can result from coagulation disturbances or maternal abuse with blunt force trauma to the abdomen (Inder et al., 2018, pp. 600–601).
    - Incidence has been underestimated mainly because these hemorrhages appear to be asymptomatic (Inder et al., 2018, p. 596)

○ **Clinical Presentation**
- Large infants above 4,000 g
- 1 minute Apgar score of 1
- Stupor, coma
- Bradycardia
- Ataxic respirations, respiratory arrest, facial paresis, seizures
- Nuchal rigidity with retrocollis or opisthotonos,
- Unequal pupils, skew deviation of eyes with lateral that is not altered by the "doll's eyes" maneuver, ocular bobbing (Inder et al., 2018, pp. 601–602).

○ **Diagnosis**
- MRI is the most effective, however CT is useful for rapid diagnosis
- Lateral skull x-rays, and cranial US are also used (Inder et al., 2018, pp. 602).

○ **Treatment**
- Rapid surgical evacuation of blood with the more severe life-threatening lacerations.
- Close surveillance in the absence of neurological symptoms.
- Subdural taps can be used to decrease signs of increased ICP (Inder et al., 2018, p. 605).

- Subarachnoid hemorrhage
  - ○ **Incidence and Etiology**
    - Primary subarachnoid hemorrhage: hemorrhage within the subarachnoid space that is not a secondary extension from subdural, intraventricular, or cerebellar hemorrhages. Most commonly the blood is found in the pia–arachnoid space over the cerebral convexities. Especially posterior and in the posterior fossa.
    - Most frequent bleed and more common in premature infants than term infants.
    - Pathogenesis is not clear. Believed to be related to trauma or circulatory events related to prematurity (Inder et al., 2018, p. 605–606).

  - ○ **Clinical presentation**
    - Minimal or no clinical signs
    - Hydrocephalus can occur
    - Seizures can occur in term infants and their onset most commonly occurs on day 2.
    - Catastrophic deterioration is very rare but can occur. Usually, these infants have sustained a severe perinatal asphyxia or an element of trauma (Inder et al., 2018, p. 606).

  - ○ **Diagnosis**
    - MRI, CT
    - Ultrasonography is insensitive in detecting subarachnoid hemorrhage because of the normal increase in echogenicity around the periphery of the brain (Neil & Inder, 2018, pg. 947).

  - ○ **Treatment and Outcomes**
    - The management is essentially that of posthemorrhagic hydrocephalus.
    - The general prognosis for infants with subarachnoid hemorrhage without traumatic or hypoxic injury is good. The infant with minimal signs in the neonatal period does well uniformly.
    - The rare patient with a catastrophic course with massive subarachnoid hemorrhage of unknown origin either suffers serious neurological residua, generally hydrocephalus, or dies (Inder et al., 2018, p. 607).

- Intracerebellar hemorrhage
  - ○ **Incidence and Etiology**
    - Occurs more commonly in preterm infants than term, especially in the very preterm infant and less than 750 g
    - Occurs 2% to 19% in the very premature infant
    - Four major categories
      - Primary cerebellar hemorrhage—it has wide range of severity, from mild to near total destruction of cerebellum. These hemorrhages can occur unilaterally or bilaterally. The hemorrhages are followed by cerebellar atrophy and reductions in cerebellar volumes.
      - Cerebellar infarction—complication of extreme preterm birth. Typically involve bilateral inferior parts of the cerebellar hemispheres and often occurs in conjunction with supratentorial white matter injury.
      - Extension of blood from intraventricular or subarachnoid spaces—IVH accompanies 95% of cerebellar hemorrhages. It can result in injury to the underlying structures and impair the immature and rapidly developing cerebellum.
      - Traumatic injury—laceration of the cerebellum or of cerebellar bridging veins. In preterm infants, the compliant skull is vulnerable to external forces that can affect the flow of venous blood and venous pressure to the cerebellum (Limperopoulos et al., 2018, p. 623–625).
  - ○ **Clinical Presentation**
    - Symptoms most commonly occur within the first 24 hours of life with the larger hemorrhages. Symptoms are consistent with brainstem compression such as apnea, respiratory irregularities, bradycardia, full fontanel, separated sutures, and moderately dilated ventricles on MRI/CT scan or cranial ultrasound (CUS). Other symptoms include skew deviation of the eyes, opisthotonos, and seizures.
    - With smaller bleeds, signs can be subtle or nonexistent. Clinical seizures and unexplained motor agitation have been seen.
    - Thrombocytopenia
    - Breech extraction of difficult forceps extraction (Limperopoulos et al., 2018, p. 632–633)
  - ○ **Diagnosis**
    - MRI
    - Cranial US through the mastoid window
  - ○ **Treatment**
    - The need for neurosurgical evaluation in infants who deteriorate quickly. These infants may need a shunt or hematoma evacuation (Limperopoulos et al., 2018, p. 635).
- Intraventricular–periventricular hemorrhages
  - ○ **Incidence and Etiology**
    - Autoregulation
      - Another factor that puts these premature infants at higher risk for hemorrhages is the lack of ability to autoregulate. This concept refers to local control of blood flow in the brain. Sustaining consistent blood flow to the brain is vital in regulating pressure in these fragile vessels. This is also known as a pressure passive state, unprotected from wide swings or changes. The more premature an infant is, the more time spent in a pressure passive state (De Vries, 2015, p. 890; Neil & Volpe, 2018, p. 445).
      - Other factors that raise the risks for IVH are related to common premature problems like hypovolemia, hypoglycemia, hypercarbia, hypoxia, and acidosis. These states all affect cerebral autoregulation, thus increasing the risk for devastating hemorrhages (Neil & Volpe, 2018, pg. 445; Inder et al., 2018, p. 651) .
    - Grades of hemorrhages
      - Germinal matrix
        - Highly cellular, gelatinous in texture, active with cellular proliferation and richly vascularized.
        - Premature infants are at risk due to the primitive and highly vascular nature of the germinal matrix.
        - Venous drainage from the deep white matter flows into the germinal matrix and into the terminal vein, which is positioned just below the germinal matrix. Eventually terminating in the great cerebral vein of Galen.
        - Is the most common form of intracranial hemorrhage in the neonatal period.
        - Four classifications of IVH are:
      - Grade I
        - Described as having a hemorrhage into the subependymal germinal matrix where a hematoma forms. The site and size can vary depending on gestational age.
      - Grade II
        - Occurs in the lateral ventricle. Blood fills less than 50% of the ventricles and the hematoma ruptures and bleeding begins to flow into the ventricles. No ventricular dilation present
      - Grade III
        - Blood fills more than 50% of the ventricle, ventricles begin to dilate and affect the brain material
      - Grade IV
        - Is an infarct or stroke in the periventricular white matter
        - Changes in systemic and cerebral hemodynamics precede the bleeding and have revealed a pattern of hypoperfusion–reperfusion cycle. This is an important causative pathway
        - Associated with large asymmetrical IVH, they usually occur on the same side as the large IVH and in some cases develop and progress after the occurrence of the IVH (De Vries, 2015, pp. 887; Inder et al., 2018, pp. 637–639, 645, 652).
  - ○ **Clinical Presentation and Assciated Findings**
    - Catastrophic syndrome: falling hematocrit, bulging anterior fontanel, hypotension, bradycardia, apnea, temperature instability, metabolic acidosis, inappropriate antidiuretic hormone secretion, generalized tonic seizures, pupils fixed to light, flaccid quadriparesis, and decerebrate posturing.

- Saltatory syndrome: altered level of consciousness, decrease in quantity and quality of spontaneous and elicited movements, hypotonia, subtle deviation from the normal of eye position and movements.
- Clinically silent syndrome: neurologic signs may be so subtle they can be easily overlooked. Most valuable sign can be an unexplained drop in hematocrit or failure of hematocrit to rise after transfusion. Twenty-five percent to 50% of infants with IVH may fail to have any clinical signs indicative of a hemorrhage (Inder et al., 2018, pp. 665–666).

○ **Diagnosis**
- Ultrasound scan is effective in identification of all degrees of severity of IVH from isolated germinal matrix hemorrhage to major degrees, with or without periventricular hemorrhagic infarction. The physical basis of the dense echoes that correlate with the hemorrhage is probably the formation of fibrin mesh within the clot (Inder et al., 2018, p. 666).
- A primary guideline for CUS screening in the United States is the Practice Parameter for Neuroimaging of the Neonate in 2002, which recommends screening with CUS for all infants with estimated gestational age (EGA) less than 30 weeks at 7 to 14 days, and optimally again at 36 to 40 weeks.
  - Studies have shown that a majority of all hemorrhages occur within the first week of life and a single scan at the end of that week show 90% of all hemorrhages as well as their maximum extent.
  - Many hemorrhages develop within the first 48 hours of life and progress over 1 to 2 days, and only 10% of GMH-IVH occurs outside the first 7 days of age.
  - The more severe the hemorrhage, the higher the risk is for post hemorrhagic ventricular dilation to occur (De Vries, 2015, pp. 886–8912; Inder et al., 2018, pp. 666–669).

○ **Treatment**
- Prevention is the best treatment. This included minimal handling, prevention of fluctuations: CO_2 levels, blood volume, fluid administration, blood pressure, and prevention of breathing over the vent, optimizing coagulation therapies, neutral positioning of head within the first 72 hours, minimal tracheal suctioning, and prophylactic indomethacin administration (Inder et al., 2018, p. 673–682).
- These grades can occur unilaterally or bilaterally, varying in degrees of severity and long-term developmental effects (Inder et al., 2018, p. 644).

- Outcomes of hemorrhages
  ○ Posthemorrhagic hydrocephalus
  - How quick and likelihood of the hydrocephalus development is directly related to the quantity of intraventricular blood present. Hypothetically with larger IVHs, it may develop over days and with the smaller grade IVHs it may develop over weeks (Inder et al., 2018, p. 643).
  - Usually develops within 1 to 3 weeks of hemorrhage (Inder et al., 2018, p. 683)
  ○ Periventricular leukomalacia

- Areas of necrosis that form cysts in the deep white matter and often occur adjacent to the lateral ventricles
- Characterized as areas of paucity of white matter, thinning of the corpus callosum, ventriculomegaly, and delayed myelination
- Deep white matter is prone to necrosis due to presumed vascular end zones.
- Studies have shown that hypoxia, hypoxia–ischemia, infection, inflammatory factors, oxidative stress, or excitotoxic factors most commonly caused white matter damage.
- The major long-term morbidity seen with PVL is spastic diplegia. Mainly there is greater spastic paresis on the lower extremities. In the more severe forms, the upper extremities are effected as well as visual and cognitive deficits (Huppi & Gressens, 2015, pp. 866–881).

○ Cerebral palsy (CP)
- Cerebral palsy (CP) refers to a group of nonprogressive, but often changing, motor impairment syndromes secondary to lesions of the developing brain (Payne & Wilson-Costello, 2015, p. 1021).
  - Decreased gestational age ~100 out of every 1,000 births of infants <31 weeks are at higher risk, compared to 10 out of every 1,000 infants between 32 and 36 weeks and one out of every 1,000 term infants (≥37 weeks; Payne & Wilson-Costello, 2015, p. 1022).
- Two common categories:
  - Diplegia: affects symmetrical parts of the body
  - Hemiplegia—referring to spasticity isolated to one side of the body
- Earliest ability to diagnose is around is around 3 to 5 years of age.

Hypoxic-Ischemic Injury

- **Incidence and Etiology**
  ○ Hypoxic-ischemic injury (HII) following severe perinatal asphyxia (also described in the literature as hypoxic-ischemic encephalopathy, perinatal hypoxia-ischemia or asphyxia neonatorum) has an incidence of 1 to 2 per 1000 live birth (Groenendaal & De Vries, 2015, p. 904).
  ○ Worldwide, hypoxic–ischemic injury (HII) is the leading cause of neonatal brain injury and neonatal mortality. Intrapartum hypoxic events caused an estimated 717,000 deaths in 2010 (~1 in 5 of all neonatal deaths worldwide) (McAdams & Traudt, 2018, p. 897). Fully 56% of all cases of newborn encephalopathy were related to hypoxic-ischemic injury that occurred during the intrapartum period (Inder & Volpe, 2018, p. 510).
  ○ The etiology of HII is multifactorial, but typically results from a serious hypoxic–ischemic event (acute or prolonged) occurring before or during labor or at delivery (McAdams & Traudt, 2018, p. 897) Neonatal hypoxia-ischemia is characterized in most cases by a combination of cerebral hypoxia (and ischemia during bradycardia). Hypoxemia leads to brain injury principally by causing myocardial disturbance and loss of cerebrovascular autoregulation, with ischemia the

major consequence (Groenendaal & De Vries, 2015, p 907; Inder & Volpe, 2018, p. 510).

○ Three features are considered to be when considering the etiology of HII: (1) evidence of fetal distress and/or fetal risk for hypoxia-ischemia (e.g., fetal heart rate (FHR) abnormalities, sentinel event, fetal acidemia); (2) the need for resuscitation and/or low Apgar scores; and (3) an overt neonatal neurological syndrome in the first hours or day of life. (Inder & Volpe, 2018, p.512).

○ Hypoxic-ischemic injury may occur at any time during pregnancy, the birth process, or the neonatal period. The pattern of brain damage is reflected by the gestational age of the fetus at the time that the injury occurs (Groenendaal & De Vries, 2015, p. 904)

  ■ The principle intrapartum events leading to hypoxic-ischemic fetal insults include acute placental or umbilical cord disturbances, such as abruptio placentae or cord prolapse, prolonged labor with transverse arrest, difficult forceps extractions or rotational maneuvers (Inder & Volpe, 2018, p. 511)

  ■ Underlying associated factors include maternal problems associated with poor placental perfusion (e.g., maternal hypotension, pre- eclampsia, chronic vascular disease), primary placental perfusion problems (tight nuchal cord, prolapsed cord, true knot, abruptio placenta, or uterine rupture), and fetal oxygenation/perfusion problems (e.g., feto-maternal hemorrhage, fetal thrombosis) (McAdams & Traudt, 2018, p. 897)

○ Selective neuronal necrosis is the most common variety of injury observed in neonatal hypoxic-ischemic encephalopathy and refers to necrosis of neurons in a characteristic, although often widespread, distribution (Inder et al., 2018, p. 500)

○ An acute hypoxic-ischemic insult leads to events that can be broadly categorized as early (primary) and delayed (secondary) neuronal death.

  ■ Early or primary neuronal damage occurs as a result of cytotoxic changes caused by failure of the microcirculation, inhibition of energy-producing molecular processes, increasing extracellular acidosis.

  ■ Recovery and reperfusion fuel the pathways to late (secondary) neuronal damage through a relatively large number of pathophysiologic mechanisms (Groenendaal & De Vries, 2015, p. 907)

• **Clinical Presentation**

○ At birth, neonates with HII are depressed and manifest clinical symptoms consistent with neurologic injury within the first few hours after delivery. The clinical presentation of affected neonates may evolve over a period of 72 hours and is often categorized using Sarnat staging, a classification scale originally based on the assessment of neonates over 36 weeks' gestation (McAdams & Traudt, 2018, p. 898; Groenendaal & De Vries, 2015, p. 904)

  ■ Sarnat stage 1 (mild encephalopathy), infants appear hyperalert with wide-open eyes, often with a "stunned look" or a blank stare, uninhibited Moro and stretch reflexes, and a normal electroencephalogram.

  ■ Sarnat stage 2 (moderate encephalopathy) present obtunded with low tone, a weak suck, constricted pupils, a decreased Moro reflex, and often have clinical seizures. The electroencephalography (EEG) showed a periodic pattern sometimes preceded by continuous delta activity.

  ■ Sarnat stage 3 (severe encephalopathy), appear stuporous with flaccid tone, intermittent decerebrate posturing (rare), absent reflexes (suck, gag, and Moro), and poorly reactive pupils (McAdams & Traudt, 2018, p. 898; Inder & Volpe, 2018, p. 513).

○ Clinical seizure-like activity often occurs by 6 to 12 hours after birth in approximately 50% to 60% of the infants who ultimately have seizures (Inder & Volpe, 2018, p. 514; McAdams & Traudt, 2018, p. 898).

  ■ Seizures occur in many infants who have sustained a significant hypoxic-ischemic insult; indeed, seizure is a feature of moderate and severe HII. In general, the more severe or prolonged the hypoxia-ischemia, the more seizure activity the infant will have (Groenendaal & De Vries, 2015, p. 920).

• **Diagnosis**

○ The recognition of neonatal HII depends principally on information gained from a careful history and a thorough neurological examination (Inder & Volpe, 2018, p. 516; McAdams & Traudt, 2018, p. 897).

  ■ The neurological examination plays two critical roles: A systematic exam before 6 hours of age will allow recognition of any neonatal HII that can lead to implementation of neuroprotective strategies, such as therapeutic hypothermia. Second, the regular and systematic neurological examination of the infant over the first week of life carries important information for prognosis (Inder & Volpe, 2018, p. 516).

○ Low Apgar scores (<5) at 5 and 10 minutes of age are consistent with an acute peripartum or intrapartum event resulting in HII. Neonates with HII who sustained an intrapartum hypoxic event typically have a fetal umbilical artery pH of less than 7.0 or base deficit greater than or equal to 12–15 mmol/L or both (McAdams & Traudt, 2018, p. 897).

○ Multisystem organ failure is common in babies with HII, evidenced by metabolic and hematologic abnormalities, hepatic, renal, gastrointestinal, and cardiac dysfunction (McAdams & Traudt, 2018, p. 898).

  ■ The diving reflex occurs during experimental asphyxia to maintain blood flow to vital organs such as the brain at the expense of less-vital organs. This is the basis of systemic complications after a clinically significant hypoxic-ischemic insult, and the heart, kidneys, and liver are the most vulnerable organs. Almost all babies with HII show compromise in at least one organ system outside the brain (Groenendaal & De Vries, 2015, p. 918–919).

○ Certain metabolic derangements may contribute significantly to the severity and qualitative aspects of the neurological syndrome, and the diagnostic evaluation should include evaluation of such derangements. Hypoglycemia, hyperammonemia, hypocalcemia, hyponatremia (inappropriate secretion of antidiuretic hormone [ADH]), hypoxemia, and acidosis are among the metabolic complications that may occur (Inder & Volpe, 2018, p. 516).

○ Monitoring for the presence of electrographic seizures is strongly recommended. Continuous video-electro-encephalogram(cEEG) is currently the gold standard for identifying neonatal seizures; however, ampli-tude-integrated electroencephalography (aEEG) is a commonly used monitoring tool for assessing cortical electrical activity trends and detecting electrographic seizures (McAdams & Traudt, 2018, p. 899).

○ Cranial ultrasound may be the only imaging modality possible if an infant is too clinically unstable to trans-port from the neonatal intensive care unit; however, it has a poor reputation when it comes to assessment of abnormalities of the brain of the full-term infant with HII. Cranial ultrasound lacks sensitivity in defining the full extent of the cerebral lesions, even in severe encephalopathy, and particularly in the first 24 hours. (Groenendaal & De Vries, 2015, p. 916; Inder & Volpe, 2018, p. 520).

○ Computed tomography is less sensitive than MRI for detecting changes in the central gray nuclei, which is the most common problem in full-term infants with HII (Groenendaal & De Vries, 2015, p. 916).

○ MRI is the study of choice for neonates with HII as it is able to show different patterns of injury MRI pro-vides the highest sensitivity for both anatomical and functional detail and also offers an array of imaging options that can be tailored to the specific clinical question.
  ■ Conventional MRI shows the abnormalities in the first 3 to 4 days, but generally not on the first day. MRI done in the first week after birth (after rewarming, day 4–5) can assess for injury patterns consistent with HII and rule out other differential diagnoses (McAdams & Traudt, 2018, p. 899; Inder & Volpe, 2018, pp. 519, 524).

○ MRI performed in the newborn period has a high pre-dictive value in neonates, with and without therapeu-tic hypothermia treatment, for subsequent neurologic impairment at 18 months of age (McAdams & Traudt, 2018, p. 899).

• Treatment & Outcomes
  ○ The emphasis on management is in terms of the follow-ing: *prevention* of peripartum hypoxic-ischemic insult; recognition of peripartum hypoxic-ischemic insult; stabilization of systemic physiology, including respira-tory, cardiovascular and metabolic; control of seizures; and commencement of neuroprotective therapy; (thera-peutic hypothermia), if indicated (Inder & Volpe, 2018, p. 548). Prevention of fetal asphyxia is far preferable to the prospect of managing the newborn who has suf-fered a hypoxic-ischemic insult in labor (Groenendaal & De Vries, 2015, p. 918).
  ○ Initial management steps should focus on promoting adequate oxygenation, ventilation (i.e., securing an airway), and circulation. Clinical and electrographic seizure activity should be assessed (e.g., with cEEG or aEEG) and controlled to limit further neurologic injury. Neonates with HII often have renal injury manifesting with oliguria or anuria with elevated creatinine levels. Close monitoring of electrolytes and fluid restriction to limit edema is recommended (McAdams & Traudt, 2018, p. 901).
  ○ Phenobarbital remains the preferred drug for the treatment of seizures in neonatal HII (Inder & Volpe,

2018, p. 554; Groenendaal & De Vries, 2015, p. 920). Seizures are associated with a markedly accelerated cerebral metabolic rate, and this acceleration may lead to a rapid fall in brain glucose, an increase in lactate, and a decrease in high-energy phosphate compounds. Moreover, the excessive synaptic release of certain exci-totoxic amino acids (e.g., glutamate) also may lead to cellular injury (Inder & Volpe, 2018, p. 554).

○ Available clinical and preclinical evidence confirms that moderate therapeutic hypothermia should be implemented as soon as possible as a standard-of-care for infants with moderate and severe HII (McAdams & Traudt, 2018, p. 901; Inder & Volpe, 2018, p. 558; Groenendaal & De Vries, 2015, p. 904).

○ The selection of infants that may benefit from hypother-mia therapy has been investigated and the following indications for the initiation of hypothermia endorsed by the American Academy of Pediatrics
  ■ More than 35 weeks gestational age
  ■ Less than 6 hours of age
  ■ Evidence of asphyxia as defined by the presence of at least 1 to 2 of the following:
    • Apgar score less than 6 at 10 minutes or contin-ued need for resuscitation with positive pressure ventilation or chest compressions at 10 minutes
    • Any acute perinatal sentinel events that may result in HII (e.g., abruptio placentae, cord pro-lapse, severe FHR abnormality)
    • Cord pH < 7.0 or base excess of −16 mmol/L or less; If cord pH is not available, arterial pH < 7.0 or base excess less than −16 mmol/L within 60 minutes of birth
  ■ Presence of moderate/severe neonatal encephalop-athy on clinical examination (Inder & Volpe, 2018, pp. 556–557)

○ Following 72 hours of cooling, infants should be *slowly* rewarmed (0.5°/hour). This rate is based on animal data showing increased seizures and increased cortical apoptosis with rapid rewarming (Inder & Volpe, 2018, p. 558).

○ Timing of hypothermia for neuroprotection is based on this "therapeutic window" of 6 hours before the onset of secondary energy failure. Its effect is thought to be related to reduction of cerebral metabolism and adenosine triphosphate (ATP) consumption and downregulating many intracerebral metabolic processes associated with rapid expression of early gene activation. (Groenendaal & De Vries, 2015, pp. 907, 921).

○ The long-term neurological sequelae depend on the topography of the neuronal injury (Inder & Volpe, 2018, p. 534). Unfortunately, despite treatment with thera-peutic hypothermia, 44% of neonates with moderate-to-severe encephalopathy will still die or have major long-term neurodevelopmental disabilities (McAdams & Traudt, 2018, p. 902; Groenendaal & De Vries, 2015, p. 924).

Neonatal Seizures

• **Incidence and Etiology**
  ○ Seizures in the neonate occur in 2 to 4 per 1000 live births and are a cause of neonatal morbidity and mor-tality (Natarajan & Gospe, 2018, p 961). Using clinical

criteria, seizure incidences ranged from 0.5% in term infants to 22.2% in preterm neonates (Scher, 2015, p. 935).

○ The incidence of seizures varies with gestational age and birthweight and is most common in the very low birthweight (VLBW) infant. Estimated incidences are 58/100 live births in the VLBW infant and 1 to 3.5/100 live births in the term infant (Abend, Jensen, Inder, & Volpe, 2018, p. 275).

○ A *seizure* is defined clinically as a paroxysmal alteration in neurological function (i.e., behavioral, motor, or autonomic function). Such a definition includes clinical phenomena that are associated temporally with seizure activity identifiable on an EEG and, therefore, are clearly epileptic (Abend et al., 2018, p. 283).

  ■ Although the fundamental mechanisms of neonatal seizures are not entirely understood, current data suggest that excessive depolarization may occur because of the imbalance of neural excitation over inhibition (Abend et al., 2018, p. 275).

○ Neonatal seizures are not disease specific and can be associated with a variety of medical conditions that occur before, during, or after parturition. Seizures may occur as part of an asphyxial brain disorder that is expressed after birth from intrapartum, peripartum or antepartum causes. (Scher, 2015, p. 936).

○ Examples may include asphyxia-related events, metabolic derangements such as hypoglycemia, hypocalcemia, or hypo- and hypernatremia. Cerebrovascular lesions, meningitis, and CNS malformations may also lead to seizures. More esoteric causes include progressive neonatal epileptic syndrome (such as benign familial neonatal seisures) and inborn errors of metabolism are rare. Finally, drug intoxication and/or withdrawal may induce seizures. (Scher, 2015, p. 936–942; Natarajan & Gospe, 2018, p. 964–967).

○ There is no agreement in the literature over whether neonatal seizures themselves can lead to damage of the immature neonatal brain. Electroclinical and electrographic neonatal seizures produce an increase in cerebral blood flow velocity which disturbs cerebral metabolism (Groenendaal & De Vries, 2015, p 914). Seizures are associated with a markedly accelerated cerebral metabolic rate, which may lead to a rapid fall in brain glucose, an increase in lactate, and a decrease in high-energy phosphate compounds. Moreover, the excessive synaptic release of certain excitotoxic amino acids (e.g., glutamate) also may lead to cellular injury (Inder & Volpe, 2018, p. 554).

  ■ Direct effects of the seizure state may have adverse effects on the developing brain. Seizures can disrupt a cascade of biochemical and molecular pathways normally responsible for the plasticity or activity-dependent development of the maturing nervous system. Seizures may disrupt the processes of cell division, migration, sequential expression of receptor formation, and stabilization of synapses, contributing to neurologic sequelae. (Scher, 2015, p. 947).

- **Clinical Presentation**
  ○ Clinical criteria for neonatal seizure diagnosis were historically subdivided into five clinical categories: focal clonic, multifocal or migratory clonic, tonic, myoclonic, and subtle seizures. (Scher, 2015, p. 927).

○ A *clonic seizure* is defined as a seizure characterized by rhythmic movements of muscle groups which consist of a rapid phase followed by a slow return movement. Clonic seizures appear as repetitive and rhythmic jerking movements that can affect any part of the body including the face, extremities, and even diaphragmatic or pharyngeal muscles. (Abend et al., 2018, p. 286; Natarajan & Gospe, 2018, p. 962).

  ■ Rhythmic movements of muscle groups in a focal distribution that consist of a rapid phase followed by a slow return movement are clonic seizures, to be distinguished from the symmetric movements of jitteriness. Gentle flexion of the affected body part easily suppresses the tremor, whereas clonic seizures persist. (Scher, 2015, p. 928).

○ *Multifocal or migratory clonic seizures* spread over body parts either in a random or anatomic fashion. Such seizure movements may alternate from side to side and appear asynchronously between the two halves of the body (Scher, 2015, p. 930). The migration most often "marches" through the body (e.g., left arm jerking may be followed by right leg jerking) (Abend et al., 2018, p. 286–287).

○ *Tonic seizures* are defined as a sustained flexion or extension of axial or appendicular muscle group. (Abend et al., 2018, p. 287). This can affect limbs but also the eye muscles with sustained eye deviation or the head, resulting in head version. Tonic seizures may be epileptic or nonepileptic, with bilateral tonic extension not having a correlate on EEG (Natarajan & Gospe, 2018, p. 962).

○ *Myoclonic seizures* are demonstrated by movements which are are rapid, lightning fast jerks. Myoclonus can occur at multiple levels of the nervous system: cortical regions, brainstem, and spinal cord (Natarajan & Gospe, 2018, p. 962). Myoclonus lacks the slow return phase of the clonic movement complex (Scher, 2015, p. 930).

  ■ There are three categories of myoclonic seizures: focal, multifocal, and generalized myoclonic seizures Focal myoclonic seizures typically involve flexor muscles of an upper extremity. Multifocal myoclonic seizures characterized by asynchronous twitching of several parts of the body. Generalized myoclonic seizures are characterized by bilateral jerks of flexion of upper and occasionally of lower limbs. (Abend et al., 2018, p. 287).

○ *Subtle seizure* activity is the most frequently observed category of neonatal seizures and includes repetitive bucco-lingual movements, orbital-ocular movements, unusual bicycling or pedaling, and autonomic findings (Scher, 2015, p 927; Abend et al., 2018, p. 285). Subtle seizures are notoriously difficult to determine clinically, where often one must first be cognizant of the neonate's typical behaviors, movements, and autonomic findings and then detect unexplained alterations of these patterns. Repetitive movements such as bicycling, pedaling, as well as ocular, oral, or buccal–lingual movements are in this category (Natarajan & Gospe, 2018, p. 963).

- **Diagnosis**
  ○ Neonatal seizures are often brief and subtle in appearance, thus raising diagnostic uncertainty when unusual movements are present. As newborns may have

behaviors that mimic movements concerning for seizure, and those at high risk of seizures may develop movements that are nonepileptic in addition to seizures, further testing is imperative to limit overtreatment as well as under-recognition of events (Natarajan & Gospe, 2018, p. 961; Inder & Volpe, 2018, p. 514).

○ Conventional EEG, the gold standard for neonatal seizure detection, is an invaluable tool for seizure detection. Continuous monitoring of neonates with EEG is recommended in certain populations including instances where one may suspect neonatal seizures to occur, such as in acute brain injury secondary to perinatal asphyxia, in neonates with clinically suspected seizures, or when neonatal epilepsy is suspected. (Natarajan & Gospe, 2018, pp. 963–964).

○ Many institutions incorporate amplitude-integrated EEG (aEEG) to aid in detection of seizures. Advantages of aEEG include bedside availability and interpretation, as well as reduced cost as compared with continuous EEG monitoring. Disadvantages of aEEG include limitations due to being prone to artifactual signals from movement, high-frequency oscillator ventilation, or extracorporeal membrane oxygenation (ECMO) (Natarajan & Gospe, 2018, p. 964)

   ■ Because subtle seizures are clinically difficult to detect, synchronized video/EEG/polygraphic recordings are recommended to document temporal relationships between clinical behavior and electrographic events (Scher, 2015, p. 928).

- **Treatment and Outcomes**
  ○ The initial antiepileptic drug (AED) most often used is phenobarbital, administered intravenously in a loading dose of 20 mg/kg. This dosing is necessary to achieve a blood level of approximately 20 µg/mL which achieves a clearly measurable anticonvulsant effect in the newborn. Total loading doses of phenobarbital in excess of 40 to 50 mg/kg generally do not provide extra benefit (Abend et al., 2018, pp. 311–312; Scher, 2015, p. 944; Natarajan & Gospe, 2018, p.968; Inder & Volpe, 2018, p. 554)

  ○ Treatment choices beyond phenobarbital vary greatly between providers. The best evidence is for phenytoin or fosphenytoin. (Natarajan & Gospe, 2018, p. 968). These drugs are often used as second line medications for infants who continues to experience electrographic or clinical seizures after as much as 40 mg/kg of phenobarbital or in the severely asphyxiated infant in whom less than the full phenobarbital loading dose is deemed appropriate because of cardiopulmonary concerns (Abend et al., 2018, p. 313).

    ■ Fosphenytoin is dosed in *phenytoin equivalents* (1.5 mg of fosphenytoin yields approximately 1 mg of phenytoin), and the effective dose is essentially identical to that described for phenytoin. The 20 mg/kg loading dose of phenytoin results in a therpeatuic blood level of approximately 15 to 20 ug/kg (Abend et al., 2018, p. 313).

  ○ Approximately 20% or more of newborns with electrographic seizures do not respond to the sequential administration of phenobarbital and phenytoin (Abend et al., 2018, p. 314). Benzodiazepines, such as midazolam, diazepam, or lorazepam, may also be used to control refractory neonatal seizures (Natarajan & Gospe, 2018, p. 968; Scher, 2015, p. 944).

○ As a newer anticonvulsant medication, levetiracetam has become a medication used for the treatment of refractory neonatal seizures. In some centers, it is used as a second-line agent before using phenytoin, benzodiazepines, or lidocaine. Although levetiracetam use is increasing, few data are available regarding efficacy (Abend et al., 2018, p. 315; Natarajan & Gospe, 2018, p. 968–969; Scher, 2015, p. 944).

   ■ Other anticonvulsants used to treat seizures include lidocaine, thiopentone, sodium valproate, and lamotrigine (Groenendaal & De Vries, 2015, p. 920)

○ The optimal duration of anticonvulsant therapy for newborns with seizures relates principally to the likelihood of seizure recurrence if the drugs are discontinued. (Abend et al., 2018, p. 317). It is now generally recommended that, when possible, AEDs be discontinued in the neonatal intensive care unit (NICU), given the low rate of seizure recurrence after AED withdrawal. There is the additional concern of the effects of AEDs on the immature brain (Natarajan & Gospe, 2018, p. 969; Abend et al., 2018, p. 318).

○ The etiology of a newborn's seizure largely accounts for the overall outcome. (Natarajan & Gospe, 2018, p 969). The mortality rate of infants who present with clinical neonatal seizures has declined over time. The incidence of adverse neurologic sequelae, however, remains high for approximately two thirds of survivors. (Scher, 2015, p. 947).

   ■ Newborns with seizures acutely in the neonatal period remain at an approximate 25% risk for developing epilepsy, defined as recurrent unprovoked seizures, in later life. Neonates with refractory seizures, requiring multiple AEDs, severe brain injury, or those with persistent interictal epileptiform discharges on EEG have the highest risk (Natarajan & Gospe, 2018, p. 970).

   ■ The incidence of neurological sequelae in infants with seizures is as much as 40-fold greater than the incidence in those without seizures (Inder & Volpe, 2018, p. 540).

Nonepileptic Neonatal Movements

- **Incidence and Etiology**
  ○ Infants are prone to a variety of movements that can raise concern for seizures but are actually nonneurologic in nature. Approximately forty-four percent of healthy term infants have been noted to experience some such movements (Natarajan & Gospe, 2018, pp. 962–963).

  ○ These nonepileptic movements can be from maternal medications such as selective serotonin repute inhibitors (SSRIs) or illicit drug usage such as cocaine and marijuana. They can also be caused by metabolic derangements such as hypoglycemia or hypocalcemia, as well as intracranial hemorrhage and/or hypothermia.

- **Clinical presentation**
  ○ Tremors can mimic subtle seizure activities like bicycling and chewing. The difference between tremors and seizures is there are equal phases and amplitude of flexion and extension. Tremors can be asymmetric and spontaneous, but can occur with tactile and environmental stimulation (Inder et al., 2018, p. 288).

○ Jittery movements are rhythmic-like tremulous movement patterns that are characterized by trembling of the hands and feet. There are no eye movements involved. A distinguishing feature is that these these movements can be stopped with passive flexion of the affected extremity (Verklan, 2015, p. 760).

○ Myoclonus is defined as an sequence of repetitive nonrhythmic movement cause by sudden involuntary contraction or relaxation of the muscles. Preterm infants are most vulnerable to this nonepileptic movement. Mostly noted while infant is asleep and resolved when awake (Natarajan & Gospe, 2018, pp. 962–963).

○ Dyskinesias are Involuntary movements that appear as abnormal posturing. Injury and are commonly mistaken for seizures in the neonatal period. Dystonia is the involuntary sustained or intermittent co-contraction of agonist and antagonist muscles resulting in abnormal posture (Natarajan & Gospe, 2018, p. 963).

- **Diagnosis**
  ○ Continuous video EEG (Natarajan & Gospe, 2018, p. 963)
- **Treatment**
  ○ Most outgrow these movements as CNS matures.
  ○ When properly diagnosed, most infants do not need medical intervention and will outgrow these movements as the CNS matures.

CONCLUSION

The developing neurological system is fragile, but postnatal function depends heavily on uncompromised fetal development. Mitigating influences that can lead to neurological dysfunction are often beyond our control. However, clinicians should maintain a high level of understanding regarding the physiological and pathophysiological processes of the neonatal neurological system to aid in appropriately diagnosing and managing the various types of neurological insults. Health team members should also assess parents and caregivers for altered psychosocial integrity, knowledge deficits, and ineffective coping skills related to the uncertainty and/or finality of the short-term and long-term outcomes of neurological dysfunction.

REVIEW QUESTIONS

1. Holoprosencephaly is primarily a disorder of incomplete:
   A. cleavage
   B. migration
   C. symbiosis

2. Development of an obstruction at any location of the cerebral spinal fluid (CSF) pathway will result in a/an:
   A. cobblestone lissencephaly
   B. hydrocephalus variants
   C. narrow squamosal sutures

3. An infant presents with respiratory distress, hypotonia, a tent-shaped upper lip, and arthrogryposis. The NNP suspects a neuromuscular disorder and knows the most common disorder is:
   A. amyotonic dysratrophy
   B. myotonic dystrophy
   C. spinal muscular atrophy

4. The NNP reviews a cerebral ultrasound of a preterm infant's ventricules and notes that more than 50% of the ventricle appears to be filled with blood. This equates to a diagnosis of intraventricular hemorrhage grade:
   A. I
   B. II
   C. III

5. One of the recognized methods to reduce the incidence and risk of intraventricular hemorrhage (IVH) is to:
   A. delay cord clamping at delivery
   B. treat pneumothoracies quickly
   C. use asynchronous ventilation

REFERENCES

Abend, N., Jense, F., Inder, T., & Volpe, J. (2018). Neonatal seizures. In J. Volpe, T. Inder, B. Darras, L. deVries, A. Plessis, … J. Perlman (Eds.). *Volpe's neurology of the newborn* (6th ed., pp. 275–321.e14). Philadelphia, PA: Elsevier.

Bass, N., Lotze, T. E., & Miller, G. (2015). Hypotonia and neuromuscular disease in the neonate. In R. Martin, A. Fanaroff, & M. Walsh (Eds.), *Fanaroff and Martin's neonatal-perinatal medicine: Diseases of the fetus and infant* (10th ed., pp. 1018–1031). Philadelphia, PA: Elsevier.

Blackburn, S. (2013). *Maternal, fetal, & neonatal physiology: A clinical perspective* (4th ed., pp. 509–554). Maryland Heights, MO. Elsevier/Saunders.

Darras, B., & Volpe, J (2018) Evaluation, special studies. In J. Volpe, T. Inder, B. Darras, L. deVries, A. Plessis, … J. Perlman (Eds.). *Volpe's neurology of the newborn* (6th ed., pp. 861–873). Philadelphia, PA: Elsevier.

De Vries, L. (2015). Intracranial hemorrhage and vascular lesions of the neonate. In R. Martin, A. Fanaroff, & M. Walsh (Eds.), *Fanaroff and Martin's neonatal-perinatal medicine: Diseases of the fetus and infant* (10th ed. pp. 1018–1031). Philadelphia, PA: Elsevier.

du Plessis, A., & Volpe, J. (2018). Prosencephalic development. In J. Volpe, T. Inder, B. Darras, L. deVries, A. Plessis, . . . J. Perlman (Eds.), *Volpe's neurology of the newborn* (6th ed., pp. 34–57). Philadelphia, PA. Elsevier.

duPlessis, A., Robinson, S., & Volpe, J. (2018). Congenital hydrocephalus. In J. Volpe, T. Inder, B. Darras, L. deVries, A. Plessis, . . . J. Perlman (Eds.), *Volpe's neurology of the newborn* (6th ed., pp. 58–72). Philadelphia, PA: Elsevier.

Evans, K., Hing, A., & Cunningham, M. (2018). Craniofacial malformations. In C. Gleason & S. Juul (Eds.), *Avery's diseases of the newborn* (10th ed., pp. 1417–1437.e2). Philadelphia, PA: Elsevier.

Gressens, P., & Hüppi, P. (2015). Normal and abnormal brain development. In R. Martin, A. Fanaroff, & M. Walsh (Eds.), *Fanaroff and Martin's neonatal-perinatal medicine: Diseases of the fetus and infant* (10th ed., pp. 836–865). Philadelphia, PA: Elsevier.

Groenendaal, F., & De Vries, L. (2015). Hypoxic-ischemic encephalopathy. In R. Martin, A. Fanaroff, & M. Walsh (Eds.), *Fanaroff and Martin's neonatal-perinatal medicine: Diseases of the fetus and infant* (10th ed., pp. 1018–1031). Philadelphia, PA: Elsevier.

Huang, S., & Doherty, D. (2018). Congenital malformations of the central nervous system. In C. Gleason & S. Juul (Eds.), *Avery's diseases of the newborn* (10th ed., pp. 857–878.e5). Philadelphia, PA. Elsevier.

Hüppi, P., & Gressens, P. (2015). White matter damage and encephalopathy of prematurity. In R. Martin, A. Fanaroff, & M. Walsh (Eds.), *Fanaroff and Martin's neonatal-perinatal medicine: Diseases of the fetus and infant* (10th ed., pp. 866–883). Philadelphia, PA: Elsevier.

Inder, T., Perlman, J., & Volpe, J. (2018). Intracranial hemorrhage: Subdural, subarachnoid, intraventricular (term infant), miscellaneous In J. Volpe, T. Inder, B. Darras, L. deVries, A. Plessis, . . . J. Perlman (Eds.), *Volpe's neurology of the newborn* (6th ed., pp. 593–622.e7). Philadelphia, PA: Elsevier.

Inder, T., & Volpe, J. (2018). Hypoxic-ischemic injury in the term infant: Clinical-neurological features, diagnosis, imaging, prognosis, therapy. In J. Volpe, T. Inder, B. Darras, L. deVries, A. Plessis, . . . J. Perlman (Eds.), *Volpe's neurology of the newborn* (6th ed., pp. 593–622.e7). Philadelphia, PA: Elsevier.

Johnson, P. (2018). Head, eyes, ears, nose, mouth, and neck assesssment. In E. P. Tappero & M. E. Honeyfield (Eds.), *Physical assessment of the newborn* (6th ed., pp. 61–77). New York, NY: Springer Publishing Company.

Juul, S., Fleiss, B., McAdams, M., & Gressens, P. (2018). Neuroprotection strategies for the newborn. In C. Gleason & S. Juul (Eds.), *Avery's diseases of the newborn* (10th ed., pp.987–909.e4). Philadelphia, PA: Elsevier.

Limperopoulos, C., du Plessis, A., & Volpe, J. (2018). Cerebellar hemorrhage. In J. Volpe, T. Inder, B. Darras, L. deVries, A. Plessis, . . . J. Perlman (Eds.). *Volpe's neurology of the newborn* (6th ed., pp. 623–636). Philadelphia, PA: Elsevier.

McAdams, R., & Traudt, C. (2018). Brain injury in the term infant. In C. Gleason & S. Juul (Eds.), *Avery's diseases of the newborn* (10th ed., pp. 987–909.e4). Philadelphia, PA: Elsevier.

Natarajan, N., & Gospe, S. (2018). Neonatal seizures. In C. Gleason & S. Juul (Eds.), *Avery's diseases of the newborn* (10th ed., pp. 987–909.e4). Philadelphia, PA: Elsevier.

Neil, J., & Volpe, J. (2018). Encephalopathy of prematurity: Clinical-neurological features, diagnosis, imaging, prognosis, therapy. In J. Volpe, T. Inder, B. Darras, L. deVries, A. Plessis, . . . J. Perlman (Eds.), *Volpe's neurology of the newborn* (6th ed., pp. 425–457.e11). Philadelphia, PA: Elsevier.

Parsons, J., Seay, A., & Jacobson, M. (2016). Neurologic disorders. In S. Gardner, B. Carter, M. Hines, & J. Hernandez (Eds.), *Merenstein & Gardner's handbook of neonatal intensive care* (8th ed., pp. 727–762.e3). St. Louis, MO. Elsevier.

Robinson, S., & Cohen, A. (2015). Disorders in head shape and size. In R. Martin, A. Fanaroff, & M. Walsh (Eds.), *Fanaroff and Martin's Neonatal-perinatal medicine: Diseases of the fetus and infant* (10th ed., pp. 964–989). Philadelphia, PA: Elsevier.

Scher, M. (2015). Neonatal seizures. In R. Martin, A. Fanaroff, & M. Walsh (Eds.), *Fanaroff and Martin's neonatal-perinatal medicine: Diseases of the fetus and infant* (10th ed., pp. 1018–1031). Philadelphia, PA: Elsevier.

Verklan, M. (2015). Neurologic disorders. In T. Verklan & M. Walden (Eds.), *Core curriculum for neonatal intensive care nursing* (5th ed., pp. 734–766). St. Louis, MO: Elsevier.

Wilson-Costello, D., & Payne, A. (2015). Early childhood neurodevelopmental outcomes of high-risk neonates. In R. Martin, A. Fanaroff, & M. Walsh (Eds.), *Fanaroff and Martin's neonatal-perinatal medicine: Diseases of the fetus and infant* (10th ed., pp. 1018–1031). Philadelphia, PA: Elsevier.

16 THE CARDIAC SYSTEM

Karen Wright
Jacqueline Hoffman

INTRODUCTION

Congenital heart disease (CHD) is one of the more common birth defects, occurring in six to 13 per 1,000 births as the result of genetic or environmental factors. Of these infants, 25% have critical CHD requiring intervention. A delay in diagnosis of critical CHD compromises neonatal outcome. CHD is the most common genetic anomaly and the leading noninfectious cause of death during the first year of life. Cardiac development is a complex multifactorial process involving a convergence of risk factors resulting in CHD. Congenital disorders of the cardiac system, if left untreated, will compromise neonatal well-being and survival.

CARDIAC SYSTEM DEVELOPMENT

The cardiac tract arises as a complex process derived from embryogenic cells from multiple origins. The fetus is dependent. Disorders of cardiac development result in abnormal fetal "programming" of tissues and may result in long-term neurobehavioral consequences as well as later health concerns.

- Cardiac development is a complex process occurring early in gestation and in general, prior to when pregnancy is known (Figure 16.1). The heart is one of the first organs to be functional in life and arises from the cardiogenic mesoderm (Swanson & Erickson, 2016, pp. 644–645).
- The primary concepts of cardiac development are:
  - Gastrulation—the arrangement of the three germ layers
  - Establishment of the first and second heart fields
  - Development of the heart tube
  - Cardiac looping, convergence, and wedging
  - Evolution of septa (common atrium, atrioventricular [AV] canal)
  - Development of the outflow tract
  - Formation of cardiac valves
  - Design of the coronary arteries and aortic arches
  - Arrangement of the conduction system (Swanson & Erickson, 2016, pp. 644–645)

Gestational Weeks 3 to 12

- Between days 16 and 18, progenitor cells from the endoderm form the splanchnic mesoderm from which the cardiac tube is formed. Fetal development of the heart begins with the cardiac tube from which the cardiac structures arise.
  - The top (cephalic) part of the heart tube gives rise to the aortic arches, and from the bottom (caudal) portion, the ventricles. By day 19, angiogenic cells form the two endocardial tubes which, develop synchronously. Near day 21, the tubes migrate together in a cranial–caudal progression, then fuse and form in a single tube. The inside of the endocardial tube becomes the endocardium and the outside the myocardium (muscular wall) of the heart.
  - The heartbeat begins at 22 to 23 days of life and begins pumping blood during week 4. The heart begins as a heart tube, which undergoes complex developmental tasks such as looping, shifting, and septation to result in a circulatory pattern. Venous-arterial communication evolves from a primitive to a complex state.
  - Complete cardiac development occurs at 6 weeks of embryologic age (Blackburn, 2018, p. 269; Swanson & Erickson, 2016, p. 644).
  - Disorders of this period include transposition of the great arteries and dextrocardia (Sadowski, 2015, pp. 536–538).

Gestational Weeks 4 to 6

- Septation of the primordial atrium begins by the end of the fourth week. The atrial septum is derived from the septum primum and the septum secundum. The foramen ovale (FO) forms as a result of the septum secundum overlapping the foramen secundum.
- Ventricular septation from the endocardial cushions is coordinated with formation of AV valves and semilunar valves. Spiraling of the truncus arteriosus and the bulbis cordis results in a single trunk separating into two vessels—the aorta and pulmonary artery (PA). The aortic and aortic branches develop during this time (Blackburn, 2018, p. 269; Swanson & Erickson, 2016, p. 644).
- Disorders arising from this developmental period:
  - Failure of the AV valves to form result in tricuspid and mitral valve abnormalities.
  - Failure of proper formation of the septum results in ventricular septal defect (VSD), atrial septal defects (ASD), endocardiac cushion defect.
  - Failure of the vessels to form and separate result in interrupted arch, and coarctation of the aorta (COA; Sadowski, 2015, pp. 538–539).

INCIDENCE AND RISK FACTORS FOR THE DEVELOPMENT OF CHD

- Cardiac development that is abnormal results in CHD. Prenatal diagnosis often occurs due to the widespread use of antenatal ultrasound, suggesting cardiac anomalies 39% of the time. Ultrasound leads to fetal echocardiography for diagnosis of CHD.
  - The timing for fetal echocardiography should be between 18 and 20 weeks gestational age.

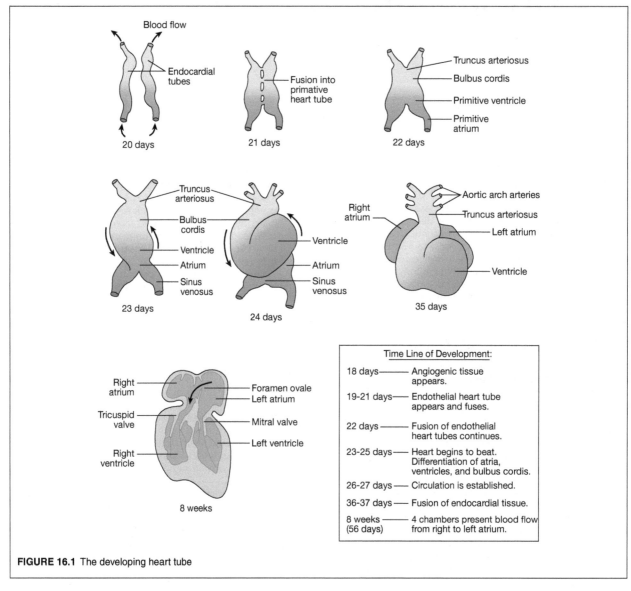

FIGURE 16.1 The developing heart tube

○ Only 39% of CHD is diagnosed prenatally despite prenatal ultrasound. Prenatal diagnosis of congenital heart defects improves patient outcomes and decreases morbidity and mortality, allowing for interventions at delivery if needed (Swanson & Erickson, 2016, pp. 647–649).

• The incidence of CHD in live-born infants is six to eight per 1,000 live births, or approximately 1% of live births, and remains constant. In general, risk factors are not evident, however certain maternal and fetal conditions are associated with risk of CHD (Sadowski, 2015, pp. 544–545; Swanson & Erickson, 2016, pp. 645, 647–649).

Maternal Health

• Maternal diabetes prior to conception adds two to four times the risk of CHD. Elevated insulin levels result in hypertrophic cardiac tissue (Martin, Fanaroff, & Walsh, 2015, p. 1212).

○ Maternal presence of anti-Ro or anti-La antibodies related to maternal systemic lupus erythematosus results in placental passage of immunoglobulin C antibody, which deposits compliment near the AV node, resulting in fetal heart block or possible hydrops (Martin et al., 2015, p. 1212).

○ Women with diabetes mellitus, especially those who are dependent on insulin, have a five-times greater risk of delivering an infant with a CHD.

   ■ The defects most commonly identified in infants of diabetic mothers are transposition of the great vessels (TGV), VSD, cardiomyopathy, and a variety of complex CHDs (Sadowski, 2015, p. 537).

• Maternal lupus disease is associated with fetal and neonatal complete congenital heart block and dilated cardiomyopathy (Sadowski, 2015, p. 537).

• Maternal infections with viral or bacterial illnesses can be associated with an increased risk of CHD.

○ Rubella and cytomegalovirus (CMV) are strongly associated with persistent ductus arteriosus (PDA), ASDs, and VSD.
○ Maternal influenza is connected with right ventricular outflow tract obstruction (RVOT) defects (Sadowski, 2015, pp. 537–538).

Maternal Substance Ingestion

• Cardiac teratogens include alcohol, tobacco, anticonvulsants, anticoagulants, lithium, amphetamines, and selective serotonin reuptake inhibitors (SSRIs; Sadowski, 2015, pp. 536–537).

Genetic Factors

• The single greatest risk factor for CHD is genetic (Swanson & Erickson, 2016, p. 647). Overall incidence of CHD in patients with a chromosome aberration is 30% (Sadowski, 2015, p. 535).
○ Incidence of CHD varies with each chromosomal aberration. Syndromes that should raise suspicion for CHD include the trisomies 13, 18, and 21; Turner syndrome; microdeletion syndromes (e.g., DiGeorge and Noonan syndromes), Beckwith–Wiedemann, VACTERL (vertebral anomalies, anal atresia, tracheo-esophageal fistula, renal anomalies, and limb abnormalities), and CHARGE (colaboma, heart defects, atresia choanae, growth retardation, genital abnormalities, and ear abnormalities) syndromes (Sadowski, 2015, pp. 535–536; Swanson & Erickson, 2016, p. 647, 649).

Family History

• Familial history of CHD increases the incidence, with higher incidence in closer relatives (parents and siblings; Swanson & Erickson, 2016, pp. 647–649). The risk of CHD in a newborn with a sibling with CHD is more than double (Scholz & Reinking, 2017, p. 803).

Gender

• Male infants are more likely to experience contraction of the aorta (COA), aortic stenosis (AS), TGV, and hypoplastic left heart syndrome (HLHS).
• Female infants are more likely to experience ASD and PDA.

Gestational Age

• Infants born prematurely are more likely to experience PDA, VSD, and AV canal defects.
• The majority of infants with CHD are born at term (Sadowski, 2015, pp. 537–538).

CLINICAL PRESENTATION OF AN INFANT WITH CHD

• The time and presentation of CHD depend on the severity and physiology of the underlying disorder. CHD may present at delivery through the first few weeks of life. Birth transition and ductal closure, in conjunction with cardiopulmonary physiology, impact the presentation of the disorder (Breinholt, 2017, p. 512).
• The critical findings of CHD are cyanosis, respiratory distress, congestive heart failure (CHF), diminished cardiac output, abnormal cardiac rhythm, and cardiac murmurs (Swanson & Erickson, 2016, p. 650).

Differential Diagnosis

• Differential diagnosis of CHD disease is a clinical challenge in the NICU due to the similarity in presentation to intrapulmonary right-to-left shunting. Pulmonary etiologies that are similar to CHD in presentation include pulmonary hypertension, pneumonia, respiratory distress syndrome (RDS), congenital diaphragmatic hernia, pneumothorax, and airway obstruction. Overall considerations for differential diagnosis of CHD include:
○ Persistent pulmonary hypertension of the newborn
○ Respiratory etiologies (RDS, aspiration)
○ Central nervous system disorders (lesions, neuromuscular disease)
○ Chest compression (congenital diaphragmatic hernia [CDH], pneumothorax)
○ Septicemia
○ Airway obstruction (Pierre Robin, tracheal stenosis, thoracic dystrophies)
○ Methemoglobinemia (Breinholt, 2017, p. 515)

Physical Examination

• A complete physical examination will provide clues to cardiac pathology. Physical examination of the newborn is holistic and not necessarily focused only on heart sounds.

Neurologic Assessment

• The assessment of the neonate should begin with a general observation of the infant's overall appearance and behavior. A newborn with CHD may exhibit decreased activity and/or appear flaccid (Vargo, 2018, p. 96).

Cardiac/Perfusion Assessment

COLOR
• Cyanosis is a bluish color of the lips, tongue, mucous membranes, skin, earlobes, and nail beds due to deoxygenated venous blood (Vargo, 2018, p. 96). Cyanosis occurs when blood shunts "right to left," causing deoxygenated blood to enter the system and bypass the lungs for oxygenation. Cyanosis is visible after 3 g/dL of desaturated hemoglobin is present in the arterial system.
• Central cyanosis must be differentiated from noncardiac etiologies, such as:
○ Acrocyanosis, which refers to bluish hands and feet and is a normal finding
○ Pulmonary hypertension or respiratory disease, which may result in cyanosis secondary to cardiac right-to-left shunting.
○ Central nervous system disorders that result in hypoxemia
○ Methemoglobinemia, which is not due to hypoxemia but, rather a blood disorder (Scholz & Reinking, 2017, p. 803; Swanson & Erickson, 2016, p. 651; Vargo, 2018, p. 96).
• Pallor and mottling should also be considered, as infants with CHD may appear pale due to vasoconstriction and/or shunting (Vargo, 2018, pp. 96–97).
• Capillary refill should be less than 3 seconds to be considered normal (Vargo, 2018, p. 97).

PULSES

- The character of the peripheral pulses including rate, rhythm, volume, and character should all be examined. Pulses represent an approximate determination of cardiac output. The axillary, palmar, brachial, radial, femoral, popliteal, posterior tibial, and dorsalis pedis may be palpated using the index finger (Vargo, 2018, p. 97).
  - Two methods to grade
    - From 0 (absent) to 6 (strong; Sadowski, 2015, p. 549)
    - From 0 (absent) to 3+ (full or bounding; Vargo, 2018, p. 97).
- Abnormalities in peripheral pulses may be present. It is helpful to compare upper to lower and side to side for discrepancies:
  - Weak pulses indicate shock, myocardial failure, or left outflow obstructions.
  - Bounding pulses indicate cardiac runoff (surplus) such as PDA, aortic insufficiency, systemic to pulmonary shunts (Sadowski, 2015, p. 549).

CARDIAC SOUNDS

- Murmurs are common and may be normal or abnormal. All neonates at one time have a murmur due to closure of the PDA. Auscultation of a murmur requires consideration and evaluation. Most innocent murmurs are systolic.
- Loudness or intensity of the murmur should be determined and recorded by the "grade":
  - Grade I: barely audible, audible only after a period of careful auscultation
  - Grade II: soft, but audible immediately
  - Grade III: of moderate intensity (but not associated with a thrill)
  - Grade IV: louder (may be associated with a thrill)
  - Grade V: very loud; can be heard with the stethoscope rim barely on the chest (may be associated with a thrill)
  - Grade VI: extremely loud; can be heard with the stethoscope just slightly removed from the chest (may be associated with a thrill; Vargo, 2018, p. 103)
- If a murmur is not heard, the infant may still have severe heart disease.
- Significant murmurs indicative of disease (pathologic) appear associated with the associated physiology. Diastolic murmurs are considered pathologic, and the severity of the murmur can be diagnostic.
  - Valvular stenosis or insufficiency generally occurs shortly after birth. Systolic murmurs (occuring during systole) are heard in mitral, tricuspid insufficiency, VSD, tetrology of Fallot (TOF), ASD, and total anomalous pulmonary venous return (TAPVR; Erickson & Swanson, 2016, p. 650).
- In the newborn with suspected CHD, listen with a stethoscope over the fontanelle and liver for a continuous bruit murmur, indicating an arteriovenous malformation (AVF; Scholz & Reinking, 2017, p. 803).

Respiratory Assessment

- Respiratory distress, such as grunting, flaring, and retractions, is not normally found in infants with CHD. Cyanosis from CHD will not be impacted by inspired oxygen (if a right-to-left shunt is present).
  - If respiratory distress is present with CHD, it would most often occur with pulmonary over circulation which is not draining due to pulmonary vein or left heart anomalies, as in pulmonary edema. In these cases, infants do exhibit respiratory distress (grunting,

flaring, and retractions); a chest x-ray will be helpful for these cases, but not diagnostic of CHD.
- Diaphoresis may be evident if the infant is in CHF due to stimulation of the autonomic nervous system resulting in an increase in metabolic demands (Swanson & Erickson, 2016, p. 650).

Abdominal Assessment

- Hepatomegally due to systemic venous overload and hepatic venous congestion (Swanson & Erickson, 2016, p. 650).

Vital Signs

HEART RATE
- Full term: 80 to 160 beats per minute (bpm), at rest 120 to 140 bpm (Tappero, 2018, p. 100)

RESPIRATORY RATE
- 30 to 60 breaths per minute (Tappero, 2018, p. 81).

BLOOD PRESSURE
- Blood pressure varies by gestational age, wellness, temperature, postnatal age, behavior state, and cuff size.
  - Blood pressure differences between upper and lower extremities are due to aortic arch abnormalities.
  - Cuff should be 25% larger than the arm width for accuracy (Sadowski, 2015, p. 549).
  - Term infant average systolic pressure is 56 to 77 mm Hg; average diastolic pressure is 33 to 50 mm Hg. MAP is 42 to 60 mm Hg (Sandowski, 2015, p. 543).

Diagnostic Testing

- Ability to oxygenate is determined by the hyperoxia test, which is conducted by obtaining an arterial pO2 in room air and in 100% oxygen, allowing 10 minutes in each prior to the test and comparison of the values.
  - Evaluate pre- and post ductal pO2s; preductal is right radial or temporal artery, post ductal is umbilical artery catheter; obtain simultaneously for most accurate comparison; results will be preductal <100 mmHg for cardiac disease and >100 mmHg for pulmonary disease (Sadowski, 2015, p. 561; Swanson & Erickson, 2016, p. 653).
  - May begin with pre- and post ductal pulse oximetry (Sadowski, 2015, p. 561).
  - Assists differential diagnosis of congenital heart defect versus respiratory etiology (Sadowski, 2015, p. 561).
- Obtaining a chest X-ray assists with identification of pulmonary findings. The chest x-ray allows evaluation of visible cardiac characteristics such as abnormal shape, size, and position. Cardiac shapes may indicate underlying disease (egg on a string—transposition), (boot-shaped—TOF). Increased pulmonary vascular markings as seen in lesions with increased blood flow, such as PDA (Sadowski, 2015, p. 561).
- Electrocardiography (EKG) used to evaluate arrhythmias but is not as useful for detecting structural heart disease. An EKG can add definition to the type of structural heart disease or may appear normal, even if there are structural cardiac defects. EKG is helpful to evaluate cardiac defects

with abnormalities of the conduction system, such as sinus node dysfunction, heart block, or accessory pathways (Swanson & Ericson, 2016, p. 654).

- ○ Stand T-wave changes indicate myocardial ischemia (Sadowski, 2015, p. 561).
- ○ Normal heart rate is 120 to 160 for 0 to 7 days of life. Premature infants have a higher resting heart rate (Sadowski, 2015, p. 561).
- ○ Normal complex is P wave then QRS wave (Sadowski, 2015, p. 561).
- ○ Normal P wave 0.04 second to 0.08 second; PR interval 0.09 to 0.12 second (Sadowski, 2015, p. 561).
- Echocardiography with Doppler is the gold standard for evaluating cardiovascular anatomy and function. Using two-dimensional echocardiography, the anatomy, physiologic pressure gradients, and cardiac function can be evaluated (Swanson & Erickson, 2016, p. 564). Enhanced echocardiograph includes contrast (to evaluate flow), color flow (to evaluate patterns and direction of blood flow), two-dimensional (evaluating anatomic relationships), and 3-D (cross-sectional images (Sadowski, 2015, p. 561–562).

Laboratory Assessment

- Lab work may be useful to determine the diagnosis of CHD versus other etiologies.
  - ○ Arterial blood gasses with a normal pCO_2 may be present with CHD unless coinciding respiratory distress or CHF is present. A blood gas revealing a metabolic acidosis may indicate low cardiac output and decreased tissue perfusion.
  - ○ An elevated lactate level indicates poor tissue perfusion and may reflect low cardiac output.
  - ○ A metabolic panel is helpful for evaluating renal function by following blood urea nitrogen (BUN) and creatinine levels.
  - ○ Hypoglycemia may be a secondary effect of CHD due to genetic abnormalities, medications treating CHD, and poor feeding. Diuretic therapy for CHF warrants monitoring of sodium, potassium, and chloride levels.
  - ○ A complete blood count (CBC) is useful to detect significant anemia as well as assist with the differential or coinciding diagnosis of sepsis. Decreased hemoglobin worsens hypoxemia and increases the workload of the heart in infants with CHD (Swanson & Erickson, 2016, p. 654).

CYANOTIC HEART DEFECTS

- Right-to-left shunting due to CHD results in cyanosis due to the mixture of pulmonary and systemic venous return. These babies may present clinically with tachypnea, poor feeding, hepatomegaly, and pulmonary edema. Cyanotic defects decreasing pulmonary blood flow result in CHF-like symptoms (Scholz & Reinking, 2017, p. 808; Swanson & Ericson, 2016, p. 650).

Ebstein's Anomaly

DEFINITION AND PATHOPHYSIOLOGY

- In fetal life, Ebstein's anomaly results from a lack of formation of the tricuspid valve, resulting in a hypoplastic right ventricle. Ebstein's anomaly is uncommon and involves a displaced tricuspid valve is with a tethered leaflet with functional pulmonary atresia and right-to-left atrial shunting; right ventricle pumps inefficiently (Ashwath & Snyder, 2013, p. 1234). The valve is displaced into the right ventricle resulting in a smaller right ventricle and a decrease in ventricular output. The displaced tricuspid valve allows regurgitation of blood, resulting in a negative impact of blood allowed systemically through the PA. With severe tricuspid atresia (TA; regurgitation), only an insignificant amount of blood is passed into the pulmonary arteries. This results in a **ductal dependent lesion,** which may be severe with severe valvular displacement (Swanson & Ericson, 2016, pp. 668–669; Ashwath & Snyder, 2013, p. 1234).

Diagnosis

- Clinical presentation is cyanosis ranging from mild to severe based on the degree of right-to-left shunting at the FO and is able to be sent to the PA. Heart sounds are of a holosystolic murmur varying from grade I to VI based on the degree of tricuspid regurgitation. Diminished S2 and diastolic murmurs may be heard. Symptoms of CHF are due to volume overload (Swanson & Ericson, 2016, p. 669).
- Diagnostic evaluation includes arterial blood gases, which will report low PAO_2 levels of 20 or above; and echocardiography to evaluate valvular displacement, presence of pulmonary atresia, and shunting (Ashwath & Snyder, 2013, p. 1234; Swanson & Ericson, 2016, p. 669). Lactate levels are normal unless cardiac output is diminished. Chest x-ray is marked abnormal for cardiomegaly and decreased pulmonary vascularity. Cardiomegaly may be profound related to the severity of tricuspid insufficiency. Electrocardiograms are positive for abnormal P waves, supraventricular tachycardia (SVT), and right bundle branch block (Swanson & Ericson, 2016, p. 669). May be associated with Wolff–Parkinson–White syndrome, COA, ASD, and PA (Ashwath & Snyder, 2013, p. 1234).

Management

- Medical management involves giving a large amount of oxygen to keep oxygen saturations greater than 75%, indicating adequate pulmonary blood flow. Prostaglandin E1 (PG-E1) may be needed to increase pulmonary blood flow and help relieve hypoxemia. Inhaled nitric oxide as a selective pulmonary vasodilator and sildenafil (vasodilator) to decrease right ventricular afterload (Swanson & Ericson, 2016). Extracorporeal membranous oxygenation (ECMO) may be indicated. Surgical management is indicated for infants demonstrating severe illness. The surgical procedure is annuloplasty (repair of the leaking mitral valve) and repositioning of the valve to minimize mitral regurgitation and plication (Swanson & Ericson, 2016, p. 670). A Blalock–Taussig (BT; pathway between the right subclavian and pulmonary arteries) shunt may be needed in severe cases, followed by a Glenn (connect inferior vena cava to the PA), then Fontan surgery (single ventricle; Ashwath & Snyder, 2013, p 1237).

Outcomes

- The most successful neonatal outcomes come from either subsequent single palliative care excluding the right ventricle and forming a single ventricle, or cardiac transplant. Replacement of the valve has not been useful in neonates (Martin et al., 2015, p. 1234).

Tetralogy of Fallot (Figure 16.2)

DEFINITION AND PATHOPHYSIOLOGY

- The cause TOF is unknown, but considered to be genetic. TOF is characterized by four (Fallot) related disorders:
  - Pulmonary stenosis (PS)/RVOT (severity directly impacts clinical presentation).
  - VSD
  - Overriding aorta (OA)
  - Right ventricular hypertrophy (RVH). A complete RVOT (pulmonary atresia) is a critical form of TOF (Scholz & Reinking, 2017, p. 815). A large VSD lessens symptomatic CHF. PS varies greatly with TOF. Most babies do not have pulmonary overcirculation, but a few do (Swanson & Ericson, 2016, p. 472).
- TOF is the most common cyanotic congenital heart defect, occurring in about three in 10,000 live births, and causes 7% to 10% of all congenital cardiac malformations. TOF presentation relates to the degree of PS (Swanson & Ericson, 2016, p. 674).

Diagnosis

- Diagnosis of TOF is by echocardiogram, which aids in determining the degree of PS, the size of the VSD, and the direction of blood flow across the septum. Blood gasses will show a normal pCO_2 and pH, and the pO_2 will be low based on the degree of right-to-left shunting. The chest X-ray is a "boot-shaped" heart without cardiomegaly. The pulmonary vascularity is more commonly diminished. The electrocardiogram is nonspecific, and shows RVH. A CBC will provide information about possible coinciding anemia or sepsis (Swanson & Ericson, 2016, p. 673).

Management

- Medical management of TOF is generally nonemergent unless there is severe PS. TOF *may be ductal dependent*, requiring continuous PG-E1 infusion (vasodilator) to maintain ductal patency. Episodes of hypoxia may be measured with oxygen and morphine. Surgery is completed during the first year of life to patch the pulmonary valve. If there are periods of severe hypoxia, a BT shunt will be performed (Swanson & Ericson, 2016, pp. 673–674).

Outcomes

- The outcome of TOF is based largely on the size of the PA. Repair of TOF is achievable in the presence of a normal-sized PA. Neonates with cyanotic TOF require a BT shunt and repair during the newborn period (Martin et al., 2015, p. 1232).

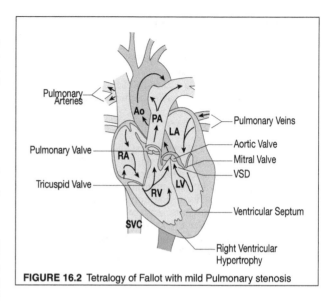

FIGURE 16.2 Tetralogy of Fallot with mild Pulmonary stenosis

Truncus Arteriosus

DEFINITION AND PATHOPHYSIOLOGY

- In truncus arteriosus (TA), during embryology, the outflow track fails to divide into the aorta and PA, both of which arise from the semilunar valve. The result is a single trunk responsible for pulmonary, systemic, and coronary circulation (Scholz & Reinking, 2017, p. 814). One great artery overrides the VSD and either divides into right and left arteries (Type 1 and Type 2), or have separate origins (Type 3; Sadowski, 2015, p. 589) and results in pulmonary overcirculation causing left ventricular hypertrophy (Ashwath & Snyder, 2013, p. 1236).
- TA is associated with extracardiac anomalies in 20% to 40% of cases, such as dysplastic valves, PS, truncal valve stenosis, and aortic arch interruption (AAI; Ashwath & Snyder, 2013, p. 1236). Thirty-five percent to 40% of neonates with TA have 22q11 deletion syndrome (DiGeorge; Swanson & Ericson, 2016, p. 678).
- Clinical presentation varies from mild desaturation to cyanosis based on the amount of pulmonary blood flow. A pansystolic, lower left sternal border murmur may be heard with a wide pulse pressure. Based on acidosis, murmur (Swanson & Ericson, 2016, p. 678), CHF symptoms may be present based on the amount of pulmonary blood flow. In basic truncus, the pulse oximetry is close to 85% until pulmonary vascular resistance falls and pulmonary blood flow increases. A desaturated infant may be due to increased pulmonary vascular resistance. Poor perfusion and bounding pulses may also be present (Ashwath & Snyder, 2013, p. 1238).

Diagnosis

- Diagnosis is by echocardiography and Doppler flow, noting the number of truncal valve leaflets and valve stenosis. Arterial blood gases may demonstrate a normal pH and pCO_2, and pO_2 may or may not be normal based on pulmonary blood flow. Chest x-ray will demonstrate cardiomegaly with displaced pulmonary arteries. Electrocardiogram will show combined ventricular hypertrophy and atrial enlargement. CBC will evaluate the hematocrit and possible origin for sepsis (Swanson & Ericson, 2016, p. 679).

Management

- Medical management involves treating CHF. Calcium levels should be monitored due to the possibility of DiGeorge syndrome. Surgical treatment involves separating the pulmonary arteries and patching the VSD. A right ventricular homograph (skin from another human) conduit connected to the PA valve (Swanson & Ericson, 2016, p. 679). Diuretics and digoxin, avoid oxygen to decrease pulmonary over-circulation, monitor calcium levels (Ashwath & Snyder, 2013, p. 1236).

Outcomes

- The mortality rate for TA is 10% to 30% based on the severity of the disease and degree of truncal valve regurgitation or stenosis and associated genetic anomalies (Swanson & Ericson, 2016, p. 679).

d-Transposition of the Great Vessels (Figure 16.3)

DEFINITION AND PATHOPHYSIOLOGY

- The most common cyanotic cardiac defect in the newborn is TGV, specifically *d* Transposition of the Great Vessels (d-TOV), or complete transposition, in which the aorta is left of the PA (Sadowski, 2015, p. 567). In TOV, deoxygenated blood returns to the right ventricle and is circulated by the aorta, and oxygenated blood returns to the left ventricle, then to the lungs, resulting in parallel circulation, hypoxia, and cyanosis if there is not a connection between systems (Ashwath & Snyder, 2013, p. 1230; Scholz & Reinking, 2017, p. 812). Opportunities for mixing blood include the ASD (best and needed for survival), PDA, and VSD if present (Ashwath & Snyder, 2013, p. 1230).
- TOV is more common in males and accounts for 5% of all CHD. The associated anomalies make a tremendous impact on the presentation of the disorder due to the opportunities for mixing blood. Associated defects include a VSD (25%), but with that may have COA or AAI (Ashwath & Snyder, 2013, p. 1230). Genetic abnormalities are not normally associated (Scholz & Reinking, 2017, p. 812; Swanson & Ericson, 2016, p. 671).
- Presentation of *d*-TOV depends on the degree of communication between the systems. TOV presents as cyanosis and tachypnea with increased work of breathing (WOB), a holosystolic murmur (with VSD) or no murmur (Ashwath & Snyder, 2013, p. 1230).

Diagnosis

- Diagnosis of *d*-TOV is by echocardiography, which also identifies associated defects (VSD, COA, IAA; Ashwath & Snyder, 2013, p. 627), and to determine the size of the ASD and PDA. Arterial blood gases reveal a low paO_2 if there is an intact septum without a VSD. A chest x-ray will demonstrate a cardiac silhouette in the shape of an "egg on a string" due to narrowing of the mediastinum, but it is not diagnostic. Pulmonary vascularity may be increased or decreased. An electrocardiogram may be normal or have RVH. Lactic acid levels should be normal (Scholz & Reinking, 2017, p. 812; Swanson & Ericson, 2016, p. 627).

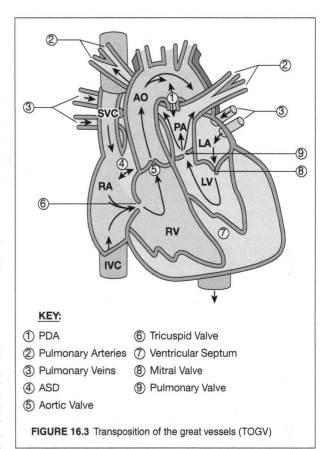

KEY:

① PDA	⑥ Tricuspid Valve
② Pulmonary Arteries	⑦ Ventricular Septum
③ Pulmonary Veins	⑧ Mitral Valve
④ ASD	⑨ Pulmonary Valve
⑤ Aortic Valve	

FIGURE 16.3 Transposition of the great vessels (TOGV)

Management

- Medical management of *d*-TOV is to infuse PG-E1 continuously to maintain a PDA and treat metabolic acidosis as *d*-TOGV may be *ductal dependent* to improve oxygenation and atrial shunting. Surgical treatment involves the arterial switch procedure whereby the PA is anastomosed to the right ventricle, and conversion of the pulmonary valve to become the functional aortic valve. Atrial balloon septostomy improves mixing by tearing the FO into an ASD for patients with a small patent FO, or with hypoxia and acidosis with a patent ductus. Surgical management is usually completed within 1 week of delivery and is the arterial switch procedure in which the aorta and PA are switched (Ashwath & Snyder, 2013, p. 1231).

Outcomes

Infants who are not preterm or without RVH experience favorable outcomes with the arterial switch procedure (Martinet al., 2015, p. 1231).

Total Anomalous Pulmonary Venous Connections

DEFINITION AND PATHOPHYSIOLOGY

- TAPV is a collection of congenital heart defects involving the anatomy of the pulmonary veins which return to the right heart circulation instead of normally returning to the left atrium. During fetal life, the pulmonary venous system development results in the absence of communication between the common pulmonary vein and the splanchnic plexus into the dorsal wall of the left atrium (Ashwath & Snyder, 2013, pp. 1235–1236).

- There are four types of pulmonary venous return:
  - ○ Supracardiac (55% and most common; routes into the superior vena cava [SVC] and RA)
  - ○ Infracardiac (13%; routes through the diaphragm and liver into the IVC to RA)
  - ○ Cardiac (routes pulmonary veins through coronary sinus or RA)
  - ○ Mixed type (5%; routes left pulmonary veins through systemic veins and right pulmonary veins to the RA). (ASD or patent foramen ovale [PFO] needed for survival; associated with left heart defects, TOGV, and TOF, and heterotaxy (Ashwath & Snyder, 2013, pp. 1234–1235).
- The clinical presentation varies because there are different variations, all present differently and at different times in the neonatal period (Ashwath & Snyder, 2013, p. 1234). The cyanosis of newborn varies with saturations less than 80%. If there is obstructive TAPVR the result is venous congestion and decreased pulmonary blood flow. Murmurs are not usually present with TAPVR unless the infant is in CHF. Less severe types of TAPVR are usually asymptomatic in the neonatal period (if unobstructed); infracardiac presents in neonatal period (Ashwath & Snyder, 2013, p. 1234).

Diagnosis

- Diagnosis of TAPVR is by echocardiogram with two-dimensional imaging and color flow to map the blood flow. Chest x-ray demonstrates a snowman sign, although this is not diagnostic. An electrocardiogram may show RVH and right atrial enlargement (Ashwath & Snyder, 2013, p. 1234).

Management

- Medical management of obstructive TAPVR is respiratory, metabolic support, and possibly ECMO until surgical anastomosis (Ashwath & Snyder, 2013, p. 1234). Obstructive TAPVR requires immediate surgery to increase blood flow, and is based on the type of TAPVR. Surgery may involve re-implantation of the common vein or directing the anomalous veins to the left atrium (Swanson & Ericson, 2016, p. 676).

Outcomes

- The prognosis of TAPVR is good prognosis unless pulmonary veins are hypoplastic (Ashwath & Snyder, 2013, p. 1234). Complications that may occur include dysrhythmias and pulmonary venous obstruction. The mortality rate of TAPVR varies from 10% to 25% (Swanson & Ericson, 2016, p. 676).

Tricuspid Atresia

DEFINITION AND PATHOPHYSIOLOGY
- In TA, the right atrium and right ventricle are not connected due to agenesis of tricuspid valve resulting in right ventricular hypoplasia and PA hypoplasia with VSD (Ashwath & Snyder, 2013, p. 1231) and possible hypoplastic

right ventricle (Sadowski, 2015, p. 567). Blood shunts across the ASD and blood goes to the lungs via left-to-right shunting via the PDA or a VSD with relative hypoxia (Ashwath & Snyder, 2013, p. 1231).
- TA may be associated with transposition of the great arteries (30%–50%; Swanson & Ericson, 2016, p. 677) and COA and relies on the presence of an ASD for neonatal survival at birth (Ashwath & Snyder, 2013, p. 1232).
- Presents as varied cyanosis with ductal closure and based on pulmonary blood flow. Murmurs from an associated VSD or PDA may be audible. Symptoms of CHF may also be present (Swanson & Ericson, 2016, p. 677), possible murmur, possible hepatomegaly (Ashwath & Snyder, 2013, p. 1232).

Diagnosis

- Diagnosis by echocardiogram demonstrating a large right atrium, an absent tricuspid valve, and the presence of right-to-left shunting across the atria, as well as a coexisting VSD or PDA. A chest x-ray may be normal or show cardiomegaly. Pulmonary vascularity varies based on the amount of pulmonary blood flow. An electrocardiogram will have left-axis deviation with a counterclockwise loop. Arterial blood gases with show a normal pH and pCO_2, with a low to normal pO_2 based on the amount of shunting that is present. A CBC will determine if anemia is present and aid in screening of coinciding sepsis (Swanson & Ericson, 2016, p. 677).

Management

- Medical treatment of TA involves maintaining pulmonary blood flow across the PDA with a PG-E1 infusion, so *may be ductal dependent*. Surgery is to remodel to a single left ventricle system for cardiac output. The infant may need a BT shunt to assure pulmonary blood flow, and PA banding if there is excessive pulmonary circulation. Finally, a Glenn and Fontan (diversion of IVC and SVC blood to the PA) may also be necessary (Swanson & Ericson, 2016, p. 677).

Outcomes

- Excellent prognosis with a Fontan repair (Martin et al., 2015, p. 1233).

Prostaglandin E1 (Alprostadil) Use in Cyanotic Heart Disease

- PGE1 (Alprostadil) is a smooth muscle vasodilator, as is the ductus arteriosis (DA). During fetal life, the placenta is the source of PGE_1 (Ashwath & Snyder, 2013, p. 1275). The action of PGE1 is to establish ductal patency and promote shunting of blood from the PA (oxygenated) to the aorta (less oxygenated) establishing a flow that is right to left (Ashwath & Snyder, 2013). PGE_1 increases blood flow through the PA, which promotes shunting across the atria (Ashwath & Snyder, 2013, p. 1275).
- In infants with suspected CHD, begin PGE1 empirically until diagnosis is confirmed and continue until corrective treatments are completed (Ashwath & Snyder, 2013, p. 1275)
- PG E1 dose is peripheral intravenous (IV) or umbilical venous catheter (UVC) based on clinical situation. A larger ductus on echocardiogram indicates a lower continuous

dose (0.01 mdg/kg/min) is needed, while a smaller ductus indicates a higher dose (0.05 mcg/kg/min) is indicated, then titrate the dose to the lowest possible dose needed to avoid side effects. The maximum dose is 0.10 mcg/kg/min (Ashwath & Snyder, 2013, p. 1275).

- Apnea is the major side effect of PGE_1 and should be prepared for respiratory assistance prior to beginning infusion. Other side effects include hypotension and tachycardia. Long-term use of PGE1 will result in periosteal thickening or gastric outlet thickening (Ashwath & Snyder, 2013, p.1275).
- Prior to transport consider intubation of the infant receiving continuous PG E1.

ACYANOTIC DEFECTS

Ventricular Septal Defect (VSD)

DEFINITION AND PATHOPHYSIOLOGY

- A VSD may be isolated, or part of congenital cardiac disease and they are the most common congenital heart defect. Openings in the septum dividing the right and left ventricle (Ashwath & Snyder, 2013, p. 1242). There are multiple types of VSD based on size and location. VSDs may impact valve function and may result in complications if left patent. Shunting of the VSD is left to right. A small VSD is not clinically significant, while a large VSD may result in clinical symptoms by sending blood back to the lungs, resulting in pulmonary overcirculation, CHF, respiratory distress, and pulmonary edema. The severity is related to the severity of pulmonary vascular resistance. Infants may also experience poor growth. VSDs are associated with COA.
- The four types of VSD are:
  - ○ Inlet
  - ○ Muscular (60%)
  - ○ Perimembranous (membranous, infracristal) infracristal
  - ○ Outlet (Scholz & Reinking, 2017, p. 806; Swanson & Ericson, 2016, p. 662)
- Clinical presentation is related to the size of the VSD. VSDs are acyanotic and present with a grade II, holosystolic, harsh murmur (Ashwath & Snyder, 2016, p. 1243). The murmur may not be audible until pulmonary vascular resistance decreases. Larger VSDs result in symptoms of CHF (Ashwath & Snyder, 2013, p. 1243; Swanson & Ericson, 2016, p. 662).

Diagnosis

- Postnatal diagnosis involves chest x-ray, which may show normal heart size or cardiomegaly and increased pulmonary vascular markings (Ashwath & Snyder, 2013, p. 1243; Swanson & Ericson, 2016, p. 662). An electrocardiogram is usually normal, or may indicate biventricular hypertrophy. A VSD is diagnosed by two-dimensional echocardiography and color flow for multiple VSDs (Ashwath & Snyder, 2013, p. 1243; Swanson & Ericson, 2016, p. 662).

Management

- Management of VSD involves medical or surgical management. Medical management is pharmacologic to control CHF and includes digoxin, diuretics, afterload reducers (Enalopril), and nutritional caloric supplementation for optimal nutrition. If the infant is not growing due to the VSD, surgical approach is indicated. Monitor weight gain. If the infant has poor growth, surgery may be indicated. Surgical repair is through the right atrium and tricuspid valve. Pulmonary artery banding may be necessary to palliative reduction in pulmonary blood flow. VSDs may be complicated by continual shunting, conduction abnormalities, or aortic or tricuspid insufficiency. Monitoring growth and nutrition is indicated (Scholz & Reinking, 2017, p. 808; Swanson & Ericson, 2016, p. 662).

Outcomes

- Spontaneous closure of VSDs is common. However, large a large VSD may instigate CHF and result in pulmonary vascular occlusive disease. Half of small VSDs close spontaneously (Ashwath & Snyder, 2013, p. 1243).

COA (Interrupted Aortic Arch)

DEFINITION AND PATHOPHYSIOLOGY

- COA is obstruction or constriction of the aortic arch near the PDA, but can occur anywhere above the aortic valve and anywhere from transverse arch to the bifurcation of the iliac arteries. Coarctation generally develops postnatally but may be detected prenatally. The incidence is 7% of cardiac lesions and is associated with Turner syndrome (Ashwath & Snyder, 2013, p. 1239, Swanson & Ericson, 2016, p. 663). More severe obstruction results in left ventricular (LV) failure or poor cardiac output (Ashwath & Snyder, 2013, p. 1239). There are three types of coarctation based on location (Figure 16.4):
  - ○ Type A (before subclavian)
  - ○ Type B (between left carotid artery and left subclavian)
  - ○ Type C (between right and left carotids; Ashwath & Snyder, 2013, p. 1239).
- Coarctation of the aorta is a *ductal dependent* lesion that affects blood supply to the descending aorta and is associated with bicuspid aortic valve, VSD, VSD are and with interrupted aortic arch, aortopulmonary window, TA, transposition of the great arteries, and DiGeorge (Ashwath & Snyder, p. 1239). The incidence of coarctation of the aorta is twice as high in males than in females. COA is associated with Turner syndrome (Scholz & Reinking, 2017, p. 823).
- The clinical presentation is directly impacted by the degree of aortic narrowing. COA presents as critical illness after ductal closure, due to obstructed left ventricular blood flow and poor cardiac output past the obstruction. The hallmark of COA is diminished femoral pulses. Signs and symptoms of newborns with coarctation are due to CHF and poor cardiac output. Coarctation may or may not present with an audible grade 1 to 1v soft systolic murmur audible in the left sternal border (Scholz & Reinking, 2017, p. 823; Swanson & Ericson, 2016, p. 664).

Diagnosis

- Diagnosis by echocardiography to visualize arch. Right-to-left shunting is found at the DA indicates a larger (Ashwath & Snyder, 2013, p. 1240). A chest x-ray will be positive for cardiomegaly and increased cardiac markings. Echocardiography is used to identify aortic narrowing and any additional left-sided obstructive lesions. EKG will be

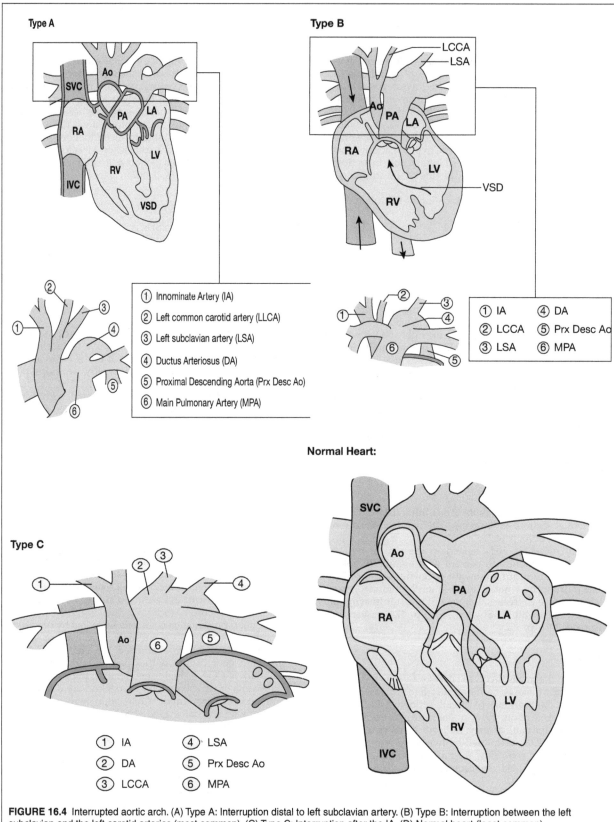

Type A

Type B

Ao
SVC
PA LA
RA
LV
RV
IVC
VSD

LCCA
LSA
Ao PA LA
RA
LV
RV
VSD

① Innominate Artery (IA)
② Left common carotid artery (LLCA)
③ Left subclavian artery (LSA)
④ Ductus Arteriosus (DA)
⑤ Proximal Descending Aorta (Prx Desc Ao)
⑥ Main Pulmonary Artery (MPA)

① IA ④ DA
② LCCA ⑤ Prx Desc Ao
③ LSA ⑥ MPA

Normal Heart:

SVC
Ao
PA
RA
LA
LV
RV
IVC

Type C

① IA ④ LSA
② DA ⑤ Prx Desc Ao
③ LCCA ⑥ MPA

Ao

FIGURE 16.4 Interrupted aortic arch. (A) Type A: Interruption distal to left subclavian artery. (B) Type B: Interruption between the left subclavian and the left carotid arteries (most common). (C) Type C: Interruption after the IA. (D) Normal heart (least common).

positive for RVH (Scholz & Reinking, 2017, p. 824). Pulse oximetry and arterial blood gas measurements document shunting (Ashwath & Snyder, 2013, p. 1240).

Management

- Medical management involves continuous prostagladin infusion for infants with poor perfusion or signs of CHF prior to surgery (Ashwath & Snyder, 2013, p. 1240). Continuous inotropes such as dopamine and dobutamine are suggested for cardiovascular support, and metabolic acidosis should be corrected (Scholz & Reinking, 2017, p. 824). Surgical repair determined by severity and of symptomatic infants by end-to-end anastomosis is completed as well as closure of the VSD (Ashwath & Snyder, 2013, p. 1240; Scholz & Reinking, 2017, p. 824).

Outcomes

- The mortality rate after surgical repair of COA is just above 5%. Ten percent to 15% of COA recurs and is managed with balloon angioplasty (Scholz & Reinking, 2017, p. 824).

Atrial Septal Defect

DEFINITION AND PATHOPHYSIOLOGY

- An ASD may be part of complex cardiac disease or isolated. During fetal life, the atrial opening between the left and right atria is patent. The opening between the atria is patent in fetal life (patent foramen ovale [PFO]; Swanson & Ericson, 2016, p. 661) or ASD may be ostium primum, secundum (most), or endocardial cushion (Sadowski, 2015, pp. 557–558; Swanson & Ericson, 2016, p. 661). If the opening is less than 6 mm in a term infant, it will likely close spontaneously and considered to be a PFO (Scholz & Reinking, 2017, p. 805). The ASD is generally not diagnosed prenatally due to the presence of the PFO (Swanson & Ericson, 2016, p. 661). The four most common types of ASD are:
  - ○ Secundum (most common; associated with Holt–Oram)
  - ○ Primum (associated with AV canal)
  - ○ Sinus venosus (a variation of anomalous venous return)
  - ○ Coronary sinus (Scholz & Reinking, 2017, p. 809)
- The clinical presentation of ASD is acyanotic because the shunting of blood is primarily left to right atrium. Oxygen saturation is normal and a large amount of left-to-right shunting results in a large ejection murmur as in mild PS. A large ASD does not cause CHF (Swanson & Ericson, 2016, p. 661).

Diagnosis

- Diagnosis is by echocardiography. Arterial blood gas values are normal with an ASD. Electrolytes and renal function labs should be normal, and a chest x-ray should be normal. An ASD may result in cardiomegaly later in life. An electrocardiogram would be normal (Swanson & Ericson, 2016, p. 661).

Outcomes

- Most ASDs (80%) close spontaneously by 2 years of life. Surgical management is indicated for a primum ASD,

sinus venosus, or secundum ASD later in life. Cardiac catheterization may be an option to insert a device to "plug the hole." Surgery is generally for older children by suture closure or patch of the defect (Swanson & Ericson, 2016, p. 661).

Hypoplastic Left Heart Syndrome

DEFINITION AND PATHOPHYSIOLOGY (FIGURE 16.5)

- A popular theory is that HLHS may result from in utero obstruction of blood flow to the left ventricle, thus preventing the growth of the ventricle and nearby vascular structures. HLHS is usually diagnosed prenatally whenever four chambers are not viewed (Scholz & Reinking, 2017, p. 819). HLHS is characterized by coinciding spectrum disorders:
  - ○ Aortic valve atresia
  - ○ Mitral valve atresia
  - ○ Severe left ventricular hypoplasia
  - ○ Aortic hypoplasia and COA (Ashwath & Snyder, 2013, p. 1240; Swanson & Ericson, 2016, p. 679)
- An ASD is required to mix blood and decrease pulmonary edema. If the ASD is too small, it is life threatening (Swanson & Ericson, 2016, p. 679). The only available circulation is blood traveling from the PA through the DA to the aorta. HLHS is critically *ductal dependent* to prevent systemic hypoperfusion, acidosis, and organ perfusion (Ashwath & Snyder, 2013, p. 1240). Too much blood sent to the lungs will result in poor perfusion, and too little blood to the lungs results in hypoxia (Swanson & Ericson, 2016, p. 679).
- HLHS is associated with multiple associations such as Turner syndrome, trisomy 9, trisomy 13, trisomy18, Holt–Oram, Smith–Lemli–Optiz, and Jacobsen syndrome (Swanson & Ericson, 2016, p. 679).
- HLHS presents as tachypnea and cyanosis and may or may not have a murmur. Perfusion and palpable pulses diminish with ductal closure (Ashwath & Snyder, 2013). Oxygen saturations may be low with poor systemic perfusion. Listening to heart sounds may reveal a single S1 and S2. If too much blood is sent to the lungs, infants will show signs of CHF, and if too little, hypoxia (Swanson & Ericson, 2016, p. 679).

Diagnosis

- Diagnosis by echocardiography showing right ventricular dilatation, a small left ventricle, and a hypoplastic mitral and aortic valve. The echocardiogram will also be useful for determining the size of the ASD and PDA, as well as cardiac function. A chest x-ray will show cardiomegaly and pulmonary vascular markings with pulmonary edema. The electrocardiogram will be abnormal with RVH and right axis deviation. Arterial blood gasses should indicate a normal pH with low pO_2 and normal pCO_2. A CBC should be done to evaluate for anemia which can aggravate hypoxia (Swanson & Ericson, 2016, p. 679).

Management

- Medical management of HLHS includes preventing excessive pulmonary blood flow and a continuous infusion of PG-E1 to maintain ductal patency. Because oxygen is a vasodilator, it should be avoided with HLHS. Volume expansion and inotropes help balance pulmonary and systemic circulation. Milrinone is an afterload reducer and pulmonary vasodilator. If ventricular function is decreased and blood pressure (BP) is stable (Scholz & Reinking, 2017, p. 820). If this is not achieved, surgical management indicated. The Norwood procedure increases systemic blood flow and decreases excessive pulmonary blood flow in three surgical steps:

○ Norwood procedure—enlarges ASD, ligates PDA, anastomoses PA to ascending aorta, reconstructs the aortic arch, and BT shunt (aorta to PA)
○ Glenn procedure—connects superior vena cava to the PA (5–9 months of age)
○ Fontan procedure—connects inferior vena cava to the PA (3–5 years of age) (Scholz & Reinking, 2017, p. 805; Swanson & Ericson, 2016, p. 679)

Outcomes

• Cardiac transplantation is sometimes an option for HLHS babies as primary palliation. A Norwood procedure is performed during the wait for transplantation and the availability of a donor heart.

The current prognosis for cardiac transplantation in infants has improved to 66% for 10 years. However, the number of available donors has not risen (Scholz & Reinking, 2017, p. 805).

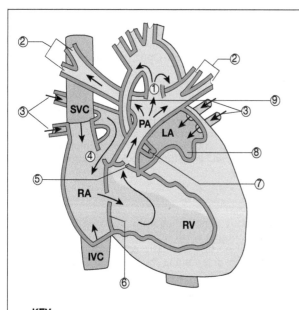

KEY:

① Large PDA   ⑥ Tricuspid Valve
② Pulmonary Arteries   ⑦ AV atresia
③ Pulmonary Veins   ⑧ Hypoplastiv LV with mitral valve atresia
④ ASD   ⑨ Hypoplastiv aortic arch and ascending aorta
⑤ Pulmonary Valve

FIGURE 16.5 Hypoplastic left heart syndrome

Atrioventricular Canal Defects (AV canal)

DEFINITION AND PATHOPHYSIOLOGY

• AV canal defects are also known as endocardial cushion defects. The endocardial cushion fails to form the center of the heart. May be a large defect severe (complete AV canal), (common AV canal and large VSD), transitional (less severe and small ASD and VSD), and small (common AV valves, cleft of the mitral valves, no VSD; Ashwath & Snyder, 2013, p. 1243).
• There is a strong association between AV canal and trisomy 21 (Ashwath & Snyder, 2013, p. 1243).
• Presents as desaturation and cyanosis due to right-to-left shunting, until PVR decreases and flow is reversed (left to right) as in CHF. Murmur may or may not be audible (Ashwath & Snyder, 2013, p. 1243)

DIAGNOSIS

• Diagnosis of AV canal is by echocardiogram to determine the type of AV canal, ventricular size, valvular insufficiency, and identify associated anomalies. An EKG will shoe a QRS axis deviation and RVH. Chest x-ray findings are based on the degree of RVOT/PS (Ashwath & Snyder, 2013, p. 1244; Scholz & Reinking, 2017, p. 809).

Management

• Medical management involves addressing cyanosis with supplemental oxygen to keep saturations >75%, or care of CHF, which may involve furosemide, digoxin, and an afterload reducer. However, avoid oxygen in the presence of CHF as it may increase pulmonary blood flow. Surgical correction at 2 to 6 months or if pulmonary hypertension (Ashwath & Snyder, 2013, p. 1244). Babies with complete AV canal are repaired at 4–6 months of life. The development of CHF may prompt an earlier repair (Scholz & Reinking, 2017, p. 810).

Outcomes

• Excellent prognosis with elective repair, however, a long-term problem may be AV valve function (Martin et al., 2015, p. 1244).

Aortic Stenosis (AS)

DEFINITION AND PATHOPHYSIOLOGY

• The aortic arches form during week 4. Stenosis, or narrowing of the aortic valve, may be mild, severe, or obstructed below the valve (subvalvular) or above the valve (supravalvular; Ashwath & Snyder, 2013, p. 1237). AS is a valvular disease resulting in left-sided outflow obstruction with subsequent shock and poor perfusion. The most common type is bicuspid aortic valve disease. Due to stenosis, the leaflets of the valve are thick and immobile causing outflow obstruction. As the stenosis progresses, pumping blood becomes more difficult for the left ventricle. When AS become or severe, or critical, it results in decreased systemic output and cardiogenic shock (Scholz & Reinking, 2017, p. 811).
• The incidence is 1% to 3%, and males are affected three times more often than females. This disorder is considered to be related to the NOTCH1 gene. AS is associated with Williams syndrome (Scholz & Reinking, 2017, p. 811).

- The clinical presentation of AS is based on severity and location. Shock with poor perfusion due to decreased blood flow in *critical* AS is similar to HLHS. Inadvertent closure of the ductus arteriosus results in worsening cardiogenic shock, acidosis, and multi-organ failure. Harsh midsystolic murmur audible with systolic ejection click. A palpable thrill at the suprasternal notch should be evident (Scholz & Reinking, 2017, p. 811). Pulse oximetry will demonstrate a gradient between the upper and lower extremities due to right to left shunting or show signs of CHF (Ashwath & Snyder, 2013, p. 1238).

Diagnosis

- Diagnosis is by echocardiogram to visualize the aorta, determine aortic valve anatomy, and size degree of blood flow of the aorta. An ECG would be normal. A chest x-ray may show pulmonary edema. Electrolytes and blood gases may show acidosis if AS decreases perfusion (Scholz & Reinking, 2017, p. 811).

Management

- If AS is mild or moderate and without illness, no treatment is needed other than follow-up. Medical management of AS requires continuous PG-E1 to prevent cardiogenic shock (Ashwath & Snyder, 2013, p. 1238). If the newborn demonstrates signs of CHF, a balloon or surgical valvotomy may be emergently indicated. The newborn may also need a Norwood procedure to provide alternative circulation to bypass the left ventricle (Scholz & Reinking, 2017, p. 811).

Outcomes

- Mild AS requires no intervention, but moderate to severe AS requires monitoring for CHF (Martin, Fanaroff, & Walsh, 2015, p. 1238).

Patent Ductus Arteriosus

DEFINITION AND PATHOPHYSIOLOGY

- During fetal life, the ductus arteriosus allows blood to flow from the right ventricle and PA to the descending aorta then the placenta and is a normal finding. After birth, as PA pressures decrease and systemic BP increases (aortic pressure), blood flows from right to left across the PDA (Beniz, 2013, p. 1224; Swanson & Ericson, 2016, pp. 657–658). Flow is reversed to this after birth due to decreased pulmonary vascular resistance and increases as pulmonary vascular resistance drops (i.e., lung disease improves), resulting in pulmonary edema (Beniz, 2013, p. 1224; Swanson & Ericson, 2016, pp. 657–658). Closes in 48 to 72 hours of life in term, healthy newborns (Beniz, 2013, p. 1224).
- The incidence is 100% in the developing fetus as this is a normal finding in embryologic life. The incidence of PDA related to cardiac disease is 3.6%. Persistent PDA is more common in females and may be linked to Chromosome 12 (Scholz & Reinking, 2017, p. 806).
- Clinical presentation stems from left-to-right shunting, which may also decrease cardiac output and increase the workload of the left side of the heart and result in decreased blood flow to vital organs (Beniz, 2013, p.1225) and presents as an left upper quadrant (LUQ) systolic "machinery" murmur, bounding pulses, visible precordium, widened pulse

pressure, worsening respiratory status due to pulmonary edema (Beniz, 2013, p. 1224), wide pulse pressure (Scholz & Reinking, 2017, p. 806; Swanson & Ericson, 2016, p. 658).

Diagnosis

- Postnatal diagnosis is primarily by Doppler echocardiogram to determine the significance of a left-to-right shunt and rules out ductal dependence. Arterial blood gases are usually normal. A significantly large PDA may result in a mixed acidosis, electrolyte abnormalities (if managed by diuretics), and renal function. A chest x-ray may be normal or may have increased pulmonary vascularity if the PDA is large with eventual cardiomegaly. An electrocardiogram may be normal or show ventricular hypertrophy. Echocardiography determines the size and significance of the PDA and rules out ductal dependent lesions (Swanson & Ericson, 2016, p. 659).

Management

- Management of a PDA may be medical or surgical. Medical management is determined by symptomatology. If the newborn is asymptomatic, monitoring for CHF, oxygen need, and failure to thrive is indicated. Often fluid restriction and observation are the approach to management of the PDA. Severe symptoms require ductal closure either pharmacologically (indomethacin, ibuprophen) or surgical ligation. Medications for ductal closure require monitoring of urine output and creatinine, which may indicate the need to discontinue the medication. Surgical ligation is usually performed by an incision of the lateral thorax if the infant can tolerate the procedure and has failed medical management (Swanson & Ericson, 2016, p. 660).

Outcomes

- Prognosis is excellent with management, mortality from surgery is <1% mortality (Beniz, 2013, p. 1226).

Congestive Heart Failure

DEFINITION AND PATHOPHYSIOLOGY

- Embryology is based on the underlying disorder or source of the problem. CHF may be caused by pressure overload (AS, COA), volume overload (left-to-right shunting such as PDA, TA, TOF, VSD, AV canal, single ventricle, arteriovenous malformation [AVM]), a combination of pressure and volume overload (interrupted aortic arch [IAA], COA with VSD, AS) or myocardial dysfunction (inborn errors of metabolism genetic disorders, myocarditis, tachyarrhythmias, perinatal asphyxia, sepsis, premature closure of the PDA) (Eichenwald, Hansen & Martin, 2017, p. 392).
- CHF may be subtle or obvious in the newborn and should be suspected in infants with a known VSD. The clinical presentation of CHF is hallmarked by decreased cardiac output and decreased tissue perfusion. Infants with CHF may have tachypnea, sinus tachycardia (to increase cardiac output), and hepatomegaly. Worsening CHF may involve retractions and grunting. Grunting respirations are a particularly concerning sign in a newborn and often accompany severe heart failure and decreased systemic perfusion (Scholz & Reinking, 2017, p. 803). Later symptoms of CHF include poor feeding and growth. As CHF

progresses, the newborn may have decreased peripheral pulses, decreased urine output, and edema (Swanson & Ericson, 2016, p. 652).

Diagnosis

- Diagnosis by echocardiogram chest x-ray, metabolic acidosis (Swanson, & Ericson, 2016). Discharge pulse oximetry is useful to find infants with subtle CHF (Scholz & Reinking, 2017, p. 803).

Management

- Medical management is to decrease oxygen consumption (neutral thermal environment [NTE], O₂, assisted ventilation) (Sadowski, 2015, p. 575). Fluid restriction, increased calories without volume (Sadowski, 2015, p. 575), monitor weight gain (Swanson & Ericson, 2016). Pharmacologic management: PGE1 if CHF is due to a ductal dependent lesion, diuretic therapy, inotropes, digoxin, afterload reducers (Swanson & Ericson, 2016).

Outcomes

- The outcome of CHF is based on the underlying cause.

NEONATAL SHOCK AND HYPOTENSION OR CARDIOVASCULAR COMPROMISE

- There are three phases of neonatal shock: (a) compensatory, involving perfusion of vital organs versus nonvital organs by vasodilatation and vasoconstriction; (b) uncompensated, with the development of hypotension, decreased cardiac output, and poor perfusion to vital organs; and (c) irreversible shock, resulting in permanent organ damage (Scholz & Reinking, 2017, p. 749).
- Shock results as a result of hypovolemia, myocardial dysfunction, and abnormal peripheral vasoregulation (Scholz & Reinking, 2017, p. 749).
- Hypovolemia is a decrease in circulating blood volume due to conditions resulting in an nonspecific inflammatory response (sepsis, asphyxia, major surgery) and afterload reducers (PGE1, milrinone) (Scholz & Reinking, 2017, p. 750).
- Dysfunction of systole or diastole may result in failed circulation (Scholz & Reinking, 2017, p. 750).

Diagnosis

- The is no standard method for diagnosing circulatory compromise, although BP is the standard parameter for diagnosis and treatment. Continuous BP measurement is crucial for managing neonatal shock and hypotension (Scholz & Reinking, 2017, p. 754).
- Other observations for the diagnosis of circulatory compromise include heart rate, slow skin capillary refill time, increased core temperature gradient, low urine output, and acidosis with increased lactate production (Scholz & Reinking, 2017, p. 754).

Management

- Management is based on the underlying cause. Delayed cord clamping improves hemodynamics. Hypovolemia

treatment is based on volume administration. Volume administration with myocardial dysfunction may increase morbidity and mortality, indicating that volume administration is cautious. The exception to this is volume administration to infants with neonatal sepsis, and in that situation decreases mortality. Isotonic saline administration has been demonstrated to be effective. If the infant has a history of blood loss, packed red blood cells with a hematocrit of 55% or greater following the administration of a crystalloid (normal saline) is indicated (Scholz & Reinking, 2017, p. 759).

- Dopamine is an endogenous catecholamine that produces a cardiovascular response based on the dose administered intravenously, stimulating a response from dopaminergic, α-adrenergic, β-adrenergic, and serotoninergic receptors impacts preload, myocardial contractility, and afterload (peripheral systemic vascular resistance) resulting in increased BP.
  - ○ The dosage range recommended is 2 to 20 μg dopamine per kilogram per minute (Scholz & Reinking, 2017, p. 760).
- Dobutamine is a cardioselective sympathomimetic amine with significant α-adrenoreceptor–mediated and β-adrenoreceptor and direct inotrope, which decreases total peripheral vascular resistance. Dobutamine works best for newborns with primary cardiac dysfunction and elevated pulmonary vascular resistance. Dobutamine added to dopamine for infants with respiratory distress syndrome improves increases BP (Scholz & Reinking, 2017, p. 761).
- Epinephrine is an α- and β-adrenergic agonist and sympathomimetic agent that increases BP and cerebral vascular blood flow (Scholz & Reinking, 2017, p. 763).
- Milrinone is a phosphodiesterase 3 inhibitor which reduces afterload in neonates with CHD or with low cardiac output. It has be shown to improve the oxygenation index of infants with persistent pulmonary hypertension of the newborn [PPHN] (Scholz & Reinking, 2017, p. 763).
- Vasopressin is a synthetic antidiuretic hormone that impacts the cardiovascular system by vasoconstriction. The benefits of vasopressin are similar to dopamine (Scholz & Reinking, 2017, p. 763).
- Hydrocortisone is a glucocorticoid steroid that improves BP, but due to the potential for adverse effects, is not a first-line treatment for neonatal hypotension but rather a rescue treatment. Hydrocortisone stabilizes cardiovascular status in the infant with vasopressor resistant hypotension (Scholz & Reinking, 2017, 764).
- Supportive measures to support the neonate during cardiovascular compromise include maintaining intravascular volume, arterial pH, and serum calcium levels. Positive pressure ventilation may decrease ventricular afterload and decreases work of breathing, which uses cardiac output (Scholz & Reinking, 2017, pp. 766–767).

Outcomes

- Outcome is based on the underlying cause of cardiovascular compromise.

RHYTHM DISTURBANCES IN NEONATES

Definition and Pathophysiology

- Arrhythmias in neonates may have normal and abnormal variations. The beginning of electrical activity in neonates is the sinus node with input from the sympathetic and parasympathetic nervous system. Conduction between the atria and ventricles is linked by the bundle of His.

- The normal pathway is sinus node ® atrial myocardium ® AV node ® bundle of His ® right and left bundle branches ® ventricular myocardium ® depolarization. Accessory pathways provide one direction (concealed pathway) or bidirectional (manifest pathway) conduction pathways. Newborns are sensitive to vagal stimulation, which fluctuates from bradycardia and tachycardia, based on newborn activity.

- The sinus node has inputs from both sympathetic and parasympathetic nervous systems. The balance of the two inputs determines the heart rate at any given moment. At rest and during sleep, vagal nerve stimulation is increased, causing slowing of the heart rate and potentially sinus bradycardia. During periods of stress, stimulation, or activity, sympathetic tone predominates, leading to an increase in heart rate and potentially sinus tachycardia.

- Tachyarrythmias originate from areas other than the sinus node, such as conduction via the conduct through the AV node, bundle of His and right and left bundle branches, and result in P-wave changes. Prolonged arrhythmias may result in cardiac failure or sudden death (Ashwath & Snyder, 2013, pp. 1261–1262).

- Normal sinus rhythm or resting heart rate in newborns is 90 to 60 bpm.

- Sinus bradycardia is a heart rate below 60 beats per minute
  - Usually episodic and is usually a physiologic response and not usually cardiac dysfunction. In neonates may be caused by increased vagal tone from intubation, gastroesophageal reflux, apnea, suctioning, seizures, and more uncommonly, increased intracranial pressure, abdominal pressure, or medications. With sinus bradycardia, the need for ventilation must be ruled out first.

- Sinus tachycardia is a heart rate >160–180 beats per minute.
  - May be a result of anemia, fever, agitation, infection, pain. But SVT must be considered and ruled out if rate is >220 bpm, or if the P wave is abnormal, the PR is prolonged, or an echocardiogram is normal (Ashwath & Snyder, 2013, p. 1260).

- Premature atrial contractions (PACs) are early depolarization of the atria but are not from the sinus node.
  - True PACs are followed by a QRS complex, and not just P waves. Bigeminy refers to EKGs characteristic of a PAC every other beats. Premature atrial contractions (PACs) are generally asymptomatic (Ashwath & Snyder, 2013, p. 1261).

- Atrial flutter is a type of reentry tachycardia via the atrial myocardium at the tricuspid valve.
  - The rate of neonatal *atrial* flutter is 300 to 600 bpm with a lower ventricular rate (2:1, 3:1, or 4:1), protected by the AV node. Ventricular beats may exceed 200, resulting in the need for intervention (Ashwath & Snyder, 2013, p. 1262).

- Atrial fibrillation (AFib) is a continuous dysrhythmia rarely seen in neonates and associated with CHD such as Ebstein anomaly and Wolff–Parkinson–White.
  - It differs from atrial ectopic tachycardia (AET) in that AFib is an organized dysrhythmia (Ashwath & Snyder, 2013, p. 1262).

- Supraventricular tachycardia is usually reentrant SVT, which uses nonconducting tissue pathways resulting in an electrical loop, which results in tachycardia resulting in narrow complexes.
  - This is usually caused by an accessory pathway, but can be due to reentry at the AV node (rarely in neonates). Wolff–Parkinson–White is a manifest (atria to ventricle, one-way) accessory pathway and is generally sporadic (Ashwath & Snyder, 2013, p. 1262).

- A premature ventricular contraction (PVC) is an early beat due to spontaneous ventricular depolarization of the ventricles.
  - If the heart is structurally normal, the baby is asymptomatic, negative family history, and they disappear at higher beats per minutes, PVCs can be considered benign (Ashwath & Snyder, 2013, p. 1286).

- Ventricular tachycardia (VT) is an abnormal tachycardia arrhythmia but idoventricular rhythm appears the same but is a benign rhythm.
  - VT originates below the bundle of HIS and may impact the baby's hemodynamic and cardiac function and requires intervention (Ashwath & Snyder, 2013, p. 1288).

- Complete AV heart block (third-degree block) indicates a dysfunctional AV node, making the atria and ventricles independent of each other.
  - Complete heart block is associated with maternal lupus erythematosus (Swanson & Erickson, 2016, pp. 684–685). Other types of heart block are type I (prolonged PR interval >200 msec) and type 2 (prolonged P-wave conduction without a prolonged PR interval), which requires pacing (Ashwath & Snyder, 2013, p. 1271).

Diagnosis

- Diagnosis of arrhythmias is by EKG considering atrial and ventricular rates, rhythm, and QRS characteristics. EKG ensures that there is no evidence of a pathologic arrhythmia such as heart block (bradycardia) or SVT (tachycardia; Ashwath & Snyder, 2013, p. 1260). Bedside monitoring may have artifact requiring a 12-lead EKG for confirmation (Swanson & Erickson, 2016, p. 681).

Management

- The majority of arrhythmias do not require urgent management. Urgent or chronic arrhythmias may be treated in a variety of ways. Treat the underlying cause such as infection or anemia, or no treatment. For bradycardias, evaluate for the need for resuscitation.
  - Adenosine—is a purinergic antidysrhythmic nucleotide given by rapid IV due to short half-life and blocks the AV node and diagnoses SVT. Also used for atrial flutter (in symptomatic patients) and SVT. Dose 0.05 to 0.1 mg/kg, increase by 0.05 to 0.1 mg/kg for nonresponsive SVT (Swanson & Erickson, 2016, pp. 683, 657).
  - Amiodarone—is an anti-arrhythmic drug used for refractory SVT if adenosine fails. Dose 10 to 15 mg/kg/day in one to two divided doses (Swanson & Erickson, 2016, p. 649).
  - Cardioversion—*synchronized* direct current used for hemodynamically unstable patients; used for atrial fibrillation (AFib), ventricular fibrillation (VFib), atrial flutter. Dose 0.5 to 2 J/kg used with paddles front to back with infant side lying (Ashwath & Snyder, 2013, p. 1262).
  - Isoproterenol—is a nonselective ® adrenoreceptor agonist for bradycardia, heart block. 0.05 mcg/kg/min given by IV infusion (Swanson & Erickson, 2016, p. 658).

○ Digoxin—is a cardiac glycoside used to increase the ventricular rate for bradycardia due to CHF or AFib. Dose divided doses–preterm infant PO route: 20–30 mcg/kg; term infant PO route: 25–35 mcg/kg given PO or IV (digitalizing); preterm infant PO route: 5 to 7.5 mcg/kg/day; term infant PO route: 6 to 10 mcg/kg/day (maintenance; Swanson & Erickson, 2016, p. 649).

○ Lidocaine—is an antiarrhythmic given for ventricular tachycardia. Dose IV bolus 1 to 2 mg/kg and IV infusion. Dose: IV bolus: 1 to 2 mg/kg IV drip: 20 to 50 mcg/kg/minute (Swanson & Erickson, 2016, p. 658).

○ Propranolol—is a beta-adrenergic blocker supporting the autonomic nervous system for prolonged SVT or atrial flutter. Dose dysrhythmias: 0.25 mg/kg/dose TID–QID (max daily dose 5 mg/kg/day) 30 to 60 min (Swanson & Erickson, 2016, p. 658).

Outcomes

• Neonatal arrythmia outcomes are based on the arrhythmia type and underlying cause of the arrhythmia.

HYPERTENSION

Definition and Pathophysiology

• Occurrence: 1 to 2% in term and preterm infants (Martin et al., 2015, p. 1687)
• Factors affecting accuracy: BP cuff size that is too small, infant activity, temperature, pain, weight, gestational/chronological age (Martin et al., 2015, p. 1686). After birth, the BP is expected to decrease over the first few hours due to fluid shifts and then gradually rises by 6 days of age (Tappero, 2018, p. 107).
• BP is most often monitored by indwelling arterial catheters in the unstable infant or by oscillometric methods. Four-extremity BP should be done if concern of cardiac etiology (Tappero, 2018, p. 108).
• Pulse pressure is the difference between the systolic and diastolic BPs; normal: 25 to 30 mmHg in term neonate, 15 to 25 mmHg in preterm neonate (Tappero, 2018, p. 108).
• Differential diagnosis: renal/renovascular disorders (most common), cardiac disorders (arch abnormalities including coarctation of aorta, PDA), neurologic disorders (seizures, pain), adverse effects of meds, BPD (Tappero, 2018, p. 108).
• Renal arterial thromboembolism secondary to umbilical artery catheter (UAC) is most common cause of renovascular hypertension (HTN); infant of diabetic mother (IDM), sepsis, dehydration, perinatal asphyxia place the infant with a UAC at higher risk for thrombotic events (Martin et al., 2015, p. 1686).
• Clinical presentation other than elevated BP during routine vital signs varies depending on etiology. Cardiorespiratory symptoms may include tachypnea, changes in perfusion, vasomotor instability, CHF, and/or hepatosplenomegaly. Clinical signs of hypertensive crisis may include cardiopulmonary failure, neurologic dysfunction, and concerns for acute kidney injury (Martin et al., 2015, pp. 1686–1687).

Diagnosis

• Diagnostic evaluation includes history and physical examination; clinical findings for infant with COA and PDA are discussed previously. Laboratory evaluation should include basic metabolic panel for evaluation of electrolytes and renal function and a urinalysis. Other laboratory evaluation may include evaluation of renin, aldosterone, cortisol, and thyroid function. Ultrasound of the abdomen/kidneys with Doppler flow study should be done to evaluate for renal or renovascular abnormalities. In more difficult cases, CT, MRI with angiography, or echocardiography may help with establishing diagnosis (Martin et al., 2015, p. 1688).

Management

• Aimed toward the underlying cause. Placement of an arterial line may be needed for close monitoring of BP. There are various antihypertensive agents that can be considered, including vasodilators, calcium channel blockers, and alpha/beta blockers. The goal of antihypertensive agents is a gradual decrease in BP not dropping below the 95th percentile for the first 24 to 48 hour of treatment. IV therapy preferred initially with switch to oral agents once BP more stable (Martin et al., 2015, p. 1688–1689).

Outcomes

• Depends on etiology. Hypertension related to BPD and complications from UAC typically resolve over time. Infants with renal abnormalities can have hypertensive issues that persist. Risk for development of late-onset hypertension and chronic kidney disease needs to be monitored for through adolescence (Martin et al., 2015, p. 1689).

CONCLUSION

CHD is the most universal congenital disorder in neonates. Critical CHD requiring clinical intervention comprises 25% of CHD and is a preeminent cause of infant mortality during the neonatal period. CHD can appear as shock, cyanosis, respiratory distress, or contrarily with subtle signs and symptoms. Delay in the recognition and management of CHD increases the risk of morbidity and mortality. Recognizing risk factors, clinical presentation, and inclusion of CHD as an in tandem differential diagnosis in the consideration of neonatal management decisions is key. Finally, consider that CHD may not be evident until day 3 to 5 of life or later due to corresponding physiologic changes. Pulse oximetry screening for hypoxemia is indicated for all newborns to detect imminent critical CHD lesions prior to hospital discharge.

REVIEW QUESTIONS

1. When monitoring the status of an infant with diagnosed tetrology of Fallot, the NNP understands the severity of the diagnosis relates to the severity of the:
   A. overriding aorta
   B. pulmonary stenosis
   C. septal defect

2. The characteristic clinical presentation of central cyanosis is:
   A. bluish mucous membranes
   B. circumoral cyanosis
   C. dusky hands and feet

3. A newborn presents with respiratory distress and pallor with tachycardia of 230 beats per minute. Electrocardiogram is consistent with supraventricular tachycardia (SVT). Prompt treatment is required due to the risk of prolonged arrhythmia resulting in:
   A. spontaneous cardio-version shock
   B. prolonged acidosis and hypotension
   C. cardiac failure and sudden death

4. A former 32-week female infant now at 1 week of age demonstrates clinical changes with increased oxygen need, a systolic "machinery" murmur in the left upper quadrant, bounding peripheral pulses, palmar pulses, and scattered rales on pulmonary auscultation. The NNP recognizes these findings as consistent with a:
   A. patent ductus arteriosus (PDA)
   B. Tetralogy of Fallot (TOF)
   C. ventricular septal defect (VSD)

5. A fetus who is at risk for heart block and possible hydrops is one whose mother has a/an:
   A. autoimmune disease
   B. concurrent viral infection
   C. type 1 diabetes mellitus

REFERENCES

Ashwath, R., & Snyder, C. (2013). Congenital defects of the cardiovascular system. In A. A. Fanaroff & J. M. Fanaroff (Eds.), *Klaus and Fanaroff's care of the high-risk neonate* (6th ed., pp. 1230–1247). Philadelphia, PA: Elsevier Saunders.

Beniz, W. (2013). Patent ductus arteriosus. In A. A. Fanaroff & J. M. Fanaroff (Eds.), *Klaus and Fanaroff's care of the high-risk neonate* (6th ed., pp. 1223–1228). Philadelphia, PA: Elsevier Saunders.

Blackburn, S. (2018). Cardiovascular system. In S. Blackburn (Ed.), *Maternal, fetal, & neonatal physiology: A clinical perspective* (5th ed., pp. 251–296) Maryland Heights, MO. Elsevier.

Breinholt, J. (2017). Cardiac disorders. In E. C. Eichenwald, A. R. Hansen, C. Martin, & A. R. Stark (Eds.), *Cloherty and Stark's manual of neonatal care* (8th ed., pp. 510–575). Philadelphia, PA: Wolters Kluwer.

Martin, R, Fanaroff, M., & Walsh, M. (2015). *Neonatal-perinatal medicine. Disease of the fetus and infant* (10th ed., pp. 1188–1290). St. Louis, MO: Elsevier.

Sadowski, S. (2015). Cardiovascular disorders. In M. T. Verklan & M. Walden (Eds.), *Core curriculum for neonatal intensive care nursing* (5th ed., pp. 534–588). St. Louis, MO: Elsevier Saunders.

Scholz, T., & Reinking, B. (2017). Congenital heart disease. In S. Gleason & S. Juul (Eds.), *Avery's diseases of the newborn* (10th ed., pp. 1032–1038). Philadelphia, PA: Elsevier.

Swanson, T., & Erickson, L. (2016). Cardiovascular diseases and surgical interventions. In S. Gardner, B. Carter, M. Hines, & J. Hernandez (Eds.), *Merenstein & Gardner's handbook of neonatal intensive care* (8th ed., pp. 644–688.e2). St. Louis, MO: Elsevier.

Tappero, E. P., & Honeyfield, M. E. (2018). *Physical assessment of the newborn: A comprehensive approach to the art of physical examination* (8th ed.). Petaluma, CA: NICU Ink Book.

Vargo, L. (2018). Cardiovascular assessment. In E. P. Tappero & M. E. Honeyfield (Eds.), *Physical assessment of the newborn* (6th ed., pp. 93–110). New York, NY: Springer Publishing Company.

17 THE PULMONARY SYSTEM

Janice Wilson
Barbara Snapp
Mary Walters

INTRODUCTION

Respiratory disorders account for the majority of admissions to NICUs (Fraser, 2015, p. 447), therefore, the understanding of lung development, physiology, function, and mechanics, as well as the understanding of disorders that contribute to pulmonary dysfunction are critical to the care of all newborns (Kallapur & Jobe, 2015, p. 1042; Keszler & Abubakar, 2017, p. 8).

Lung Development

- Lung development is a complex interrelationship between genetic signaling, physical, biochemical, hormonal, and structural factors. Lung development and maturation are reflected in five overlapping anatomic phases (Fraser, 2015, pp. 447–448; Kallapur & Jobe, 2015, pp. 1042–1046; Keszler & Abubakar, 2017, p. 9).

Phases of Lung Development

- Embryonic phase—(weeks 3–6): Proximal airways. The lung bud develops within mesenchyme from the primitive embryonic foregut. The single lung bud divides into the right and left lung buds as well as the trachea. Rudimentary airway branching, pulmonary vein, and pulmonary artery formation occur during this stage. Abnormal development during the embryonic phase can result in tracheal agenesis, tracheal stenosis, tracheoesophageal fistula (TEF), and pulmonary sequestration (Joyner, 2019, p. 2; Keszler & Abubakar, 2017, p. 9).
- Pseudoglandular phase—(weeks 6–16): During this phase, 20 generations of conducting airways are formed. Simultaneously, the lymphatic vessels and bronchial capillaries also develop (Keszler & Abubakar, 2017, p. 9). The lung at this stage has the "gland-like" (Pseudoglandular) appearance of an exocrine organ due to the surrounding loose mesenchyme tissue. Abnormal development during this phase can result in bronchogenic cysts, congenital lobar emphysema, and congenital diaphragmatic hernia (CDH; Joyner, 2019, pp. 2–3, Kallapur & Jobe, 2015, p. 1042, Keszler & Abubakar, 2017, p. 9).
- Canalicular phase—(weeks 16–26): The acinar or respiratory units develop, which includes airway generations from 21 to 23. Pulmonary capillaries grow closer to the primitive acinus or respiratory unit. Cuboidal cells develop into Type I cells (those responsible for gas exchange) and Type II cells (those responsible for surfactant production and secretion). Gas exchange may occur near the end of this stage, but is dependent on the approximation of the capillaries to the acinar units (Joyner, 2019, pp. 3–4, Kallapur & Jobe, 2017, p. 1044, Keszler & Abukakar, 2017, p. 9).
- Terminal sac or saccular phase—(weeks 26–36): The primitive acini develop into saccules that continue to septate via the development of secondary crests. The saccules will develop into alveoli. The capillary network moves closer to the alveoli facilitating rudimentary gas exchange. Type II cells increase production and release of surfactant. As lung size increases an increase in the surface area responsible for gas exchange occurs. Infants delivered during this phase may develop respiratory distress syndrome (RDS; surfactant deficiency), pulmonary insufficiency (reduced surface area, increased distance between alveoli and capillaries, immature lung mechanics), pulmonary interstitial emphysema (PIE), and bronchopulmonary dysplasia (BPD; Joyner, 2019, pp. 4–5, Kallapur & Jobe, 2015, p. 1045; Keszler & Abubakar, 2017, p. 9).
- Alveolar phase—(36 weeks to age 3): Alveoli continue to increase in number and maturity and may continue to develop into early adulthood (Joyner, 2019, p. 6, Keszler & Abubakar, 2017, p. 9). Several factors can influence alveolarization (Box 17.1). Continued alveolarization past the newborn period may assist in normalization of lung function of infants born prematurely (Kallapur & Jobe, 2015, p. 1046).

Box 17.1 Factors that facilitate or impede alveolarization

Factors That Impede Alveolarization
Mechanical ventilation
Antenatal/postnatal administration of glucocorticoids
Chorioamnionitis
Pro-inflammatory mediators
Hyperoxia
Hypoxia
Poor nutrition

Factors That Facilitate Alveolarization
Retinoids (Vitamin A)
Thyroxin

Source: Reproduced with permission from Kallapur, S. G., & Jobe, A. H. (2015). Lung development and maturation. In R. J. Martin, A. A. Fanaroff, & M. C. Walsh (Eds.), *Fanaroff and Martin's neonatal-perinatal medicine diseases of the fetus and infant* (10th ed., pp. 1042–1059). Philadelphia, PA: Saunders.

The Role Of Surfactant

- Surfactant is produced in type II alveolar cells. It is packaged and stored in the lamellar bodies. Lamellar bodies are extruded into the alveoli by exocytosis forming tubular myelin. Tubular myelin is a lattice-like structure with the hydrophobic end of the phospholipid extending into the alveolar air and the hydrophilic end binding with water at the air–liquid interface. This process reduces surface tension. Surfactant components are also "recycled" by the lamellar bodies or broken down by lysosomes (Fraser, 2015, p. 448; Suresh, Soll, & Mandy, 2017, pp. 338–339).
  - Surfactant is a combination of phospholipids (80%) and proteins (12%; Fraser, 2015, p. 448; Suresh et al., 2017, p. 338). The primary phospholipids in surfactant are dipalmitoyl phosphatidylcholine (DPPC at 60%) unsaturated phosphatidylcholine (25%), phosphatidyl glycerol (15%), and phosphatidylinositol (Suresh et al., 2017, p. 338). Surfactant production begins as early as 20 weeks and increases to mature levels as the fetus approaches term.
- Phospholipids (primarily DPPC) are responsible for the reduction of alveolar surface tension and stabilization of the alveolar membrane, preventing alveolar collapse at the end of expiration (Fraser, 2015, p. 448; Suresh et al., 2017, p. 338).
  - There are four surfactant proteins; two are hydrophilic (surfactant proteins A and D or SP-A and SP-D) and two are hydrophobic (surfactant proteins B and C or SP-B and SP-C). See Table 17.1.
- Genetic mutations may result in SP-B deficiency and cause respiratory distress that is fatal in the newborn period. If SP-B is deficient, SP-C production is also reduced. Genetic mutations that result in SP-C deficiency can result in respiratory distress and or interstitial lung disease in infancy and childhood (Kallapur & Jobe, 2015, p. 1049).
  - The ATP-binding cassette transporter gene (*ABCA3*) is responsible for lipid transport in the lamellar bodies.

Genetic aberrancies in *ABCA3* gene can result in severe RDS, similar to SP-B deficiency (Kallapur & Jobe, 2015, p. 1049).

The Role of Fetal Lung Fluid and Fetal Breathing

- Fetal lung fluid is produced at 4 to 5 mL per kg per hour and is facilitated by the active transport of chloride from the interstitium. Fetal lung fluid and its constituents like phospholipids contribute to the amniotic fluid volume and as such can be evaluated as a test of fetal lung maturity (Joyner, 2019, p. 8; Kallapur & Jobe, 2015, pp. 1047 and 1049).
- The lecithin–sphyngomyelin (L-S) ratio and the phosphatidyglycerol (PG) levels can be used to assess lung maturity. Lecithin (phosphatidylcholine) is produced by the fetal lung. Sphyngomyelin is a non-fetal membrane lipid found in amniotic fluid and begins to fall by 32 weeks. An L-S of 2:1 is indicative of fetal lung maturity. Its use is not accurate in infants of diabetic mothers. PG increases in production at around 35 weeks. The presence of PG indicates lung maturity (Fraser, 2015, p. 448; Hansen & Levin, 2019, pp. 411–412; Kallapur & Jobe, 2015, p. 1049).
- Chronic stress (fetal, maternal, placental) can facilitate early lung maturation. Growth restriction and preeclampsia do not facilitate lung maturation (Kallapur & Jobe, 2015, p. 1049).
- Fetal breathing movements (FBMs) can be seen as early as 11 weeks and are important for lung development. With fetal breathing, lung fluid moves up the trachea and is swallowed and some makes it way out into the amniotic fluid. Fetal tracheal pressure is higher than amniotic fluid pressure maintaining a distending pressure, which promotes lung development. FBM increases cardiac output and blood flow to the heart and placenta. Decreased movement of the diaphragm has been associated with the development of pulmonary hypoplasia (Kallapur & Jobe, 2015, p. 1047; Patrinos, 2015, p. 1137).

TABLE 17.1 Surfactant Proteins

Surfactant Protein Type	Surfactant Protein Function(s)	Present in Commercial Surfactants (yes/no)
SP-A Hydrophilic (water soluble)	Active in lung host defense mechanisms and regulation of lung inflammation. Binds to pathogens and facilitates phagocytosis by macrophages	No
SP-B Hydrophobic (water insoluble)	Co-secreted with phospholipids. Works in conjunction with phospholipids in stabilizing the alveolar membrane. Important in formation of tubular myelin and in surfactant recycling	Yes
SP-C Hydrophobic (water insoluble)	Assists with surfactant dispersal, spreading, and recycling of surfactant in conjunction with SP-B	Yes
SP-D Hydrophilic (water soluble)	Performs lung host defense support similar to SP-A	No

Sources: Data from Kallapur, S. G., & Jobe, A. H. (2015). Lung development and maturation. In R. J. Martin, A. A. Fanaroff, & M. C. Walsh (Eds.), *Fanaroff and Martin's neonatal-perinatal medicine diseases of the fetus and infant* (10th ed., pp. 1042–1059). Philadelphia, PA: Saunders; Suresh, G. K., Soll, R. F., Mandy, G. T. (2017). Pharmacologic therapies I: Surfactant therapy. In J. Goldsmith, E. Karotkin, M. Keszler, & G. Suresh (Eds.), *Assisted ventilation of the neonate* (6th ed., pp. 338–348). Philadelphia, PA: Elsevier; Fraser, D. (2015). Respiratory distress. In M. T. Verklan & M. Walden (Eds.), *Core curriculum for neonatal intensive care nurses* (5th ed., pp. 447–477). St. Louis, MO: Elsevier.

TABLE 17.2 American College of Obstetricians and Gynecologists (ACOG) Antenatal Steroid Recommendations

Gestational Age	ACOG Recommendation	Betamethasone	Dexamethasone
23 and 0/7 weeks (with or without PROM)	May be considered for women at risk for preterm delivery in 7 days	2 doses of 12 mg IM 24 hours apart	4 doses of 6 mg IM every 12 hours
24 and 0/7 weeks to 33 and 6/7 weeks (with or without PROM)	Is recommended to be given to women at risk for preterm delivery in 7 days	2 doses of 12 mg IM 24 hours apart	4 doses of 6 mg IM every 12 hours
34 and 4/7 weeks to 36 and 6/7 weeks (with or without PROM)	May be considered for women at risk for preterm delivery in 7 days	2 doses of 12 mg IM 24 hours apart	4 doses of 6 mg IM every 12 hours
<34 and 0/7 weeks with course of steroids more than 14 days previously	Single repeat course should be considered for women at risk for preterm delivery in 7 days.	2 doses of 12 mg IM 24 hours apart	4 doses of 6 mg IM every 12 hours

Source: Data from Hansen, A., & Levin, J. (2019). Neonatal pulmonary disorders. In B. K. Walsh (Ed.), *Neonatal and pediatric respiratory care* (5th ed., pp. 407–452). St. Louis, MO: Elsevier.

PROM, premature rupture of membranes

The Role Of Antenatal Steroids

- Treatment with maternal corticosteroids less than 24 hours before preterm delivery is associated with a decrease in mortality, RDS and intraventricular hemorrhage (IVH) and is considered the standard of care for mothers at risk for preterm delivery (Fraser, 2015, p. 449; Hamar & Hansen, 2019, pp. 28, 412; Kallapur & Jobe, 2015, p. 1056). Antenatal steroid recommendations can be found in Table 17.2.
- Maximum benefit of steroids to the fetus is at 48 hours after administration with a result in the increase in production of proteins that control the manufacture of surfactant by the type II cells in the fetal lung. Steroid administration should be considered when preterm delivery is anticipated with seven days (Hamar & Hansen, 2019, p. 28, Zanelli & Kaufman, 2019, pp. 249–250).
- Multiple repeated courses of antenatal asteroids are not recommended due to an associated increased risk of negative neurodevelopmental (Hamar & Hansen, 2019, p. 28).
  - ○ A second dose of steroids may be considered if more than 7 days to 2 weeks have passed since the first dose, and if preterm delivery is still a risk (Hamar & Hansen, 2019, p. 28, Zanelli & Kaufman, 2019, pp. 249–250).

CONGENITAL/DEVELOPMENTAL RESPIRATORY DISORDERS

Pulmonary Hypoplasia

DEFINITION AND PATHOPHYSIOLOGY

- Pulmonary hypoplasia (PH) is part of a subset of pulmonary underdevelopment diseases, which include pulmonary agenesis and pulmonary aplasia, decreased numbers of alveoli, bronchioles, and arterioles. It can be either unilateral or bilateral (Jensen, Mong, Biko, Maschhoff, & Kirpalani, 2017, p. 77; Joyner, 2019, pp. 6–7; Verklan, 2004, p. 70).
  - ○ Primary hypoplasia is a result of intrinsic failure of normal lung development (Blackburn, 2013, p. 313;

Crowley, 2015, pp. 1113–1114; Fraser, 2015, p. 470; Pappas & Robey, 2015, p. 90).
  - ○ Secondary hypoplasia is a result of abnormal processes that interfere with lung development.
    - ▪ Oligohydramnios resulting from renal anomalies (Potter Sequence), early amniotic fluid leak/loss, and/or placental abnormalities
    - ▪ Intrauterine growth retardation (IUGR)
    - ▪ Space occupying lesions that compress the lungs inhibiting growth such as CDH, cardiomegaly, and/or cystic lung diseases
    - ▪ Abnormal diaphragmatic movement secondary to a central or peripheral nervous system disorder or musculoskeletal disease. The inhibition of fetal breathing movement (FBM) and lack of chest wall expansion will restrict normal growth (Blackburn, 2013, p. 313; Crowley, 2015, pp. 1113–1114; Fraser, 2015, pp. 470–471; Jensen et al., 2017, pp. 77–78; Pappas & Robey, 2015, p. 90; Van Marter & McPherson, 2017, p. 469; Verklan, 2015, p. 90).

DIAGNOSIS

- Antenatal assessments can be helpful in identification of PH. Antenatal ultrasound (US) evaluation of thoracic circumference (TC), TC to abdominal circumference, and thoracic to heart area can be evaluated. It is more useful with secondary versus primary hypoplasia. This is more reflective of chest wall measurement and not lung measurement. Antenatal three-dimensional MRI has been used to evaluate lung volume (Crowley, 2015, pp. 1113–1114).
- A high index of suspicion for PH should be considered in infants with fetal growth restriction (FGR), altered FBM, prolonged polyhydramnios, decreased nutrient supply, nicotine exposure, and preterm birth (Blackburn, 2013, p. 313; Fraser, 2015, p. 471; Keszler & Chatburn, 2017, p. 147).
- The most common presentation is severe respiratory distress.
  - ○ Infants with pulmonary hypoplasia may exhibit hypoxia, hypercapnia, and are at risk for pulmonary air leak syndrome (pneumothorax).

○ Chest radiographs are compatible with decreased thoracic volume.
○ Abnormal pulmonary vasculature development may lead to persistent pulmonary hypertension of the newborn (PPHN) symptoms.
○ Poor lung compliance requiring higher pressures to ventilate (Fraser, 2015, pp. 459, 471; Keszler & Chatburn, 2017, p. 147; Pappas & Robey, 2015, p. 90).

INFANTS AT RISK
- Infants with FGR, altered FBM, prolonged polyhydramnios, decreased nutrient supply, nicotine exposure, and preterm birth (Blackburn, 2013, p. 313; Fraser, 2015, p. 471; Keszler & Chatburn, 2017, p. 147).
- Antenatal US evaluation of TC, TC to abdominal circumference, and thoracic to heart area can be evaluated. It is more useful with secondary versus primary hypoplasia. This is more reflective of chest wall measurement and not lung measurement (Crowley, 2015, pp. 1113–1114).
- Antenatal three-dimensional MRI has been used to evaluate lung volume.

MANAGEMENT
- Intubation and assisted ventilation
  ○ Avoid hypoxia, hyperoxia, hypercarbia, hypocarbia, and acidosis
  ○ Minimize overexpansion and consider high-frequency oscillatory ventilation (HFOV) if peak inspiratory pressure (PIP) is greater than 25 cm H_2O (Fraser, 2015, p. 471; Keszler & Chatburn, 2017, p. 147; Mammel & Courtney, 2017, p. 222; Pappas & Robey, 2015, p. 90).
  ○ Surfactant administration
  ○ Consider the use of inhaled nitric oxide (iNO) if PPHN is present (Fraser, 2015, p. 471; Mammel & Courtney, 2017, p. 22).
  ○ Implementation of pain management and sedation protocols
  ○ Hemodynamic support (volume expansion, inotropes and vasopressors)
  ○ Extracorporeal Membrane Oxygenation (ECMO) [Fraser, 2015, p. 471].
- The mortality rate is high and the degree of hypoplasia dictates outcome. Infants who survive are at an elevated risk for the development of chronic lung disease (CLD). While postnatal lung growth is rare, it is possible if treatment and supportive care are successful (Crowley, 2015, pp. 1113–1114; Fraser, 2015, p. 471).

Congenital Diaphragmatic Hernia (CDH)

DEFINITION AND PATHOPHYSIOLOGY
- CDH results from a developmental defect in the formation of the fetal diaphragm allowing abdominal contents to herniate into the thoracic cavity creating a mass effect that impedes lung development (Bradshaw, 2015, pp. 618–619; Hansen & Levin, 2019, p. 459; Jensen et al., 2017, p. 79; Yoder, 2017, pp. 236, 288).
  ○ Posterolateral defects (Bochdalek) are the most common. Anterior defects (Morgagni) are less common and central defects are rare (Bradshaw, 2015, p. 618; Crowley, 2015, p. 1115; Jensen et al., 2017, p. 79; Madenci, Rice-Townsend & Weldon, 2019, p. 459).

- Overall incidence has been estimated at 1:2,000 to 4,000 live births with the left side more commonly affected. Most are diagnosed antenatally.
- CDH can be an isolated occurrence but approximately 50% are associated with other anomalies (cardiac, urogenital, chromosomal, and musculoskeletal; Jensen et al., 2017, p. 79).
- Pulmonary hypoplasia is common, secondary to lung compression of the herniated contents (Bean, Arensman, Srinivasan, Maheshwari, & Ambalavanan, 2017, p. 400; Blackburn, 2013, p. 313; Crowley, 2015, p. 1115; Jensen et al., 2017, p. 79; Madenci et al., 2019, p. 459; Owen, Weiner & Davis, 2017, p. 288; Yoder, 2017, p. 236).
- Severity of respiratory distress is related to severity of the defect and degree of hypoplasia (Bradshaw, 2015, p. 619; Yoder, 2017, pp. 236–237).
- These infants are also at high risk for pneumothoraces (Bradshaw, 2015, p. 619).

DIAGNOSIS
- Measurement of the lung to head ratio (LHR) on prenatal US can predict the severity of pulmonary hypoplasia. Infants with low observed to expected (O/E) LHRs are at highest risk for significant pulmonary hypoplasia.
- If undiagnosed antenatally, infants can present with severe respiratory distress, cyanosis, and scaphoid abdomen.
- Breath sounds are diminished or absent on the affected side and cardiac sounds may be shifted toward the opposite side. Bowel sounds may be heard over chest on the affected side.
- Chest radiographs are consistent with abdominal contents in the thorax, shift of mediastinal structures to the unaffected side, and the abdomen may be gasless (Bradshaw, 2015, p. 618; Crowley, 2015, p. 1115; Ehret, 2015, pp. 264–265; Madenci et al., 2019, p. 460).

MANAGEMENT
- Treatment is supportive and aimed at preventing respiratory failure (Fraser, 2015, p. 619; Madenci et al., 2019, p. 460).
- Immediate intubation and positive pressure ventilation are required.
  ○ Avoid bag mask ventilation. Swallowed air leads to gastric distention, and further compression of the lung by the herniated portions of the gastrointestinal (GI) system. The use of cuffed endotracheal tubes may further reduce gastric distention (Blackburn, 2013, p. 313; Bradshaw, 2015, p. 619; DiBlasi & Gallagher, 2017, p. 296; Eichenwald, 2017, p. 402; Madenci et al., 2019, p. 460; Owen et al., 2017, p. 288).
  ○ Ventilation strategies that minimize barotrauma (HFOV), use of PIPs less than 25 cm H_2O, permissive hypercapnia, preductal saturation levels greater than or equal to 85%, pH greater than or equal to 7.25 (Bradshaw, 2015, p. 619; Crowley, 2015, p. 1116; Madenci et al., 2019, p. 460; Mammel & Courtney, 2017, p. 222; Yoder, 2017, p. 237).
- Gastric decompression via nasogastric tube (NG) tube under continuous suction
  ○ It is advisable to perform decompression maneuvers prior to intubation to further minimize unintentional distention with air (Madenci et al., 2019, p. 460).
  ○ Minimizes gastric distention, and further elevation of the diaphragm and compression of the lung (Blackburn,

2013, p. 313; Bradshaw, 2015, p. 619; DiBlasi & Gallagher, 2017, p. 296; Eichenwald, 2017, p. 402; Owen et al., 2017, p. 288).

- Hemodynamic support and treatment of PPHN
  - Inotropes, pulmonary vasodilators, and volume expanders to maintain systemic blood pressure and decrease right to left shunting (Bradshaw, 2015, p. 619; Madenci et al., 2019, p. 460; Owen et al., 2017, g. 288).
  - iNO may be used in infant's with severe hypoxemia. iNO dilates the pulmonary arteries, decreases pulmonary vascular resistance (PVR), and decreases right-to-left shunting across the ductus arteriosus (Bradshaw, 2015, p. 619; Kinsella, 2017, p. 359; Madenci et al., 2019, p. 460).
    - Additional vasodilator therapies include vasopressin, milrinone, and sildenafil (Madenci et al., 2019, p. 460; Yoder, 2017, p. 238).
  - Pulmonary arterial tension complicates most CDH cases and ECMO may be necessary (Bradshaw, 2015, p. 619; Jensen et al., 2017, p. 79; Madenci et al., 2019, p. 460).
- Pain management and sedation are critical to the care of CDH infants (Bradshaw, 2015, p. 620).
- Surgical repair can be done, when physiological stability has been achieved. CDH is no longer considered a surgical emergency and immediate surgical repair is thought to be detrimental (Bradshaw, 2015, p. 619; Madenci et al., 2019, p. 460; Yoder, 2017, p. 236).
- Overall prognosis is related to the degree of pulmonary hypoplasia. Surgical repair does not reverse the complications of CDH (Bradshaw, 2015, p. 619; Madenci et al., 2019, p. 460).
  - Mortality is high with larger defects, when the liver is involved in the defect, with the presence of other defects and with severe hypoplasia. (Blackburn, 2013, p. 313; Crowley, 2015, p. 1116; Owen et al., 2017, p. 288).
  - Survival is highest in tertiary centers and with use of multidisciplinary standardized treatment guidelines (Bradshaw, 2015, p. 619; Crowley, 2015, p. 1116).
  - CDH infants are at a higher risk of long term pulmonary, GI, neurologic, and skeletal systems morbidities

due to delayed lung maturation, altered pulmonary vasculature, and defects in surfactant maturation (Bradshaw, 2015, p. 620).

Esophageal Atresia (EA) and Tracheal–Esophageal Fistula (TEF)

DEFINITION AND PATHOPHYSIOLOGY

- Esophageal atresia is an anatomic interruption of the esophagus.
- Tracheoesophageal fistula is a subset of combined anomalies of the esophagus and trachea due to the abnormal development of the embryonic foregut. EA and TEF can occur as separate defects, or more commonly, in association with one another (Bradshaw, 2015, p. 594; Clemmens & Piccione, 2017, p. 120; Ringer & Hansen, 2017, pp. 947–948).
- The incidence of esophageal atresia (EA)/TEF is roughly 1 to 2 per 5,000 live births and is higher in White populations than in non-White (Bradshaw, 2015, p. 594; Parry, 2015, pp. 1395–1396) with a male predisposition (Madenci et al., 2019, p. 457).
  - There is an association with trisomy 13, 18, 21 as well as with Pierre–Robin, DiGeorge, Fanconi, and polysplenia syndromes.
  - Infants with EA/TEF have a higher incidence of defects in VACTERL Association and CHARGE Syndrome (Bradshaw, 2015, p. 595; Madenci et al., 2019, p. 457; Parry, 2015, pp. 1395–1396; Ringer & Hansen, 2017, p. 948).
- The most common type of defect is the presence of a proximal blind esophageal pouch/atresia with a more distal fistulous attachment of the trachea to the esophagus (Bradshaw, 2015, p. 594; Clemmens & Piccione, 2017, p. 120; Madenci et al., 2019, p. 457; Parry, 2015, pp. 1395–1396). See Table 17.3 for the description of the five EA/TEF types.

DIAGNOSIS

- EA can be diagnosed antenatally. EA may result in obstruction to the swallowing of amniotic fluid resulting in polyhydramnios. Prenatal imaging may demonstrate a small stomach. EA should be suspected in the presence of polyhydramnios and small stomach size (Madenci, et al., 2019, p. 457).

TABLE 17.3 Types of EA/TEF

EA/TEF Description	Type by Alphabetical Designation
Isolated EA with no associated fistula	Type A
Proximal TEF with distal EA	Type B
EA with distal TEF Most common type of EA/TEF	Type C
Both proximal and distal TEF present Most rare type of EA/TEF	Type D
Isolated TEF (also known as "H" type)	Type E

EA, esophageal atresia; TEF, tracheoesophageal fistula.

Sources: (Data from (Bradshaw, W. T. (2015). Gastrointestinal disorders. In M. T. Verklan & M. Walden (Eds.), *Core curriculum for neonatal intensive care nursing* (5th ed., pp. 583–631). St. Louis, MO: Elsevier; Madenci, A. L., Rice-Townsend, S. E., & Weldon, C. B. (2019). Surgical disorders in childhood that affect respiratory care. In B. K. Walsh (Ed.), *Neonatal and pediatric respiratory care* (5th ed., pp. 453–468). St. Louis, MO: Elsevier; Parry, R. L. (2015). Selected gastrointestinal anomalies in the neonate. In R. Martin, A. Fanaroff, & M. Walsh (Eds.), *Fanaroff and Martin's neonatal-perinatal medicine: Diseases of the fetus and infant* (10th ed., pp. 1395–1422). Philadelphia, PA: Elsevier Saunders).

- The inability to pass/advance an orogastric (OG) or NG may be indicative of the presence of the defect.
- Varying degrees of respiratory distress are evident, depending on the degree of pulmonary involvement and the type of tracheoesophageal anomaly. Excessive salivation, coughing, cyanosis, vomiting after feeding, abdominal distention are commonly seen symptoms (Bradshaw, 2015, p. 595; Madenci et al., 2019, p. 457; Parry, 2015, p. 139; Ringer & Hansen, 2017, p. 948).
- Chest radiographs, in most common type, are consistent with the OG/NG tube being visibly coiled in blind proximal pouch (Madenci et al., 2019, p. 457; Ringer & Hansen, 2017, p. 948).
  - When EA is found, the absence or presence of a distal TEF is confirmed by air in the stomach and intestinal tract.
    - Absence of air in the abdomen indicates a pure EA or an EA with an isolated upper pouch TEF
    - Presence of air in the abdomen indicates a TEF patent to the distal esophagus. These infants may experience respiratory distress as a result of aspiration of gastric contents into the trachea. The primary goal then becomes surgical intervention to divide and close the TEF (Flynn-O'Brien, Rice-Townsend, & Ledbetter, 2018, p. 1042.
- Contrast studies and or bronchoscopy/esophagoscopy may be required to confirm the rarer types (Parry, 2015, p. 1396; Ringer & Hansen, 2017, p. 948). The use of contrast studies increases the risk chemical pneumonitis secondary to aspiration of the contrast material (Bradshaw, 2015, p. 595).

MANAGEMENT
- Prematurity or the presence of associated defects may delay repair (Ringer & Hansen, 2017, p. 949).
- Supporting spontaneous respirations on room air is preferred (Madenci et al., 2019, p. 457).
- Mechanical ventilation should be avoided if possible. The introduction of positive pressure may create increased abdominal distention and subsequent respiratory compromise (Ringer & Hansen, 2017, p. 948).
  - Ventilatory support may be necessary with severe respiratory distress and low birth weight. Clinical condition largely dictates timing of surgical repair (Madenci et al., 2019, p. 457).
  - HFOV is recommended if ventilation is required to minimize GI distention.
- A suction catheter/OG or a Replogle tube place on continuous suction is necessary to minimize secretion aspiration and subsequent pneumonia (Bradshaw, 2015, p. 595; Madenci et al., 2019, p. 457; Ringer & Hansen, 2017, p. 948).
- Elevation of the head of the bed may help to minimize aspiration of gastric contents in EA with TEF (Bradshaw, 2015, p. 595; Ringer & Hansen, 2017, p. 948).
- Comfort measures to prevent crying which leads to swallowed air, abdominal distention, and increased risk of reflux (Bradshaw, 2015, p. 595).
- Surgical therapy in a stable, adequately sized term infant involves placement of a gastrostomy tube, division of the fistula, and primary anastomosis of the proximal and distal ends of the esophagus. Repair may need to be staged depending on the length of atretic segment until a primary anastomosis of the esophagus can be performed. Implementation of pain management and

sedation protocols postoperatively is critical to appropriate care (Bradshaw, 2015, p. 595; Madenci et al., 2019, p. 458; Parry, 2015, p. 1397, Ringer & Hansen, 2017, p. 949).
- If TEF is present with EA the administration of a gastric acid reduction medication may reduce chemical pneumonitis. Antibiotics may be required when pneumonia/pneumonitis is evident.
- Survival rate is greater than 95%. The highest mortality rates are seen in low birth weight infants, infants with associated anomalies, cardiac comorbidities, and/or the presence of pneumonia (Bradshaw, 2015, p. 595; Madenci et al., 2019, p. 459; Parry, 2015, p. 1400).
- Postoperative anastomotic leaks and strictures, recurrent fistulas can occur (Bradshaw, 2015, p. 596; Madenci et al., 2019, p. 459).
- Esophageal dysmotility, dysphagia, gastroesophageal reflux (GER), bronchospastic airway symptoms (stridor, brassy cough), and some degree of tracheolmalacia may be seen (Bradshaw, 2015, p. 596; Clemmens & Piccione, 2017, p. 120; Madenci et al., 2019, p. 459).

CONGENITAL CYSTIC LUNG LESIONS

Bronchogenic Cyst

DEFINITION AND PATHOPHYSIOLOGY
- Bronchogenic cysts occur due to the abnormal budding of the embryonic foregut or maldevelopment of the tracheobronchial tree.
- Cysts are usually single in nature and commonly located near the carina, but may be found in the parenchyma, pleura, and diaphragm. They can enlarge over time and become infected (Bean et al., 2017, p. 402; Crowley, 2015, p. 1121).

DIAGNOSIS
- Bronchogenic cyst may be diagnosed antenatally by US or fetal MRI.
- Postnatally the chest x-ray may demonstrate fluid-filled cysts or air-fluid levels in cysts within the airway and CT scan and bronchoscopy may confirm the diagnosis.
- Symptoms are related to airway compression/obstruction.
  - Symptoms of respiratory distress and stridor may occur later in the neonatal period or childhood (Bean et al, 2017, p. 402; Crowley, 2015, p. 1121).

MANAGEMENT
- Respiratory support may include supplemental oxygen, intubation, and ventilation (Bean et al., 2017, p. 402) depending on whether airway obstruction is complete or partial or if the airway is displaced anteriorly or posteriorly (Keller, Hirose, & Farmer, 2018, p. 702).
- Treatment for bronchogenic cyst consists of surgical resection and can be done thoracoscopically. Partial or total lobectomy yields uniformly good results. Early excision aims to prevent malignant changes over time (Keller et a., 2018, p. 702; Madenci et al., 2019, p. 463).

OUTCOMES
- Outcomes are excellent after excision with no long-term complications (Crowley, 2015, p. 1121). Without excision

there is a risk of bleeding, rupture, infection, and malignancy (Madenci et al., 2019, p. 463).

Congenital Pulmonary Airway Malformation (CPAM)

DEFINITION AND PATHOPHYSIOLOGY
- Formerly known as cystic adenomatoid malformations (CCAMs) but revisions were made to the classification system to include less common proximal and distal malformations (Keller et al., 2018, p. 708.)
- It is the most common congenital cystic lung disease, with an incidence of 1 in an 11,000 to 30,000 births.
- The malformation is due to the abnormal branching of the fetal bronchial tree during the pseudoglandular period. The lesion is connected to the tracheobronchial tree and has a pulmonary blood supply. Cysts can be microcystic or macrocystic and can affect all lobes (Bean et al., 2017, p. 401); (Crowley, 2015, pp. 1118–1119). CPAMs have been classified into four types (Table 17.4).

DIAGNOSIS
- CPAM can be diagnosed antenatally with US and prenatal MRI when mediastinal shift is noted because of mass effect and a cystic, intermediate, or solid mass is detected (Bean et al., 2017, p. 401; Keller et al., 2018, p. 710).

TABLE 17.4 Classification of CPAMs

CPAM Type	Disease Description
Type 0	Multiple small cysts, associated with other anomalies (cardiac, renal, dermal, and pulmonary hypoplasia) Involves all lobes, is the rarest and commonly lethal
Type 1	Large cysts surrounding by small cysts. Mass effect in utero can lead to hydrops and pulmonary hypoplasia. Cysts can collapse antenatal with normal growth of unaffected lobes. Most common type.
Type 2	Multiple small cysts, associated with other anomalies (renal, cardiac, CDH, Extralobar sequestrations)
Type 3	Multiple small cysts that appear as a solid mass. Associated with hydrops, polyhydramnios, and pulmonary hypoplasia.
Type 4	Large, thin-walled air-filled cysts in the lung periphery. May be asymptomatic at birth.

CPAM, congenital pulmonary airway malformation; CDH, congenital diaphragmatic hernia.

Source: Data from Crowley, M. A. (2015). Neonatal respiratory disorders. In R. J. Martin, A. A. Fanaroff, M. C. Walsh (Eds.), *Fanaroff and Martin's neonaal-perinatal medicine diseases of the fetus and infant* (10th ed., pp. 1113–1136). Philadelphia, PA: Saunders.

- Initial US evaluation of the fetus with possible CPAM should include assessment of lesion size, degree of mediastinal shift, and the presence of fluid indicating the development of fetal hydrops. Up to one-third of fetuses with a CPAM develop hydrops and polyhydramnios is common (Keller et al., 2018, p. 710).

- ○ Fetal and neonatal problems that arise as the result of a CPAM include the development of nonimmune hydrops and lung hypoplasia, which may be due to compression of the otherwise normally developing lung (Keller et al., 2018, p. 710).
- The postnatal degree of respiratory distress is related to the degree of pulmonary hypoplasia. Approximately 75% of newborns with a prenatally diagnosed CPAM are asymptomatic at birth (Bean et al., 2017, p. 401; Keller et al., 2018, p. 711).
- In non-emergent situations, a postnatal CT should be done to evaluate the mass size, which facilitates surgical removal (Crowley, 2015, p. 1120).

MANAGEMENT
- Antenatal steroids may reduce the size of microcystic lesions and resolve hydrops if present. With large volume lesions, fetal surgery (excision) may be required.
- The degree of respiratory/ventilatory support will be indicted by the severity of the lesion. Severely affected infants may require inhaled nitric oxide or ECMO support. The management of pulmonary hypertension if present is critical to the prevention of hypoxemia, the maintenance of pulmonary and systemic perfusion, and to preserve end-organ function.
- Postnatally if respiratory distress is severe, immediate surgical excision is required.
- ○ In asymptomatic infants, surgical removal can be elective, however, lesion removal is recommended in order to avoid the risks of infection and later malignancy (Bean et al., 2017, p. 401; Crowley, 2015, p. 1120; Madenci, et al., 2019, p. 461; Marter & McPherson, 2017, p. 471).

OUTCOMES
- Generally, children who have undergone resection for CPAMs are healthy. Pulmonary function data demonstrate normal vital capacity, residual volume, and expiratory flows between 1 and 2 years post lobectomy (Keller et al., 2018, p. 712). However, the prognosis for infants with CPAM is related to the severity of other associated anomalies and mortality is high when associated with pulmonary hypoplasia and hydrops. Long-term ventilatory assistance may be required when CPAM is more severe.
- There is an increased risk of bronchioloalveolar carcinoma (Type 1) for lesions that are not removed (Bean et al., 2019, p. 461; Crowley, 2015, p. 1119). The intact lesion also remains a persistent reservoir for lower respiratory tract infection (Keller et al., 2018, p. 712).

Congenital Lobar Emphysema (CLE)

DEFINITION AND PATHOPHYSIOLOGY
- CLE is an obstructive lesion, thought to be caused by abnormal bronchial cartilage formation and bronchomalacia. The obstructive lesion (intrinsic or extrinsic) leads to overinflation because air is allowed to pass into the effected bronchus but is unable to leave, causing air trapping.
- CLE usually presents in the neonatal period or within the first 6 months of life. It affects males more often than females

and affects the left upper lobe most often, followed by the right middle lobe and right upper lobe (Bean et al., 2017, p. 401; Crowley, 2015, p. 1121; Keller et al., 2018, p. 714).

DIAGNOSIS

- The severity of respiratory distress symptoms is dictated by the size of the lesion, the compression of the surrounding tissue, and the extent of mediastinal shift (Keller et al., 2018, p. 714).
- Chest radiographs are consistent with hyperinflation, widened rib space, shift of the mediastinal structures, and collapse of the unaffected lung. Lung markings are visible through the emphysematous area.
- Bronchoscopy or CT scan may help to confirm the diagnosis (Bean et al., 2017, p. 401; Crowley, 2015, p. 1121; Madenci, et al., 2019, p. 462).

MANAGEMENT

- Intubation may be required if respiratory distress is severe.
- Thoracotomy and removal of the affected lung lobe are recommended if the lesion is severe. Removal of the lesion releases compression of the lung by the emphysematous lesion (Madenci, et al., 2019, p. 462).

OUTCOMES

- Long-term prognosis is good once the affected segment is removed (Crowley, 2015, p. 1122). Compensatory lung growth will present on the affected side; however, airway obstruction continues to be a feature of the disease on pulmonary function tests. Although these findings could be consistent with either compensatory lung growth exceeding airway growth (dysanapsis) or intrinsic, diffuse airway abnormality (Keller et al., 2018, p. 714).

Bronchopulmonary Sequestration (BPS)

DEFINITION AND PATHOPHYSIOLOGY

- BPS lesions are thought to arise from the primitive foregut. The defect consists of microscopic cystic masses of nonfunctioning lung tissue that do not attach to the bronchopulmonary tree. It has a systemic arterial blood supply and it occurs in the lower lobes more often than the upper lobes.
- It affects males more often than females and is associated with other congenital anomalies (congenital diahragmatic hernia [CDH], vertebral anomalies, congenital heart disease [CHD]). Fetal hydrops may develop secondary to a mass effect (Bean et al., 2017, p. 401; Crowley, 2015, pp. 1120–1121).
- BPS can be intralobar or extralobar.
  - ○ Intralobar lesions are integral to the lung pleura and drain via the pulmonary venous system. Intralobar lesions usually require lobectomy for removal, because they are invested within the lung (Keller et al., 2018, p. 712).
  - ○ Extralobar lesions are more remote and may be covered in their own pleura and systemic (80% of the time) venous drainage, and they are therefore separate from the lung. The extralobar type is more commonly associated with other anomalies as noted above (Bean et al.,

2017, p. 401; Crowley, 2015, pp. 1120–1121, Keller et al., 2018, p. 712).

DIAGNOSIS

- BPS can be identified antenatally and may look similar to CPAM. Color Doppler can identify the systemic arterial blood supply (Crowley, 2015, p. 1120).
- Postnatal US can also be useful in demonstrating the lesion (most easily seen if it is located at the lung base), and CT and or MRI may help define the systemic arterial blood supply (Crowley, 2015, p. 1120; Keller, Hirose, & Farmer, 2018, p. 712; Madenci et al., 2019, p. 462).
- The degree of respiratory distress will dictate severity of the disease. Distress at birth can be severe, particularly with large lesions complicated by a pleural effusion hydrops fetalis, or pulmonary hypoplasia (Keller et al., 2018, p. 712).
  - ○ Chest x-rays are often consistent with a left posterior thoracic mass.
- If asymptomatic at birth, they may present later in infancy with atelectasis, high output congestive heart failure (CHF), bleeding, and recurrent pneumonia (Crowley, 2015, p. 1121; Madenci, et al., 2019, p. 462).

MANAGEMENT

- If symptoms are severe, intubation and ventilatory support minimizing overdistention (HFOV) may be required. Urgent excision of the lesion is required.
  - ○ Because the lesion is completely separate from lung, sequestrectomy is not a complex operation and can be done thorascopically. However, the feeding vessels can be very large in more severe cases, mandating a thoracotomy (Keller et al., 2018, p. 712.)
- In asymptomatic patients, removal of the lesion can be elective, although there is controversy in this practice. The primary risk associated with an unresected BPS is recurrent infection (Keller et al., 2018, p. 713).

OUTCOMES

- Long-term pulmonary outcomes are dictated by the size and location of the lesion, associated anomalies, and the degree of pulmonary hypoplasia.
  - ○ BPS has a higher incidence of malignancy development (Crowley, 2015, p. 1121).

ACQUIRED RESPIRATORY DISORDERS

Respiratory Distress Syndrome (RDS)

DEFINITION AND PATHOPHYSIOLOGY

- Insufficient or inactivated pulmonary surfactant leads to hypoxia, hypoventilation, and progressive atelectasis (Blackburn, 2013, pp. 330–342; Fraser, 2015, p. 449; Hansen & Levin, 2019, p. 408; Jensen, et al., 2017, p. 71; Shepherd & Nelson, 2017, pp. 62–63; Yoder, 2017, pp. 229–230).
- Pulmonary edema from serum proteins leaking into the alveoli contributes to the loss of functional residual capacity (FRC) and alterations in ventilation-perfusion ratio (Blackburn, 2013, pp. 333–336; Fraser, 2015, p. 450; Hansen & Levin, 2019, p. 408; Yoder, 2017, p. 229).

○ Lung maturity or inadequate production of surfactant from type II alveolar cells is the most significant risk factor (Fraser, 2015, p. 450; Guttentag, 2017, p. 436; Hansen & Levin, 2019, p. 408; Yoder, 2017, p. 229).

○ Inflammation as with infection can negatively impact surfactant production and function (Guttentag, 2017, p. 437; Jensen et al., 2017, p. 72; Kallapur & Jobe, 2015, p. 1057).

○ Increased fetal insulin in response to maternal diabetes inhibits proteins critical for surfactant production (Blackburn, 2013, p. 318; Jensen et al., 2017, p. 71; Guttentag, 2017, p. 437).

○ Mutations in surfactant protein production or surfactant packaging can result in reduced production or functioning of surfactant (Blackburn, 2013, pp. 314–316; Fraser, 2015, p. 450; Guttentag, 2017, p. 437).

• RDS incidence is inversely proportional to gestational age (Blackburn, 2013, p. 342; Fraser, 2015, p. 449; Hansen & Levin, 2019, p. 408).

○ Incidence is higher in males (male to female ratio is 2:1) as the presence of fetal androgens inhibits surfactant phospholipid production, and is higher in Caucasian infants (Fraser, 2015, p. 450; Guttentag, 2017, p. 437).

○ Maternal administration of corticosteroids enhances lung maturity, antenatally inducing lung structural maturation by increasing the surface area for gas exchange and stimulation of surfactant production (Blackburn, 2013, p. 318; Fraser, 2015, p. 453; Hansen & Levin, 2019, pp. 409, 412; Kallapur & Jobe, 2015, p. 1057).

DIAGNOSIS

• Symptoms of RDS present soon after delivery, and respiratory difficulty increases within the first few hours of life, to include tachypnea, retractions, audible expiratory grunting, nasal flaring, cyanosis, and an increased oxygen requirement (Blackburn, 2013, p. 343; Fraser, 2015, pp. 449–451; Hansen & Levin, 2019, p. 411; Shepherd & Nelin, 2017, pp. 62–63, 71–72; Wambach & Hamvas, 2015, p. 1078).

○ Diagnostics include chest x-ray, arterial blood gas (ABG) measurements, blood cultures, and blood glucose monitoring.

○ Breath sounds may be diminished with poor air entry. Crackle, paradoxical seesaw respirations, and tachycardia may be present with disease progression, as well as pallor, central cyanosis, decreased capillary fill time, and progressive edema of the face, palms, and soles (Blackburn, 2013, p. 344; Fraser, 2015, p. 450; Hansen & Levin, 2019, p. 411).

○ A chest x-ray will present with ground glass or hazy appearance, low lung volumes, air bronchograms (more prominent as disease progresses), and micro atelectasis. Complete atelectasis is characterized as "white-out" on chest x-ray (Blackburn, 2013, p. 342; Fraser, 2015, p. 451; Guttentag, 2017, p. 439; Hansen & Levin, 2019, p. 411; Jensen et al., 2017, p. 72; Shepherd & Nelin, 2017, p. 62).

○ Hypoxemia, hypercarbia, and acidosis can be seen on blood gas analysis (Fraser, 2017, p. 450; Hansen & Levin, 2019, p. 411).

○ Oliguria is a common presentation in the first 48 hours and lung improvement is seen at 2 to 4 days with diuresis (Fraser, 2015, p. 450; Guttentag, 2017, p. 445).

• Symptoms gradually worsen and peak by two to three days, with improvement by 72 hours of life (Blackburn, 2013, p. 344; Hansen & Levin, 2019, pp. 411, 416; Wambach & Hamvas, 2015, p. 1078).

MANAGEMENT

• Exogenous surfactant administration augments endogenous surfactant production, improves lung compliance and stabilizes the alveolar membrane, reducing alveolar collapse and atelectasis (Hansen & Levin, 2019, pp. 413–414; Kallapur & Jobe, 2015, pp. 1052–1054). Treatment is supportive to prevent further lung damage until the infant can produce adequate surfactant (Blackburn, 2013, p. 344; Fraser, 2015, pp. 451–452; Hansen & Levin, 2019, pp. 411–415; Suresh et al., 2017, p. 341; Yoder, 2017, pp. 230, 233).

• Mechanical ventilation strategies help to establish and maintain FRC, recruit collapsed alveoli, and assist in improved oxygenation and ventilation (Blackburn, 2013, p. 344; Guttentag, 2017, pp. 444–445; Hansen & Levin, 2019, p. 415; Yoder, 2017, pp. 230–233).

• Caffeine therapy promotes respiratory drive (Guttentag, 2017, p. 444; Hansen & Levin, 2019, p. 415).

• Evaluation for inflammatory/infectious processes and treatment with antibiotics may be necessary. Group B *Streptococcus* (GBS) pneumonia and RDS are often indistinguishable on chest x-ray (Fraser, 2015, p. 451).

OUTCOMES

• Resolution of RDS results in minimal to no complications in infants born at or over 32 weeks' gestation (Guttentag, 2017, p. 445).

• Surfactant therapy reduces both the risk and severity of RDS and has been associated with a 30% reduction in mortality (Blackburn, 2013, pp. 344–345; Suresh et al., 2017, p. 341).

• Long-term sequelae are related to specific complications: CLD, IVH, retinopathy of prematurity (ROP), and respiratory syncytial virus (RSV) infection (Fraser, 2015, p. 453).

○ With severe RDS requiring prolonged ventilation, lung injury may be more severe, and recovery delayed (Wambach & Hamvas, 2017, p. 1078). The risk for the development of CLD is highest in the lowest birth weight groups (Fraser, 2015, p. 453; Stewart, Hernandez, & Duncan, 2017, p. 193).

○ Readmissions for the treatment of respiratory infections in the first year of life is not uncommon and lung disease may persist into adulthood (Stewart et al., 2017, p. 193).

Pneumonia

DEFINITION AND PATHOPHYSIOLOGY

• Multiple pathogens can be implicated with infection of the lung and can present early (within first 3 days of life) or late (after 3 days of life). Organisms responsible for pneumonia vary by early and late onset (see Table 17.5).

○ Congenital, or early onset, pneumonia, is acquired by vertical transmission in utero from aspiration of infected amniotic fluid, ascending infections from the birth canal, or via the transplacental route (Crowley, 2015, p. 1126; Fraser, 2015, pp. 454–455; Hansen & Levin, 2019, pp. 426–428; Jensen et al., 2017, p. 73; Wilson & Tyner, 2015; p. 700).

○ Late-onset pneumonia is common in infants requiring prolonged ventilation, and is often hospital acquired or

TABLE 17.5 Organisms Responsible for Early and Late-Onset Pneumonia

Early Onset	Late Onset
Group B *Streptococcus* (GBS)	*Staphylococcus* spp.
Escherichia coli	Coagulase-Negative Staphylococci
Klebsiella spp.	*Staphylococcus aureus, Staphylococcus epidermis*
Enterobacter spp.	*Streptococcus pneumoniae*
Group A *Streptococcus*	*Escherichia coli*
Staphylococcus aureus	*Klebsiella* spp.
Listeria Monocytogenes	*Serratia* spp.
Herpes simplex virus (type I and II)	*Enterobacter cloacae*
Adenovirus	*Pseudomonas* spp.
Enterovirus	*Candida* spp.
Mumps virus	*Bacillus cereus*
Rubella virus	*Citrobacter* spp.
Cytomegalovirus	Respiratory syncytial virus
Treponema pallidum	Adenovirus
Toxoplasma gondii	Enterovirus
Candida spp.	Parainfluenza
Mycobacterium tuberculosis	Rhinovirus
Hemophilus influenzae	Influenza viruses
Chlamydia trachomatis	Cytomegalovirus
Ureaplasma urealyticum	*Chlamydia trachomatis*

Source: Data from Fraser, D. (2015). Respiratory distress. In M. T. Verklan & M. Walden (Eds.), *Core curriculum for neonatal intensive care nurses* (5th ed., pp. 447–477). St. Louis, MO: Elsevier.

nosocomial, caused by both bacterial and viral pathogens (Fraser, 2015, pp. 454–455; Hansen & Levin, 2019, p. 426; Jensen et al., 2017, p. 73; Wilson & Tyner, 2015, p. 700).
- Pneumonia risk factors include prematurity, prolonged rupture of membranes, GBS colonization, chorioamnionitis, intrapartum maternal fever, sepsis, invasive procedures, presence of central lines, aspiration, and prolonged ventilation (Crowley, 2015, p. 1126; Fraser, 2015, p. 455; Hansen & Levin, 2019, pp. 409, 427–428; Jensen et al., 2017, p. 73).
  - ○ According to Hansen & Levin (2019, p. 426), *Escherichia coli* is the most common bacterial isolate in the premature population.

DIAGNOSIS
- Pneumonia symptoms are often indistinguishable from other respiratory diseases, RDS and sepsis. Symptoms include grunting, nasal flaring, retractions, cyanosis, and desaturations requiring supplemental oxygen, poor feeding, lethargy, irritability, temperature instability, and unwell appearance (Fraser, 2015, p. 455; Hansen & Levin, 2019, pp. 409, 427; Wilson & Tyner, 2015, p. 701).
- Chest x-ray findings may be nonspecific (unilateral or bilateral), they include alveolar infiltrates, areas of confluent opacities, diffuse interstitial pattern, and pleural effusions. Ground glass appearance and air bronchograms may be present (Crowley, 2015, p. 1126; Ehret, 2015, p. 261; Fraser, 2015, p. 455; Hansen & Levin, 2019, p. 428).
  - ○ Radiographic findings with postnatally acquired infections often change from normal to severely abnormal in a few days and may include pulmonary edema, pleural effusions, pneumatoceles, evidence of barotrauma, and cardiomegaly, depending on the severity of the disease process (Ehret, 2015, p. 261; Fraser, 2015, p. 455; Hansen & Levin, 2019, p. 428; Wilson & Tyner, 2015, p. 701).
- Infants should be evaluated for accompanying or concurrent septicemia: lethargy, temperature instability, apnea, poor feeding, and metabolic acidosis (Crowley, 2015, p. 1126; Wilson & Tyner, 2015, p. 701).

MANAGEMENT
- Ventilation, circulatory support, management of hypoxia, acidosis, hypoglycemia, and electrolytes as well as adequate nutrition helps reduce mortality and morbidity.
- Sepsis evaluation to rule out septicemia should be performed and should include a complete blood cell count with differential, blood culture, and inflammatory markers like C-reactive protein (CRP), and polymerase chain reaction (PCR) to detect herpes viruses (Fraser, 2015, p. 455; Hansen & Levin, 2019, p. 428; Wilson & Tyner, 2015, p. 701). Gram stain and culture of intubated infants, urine cultures, and cerebrospinal fluid (CSF) cultures may also be helpful in determining the origin of infection.
  - ○ Positive tracheal aspirates after 8 hours of life may correlate with tracheal colonization and not infection (Crowley, 2015, p. 1126).
- Empiric antibiotics may be started before the identification of an organism. Antibiotic choice is based on the index of suspicion.
- Suspected early-onset pneumonia is usually treated with ampicillin and gentamicin. Late-onset pneumonia is treated with vancomycin and gentamicin. Antivirals may be administered for herpes simplex or other pneumonias of viral origin.
- Blood gas evaluation is important because metabolic acidosis may be severe. Tracheal aspirates may assist in the identification of a predominant infectious organism. CSF cultures should be obtained when the infant is stable since meningitis often accompanies pneumonia (Fraser, 2015, pp. 455–456).
- Length of antibiotic treatment is dictated by the organism responsible for the infection; treatment for 10 to 14 days is usually effective (Crowley, 2015, p. 1126; Hansen & Levin, 2019, p. 428; Wilson & Tyner, 2015, p. 702).

OUTCOMES

- Outcome depends on the causative organism and response to antibiotic therapy. Complications include cardiopulmonary sequelae, systemic inflammatory response syndrome, disseminated intravascular coagulopathy, air leak, persistent pulmonary hypertension, and eventual development of CLD from prolonged ventilation (Fraser, 2015, p. 456; Hansen & Levin, 2019, p. 429).
- Rapid identification of the infecting organism and timely treatment helps to minimize morbidity and mortality (Crowley, 2015, p. 1126).

Transient Tachypnea of the Newborn (TTN)

DEFINITION AND PATHOPHYSIOLOGY

- TTN is a delayed clearance of fetal lung fluid resulting in pulmonary edema. FRC may be reduced and thoracic gas volume may be increased secondary to air trapping (Blackburn, 2013, p. 342; Fraser, 2015, p. 456; Gregory, 2017, p. 432; Jensen et al., 2017, p. 72).
  - ○ The disease is characterized by tachypnea (up to 60-140 breaths per minute), mild-to-moderate retractions, grunting, cyanosis, decreased oxygen saturation, hypercapnia, and respiratory acidosis, with a duration of 1 to 5 days (Blackburn, 2013, p. 342; Fraser, 2015, p. 456; Gregory, 2017, pp. 432–434; Hansen & Levin, 2019, p. 425; Jensen et al., 2017, p. 72; Shepherd & Nevin, 2017, p. 63).
- Risk factors include precipitous birth, preterm delivery, macrosomia, maternal diabetes, maternal asthma, multiple gestations, male gender, breech presentation, maternal sedation, and Caesarean delivery with or without labor (Blackburn, 2013, p. 320; Fraser, 2015, pp. 456–457; Gregory, 2017, p. 433; Hansen & Levin, 2019, p. 425; Jensen et al., 2017, p. 72).
  - ○ TTN usually affects late preterm or term infants, occurring in 0.3% to 0.6% of term deliveries and 1% of preterm deliveries (Gregory, 2017, p. 433).
- Delayed clearance of fetal lung fluid is thought to be related to a delayed transition of the lungs from the in utero secretory fetal lung mode to the absorptive mode, and by the absence of the hormonal changes that accompany spontaneous labor, including a surge in glucocorticoids and catecholamines. Impaired sodium channel clearance and the active transport of chloride have also been implicated (Blackburn, 2013, p. 323; Fraser, 2015, p. 456; Hansen & Levin, 2019, p. 425).

DIAGNOSIS

- A diagnosis of TTN requires the exclusion of other potential etiologies for respiratory distress occurring in the first 6 hours of life, including RDS, sepsis, pneumonia, meconium aspiration syndrome (MAS), pulmonary hypertension, cyanotic congenital heart disease, central nervous system injury, pneumothorax, congenital malformations, metabolic acidosis, and polycythemia (Blackburn, 2013, p. 342; Fraser, 2015, p. 457; Gregory, 2017, p. 433; Jensen et al., 2017, p. 72; Shepherd & Nevin, 2017, p. 62).
  - ○ TTN is commonly seen in the first 6 hours of life and can persist for up to 72 hours (Gregory, 2017, p. 433; Hansen & Levin, 2019, p. 425; Jensen et al., 2017, p. 72; Shepherd & Nevin, 2019, p. 63). Air exchange is good and breath sounds may initially be moist, but clear quickly (Blackburn, 2013, p. 342).

- ○ Chest x-rays exhibit increased pulmonary markings with perihilar streaking clearing at the periphery and fluid-filled interlobar fissures (Blackburn, 2013, p. 342; Fraser, 2015, p. 457). Hyperaeration with widened intercostal spaces, mild cardiomegaly, mild hyper expansion, mild pleural effusions, a flattened diaphragm, and occasionally air bronchograms may also be present (Blackburn, 2013, p. 342; Ehret, 2015, pp. 258–259; Fraser, 2015, p. 457; Gregory, 2017, p. 434; Hansen & Levin, 2019, pp. 425–426; Jensen et al., 2017, p. 72).
- ○ Decreased lung compliance results in tachypnea and increased work of breathing (WOB), cyanosis, grunting, retractions, and nasal flaring all beginning within a few hours of birth (Fraser, 2015, p. 456; Gregory, 2017, p. 433; Hansen & Levin, 2019, p. 425).
- ○ Infants may have a depressed diaphragm, an increased anterioposterior diameter, and a barrel-shaped chest secondary to hyperinflation (Blackburn, 2013, p. 342; Gregory, 2017, p. 433; Hansen & Levin, 2019, pp. 425–426).
- Laboratory evaluation should include serial complete blood count (CBC) and CRP levels as well as appropriate cultures to rule out possible pneumonia or sepsis (Blackburn, 2013, p. 342; Gregory, 2017, p. 434).

MANAGEMENT

- Treatment is mainly supportive and includes close observation, blood gas evaluation, and continuous positive airway pressure (CPAP) with or without supplemental oxygen therapy to prevent hypoxia.
  - ○ CPAP to improve lung recruitment may be indicated in more severe cases of TTN; however, CPAP is associated with an increased risk of air leak (Fraser, 2015, p. 457; Gregory, 2017, p. 434; Hansen & Levin, 2019, p. 426).
  - ○ If tachypnea and hypoxemia persist, evaluate for PPHN (Fraser, 2015, p. 457).
  - ○ Empiric broad-spectrum antibiotics may not be necessary if there are no risk factors for infection.
  - ○ Feedings should be held if respiratory rates are sustained consistently above 60 to 80 breaths per minute. Restricting fluid intake may decrease the duration of support when TTN is severe (Fraser, 2015, p. 457; Gregory, 2017, p. 434; Hansen & Levin, 2019, p. 426).

OUTCOMES

- TTN is usually self-limiting disease, generally improving within the first 48 to 72 hours of life, and in general there are no significant long-term negative outcomes (Fraser, 2015, p. 457; Gregory, 2017, p. 435; Hansen & Levin, 2019, p. 426; Jensen et al., 2017, p. 72; Shepherd & Nevin, 2017, p. 62).
  - ○ There may be a link between TTN and the later development of wheezing or reactive airway disease later in childhood (Crowley, 2015, p. 1128; Gregory, 2017, p. 435).

Meconium Aspiration Syndrome (MAS)

DEFINITION AND PATHOPHYSIOLOGY

- MAS is the aspiration of meconium-stained amniotic fluid (MSAF) into the lungs in term or post-term infants, when the fetus gasps in the presence of fetal stress before, during, or immediately after delivery (Blackburn, 2013, p. 347; Fraser, 2015, p. 462; Hansen & Levin, 2019, p. 429; Yoder, 2017, pp. 233–234).

○ With intrauterine stress or asphyxia, peristalsis is stimulated and the relaxation of the anal sphincter releases meconium into the amniotic fluid rarely occurs in infants less than 36 weeks gestation (Blackburn, 2013, p. 347; Fraser, 2015, p. 462; Hansen & Levin, 2019, p. 429).

○ The severity of MAS is related to the amount of fluid aspirated, the degree of asphyxial insult, and is frequently accompanied by air leak (Plosa, 2017, p. 461).

- Risk factors for MSAF are post-term (<41 weeks), small for gestational age, fetal distress, placental insufficiency, oligohydramnios, cord compression, and intrauterine hypoxia (Blackburn, 2013, p. 347; Crowley, 2015, p. 1122; Hansen & Levin, 2019, p. 430; Yoder, 2017, p. 233).

○ Delivery room management: routine suctioning at delivery of vigorous or depressed infants born through MSAF is not beneficial and is no longer recommended (Blackburn, 2013, p. 347; Hansen & Levin, 2019, p. 431; Plosa, 2017, p. 461).

- Meconium can inactivate both endogenous and exogenous surfactant, and inhibit surfactant production, causing airway obstruction, severe respiratory distress, impaired gas exchange, hypoxia, and increased PVR (Blackburn, 2013, pp. 347–348; Fraser, 2015, p. 462; Hansen & Levin, 2019, p. 430; Yoder, 2017, p. 233).

○ The *Obstructive phase* is accompanied by acute airway obstruction, markedly increased airway resistance, scattered atelectasis with V/Q mismatching, and lung hyper-expansion secondary to air trapping and ball-valve effects (Blackburn, 2013, p. 347; Fraser, 2015, p. 462; Hansen & Levin, 2019, pp. 430–432; Plosa, 2017, p. 462; Yoder, 2017, pp. 233–234).

○ The *Inflammatory phase*, from the release of cytokines and vasoactive substances, occurs 12 to 24 hours later leading to chemical pneumonitis and further alveolar involvement. Infants delivered with MSAF have an increased risk of pneumonia and PPHN (Blackburn, 2013, p. 347; Fraser, 2015, p. 462; Hansen & Levin, 2019, p. 430; Plosa, 2017, p. 464; Yoder, 2017, pp. 233–234).

DIAGNOSIS

- MAS may present with birth depression requiring vigorous resuscitation (Crowley, 2015, p. 1123; Fraser, 2015, p. 462).
- Symptoms of respiratory distress may range from mild and transient to severe and prolonged, and include grunting, flaring, retractions, tachypnea, and cyanosis (Crowley, 2015, p. 1123; Fraser, 2015, p. 463).

○ Physical examination may reveal a barrel-shaped chest secondary to hyperinflation with audible rales on auscultation (Fraser, 2015, p. 463; Hansen & Levin, 2019, 431).

▪ Physical examination consistent with meconium aspiration related to postmaturity: peeling/cracking skin, loss of weight, long meconium-stained nails, meconium-stained umbilical cord (Crowley, 2015, p. 1123; Hansen & Levin, 2019, p. 431).

▪ Diffuse, asymmetrical patchy infiltrates, areas of consolidation, hyper-expanded lucent areas mixed with areas of atelectasis, and a flattened diaphragm are classic findings on chest radiography (Blackburn, 2013, p. 347; Ehret, 2015, pp. 260–261; 463; Fraser, 2017, p. 464; Hansen & Levin, 2019, p. 431; Jensen et al., 2017, p. 72).

MANAGEMENT

- Respiratory failure requiring mechanical ventilation is common. Use of positive pressure may result in air leak because of ball-valve effects of MAS. Low levels of positive end expiratory pressure (PEEP; 4 to 5 cm H_2O) splint open partially obstructed airways and equalize $\dot{V}/Q$ matching. When airway resistance is high but lung compliance is normal, the use of a slow rate and moderate pressure or volume is indicated (Blackburn, 2013, p. 348; Eichenwald, 2017, p. 415; Fraser, 2015, p. 463; Hansen & Levin, 2019, p. 432; Yoder, 2017, pp. 232–236).

○ Infants with severe MAS may require the use of high-frequency ventilation (HFV), nitric oxide, and/or extracorporeal membrane oxygenation, if PPHN develops (Fraser, 2015, p. 463; Hansen & Levin, 2019, p. 432; Plosa, 2017, pp. 464–466; Yoder, 2017, p. 234).

- MAS management is primarily supportive and should include ventilatory/oxygen support (including close monitoring of blood gases) to maintain peripheral oxygen saturation between 95% and 99%, cardiovascular stabilization, and blood pressure support as well as avoiding hypoxia and acidosis (Crowley, 2015, p. 1125; Fraser, 2015, p. 463; Hansen & Levin, 2019, p. 431).

○ Antibiotic administration is required to treat pneumonia/sepsis (Crowley, 2015, p. 1125; Yoder, p. 233).

○ Surfactant therapy may improve lung compliance and oxygenation (Blackburn, 2013, p. 347; Fraser, 2015, p. 463; Plosa, 2017, p. 465; Suresh et al., 2017, p. 348; Yoder, 2017, p. 233). Surfactant administration is thought to reduce the severity of respiratory distress and may reduce disease progression and the need for ECMO, a last resort therapy (Hansen & Levin, 2019, p. 432).

○ May need iNO if PPHN develops (Hansen & Levin, 2019, p. 432).

○ Sedation (morphine, fentanyl, lorazepam, or midazolam) or muscle relaxation (pancuronium bromide, vecuronium) may lower the risk of air leak in severe MAS (Eichenwald, 2017, p. 415; Hansen & Levin, 2019, p. 432).

○ Non-pharmacologic interventions may help decrease agitation and limit need for sedation and include limiting stimulation by lowering environmental light, noise, and any unnecessary tactile stimulation (Hansen & Levin, 2019, p. 432).

- Recovery and weaning of respiratory support are proportional to resolution of airway obstruction, degree of inflammation, and extent of lung injury (Eichenwald, 2017, p. 415).

OUTCOMES

- Mild cases of MAS generally have excellent prognoses, unless the MAS is accompanied by PPHN or severe asphyxia (Fraser, 2015, p. 463; Hansen & Levin, 2019, p. 432).

○ MAS complicated by PPHN carries an increased risk of mortality (Hansen & Levin, 2019, p. 432; Plosa, 2017, p. 466).

○ A small number of infants who survive MAS will continue to require oxygen at 1 month and pulmonary function may be abnormal (Hansen & Levin, 2019, p. 432; Plosa, 2017, p. 466).

○ Prolonged ventilatory support resulting from PPHN may result in CLD (Crowley, 2015, p. 1125).

Pulmonary Hemorrhage

DEFINITION AND PATHOPHYSIOLOGY

- Pulmonary hemorrhage (PH) is defined as the presence of erythrocytes in the alveoli and/or the lung interstitium and occurs in 3% to 5% of preterm infants ventilated for RDS. Eighty percent of PHs in preterm infants occurs within 72 hours of birth or between day 2 and 4 of life (Fraser, 2015, p. 471; Hansen & Levin, 2019, p. 432, Plosa, 2017, p. 479).
- PH is thought to result from hemorrhagic pulmonary edema rather than direct bleeding into the lung. It results in poor lung compliance, surfactant inactivation, and pulmonary edema (Hansen & Levin, 2019, p. 443; Keszler & Chatburn, 2017, p. 146). Other mechanisms contributing to PH may include increased pulmonary capillary pressure and injury to the capillary endothelium from acute left ventricular failure; altered epithelial-endothelial barrier, and coagulation disorders, which may worsen the condition but not initiate it (Hansen & Levin, 2019, p. 444; Fraser, 2015, p. 471; Plosa, 2017, p. 478).
  - It is rarely an isolated condition and is typically exhibited by the clinical presence of hemorrhagic fluid (pink or red frothy fluid) in the trachea accompanied by respiratory decompensation requiring increased respiratory support or intubation within 60 minutes of the appearance of hemorrhagic fluid (Fraser, 2015, p. 471; Hansen & Levin, 2019, p. 443–444; Jensen et al., 2017, p. 75; Plosa, 2017, p. 478).
- Predisposing factors linked to PH include patent ductus arteriosus (PDA), exogenous surfactant administration, sepsis, severe systemic illness, extreme prematurity, coagulopathy, IVH, heart disease, perinatal asphyxia, hypothermia, male gender, and multiple birth.
  - Other causes of blood in the airway not related to PH include direct trauma to the airway, and aspiration of blood (Fraser, 2015, p. 471; Hansen & Levin, 2019, p. 443; Jensen et al., 2017, p.75; Plosa, 2017, p. 479).

DIAGNOSIS

- Acute respiratory distress symptoms include cyanosis, bradycardia, apnea, gasping, hypotension, increased WOB, hypoxia, and hypercapnia (Crowley, 2015, p. 1128; Fraser, 2015, p. 471; Hansen & Levin, 2019, p. 444).
  - The presence of the pink frothy fluid noted in airway or endotracheal tube.
  - Chest x-ray findings may be nonspecific and include the presence of fluffy infiltrates or opacification of one or both lungs with air bronchograms (Hansen & Levin, 2019, p. 444; Jensen et al., 2017, p. 75).
  - A fall in hematocrit, metabolic, or mixed acidosis coagulopathy can also be seen (Plosa, 2017, p. 480).
- An echocardiogram should be done to assess and treat PDA and evaluate ventricular function (Hansen & Levin, 2019, p. 445).

MANAGEMENT

- Ventilatory support including high mean airway pressure, high PEEP of 6 to 8 cm of H_2O, and ventilation strategy that maintains gas exchange and tamponades or minimizes further accumulation of interstitial and alveolar fluid. Aggressive airway suctioning should be avoided (Fraser, 2015, p. 471; Hansen & Levin, 2019, p. 445; Jensen et al., 2017, pp. 75, 146; Plosa, 2017, p. 480).
  - Consider surfactant administration to treat primary RDS or secondary surfactant deficiency from airway

edema caused by the hemorrhage (Hansen & Levin, 2019, p. 445; Plosa, 2017, p. 480). However, the efficacy of surfactant therapy is not well established and routine use is questionable (Hansen & Levin, 2019, p. 445; Suresh et al., 2017, p. 348).
  - Endotracheal administration of epinephrine will cause restriction of the pulmonary capillaries (Hansen & Levin, 2019, p. 445).
- Volume resuscitation, including packed red blood cell (PRBC) replacement in addition to the administration of vasoactive medications may be required (Fraser, 2015, p. 471; Hansen & Levin, 2019, p. 445; Plosa, 2017, p. 480).
- Assess for and treat PDA and clotting abnormalities (Fraser, 2015, p. 471; Hansen & Levin, 2019, p. 444).

OUTCOMES

- If the hemorrhage is isolated or small, the outcome will depend on the underlying disease. If bleeding is massive, death will quickly occur in spite of aggressive management. Mortality is 30% to 40% (Fraser, 2015, p. 471; Jensen et al., 2017, p. 75).
- PH may be associated with a higher incidence of cerebral palsy, cognitive delay, periventricular leukomalacia, and seizures, with the highest mortality rates occurring in the extremely low birth weight population (Crowley, 2015, p. 1128).

Persistent Pulmonary Hypertension

DEFINITION AND PATHOPHYSIOLOGY

- PPHN is a syndrome of acute respiratory depression from sustained elevation in PVR and pulmonary artery pressure leading to right-to-left shunting across persistent fetal channels (PDA, patent foramen ovale/PFO), decreased pulmonary perfusion, severe systemic hypoxemic respiratory failure, academia, and lactic acidosis (Blackburn, 2013, p. 348; Clemmens & Piccione, 2017, p. 125; Fraser, 2015, pp. 457–458; Hansen & Levin, 2019, p. 433; Keszler & Abubakar, 2017, p. 28; Van Marter & McPherson, 2017, p. 467).
  - Adequate oxygenation after delivery depends on lung inflation, closure of the fetal shunts, decreased PVR, and increased pulmonary blood flow (Fraser, 2015, p. 458).
- Antenatal conditions linked to PPHN include asphyxia; pulmonary parenchymal disease (pneumonia, surfactant deficiency, aspiration syndromes); abnormal pulmonary development and structure (CDH, pulmonary hypoplasia, space-occupying lesions); congenital heart disease; myocardial dysfunction; prenatal pulmonary hypertension (systemic or secondary to premature closure of the ductus arteriosus associated with maternal aspirin or nonsteroidal anti-inflammatory drugs); pneumonia, bacterial, or viral sepsis; and genetic predisposition. Contributing mechanical pathology includes low cardiac output and hyperviscosity, associated with polycythemia, and abnormal pulmonary vasoreactivity and adaptation (Fraser, 2015, p. 458; Hansen & Levin, 2019, p. 433; Keszler & Abubakar, 2017, pp. 25–28; Kinsella, 2017, p. 353, 363; Van Marter & McPherson, 2017, p. 468).
- Perinatal risk factors include MSAF, maternal fever, urinary tract infection (UTI), anemia, diabetes, or pulmonary disease, as well as selective serotonin reuptake

inhibitor exposure, hypothermia, and cesarean delivery (Fraser, 2015, p. 458; Hansen & Levin, 2019, 433; Van Marter & McPherson, 2017, p. 468).

○ PPHN is most common in full-term and post-term infants at rates of 1 to 2 per 1,000 live births (Fraser, 2015, p. 457; Hansen & Levin, 2019, p. 433; Van Marter & McPherson, 2017, p.468).

○ The most common precipitating factor for PPHN is intrauterine asphyxia (Fraser, 2015, p. 458).

DIAGNOSIS

- PPHN is suspected based on the history and clinical course.
- Respiratory distress, cyanosis with a gradient of 10% or more, between pre- and post-ductal oxygen saturation is helpful in making diagnosis (Fraser, 2015, p. 459; Hansen & Levin, 2019, p. 433; Van Marter & McPherson, 2017, p. 470).

  ○ A hyperoxia test is one of the most helpful early screens to determine if cyanosis has a cardiac or a pulmonary origin. A right to left shunt is demonstrated if PaO_2 does not increase with 100% oxygen administration, indicating either PPHN or congenital heart disease (Fraser, 2015, p. 459).

- A single or narrowly split and accentuated second heart sound can be heard as well as a systolic murmur (Van Marter & McPherson, 2017, p. 470).
- EKG findings: normal right ventricular predominance, evidence of myocardial ischemia, or infarction (Van Marter & McPherson, 2017, p. 470).
- Laboratory studies should be done to evaluate metabolic abnormalities like hypoglycemia, hypocalcemia, and metabolic acidosis. Clotting studies may be abnormal secondary to end-organ damage from asphyxia.
- The chest x-ray usually appears normal but may reveal associated pulmonary disease (Fraser, 2015, p. 459; Hansen & Levin, 2019, p. 434; Van Marter & McPherson, 2017, p. 470).
- Echocardiogram findings include intracardiac or ductal shunting, tricuspid valve regurgitation, and flattened/bowing of ventricular septum. The echocardiogram assists in the diagnosis of congenital heart disease (Fraser, 2015, p. 459; Hansen & Levin, 2019, p. 434; Kinsella, 2017, pp. 354–355, 363; Van Marter & McPherson, 2017, p. 470; Weisz & McNamara, 2017, p. 126).

MANAGEMENT

- Intubation and mechanical ventilatory support are required to improve oxygenation while minimizing hyperoxia and hyperventilation. The main goal is to correct hypoxia and acidosis as well as to promote dilation of the pulmonary vascular bed (Fraser, 2015, p. 460; Hansen & Levin, 2019, p. 435; Van Marter & McPherson, 2017, pp. 471–472; Weisz & McNamara, 2017, p. 128).

  ○ HFV, high-frequency oscillatory ventilation (HFOV) or high-frequency jet ventilation (HFJV) may be required if conventional mechanical ventilation fails (Fraser, 2015, p. 460; Hansen & Levin, 2019, p. 435).

- Maintaining post-ductal oxygen saturations between 93% and 98% may help to promote adequate tissue oxygenation, avoid hypoxia-induced vasoconstriction, and minimize free radical release secondary to hyperoxia that may also worsen PPHN (Hansen & Levin, 2019, p. 435; Van Marter & McPherson, 2017, p. 471).

  ○ High oxygen (the most potent pulmonary vasodilator) concentrations may be required to reverse hypoxemia

and pulmonary vasoconstriction (Fraser, 2015, p. 460; Steinhorn, 2015, p. 1205).

- Arterial access assists in the monitoring of blood gases and blood pressure.

  ○ Hemodynamic support to maintain systemic blood pressure and improve cardiac output may be required.

    ▪ This may include the use of volume expanders: normal saline, and packed red cells in the face of anemia (Hansen & Levin, 2019, p. 436).

    ▪ Pharmacologic management includes the use of inotropic agents like dobutamine and milrinone, or the administration of vasopressors like dopamine, epinephrine, and or vasopressin (Barrington & Dempsey, 2017, p. 363; Fraser, 2015, p. 462; Hansen & Levin, 2019, p. 436; Van Marter & McPherson, 2017, p. 474).

    ▪ Correction of hypoglycemia and hypocalcemia promotes myocardial function and improves the response to inotropic drugs (Fraser, 2015, p. 460; Hansen & Levin, 2019, p. 435; Van Marter & McPherson, 2017, p. 474).

- Administration of iNO promotes smooth muscle relaxation and pulmonary vasodilation for term- and near-term infants with minimal to no impact on systemic arterial pressure. Nitric oxide is also a naturally occurring substance that is produced by pulmonary endothelial cells. It is a selective pulmonary vasodilator that decreases PVR and can be administered via the ventilator at 1 to 20 parts per million (ppm).

  ○ Methemoglobin is by-product of iNO therapy and should be monitored regularly (Fraser, 2015, pp. 460, 462; Hansen & Levin, 2019, p. 436; Keszler & Abubakar, 2017, p. 28; Kinsella, 2017, pp. 349, 363; Van Marter & McPherson, 2017, p. 472).

  ○ Ventilatory support as well as iNO should be weaned gradually to avoid rebound hypoxemia and PPHN (Van Marter & McPherson, 2017, p. 472).

- Infants who fail ventilatory management and or iNO therapy, may require ECMO. The calculation of the oxygen index (OI) helps to identify infants who might benefit from ECMO (Hansen & Levin, 2019, p. 436; Kinsella, 2017, p. 363; Van Marter & McPherson, 2017, p. 473).

  ○ The OI index is a measure of the severity of respiratory failure and can be calculated as follows: OI = mean airway pressure $(P_{aw}) \times FiO_2/PaO_2 \times 100$. Two OIs of greater than 40 within 1 hour, one OI of 60 on HFV, or one OI of 40 combined with cardiovascular instability are indicators of the need for ECMO (Clemmens & Piccione, 2017, p. 128; Wolf & Arnold, 2017, p. 491).

- Reduction in noise, minimal stimulation and handling may facilitate shunt reduction. Administration of sedatives and analgesics (fentanyl citrate or morphine sulfate) is also useful in minimizing agitation and shunting, if there is no systemic hypotension (Barrington & Dempsey, 2017, p. 363; Hansen & Levin, 2019, p. 436; Van Marter & McPherson, 2017, p. 473).

OUTCOMES

- Infants with PPHN are at a higher risk for negative neurodevelopmental, cognitive, and audiologic (sensorineural hearing loss) impairments. Survival is dependent on the center where care is delivered, and the underlying disease proves. The combined availability of iNO and ECMO has reduced PPHN mortality and the occurrence of CLD incidence in infants with hypoxemic respiratory failure (Fraser, 2015, p. 462; Hansen & Levin, 2019, p. 436; Van Marter & McPherson, 2017, p. 477).

Pulmonary Air Leak Syndromes

DEFINITION AND PATHOPHYSIOLOGY

- Pulmonary air leaks occur secondary to alveolar distention and rupture with a common etiology of high transpulmonary pressures that damages terminal airways and alveoli and allowing air to enter the interstitium resulting in pulmonary interstitial emphysema (PIE). If transpulmonary pressures remain high air may continue to dissect along the perivascular sheaths into the visceral pleura, the hilum and pericardium resulting in pneumothorax, pneumomediastinum, and pneumopericardium (Fraser, 2015, p. 469; Hansen & Levin, 2019, p. 439; Jensen et al., 2017, pp. 74–75; Markham, 2017, p. 482).

  - The primary risk factors contributing to air leak syndromes are mechanical ventilation and underlying lung disorders, which result in decreased compliance or obstruction with air trapping (Hansen & Levin, 2019, p. 432; Jensen et al., 2017, p. 74; Markham, 2017, p. 482). Air leaks can occur spontaneously if there is unequal air distribution at birth or iatrogenically from excessive use of airway pressure during resuscitation or with assisted ventilation (Fraser, 2015, p. 469).

DIAGNOSIS

- Clinical findings can range from subtle changes in vital signs to cardiovascular collapse if the air leak is large. Symptoms include sudden respiratory deterioration (tachypnea, grunting, flaring, retractions), cyanosis, oxygen desaturation, increased oxygen requirement, hypotension, bradycardia, chest asymmetry or a barrel-shaped chest, a shifted point of maximum impulse (PMI), and distant heart sounds (Fraser, 2015, p. 469; Hansen & Levin, 2019, p. 439; Markham, 2017, p. 483).

  - Other symptoms may result from air continuing to dissect into subcutaneous tissues producing subcutaneous emphysema, pulmonary emboli, as well as pneumoperitoneum (Fraser, 2015, p. 469; Hansen & Levin, 2019, p. 439; Markham, 2017, pp. 489–490).

  - Chest radiography remains the gold standard but may not be timely. Transillumination may be helpful in emergent situations but can be prone to false negative or positive results (Ehret, 2015, pp. 262–263; Fraser, 2015, p. 469; Hansen & Levin, 2019, pp. 440–441; Shepherd & Nevin, 2017, p. 63).

MANAGEMENT

- See Table 17.6 for management overview of air leak syndromes.

TABLE 17.6 Management Overview of Air Leak Syndromes

Air Leak Syndrome	Signs and Symptoms	Diagnosis	Management
Pulmonary Interstitial Emphysema (PIE)	Respiratory distress, hypotension, bradycardia, hypercarbia, hypoxia, and acidosis	Common in first 48 hours after birth. Linear cyst-like cysts lucencies on x-ray. Cysts can be large and bleb like	Decrease P_{aw}, PEEP, and inspiratory time. High-frequency ventilation may help reduce tidal volume [TV].
Pneumothorax	Respiratory distress may be severe, cyanosis, chest asymmetry, diminished/distant breath sounds, shift in point of maximum impulse, acute deterioration of vital signs, decreased cardiac output	Hypoxia, hypercarbia, acidosis. Transillumination positive for air on affected side. Hyperlucent hemithorax on x-ray and may see shift of mediastinal structures	Thoracentesis/needle aspiration, Thoracotomy/chest tube insertion, Insertion of pigtail catheter. Ventilatory management to reduce P_{aw}, PEEP, TV, high frequency ventilation may be strategy of choice
Pneumomediastinum	Heart sounds may be distant. Cardiopulmonary decompensation is rare.	Central air collections seen on x-ray and lifting of thymus from heart (sail sign) and may be more prominent in lateral view.	Strategies to reduce P_{aw}.
Pneumopericardium	Acute hemodynamic instability, with hypotension, decreased pulse pressure, bradycardia, and cyanosis with distant heart sounds	Muffled heart sounds, with air surrounding heart on x-ray. May be identified by transillumination	Needle aspiration if cardiac tamponade is present.

P_{aw}, mean airway pressure; PEEP, positive end expiratory pressure.

Sources: Data from Fraser, D. (2015). Respiratory distress. In M. T. Verklan & M. Walden (Eds.), *Core curriculum for neonatal intensive care nurses* (5th ed., pp. 447–477). St. Louis, MO: Elsevier; Hansen, A., & Levin, J. (2019). Neonatal pulmonary disorders. In B. K. Walsh (Ed.), *Neonatal and pediatric respiratory care* (5th ed., pp. 407–452). St. Louis, MO: Elsevier; Jensen, E. A., Mong, D. A., Biko, D. M., Maschhkoff, K. L., & Kirpalani, H. (2017). Imaging: Radiography, lung ultrasound, and other imaging modalities. In J. P. Goldsmith, E. H. Karotkin, M. Keszler, & G. K. Suresh (Eds.), *Assisted ventilation of the neonate* (6th ed., pp. 67–79). Philadelphia, PA: Elsevier; Keszler, M., & Chatburn, R. L. (2017). Oxygen therapy and respiratory support, overview of assisted ventilation. In J. P. Goldsmith, E. H. Karotkin, M. Keszler, & G. K. Suresh (Eds.), *Assisted ventilation of the neonate* (6th ed., pp. 140–152). Philadelphia, PA: Elsevier; Mammel, M. C., & Courtney, S. E. (2017). High frequency ventilation. In J. P. Goldsmith, E. H. Karotkin, M. Keszler, & G. K. Suresh (Eds.), *Assisted ventilation of the neonate* (6th ed., pp. 211–228). Philadelphia, PA: Elsevier; Markham, M. (2017). Pulmonary air leak. In E. Eichenwald, A. Hansen, C. Martin, & A. Stark (Eds.), *Cloherty & Stark's manual of neonatal care* (8th ed., pp. 482–490). Philadelphia, PA: Wolters Kluwer).

OUTCOMES

- Outcomes depend on the underlying pathology. There are high mortality rates with pneumoperitoneum, bilateral pneumothoraces, and bilateral PIE (Hansen & Levin, 2019, p. 443). The risk of CLD is high with bilateral PIE (Fraser, 2015, p. 470).

Chronic Lung Disease (CLD)

- Respiratory management improved with the onset of more advantageous approaches to ventilation in the 1960s. More preterm infants survived, but with severe chronic lung damage, which was first described as bronchopulmonary dysplasia or BPD (Bancalari & Walsh, 2015, p. 1157; Blackburn, 2013, p. 345; Fraser, 2015, p. 464; Hansen & Levin, 2019, p. 416).
  - The terms CLD and BPD are used interchangeably, and the current definition focuses on specific criteria which include the need for and duration of oxygen, or ventilatory support at specific post-menstrual ages. CLD can be classified as mild, moderate, or severe and the incidence is inversely proportional to gestational age and birthweight (Bancalari & Walsh, 2015, p. 1157; Blackburn, 2013, p. 345; Fraser, 2015, p. 464; Hansen & Levin, 2019, p. 416; Karotkin & Goldsmith, 2017, p. 1; Suresh & Raghavan, 2017, p. 54). Large and small airways, alveoli, and the pulmonary vascular bed are involved.
  - Pathogenesis is multifactorial and includes gestational age, birth weight, lung immaturity, arrested lung development, and acute lung injury from maternal chorioamnionitis; barotrauma, volutrauma, and lung injury secondary to mechanical ventilation. Inflammation, oxygen toxicity (hyperoxia), excessive early IV fluid administration, PDA, intrauterine/perinatal infection, IUGR,

decreased surfactant synthesis/function, nutritional deficits, and abnormal repair processes also play a role (Blackburn, 2013, pp. 339, 345–346; Fraser, 2015, pp. 464–465; Hansen & Levin, 2019, pp. 417–419; Parad & Benjamin, 2017, pp. 447–448; Suresh & Raghavan, 2017, p. 54).

DIAGNOSIS

- CLD is a disease of exclusion. Clinical presentation typically reveals tachypnea, retractions, and rales on auscultation and inability to wean from respiratory support. ABG analysis often reflects hypoxemia, hypercarbia, and respiratory acidosis (Fraser, 2015, p. 466; Parad & Benjamin, 2017, p. 449).
  - Chest radiographs are consistent with abnormal lung parenchyma (Ehert, 2015, pp. 259–260; Hansen & Levin, 2019, p. 419; Parad & Benjamin, 2017, pp. 447–448).
    - Initial presentation includes diffuse haziness, increased density, and low to normal lung volumes.
    - Chronic changes in more severe disease include regions of opacification and hyperlucency as well as superimposed air bronchograms (Parad & Benjamin, 2017, p. 449) and may also include hyperinflation, infiltrates, blebs, and cardiomegaly (Fraser, 2015, p. 466; Hansen & Levin, 2019, p. 419).
  - Fluid intolerance often occurs, despite no change in fluid intake, as evidenced by increased edema, weight, and decreased urine output (Fraser, 2015, p. 466; Hansen & Levin, 2019, p. 423).
  - Complications of CLD include intermittent bronchospasm, recurrent respiratory tract infections, GER, and developmental delays (Fraser, 2015, p. 466; Hansen & Levin, 2019, p. 424).
  - Table 17.7 includes a summarization of CLD/BPD diagnostic criteria.

TABLE 17.7 Summarization of CLD/BPD Diagnostic Criteria

Gestational Age	<32 weeks	≥32 weeks
Timing of assessment	36 weeks post-menstrual age (PMA) or discharge to home (whichever comes first)	> 28 postnatal days, but less than 56 postnatal days, or discharge to home (whichever comes first)
	Treatment with >21% oxygen for at least 28 days PLUS the following	
Mild BPD	Breathing 21% oxygen at 36 weeks PMA or at discharge (whichever comes first)	Breathing 21% oxygen at 56 postnatal days or discharge to home (whichever comes first)
Moderate BPD	Need for <30% oxygen at 36 weeks PMA or at discharge (whichever comes First)	Need for <30% oxygen at 56 postnatal days or at discharge to home (whichever comes first)
Severe BPD	Need for ≥30% oxygen or positive pressure ventilation (PPV) or nasal continuous pressure (NCPAP) at 36 weeks PMA or at discharge (whichever comes first)	Need for ≥30% oxygen or PPPV or NCPAP at 56 postnatal days or at Discharge to home (whichever comes first)

CLD, chronic lung disease; BPD, bronchopulmonary dysplasia.

Source: Reproduced with permission from Bancalari, E. H., & Walsh, M. C. (2015). Bronchopulmonary dysplasia. In R. Martin, A. A. Fanaroff, & M. C. Walsh (Eds.), *Fanaroff and Martin's neonatal-perinatal medicine diseases of the fetus and infant* (10th ed., pp.1157–1169). Philadelphia, PA: Saunders.

MANAGEMENT

- Aggressive enteral and parenteral nutritional helps to optimize growth and repair. Infants with CLD may require higher caloric intake (150–180 kcal/kg/day), as well as a higher protein, vitamin, and mineral intake. Fortification of human milk is recommended (Ditzenberger, 2015, p. 186; Fraser, 2015, p. 468; Hansen & Levin, 2019, p. 423).
- Evaluation for cor pulmonale and right ventricle hypertrophy using serial electrocardiography and echocardiography is imperative (Fraser, 2015, p. 468).
  - ○ Fluid restriction (130–140 mL/k/day), with reduction in salt intake can help reduce pulmonary edema and right-sided heart failure (Bancalari & Walsh, 2015, p. 1164; Fraser, 2015, p. 468; Hansen & Levin, 2019, p. 421; Parad & Benjamin, 2017, p. 452).
- Diuretics can be used to treat pulmonary edema (Fraser, 2015, p. 467; Parad & Benjamin, 2017, p. 452) and include furosemide, spironolactone, chlorothiazide, hydrochlorothiazide, and hydrochlorothiazide with spironolactone (Fraser & Diehl-Jones, 2015, p. 507; Hansen & Levin, 2019, p. 424).
  - ○ If diuretics are used, serum electrolytes should be monitored for hyponatremia, hypokalemia, resultant hypochloremia, and metabolic alkalosis, which may impair growth. Supplementation of electrolytes may be needed (Fraser, 2015, p. 467; Fraser & Diehl-Jones, p. 507; Hansen & Levin, 2019, p. 424; Parad & Benjamin, 2017, pp. 452–453).
  - ○ Long-term use of furosemide is associated with hypercalciuria, bone demineralization, nephrolithiasis, and ototoxicity (Fraser, 2015, p. 467; Fraser & Diehl-Jones, 2015; p. 507; Hansen & Levin, 2019, p. 424; Parad & Benjamin, 2017, p. 453).
- Administration of bronchodilators assists in the reduction of bronchospasm and resistance to airflow related to smooth muscle hypertrophy commonly seen in CLD (Blackburn, 2013, p. 347; Hansen & Levin, 2019, p. 424).
- Caffeine citrate promotes airway bronchodilation and has a mild diuretic effect and has both a lung protective and brain-protective effect (Blackburn, 2013, p. 340; Fraser, 2015, p. 467; Fraser & Diehl-Jones, 2015, p. 506; Hansen & Levin, 2019, pp. 421, 424; Parad & Benjamin, 2017, pp. 449–450).
- Postnatal corticosteroid therapy reduces inflammation, improves lung function and facilitates weaning from the ventilator (Bancalari & Walsh, 2015, p. 1165; Blackburn, 2013, p. 347; Fraser, 2015, p. 468; Hansen & Levin, 2019, pp. 420–421; Parad & Benjamin, 2017, pp. 453–454).
  - ○ The administration of corticosteroids postnatally has not been found to have a substantial impact on long-term respiratory outcomes and is controversial because of the potential for adverse neurologic outcomes with prolonged therapy (Blackburn, 2013, p. 347; Fraser, 2015, p. 468; Fraser & Diehl-Jones, 2015, p. 507).
- Blood transfusions of PRBCs to maintain a hematocrit of 30% to 35% while still on supplemental oxygen or if ventilator support is helpful (Parad & Benjamin, 2017, p. 455).
- RSV prophylaxis is recommended (Fraser, 2015, p. 468; Hansen & Levin, 2019, p. 424).

OUTCOMES

- Overall mortality is low. Highest mortality occurs in cases of severe CLD (Bancalari & Walsh, 2015, p. 1166; Fraser, 2015, pp. 468–469; Parad & Benjamin, 2017, p. 459).

- Infants with CLD have a higher rate of readmission in the first year of life secondary to lower respiratory tract infections and reactive airway disease. CLD survivors have a higher incidence of wheezing episodes in the first 2 years of life that may require hospitalization (Bancalari & Walsh, 2015, p. 1165; Hansen & Levin, 2019, p. 424).
  - ○ Pulmonary function may be reduced and may remain abnormal into adulthood (Bancalari & Walsh, 2015, p. 1165; Fraser, 2015, p. 469).
  - ○ Cor pulmonale and pulmonary hypertension can develop secondary to severe hypoxemia and can result in respiratory failure and death (Bancalari & Walsh, 2015, p. 1165; Fraser, 2015, p. 468; Hansen & Levin, 2019, p. 425).
- Higher rates of neurological delays or deficits are seen with severe CLD. Cerebral palsy is more common, as well as sensorineural hearing loss and visual difficulties (Fraser, 2015, p. 469; Hansen & Levin, 2019, p. 425; Parad & Benjamin, 2017, p. 459).

APNEA

DEFINITION AND PATHOPHYSIOLOGY

- Apnea is defined as the cessation of breathing for 20 seconds, or less, if there is evidence of corresponding desaturations with pallor or cyanosis, bradycardia, and hypotonia (Goodwin, 2015, p. 478; Guarda & Martin, 2018).
  - ○ Periodic breathing (recurrent sequences of pauses lasting 5–10 seconds follow by 10–15 seconds of rapid respiration is considered normal in preterm and early term infants. Periodic breathing is not accompanied by cyanosis or heart rate changes; Goodwin, 2015, p. 478).
  - ○ Respiratory pauses may be caused by immature peripheral chemoreceptors unable to respond to changes in $PaCO_2$ via increased respirations. The resulting acidosis may be responsible for apnea episodes. Central chemoreceptors are found throughout the brainstem (Patrinos, 2015, p. 1138).
  - ○ Apnea in premature infants may be the result of neural immaturity and disorganization of neurotransmitters gamma-aminobutyric acid (GABA), and adenosine. Brain stem immaturity contributes to the lack of respiratory drive (Patrinos, 2015, p. 1139).

DIAGNOSIS

- Apnea is classified into three categories based on the presence or absence of upper airway obstruction (Gauda & Martin, 2018, pp. 613–614):
  - ○ Central apnea: respiratory efforts cease without evidence of obstruction.
  - ○ Obstructive apnea: breathing motions without effect due to a blocked airway
  - ○ Mixed apnea: upper airway obstruction combined with central cession of respiratory efforts. Fifty to sixty percent of apnea episodes are obstructive in origin (Goodwin, 2015, p. 480).
- Non-respiratory issues, such as systemic infections, metabolic disorders, or environmental factors such as hypothermia, may present with apnea (Gauda & Martin, 2018, p. 614).

MANAGEMENT

- All infants less than 35 weeks should be monitored for apnea and should include the use of cardiorespiratory monitors and pulse oximetry. Apnea monitors alone may not differentiate breathing efforts through an obstructed airway from normal breathing patterns; therefore, heart rate should be monitored in addition to respiration (Stark, 2015, p. 428).
- Positioning: Maintain the neck in a neutral position, use a neck roll for support as needed. Prone positioning may help decrease frequent obstructive apnea events related to impaired airway protective mechanisms (e.g., micrognathia; Goodwin, 2015, p. 483).
- Respiratory support as required.
  - ○ Adaptive backup ventilation for apnea is available using invasive or noninvasive means. If the infant is apneic or becomes hypoxic, the modality provides a preset mandatory breathing rate. Early studies show these modalities can better match the varying ventilatory needs of preterm or ill infants than conventional mandatory ventilation (Claure & Bancalari, 2018, p. 208).
  - ○ CPAP may splint upper airway and prevent obstruction (Stark, 2017, p. 430). CPAP increases end-expiratory lung volumes and splints the upper airway and compliant chest wall (Goodwin, 2015, p. 483).
- Methylxanthines stimulate the central respiratory chemoreceptors and increase ventilatory response to CO_2 through the antagonism of the neurotransmitter adenosine. Methylxanthine therapy also increases the respiratory drive and thereby reduces the number of periodic breathing events (Goodwin, 2015, pp. 483–484; Stark, 2017, p. 430).
- Apnea generally resolves by 36 to 40 weeks' postconceptional age (PCA); however, for extremely preterm infants, events may extend until 43 to 44 weeks (Gauda & Martin, 2018, p. 616).
  - ○ Home cardiorespiratory monitoring may be an option for infants with a history of apnea events who are discharged prior to 44 weeks' PCA to avoid prolonged hospital stays (Gauda & Martin, 2018, p. 616).
  - ○ Indications for home monitoring include: Premature infants with idiopathic apnea who are otherwise ready for discharge, a history of a sibling death from Sudden Infant Death Syndrome (SIDS), a sleep apnea syndrome secondary to a neurologic condition, or other conditions attributable to of a high-risk infants (Goodwin, 2015, p. 485).
    - ■ Home monitoring is not intended as a SIDS prevention in symptom-free, healthy infants. (Goodwin, 2015, p. 484).
    - ■ Over time, an absence of a clear relationship between apnea and SIDS has reduced the practice of home monitoring without a subsequent increase in the incidence of SIDS (Gauda & Martin, 2018, p. 616).
  - ○ In 80% of infants, home monitoring may be discontinued at 45 weeks' PCA (Goodwin, 2015, p. 486).

Infants discharged from a NICU often experience multiple comorbidities which complicates an analysis to determine a relationship between apnea. However, data have demonstrated a correlation between a high number of cardiorespiratory events and less favorable neurodevelopmental, especially longer (>60 seconds) events or events which require significant intervention (Gauda & Martin, 2015, p. 616).

Additional Causes of Respiratory Distress

- See Table 17.8 for summary of other disorders that contribute to respiratory distress in the neonate.

TABLE 17.8 Summary of Other Disorders That Contribute to Respiratory Distress in the Neonate

Disorder	Etiology	Diagnosis	Management	Outcomes
Heart disease (congenital)	Overall incidence is 0.6% to 0.8% and 25% of congenital defects may be critical CHD lesions. The most common lesions appear in first weeks of life and may be associated with other disorders or syndromes	Cyanosis, respiratory distress, tachypnea, murmur, CHF, difference in upper and lower extremities Hyperoxia test, Echocardiogram EKG	Respiratory support as needed. Stabilization and transport if intervention is required. Administration of prostaglandins may be required to support patency of fetal channels	Is lesion dependent
Choanalatresia	Bony abnormality causing obstruction to flow. Unilateral/bilateral Bilateral is the most common cause of complete nasal obstruction. Can be associated with other anomalies (CHARGE)	Cyanosis, respiratory distress, asphyxia. Obligate nose breathers, so minimal to no oral air intake. Symptoms may worsen with sucking. If bilateral, symptom improvement seen with crying. Failure to pass small caliber tube may be diagnostic	Bilateral and severe will require immediate repair Unilateral repair can be postponed Intubation may be required. Respiratory support as needed	Good post-surgery May need successive dilations. Tracheostomy may be needed with other associated anomalies (CHARGE)

(continued)

TABLE 17.8 Summary of Other Disorders That Contribute to Respiratory Distress in the Neonate *(cont.)*

Disorder	Etiology	Diagnosis	Management	Outcomes
Laryngomalacia	Obstructive disorder caused by flaccid larynx Common cause of neonatal stridor. Supraglottic structures collapse into laryngeal inlet during inspiration	Wheezing a stridor, with or without respiratory distress. Presence of cough or weak cry. Diagnosed via direct laryngoscopy or rigid bronchoscopy	Surgical repair only in most severe cases Prone positioning supports airway	Tracheostomy may be required in severe cases
Tracheomalacia	Airway obstruction caused by the collapse of the trachea during expiration May develop from compression of adjacent structures as with esophageal atresia, tracheo-esophageal fistula, aberrant innominate artery, vascular rings, mediastinal masses, connective tissue disorders, or prolonged mechanical ventilation	Expiratory stridor Diagnosed by bronchoscopy. May be associated with respiratory distress.	Humidification of airway to thin secretions. If severe may require tracheostomy. Respiratory support as required.	Spontaneously resolves by 6 to 12 months.
Micrognathia	Mandibular hypoplasia and can be associated with Pierre Robin Sequence	Severe respiratory distress, airway obstruction and feeding difficulties	Prone positioning, use of oral airway and if severe immediate surgical intervention. Tracheostomy may be required	If not severe, symptoms improve with normal growth
Anemia	Hematocrit (Hct) more than 1 to 2 standard deviations below mean for age. Accelerated loss/destruction of RBCs, defects in production. Decreased oxygenation and tissue perfusion	Cyanosis, pallor, tachycardia, tachypnea, apnea, respiratory distress, jaundice	Follow reticulocyte counts. Avoid hypoxia Transfuse with PRBCs if symptomatic Infants on oxygen/respiratory support may need Follow CBC and Hct for those at risk. Transfusion sooner	CHF if anemia is severe or chronic, failure to grow
Polycythemia	Venous hematocrit >65% leading to hyperviscosity. Risk factors include IUGR, SGA, LGA, IDM, and postdates, delayed cord clamping, cord stripping, maternal-fetal transfusion, twin-twin transfusion, sepsis, dehydration	Cyanosis, respiratory distress, tachypnea, heart murmur, cardiomegaly, increased PVR, renal vein thrombosis, jaundice, DIC, hypoglycemia, hypocalcemia, thrombosis, NEC, low platelets, lethargy, poor feeding, apnea, seizures. Infants are ruddy/plethoric Prominent vascular markings on x-ray. If capillary hematocrit is >65, draw central sample	Exclude other reasons for symptoms. Partial exchange transfusion. If asymptomatic, increase fluid intake and follow hematocrit	Higher risk of PPHN

(continued)

TABLE 17.8 Summary of Other Disorders That Contribute to Respiratory Distress in the Neonate *(cont.)*

Disorder	Etiology	Diagnosis	Management	Outcomes
Cystic hygroma	Most commonly seen neck mass due to development of cyst secondary to sequestrated lymph channels	Supraclavicular mass of varying size that transilluminates. Varying degrees of respiratory distress with compression of airway. Diagnosis confirmed by US, MRI/CT	Prenatal evaluation of mass size and growth. May require urgent C/S to protect airway. Needle aspiration for rapid decompression. Surgical excision is treatment of choice. Respiratory support as required	If small may spontaneously regress. If respiratory distress is severe may require tracheostomy
Diaphragmatic eventration	Congenital: Thinned or absent musculature Acquired: Phrenic nerve injury from birth trauma or cardiothoracic surgery	Doming of diaphragm, symptoms vary from mild to severe respiratory distress. Diagnosis confirmed by US or fluoroscopy—paradoxical movement of affected side	Surgical diaphragm plication or resection and repair in symptomatic congenital cases. Supportive care in acquired disorder to evaluate return of function. Respiratory support as required	In phrenic nerve damage, nerve function may return over 6 months to one year. Surgical repair is indicated if it does not

CBC, complete blood count; DIC, disseminated intra-vascular coagulopathy; IDM, infant of diabetic mother; IUGR, intrauterine growth restriction; LGA, large for gestational age; NEC, necrotizing enterocolitis; PPHN, persistent pulmonary hypertension of the newborn; PRBC, packed red blood cell; PVR, pulmonary vascular resistance; SGA, small for gestational age.

Sources: Data from Bennett, M., & Meier, S. R. (2019). Assessment of the dysmorphic infant. In E. P. Tappero & M. Honeyfield (Eds.), *Physical assessment of the newborn* (6th ed., pp. 219–237). New York NY: Springer Publishing Company; Breinholt, J. P. G. (2017). Cardiac disorders. In E. C. Eichenwald, A. R. Hansen, C. R. Martin, & A. R. Stark (Eds.), *Cloherty and Stark's manual of neonatal care* (8th ed., pp. 510–575). Philadelphia, PA: Wolters Kluwer; Diab, Y., & Luchtman-Jones, L. (2015). Hematologic and oncologic problems in the fetus and neonate. In R. J. Martin, A. A. Fanaroff, M. C. Walsh (Eds.), *Fanaroff and Martin's neonatal-perinatal medicine diseases of the fetus and infant* (10th ed., pp. 1295–1341). Philadelphia, PA: Saunders; Lissauer, T. (2015). Physical examination of the newborn. In R. J. Martin, A. A. Fanaroff, & M. C. Walsh (Eds.), *Fanaroff and Martin's neonatal-perinatal medicine diseases of the fetus and infant* (10th ed., pp. 391–406). Philadelphia, PA: Saunders; Madenci, A. L., Rice-Townsend, S. E., & Weldon, C. B. (2019). Surgical disorders in childhood that affect respiratory care. In B. K. Walsh (Ed.), *Neonatal and pediatric respiratory care* (5th ed., pp. 453–468). St. Louis, MO: Elsevier; O'Reilly, D. (2017). Polycythemia. In E. C. Eichenwald, A. R. Hansen, C. R. Martin, & A. R. Stark (Eds.), *Cloherty and Stark's manual of neonatal care* (8th ed., pp. 624–629). Philadelphia, PA: Wolters Kluwer; Otteson, T. D., & Arnold, J. E. (2015). Upper airway lesions in the neonate. In R. J. Martin, A. A. Fanaroff, & M. C. Walsh (Eds.), *Fanaroff and Martin's neonatal-perinatal medicine diseases of the fetus and infant* (10th ed., pp. 1147–1156). Philadelphia, PA: Saunders; Parikh, A. S., & Mitchell, A. L. (2017). Congenital anomalies. In R. J. Martin, A. A. Fanaroff, & M. C. Walsh (Eds.), *Fanaroff and Martin's neonatal-perinatal medicine diseases of the fetus and infant* (10th ed., pp. 436–457). Philadelphia, PA: Saunders; Patrinos, M. E. (2017). Neonatal apnea and the foundation of respiratory control. In R. J. Martin, A. A. Fanaroff, & M. C. Walsh (Eds.), *Fanaroff and Martin's neonatal-perinatal medicine diseases of the fetus and infant* (10th ed., pp. 1137–1146). Philadelphia, PA: Saunders.

NEONATAL RESPIRATORY MECHANICS AND RESPIRATORY SUPPORT

Oxygen Physiology

- At sea level, maternal hemoglobin is 96% oxygenated at 100 mmHg. Fetal tissues are ~80% oxygenated with a PaO_2 of 30 to 40 mmHg and fully oxygenated at 50 to 60 mmHg. This illustrates why oxygen supplementation can be detrimental to the tissues of preterm infants (Meschia, 2019, p. 212).
- The gradient of higher maternal oxygen level diffuses through the placenta to the hypoxic fetus. In utero, fetal hemoglobin has a greater binding capacity to attract oxygen molecules.
  - Increasing the maternal oxygen level does not significantly increase the fetal PO_2 (Meschia, 2019, p. 218). The fetus responds to variability in oxygen levels by changes in cardiac output (Meschia, 2019, p. 213).
  - Placental insufficiency decreases oxygen availability to the fetus diminishing growth resulting in intrauterine growth restriction (Greenberg, Narendran, Schibler, Warner, & Haberman, 2019, p. 1310).
- The neonate transitions over the first 3 to 6 months of life to the production of adult hemoglobin (HgA) with increased

2,3-diphosphoglycerate (DPG) production. The transition from HgF to HgA is associated with reduced oxygen affinity and rightward shift of the oxyhemoglobin dissociation curve (Rabi, Kowal, & Ambalavanan, 2018, p. 80).
  - The oxyhemoglobin dissociation curve demonstrates oxygen saturation (SO_2) and the partial pressure of oxygen (PO_2). Never static, the curve shifts to the left for well-saturated hemoglobin or to the right with less saturated hemoglobin (Meschia, 2019, p. 213).
  - The Bohr effect describes the changes in oxygenation and blood pH depending upon acidity, shifting the curve to the right with lower pH and/or hypercarbia.

Oxygen Toxicity

- Oxygen (O_2) is probably the most widely used drug in neonatology. Oxidative processes provide most of the adenosine triphosphate (ATP) needed by the body, especially for aerobic-dependent tissues known as oxyregulators, such as the brain, which cannot adapt to absence of oxygen (Vento, 2019, p. 153).
- Reactive oxygen species (ROS) are a series of molecules derived from incomplete reduction of molecular oxygen). A small percentage of electrons "leak," leaving the oxygen molecule only partly reduced. ROS can be extremely

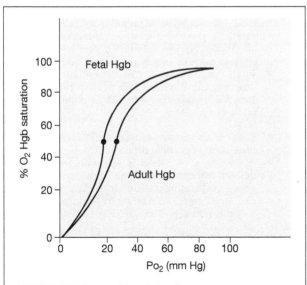

FIGURE 17.1 Oxygen Dissociation Curve

Source: Reproduced with permission from Bradshaw, W., & Tanaka. (2016). Physiologic monitoring. In S. Gardner, B. Carter, M. Hines, & J. Hernandez (Eds.), *Merenstein & Gardner's handbook of neonatal intensive care* (8th ed., pp. 126–144.e1). St. Louis, MO: Elsevier.

aggressive free radicals and can cause direct structural and/or functional damage to the body (Vento, 2019, p. 154).
  ○ The term *free radical* refers to the molecule that has escaped from the partial reduction of oxygen. Free radicals easily decompose and lead to the formation of toxic products. These products may cause damage to DNA (deoxyribonucleic acid), proteins, and lipids. Under very stressful conditions (ischemia–reperfusion, inflammation, or hyperoxia) damage caused by free radicals can lead to marked cellular dysfunction and/or cell death by necrosis or apoptosis (Vento, 2019, p. 154).
• Several examples of oxygen overuse are present in the history neonatology:
  ○ Retinopathy of prematurity: In early neonatology, oxygen was used liberally in the treatment of preterm infants with respiratory distress. This unrestricted use of oxygen resulted in a devastating eye disease, retrolental fibroplasia (RLF) or ROP. ROP occurs when the eye vessels thicken and become tortuous to the point the retina detaches with a corresponding loss of sight. Based on this discovery, oxygen use was then curtailed; however, subsequent restriction of oxygen use resulted in hypoxic states and increased respiratory failure (Vento, 2017, p. 153).
  ○ Chronic Lung Disease (CLD): High oxygen levels result in the formation of ROS and free radicals which in turn cause tissue injury and changes in lung function and the distribution of gas. These changes are a primary contributor to the development of CLD (Walsh, 2019, p. 152; Walsh & Chatburn, 2019, p. 328).

ALGORITHMS FOR OXYGEN USE
• Judicious oxygen delivery maximizes the benefits of oxygen while minimizing potential morbidities. Evidence-based oxygen use algorithms help to minimize the toxic effects of oxygen administration particularly in the very low birth weight group of infants or infants <1,500 g (Walsh, 2019, p. 152).

Fetal and Neonatal Pulmonary Mechanics
• Cord clamping initiates air breathing and lung filling for the establishment of FRC. In the newborn, the FRC is only slightly above closing volume.
• With lung expansion, surfactant is released which helps maintain FRC by homogeneously decreasing surface tension and creating a pressure gradient for lung fluid removal through the alveoli.
• In premature infants, lack of surfactant results in alveolar collapse and atelectasis causing a diminished FRC. The FRC can also be affected by disease states such as MAS, which plugs the airways resulting in air trapping and a high FRC.
• Diaphragmatic activity controls breathing while accessory muscles stabilize the chest wall. A premature infant has a more compliant chest wall, decreased intercostal muscle tone, and therefore is more prone to a concave rib cage during breathing (Keszler & Chatburn, 2017, p. 140).
  ○ Exhaustion of these muscles can lead to respiratory failure in a compromised infant (Keszler & Chatburn, 2017, p. 140).
• The neonatal chest is more cylindrical compared to the elliptical shape of the adult. Neonatal ribs have a more horizontal orientation resulting in a relative shortening of the intercostal muscles. The compliant neonatal chest wall, in combination with non-compliant lungs, fewer interalveolar communications, less alveoli and minimal surfactant production, can lead to chest wall collapse on expiration and atelectasis. This results in an increase in the WOB (intercostal/subcostal retractions) and exaggerated abdominal breathing (Keszler & Abubakar, 2017, pp. 10–11).

Respiratory Support in the Neonate

DEFINITIONS
• Oxygenation: The partial pressure of oxygen (PaO_2) within the arterial blood reflects the exchange of oxygen. Factors that impact oxygenation include percentage of oxygen delivered and mechanical mean airway pressure (Donn & Sinha, 2015, p. 1090).
• Ventilation: Ventilation refers to the removal of CO_2. Infant generated breaths contribute to CO_2 removal and pulmonary blood flow can also impact CO_2 removal.
  ○ In conventional ventilation strategies, carbon dioxide removal is most affected by tidal volume (amplitude of the breath defined by PIP minus PEEP) and frequency.
  ○ In HFV, strategies, carbon dioxide removal is a product of frequency and the square of the tidal volume (amplitude). (Donn & Sinha, 2015, p. 1100).
• PIP: the peak pressure at which each breath is delivered. It is measured in cm of H_2O (Donn & Sinha, 2015, pp. 1090–1091).
• PEEP: the amount of airway pressure in the lung at the end of expiration and is measured in cm of H_2O. It promotes and improves FRC. Lack of PEEP results in alveolar collapse, and high PEEP can result in barotrauma (Donn & Sinha, 2015, pp. 1090–1091).
• Mean airway pressure (P_{aw}) the average pressure applied to the lungs during the respiratory cycle. Mean airway pressure is affected by PEEP, PIP, inspiratory time, frequency,

and gas flow. Excessive $P_{\overline{aw}}$ can contribute to barotrauma and lung damage (Donn & Sinha, 2015, p. 1091).

- Rate or frequency of the ventilator in combination with tidal volume influences the exchange of carbon dioxide during ventilation. Tidal volume has a higher impact on minute ventilation than the rate delivered (Donn & Sinha, p. 1091).
- Inspiratory time (T_I) refers to the length of time of the inspiratory phase of the breath and as inspiratory time increases, mean airway pressure also increases (Donn & Sinha, 2015, pp. 1090–1091).
- Expiratory time (T_e) the length of time of the expiratory phase of the breath. If expiratory time is shortened, it can also contribute to an increase in mean airway pressure. Increases in expiratory time may facilitate carbon dioxide removal. Very prolonged expiratory times can result in gas/air trapping (Donn & Sinha, 2015, p. 1091).
- Tidal volume (TV or V_T): Tidal volume is the amplitude of a mechanical breath and is determined by the difference between the PIP and the PEEP. Normal neonatal tidal volumes vary but normal can be considered to be between 4 and 6 mL/kg (Donn & Sinha, 2015, p. 1091).

Assisted Ventilation

- An infant's overall history and clinical condition dictate the mode of ventilation to be used. There are many types of ventilators and respiratory support devices available. Device selection will be practitioner and institution dependent (Donn & Sinha, 2015, p. 109).

NON-INVASIVE RESPIRATORY SUPPORT—PURPOSE

- Noninvasive respiratory support provides continuous distending pressure and causes less injury to the lungs than mechanical ventilation. It is used in patients with a sustainable respiratory drive and is considered an appropriate therapy in preterm infants <29 weeks' gestation. It is most often used for oxygen requirements of 40% to 50% (Diblasi & Courtney, 2017, p. 162).
- It maintains FRC and stabilizes the chest wall through supporting better lung compliance and aids in decreasing WOB and promotes improved oxygenation. Close monitoring is necessary as it can cause abdominal distention (Diblasi & Courtney, 2017, pp. 164–165).

Non-Invasive Respiratory Support—Devices

- Nasal continuous positive airway pressure (NCPAP)
  - Heated humidified gas is delivered via short nasal prongs or nasal masks to the infant's airway at varying pressures measured in cm of H_2O pressure.
  - It can be delivered via a ventilator, a stand-alone NCPAP device, or through a "bubble" CPAP system (Donn & Sinha, 2015, p. 1088).
- High-flow nasal cannula (HFNC)
  - HFNC delivers blended heated and humidified oxygen generally at flows >1 L/min.
  - Pressure generated by HFNC may be variable and dependent on cannula size and air entrainment secondary to the leak around the cannula. This can result in both low and high distending pressures
  - It may be delivered by a standard nasal cannula. Commercial devices are also available (Donn & Sinha, 2015, p. 1089).

- Noninvasive nasal ventilation
  - Methods of noninvasive ventilation include: Nasal intermittent positive pressure ventilation (NIPPV), synchronized NIPPV (SNIPPV), and synchronized inspiratory positive airway pressure (SiPAP)
    - In all three of these methods, ventilator "breaths" augment CPAP while PEEP, peak inspiratory pressure (PIP), respiratory rate, and inspiratory time can all be manipulated.
    - SiPAP
    - SiPAP is also known as bilevel CPAP of BiPAP and is delivered by a flow driver device.
    - A baseline CPAP level is set, with the ability to deliver mandatory or "sigh" breaths set slightly above the baseline pressure level. The frequency of the "sigh" breaths can be set by setting of a respiratory rate (Donn & Sinha, 2015, p. 1089).

Invasive Mechanical Ventilation

- Indications for the use of invasive respiratory support include apnea, increased WOB (retractions, nasal flaring, tachypnea, and grunting), hypercapnia, hypoxia, inadequate respiratory effort, and overall worsening of clinical condition (falling blood pressure, respiratory failure, and bradycardia).

CONVENTIONAL METHODS OF VENTILATION

- Intermittent mandatory ventilation (IMV): Scheduled ventilator breaths. Scheduled breaths may interfere with an infant's own spontaneous breathing which can be detrimental to the infant (Keszler & Mammel, 2017, p. 180).
- Synchronized intermittent mandatory ventilation (SIMV): Ventilator breaths are scheduled but are triggered by the infant's respiratory efforts. Breaths are triggered in the presence of apnea and breaths beyond the preset number of scheduled breaths are not supported (Keszler & Mammel, 2017, pp. 182–183).
- Assist control (AC): Every breath that the infant initiates triggers a ventilator breath with a preset number of assisted breaths (Keszler & Mammel, 2017, pp. 183–184).
- Pressure support ventilation (PS): Inspiration is controlled by a preset peak pressure, with a variable V_T dependent on lung compliance and resistance (Keszler & Mammel, 2017, pp. 184–186).
- Volume-controlled ventilation (VC): Preset V_T is delivered with each breath which changes depending on lung compliance (Keszler & Morley, 2017, pp. 195–197).
- Volume guarantee (VG): A targeted V_T and peak pressure are predetermined which is automatically adjusted according to lung compliance and the infant's breathing patterns (Keszler & Morley, 2017, pp. 197–199).
- Neurally adjusted ventilator assist or NAVA ventilation recognizes diaphragmatic activity through the use a nasogastric catheter. Inflation is patient triggered by signals from the diaphragm (Diblasi & Courtney, 2017, pp. 173–174).

HIGH FREQUENCY VENTILATION

- There are three main types of high frequency ventilation (HFV): High-frequency oscillator ventilation, HFJV, and high-frequency flow interruption. All use a ventilation mode at very high rates and small tidal volumes. Currently, there are not clear randomized controlled trials, demonstrating the advantage of one form of ventilation or another (conventional mechanical ventilation [CMV] or high frequency ventilation [HFV]). User bias and level of experience often influence the choice of ventilation (Mammel & Courtney, 2017, p. 211).

○ HFOV: During HFOV, inspiration and expiration are both active through the actions of an electromagnetically operated piston which generates the oscillations. The amplitude of the oscillations within the airway determines the VTs delivered to the lungs around a constant mean airway pressure. Often used when conventional modes of ventilation fail or for use with specific diseases such as MAS or PPHN (Mammel & Courtney, 2017, p. 214).

○ High-frequency jet ventilation (HFJV): Delivers a direct pulse of pressurized gas into the endotracheal tube and the upper airway through a narrow-bore cannula or jet injector. Exhalation during HFJV is a result of passive lung recoil. It is used for air-leak and air-trapping disorders although has more widespread use for RDS depending on user experience. With HFJV, CO_2 removal can be achieved at lower peak and mean airway pressures than with either HFV or HFOV (Mammel & Courtney, 2017, p. 213).

○ High-frequency flow interruptions (HFFI): The term *flow interrupter* originally was used to describe a group of ventilators that were neither true oscillators nor true jets. HFFI ventilation has experienced a modest resurgence in the form of The Bronchotron®, a popular transport ventilator. The high-frequency gas pulses enter a piston mechanism and create pulses of gas flow by the rapid movement of a spring mechanism that balances inspiratory and expiratory pressures (Mammel & Courtney, 2017, pp. 214–215).

Inhaled Nitric Oxide

● Inhaled nitric oxide (iNO) is a potent vasodilator derived from the amino acid L-arginine. iNO binds to hemoglobin when diffused throughout the lungs. It increases oxygenation and improves pulmonary perfusion and reduces lung inflammation.

○ It is used in the treatment of respiratory failure, pulmonary hypertension and may reduce the need for extracorporeal membrane oxygenation (Kinsella, 2017, p. 349).

Extracorporeal Membrane Oxygenation (ECMO)

● ECMO is the application of a modified cardiopulmonary bypass for infants in respiratory or cardiac failure that have not responded to conventional management strategies (Wolf & Arnold, 2017, p. 491).

● Respiratory indications for use of ECMO include respiratory failure, severe air leak syndromes, MAS, PPHN, CDH, pneumonia, and RDS (Arensman, Short, and Stephens, 2017, p. 437; Wolf & Arnold, 2017, pp. 491–493).

○ Venoarterial (VA) ECMO supports the cardiac and respiratory system and is used for primary cardiac failure or respiratory failure combined with secondary cardiac failure. Blood is drained from a single vein (internal jugular, femoral) and returned to the arterial system usually via the internal carotid artery (Wolf & Arnold, 2017, pp. 493–494).

○ Venovenous (VV) ECMO supports only the respiratory system and is intended for the use is isolated respiratory therapy. It refers to drainage from a single vein (Wolf & Arnold, 2017, p. 493–494).

Respiratory Support Monitoring

PULSE OXIMETRY

● A light source (red and infrared) is transmitted to a light receiver. Hemoglobin absorbs the infrared light and deoxyhemoglobin absorbs the red light. The ratio is calculated as a percent of oxygen saturation. The percent of oxygen displayed by pulse oximetry does not equal PaO_2 (partial pressure of oxygen). Pulse oximetry is used as an oxygen monitoring tool to limit the number of blood gasses required and provide continuous observation. It measures the oxygen saturation in hemoglobin.

● Pulse oximetry has many applications: CHD screening, pre- and post-ductal monitoring for PPHN (persistent pulmonary hypertension), a transition monitor in the delivery room, car seat testing in preparation of discharge, and as a continuous screening tool for neonates.

● Disadvantages include the inability to detect changes in carbon dioxide. Also, movement, incorrect application of probe, and poor perfusion can affect pulse oximetry function (Rabi et al., 2017, pp. 89–90).

BLOOD GAS ANALYSIS

● Blood gas analysis can be performed from arterial, venous, or capillary blood samples, and can assist in the evaluation of intrapulmonary shunting, the severity/progression of disease, and the response to respiratory support therapy (Walsh, 2019, p. 119).

TRANSCUTANEOUS MONITORING

● A sensor with a built-in heating element that is applied to the skin can assist in the evaluation of the partial pressure of oxygen ($P_{TC}O_2$) and the carbon dioxide tension ($P_{TC}CO_2$).

○ Heating of the skin increases capillary blood flow with a subsequent increase in permeability to gas diffusion. Although changes in perfusion can negatively impact measurement accuracy (Smallwood, pp. 142–143).

CAPNOGRAPHY

● Capnography is a noninvasive method to evaluate exhaled carbon dioxide, using an airway adaptor or a specialized nasal cannula. This monitoring method also includes a monitoring device to measure the inhaled partial pressure of CO_2 and the total volume of exhaled CO_2 per unit of time (Smallwood, 2019, pp. 139–140).

● During mechanical ventilation it provides information about ventilation. It can assist in the confirmation of intubation, and the response to changes in respiratory support therapy.

○ End-tidal CO_2 refers to the partial pressure of CO_2 and the end of an exhalation (PetCO$_2$). Evaluation of PetCO$_2$ trends can assist in the evaluation of adequate ventilation (Smallwood, 2019, pp. 139–140).

BEDSIDE PULMONARY MECHANICS EVALUATION

● Modern mechanical ventilators are equipped to measure and display airway graphics of pressure, flow, and volume. The graphics are displayed on the ventilator screen and can assist the provider in the evaluation of the inter-action between the ventilator and the patient. They can be used to maximize ventilatory support and minimize com-plications (Hynes & Mottram, 2019, p. 66).

Respiratory Support at Discharge

- Infants may meet the basic criteria for discharge home (adequate weight gain, competent caretakers, appropri-ate outpatient follow-up, free of apneic and bradycardic events, and overall stable condition) but still require some form of respiratory support.
- Oxygen support
  - It is not uncommon for infants delivered at less than or equal to 28 weeks' gestation to require oxygen therapy at the time of discharge. The most frequent indicator for home oxygen use is CLD and/or hypoxia.
  - Other risk factors related to the need of home oxygen therapy include small for gestational age infants, con-genital anomalies requiring ventilatory support in the first 72 hours of birth and PDA.
  - The goal of home oxygen therapy is to minimize the effects of chronic hypoxemia, which include pulmo-nary vasoconstriction, and pulmonary vascular remod-eling which both can lead to pulmonary hypertension, bronchial constriction, and airway obstruction (Vento, 2017, pp. 160–161).
- Ventilatory support
  - Infants requiring long-term ventilatory support can be discharged home on mechanical ventilation.
  - Airway stabilization is critical to patient safety when mechanical ventilation is provided in the home set-ting. Tracheostomy may assist in consistent and sta-ble airway management in these infants (Rhein, 2017, p. 448).
- Patient care management at discharge must be a well-coor-dinated effort involving primary care providers, pulmon-ology specialists (as well as other specialists as required), discharge coordinators, home care staff, family caregivers and medical equipment suppliers. Plans of care need to be clearly delineated for all providers (Rhein, 2017, pp. 446–448).
- Both family and professional caretakers must be suffi-ciently educated and able to safely care for the infant. Emergency planning must be clearly mapped out and should include common scenarios that require urgent intervention, notification of community rescue and ambulance services that emergency treatment or trans-port might be required, and notification of local utilities that interruption of power will impact ventilator function (Rhein, 2017, p. 448).

CONCLUSION

Many of the pathology and management challenges faced by neonatal providers are directly related to the respiratory system and the sequelae of respiratory dysfunction. A thor-ough understanding of fetal and neonatal lung development as well as an understanding of basic respiratory physiology, and respiratory pathology is crucial to the ability to implement successful evidence-based management strategies while car-ing for this very vulnerable population.

REVIEW QUESTIONS

1. The most accurate description of surfactant and its mecha-nism of action is that:
   A. Type I cells are responsible for surfactant production and surfactant reduces alveolar surface tension, preventing alveolar collapse.
   B. Type II cells are responsible for surfactant production and surfactant reduces alveolar surface tension, preventing alveolar collapse.
   C. Type I and Type II cells are responsible for surfactant production and surfactant reduces alveolar tension, preventing alveolar collapse.

2. The most common precipitating etiology for persistent pulmonary hypertension of the newborn (PPHN) is:
   A. Abruptio placentae
   B. Intrauterine asphyxia
   C. Meconium aspiration

3. Clinical signs/symptoms of respiratory distress syndrome (RDS) most commonly present during:
   A. First few hours of life
   B. 24–28 hours of age
   C. 48–96 hours of age.

4. When using a conventional ventilator (synchronized intermittent mandatory ventilation [SIMV]), the average pressure applied to the lungs during a respiratory cycle describes the:
   A. Complete tidal volume
   B. Mean airway pressure
   C. Peak inspiratory pressure

5. The lung property which is responsible for decreasing sur-face tension and maintaining functional residual capacity (FRC) is:
   A. Atelectasis
   B. Perihilum
   C. Surfactant

REFERENCES

Arensman, R., M., Short, B., E., & Stephens, D. (2017). Extracorporeal mem-brane oxygenation. In J. P. Goldsmith, E. H. Karotkin, M. Keszler, & G. K. Suresh (Eds.), *Assisted ventilation of the neonate* (6th ed., pp. 434–445). Philadelphia, PA: Elsevier.

Bancalari, E. H., & Walsh, M. C. (2015). Bronchopulmonary dysplasia. In R. Martin, A. A. Fanaroff, & M. C. Walsh (Eds.), *Fanaroff and Martin's neonatal-perinatal medicine diseases of the fetus and infant* (10th ed., pp. 1157–1169). Philadelphia, PA: Saunders.

Barrington, K. J. (2017). Pharmacologic therapies III: Cardiovascular ther-apy and persistent pulmonary hypertension of the newborn. In J. P. Goldsmith, E. H. Karotkin, M. Keszler, & G. K. Suresh (Eds.), *Assisted ventilation of the neonate* (6th ed., pp. 362–365). Philadelphia, PA: Elsevier.

Bean, J. F., Arensman, R. M., Srinivaan, N., Maheshwari, A., & Ambalavanan, N. (2019). Medical and surgical interventions for respiratory distress and airway management. In J. P. Goldsmith, E. H. Karotkin, M. Keszler, & G. K. Suresh (Eds.), *Assisted ventilation of the neonate* (6th ed., pp. 381–406). Philadelphia, PA: Elsevier.

Blackburn, S. (2013). Respiratory system. In S. Blackburn (Ed.), *Maternal, fetal, and neonatal physiology* (4th ed., pp. 297–355). Philadelphia PA: Elsevier.

Bradshaw, W. T. (2015). Gastrointestinal disorders. In M. T. Verklan & M. Walden (Eds.), *Core curriculum for neonatal intensive care nursing* (5th ed., pp. 583–631). St. Louis, MO: Elsevier.

Claure, M., & Bancalari, E. (2017). Special techniques of respiratory support. In J. Goldsmith, E. Karotkin, M. Meszler, & G. Suresh (Eds.), *Assisted ventilation of the neonate* (6th ed., pp. 205–210.e2). Philadelphia, PA: Elsevier.

Clemmens, C., & Piccione, J. (2017). Airway evaluation: Bronchoscopy, laryngoscopy, and tracheal aspirates. In J. P. G. Goldsmith, E. H. Karotkin, M. Keszler, & G. K. Suresh (Eds.), *Assisted ventilation of the neonate* (6th ed., pp. 118–123). Philadelphia, PA: Elsevier.

Crowley, M. A. (2015). Neonatal respiratory disorders. In R. J. Martin, A. A. Fanaroff, M. C. Walsh (Eds.), *Fanaroff and Martin's neonatal-perinatal medicine diseases of the fetus and infant* (10th ed., pp. 1113–1136). Philadelphia, PA: Saunders.

Diblasi, R., & Courtney, S., E. (2017). Non-invasive respiratory support. In J. P. Goldsmith, E. H. Karotkin, M. Keszler, & G. K. Suresh (Eds.), *Assisted ventilation of the neonate* (6th ed., pp. 162–179). Philadelphia, PA: Elsevier.

DiBlasi, R., & Gallagher, J. T. (2017). Respiratory care of the newborn. In J. P. Goldsmith, E. H. Karotkin, M. Keszler, & G. K. Suresh (Eds.), *Assisted ventilation of the neonate* (6th ed., pp. 291–301). Philadelphia, PA: Elsevier.

Ditzenberger, G. R. (2015). Nutritional management. In M. T. Verklan & M. Walden (Eds.), *Core curriculum for neonatal intensive care nursing* (5th ed., pp. 172–196). St. Louis, MO: Elsevier.

Donn, S. M., & Sinha, S. K. (2015). Assisted ventilation and its complications. In R. J. Martin, A. A. Fanaroff, & M. C. Walsh (Eds.), *Fanaroff and Martin's neonatal-perinatal medicine diseases of the fetus and infant* (10th ed., pp. 1087–1112). Philadelphia, PA: Saunders.

Ehret, L. L. (2015). Radiologic evaluation. In M. T. Verklan & M. Walden (Eds.), *Core curriculum for neonatal intensive care nursing* (5th ed., pp. 253–281). St. Louis, MO: Elsevier Saunders.

Eichenwald, E. C. (2017). Mechanical ventilation. In E. Eichenwald, A. Hansen, C. Martin, & A. Stark (Eds.), *Cloherty & Stark's manual of neonatal care* (8th ed., pp. 401–418). Philadelphia, PA: Wolters Kluwer.

Flynn-O'Brien, D., Rice-Townsend, S., & Ledbetter, D. (2018). Structural anomalies of the gastrointestinal tract. In C. Gleason & S. Juul (Eds.), *Avery's diseases of the newborn* (10th ed., pp. 1039–1053.e3). Philadelphia, PA: Elsevier.

Fraser, D. (2015). Respiratory distress. In M. T. Verklan & M. Walden (Eds.), *Core curriculum for neonatal intensive care nurses* (5th ed., pp. 447–477). St. Louis, MO: Elsevier.

Fraser, D., & Diehl-Jones, W. (2015). Assisted ventilation. In M. T. Verklan & M. Walden (Eds.), *Core curriculum for neonatal intensive care nursing* (5th ed., pp. 487–511). St. Louis, MO: Elsevier Saunders.

Gauda, E. B., & Martin, R. J. (2018). Control of breathing. In C. A. Gleason & S. E. Juul (Eds.), *Avery's diseases of the newborn* (10th ed., pp. 600–617). Philadelphia, PA: Elsevier.

Goodwin, M. (2015). Apnea. In T. Verklan & M. Walden (Eds.), *Core curriculum for neonatal intensive care nursing* (5th ed., pp. 478–486). St. Louis, MO: Elsevier.

Greenberg, J. M., Narendran, V., Schibler, K. R., Warner, B. B., & Haberman, B. E. (2019). Neonatal morbidities of prenatal and perinatal origin. In R. Resnik, C. Lockwood, T. Moore, M. Greene, J. Copel, & R. Silver (Eds.), *Creasy and Resnik's maternal-fetal medicine: Principles and practice* (8th ed., pp. 1215–1239-e7). Philadelphia, PA: Elsevier Saunders.

Gregory, M. L. P. G. (2017). Transient tachypnea of the newborn. In E. Eichenwald, A. Hansen, C. Martin, & A. Stark (Eds.), *Cloherty & Stark's manual of neonatal care* (8th ed., pp. 432–435). Philadelphia, PA: Wolters Kluwer.

Guttentag, S. (2017). Respiratory distress syndrome. In E. Eichenwald, A. Hansen, C. Martin, & A. Stark (Eds.), *Cloherty & Stark's manual of neonatal care* (8th ed., pp. 436–445). Philadelphia, PA: Wolters Kluwer.

Hamar, B., & Hansen, A. (2019). Antenatal assessment and high-risk delivery. In B. K. Walsh (Ed.), *Neonatal and pediatric respiratory care* (5th ed., pp. 22–40). St. Louis, MO: Elsevier.

Hansen, A., & Levin, J. (2019). Neonatal pulmonary disorders. In B. K. Walsh (Ed.), *Neonatal and pediatric respiratory care* (5th ed., pp. 407–452). St. Louis, MO: Elsevier.

Jensen, E. A., Mong, D. A., Biko, D. M., Maschhkoff, K. L., & Kirpalani, H. (2017). Imaging: Radiography, lung ultrasound, and other imaging modalities. In J. P. Goldsmith, E. H. Karotkin, M. Keszler, & G. K. Suresh (Eds.), *Assisted ventilation of the neonate* (6th ed., pp. 67–79). Philadelphia, PA: Elsevier.

Joyner, R. L. (2019). Fetal lung development. In B. K. Walsh (Ed.), *Neonatal and pediatric respiratory care* (5th ed., pp. 2–13). St. Louis, MO: Elsevier.

Kallapur, S. G., & Jobe, A. H. (2015). Lung development and maturation. In R. J. Martin, A. A. Fanaroff, & M. C. Walsh (Eds.), *Fanaroff and Martin's neonatal-perinatal medicine diseases of the fetus and infant* (10th ed., pp. 1042–1059). Philadelphia, PA: Saunders.

Karotkin, E. H., & Goldsmith, J. P. (2017). Introduction and historical aspects. In J. P. Goldsmith, E. H. Karotkin, M. Keszler, & G. K. Suresh, (Eds.), *Assisted ventilation of the neonate* (6th ed., pp. 1–7). Philadelphia, PA: Elsevier.

Keller, B., Hirose, S., & Farmer, D. (2018). Surgical disorders of the chest and airways. In C. Gleason & S. Juul (Eds.), *Avery's diseases of the newborn* (10th ed., pp. 695–723.e9). Philadelphia, PA: Elsevier.

Keszler, M., & Abubakar, K. (2017). Physiologic principles. In J. Goldsmith, E. Karotkin, M. Keszler, & G. Suresh (Eds.), *Assisted ventilation of the neonate* (6th ed., pp. 8–30.e3). Philadelphia, PA: Elsevier.

Keszler, M., & Chatburn, R. L. (2017). Oxygen therapy and respiratory support, overview of assisted ventilation. In J. P. Goldsmith, E. H. Karotkin, M. Keszler, & G. K. Suresh (Eds.), *Assisted ventilation of the neonate* (6th ed., pp. 140–152). Philadelphia, PA: Elsevier.

Keszler, M., & Mammel, M. C. (2017). Basic modes of synchronized ventilation. In J. Goldsmith, E. Karotkin, M. Keszler, & G. Suresh (Eds.), *Assisted ventilation of the neonate* (6th ed., pp. 180–187). Philadelphia, PA: Elsevier.

Keszler, M., & Morley, C. J. (2017). In J. Goldsmith, E. Karotkin, M. Keszler, & G. Suresh (Eds.), *Assisted ventilation of the neonate* (6th ed., pp. 195–204). Philadelphia, PA: Elsevier.

Kinsella, J. P. G. (2017). Pharmacologic therapies II: Inhaled nitric oxide. In J. P. Goldsmith, E. H. Karotkin, M. Keszler, & G. K. Suresh (Eds.), *Assisted ventilation of the neonate* (6th ed., pp. 349–361). Philadelphia, PA: Elsevier.

Madenci, A. L., Rice-Townsend, S. E., & Weldon, C. B. (2019). Surgical disorders in childhood that affect respiratory care. In B. K. Walsh (Ed.), *Neonatal and pediatric respiratory care* (5th ed., pp. 453–468). St. Louis, MO: Elsevier.

Mammel, M. C., & Courtney, S. E. (2017). High frequency ventilation. In J. P. Goldsmith, E. H. Karotkin, M. Keszler, & G. K. Suresh (Eds.), *Assisted ventilation of the neonate* (6th ed., pp. 211–228). Philadelphia, PA: Elsevier.

Markham, M. (2017). Pulmonary air leak. In E. Eichenwald, A. Hansen, C. Martin, & A. Stark (Eds.), *Cloherty & Stark's manual of neonatal care* (8th ed., pp. 482–490). Philadelphia, PA: Wolters Kluwer.

Marter, L. J., & McPherson, C. C. (2017). Persistent pulmonary hypertension. In E. C. Eichenwald, A. R. Hansen, C. R. Martin, & A. R. Stark (Eds.), *Cloherty and Stark's manual of neonatal care* (8th ed., pp. 467–477). Philadelphia: Wolters Kluwer.

Meschia, G. (2019). Placenta respiratory gas exchange and fetal oxygenation. In R. Resnik, C. J. Lockwood, T. Moore, M. F. Greene, J. Copel, & R. M. Silver (Eds.), *Creasy and Resnik's maternal fetal medicine: Principles and practice* (8th ed., pp. 210–222.e1). Philadelphia, PA: Elsevier.

Owen, L. S., Weiner, G. M., & Davis, P. G. G. (2017). Delivery room stabilization and respiratory support. In J. P. Goldsmith, E. H. Karotkin, M. Keszler, & G. K. Suresh (Eds.), *Assisted ventilation of the neonate* (6th ed., pp. 275–290). Philadelphia, PA: Elsevier.

Pappas, B. E., & Robey, D. L. (2015). Neonatal delivery room resuscitation. In M. T. Verklan & M. Walden (Eds.), *Core curriculum for neonatal intensive care nursing* (5th ed., pp. 77–94). St. Louis, MO: Elsevier Saunders.

Parad, R. B., & Banjamin, J. (2017). Bronchopulmonary dysplasia/chronic lung disease. In E. Eichenwald, A. Hansen, C. Martin, & A. Stark (Eds.), *Cloherty & Stark's manual of neonatal care* (8th ed., pp. 446–460). Philadelphia, PA: Wolters Kluwer.

Parry, R. L. (2015). Selected gastrointestinal anomalies in the neonate. In R. Martin, A. Fanaroff, & M. Walsh (Eds.), *Fanaroff and Martin's neonatal-perinatal medicine: Diseases of the fetus and infant* (10th ed., pp. 1395–1422). Philadelphia, PA: Elsevier Saunders.

Patrinos, M. E. (2017). Neonatal apnea and the foundation of respiratory control. In R. J. Martin, A. A. Fanaroff, & M. C. Walsh (Eds.), *Fanaroff and Martin's neonatal-perinatal medicine diseases of the fetus and infant* (10th ed., pp. 1137–1146). Philadelphia, PA: Saunders.

Plosa, E. J. (2017). Meconium aspiration. In E. Eichenwald, A. Hansen, C. Martin, & A. Stark (Eds.), *Cloherty & Stark's manual of neonatal care* (8th ed., pp. 461–466). Philadelphia, PA: Wolters Kluwer.

Plosa, E. J. (2017). Pulmonary hemorrhage. In E. Eichenwald, A. Hansen, C. Martin, & A. Stark (Eds.), *Cloherty & Stark's manual of neonatal care* (8th ed., pp. 478–481). Philadelphia, PA: Wolters Kluwer.

Rabi, Y., Kowal, D., & Ambalavanan, N. (2017). Blood gasses: Technical aspects and interpretation. In J. Goldsmith, E. Karotkin, M. Keszler, & G. Suresh (Eds.), *Assisted ventilation of the neonate* (6th ed., pp. 80–96.e3). Philadelphia, PA: Elsevier.

Rhein, L. (2017). Discharge and transition to home care. In J. Goldsmith, E. Karotkin, M. Keszler, & G. Suresh (Eds.), *Assisted ventilation of the neonate* (6th ed., pp. 80–83). Philadelphia, PA: Elsevier.

Ringer, S. A., & Hansen, A. R. (2017). Surgical emergencies in the newborn. In E. Eichenwald, A. Hansen, C. Martin, & A. Stark (Eds.), *Cloherty &*

Stark's manual of neonatal care (8th ed., pp. 942–966). Philadelphia, PA: Wolters Kluwer.

Shepherd, E. G., & Nevin, L. D. (2017). Physical examination. In J. P. Goldsmith, E. H. Karotkin, M. Keszler, & G. K. Suresh (Eds.), *Assisted ventilation of the neonate* (6th ed., pp. 61–66). Philadelphia, PA: Elsevier.

Smallwood, C. D. (2019). Noninvasive monitoring in neonatal and pediatric care. In B. K. Walsh (Ed.), *Neonatal and pediatric respiratory care* (5th ed., pp. 135–148). St. Louis, MO: Elsevier.

Stark, A. R. (2017). Apnea. In E. C. Eichenwald, A. R. Hansen, C. R. Martin, & A. R. Stark (Eds.), *Cloherty and Stark's manual of neonatal care* (8th ed., pp. 426–435). Philadelphia, PA: Wolters Kluwer.

Steinhorn, R. H. (2015). Pulmonary vascular development. In R. Martin, A. Fanaroff, & M. Walsh (Eds.), *Fanaroff and Martin's neonatal-perinatal medicine: Diseases of the fetus and infant* (10th ed., pp. 1198–1209). Philadelphia, PA: Elsevier Saunders.

Stewart, J. E., Hernandez, F., & Duncan, A. F. (2017). Follow-Up care of very preterm and very low birth weight infants. In E. Eichenwald, A. Hansen, C. Martin, & A. Stark (Eds.), *Cloherty & Stark's manual of neonatal care* (8th ed., pp. 192–201). Philadelphia, PA: Wolters Kluwer.

Suresh, G. K., & Raghavan, A. (2017). Quality and safety in respiratory care. In J. P. Goldsmith, E. H. Karotkin, M. Keszler, & G. K. Suresh (Eds.), *Assisted ventilation of the neonate* (6th ed., pp. 49–55). Philadelphia, PA: Elsevier.

Suresh, G. K., Soll, R. F., & Mandy, G. T. (2017). Pharmacologic therapies I: Surfactant therapy. In J. Goldsmith, E. Karotkin, M. Keszler, & G. Suresh (Eds.), *Assisted ventilation of the neonate* (6th ed., pp. 338–348). Philadelphia, PA: Elsevier.

Van Marter, L. J., & McPherson, C. C. (2017). Persistent pulmonary hypertension. In E. Eichenwald, A. Hansen, C. Martin, & A. Stark (Eds.), *Cloherty & Stark's manual of neonatal care* (8th ed., pp. 467–477). Philadelphia, PA: Wolters Kluwer.

Vento, M. (2017). Oxygen therapy. In J. Goldsmith, E. Karotkin, M. Keszler, & G. Suresh (Eds.), *Assisted ventilation of the neonate* (6th ed., pp. 153–161). Philadelphia, PA: Elsevier.

Verklan, M. T. (2015). Adaptation to extrauterine life. In M. T. Verklan & M. Walden (Eds.), *Core curriculum for neonatal intensive care nursing* (5th ed., pp. 58–76). St. Louis, MO: Elsevier Saunders.

Walsh, B. K., & Chatburn, R. L. (2019). Invasive mechanical ventilation of the neonate and pediatric patient. In B. K. Walsh (Ed.), *Neonatal and pediatric respiratory care* (5th ed., pp. 301–337). St. Louis, MO: Elsevier.

Wambach, J. A., & Hamvas, A. (2015). Respiratory distress syndrome in the neonate. In R. Martin, A. Fanaroff, & M. Walsh (Eds.), *Fanaroff and Martin's neonatal-perinatal medicine: Diseases of the fetus and infant* (10th ed., pp. 1074–1086). Philadelphia, PA: Elsevier Saunders.

Weisz, D. E., & McNamara, P. G. J. (2017). Cardiovascular assessment. In J. P. Goldsmith, E. H. Karotkin, M. Keszler, & G. K. Suresh (Eds.), *Assisted ventilation of the neonate* (6th ed., pp. 124–139). Philadelphia, PA: Elsevier.

Wilson, D. J., & Tyner, C. I. (2015). Infectious disease in the neonate. In M. T. Verklan & M. Walden (Eds.), *Core curriculum for neonatal intensive care nursing* (5th ed., pp. 689–718). St. Louis, MO: Elsevier Saunders.

Wolf, G. K., & Arnold, J. H. (2017). Extracorporeal membrane oxygenation. In E. Eichenwald, A. Hansen, C. Martin, & A. Stark (Eds.), *Cloherty & Stark's manual of neonatal care* (8th ed., pp. 491–501). Philadelphia, PA: Wolters Kluwer.

Yoder, B. A. (2017). Mechanical ventilation: Disease specific strategies. In J. P. Goldsmith, E. H. Karotkin, M. Keszler, & G. K. Suresh (Eds.), *Assisted ventilation of the neonate* (6th ed., pp. 224–242). Philadelphia, PA: Elsevier.

Zanelli, S. A., & Kaufman, D. (2019). Surfactant replacement therapy. In B. K. Walsh (Ed.), *Neonatal and pediatric respiratory care* (5th ed., pp. 244–266). St. Louis, MO: Elsevier.

18 THE GASTROINTESTINAL SYSTEM

Jacqueline Hoffman
Karen Wright

INTRODUCTION

- This chapter highlights gastrointestinal (GI) disorders in the neonate and is to be used in conjunction with all recommended resources from the National Certification Corporation for more in-depth review. Failure of normal developmental processes can result in an array of congenital GI disorders located anywhere from the esophagus to the anus, such as atresia/stenosis, abdominal wall defects, nonfixation of the intestines, and anorectal malformations. Functional obstruction may also occur due to abnormal intestinal mucous gland production or lack of neuronal migration of ganglion cells. It is important for the NNP to be aware of timing of clinical presentation and the physical examination findings in order to determine the best diagnostic workup, which may end up being therapeutic as well as to assist in determining the final diagnosis.

GASTROINTESTINAL SYSTEM DEVELOPMENT

- The GI tract extends from the mouth to the anus and includes all the associated organs and glands that secrete hormones necessary for function. The fetus is dependent on placental transfer of maternal nutrients for normal fetal growth and development (see Table 18.1). Disorders of maternal nutrition results in abnormal fetal "programming" of tissues and may result in long-term neurobehavioral consequences as well as later health concerns such as hypertension, cardiovascular disease, and obesity (Ditzenberger, 2018, pp. 395, 410).
- During the embryonic stage, which extends from the third through the eighth week of gestation, anatomical development is prevalent.

- ○ The primordial gut forms by the fourth week and can be divided into three parts: foregut (some resources separate this into pharyngeal and foregut), midgut, and hindgut (see Table 18.2; Ditzenberger, 2018, pp. 402–403).
- ○ Failure of the tracheobronchial diverticulum to divide into the ventral respiratory primordium and the dorsal esophagus at 4 to 5 weeks results in tracheoesophageal fistula (TEF; Bucher, Pocatti, Lauvorn, & Carter, 2016, p. 790; Ditzenberger, 2018, pp. 403–404).
- ○ The lumen of many of the GI structures becomes temporarily obliterated due to rapid growing epithelium; recanalization of these structures must occur, otherwise, stenosis or atresia occurs.
  - Failure of the duodenum to recanalize during the sixth to seventh week results in duodenal atresia; partial recanalization results in duodenal stenosis.
  - Failure of the esophagus to recanalize during the eighth week results in esophageal atresia (EA); partial recanalization results in esophageal stenosis.
  - Failure of the hepatic bile ducts to recanalize results in biliary atresia (Ditzenberger, 2018, pp. 404–406).
- Due to rapid growth and elongation of the intestinal loops and growth of the liver during the sixth week of gestation, there is not enough room in the abdomen, leading to the intestinal loops herniating into the umbilical stalk; this is referred to as physiologic herniation. The midgut loop rotates 90° counterclockwise around the axis of the superior mesenteric artery while it is in the umbilical cord, with the caudal end being on the left and the cranial limb on the right (Bucher et al., 2016, p. 795; Ditzenberger, 2018, pp. 405–406).
- During the fetal stage, from the ninth week to birth, development of the functional components (hormones, enzymes, reflexes) are evident (see Exhibit 18.1; Ditzenberger, 2018, pp. 401–402, 408–409, 411).

TABLE 18.1 Fetal Requirements From Maternal Nutrients

Maternal Nutrient	Fetal Requirements
Protein	For rapid fetal tissue growth
Calcium, phosphorus, vitamin A	For fetal skeleton and tooth bud formation
Vitamin A	For fetal bud formation, in particular for development of enamel-forming cells in gum tissue
Vitamin D	For mineralization of fetal bone tissue and tooth buds
Iron	For fetal liver storage

Source: Data from Ditzenberger, G. (2018). Gastrointestinal and hepatic systems and perinatal nutrition. In S. Blackburn (Ed.), *Maternal, fetal, & neonatal physiology: A clinical perspective* (5th ed., pp. 387–434). Maryland Heights, MO: Elsevier.

TABLE 18.2 The Primordial Gut

Primitive Component	Neonatal Structure	Blood Supply	Defects That May Occur
Foregut	Primordial pharynx and its derivatives, lower respiratory tract, esophagus, stomach, liver, upper portion of the duodenum distal to the entry of the bile duct, liver, biliary tree, and pancreas	Supplied by celiac artery	TEF with or without EA, isolated EA, esophageal stenosis, pyloric stenosis, duodenal atresia/stenosis, biliary atresia, annular pancreas
Midgut	Small intestine (except for the upper duodenum), cecum, appendix, ascending colon, and proximal portion (1/2 to 2/3) of the transverse colon	Supplied by superior mesenteric artery	Abdominal wall defects, intestinal stenosis/atresia, malrotation
Hindgut	Distal (1/3 to 1/2) transverse colon, descending and sigmoid colons, rectum, superior part of (upper) anal canal, epithelium of the bladder and urethra	Supplied by inferior mesenteric artery	Hirschsprung disease, anorectal malformations such as persistent cloaca, imperforate anus, and anal stenosis/atresia

EA, esophageal atresia; TEF, tracheo-esophageal fistula.

EXHIBIT 18.1 Highlights of Anatomic and Hormone Development

Week 3	Week 4	Week 5	Week 6	Week 7	Week 8	Week 9-10	Week 12	2nd trimester	3rd trimester
Tubular intestine, yolk sac, and mesentery forming	Primordial gut forms. Primordium of stomach evident. Esophagus and trachea separate. **TEF, EA (4–5 wk)**	Intestine elongates into a loop, rotation begins. Pancreas present. Cloaca is divided into two parts by the urorectal septum. **Anorectal malformation (5–8 wk)**	Midgut herniates into umbilical cord; 90° counterclockwise rotation. Temporary duodenal occlusion occurs. Stomach dilates, enlarges, and rotates 90° around an anteroposterior axis.	Esophagus reaches final length. Lengthening, 90° counterclockwise rotation of intestinal loops in umbilical cord. Urorectal septum fuses with cloacal membrane. Perineum formed when urorectal and cloacal membranes fuse.	Esophagus, duodenum and small intestine recanalize. Development intestinal villi. Diaphragm complete. **Duodenal, atresia (8–10 wk) Jejunoileal atresia, primary defect (8-10 wk) Omphalocele (8-11th wk)**	Rupture of pit in anal membrane; now open communication between rectum and exterior body. Intestines reenter abdominal cavity with 180° counterclockwise rotation around superior mesenteric artery. **Gastroschisis (9-11 wk)**	Intestinal muscular layer present. Ganglion cell migration complete. Pancreatic islet cells appear. Lactase appears. **Hirschsprung disease**	Meconium present and swallowing observed Week 16. Rectal ganglion cells present by week 24. **Jejunoileal atresia, secondary defect (after 12 weeks)**	Coordination of sucking and swallowing occurs during weeks 34-36. Maturation of GI system complete by week 38.

- During the 10th week of gestation, retraction occurs with the small intestine returning to the abdominal cavity first occupying the central region of the abdomen followed by the large intestines, which rotate an additional 180° counterclockwise rotation occupying the right side of the abdomen. At this time, the duodenojejunal junction is in the left upper quadrant of the abdomen with fixation in the location of the ligament of Treitz (this becomes important to note when evaluating for malrotation/volvulus) (Bucher et al., 2016, p. 796; Ditzenberger, 2018, pp. 405–406).
- By the end of the 11th week of gestation, the cecum is fixed in the right lower quadrant and the hindgut (splenic flexure of the colon to the rectum) is fixed in the left hemiabdomen; Bucher et al., 2016, p. 796).
  ○ The hindgut ends at the cloacal membrane. Development of the hindgut and urogenital system are interrelated (Ditzenberger, 2018, p. 407).
- The intestinal length increases 100-fold during gestation with doubling in length the last trimester (Bradshaw, 2015, p. 584).

- Many of GI disorders result from abnormalities during embryogenesis and can be associated with other conditions or anomalies related to systems/organs that are also developing at the same time (see Table 18.3).
- After birth, there is coordinated function of the hormone and enzymes needed for digestion in addition to maturation of the suck–swallow mechanism (Ditzenberger, 2018, pp. 401–402).

GENERALIZATION ABOUT GASTROINTESTINAL TRACT DISORDERS

Definitions and Pathophysiology

- A *mechanical obstruction* refers to a specific point of obstruction either by abnormal tissue growths or malpositioning of the organs (Flynn-O'Brien, Rice-Townsend, & Ledbetter, 2018, p. 1039);

TABLE 18.3 Association Conditions with Gastrointesinal (GI) Defects

GI Disorder	Associated Conditions
Duodenal atresia	Fetal hydantoin syndrome, Trisomy 21
Esophageal atresia/tracheo-esophageal fistula	Apert's syndrome, CHARGE Association, Trisomy 18, VACTERL association
Hirschsprung's disease	DiGeorge syndrome, Smith–Lemli–Opitz syndrome, Trisomy 21
Intestinal malrotation	Trisomy 13, Trisomy 18
Imperforate anus	VACTERL association
Pyloric stenosis	Apert syndrome, Trisomy 18, Trisomy 21
Umbilical wall defects	Beckwith-Widemann syndrome (Chromosome 11), fetal hydantoin syndrome (umbilical hernia), Trisomy 13, Trisomy 18, Trisomy 21

- A *functional obstruction* is not associated with an anatomic malformation; it is most commonly related to a problem with bowel motility.
- An *atresia* occurs when there is complete discontinuity of the intestinal lumen, ranging from a short web segment to complete loss of a segment of the intestine and the mesentery, or to multiple areas of discontinuity resulting in multiple atresias (Flynn-O'Brien et al., 2018, p. 1049).
- A *stenosis* occurs when there is narrowing of the intestinal lumen; it remains continuous and ranges from involving a partial web to involving the entire thickness of the intestinal lumen (Fanaroff, 2013, p. 184).

Diagnosis

- Polyhydramnios and large gastric aspirates at birth suggest a more proximal obstruction; more likely to see early feeding intolerance, emesis, and a scaphoid abdomen with proximal obstructions (Bradshaw, 2015, p. 593; Bucher et al., 2016, p. 799; Fanaroff, 2013, p. 184).
- Ninety-five percent of term infants pass meconium by 24 hours; almost 100% will pass meconium by 48 hours unless there is a mechanical or functional obstruction (Bradshaw, 2015, p. 593).
  - Passage of meconium does not exclude an obstruction as it may initially be passed from the bowel distal to the site of obstruction (Fanaroff, 2013, p. 184).
- There is a direct relationship between amount of abdominal distention and the level of the obstruction; the more distal the obstruction, the greater the amount of distention (Bradshaw, 2015, p. 593).
- Bilious emesis in an otherwise healthy neonate is considered a midgut volvulus until proven otherwise, prompt diagnosis is necessary to minimize amount of necrotic bowel. When the obstruction is distal to the ampulla of Vater, bilious emesis will be present (Bradshaw, 2015, p. 593; Bucher et al., 2016, p. 184).

Management

- Generalized preoperative management: NPO, gastric decompression such as replogle to suction (decreases risk of emesis and aspiration, improves bowel wall perfusion), parenteral fluid support, correction of electrolytes if emesis has been ongoing, surgical consult, and antibiotic therapy to provide coverage for enteric organisms (Bradshaw, 2015, pp. 593–594; Bucher et al., 2016, pp. 791–807; Fanaroff, 2013, pp. 186–190).

Outcomes

- Prognosis will depend on presence of additional anomalies, amount of bowel loss (if any), and other long-term complications (Bradshaw, 2015, pp. 593–594; Bucher et al., 2016, pp. 791–807; Fanaroff, 2013, pp. 186–190).

ABNORMALITIES IN THE DEVELOPMENT OF THE FOREGUT

Esophageal Atresia /Tracheo-esophageal Fistula

DEFINITION AND PATHOPHYSIOLOGY

- EA is an interruption in the esophagus resulting in a blind pouch. There are four variations seen in the neonate with an EA: most commonly (85%–90%), the neonate with an EA will have an associated distal TEF, 8% will have only an isolated EA, and less commonly, the remaining will have an EA with a proximal TEF or with a double (proximal and distal) TEF (Bradshaw, 2015, p. 594; Bucher et al., 2016, p. 790; Ringer & Hansen, 2017, pp. 947–948; see Figure 18.1).
- TEF is an abnormal connection between the esophagus and the trachea; only 5% will have only the abnormal connection between a normal esophagus and trachea "H-type" (Bradshaw, 2015, p. 594; Bucher et al., 2016, p. 790; see Figure 18.1).
- The spectrum of EA/TEF defects occurs during week 4 of gestation when there is failure in normal development of the esophagus and/or incomplete separation of the trachea from the esophagus in the primitive foregut. This may occur due to hedgehog signaling abnormalities, other genetic alterations, or environmental insults (Bradshaw, 2015, p. 594; Bucher et al., 2016, p. 790).
  - Associated anomalies are common (50–70%) as this defect occurs during a critical period of organogenesis.
    - VACTERL (Vertebrae, imperforate Anus, Cardiac system (typically ASD/VSD), Trachea, Esophagus, Renal [urinary tract], Limbs).
    - Esophageal anomalies are also seen in CHARGE association (Coloboma, Heart defects, Atresia choanae, growth Retardation, Genital abnormalities, and Ear abnormalities). Up to one-third of infants with TEF may have severe tracheomalacia (Bradshaw, 2015, p. 595; Bucher et al., 2016, p. 791; Fanaroff, 2013, p. 186).

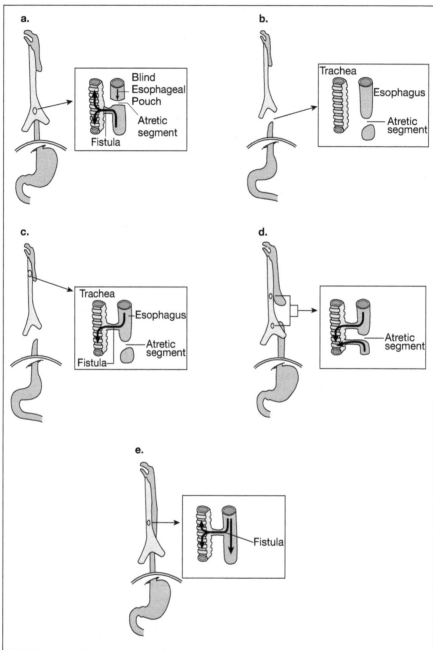

FIGURE 18.1 Five types of esophageal atresia (EA)/tracheo-esophageal fistula (TEF). (A) EA with distal TEF (85%). (B) Isolated EA (8%). (C) EA with proximal TEF (1%). (D) EA with double TEF (1%). (E) Isolated TEF (5%).

DIAGNOSIS

- Prenatal findings may include small or absent stomach on fetal ultrasound (US) [especially after 14 weeks' gestation] and concomitant polyhydramnios.
- EA is postnatally diagnosed by inability to pass a catheter to the stomach; x-ray will show the catheter coiled in the proximal esophageal pouch typically at the second or third thoracic vertebrae, above the carina. Air in the GI tract on x-ray indicates the presence of an EA with distal TEF, an EA with double TEF, or an isolated TEF. A gasless abdomen on x-ray with a scaphoid-appearing abdomen indicates the presence of an EA with proximal TEF or an isolated EA (Bradshaw, 2015, p. 595; Bucher et al., 2016, p. 790; Fanaroff, 2013, pp. 185–186; Ringer & Hansen, 2017, pp. 947–948).

- Clinical presentation depends on the type of defect and may include excessive oral secretions, drooling, coughing/choking, and regurgitation of undigested formula/breast milk.
  - ○ Respiratory distress is due to airway obstruction from excess oral secretions, from aspiration of saliva/feeds, or from reflux of gastric contents up the distal esophagus into the lungs through the abnormal connection. If there is recurrent pneumonia with coughing/choking during feedings in the infant that a catheter can be passed, think "H-type" TEF (Bradshaw, 2015, p. 595; Bucher et al., 2016, p. 790; Flynn-O'Brien et al., 2018, p. 1042).

MANAGEMENT
PREOPERATIVE

- Placement of a replogle catheter into the proximal esophageal pouch to low continuous suction to prevent aspiration of oral secretions.
- Elevation of head to minimize aspiration of oral secretions that accumulate in the proximal esophageal pouch as well as minimize gastric reflux through the fistula into the lungs.
- Comfort measures to minimize crying; crying increases air in stomach, abdominal distention, and may be associated with increased risk for aspiration of gastric contents into the trachea.
- Avoid continuous positive airway pressure (CPAP), use low mean airway pressure if on conventional ventilation or use high-frequency oscillatory ventilation (HFOV) to minimize shunting of tidal volume from the trachea to the stomach; if respiratory support is required, these infants require surgery sooner for ligation of TEF; placement of gastrostomy is needed if there is increased abdominal distention compromising effective ventilation (Bradshaw, 2015, p. 595; Bucher et al., 2016, p. 791; Ringer & Hansen, 2017, p. 948).
- Evaluate for other anomalies
  - ○ Echocardiogram should be done prior to surgery as presence of cardiac defect may influence the surgical approach; abdominal US of kidneys/genitourinary tract, plain radiographs of the spine and limbs can be done after surgery (Bradshaw, 2015, p. 595; Bucher et al., 2016, p. 791; Flynn-O'Brien et al., 2018, p. 1043; Ringer & Hansen, 2017, p. 948).

SURGICAL INTERVENTIONS

- Complete repair if possible is preferred (division and ligation of fistula with primary anastomosis of esophageal segments).
- Staged repair with early placement of a gastrostomy tube for decompression and feeding, and division of fistula when the gap is too large between the two esophageal segments is recommended in the very premature infant, the infant with pneumonia or the infant with other coexisting morbidities.
- In rare cases, esophageal replacement using gastric or colon segment is done if the gap between the two esophageal segments is too wide.
- If severe congenital heart defects (CHDs) or lethal chromosomal defects are present, palliation with cervical esophagostomy and gastrostomy may be done; later it can be determined if further surgical interventions are warranted (Bradshaw, 2015, pp. 595–596; Bucher et al., 2016, pp. 791–792; Ringer & Hansen, 2017, p. 949).

POSTOPERATIVE MANAGEMENT

- Protect the anastomosis site to prevent suture disruption leading to anastomosis leak or recurrent fistula
  - ○ ventilate using lowest mean airway pressure possible
  - ○ suction length of endotracheal tube only; or if suctioning posterior pharynx, use a premeasured catheter
  - ○ do not extubate until certain that respiratory status is stable with minimal risk for requiring re-intubation
  - ○ if self-extubates or fails elective extubation, only skilled personnel should intubate;
  - ○ do not replace orogastric/nasogastric tube placed during surgery if accidental dislodgement occurs
- Monitor chest tube and gastric drainage; chest tube drainage suggests leakage from the esophageal anastomosis.
- Head of bed elevated to prevent aspiration; consider gastric acid blocker to minimize reflux sequela.
- Total parenteral nutrition (hyperalimentation/lipids) preferably via central line
- Enteral nutrition is typically started after esophagram confirms anastomosis site has healed with no leaking (usually at least 7–10 days postoperatively).
- Pain management (Bradshaw, 2015, p. 596; Bucher et al., 2016, pp. 791–792; Flynn-O'Brien et al., 2018, p. 1044; Ringer & Hansen, 2017, p. 948).

POSTOPERATIVE COMPLICATIONS

- Strictures requiring periodic esophageal dilation; may be exacerbated by gastroesophageal reflux (GER).
  - ○ GER may be lessened with elevation of head of bed, slow low-volume feeds, administration of histamine (H2) antagonists or proton pump inhibitors (PPIs).
- Dysmotility in the distal esophageal segment may require gastrostomy feeds to minimize vomiting and aspiration.
- Anastomosis site problems such as leak or recurrent fistula (usually as a result of a leak)
  - ○ Correct with delay in feeds/provide parenteral nutrition, maintain chest tube, determine if antibiotic therapy needed, allow time for healing.
- Tracheomalacia due to compression of the posterior trachea by the proximal esophageal pouch leading to deformation and softening of the tracheal cartilages
- Aspiration leading to pneumonia
- Sepsis
- Recurrent laryngeal nerve injury and vocal cord dysfunction
- Unilateral diaphragmatic paralysis (Bradshaw, 2015, p. 596; Bucher et al., 2016, pp. 792–793)

OUTCOMES

- Final stage of anastomosis of the proximal and distal esophagus segments typically is done at 6 to 12 months of age; until that time, the infant will require a mechanism to keep the esophageal pouch emptied (continuous suction of proximal pouch or esophagostomy).
- Long-term survival depends on presence/types of comorbidities such as prematurity with respiratory distress syndrome (RDS), CHD, or presence of lethal chromosomal defects (Bradshaw, 2015, pp. 595–596; Bucher et al., 2016, p. 791).

Pyloric Stenosis

DEFINITION AND PATHOPHYSIOLOGY

- Stricture of the outlet from the stomach to the small intestine due to hypertrophy mainly of the circular muscles of the pylorus; this results in obstruction of the passage of liquids (human milk or formula; Bradshaw, 2015, p. 596).

- Exact etiology is unknown. There is an increased association in infants whose mothers during the third trimester had increased gastrin secretion and in infants who received prostaglandin E. There has been some suggested association in infants who receive erythromycin in the first 6 weeks of life. There is a proposed genetic component as 10% to 20% of affected infants are born to mothers who had same disorder and a higher rate of occurrence in monozygotic twins. More common in first-born, males, and Whites (Bradshaw, 2015, p. 596; Flynn-O'Brien et al., 2018, p. 1047).
- Commonly associated with Trisomies 18 and 21, and Apert syndrome; otherwise, associated anomalies are uncommon (Bradshaw, 2015, p. 596).

DIAGNOSIS

- Clinical presentation does not typically occur until after 2 to 3 weeks of life (can present as early as 1 week and as late as 5 months of age) with nonbilious emesis that over time due to progressive gastric outlet obstruction becomes projectile.
  - On palpation, a small, firm, mobile oval-shaped pyloric mass, "olive," in the right upper quadrant can be felt (Bradshaw, 2015, p. 597; Flynn-O'Brien et al., 2018, p. 1047; Ringer & Hansen, 2017, p. 957).
- Ultrasound confirms the diagnosis in majority of cases.
  - Diagnosis is by abdominal radiography showing distended stomach with little or no abdominal gas pattern below the duodenum.
  - If diagnosis still unclear, a contrast upper GI can be done which will show delayed or no gastric emptying with an elongated pyloric channel referred to as "string sign" (Bradshaw, 2015, p. 597).

MANAGEMENT

- Preoperative management includes gastric decompression, correcting any electrolyte or acid–base abnormalities, and fluid resuscitation as a result of persistent vomiting (Bradshaw, 2015, p. 597; Flynn-O'Brien et al., 2018, p. 1047).
- Surgical repair is most often a pyloromyotomy, where an incision is made into the circular and longitudinal muscles of the pylorus releasing the stricture.
- Postoperative management includes:
  - Never place or replace an orogastric or nasogastric feeding tube postoperatively as perforation of the surgical repair site may occur.
  - NPO until awake and then feedings are progressed over 24 hours. Persistent emesis the first couple of days postoperative may occur until normal gastric emptying times resume; this may alarm parents as the infant does not seem improved after surgery (Bradshaw, 2015, p. 597).

OUTCOMES

- Prognosis is excellent with no residual effects; strictures are uncommon.

Duodenal Atresia

DEFINITION AND PATHOPHYSIOLOGY

- Duodenal atresia occurs when there is failure of vacuolization (during weeks 5–6 of gestation) and recanalization of the intestinal lumen (weeks 8–10 of gestation; Bradshaw, 2015, p. 597; Bucher et al., 2016, pp. 798–799).

- Prenatal findings include dilated stomach and duodenum on fetal US, the classic "double bubble" echogenicity, more commonly noted in third trimester when the duodenum becomes more dilated; there may also be polyhydramnios (Bradshaw, 2015, p. 597; Fanaroff, 2013, p. 187; Ringer & Hansen, 2017, p. 954).
- Congenital obstruction of the duodenum is the most common portion of the bowel involved when considering the group of intestinal atresias. Partial or complete obstruction of the duodenum can be caused by extrinsic lesions, such as malrotation, or by intrinsic lesions, such as duodenal stenosis or atresia (Bucher et al., 2016, p. 798; Fanaroff, 2013, p. 187).
- There are three common types (see Figure 18.2)
  - Type 1: membranous web, often associated with common bile duct abnormalities
  - Type 2: fibrous atretic cord connecting the two segments of the duodenum
  - Type 3: complete separation of the two atretic ends of the duodenum; may be associated with annular pancreas (Bradshaw, 2015, p. 597):
- Associated anomalies are commonly associated, including Down syndrome (up to 30%), CHDs (up to 30%), and other GI anomalies including annular pancreas, malrotation of the small intestine, small-bowel atresia, and imperforate anus (Bradshaw, 2015, p. 597; Bucher et al., 2016, p. 799; Ditzenberger, 2018, p. 403; Flynn-O'Brien et al., 2018, p. 1049; Ringer & Hansen, 2017, p. 954).

DIAGNOSIS

- Clinical presentation includes bilious emesis (obstruction usually distal to the ampulla of Vater) within a few hours to 24 hours after birth, minimal abdominal distention limited to the upper abdomen, and failure to pass meconium (Bradshaw, 2015, pp. 597–598; Ringer & Hansen, 2017, p. 954).
  - Radiography that demonstrates the classic "double bubble," air in the stomach, and upper duodenum but no air distally in the small or large intestine is diagnostic.
  - "Double bubble" with air present distally suggests duodenal stenosis (Bradshaw, 2015, p. 598; Bucher et al., 2016, p. 799; Ringer & Hansen, 2017, p. 954).

MANAGEMENT

- Preoperative management to include generalized preoperative management and evaluate for other anomalies (e.g., send chromosomes if dysmorphic features consistent with Trisomy 21 or echocardiogram to rule out CHD).
- Surgical management includes excision of the atretic portion with primary end-to-end anastomoses (duodenoduodenostomy). If the duodenal obstruction is related to annular pancreas or other causes compressing the duodenum, surgery goal is to remove or redirect the tissue causing the duodenal obstruction.
- Postoperative management includes using a replogle to suction until return of bowel function, then initiation of enteral nutrition slowly due to delayed gastric emptying and microcolon distal to the repair site resulting in feeding intolerance (Bradshaw, 2015, p. 598; Bucher et al., 2016, pp. 799–800).

OUTCOMES

- Prognosis is generally good with long-term outcomes determined by associated anomalies. Early complications may include anastomotic leak and stricture; potential long-term problems may include dysmotility of the stomach and duodenum (Bucher et al., 2016, p. 800; Flynn-O'Brien et al., 2018, p. 1050).

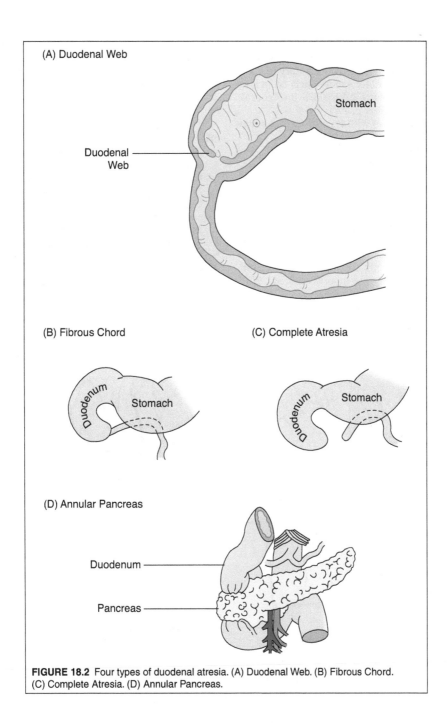

(A) Duodenal Web

Stomach

Duodenal Web

(B) Fibrous Chord

Duodenum   Stomach

(C) Complete Atresia

Duodenum   Stomach

(D) Annular Pancreas

Duodenum

Pancreas

FIGURE 18.2 Four types of duodenal atresia. (A) Duodenal Web. (B) Fibrous Chord. (C) Complete Atresia. (D) Annular Pancreas.

ABNORMALITIES IN THE DEVELOPMENT OF THE MIDGUT

Jejunal and Ileal Atresias

DEFINITION AND PATHOPHYSIOLOGY

- Congenital obstruction of the jejunum, the ileum, or both as a result of a primary or secondary defect. The ileum is involved more commonly in comparison to the jejunum (Ditzenberger, 2018, p. 407; Fanaroff, 2013, p. 187; Ringer & Hansen, 2017, p. 953).

- Jejunal/ileal atresia occurs as a primary defect when there is complete failure of recanalization of the intestinal lumen (weeks 8–10 of gestation). If partial recanalization occurs, this results in stenosis instead of atresia (Bradshaw, 2015, p. 598; Bucher et al., 2016, p. 799; Ringer & Hansen, 2017, p. 954).

- Jejunal/ileal atresia occurs more commonly due to a secondary defect when an intrauterine accident occurs, either as a vascular mesenteric insult interrupting the blood supply (infarction) with subsequent necrosis and reabsorption of the affected segment(s) OR secondary to a segmental volvulus. Secondary defects more likely occur after 12 weeks of gestation (Bradshaw, 2015, p. 598; Bucher et al., 2016, p. 799; Ditzenberger, 2018, p. 407)

- There are four common types with type III further subdivided (see Figure 18.3):
  - ○ Type I: Membranous web with intact mesentery
  - ○ Type II: Fibrous atretic cord connecting the two segments with intact mesentery
  - ○ Type IIIa: The two segments are separated by a v-shaped mesenteric defect.
  - ○ Type IIIb: The two segments are separated by a v-shaped mesenteric defect; the distal small intestine twists around the ileocecal artery; this type is referred to as the apple-peel defect.
  - ○ Type IV: Multiple segments are atretic and discontinuous, appearing like sausage links (Bradshaw, 2015, p. 598; Bucher et al., 2016, p. 799).

- Not commonly associated with major congenital anomalies or syndromes, however, association with anomalies of the GI tract may be seen including malrotation, meconium peritonitis, and meconium ileus (Bradshaw, 2015, p. 598; Bucher et al., 2016, p. 799; Ditzenberger, 2018, p. 407).

DIAGNOSIS

- Prenatal findings may include presence of polyhydramnios and distended intestinal loops on fetal US. If in utero bowel perforation occurred, peritoneal calcifications may be visible (Bradshaw, 2015, p. 698).
- Clinical presentation includes failure to pass meconium, abdominal distention, and bilious emesis within the first 24 to 36 hours of life (Bradshaw, 2015, p. 598; Bucher et al., 2016, p. 799; Ringer & Hansen, 2017, p. 953).
- Contrast enema is the gold standard for diagnosis. A contrast enema will reveal a micro-colon as a result of lack of use and no reflux of the contrast material into the proximal bowel reflecting the area where the atresia occurs.

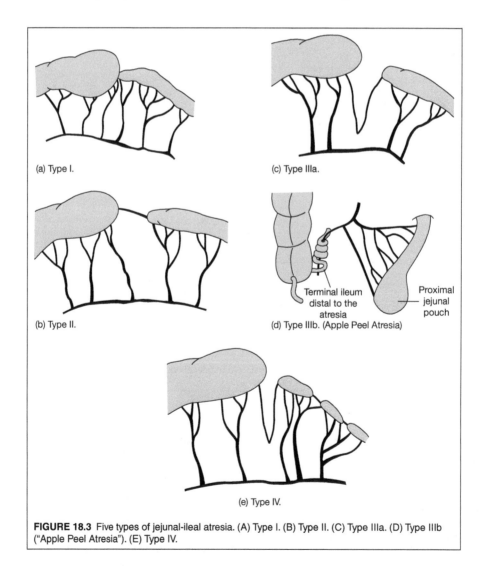

(a) Type I.

(b) Type II.

(c) Type IIIa.

(d) Type IIIb. (Apple Peel Atresia)

Terminal ileum distal to the atresia

Proximal jejunal pouch

(e) Type IV.

FIGURE 18.3 Five types of jejunal-ileal atresia. (A) Type I. (B) Type II. (C) Type IIIa. (D) Type IIIb ("Apple Peel Atresia"). (E) Type IV.

○ Abdominal x-rays are often nonspecific showing multiple dilated bowel loops with absence of air in the distal bowel reflecting some type of distal intestinal obstruction. If proximal jejunal atresia, the classic "triple" bubble will be seen (dilated stomach, dilated duodenum, dilated proximal jejunum); (Bradshaw, 2015, p. 598; Bucher et al., 2016, p. 799).

MANAGEMENT

- Preoperative management to include generalized preoperative management consistent with previously discussed pathologies secondary to GI obstructions.
- Surgery is dependent on location of the atresia and amount of intestinal involvement. The atretic intestinal portion may be tapered and connected to the distal segment with an end-to-oblique-side anastomosis, resection proximally to the point of normal bowel dimensions with an end-to-end anastomosis, or resection of the atretic area, creation of ileostomy and later reconnection (Bradshaw, 2015, p. 599; Bucher et al., 2016, pp. 799–700).
- Postoperative management similar to duodenal atresia:
  ○ Replogle to suction until return of GI function
  ○ Slow initiation of breast milk or elemental formula feeds due to common occurrence of delayed gastric emptying and microcolon distal to repair site resulting in dysmotility and feeding intolerance
  ○ Parenteral nutrition (PN) through central line such as PICC or Broviac, until able to tolerate full enteral feeds
  ○ Pain management
  ○ Antibiotics postoperatively to prevent sepsis (Bradshaw, 2015, p. 599–600; Bucher et al., 2016, p. 800)
- If there is a proximal ileostomy, high ostomy output is common due to lack of absorptive capacity which may limit advancement of feeding volume and require fluid and electrolyte replacement parenterally. Proximal output can be refed to the distal mucous fistula to promote function of the distal microcolon (Bucher et al., 2016, p. 800).

OUTCOMES

- Prognosis is related to the type of defect.
  ○ Mortality and morbidity (in particular, short bowel syndrome [SBS]) are higher with types III and IV defects. With types I and II, prognosis is generally good.
  ○ Common postoperative complications may include anastomotic leak, stricture, ileus with prolonged intestinal dysfunction, and risk for peritonitis (Bradshaw, 2015, p. 599; Bucher et al., 2016, p. 800).

Malrotation/Volvulus

DEFINITION AND PATHOPHYSIOLOGY

- Malrotation describes failure of the normal rotation and retroperitoneal fixation of the intestines that normally occurs during weeks 6 to 11 of gestation during the return from the extracoelomic position of the embryonic intestine to the fetal abdominal cavity. The hedgehog signaling pathway is responsible for transmitting information to embryonic cells required for proper cell differentiation. It is felt that abnormal hedgehog signaling can result in rotation and fixation abnormalities (Bradshaw, 2015, p. 600; Bucher et al., 2016, pp. 795–796; Fanaroff, 2013, p. 188).

- Normal rotation of the intestines occurs during physiologic midgut herniation and upon return to the abdominal cavity during weeks 10 to 12 of gestation, at which time there is fixation to the retroperitoneum in a precise pattern. Normal position of the intestines is the distal duodenum crossing to the left of the vertebral column joining the jejunum to a normally positioned ligament of Treitz; the cecum and ascending colon attaching to the right-lateral posterior body wall, whereas attaching of the descending colon is to the left-lateral body wall. The blood supply to the entire midgut is attached to the retroperitoneum from the ligament of Treitz in the upper left quadrant of the abdomen to the cecum in the right lower quadrant (Fanaroff, 2013, p. 188; Flynn-O'Brien et al., 2018, p. 1048).
  ○ Partial malrotation involves only one segment being improperly fixed.
  ○ Mixed rotation results when the midgut only rotates 180° leading to the terminal ileum reentering first, resulting is the cecum being subpyloric and fixed to the abdominal wall; this results in compression of the duodenum. If the initial rotation is clockwise, the transverse colon ends up behind the duodenum (Ditzenberger, 2018, p. 407).
  ○ With complete nonrotation, the midgut only rotates 90° and the entire intestines return en masse to the abdomen resulting in the entire small bowel lying on the right side of the abdomen and the colon lying on the left; commonly coined left-sided colon. The intestines are loosely suspended by the superior mesenteric artery and vein but are not fixed to the retroperitoneal surface; in this case, the intestines are basically free-floating, resulting in high risk for volvulus (Bucher et al., 2016, pp. 795–796; Ditzenberger, 2018, p. 407).
- Volvulus is twisting of the unfixed intestine, most commonly around the superior mesenteric artery, leading to compromise of the blood supply with rapidly evolving ischemia, bowel infarction, and necrosis, and potential loss of the entire midgut (see Figure 18.4).
- Associated with other GI abnormalities including intestinal atresia, Ladd's bands causing duodenal obstruction, and abdominal wall defects including congenital diaphragmatic hernia. Seen more commonly in males compared to females (Bradshaw, 2015, p. 600; Bucher et al., 2016, p. 796; Ringer & Hansen, 2017, p. 955).

DIAGNOSIS

- Clinical presentation of malrotation *with volvulus* is sudden onset of bilious emesis in an otherwise healthy infant who has been stooling and feeding normally. Majority of infants will become symptomatic within the first week of life, the remaining present within the first month of life; presentation after 1 month of life is less common. In cases where there is intermittent kinking of the bowel, these infants will have intermittent bilious emesis, abdominal tenderness, and poor growth. As bowel ischemia increases, the infant becomes more symptomatic with abdominal distention, lethargy, pain, bloody emesis and/or stool, and signs of hypovolemia and sepsis (Bradshaw, 2015, p. 600; Bucher et al., 2016, p. 797; Ringer & Hansen, 2017, p. 955).
- Clinical presentation of malrotation *without volvulus* is similar to infants with proximal intestinal obstruction, including symptoms of feeding intolerance followed by bilious emesis; the abdomen may be scaphoid on exam in cases (Bucher et al., 2016, p. 797).

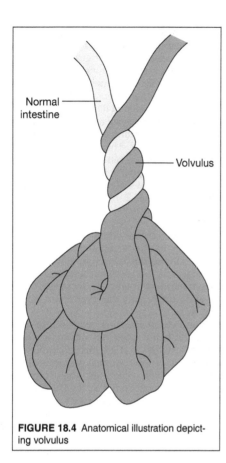

FIGURE 18.4 Anatomical illustration depicting volvulus

- A barium enema may show obstruction with failure of barium to pass beyond the transverse colon; it may show the cecum in the abnormal position confirming malrotation but provides no information about the presence or absence of a volvulus.
- Abdominal radiograph may show a pattern of obstruction with a dilated stomach and proximal duodenum, but it does not confirm or rule out malrotation; if the malrotation is intermittent, the abdominal x-ray may be normal (Bradshaw, 2015, p. 600; Bucher et al., 2016, p. 797).
- Abdominal US can be helpful if there is malrotation with volvulus which shows the twisting of the mesentery and the abnormal relationship of the mesenteric vessels, but it is user dependent (Bucher et al., 2016, p. 797).
- Gold standard for diagnosis is an upper GI that shows absent or abnormal position of the ligament of Treitz (confirms malrotation); presence of what appears as a bird's beak, suggests complete midgut obstruction (Bradshaw, 2015, p. 600; Bucher et al., 2016, p. 797; Ringer & Hansen, 2017, p. 955).
- If there is any doubt after doing diagnostic workup of malrotation with volvulus, an exploratory laparotomy is mandatory as a missed diagnosis may lead to significant loss of bowel (Fanaroff, 2013, p. 188).

MANAGEMENT
- Preoperative management includes generalized preoperative management. This is a surgical emergency and loss of bowel due to ischemia can occur in as little as 4 hours

(Bradshaw, 2015, p. 600; Bucher et al., 2016, p. 797; Flynn-O'Brien et al., 2017, p. 1049).
- Surgery is dependent on the pathology and amount of intestinal involvement. The volvulus is untwisted to allow perfusion to the bowel to be reestablished, any necrotic intestinal segments are excised with creation of an ileostomy, if Ladd's bands are present they are divided to relieve any potential duodenal obstruction, there is correction of the malrotation with the small intestine returned to the right and the large intestine returned to the left with attachment to the posterior wall, and an appendectomy is done. Removal of the appendix is done because the final location postoperatively is unpredictable making the diagnosis of appendicitis later in life problematic.
  ○ In the event of significant intestinal ischemia, marginal areas are not excised and in 24 to 48 hours the marginal area is reevaluated for additional need for resection; this approach allows the marginally viable intestinal portion the time to see if recovery is possible and hopefully result is less total bowel resection (Bradshaw, 2015, p. 600; Bucher et al., 2016, pp. 797–798).
- Postoperative management includes replogle to suction until return of bowel function (typically 4–6 days average); parenteral support is continued until full feedings obtained (Bucher et al., 2016, p. 798).
  ○ A major postoperative complication with midgut volvulus is SBS, which may lead to the infant being PN-dependent and all of the associated morbidities related to long-term parenteral needs (Bradshaw, 2015, p. 600; Bucher et al., 2016, p. 798).

OUTCOMES
- Prognosis is dependent on amount of intestinal resection and presence of other anomalies. Mortality is increased in the presence of intestinal necrosis or prematurity.

Gastroschisis

DEFINITION AND PATHOPHYSIOLOGY
- Herniation of abdominal contents through a full-thickness anterior abdominal wall defect usually to the right of an intact umbilical ring and cord. Due to lack of covering, the abdominal contents are exposed to the amniotic fluid (Bradshaw, 2015, p. 590; Bucher et al., 2016, p. 812).
- There are several theories as to the cause of the defect:
  ○ Occurs due to a vascular accident involving the right omphalomesenteric artery that weakens the anterior abdominal wall during the seventh week of gestation (Bucher et al., 2016, p. 812; Wolf, 2019, p. 400).
  ○ Failure of differentiation of the lateral fold somatopleure after return of the bowel to the peritoneal cavity and before the umbilical ring has formed (Ditzenberger, 2018, p. 407; Ledbetter, Chabra & Javid, 2018, p. 1072).
  ○ Failure in formation of the umbilical coelom at the base of the umbilical cord due to rupture of the amniotic membrane (Ditzenberger, 2018, p. 407; Ledbetter et al., 2018, p. 1072).
  ○ Intrauterine rupture of the incarcerated hernia into the umbilical cord (Ditzenberger, 2018, p. 407).
  ○ Alterations in the normal involution of the second umbilical vein or ischemic damage leading to weakness in the abdominal wall (Ditzenberger, 2018, p. 407; Wolf, 2019, p. 400).

- Occurs three to four times more frequently than an ompha-locele; this defect is associated with preterm birth and small-for-gestational age (Bucher et al., 2016, p. 812).
- Not commonly associated with major congenital anomalies or syndromes, however, association with anomalies of the GI tract is common. Malrotation is usually seen in **all** of these infants, up to 25% may have an associated intestinal atresia/stenosis as a result of the initial vascular accident or from constriction of the fascial defect compromising the affected bowel segment (Bradshaw, 2015, p. 590; Bucher et al., 2016, p. 812; Ledbetter et al., 2018, p. 1072; Ringer & Hansen, 2017, p. 958).

DIAGNOSIS
- Prenatal findings may include elevated serum alpha-fetoprotein; fetal US can confirm diagnosis early in the second trimester with multiple loops of bowel seen freely floating in the amniotic fluid with a typical "cauliflower" appearance (Bradshaw, 2015, p. 591; Wolf, 2019, p. 400). Early delivery may be warranted if there is progressive bowel distention or thickening suggesting intestinal obstruction or severe inflammation. There is minimal risk of bowel injury during vaginal delivery; therefore, vaginal delivery is not contraindicated.
- Clinical presentation includes eviscerated intestinal viscera, typically small and large intestines, that may be matted, thickened, and edematous, with no membranous sac; intact umbilical cord generally to the right of the umbilical cord (Bradshaw, 2015, p. 591; Bucher et al., 2016, p. 813; Ledbetter et al., 2018, p. 1071).

MANAGEMENT
PREOPERATIVELY
- Place in bowel bag to maintain sterile environment and allow visualization of the exposed viscera; covering defect also minimizes heat and fluid losses.
  - ○ Increased insensible water loss due to the exposed bowel may require up to three times maintenance volume.
- Alternative option is wrapping in warm–saline-soaked gauze and covering with plastic wrap, taking caution to prevent kinking of the mesenteric blood supply; gauze dressing will adhere to the viscera and cause tissue trauma when removed if not kept moistened; increased risk of hypothermia as saline cools over time.
- Minimize handling of viscera to prevent damage; handle with sterile gloves.
- Place infant with right side slightly angled down to prevent kinking of the viscera resulting in vascular compromise.
- Maintain NPO with gastric decompression to prevent restriction of intestinal blood flow due to intestinal distention.
- Provision of PN important to provide protein.
- Latex-free products should be used in all infants with congenital conditions that may require multiple procedures to minimize excessive exposure to latex and potential for development of allergies.
- Broad spectrum antibiotics (Bradshaw, 2015, pp. 591–592; Bucher et al., 2016, p. 813; Ledbetter et al., 2018, pp. 1072–1073; Ringer & Hansen, 2017, p. 955).

SURGICAL INTERVENTION
- Primary repair with return of all contents back into the peritoneal cavity with closure of the fascia and skin is the preferred method. If defect is too large or during primary repair there is impediment of intestinal blood supply from increased intra-abdominal pressure or impaired venous return, a staged repair should be done.
- There are three options for staged repair:
  - ○ One intervention involves placement of a prosthetic sac or "silo" that is sutured to the edge of the defect or secured underneath the fascia. Support of the silo at a 90° angle promotes reduction of defect by gravity and decreases the risk of vascular compromise.
  - ○ A second intervention is to apply a spring-loaded silo over the exposed viscera under the fascia; this approach is associated with fewer complications, fewer ventilator days, and shorted length of stay.
  - ○ The third intervention for staged repair involves placement of an umbilical turban with coiling of the umbilical cord over the defect; this allows epithelization to take place but may result in an umbilical hernia.
  - ○ Regardless of the approach, reduction occurs by gravity with the application of gentle pressure during daily or twice daily reduction; this gentle reduction allows the respiratory and vascular systems to slowly adjust to the increased pressure of the organs. Once the intestines are at the level of the fascia, the silo is removed, and the fascia is closed. Final closure of the defect and abdominal wall is attempted by 10 days, after this time infection risk and dehiscence of silo become major concerns (Bradshaw, 2015, pp. 592–593; Bucher et al., 2016, pp. 814–815; Ledbetter et al., 2018, pp. 1073–1074).

POSTOPERATIVE MANAGEMENT
- In the immediate postoperative period, there is a risk for intestinal obstruction, abdominal compartment syndrome, sepsis, skin necrosis over the repaired defect, and risk for complications if diminished venous return distal to the repair. Monitoring of oxygen saturations, urine output, and blood pressure continuously is imperative to detect compromise, especially after primary repair (Bradshaw, 2015, p. 593; Bucher et al., 2016, pp. 815–816).
- Maintain NPO with gastric decompression until gastric output is minimal and bowel sounds indicate readiness to begin feeds.
  - ○ Infants with gastroschisis may have a prolonged ileus, making feeding advancement a challenge. Low-osmolality feeds preferred; soy or elemental formulas may be needed for continued feeding intolerance or absorption.
- PN through central line such as PICC or Broviac, until able to tolerate full enteral feeds.
- Pain management
- Aseptic dressing changes and antibiotics postoperatively to prevent sepsis (Bradshaw, 2015, p. 593; Bucher et al., 2016, pp. 815–816).

OUTCOMES
- Prognosis is dependent on the size of the defect (large defects have higher mortality risk) and associated GI anomalies.
  - ○ The amount of intestinal dysfunction impacts the morbidity (impaired absorption, reduced enzymes, and significant dysmotility may result in SBS). Long-term complications include intestinal stricture, incisional hernia and adhesive bowel obstruction (Bucher et al., 2016, pp. 815–816; Ledbetter et al., 2018, p. 1074).

Omphalocele

DEFINITION AND PATHOPHYSIOLOGY

- A developmental defect that is felt to occur as a result of a primary folding abnormality of the germ disc during weeks 4 to 7 of gestation. There is a concomitant failure of the intestines to return during midgut herniation during weeks 8 to 11 of gestation (bowel-containing omphalocele) and an associated failure of the ventral abdominal musculature at the junction of the umbilical cord to close (Bradshaw, 2015, p. 580; Bucher et al., 2016, p. 812; Ditzenberger, 2018, p. 407; Ledbetter et al., 2018, p. 1074).
- A midline ventral wall defect with herniation of the abdominal viscera through the umbilical ring into the umbilical cord with a thin, avascular membranous sac; this covering consists of the peritoneum on the inside, amnion on the outside, and Wharton's jelly between these two layers. The umbilical cord passes through the mass and actually inserts into the membrane as opposed to the abdominal wall. The umbilical arteries and vein are inserted into the apex of the defect (Bradshaw, 2015, p. 589; Bucher et al., 2016, p. 812; Ditzenberger, 2018, p. 407; Ledbetter et al., 2018, p. 1074; Wolf, 2019, p. 404).
- High association (up to 80%) with other congenital anomalies. Chromosomal defects (including trisomies 13, 18, and 21) and CHD are seen in approximately 50% of infants with this defect. May also be associated with other midline defects such as genitourinary, craniofacial, musculoskeletal (including limb), or vertebral defects. Omphalocele can be present in several recognizable syndromes, including Beckwith–Wiedemann syndrome, cloacal entropy, OEIS complex (omphalocele, entropy, imperforate anus and spinal anomalies), and pentalogy of Cantrell (Bucher et al., 2016, p. 813; Ditzenberger, 2018, p. 407; Ledbetter et al., 2018, p. 1074; Ringer & Hansen, 2017, p. 957; Wolf, 2019, p. 404).

DIAGNOSIS

- Prenatal findings: serum alpha-fetoprotein may not be uniformly elevated as seen with gastroschisis defect; fetal US provides definitive diagnosis after the first trimester. If detected on fetal US, evaluate for other potential anomalies, especially if there is absence of the liver within the omphalocele as this is associated with aneuploidy. Fetal echo should be done. Liver herniation or herniation of other abdominal contents may warrant a cesarean section to minimize potential trauma; otherwise, as with gastroschisis, vaginal delivery can be considered (Bradshaw, 2015, p. 590; Bucher et al., 2016, p. 813; Ledbetter et al., 2018, pp. 1074–1075; Wolf, 2019, p. 404).
- Clinical presentation of defect ranging from small to large mass at the base of the umbilical cord. The defect may be covered by an intact thin, avascular membrane or the membrane may have ruptured, leaving the herniated contents exposed to the amniotic fluid as in a gastroschisis. Herniated contents can range from a few loops of intestines to potentially any abdominal organ being present, including the liver, spleen, stomach, bladder, and reproductive organs. There is a larger fascia defect with an omphalocele compared to a gastroschisis (Bradshaw, 2015, p. 590; Ditzenberger, 2018, p. 407; Ringer & Hansen, 2017, p. 957).
  - ○ Care should be taken always to examine any thickened umbilical cord closely prior to placing a cord clamp, as it may be a small omphalocele (Bradshaw, 2015, p. 590).

MANAGEMENT
PREOPERATIVELY

- As with gastroschisis, place in bowel bag to maintain sterile environment. Handle carefully to prevent tearing of the membrane (Ledbetter et al., 2018, p. 1075).
- Alternative options include covering with a nonadherent dressing to protect the sac or wrapping in warm–saline-soaked gauze and covering with plastic wrap; a gauze dressing will adhere to the viscera and cause tissue trauma when removed if not kept moistened, however, there is an increased risk of hypothermia as saline cools over time. Do not attempt to reduce the sac as it may rupture, interfere with venous return, or cause respiratory compromise (Bucher et al., 2016, p. 813; Ledbetter et al., 2018, p. 1075; Ringer & Hansen, 2017, p. 957).
- Minimize handling of viscera to prevent damage; handle with sterile gloves (Bradshaw 2015, p. 592; Bucher et al., 2016, p. 813).
- Evaluate for other potential anomalies:
  - ○ Echocardiogram to rule out CHD
  - ○ Chest and abdomen radiograph to assess bony structures and for other anomalies:
    - Abdominal US to assess structures and integrity of urinary tract
    - If uncorrectable due to congenital anomalies, provide palliative care (Bucher et al., 2016, pp. 813–814).
- Maintain NPO with gastric decompression to prevent restriction of intestinal blood flow due to intestinal distention (Bradshaw, 2015, p. 592; Ledbetter et al., 2018, p. 1073).
- Provision of PN; less evaporative and heat losses if intact sac so may not need as much volume support compared to if the sac is ruptured (Bucher et al., 2016, p. 813).
- Latex-free products
- Broad spectrum antibiotics (Ringer & Hansen, 2017, p. 957).

SURGICAL REPAIR

- Surgery more emergent if sac is ruptured (Ringer & Hansen, 2017, p. 958).
- Primary repair with removal of sac, return of all contents back into the peritoneal cavity, and closure of the fascia and skin, is the preferred method (Bradshaw, 2015, p. 592; Bucher et al., 2016, p. 814).
- If the defect is too large or during primary repair there is impediment of intestinal blood supply from increased intra-abdominal pressure or impaired venous return, OR if the infant has uncorrectable congenital anomalies, the defect is painted with an escharotic agent, with epithelization occurring within 10 to 20 weeks (Bradshaw, 2015, p. 592; Bucher et al., 2016, p. 814).
  - ○ If painting with escharotic agent, assess for potential adverse systemic effects from the agent used (Bradshaw, 2015, p. 593).

POSTOPERATIVE MANAGEMENT

- If primary repair done, in the immediate postoperative period there is a risk for intestinal obstruction, abdominal compartment syndrome, sepsis, and risk for complications if diminished venous return distal to the repair (Bradshaw, 2015, p. 593; Bucher et al., 2016, p. 815). Monitoring of oxygen saturations, urine output, and blood pressure continuously is imperative to detect compromise.

- Maintain NPO with gastric decompression until gastric output is minimal and bowel sounds indicate readiness to begin feeds.
  - ○ Feeding advancement is typically not a problem unless the sac was not intact and then, like infants with gastroschisis, there may be a prolonged ileus, making feeding advancement a challenge.
- PN through central line such as PICC or Broviac, until able to tolerate full enteral feeds
- Pain management
- Aseptic dressing changes and antibiotics postoperatively to minimize risk of sepsis (Bradshaw, 2015, p. 593; Bucher et al., 2016, pp. 815–816).

OUTCOMES
- Prognosis is related to the size of the defect, the severity of associated congenital anomalies, and if there are any challenges to closing the defect (Bradshaw, 2015, p. 590; Bucher et al., 2016, p. 816; Ledbetter et al., 2018, p. 1075).
  - ○ Possible short- and long-term complications include intestinal stricture, incisional hernia, and adhesive bowel obstruction (Bucher et al., 2016, p. 816).

ABNORMALITIES INVOLVING THE HINDGUT

Hirschsprung Disease (congenital megacolon, aganglionic megacolon)

DEFINITION AND PATHOPHYSIOLOGY
- Congenital absence of the ganglion cells of a segment of the colon resulting in a functional obstruction. More commonly affects the rectum or the rectosigmoid portion of the colon; less commonly may extend to proximal colon. It is the most common cause of large bowel obstruction in the newborn (Bradshaw, 2015, p. 604).
- Caused by failure of the ganglion cells prior to 12 weeks of gestation to migrate cephalocaudally, resulting in partial or complete aganglionosis of the submucosal and mesenteric plexuses of the colon. Absence of ganglion cells prevents the inhibitory relaxation normally regulated by parasympathetic nerves, leading to functional obstruction because the affected segment is unable to relax and becomes dysfunctional.
- There is increased hypertrophy of the normally innervated proximal portion of the colon as it attempts to overcome the functional obstruction. The presence of ganglion cells to the area of no ganglion cells is referred to as the transition zone. The time at which migration of the ganglion cells stopped determines the length of bowel involved (Bradshaw, 2015, p. 604; Bucher et al., 2016, p. 806; Flynn-O'Brien et al., 2018, p. 1051).
- There are at least eight genomes associated with Hirschsprung disease, explaining family history in up to one-third of cases. Almost 20% of patients with Hirschsprung disease may have chromosomal abnormalities, most commonly Trisomy 21 (Bradshaw, 2015, p. 604; Bucher et al., 2016, p. 807; Flynn-O'Brien et al., 2018, p. 1052).
- The oral, facial, and cranial ganglia arise from the same neural crest as the ganglionic plexus of the bowel, so other associated anomalies may also be present, such as sensorineural deafness with central alveolar hypoventilation, ocular neuropathies, systemic anomalies associated with Smith–Lemli–Opitz syndrome, and cardiovascular with skeletal and limb anomalies seen in DiGeorge syndrome. Colonic atresia and imperforate anus may also be present. Males are affected four times more often than females (Bradshaw, 2015, p. 604; Bucher et al., 2016, p. 807; Flynn-O'Brien et al., 2018, p. 1052).

DIAGNOSIS
- Clinical presentation in the newborn includes failure to pass meconium spontaneously by 48 hours of age, increased abdominal distention, and bilious emesis. Rectal stimulation often results in passage of stool. If the obstruction continues, risk for enterocolitis increases evidenced by diarrhea, obstipation, progressive abdominal distention, vomiting, poor feeding with failure to thrive, lethargy, and fever. Hirschsprung disease in some cases does not present until older infancy or childhood with chronic constipation problems (Bradshaw, 2015, p. 604; Bucher et al., 2016, p. 807; Fanaroff, 2013, p. 190; Flynn-O'Brien et al., 2018, p. 1051; Ringer & Hansen, 2017, p. 956).
- Rectal biopsy is the gold standard to confirm diagnosis demonstrating absence of ganglion cells and hypertrophic nonmyelinated axons in the nerve plexus. Histochemical tests of the biopsy samples show an increase in acetylcholine. Suction or punch biopsy can be done at the bedside; however, full thickness biopsy needs to be done under general anesthesia (Bradshaw, 2015, p. 604–605; Flynn-O'Brien et al., 2018, p. 1052; Ringer & Hansen, 2017, p. 952).
- A contrast barium enema suggests the diagnosis showing the contracted rectosigmoid colon with contrast material entering the proximal dilated bowel; in newborns, the conical tapering demonstrating the transition zone is not always evident. Barium retained for greater than 24 hours after a contrast enema is suggestive of Hirschsprung disease.
- Abdominal x-ray demonstrates proximal bowel distention with absence of air at the point of the obstruction to the rectum demonstrating a bowel obstruction (Bradshaw, 2015, p. 604; Fanaroff, 2013, p. 190; Ringer & Hansen, 2017, p.952).

MANAGEMENT
- Medical management includes gentle rectal irrigations with warm saline solution twice a day to empty the colon and minimize the risk for enterocolitis until surgery.
  - ○ If the rectal irrigations evacuate stool, feedings can continue.
  - ○ If unable to evacuate stool and increased abdominal distention with emesis, feedings are stopped, and preoperative management includes generalized preoperative management for bowel obstruction (Bradshaw, 2015, p. 605; Bucher et al., 2016, p. 807–808; Ringer & Hansen, 2017, p. 952).
- Surgery goal is to bring the normal ganglionated bowel down to the anus using a pull-down procedure. If the infant develops enterocolitis, is preterm, is less than 2 kg, or has significant proximal bowel distention, the abnormally innervated area of the colon is removed, a colostomy is done with a pull-through procedure done later (Bradshaw, 2015, p. 605; Bucher et al., 2016, p. 808; Fanaroff, 2013, p. 190; Flynn-O'Brien et al., 2018, p. 1052).
- Postoperative management is similar to other GI obstruction disorders; in addition, these infants receive routine rectal

irrigations with normal saline postoperatively to decrease the risk for recurrent enterocolitis (Bradshaw, 2015, p. 605).

- ○ Postoperatively if colostomy required, need to monitor for prolapse, skin dehiscence with excoriation, and stomal ulceration and bleeding.
- ○ Approximately 2 weeks postoperatively following primary pull-through, a series of anal dilations occur in those infants that had a primary pull-through procedure.

- Diet adjustments may need to be made to improve stool consistency; in some cases, loperamide (Imodium) may be required to reduce stool frequency or kaolin–pectin suspensions to solidify stools (Bradshaw, 2015, p. 605; Bucher et al., 2016, p. 809).

OUTCOMES

- Prognosis is based on time of diagnosis, development of enterocolitis, and amount of bowel affected. Postoperative complications may include anastomotic leak or stricture. Morbidity associated with continued elimination problems despite removal of the aganglionic segment can be seen; surgical intervention is not curative as despite surgical resection, there is still an abnormally innervated anal sphincter. These infants remain at risk for persistent constipation, encopresis, and life-threatening enterocolitis with functional outcomes not known until the child reaches the age of toilet-training.
  - ○ Mortality is increased with delayed diagnosis, especially if enterocolitis develops as bacterial translocation can lead to overwhelming systemic sepsis (Bradshaw, 2015, p. 605; Flynn-O'Brien et al., 2018, p. 1052; Ringer & Hansen, 2017, p. 956).

Anorectal Malformations

DEFINITION AND PATHOPHYSIOLOGY

- A broad spectrum of anomalies characterized by an absent or abnormally located anus outside the normal sphincter muscles. This can be a stenotic or atretic anal canal that may be isolated, include a fistulous communication between the urogenital tract or vagina and the rectum, or in females a complex persistent cloaca (Bradshaw, 2015, p. 605; Bucher et al., 2016, p. 809; Flynn-O'Brien et al., 2018, p. 1052).
- Caused by failure of differentiation of the urogenital sinus and cloaca during early embryonic development (Bradshaw, 2015, p. 606). Persistent cloaca in females is the result of arrest of development during weeks 4 to 6 of gestation of the gut and the complete separation from the urogenital tract. If the disruption of the cloacal membrane occurs before the urorectal septum has separated the urinary bladder from the hindgut, cloacal exstrophy occurs. Whereas, if the disruption of the cloacal membrane occurs after septation, exstrophy of the bladder occurs (Bucher et al., 2016, p. 810).
- Imperforate anus is classified based on the level of the defect:
  - ○ High lesions are above the levator muscle component of the anal sphincter muscle complex (can be estimated by drawing an imaginary pubococcygeal line); a low defect occurs below this area. High defects are more common in contrast to low lesions, are more common in males, generally more complex with rectourinary or rectovaginal fistulas, more likely to be associated with

other malformations, and more likely to have incontinence if sacral anomaly present due to lack of innervation to the bowel and/or bladder.
  - ○ Low lesions occur in both sexes equally and commonly may have a perineal fistula (Bradshaw, 2015, pp. 605–606; Bucher et al., 2016, p. 810; Ringer & Hansen, 2017, p. 955).

- There is a common association of VACTERL anomalies and Trisomy 21 with anorectal malformations. There is also a high incidence of cryptorchidism in males and spinal dysraphism. Imaging of the spine should be done as well as other evaluation based on physical exam (Bradshaw, 2015, p. 606; Bucher et al., 2016, p. 810).

DIAGNOSIS

- Clinical presentation may include absence of an anal opening with imperforate anus. In the case of anal stenosis or an anal membrane there is visually a normal appearing rectum, but failure to pass meconium with increasing abdominal distention prompts further evaluation (Bradshaw, 2015, p. 606).
- Diagnosis of imperforate anus is based on physical examination reflecting absence of an anal opening. Presence of a fistula needs to be determined. A fistula may not be evident until up to 24 hours of life; presence of meconium in the urine is diagnostic for a rectourinary fistula and presence of meconium in the vaginal vault is diagnostic for a rectovaginal fistula (Bucher et al., 2016, p. 810; Ringer & Hansen, 2017, p. 955)
- Abdominal radiograph shows increased bowel gas pattern with lack of air in the rectum (Bucher et al., 2016, p. 810). An inverted lateral radiograph is sometimes done in an attempt to determine the level of the air-filled rectal pouch (Bradshaw, 2015, p. 606).
- A perineal US may be helpful in determining the termination of the rectum and its distance from the skin (Bucher et al., 2016, p. 810).
- A contrast study of the urethra in males will determine if fistula is present or not and a contrast genitogram in females will determine the anatomic relationships of a persistent cloaca (Bucher et al., 2016, p. 810).

MANAGEMENT

- Preoperative management includes generalized preoperative management while evaluation is underway. An echocardiogram, spine radiographs, and renal/spinal USs should be done to rule out other anomalies that are commonly seen. Infants with a fistula are at high risk for developing a hyperchloremic acidosis due to colonic absorption of urine (Bucher et al., 2016, pp. 810–811).
- Surgery is always necessary, but the procedure is dependent on the level of the defect.
  - ○ Intermediate and high defects require a colostomy with pull-through procedure done later (ranges from 3 to 8 months). Colostomy closure is done about 6 to 8 weeks after anorectoplasty if no stricture present.
  - ○ Low defects have good outcome with anoplasty that may be done in the newborn period or by first month of life. With low defects if there is no associated fistula, a colostomy will be required temporarily.
  - ○ If there is a perineal fistula and early repair not possible, dilation twice daily is done to promote elimination of stool until able to have a surgical procedure performed (Bradshaw, 2015, p. 606; Bucher et al., 2016, p. 811).

- Postoperative management includes stoma care and parent teaching if colostomy has been done with later definitive repair. Anal dilation is started 2 weeks postoperatively to prevent anal stenosis, and may be continued for several months. If the fistula has not been divided, antibiotic prophylaxis for urinary tract infections should be administered and bicarbonate supplementation may be necessary (Bradshaw, 2015, pp. 606–607; Bucher et al., 2016, pp. 811–812).

OUTCOMES

- Prognosis is generally excellent with low defects; there is an increased risk of constipation that may require anal dilation if related to a stricture and in rare cases, revision of the anoplasty may be required. Prognosis for infants with high defects is determined by the amount of sphincter muscle development and innervation with bowel incontinence strongly associated long term. Long-term complications may also include urinary incontinence, ejaculatory dysfunction, and erectile dysfunction (Bradshaw, 2015, p. 606; Bucher et al., 2016, p. 812; Flynn-O'Brien et al., 2018, p. 1053).

DISORDERS INVOLVING THE SMALL/LARGE INTESTINE

Meconium Ileus

DEFINITION AND PATHOPHYSIOLOGY

- Mechanical obstruction of the distal lumen of the *ileum* due to thick, tenacious meconium; the proximal segment of the bowel is dilated. More complex forms may be associated with volvulus, intestinal atresia, or perforation with meconium peritonitis (Bradshaw, 2015, p. 601; Bucher et al., 2016, p. 803; Ringer & Hansen, 2017, p. 954).
- Ninety percent of infants with meconium ileus have cystic fibrosis (CF) due to an autosomal recessive gene defect that results in alteration of the chloride channel transporter and transport of fluid across the epithelial cells (Bucher et al., 2016, p. 803; Ringer & Hansen, 2017, p.954).
- Two implicating factors: hyposecretion of pancreatic enzymes or abnormal viscid secretions from the mucous glands of the intestines. Pancreatic enzymes are necessary for digestion of intestinal contents, when lacking there are abnormal amounts of proteins and glycoproteins causing the meconium/stool to be thick and viscid (Bradshaw, 2015, p. 601; Bucher et al., 2016, p. 803). In patients with CF, there are gene mutations in the CF transmembrane regulator (CFTR) that affect transport of bicarbonate and chloride resulting in the characteristic meconium that adheres to the intralumen of the bowel wall resulting in obstruction (Flynn-O'Brien et al., 2018, p. 1050).

DIAGNOSIS

- Prenatal findings may include polyhydramnios, ascites, hyperechoic appearance, or dilation of the bowel; pathognomonic for meconium ileus is in utero meconium peritonitis with perforation noted as intra-abdominal calcifications (Bucher et al., 2016, p. 803; Fanaroff, 2013, p. 189). Meconium ileus may be suspected prenatally when there is a family history of CF or when parents are carriers of the CFTR mutations; in these cases, diagnosis can be confirmed by fetal DNA analysis (Flynn-O'Brien et al., 2018, p. 1050).

- Clinical presentation with uncomplicated meconium ileus presents by 24 to 48 hours of life with bilious emesis, progressive abdominal distention, failure to pass meconium despite digital stimulation, and a dough-like sensation on palpation due to the thickened meconium in the distal bowel. May manifest more abruptly and progress more quickly in complex forms with abdominal distention within the first 24 hours of life, an erythematous edematous abdomen, and respiratory distress (Bradshaw, 2015, p. 601; Bucher et al., 2016, pp. 803–804; Fanaroff, 2013, p. 189; Ringer & Hansen, 2017, p. 954).

DIAGNOSIS

- Gold standard for diagnosis is a water-soluble contrast enema showing a microcolon and pellets of meconium at the site of the distal obstruction. In up to 60% of the cases, fluid is drawn into the intestine during the contrast study, dislodging the meconium and allowing normal intestinal activity (Bradshaw, 2015, p. 601; Bucher et al., 2016, p. 805; Ringer & Hansen, 2017, p. 954).
- On abdominal x-ray there are distended loops of bowel with few air–fluid levels due to the viscous nature of the meconium; in addition, the distal intestine may have a "soap bubble" appearance as tiny air bubbles are mixed within the meconium (Bradshaw, 2015, p. 601; Bucher et al., 2016, p. 805; Fanaroff, 2013, p. 189; Ringer & Hansen, 2017, p. 954).
  - In complex cases, there may be scattered calcification if an intrauterine perforation occurred (Bradshaw, 2015, p. 601; Bucher et al., 2016, p. 805).

MANAGEMENT

- Medical management includes replogle to low suction, parenteral fluid support, and water-contrast enema (Gastrografin or Hypaque are common agents used).
- Maintenance fluids up to one- and one-half normal needs are required due to rapid fluid shifts from the contrast agents that can lead to hypovolemic shock; this is seen more commonly with use of hyperosmolar agents. Additional enemas may be required if meconium is not passed (Bradshaw, 2015, p. 602; Bucher et al., 2016, p. 805; Ringer & Hansen, 2017, pp. 954, 956).
  - It is important to monitor for the first 48 hours after the enema for potential intestinal perforation; the risk for perforation increases with each successive enema (Bradshaw, 2015, p. 602; Bucher et al., 2016, p. 805).
  - In some cases, *N-acetylcysteine* (Mucomyst) enema(s) are used to break up the abnormal meconium and relieve the obstruction (Flynn-O'Brien et al., 2018, p. 1051).
- Surgery is required to relieve the intestinal obstruction if the contrast enema(s) fails to relieve the meconium obstruction (Bradshaw, 2015, p. 602; Flynn-O'Brien et al., 2018, p. 1051; Ringer & Hansen, 2017, p. 956).
- With simple cases, a T-tube enterostomy is done to allow continued irrigations after surgery. With complex cases, resection of compromised intestinal segment with end-to-end anastomosis or creation of an ostomy and later connection is done (Bradshaw, 2015, p. 602; Bucher et al., 2016, p. 805; Flynn-O'Brien et al., 2018, p. 1051).
- Postoperative management is similar to duodenal and small intestine obstructions. In addition, these infants may require irrigation of the T-tube enterostomy or the distal stoma with N-acetylcysteine or pancreatic enzymes, typically started after a couple of days post-operatively.

- Due to high association with CF, chest physiotherapy (CPT), supplemental humidity and aerosolized mucolytic agents, such as Mucomyst, are provided to prevent atelectasis and pneumonia. These infants also require supplementation of feedings with pancreatic enzymes.
- Parental education on pulmonary hygiene, infection prevention, nutritional supplements, and genetic counseling is important (Bradshaw, 2015, pp. 602–603).

OUTCOMES
- Prognosis is dependent on the presence of associated anomalies and the number and degree of organs involved as a result of CF (Bradshaw, 2015, p. 601; Bucher et al., 2016, p. 806).

Meconium Plug

DEFINITION AND PATHOPHYSIOLOGY
- Mechanical obstruction of the distal lumen of the *colon* due to thick, tenacious meconium in the absence of enzymatic deficiency or abnormalities of the ganglion cells (Bradshaw, 2015, p. 603; Bucher et al., 2016, p. 803).
  - With Hirschsprung disease or meconium ileus associated with CF, these infants may have a meconium plug but there is an underlying disorder causing the plug.
- Results from colonic dysmotility and meconium clearance and is more commonly associated with both maternal and neonatal conditions:
  - Maternal diabetes due to increased fetal glycogen production, which results in decreased bowel motility
  - Maternal magnesium therapy due to myoneural depression, which results in decreased bowel motility
  - Neonatal central nervous system disease with hypotonia
  - Neonatal sepsis
  - Prematurity (Bradshaw, 2015, p. 603; Fanaroff, 2013, p. 189; Ringer & Hansen, 2017, p. 956)

DIAGNOSIS
- Clinical presentation includes failure to pass meconium by 48 hours of life, hyperactive bowel sounds, increasing abdominal distention, and a late sign is bilious emesis. Seventy-five percent of newborns expel the plug spontaneously (Bradshaw, 2015, p. 603; Fanaroff, 2013, p. 189).
- The gold standard is performing a water-soluble contrast enema which can be both diagnostic and therapeutic. A contrast enema will outline the intraluminal plug leading often to expulsion of the meconium plug (Bradshaw, 2015, p. 603; Fanaroff, 2013, p. 189).
- Rectal examination should be done prior to diagnostic work-up and often prompts the passage of the characteristic yellowish-white, gelatinous plug.
- An abdominal x-ray is nonspecific with multiple dilated loops of bowel, with no air in the rectum consistent with bowel obstruction (Bradshaw, 2015, p. 603).

MANAGEMENT
- Medical management includes rectal stimulation, which may expel the plug in some circumstances, and enemas of warm saline, meglumine diatrizoate, or acetylcysteine.
- Surgery is rare and indicated when medical management does not result in expulsion of the plug.

- If the symptoms persist or recur, must consider CF and Hirschsprung disease requiring additional workup (Bradshaw, 2015, p. 603–604; Fanaroff, 2013, p. 189).

OUTCOMES
- Prognosis is excellent if no associated conditions exist (Bradshaw, 2015, p. 603).

Small Left Colon Syndrome

DEFINITION AND PATHOPHYSIOLOGY
- A form of meconium plug syndrome. A functional distal bowel obstruction caused by transient dysmotility in the descending colon results in normal meconium becoming impacted in the distal portion of the colon. In meconium plug syndrome, the obstruction is generally in the sigmoid colon. In small left colon, the site of obstruction is the splenic flexure which is small in caliber (Gorman, 2017, p. 919).
- Up to 50% of cases of small left colon syndrome is seen in infants of diabetic mothers (Gorman, 2017, p. 919).

DIAGNOSIS
- Clinical presentation includes failure to pass meconium within the first 24 to 36 hours of life and generalized abdominal distention with bilious emesis (Ehret, 2015, p. 274; Fanaroff, 2015, p. 190).
- Gold standard for diagnosis is water-contrast enema; this procedure may also be therapeutic resulting in evacuation of stool (Ehret, 2015, p. 274).
- Abdominal radiography may show dilation of the proximal colon with abrupt narrowing of the distal colon usually at the splenic flexure (Fanaroff, 2013, p. 190).

MANAGEMENT
- Medical management is conservative treatment with enemas (Lee-Parritz & Cloherty, 2012, p. 22).

OUTCOMES
- Prognosis is excellent with resolution of stooling difficulties occurring in the first month of life (Fanaroff, 2013, p. 190).

ACQUIRED DISORDERS OF THE GASTROINTESTINAL TRACT

Necrotizing Enterocolitis (NEC)

DEFINITION AND PATHOPHYSIOLOGY
- The most common acquired disease, mainly of preterm infants, characterized by inflammation of the bowel wall and necrosis. The terminal ileum and proximal ascending colon are the most frequent involved sites (Bucher et al., 2016, p. 801; Weitkamp, Premkumar, & Martin, 2017, p. 340).
- NEC is a multifactorial disease resulting from complex interactions between intestinal immaturity, abnormal microbial colonization with poor host response to injury, and feedings. The interplay of these result in mucosal injury, intestinal inflammation, and ischemia progressing to necrosis, and bacterial translocation across the compromised intestinal barrier with a proinflammatory response (Bucher et al., 2016, p. 801; Ditzenberger, 2018, p. 427, 475; Javid, Riggle, & Smith, 2018, p. 1091; Weitkamp et al., 2017, p. 354).

○ The innermost intestinal mucosa is affected first, but as the disease progresses, the muscular and subserosal layers of the intestine become involved. Proliferation of colonizing bacteria leads to the release of endotoxins and cytokines. Bacterial fermentation leads to gaseous distention further compromising intestinal blood flow (Bucher et al., 2016, p. 801; Ditzenberger, 2018, p. 427; Javid et al., 2018, pp. 1091–1092; Weitkamp et al., 2017, p. 355).

- Although enteral feedings appear to be a key trigger, keeping a preterm infant NPO actually increases the incidence of NEC and is not protective (Wilson-Costello, Kleigman, & Fanaroff, 2013, pp. 193–194).
- Risk factors in preterm infants include:
  ○ Prematurity is the single greatest risk factor, with increasing risk with decreasing gestational age.
  ○ Immaturity of the intestinal tract related to decreased immunologic factors, increased gastric pH, immature intestinal epithelial barrier allowing translocation to occur and dysmotility of the intestine.

○ Up to 90% of infants who develop NEC have been fed. It is hypothesized that the presence of feeds and oral medication increase intestinal oxygen demand during absorption resulting in tissue hypoxia; in addition, fluid shifts into the intestine occur resulting in decreased intestinal blood flow and intestinal ischemia (Bradshaw, 2015, p. 607; Bucher et al., 2016, pp. 801–802; Javid et al., 2018, pp. 1090–1091; Weitkamp et al., 2017, p. 355).

- Risk factors in term infants include:
  ○ Presence of cyanotic CHD (Figure 18.5), polycythemia, sepsis, hypotension, asphyxia, intrauterine growth restriction, cocaine exposure in utero, and a history of gastroschisis (Javid et al., 2018, p. 1090; Weitkamp et al., 2017, pp. 354–355).
- Transfusion-related NEC is a distinct entity that can also lead to NEC (Ditzenberger, 2018, p. 245, 434). That phenomenon requires separate discussion and will not be covered in this chapter.

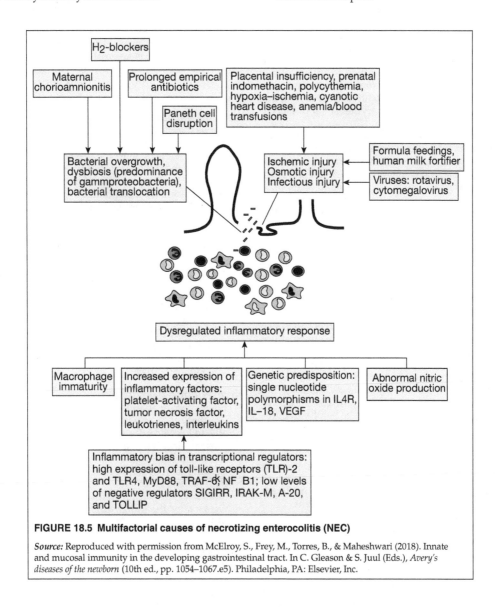

FIGURE 18.5 Multifactorial causes of necrotizing enterocolitis (NEC)

Source: Reproduced with permission from McElroy, S., Frey, M., Torres, B., & Maheshwari (2018). Innate and mucosal immunity in the developing gastrointestinal tract. In C. Gleason & S. Juul (Eds.), *Avery's diseases of the newborn* (10th ed., pp. 1054–1067.e5). Philadelphia, PA: Elsevier, Inc.

- Preventative measures include prevention of preterm birth, and antenatal steroids with threatened preterm delivery (Weitkamp et al., 2017, p. 364; Wilson-Costellom et al., 2013, p. 195).
- Measures associated with lowering risk of NEC include exclusive human milk diet, standardized feeding protocol especially in the very low birth weight (VLBW) population, and avoiding use of H2-blockers (this allows the acidic environment to remain). There is some potential benefit with the use of *Bifidobacterium* probiotics (Bradshaw, 2015, p. 607; Bucher et al., 2016, pp. 801–802; Javid et al., 2018, pp. 1095–1096; Weitkamp et al., 2017, p. 364).

DIAGNOSIS

- Postnatal onset is inversely related to birthweight and gestational age, with a mean gestation age for presentation of NEC typically between 30 and 32 weeks (Weitkamp et al., 2017, p. 354).
- Clinical presentation varies from a subtle course to an overwhelming fulminant course associated with high rate of mortality and morbidity.
  - A subtle presentation may include general systemic signs mistaken for sepsis including lethargy, temperature instability, increased apnea and bradycardia events, poor feeding, in addition to GI symptoms including feeding intolerance (emesis, increased gastric aspirates), abdominal distention with or without tenderness, abdominal wall erythema, and bloody stools.
  - If undetected, the clinical course will progress, displaying increased systemic signs such as respiratory distress, decreased perfusion, hypotension, metabolic acidosis, oliguria, and coagulopathies (Bradshaw, 2015, p. 608; Bucher et al., 2016, p. 802; Weitkamp et al., 2017, pp. 342–343).
- Laboratory findings are nonspecific; however, a common triad is thrombocytopenia, persistent metabolic acidosis, and refractory hyponatremia (Bradshaw, 2015, p. 608; Bucher et al., 2016, p. 802; Weitkamp et al., 2017, p. 357).
- Radiological findings are diagnostic with presence of pneumatosis intestinalis (hallmark finding of hydrogen gas in the bowel wall), portal venous gas, and/or pneumoperitoneum.
  - A fixed bowel loop on serial studies and stacking of intestinal loops supports the concern for NEC. Presence of periumbilical air collection noted in an anterior–posterior x-ray is referred to as the "football sign."
  - Ultrasound can also be used to evaluate for the presence of portal venous gas and pneumatosis (Javid et al., 2018, pp. 1092–1093; Weitkamp et al., 2017, p. 357).
- Bell staging is an important tool that allows comparison of infants across clinical sites but can also be helpful in guiding management
  - Stage 1 (*suspected*)—clinical signs and symptoms as discussed above and inconclusive radiologic findings
  - Stage 2 (*definite*)—clinical signs and symptoms with presence of *pneumatosis or portal venous gas* on x-ray; further divided into *2A* for mildly ill infant and *2B* for moderately ill infant with systemic clinical signs
  - Stage 3 (*advanced*)—also divided into two stages; *3A* for same as stage 2B but now critically ill infant with concern for impending perforation, *3B* proven intestinal perforation with *pneumoperitoneum* on x-ray (Javid et al., 2018, pp. 1092–1093; Weitkamp et al., 2017, p. 357; Wilson-Costello et al., 2013, p. 194).

MANAGEMENT
MEDICAL MANAGEMENT

- Medical management is geared toward supportive care.
  - Stage 1 NEC management includes bowel rest (NPO), fluid resuscitation, replogle to suction to decompress and allow better intestinal bowel wall perfusion, monitoring labs (complete blood count [CBC], electrolytes), blood culture with broad spectrum antibiotics to cover enteric flora, abdominal x-rays every 4 to 8 hours (for progression of disease), and discussion with pediatric surgery specialists.
  - Management for Stage 2 NEC includes the same medical management as Stage 1, in addition lateral decubitus x-rays should be done due to increased risk for pneumoperitoneum now that there is pneumatosis intestinalis and/or portal venous air, addition of anaerobic agent should be considered, placement of central line once blood cultures remain negative at 48 hours, supportive care, and official pediatric surgery consultation.
  - Management for Stage 3: NEC includes supportive care (treatment of coagulopathies and hypotension, may need intubation and mechanical ventilation) and pediatric surgery consultation with intervention. Medical management is successful in more than 50% of infants (Bradshaw, 2015, pp. 608–609; Bucher et al., 2016, p. 802; Javid et al. 2018, p. 1094; Weitkamp et al., 2017, p. 360).

SURGICAL MANAGEMENT

- Surgery indicated if abdominal free air present; may also be indicated if the clinical picture is worsening despite medical management, for the presence of portal venous gas, or if there is a persistent fixed intestinal loop on serial x-rays in the symptomatic infant.
  - Surgery goal traditionally has been to excise necrotic bowel while preserving as much viable intestine as possible and creation on an ostomy. If there is extensive involvement, no or minimal intestinal excision is done with a second operation in 24 to 48 hours to determine if some of the questionable areas are viable
  - If the infant is extremely unstable or in extremely low birth weight (ELBW) infants, a peritoneal drain may be placed as a temporizing measure; in some cases, additional surgery may be initially everted but there is a suggested increased incidence of strictures (as the inflamed intestine heals, there is scarring of the intestinal wall; Bradshaw, 2015, p. 609; Bucher et al., 2016, pp. 802–803; Javid et al., 2018, pp. 1094–1095; Weitkamp et al., 2017, p. 363).

POSTOPERATIVE MANAGEMENT

- Bowel rest for 10 to 14 days
- PN through a central line such as PICC or Broviac until able to tolerate full enteral feeds; once intestinal motility is present, slow introduction of low osmolar elemental feeds can be started.
- Continuation of antibiotics
- Pain management
- Stoma closure with reanastomosis is typically done 6 to 8 weeks after the initial surgery (Bradshaw, 2015, pp. 609–610; Weitkamp et al., 2017, p. 363)

OUTCOMES

- Prognosis is dependent on numerous factors. There are decreased mortality rates in agencies that have

TABLE 18.4 Implications of Intestinal Loss

Area of Intestine	Function	Complications Associated With Loss
Jejunum	Digestion and absorption	Nutritional deficiencies, steatorrhea, cholestasis
Ileum	Absorption of fat-soluble vitamins, vitamin B12, and bile salts	Metabolic and nutritional consequences

standardized therapeutic protocols defining medical and surgical management and with early diagnosis (Weitkamp et al., 2017, p. 363).

- Infants with Stage 2B and higher have an overall higher incidence of mortality, growth delay, and poor neurodevelopmental outcomes. Infants that required surgical intervention also have increased mortality secondary to sepsis, respiratory failure, and parental nutrition–associated liver disease (PNALD); (Weitkamp et al., 2017, p. 363).
  - ○ Up to one-third of infants treated medically develop an intestinal stricture in the large bowel as a result of cicatricial scarring of the previous inflamed bowel. Additional morbidity in the immediate postoperative period includes stoma prolapse or retraction, wound dehiscence, sepsis, and recurrent NEC.
- Long-term morbidity can include SBS (if less than 40 cm of bowel remains with no ileocecal value, of if <20 cm with presence of ileocecal valve which will be discussed later in this chapter), malabsorption and chronic diarrhea, cholestasis secondary to long-term PN, failure to thrive, metabolic bone disease, and increased risk of impaired neurodevelopmental outcome (Bradshaw, 2015, p. 608; Bucher et al., 2016, p. 803; Javid et al., 2018, p. 1095; Weitkamp et al., 2017, pp. 363–364). There is a risk for recurrent NEC in up to 6% of infants, however, in these cases medical management is usually successful (Javid et al., 2018, p. 1095).

Spontaneous Intestinal Perforation (SIP)

DEFINITION AND PATHOPHYSIOLOGY

- SIP is an isolated perforation not associated with intestinal ischemia or necrosis. This is a distinctly different disease process compared to NEC (Javid et al., 2018, p. 1090; Weitkamp et al., 2017, p. 358).
- SIP is associated with the presence of an umbilical artery catheter (UAC), early administration of indomethacin or ibuprofen, early administration of postnatal steroids, or having a patent ductus arteriosis (PDA) or intraventricular hemorrhage (IVH) in the extremely preterm infant. There is an association with a history of maternal chorioamnionitis in some of the cases (Bradshaw, 2015, p. 607; Fanaroff, 2013, p. 193; Weitkamp et al., 2017, p. 358).

DIAGNOSIS

- Clinical presentation is usually in the first 1 to 2 weeks of life with acute abdominal distention, often with a blue discoloration of the abdominal wall as a result of meconium butting up against the thin, abdominal wall. Less hemodynamic instability and less metabolic acidosis compared to NEC. The onset of presentation is much earlier than seen with NEC.
- Gold standard for diagnosis is the clinical presentation with abdominal radiography (anterior–posterior, left

lateral decubitus, or cross-table lateral imaging) showing a pneumoperitoneum (Bradshaw, 2015, p. 607; Javid et al., 2018, p. 193; Weitkamp et al., 2017, p. 358).

MANAGEMENT

- Preoperative management includes NPO with replogle to low suction, supportive care for respiratory or cardiac instability, and antibiotic therapy including an anaerobic agent.
- Surgical options include the placement of a peritoneal drain (if the infant is unstable) or laparotomy with resection of the segment of the bowel with the perforation. An end-to-end anastomosis may be done, or an ostomy created with reconnection planned in the future when the infant is older (Fanaroff, 2013, p. 193; Weitkamp et al., 2017, p. 357).

OUTCOMES

- Prognosis is good with lower mortality and morbidity as well as neurodevelopmental impairment compared to intestinal perforation from NEC (Javid et al., 2018, p. 1090).

Short Bowel Syndrome (SBS)

DEFINITION AND PATHOPHYSIOLOGY

- Normal GI function consists of digestion and absorption of nutrients. Carbohydrates, proteins, and fats must be broken down into smaller molecules of monosaccharides, oligopeptides, amino acids and free fatty acids, and monoglycerides so that absorption into the intestinal epithelial cells and into the portal circulation can occur. Understanding this process makes the understanding of alterations in digestion or absorption with loss of bowel clearer (Dimmitt, Sellers, & Sibley, 2017, p. 1032).
- Following surgical resection, malabsorption and malnutrition as a result of loss of intestine absorptive surface area may result in SBS. The amount of malabsorption and malnutrition is dependent on:
  - ○ how much and what segments of the intestine remain as this will determine the amount of surface area for absorption and which functions of the resected segment were lost, and
  - ○ whether or not the ileocecal valve was able to be preserved. The ileocecal valve slows down transit time to increase absorption and prevents bacterial colonic overgrowth in the small intestine (Bradshaw, 2015, pp. 610–611).

DIAGNOSIS

- Diagnosis of SBS varies and may be based on length of remaining bowel or on the presence of intestinal failure. Intestinal failure due to inadequate length or function occurs with any length of remaining bowel that is unable to meet fluid, electrolyte, and energy requirements of the infant. Intestinal adaptation involves significant structural and functional alterations, the progress of which is often unpredictable and individualized (Javid et al., 2018, p. 1096).

MANAGEMENT
- Medical management is complex and requires multidisciplinary care. Management includes parenteral nutrition and providing as much enteral nutrition as possible, even if only small amounts. Cycling of PN may be necessary if infant develops cholestasis. Skin care is important at the ostomy site and after reanastomosis in the perianal area due to diarrhea. Speech involvement is important to provide appropriate oral stimulation (Bradshaw, 2015, p. 611).
- When medical management fails, surgical bowel lengthening procedures to increase intestinal surface area or to decrease motility may be attempted. Small-bowel transplant is considered when other surgical procedures fail, and the patient cannot attain enteral autonomy (Bradshaw, 2015, p. 611; Javid et al., 2018, p. 1097).
- Following surgery, the remaining bowel will over 1 to 2 years make adaptive changes that leads to increased digestion and absorption of nutrients. Initially the proximal bowel dilates to increase the mucosa surface area for absorption. In addition, there is increased crypt depth, increased villous height, and an increase in the number of enterocytes to allow for mucosal hyperplasia. This period of adaptation may continue over several years. Adaptation occurs less in the jejunum compared to the ileum, however, other areas of the intestine can perform the functions lost by the jejunum therefore, these infants tend to do better than infants with loss of the ileum (see Table 18.4; Bradshaw, 2015, p. 610; Javid et al., 2018, p. 1096).

OUTCOMES
- The past decade has demonstrated significant improvements in long-term survival of children with SBS. These improvements are multifactorial and include improved delivery of parenteral nutrition, prevention of infection, and innovative bowel-lengthening techniques (Javid et al., 2018, p. 1096).
- Survival is possible with as little as 15 cm small bowel with an intact ileocecal valve or with 30 to-45 cm small bowel with absence of the ileocecal valve (Bradshaw, 2015, p. 611). Eventual tolerance of full feeds is possible with as little as 25 cm small bowel with an intact ileocecal valve or with more than 40 cm and no ileocecal valve (Ditzenberger, 2018, p. 425).

OTHER CONCERNS INVOLVING THE GI TRACT

Inguinal Hernia

DEFINITION AND PATHOPHYSIOLOGY
- Bulging of the intrabdominal contents through the normal internal and external ring openings of the abdominal wall muscles in the groin.
  - If only fluid protrudes through the opening, it is a hydrocele (Ledbetter et al., 2018, p. 1077).
- Inguinal hernia occurs when the tunica vaginalis and the peritoneal cavity fail to close, resulting in a persistent processus vaginalis.
- Inguinal hernias occur more commonly in preterm, small-for-gestational age and male infants. Occurs more frequently on the right side compared to the left, however can be bilateral (Fanaroff, 2013, p. 191; Ledbetter et al., 2018, p. 1077; Ringer & Hansen, 2017, pp. 960–961).

DIAGNOSIS
- Clinical presentation of inguinal hernias includes a bulge in the groin that can extend into the scrotum in males or labia in females (Ledbetter et al., 2018, p. 1077). Hydroceles can be differentiated by transillumination of the scrotal sac.

MANAGEMENT
- Surgery indicated if the hernia contents become strangulated or prior to discharge as these do not spontaneously heal but get larger over time (Ledbetter et al., 2018, p. 1077).
  - With strangulation (incarceration), sedation to relax infant with steady firm pressure and elevation of feet may reduce the hernia back into the abdomen; once edema has resolved, surgery should be done promptly (Ringer & Hansen, 2017, p. 961).
  - Hydroceles usually resolve by 1 year of age if they are present at birth (Ledbetter et al., 2018, p. 1077).

OUTCOMES
- Prognosis excellent if not incarcerated. Most common complication postoperatively is apnea (Fanaroff, 2013, p. 191; Ringer & Hansen, 2017, p. 961).

Gastroesophageal Reflux

DEFINITION AND PATHOPHYSIOLOGY
- GER is the physiologic movement of gastric contents up into the esophagus, with or without regurgitation. Gastroesophageal reflux disease (GERD) is the pathologic passage of those gastric contents into the esophagus that is associated with failure to grow, a variety of significant symptoms, and complications such as respiratory distress or esophagitis.
- There are several factors in the neonate and infant correlated with reflux including a shorter and narrower esophagus, relaxation of the lower esophageal segment, delayed esophageal clearance, excessive air in the stomach, delayed gastric emptying, and/or decreased esophageal motility (Bradshaw, 2015, p. 615; Ditzenberger, 2018, p. 427; Richards & Goldin, 2017, pp. 1079–1080).
  - The lower esophageal segment forms a pressure barrier between the esophagus and the stomach and in the neonate is positioned primarily above the diaphragm allowing reflux to occur (Ditzenberger, 2018, p. 427).
- More common in preterm than term infants, in infants with neurologic or GI disorders, in infants with brochopulmonary dysplasia (BPD) or as adverse effect of some medications such as methylxanthines (Bradshaw, 2015, p. 615).

DIAGNOSIS

- Clinical presentation includes feeding difficulties, fussiness or irritability, or back arching (Bradshaw, 2015, p. 615). It is important to rule out other underlying causes that may cause these symptoms, such as cow's milk protein allergy, neurologic disorders, excessive gassiness, or constipation (Richards & Goldin, 2017, p. 1079).
- Diagnosis is most often based on physical symptoms.
  - ○ Upper GI series may miss reflux events since they can be transient (false negative).
  - ○ Esophageal pH probe studies do not detect nonacid reflux, which is more common in neonates due to milk-based diet.
  - ○ Endoscopy is helpful in identifying esophageal erosion (Bradshaw, 2015, p. 616).

MANAGEMENT

- Medical management strategies include elevating head of bed at least 45° and trying to keep upright for 30 minutes after feedings, positioning prone if severe reflux or right-side down, administering gavage feedings over a longer time period, small frequent feeds if oral feeding, frequent burping, and thickening of feeds (Bradshaw, 2015, p. 616; Parad & Benjamin, 2017, p. 458).
  - ○ There are currently no approved U.S. Food and Drug Administration (FDA) medications for pharmacologic management of GER in infants. Medications that have been trialed, such as metoclopramide, a prokinetic, have been associated with significant adverse reactions and should not be used (Anderson, Poindexter, & Martin, 2018, p. 280; Richards & Goldin, 2017, pp. 1081–1081). PPIs in the infant with documented esophagitis may be trialed and if no improvement in irritability, should be discontinued (Richards & Goldin, 2017, p. 1081).
- When conservative and pharmacologic management fails and the infant develops consequences from GERD such as development of strictures, erosive esophagitis, failure to thrive, aspiration, recurrent pneumonia, wheezing, and asthma, the most common surgical procedure considered is a Nissen fundoplication (Bradshaw, 2015, p. 616; Richards & Goldin, 2017, pp. 1079, 1082).

OUTCOMES

- Prognosis is good as it typically self-resolves in majority of infants by 1 to 1 1/2 years of age. A small percentage of infants require prolonged medical management or even surgery.
  - ○ In infants with GERD, morbidity includes worsening of BPD, aspiration, esophagitis, strictures, and failure to thrive (Bradshaw, 2015, p. 616; Ditzenberger, 2018, p. 427).

CONCLUSION

Gastrointestinal obstructions are one GI disorder that may be seen in the neonate and can occur anywhere from the esophagus to the anus. Most GI obstructions are not considered surgical emergencies except for malrotation with volvulus. It is often difficult to differentiate between the different disorders; however, a thorough history and physical examination may help guide the diagnostic workup.

REVIEW QUESTIONS

1. A 12-hour-old term infant who has not stooled since delivery and no has persistent increasing emesis. On physical examination there is mild upper abdominal distention, otherwise the abdomen is soft with no tenderness. An x-ray is obtained and shown here. The most likely diagnosis based on the radiograph is:

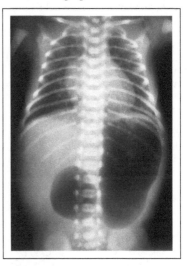

   A. duodenal atresia
   B. ileal closure
   C. jejunal stenosis

2. The NNP is called to evaluate a former 26-week infant who is now 28 5/7 weeks' corrected age who has demonstrated clinical changes including increased oxygen needs, more frequent apnea and bradycardia events, and recurrent emesis with feedings. An abdominal x-ray is ordered and pictured here. The changes in the infant's condition and the findings on this radiograph raise concern for the infant having:

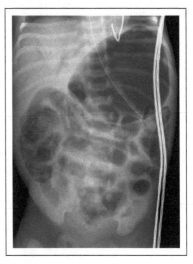

   A. malrotation with volvulus
   B. necrotizing enterocolitis
   C. obstruction of the colon

3. The NNP is consulted regarding a 3-day-old term infant who has a sudden onset of bilious emesis after feeding and stooling well. Pregnancy and delivery history are unremarkable and the infant is otherwise healthy. The correct diagnosis, until proven otherwise, is a/an:
   A. cystic fibrosis-related meconium plug
   B. malrotation and/or mid-gut volvulus
   C. onset of allergic colonic enterocolitis

4. A large-for-gestational-age term infant has not stooled by 48 hours of age, and a contrast enema shows retained barium after 36 hours. An appropriate intervention would be to perform a:
   A. decubitus radiograph
   B. repeat contrast study
   C. warm saline enema

5. Following bowel resection after necrotizing enterocolitis (NEC), infants who tend to recover more fully are those with an intact:
   A. duodenum
   B. ileum
   C. jejunum

REFERENCES

Anderson, D. M., Poindexter, B. B., & Martin, C. R. (2017). Nutrition. In E. Eichenwald, A. Hansen, C. Martin, & A. Stark (Eds.), *Cloherty and Stark's manual of neonatal care* (8th ed., pp. 280). Philadelphia, PA: Wolters Kluwer.

Bradshaw, W. T. (2015). Gastrointestinal disorders. In M. T. Verklan & M. Walden (Eds.), *Core curriculum for neonatal intensive care nursing* (5th ed., pp. 583–631). St. Louis, MO: Elsevier Saunders.

Bucher, B. T., Pocatti, A. S., Lauvorn, H. N., & Carter, B. S. (2016). Neonatal surgery. In S. L. Gardner, B. S. Carter, M. E. Hines., & J. A. Hernandez (Eds.), *Merenstein & Gardner's handbook of neonatal intensive care* (8th ed., pp.790–816). St. Louis, MO: Elsevier.

Dimmitt, R., Sellers, Z. K., & Sibley, E. (2018). Gastrointestinal tract development. In C. Gleason & S. Juul (Eds.), *Avery's diseases of the newborn* (10th ed., pp. 1032–1038). Philadelphia, PA: Elsevier.

Ditzenberger, G. (2018). Gastrointestinal and hepatic systems and perinatal nutrition. In S. Blackburn (Ed.), *Maternal, fetal, & neonatal physiology: A clinical perspective* (5th ed., pp. 387–434). Maryland Heights, MO: Elsevier.

Ehret, L. (2015). Radiologic evaluation. In T. Verklan & M. Walden (Eds.), *Core curriculum for neonatal intensive care nursing* (5th ed., pp. 253–281). St. Louis, MO: Elsevier.

Fanaroff, A. (2013). Part two: Selected disorders of the gastrointestinal tract. In A. A. Fanaroff & J. M. Fanaroff (Eds.), *Klaus and Fanaroff's care of the high-risk neonate* (6th ed., pp. 184–200). Philadelphia, PA: Elsevier Saunders.

Flynn-O'Brien, K., Rice-Townsend, S., & Ledbetter, D. (2018). Structural anomalies of the gastrointestinal tract. In C. Gleason & S. Juul (Eds.), *Avery's diseases of the newborn* (10th ed., pp. 1039–1053). Philadelphia, PA: Elsevier.

Gorman, T. (2017). Neonatal effects of maternal diabetes. In E. Eichenwald, A. Hansen, C. Martin, & A. Stark (Eds.), *Cloherty and Stark's manual of neonatal care* (8th ed., pp. 910–922). Philadelphia, PA: Wolters Kluwer.

Javid, J., Riggle, K. M., & Smith, C. (2018). Necrotizing enterocolitis and short bowel syndrome. In C. Gleason & S. Juul (Eds.), *Avery's diseases of the newborn* (10th ed., pp. 1090–1097). Philadelphia, PA: Elsevier.

Ledbetter, D. J., Chabra, S., & Javid, P. J. (2018). Abdominal wall defects. In C. Gleason & S. Juul (Eds.), *Avery's diseases of the newborn* (10th ed., pp. 1068–1078). Philadelphia, PA: Elsevier.

Lee-Parritz, A., & Cloherty, J. P. (2012). Diabetes mellitus. In J. P. Cloherty, E. C. Eichenwald, A. R. Hansen, & A. R. Stark (Eds.), *Manual of neonatal care* (7th ed., pp. 11–23). Philadelphia, PA: Lippincott Williams & Wilkins.

McElroy, S., Frey, M., Torres, B., & Maheshwari (2018). Innate and mucosal immunity in the developing gastrointestinal tract. In C. Gleason & S. Juul (Eds.), *Avery's diseases of the newborn* (10th ed., pp. 1054–1067.e5). Philadelphia, PA: Elsevier.

Parad, R., & Benjamin, J. (2017). Bronchopulmonary dysplasia/Chronic lung disease. In E. Eichenwald, A. Hansen, C. Martin, & A. Stark (Eds.), *Cloherty and Stark's manual of neonatal care* (8th ed., pp. 446–460). Philadelphia, PA: Wolters Kluwer.

Richards, M. K., & Goldin, A. B. (2018). Neonatal gastrointestinal reflux. In C. Gleason & S. Juul (Eds.), *Avery's diseases of the newborn* (10th ed., pp. 1079–1083). Philadelphia, PA: Elsevier.

Ringer, S., & Hansen, A. (2017). Surgical emergencies in the newborn. In E. Eichenwald, A. Hansen, C. Martin, & A. Stark (Eds.), *Cloherty and Stark's manual of neonatal care* (8th ed., pp. 942–966). Philadelphia, PA: Wolters Kluwer.

Weitkamp, J., Premkumar, M., & Martin, C. (2017). Necrotizing enterocolitis. In E. Eichenwald, A. Hansen, C. Martin, & A. Stark (Eds.), *Cloherty and Stark's manual of neonatal care* (8th ed., pp. 353–365). Philadelphia, PA: Wolters Kluwer.

Wilson-Costello, D., Kliegman, R. M., & Fanaroff, A. A. (2013). Part three: Necrotizing enterocolitis. In A. A. Fanaroff & J. M. Fanaroff (Eds.), *Klaus and Fanaroff's care of the high-risk neonate* (6th ed., pp. 184–200). Philadelphia, PA: Elsevier Saunders.

Wolf, R. (2019). Abdominal imaging. In R. Resnik, C. Lockwood, T. Moore, M. Greene, J. Copel, & R. Silver (Eds.), *Creasy and Resnik's maternal-fetal medicine: Principles and practice* (8th ed., pp. 393–413.e11). Philadelphia, PA. Elsevier.

19 THE RENAL SYSTEM

Cheryl A. Carlson
Lori Baas Rubarth

INTRODUCTION

In the past 25 years, the field of neonatal nephrology has expanded in conjunction with that of neonatology, influenced by the development of therapies and interventions to promote survival among the smallest of infants. The expanded understanding of acute kidney injury (AKI) and therefore increase in incidence has necessitated the development of preventative approaches. The improved survival of infants who develop significant chronic lung disease has led to new renal-focused complications. Finally, the use of prenatal ultrasounds has created new paradigms for prenatal management of renal tract anomalies (Vogt & Dell, 2015, p. 1676). This chapter provides a brief review of the embryology, physiology, and pathophysiology of the renal system.

ANATOMY AND PHYSIOLOGY

Kidney

- The kidney is located in the retroperitoneal space on both sides of the vertebral column.
- The kidney is approximately 4.0 to 5.0 cm in length in a full-term infant; length is related to gestational age in millimeters (Cavaliere, 2019, p. 122).
- The kidney develops from the pronephros, mesonephros, and metanephros into the true kidney, which begins functioning at about 9 to 10 weeks of gestation. Nephrogenesis, the process of nephron formation, is complete by about 34 to 36 weeks of gestation, with the critical time between 31 and 36 weeks. Once nephrogenesis is complete, the kidney contains 800,000 to 1.2 million nephrons and there is only growth of individual nephrons after completion of nephrogenesis (Blackburn, 2013, p. 370; Engen & Hingorani, 2018, p. 1250; McAleer, 2018, p. 1248; Sherman, 2015, pp. 719–720; Vogt & Dell, 2015, p. 1677).
  - The metanephros' origins are in the pelvis and then ascends to the abdomen between the fifth and ninth week of gestation (Merguerian & Rowe, 2018, p. 12611).
- The nephron is the functional unit of the kidney, with each kidney containing a glomerulus, renal tubules, and the collecting system (Blackburn, 2013, p. 371; Merguerian & Rowe, 2018, p. 1261).
  - The glomerulus lies within Bowman's capsule and filters plasma, allowing nonprotein components of the plasma to pass into Bowman's capsule and then into the renal tubule system.
  - The renal tubular system is a filtration system that allows plasma to pass through the renal tubule system.
  - The proximal tubules lie in the cortex of the kidney and continue to become the loop of Henle, which descends into the renal medulla making a loop and ascending back into the cortex.
  - The tubule then becomes the distal convoluted tubule, which joins those from other nephrons to form the collecting tubules and collecting duct (Blackburn, 2013; Merguerian & Rowe, 2018, p. 1301). The tubules and loop continue to grow after birth.
- Renal blood flow is dependent on cardiac output. Renal arteries come off the aorta at L1–L2.
- Circulation of the nephrons is supported by two capillary beds—the afferent arterioles that supply oxygenated blood to the glomerulus and the efferent arterioles that drain blood unable to enter Bowman's capsule continuing to form the peritubular capillary system.
  - The peritubular capillary system follows along the renal tubular system allowing for the specific functions of the tubular system. Venous blood leaves the kidneys through the renal veins emptying into the inferior vena cava.
- Bladder formation begins between 4 and 6 weeks of gestation. The ureters go from kidneys to bladder and are functionally open at about 9 weeks of gestation. The urethra's development is complete by 12 to 13 weeks of gestation (Vogt & Dell, 2015, p. 1679).
- The glomerular filtration rate (GFR) is the amount of filtrate formed within the glomerulus each minute (Blackburn, 2013, p. 358).
  - The GFR is calculated using serum and urinary creatinine levels. The GFR is low in utero and increases initially due to increases in glomerular perfusion pressure, after which the increase in GFR is related to the increase in renal blood flow.
  - The major determinate of GFR is blood pressure in the peritubular capillary system. Other factors that influence the GFR are: (a) hydrostatic pressure in the glomerular capillaries and Bowman's capsule, and (b) the colloid osmotic pressure within the capillaries. The average rates of GFR are the following (Samuels, Munoz, & Swinford, 2017, p. 376; Vogt & Dell, 2015, p. 1680):
    1. Preterm less than 34 weeks: 13 to 15 mL/min/1.73 m^2
    2. Term infant at birth: 15 to 60 mL/min/1.73 m^2
    3. Term infants at 2 weeks: 63 to 80 mL/min/1.73 m^2
    4. Adult levels by 2 years of age: 120 mL/min/1.73m^2 (Vogt & Dell, 2015, p. 1680)

Roles of Renal Tubules (Blackburn, 2018, p 358)

- **Filtration**: process where the plasma filtrated from the vascular space in the afferent arterioles into Bowman's capsule forms filtrate in the renal tubules in the glomerulus.
- **Reabsorption:** movement of substances from the renal tubules across the tubular epithelium into the peritubular capillaries.
- **Secretion:** movement of substances from the peritubular capillaries across the tubular epithelium into the renal tubules.
- **Excretion**: loss of metabolic wastes and toxins, as well as the fluid that makes up urine. Substances such as urea, creatinine, uric acid, urates, and toxins are filtered in the glomerulus and not reabsorbed, allowing for their excretion in the urine.

Tubular Function

- Proximal tubules are re-absorptive generally and will reabsorb water, sodium, potassium glucose, amino acids, bicarbonate, phosphorous, magnesium, chloride, and calcium. Substances such as organic acids and hydrogen ions are secreted.
- Distal convoluted tubules secrete potassium and hydrogen ions, with water reabsorption in the presence of arginine vasopressin. Reabsorption of sodium is variable and dependent on the presence of aldosterone.
- Loop of Henle and collecting ducts dilute or concentrate urine. Preterm infants have a decreased ability to concentrate urine and respond to a fluid load (Vogt & Dell, 2015, p. 615).

Urine Formation

- Formed from filtrate in Bowman's capsule
- Movement of substances between the tubular lumens and the plasma in the peritubular capillaries
- Renal blood flow and GFR affects the function of the renal tubules.

Hormonal Regulation

- The kidney is responsible for maintaining both systemic blood pressure and renal blood flow.
- Autoregulation of renal blood flow is accomplished through the vasorelaxation and vasoconstriction of the afferent and efferent arterioles to maintain a constant blood supply to the kidneys, despite variations in systemic blood pressure (hypotension or hypertension).
  - ○ Regulated by the renin–angiotensin–aldosterone–antidiuretic hormone (ADH) system and atrial and B natriuretic factors
  - ○ Other vaso-reactive factors affecting renal blood flow include endothelin, nitric oxide, and prostaglandins.
- Renal perfusion is measured indirectly by monitoring the concentration of sodium chloride by the macula densa cells in the ascending loop of Henle.
  - ○ A decrease in sodium chloride will cause a relaxation of the afferent arteriole, allowing for increased blood flow into the glomerulus.
  - ○ The macula densa cells will stimulate the juxtaglomerular cells, located in the afferent and efferent arterioles.
  - ○ This will release renin, activating the renin–angiotensin–aldosterone–ADH system.

The Goal of the Renin–Angiotensin–Aldosterone-ADH System

- The goal is to maintain adequate renal perfusion and blood flow to vital organs by increasing sodium chloride and water reabsorption by the peritubular capillaries to increase intravascular volume, increasing cardiac output and blood pressure.
- **Renin** is released in response to decreased renal blood flow; will convert angiotensinogen released from the liver to angiotensin I
- **Angiotensin** I will undergo further conversion to angiotensin II, in the lungs and renal endothelium under the actions of angiotensin-converting enzyme (ACE)
- **Angiotensin II** is a potent vasoconstrictor of peripheral blood vessels and the efferent arteriole that increases tubular sodium, chloride, and water reabsorption in the renal tubules.
- **Aldosterone,** a mineral–corticoid hormone, is released by the adrenal cortex in response to angiotensin II, adrenocorticotrophic hormone, or hyperkalemia. Aldosterone increases intravascular volume through sodium, chloride, and water reabsorption and excretion of potassium and hydrogen ions.
- **Arginine vasopressin** or **ADH** is produced in the hypothalamus, stored in the posterior pituitary, and released in response to decreased intravascular volume or an increase in plasma osmolality and angiotensin II.
  - ○ Arginine vasopressin increases the permeability of the collecting ducts to water and allows increased water reabsorption into the peritubular capillaries, increasing intravascular volume.
- **Atrial natriuretic protein (ANP)** and **B natriuretic protein (BNP)** reverse the renin–angiotensin–aldosterone–ADH system.
  - ○ ANP is secreted by the cardiac atria myocytes in response to increased intravascular volume; BNP is released in response to left ventricular dilation. It acts by decreasing renin level, decreasing conversion of angiotensin I to angiotensin II, and decreasing release of aldosterone.
  - ○ Overall effect is peripheral vasodilation, decreased blood pressure, decreased intravascular volume and increase in diuresis (Blackburn, 2013, pp 361–362; McAleer, 2018, p. 1247).

Major Functions of the Kidney

- At birth, the kidneys become the major homeostatic organs, replacing the placenta in functions such as:
  - ○ Removal of metabolic wastes
  - ○ Regulation of fluid volume and electrolyte composition
  - ○ Acidbase homeostasis
  - ○ Regulation of blood pressure
  - ○ Regulation of red blood cell production through release of erythropoietin, a hormone that stimulates the production of erythrocytes by the bone marrow
  - ○ Regulation of calcium, phosphorous, and magnesium homeostasis through metabolism of vitamin D into active metabolite (Samuels et al., 2017, p. 368)

Newborn Renal Function

- There are gestational age differences in renal function due to tubular developmental and functional maturity at birth.

Renal function will improve with an increase in renal blood flow, GFR, and tubular function due to postnatal transition in all infants, in spite of gestational age at birth (Blackburn, 2013, pp. 372–375; McAleer, 2018, pp. 1247–1248).

- Asphyxia or ischemic damage may occur prenatally, during birth, or after birth, further affecting renal function (Askenazi, Selewski, Willig, & Warady, 2018, pp.1282–1289).
- Overall differences in newborn and adult kidney function (Blackburn, 2013, p. 372; McAleer, 2018, pp. 1247–1248):
  o Decreased renal blood flow in neonate
  o Reduced GFR, especially in preterm infants <34 weeks gestation due to immature renal development and function
  o Reduced ability to excrete fluid and solute
  o Altered tubular function in term infants after birth
  o Decreased response of renal tubules to aldosterone especially in preterm infants

ASSESSMENT OF INFANT WITH ABNORMAL KIDNEY FUNCTION

Family and Prenatal History

- Family history of renal disorders including urinary tract abnormalities, polycystic kidney disease, or familial diseases such as autosomal recessive polycystic kidney Ddisease (ARPKD) or congenital nephrotic syndrome. Prenatal ultrasound can be used to evaluate fetal kidney and urinary tract.
- Prenatal history includes maternal disease state, medications during pregnancy and labor, amniotic fluid volume, and prenatal ultrasound.
  o Elevated maternal serum or amniotic alpha-fetoprotein levels may indicate obstructive uropathy, renal agenesis, or congenital nephrotic syndrome.
  o Oligohydramnios can be associated with decreased fetal urine output, renal agenesis, dysplasia, polycystic kidney disease, or urinary tract obstruction.
  o Polyhydramnios may be due to renal tubular dysfunction and decreased ability to concentrate urine.
  o Maternal use of ACE inhibitors, indomethacin (nonsteroidal anti-inflammatory drugs [NSAIDs]), or angiotensin receptor blockers will affect renal capillary pressure, leading to a decrease in GFR.
  o Perinatal asphyxia/depression during or after delivery is associated with hypoxic or ischemic damage to the kidneys (Vogt & Dell, 2015, pp. 1684–1685).

Physical Assessment

- Presence of abdominal mass on examination
- Abdominal wall defects
- Abnormal facies, ear malformations
- Abnormal genitalia
- Hypospadias/epispadias
- Single umbilical artery
- Palpation of bladder (Cavaliere, 2019, p. 122)

Clinical Assessment

- Signs of volume depletion or volume overload
- Heart rate and blood pressure

- Urine output (Samuels et al., 2017, p. 370)
  o Approximately 90% of newborns will void in first 24 hours and 99% by 48 hours of age.
  o Range of urine formation 0.5 to 5 mL/kg/hour
- Presence of edema
- Total fluid intake including medications and flush volume

Laboratory Assessment

- Serum electrolytes
  o Blood urea nitrogen (BUN) may be elevated in AKI or in hypercatabolic states or with increased protein intake (BUN >29 mg/dL or increase of 1 mg/dL/day).
  o Creatinine initially reflective of maternal renal function and depending on gestational age will either remain the same and then decrease as kidneys mature. An increase in serum creatinine is suggestive of renal dysfunction (creatinine >1.5 mg/dL or increase of >0.2 mg/dL/day).
    ▪ Preterm infants will often have increased creatinine levels over the first week of life due to decreased GFR.
  o BUN/creatinine ratio
    ▪ Prerenal azotemia—disproportionate rise
    ▪ Intrinsic AKI—proportionate rise
  o Sodium maybe decreased due to fluid overload from decreased urine output or loss of sodium in the urine
  o Potassium is often elevated in AKI due to decreased renal excretion.
  o Calcium and phosphorous levels may be abnormal due to renal tubular dysfunction (Samuels et al., 2017, p. 377).
- Complete blood count and differential to evaluate for sepsis
- Urinalysis and culture
- Urine electrolytes if significant serum electrolyte abnormalities
- Serum albumin
- Renal and bladder ultrasound
- Urinalysis (Samuels et al., 2017, p. 372; Vogt & Dell, 2015, p. 1680):
  o Specific gravity should be about 1.021 to 1.025 in full-term infants due to limited concentrating ability.
  o Protein excretion will vary with gestational age and is higher in preterm infants <34 weeks' gestation. In term infants, protein excretion after 2 weeks of life is minimal. If present, associated with damage to the glomerulus.
  o Glycosuria is common in preterm infants <34 weeks due to decreased tubular resorption of glucose in infants that is increased with lower gestational ages.
  o Hematuria is an abnormal presentation and may indicate intrinsic kidney injury due to acute tubular necrosis (ATN).
- Calculation of fractional excretion of sodium (FENa%); Askenazi et al., 2018, p. 1287; Vogt & Dell, 2015, p. 1685)
  o Amount of urinary sodium excretion is a percentage of the filtered sodium, reflecting the balance between glomerular filtration and tubular reabsorption of sodium (Doherty, 2017, p. 299).
  o FENa (%) = (urine Na × plasma creatinine)/plasma Na × urine creatinine) × 100%
    ▪ FENa >3.0% indicative of intrinsic renal injury
    ▪ FENa <2.5% indicative of pre-renal injury

■ FENa values not helpful in preterm infants less than 32 weeks gestation due to normal baseline values being as high as 6%: May be as high as 15% in very low birth weight (VLBW) infants during the first week of life, decreases by 1 month of age.

ACUTE KIDNEY INJURY

AKI—deterioration of renal function that occurs over hours to days presenting as mild renal dysfunction to complete anuric renal failure.

Definition and Etiology

- Serum creatinine greater than 1.5 mg/dL has been used, but there are difficulties in defining AKI due to wide variability of serum creatinine levels in neonates due to gestational age changes, low GFR, and initial levels reflective of maternal creatinine levels.
  - ○ Other markers of renal function include urine output, urine and serum neutrophil gelatinase–associated lipocalin (NGAL), serum cystatin C, and urine interleukin-18. Further research is needed as these values will vary based on gender, gestational age, and day of life. With further research the goal is to use these biological markers to detect injury early and determine the cause and tissue injured (Askenazi et al., 2018, p. 1281; Vogt & Dell, 2015, p. 1684)
- Most common cause of AKI in neonates related to hypoperfusion or decreased blood flow to the kidney.
  - ○ May be due to neonatal asphyxia causing both anoxic and ischemic damage to kidney, blood loss, fluids loss from intravascular compartment due to sepsis or third space losses, dehydration, or shock. Tubular function and reabsorption are intact in most cases of prerenal azotemia.

PRERENAL

- Prerenal azotemia accounts for up to 85% of AKI. Potential causes include:
  - ○ Hypotension/hypoperfusion
  - ○ Congestive heart failure
  - ○ Respiratory distress/hypoxia
  - ○ Dehydration
  - ○ Hypoalbuminemia
  - ○ Nephrotoxic medications such as ACE inhibitors, intrautero exposure to NSAIDs, COX2 inhibitors, angiotensin receptor antagonists, aminoglycosides (Askenazi et al., 2018, p. 1283–1285; Vogt & Dell, 2015, p. 1684)

INTRINSIC

- AKI may result as a prolongation of prerenal causes of renal injury, ischemic injury, or injury as a result of obstructive causes of renal injury (Askenazi et al., 2018, p. 1285).
  - ○ Congenital abnormalities
  - ○ Inflammation/infection due to congenital viral or yeast infections
  - ○ Vascular/ischemia hypoperfusion such as aortic or artery thrombosis
  - ○ Nephrotoxic medications either in utero or postnatal administration
  - ○ ATN may be due to perinatal asphyxia or secondary to nephrotoxic medications.

- Intrinsic damage can be divided into several phases, which is helpful in the diagnosis, management, and prognosis of the disorder. These are divided as early, initiation, maintenance, and recovery phases (Askenazi et al., 2018, p. 1284).
  - ○ **Early** (prerenal) phase may be associated with hypoperfusion of the kidney due to prerenal causes.
  - ○ **Initiation** phase includes the initial insult and the effect on the GFR.
  - ○ **Maintenance** phase—tubular dysfunction and low GFR is seen in the maintenance phase and the duration will depend on the extent and duration of the initial insult.
  - ○ **Recovery** phase can take months, during which there is a gradual improvement in GFR and tubular function.

POSTRENAL

- AKI is primarily due to obstructive kidney dysfunction occurring in utero, though postnatal causes include renal calculi or fungal balls.
  - ○ Posterior urethral valves (PUVs)
  - ○ Bilateral ureteropelvic junction obstruction (UPJO)
  - ○ Bilateral ureterovesical junction obstruction
  - ○ Neurogenic bladder
  - ○ Obstructive nephrolithiasis (Askenazi et al., 2018, p. 1286).

Incidence

- Variable due to different diagnostic criteria, ranging from 8% to 24% (Askenazi et al., 2018, p. 1282; Vogt & Dell, 2015, p. 1684).
- Risk factors include:
  - ○ VLBW and extremely low birth weight (ELBW)
  - ○ Low 5-minute Apgar score
  - ○ Maternal medications, especially antibiotics and NSAIDs
  - ○ Intubation at birth
  - ○ Respiratory distress syndrome (RDS)
  - ○ Patent ductus arteriosus (PDA)
  - ○ Phototherapy
  - ○ Neonatal drug administration (NSAIDs, antibiotics, and diuretics)
  - ○ Congenital diaphragmatic hernia
  - ○ Extracorporeal membrane oxygenation (Askenazi et al., 2018, p. 1282; Vogt, & Dell, 2015, p. 1684)

Clinical Presentation

- Oliguria
- Systemic hypotension
- Volume overload or dehydration
- Decreased activity (Vogt & Dell, 2015, p. 1684).

LABORATORY CHANGES

- Elevated serum creatinine
- Hyperkalemia
  - ○ Defined as a serum level obtained by a central sample that is >6 to 6.5 mEq/L
  - ○ Remove all potassium from intravenous (IV) fluids.
  - ○ Therapies that cause a temporary increase in uptake of potassium (K^+) by the cells (Askenazi et al., 2018, p. 1288):
    - ■ Calcium gluconate (100%) 1 to 2 mL/kg is used to decrease the effects of elevated potassium on cardiac muscle cells' excitability.

- Sodium bicarbonate is used to correct metabolic acidosis increasing the serum pH which will shift the K^+ into the cells temporarily, though efficacy in acute AKI is controversial (Askenazi et al., 2018, p. 1288).
  - Glucose and insulin solution can be used to shift K+ back into the cells temporarily.
  - Albuterol increases cellular uptake of potassium through Na^+/K^+ ATPase activity and increase in insulin levels (Samuels et al., 2017, p. 384).
  ○ Furosemide 1 mg/kg given intermittently or as continuous infusion to decrease fluid overload, if there is urine output
  ○ Sodium polystyrene sulfonate (Kayexalate) rectal administration to draw potassium from colon. Not recommended for use in premature infants or low birth weight infants due to the risk of rectal perforation with insertion of rectal/enema tube.
  ○ Metabolic acidosis may develop acutely in severe AKI due to decreased tubular reabsorption of bicarbonate and decreased excretion of hydrogen (H^+) ion (Askenazi et al., 2018, p. 1289).
    - Judicious use of sodium bicarbonate in treatment is important due to increased risk of fluid overload with the use of large doses.
- Metabolic acidosis
- Hypocalcemia
  ○ May be a result of increased calcium deposition in injured tissues, resistance to parathyroid hormone (PTH) and skeletal release of calcium, due to decrease in vitamin D metabolism in injured kidney (Askenazi et al., 2018, p. 1289). Also seen in nephrotoxic AKI especially due to aminoglycoside toxicity. Associated with hyperphosphatemia.
- Hypomagnesemia
  ○ May be a result of tubular loss; can also cause abnormal parathyroid activity.
    - Dialysis if failure to decrease serum potassium and other electrolyte imbalances due to tubular damage (Vogt & Dell, 2015, p. 1685)
      • Peritoneal dialysis requires placement of peritoneal catheter and is most commonly used in neonates due to the large area for dialysate insertion and no need for vascular access or use of anticoagulation.
      • Hemodialysis or continuous renal replacement therapy (CRRT) requires vascular access using large diameter catheters placed in the internal jugular or femoral vein. The extracorporeal circuit requires reliable vascular access, frequent monitoring of anticoagulants and temperature, and carries the risk of rapid fluid shifts. Limited use in infants weighing less than 2.5 kg. Management includes access, frequent monitoring of anticoagulants and temperature, and the risk of rapid fluid shift.
- Hyperphosphatemia
- Prolonged half-life for renally excreted medications
- Newer diagnostic techniques will lead to quicker identification of kidney injury and differentiate between functional and/or structural damage (Vogt & Dell, 2015, p. 1684).

Management of AKI

- Initial management for prerenal kidney injury is a fluid challenge with an isotonic solution such as normal saline 10 to 20 mL/kg over 30 minutes to replace intravascular volume and determine intravascular fluid loss.
- Renal ultrasound should be completed to assess presence of urine in bladder, renal blood flow, and presence of obstruction to urine output.
- Use of low-dose dopamine may increase renal blood flow but has not been shown to improve overall survival (Askenazi et al., 2018, p.1287).
- Treat underlying condition as indicated.
- Avoid nephrotoxic drugs and follow serum drug levels in those with kidney injury if these drugs are used (i.e., gentamicin, vancomycin).
- Furosemide for fluid overload may be helpful, but it has not been shown to prevent or change the course of AKI (Askenazi et al., 2018, p. 1287).
- Fluid management should be based on individual infant's fluid and electrolyte status (Askenazi et al., 2018, p. 1288).
  ○ Fluid restriction with low-output renal injury
  ○ Fluid replacement with high-output renal injury
- Electrolyte supplementation is based on individual needs.
  ○ No additional potassium, magnesium, or phosphate should be added during oliguric phase due to tubular dysfunction.
  ○ Supplementation of electrolytes is dependent on serum and urine electrolytes during high-output phase.

Outcomes

- Prompt recognition and treatment will improve prognosis. Risk of progressive renal disease and chronic kidney disease, hypertension, and renal tubular acidosis with impairment of renal tubular growth has been recognized in long-term survivors of AKI (Vogt & Dell, 2015, p. 1687).

Prevention of AKI

- Importance of family history and history of current pregnancy and medications used to determine risk of AKI in neonate (Askenazi et al., 2018 p. 1286)
- Maintenance of circulatory volume—monitor blood pressure, heart rate, and urine output to prevent hypoperfusion of the kidney.
- Fluid and electrolyte management—follow serum electrolytes, urine electrolytes as indicated, and accurate volume intake and output.
- Prompt diagnosis and treatment of respiratory, infectious, or hemodynamic conditions
- Monitor nephrotoxic medications through serum levels and avoid use in infants at risk if possible (i.e., aminoglycoside antibiotics, indomethacin, IV contrast, diuretic).

BILATERAL RENAL AGENESIS (ALSO CALLED "POTTER SEQUENCE")

Definition and Etiology

- Bilateral renal agenesis is the failure of renal development or the complete absence of the kidneys (Engen & Hingorani, 2018; Samuels et al., 2017, p. 386).

Incidence

- There is an incidence of about 1:3,000 to 5,000 births with a slight male predominance (Engen & Hingorani, 2018, pp. 1250–1251; Sherman, 2015, p. 729; Vogt & Dell, 2015, p. 1690)

Clinical Presentation

- Potter faces (or "squished face") is a unique appearance of the face and body of the fetus/infant due to fetal compression in utero. The infant has a flat face and a "pushed in" or blunted nose with a depressed nasal bridge. These infants may have micrognathia or receded chin, with wide-spaced eyes, epicanthal folds, low-set or malformed ears, and wrinkled skin (Engen & Hingorani, 2018, p. 1251; Samuels et al., 2017, p. 386; Sherman, 2015, p. 729; Vogt & Dell, 2015, p. 1690).
- Table 19.1 lists signs and symptoms of Potter sequence

TABLE 19.1 Clinical Presentation of Potter Sequence

Prenatal	Newborn
Oligohydramnios	Anuria or oliguria
Breech position (more common)	Potter facies or "squished face"
intrauterine growth restriction (↓ growth)	Abnormal genital development
Fetal compression	Leg deformities
	GI defects
	Broad, flat hands
	Contractures
	Respiratory distress due to pulmonary hypoplasia
	No kidneys on palpation

Diagnosis

- The diagnosis of bilateral renal agenesis can be accomplished by renal ultrasound either prenatally or after birth. The kidneys can also be evaluated using radionuclide scintography (radioisotope renal scan) after birth (Bates & Schwaderer, 2018, pp. 1278–1279).

Complications

- Due to the compression of the fetus and oligohydramnios, the infant's lungs are hypoplastic, causing respiratory failure. With early ventilation and stiff lungs, the infant can develop a pneumothorax. Acute renal failure occurs due to the lack of kidney development or complete agenesis (Engen & Hingorani, 2018, p. 1251; Sherman, 2015, p. 729).

Management

- Options for treatment include: (a) providing comfort measures due to pulmonary hypoplasia and poor outcome, (b) peritoneal dialysis if pulmonary hypoplasia is not severe, and/or (c) renal transplant, which can be considered if death does not occur within the first few days of life (Engen & Hingorani, 2018, p. 1251; Samuels et al., 2017, p. 386).

Outcomes

- The mortality rate is almost always 100%, incompatible with life, due to lack of kidney function, resulting in pulmonary hypoplasia (Engen & Hingorani, 2018, p. 1251). Most infants die within 24 to 48 hours after birth and the stillborn rate is about 40% (Engen & Hingorani, 2018, p. 1251).

UNILATERAL RENAL AGENESIS (CONGENITAL SINGLE KIDNEY)

Definition

- This disorder is similar to bilateral renal agenesis, but diagnosed later in childhood or adulthood due to one healthy kidney; therefore, the newborn is asymptomatic (Engen & Hingorani, 2018, p. 1250; Sherman, 2015, p. 729).

Incidence

- Is about 1:500 to 3,200 live births (Engen & Hingorani, 2018, p. 1250; Sherman, 2015, p. 729; Vogt & Dell, 2015, p. 1690).

Complications and Outcomes

- Many of these infants will have other developmental anomalies, including genital tract anomalies like bicornate or unicornate uterus in females, or anomalies of the cardiovascular or musculoskeletal systems (Engen & Hingorani, 2018, p. 1250). There is also increased risk of chronic kidney disease (CKD) in late childhood or adulthood in the remaining kidney (Engen & Hingorani, 2018).

POLYCYSTIC KIDNEY DISEASE (PKD)

Definition and Etiology

- PKD is an autosomal recessive cystic kidney disorder, which usually occurs in both kidneys soon after birth (Sherman, 2015, p. 730). It can have delayed presentation until later childhood (autosomal dominant version), but the autosomal recessive type occurs in the neonate (Vogt & Dell, 2015, p. 1695).
  - The disorder requires each parent to have the abnormal gene with a 25% chance of passing it on to each child. The autosomal recessive type of PKD is linked to a specific gene, *PKHD1* gene on chromosome 6p21 (Engen & Hingorani, 2018, p. 1255; Samuels et al., 2017, p. 399; Vogt & Dell, 2015, p. 1695).

Incidence

- Incidence of autosomal recessive PKD is about 1:20,000 to 40,000 live births, with equal incidence in both males and females (Engen & Hingorani, 2018, p. 1255; Vogt & Dell, 2015, p. 1695).

Clinical Presentation

- Prenatally, infants with bilateral polycystic kidneys may have a history of oligohydramnios depending on the extent of renal failure prior to birth. After birth, these infants will have palpable flank masses bilaterally with oliguria or decreased urine output. The large flank masses can result in abdominal distension and a palpable liver. With the oligohydramnios, there are hypoplastic lungs resulting in respiratory distress. Other signs of renal failure are elevated BUN and creatinine, elevated K+ and phosphorus/phosphate (PO_4), low serum calcium (Ca++), hypertension, hematuria, and proteinuria (Engen & Hingorani, 2018, p. 1255; Samuels et al., 2017, p. 399; Vogt & Dell, 2015, pp. 1695–1696).

Diagnosis

- A renal ultrasound can diagnose this disorder by noting enlarged, nodular, or cystic kidneys (Bates & Schwaderer, 2018, pp. 1278–1279). Abdominal x-rays can also assist with diagnosis by seeing cystic areas on the kidneys (Vogt & Dell, 2015, p. 1696).

Complications

- Those that result from PKD are renal failure, hypertension, frequent urination, urinary tract infections (UTI), esophageal varices, congestive heart failure from fluid overload, and portal hypertension leading to hepatic failure. Liver involvement occurs in about 40% of infants with the recessive type of PKD (Samuels et al., 2017, p. 400; Vogt & Dell, 2015, p. 1695).

Management

- The management of PKD includes genetic counseling of the parents. Management of fluid overload and electrolyte abnormalities are treated with diuretics, anti-hypertensives, and supplementation with dialysis (Vogt & Dell, 2015, pp. 1695–1696). Management of renal failure includes dialysis, kidney transplant, or supportive care (Samuels et al., 2017, p. 399). Renal and respiratory monitoring is needed for infants with PKD to evaluate the degree of renal and respiratory involvement (Engen & Hingorani, 2018, p. 1255; Samuels et al., 2017, p. 399; Vogt & Dell, 2015, pp. 1695–1696).

Outcomes

- Infants with severe renal or respiratory involvement may die in the neonatal period and survival rates have improved with aggressive treatment to 70% to 75% (Engen & Hingorani, 2018, p. 1256; Samuels et al., 2017, p. 399; Vogt & Dell, 2015, p. 1696). If infants survive the neonatal period, they may develop renal insufficiency in childhood or adolescence (Engen & Hingorani, 2018, p. 1256; Samuels et al., 2017, p. 399; Vogt & Dell, 2015, p. 1696).

MULTICYSTIC DYSPLASTIC KIDNEY DISEASE (MCDK)

Definition and Etiology

- MCDK disease is a nongenetic, developmental renal disorder which usually occurs in only one kidney. The cysts are described as "grape-like" clusters (Sherman, 2015, p. 730). The parenchyma of the kidney is abnormal with few normal nephrons. The proximal ureter is usually stenotic or nonpatent, which contributes to renal failure in that kidney (Engen & Hingorani, 2018, p. 1252–1253).

Incidence

- The incidence of MCDK disease is 1:4,300 infants with a small male predominance (Engen & Hingorani, 2018, p. 1252).

Clinical Presentation

- These infants may present with a history of oligohydramnios depending on the extent of renal involvement. After birth, the infant may present with an abdominal mass which is usually unilateral, of irregular shape, and usually on the left side. The other kidney is usually noncystic, but there is a risk of UPJO. This disorder is one of the most common causes of an abdominal mass in a newborn infant. The normal kidney in these infants is often larger than normal (Engen & Hingorani, 2018, pp. 1252–1253).

Diagnosis

- MCDK disease is diagnosed mainly by renal ultrasound (or fetal ultrasound) (Samuels et al., 2017, p. 380). Visualization of the multiple "grape-like" cysts is diagnostic (Samuels et al., 2017, p. 380). The ureter is usually atretic. There is no communication between the dysplastic tissue and the renal pelvis in the non-functioning kidney. A renal scan may not be needed for accurate visualization (Engen & Hingorani, 2018, p. 1252). A voiding cysto-urethrogram (VCUG) is controversial (Bates & Schwaderer, 2018, pp. 1278–1279; Engen & Hingorani, 2018, p. 1252).

Complications

- Complications of MCDK disorders are hypertension, infection, hematuria with or without proteinuria, and pain.

Management

- Management of MCDK disease has two possible plans: (a) nonoperative plan with close follow-up, or (b) operative plan with removal of the cystic, nonfunctional kidney (nephrectomy; Samuels et al., 2017, p. 381).

Outcomes

- If the multicystic kidneys occur in both kidneys (bilateral), then the infant will die without dialysis and kidney transplant. If the multicystic kidney occurs in just one kidney (unilateral), then the infant survives. A possible malignancy may occur later in life within the nonfunctional kidney, necessitating removal. Otherwise, the unilateral kidneys may regress by about 5 years of age (Engen & Hingorani, 2018, p. 1253; Sherman, 2015).

HYDRONEPHROSIS/HYDROURETER

Definition and Etiology

- Hydronephrosis is damage to the kidney from a congenital obstruction in the urinary tract, resulting in backup of urine into the kidneys, which dilates the renal pelvis and calyces and may also dilate the ureters (hydroureters). Etiology of the obstruction is unknown.
- Four causes of obstruction to urine flow:
  - Ureteropelvic Junction Obstruction
    - UPJO is one of the most common causes of hydronephrosis (Merguerian & Rowe, 2018, p. 1265; Sherman, 2015, p. 731). It is more common in males (Sherman, 2015, p. 731).
  - Posterior Urethral Valves
    - PUV is the most common lower urinary tract/bladder obstruction in males (Sherman, 2015, p. 731). The obstruction is due to a membrane, not really a valve, which causes an obstruction or partial obstruction with urine backing up into the kidneys and ureters causing hydroureters and hydronephrosis in utero and neonatal life (Merguerian & Rowe, 2018, p. 1268; Sherman, 2015, p. 731).
  - Vesicoureteral Reflux (VUR)
    - VUR is a condition that results in urine flowing backwards from the bladder into the ureters, causing hydroureters and possibly hydronephrosis. VUR predisposes the infant to a UTI and/or pyelonephritis (Kenagy & Vogt, 2013, p. 431; Wang, Djahangirian, & Wehbi, 2018, p. 1309).
  - Prune Belly Syndrome (see discussion in the separate section later in this chapter)

Clinical Presentation

- Prenatally, infants with hydronephrosis from any of these causes can have oligohydramnios, depending on the extent of renal damage or obstruction. Mild hydronephrosis may not have oligohydramnios, and often the hydronephrosis can disappear after birth, depending on the cause.
- After birth, infants with moderate to severe hydronephrosis will have oliguria, enlarged kidney(s), and abdominal distension. A poor urinary stream is almost definitive of posterior, urethral valves in male infants.
- With the lower urinary tract obstruction, a distended and palpable bladder may be noted (Sherman, 2015, p. 731). Other possible clinical signs would be proteinuria, hematuria, leukocyturia (UTI), increased BUN, and increased creatinine. There is also an increase in other associated anomalies and a thorough assessment must be completed.

Incidence

- About 1:1,000 fetuses have a congenital UPJO, which results in hydronephrosis with hydroureter either unilaterally or bilaterally; though unilateral hydronephrosis is more common (Engen & Hingorani, 2018; Merguerian & Rowe, 2018, p. 1265; Samuels et al., 2017, p. 380; Sherman, 2015, p. 731).
- PUVs occur only in males, with an incidence of 1:5,000 to 8,000 live births (Sherman, 2015, p. 731; Vogt & Dell, 2015, p. 1694).

Diagnosis

- Diagnosis of hydronephrosis can be made with a renal ultrasound (before or after birth) or by a renal scan (Bates & Schwaderer, 2018, pp. 1278–1279; Samuels et al., 2017, p. 380).
- A VCUG is usually done to rule out obstruction, especially with VUR or PUV (Merguerian & Rowe, 2018, p. 1268; Samuels et al., 2017, p. 379; Sherman, 2015, p. 731). An intravenous pyelogram (IVP) can also be done to view obstructions in the urinary tract. Both of these tests involve the use of contrast media and radiation.

Complications

- Hydronephrosis can result in damage to the renal parenchyma due to the backup of urine into the kidney. Hypertension can also be a complication of kidney damage. UTI is common with VUR from the urine refluxing from the bladder (Merguerian & Rowe, 2018, p. 1268; Samuels et al., 2017, p. 379; Sherman, 2015, p. 731).

Management

- The management of hydronephrosis involves getting rid of the obstruction and facilitating urine passage through the urinary tract, mainly with surgical correction.
  - Pyeloplasty is surgical correction of the obstruction seen at the ureteropelvic junction (UPJ) (Merguerian & Rowe, 2018, p. 1265).
  - Management for PUV is to catheterize the infant, relieving the obstruction of the "valves" or membranes in the urethra. Direct transurethral ablation surgery can also be used to relieve the obstruction as a more permanent solution.
  - Surgical repair with antibiotic prophylaxis for the prevention of UTI is the treatment of choice for VUR (Sherman, 2015, p. 731).

Outcomes

- The outcome for hydronephrosis depends on the extent of kidney damage and whether there is any pulmonary involvement causing respiratory distress or lung hypoplasia (Merguerian & Rowe, 2018, p. 1268; Samuels et al., 2017, p. 386). Prompt treatment improves the prognosis with many infants, and the outcome with prenatally diagnosed hydronephrosis often results in spontaneous resolution (Vogt & Dell, 2015, p. 1694).
- Infants with PUV usually do well with some incontinence in about half of the infants, which improves with age; others may develop some renal insufficiency and chronic

or progressive renal disease (Merguerian & Rowe, 2018, p. 1268).

- If surgery is not successful, the infant may require a kidney transplant (Merguerian & Rowe, 2018, p. 1268; Samuels et al., 2017, p. 379).

RENAL VEIN THROMBOSIS (RVT)

Definition and Etiology

- RVT is the most common cause of thrombosis in newborns unrelated to catheter placement (Diab & Luchtman-Jones, 2015, p. 1336; Letterio, Ahuja, & Petrosiute, 2013, p. 470; Sparger & Gupta, 2017, p. 597). The thrombosis is usually unilaterally, and more often on the left side (Askenazi et al., 2018, p. 1292; Diab & Luchtman-Jones, 2015, p. 1336).
- There are many disorders or treatments that may contribute to RVT, including a high hematocrit at birth (Letterio et al., 2013, p. 470; Samuels et al., 2017, p. 393).
  ○ Prenatal conditions include maternal diabetes (IDM), maternal pre-eclampsia/eclampsia, or perinatal asphyxia (Letterio et al., 2013, p. 470; Samuels et al., 2017, p. 393).
  ○ Blood clots are more prevalent with polycythemia and/or hyperviscosity of the blood. Blood clots can result from the use of umbilical venous catheterization (UVC) or from abnormal coagulation factors or disseminated intravascular coagulation (DIC; Letterio et al., 2013, p. 470).
  ○ Severe dehydration can also cause thicker blood. Cyanotic congenital heart disease can also result in polycythemia because of the low oxygen level to the tissues (Diab & Luchtman-Jones, 2015, p. 1336; Letterio et al., 2013, p. 470).
  ○ Hypovolemia or low blood volume leads to low blood pressure (hypotension).

Incidence

- About 1% to 2% of neonatal deaths are the result of RVT and they occur in about 2.4 per 1,000 neonatal admissions to the NICU or 2.2 cases per 100,000 live births, with most associated with the use of umbilical catheters (Askenazi et al., 2018, p. 1292; Letterio et al., 2013, p. 470).
- There is a slight male predominance, with other authors stating no sexual preference. Most infants with RVT are term and large for gestational age (LGA) (Askenazi et al., 2018, p. 1292; Diab & Luchtman-Jones, 2015, p. 1336; Letterio et al., 2013, p. 470).

Clinical Presentation

- Infants with RVT usually present with an abdominal flank mass (larger than normal kidneys), either unilateral or bilateral, with possible abdominal distension, but with significant hematuria and thrombocytopenia (Diab & Luchtman-Jones, 2015, p. 1336; Merguerian & Rowe, 2018; Samuels et al., 2017, p. 393; Vogt & Dell, 2015, pp. 1336–1337).
- Blood loss results in anemia, metabolic acidosis, and hypertension. Oliguria or anuria will result if kidney failure occurs.

- If clots occur with umbilical venous catheters, they often occur in the inferior vena cava (IVC) and edema distal to the clot can be the result (Samuels et al., 2017, p. 393).

Diagnosis

- RVT is usually diagnosed by renal ultrasound (with or without color Doppler flow studies) (Askenazi et al., 2018, p. 1292; Diab & Luchtman-Jones, 2015, p. 1336; Letterio et al., 2013, p. 470; Samuels et al., 2017, p. 393).
- Contrast angiography has been the gold standard for diagnosis, but the radiation exposure makes it dangerous to newborns (Bates & Schwaderer, 2018, pp. 1278–1279; Letterio et al., 2013, p. 470; Merguerian & Rowe, 2018, p. 1264).

Complications

- RVT can result in renal tubular dysfunction leading to renal failure and atrophy of the kidney. Prolonged lack of blood flow to the lower extremities can result in hypertension, adrenal hemorrhage, chronic renal insufficiency, and death (Diab & Luchtman-Jones, 2015, p. 1336).

Management

- Treatment of the underlying cause is most important with this diagnosis.
  ○ Treatment of RVT is supportive care only if the thrombi is unilateral and not a large clot (Diab & Luchtman-Jones, 2015, p. 1336; Samuels et al., 2017, p. 395). Removal of the catheter is usually essential and may resolve the clot (Letterio et al., 2013, p. 470).
  ○ If clots are bilateral or in the IVC, then heparin or tissue plasminogen activator (t-PA) are used to try to break up the clot and reestablish circulation from the lower part off the body (Diab & Luchtman-Jones, 2015, p. 1336; Samuels et al., 2017, p. 395).
  ○ Surgical excision of the clot is considered if (a) renal failure is apparent, (b) the thrombosis was the result of a UVC, or (c) the thrombosis is bilateral and resistant to heparin or t-PA (Letterio et al., 2013, p. 470; Samuels et al., 2017, p. 395)

Outcomes

- Many of the kidneys of infants with an RVT will atrophy, becoming smaller, and infants may develop hypertension due to damage to the kidney (Askenazi et al., 2018, p. 1292; Merguerian & Rowe, 2018, p. 1293). Mortality or death rarely occurs, but the affected kidney often develops atrophy (Sparger & Gupta, 2017, p. 597; Vogt & Dell, 2015, p. 1337). Mortality rate has been noted to be about 3% (Askenazi et al., 2018, p. 1293).

RENAL ARTERY THROMBOSIS (RAT)

Definition and Etiology

- RAT is the result of a clot in the renal artery, blocking blood flow to the kidneys.

- RATs frequently occur after or during the use of an umbilical artery catheter (UAC) (Diab & Luchtman-Jones, 2015, p. 1336). The thromboses can also occur with coagulation disorders or severe hypotension (Samuels et al., 2017, p. 393).

Clinical Presentation

- Infants with a RAT can be asymptomatic or present with systemic hypertension, hematuria, thrombocytopenia, oliguria, or anuria, and can present with a lack of blood flow to the lower abdomen and the lower extremities (Diab & Luchtman-Jones, 2015, p. 1336).

Diagnosis

- Magnetic resonance (MR) angiography or renal ultrasound with color Doppler flow studies are both used to diagnose an arterial thrombosis (Bates & Schwaderer, 2018, pp. 1278–1279; Diab & Luchtman-Jones, 2015, p. 1336).

Management

- Management of RAT initially involves removal of the arterial catheter, and then can involve removal of the clot, thrombolytic agents (heparin or t-PA), or supportive care with antihypertensives, especially if affecting only one kidney or a unilateral clot (Diab & Luchtman-Jones, 2015, p. 1336; Samuels et al., 2017, p. 393). Peritoneal dialysis with a possible transplant may become necessary if kidney failure becomes permanent.

URINARY TRACT INFECTIONS (UTI)

Definition and Etiology

- UTI is an infection of the urinary tract with a bacteria, virus, or fungus.
- The cause of a UTI can be an abnormality of the urinary tract, which facilitates colonization or infection due to either reflux or an obstruction (Leonard & Dobbs, 2015, p. 739).
- Some of the main bacteria causing sepsis are the following: *Escherichia coli* (*E.coli*) is the most common bacteria causing a UTI; *Klebsiella* species (Gram-negative bacilli) can also be a contributing bacterium, and some Gram-positive bacteria are also seen in neonates (e.g,. coagulase-negative Staphylococci or Group B *beta-hemolytic streptococcus* [GBS]) (Leonard & Dobbs, 2015, p. 739; Samuels et al., 2017, p. 397; Wang et al., 2018, p. 1308)
- Risk factors for a UTI are uncircumcised males, a maternal history of UTI, or VUR (Wang et al., 2018, p. 1309).

Incidence

- Zero to 1% of infants will develop a UTI during the first three days of life in the United States, but the rates are higher in premature infants and in male infants (Leonard & Dobbs, 2015, p. 739; Wang et al., 2018, p. 1308). There is also a prevalence rate of 5% to 20% in children under 2 months of age with a fever and no other known source of infection (Wang et al., 2018, p. 1308).

Clinical Presentation

- Infants with a UTI can be asymptomatic or have very nonspecific signs of sepsis. Infants may have poor feeding, respiratory distress, or lethargy (Wang et al., 2018, p. 1309). It is rare for infants to have a UTI before 48 hours of life (Samuels et al., 2017, p. 397). A fever with UTI results in an increased incidence of bacteremia, so a blood culture MUST be obtained! (Samuels et al., 2017, p. 397; Wang et al., 2018, p. 1310).

Diagnosis

The definitive diagnostic test is a positive urine culture (obtained by sterile bladder tap) or a Gram stain with a high colony count (Leonard & Dobbs, 2015, p. 739; Wang et al., 2018, p. 1311). A renal ultrasound showing urinary tract abnormalities would assist with the diagnosis of a continuing UTI (Bates & Schwaderer, 2018, pp. 1278–1279). A VCUG is used to diagnose a possible VUR (Leonard & Dobbs, 2015, p. 740).

Management

- Antibiotics should be given for a minimum of 10 to 14 days, depending on symptoms and resolution of the urine culture (Wang et al., 2018, p. 1311). Follow-up of urine cultures is required after antibiotics are discontinued and supportive care is essential, which may include continuous antibiotic prophylaxis (Wang et al., 2018, pp. 1311–1312)

Outcomes

- Infants with a UTI can have renal scarring, a reoccurrence of the UTI, systemic sepsis, or meningitis (Wang et al., 2018, pp. 1308–1311).
- There are excellent outcomes for infants with a UTI if they are treated promptly and adequately (Wang et al., 2018, p. 1313).

ECTOPIC KIDNEY OR SUPERNUMERARY KIDNEY

Definition and Etiology

- A kidney that does not migrate to normal kidney position during fetal development. Ectopic kidneys are associated with other genital or cloacal anomalies, especially in females (Merguerian & Rowe, 2018, p. 1262).
- Horseshoe kidney is a U-shaped kidney, where there are two kidneys which are connected at the bottom in the midline of the abdomen. This type of kidney results in a higher incidence of Wilms tumor in childhood.
- Crossed renal ectopia refers to kidneys which have ureters entering the bladder from the wrong side.
- A supernumerary kidney is a rare phenomenon where the extra kidney and its collecting system is somewhere in the abdomen, but not related to the functioning kidneys (Merguerian & Rowe, 2018, p. 1262).

Incidence

- An ectopic kidney occurs in about 1 in 700 infants as seen on a fetal ultrasound (Merguerian & Rowe, 2018, p. 1262). The incidence of a horseshoe kidney is about 1 in 400 infants (Engen & Hingorani, 2018, p. 1252).

Clinical Presentation

- Typically asymptomatic; approximately 90% of patients are never diagnosed (Engen & Hingorani, 2018, p. 1251).
- Usually only diagnosed if the ectopic/supernumerary kidney becomes infected or obstructed (Merguerian & Rowe, 2018, p. 1262)

Management

- Surgical removal may be necessary if supernumerary and/or if malignancy occurs (Merguerian & Rowe, 2018, p. 1262).

Outcomes

- Prognosis for the ectopic kidney is good, with no evidence of adverse effects on blood pressure or renal function (Merguerian & Rowe, 2018, p. 1262).
- It is not associated with hypertension, proteinuria, or chronic kidney disease. Patients are typically not followed unless there is evidence of reflux or obstruction (Engen & Hingorani, 2018, p. 1252).

PRUNE BELLY SYNDROME (EAGLE-BARRETT SYNDROME)

Definition and Etiology

- Prune belly syndrome is also called Eagle-Barrett syndrome, and includes a triad of three abnormalities: (a) lack of abdominal wall muscles, causing wrinkled, abdominal skin with a "prune-like" appearance; (b) hydronephrosis with a dilated bladder without obstruction; and (c) bilateral cryptorchidism (Merguerian & Rowe, 2018, p. 1271; Sherman, 2015, p. 731).
- Causes of the prune belly association are an obstructive uropathy or mesenchymal dysplasia, and often with dysplastic kidneys; though no genetic abnormality noted, there may be some variation in genetic phenotype presentations in the infant (Blackburn, 2013, p. 371; Bradshaw, 2015, p. 617).

Incidence

- Incidence of prune belly syndrome is approximately 1 in 35,000 to 50,000 live births with a definitive, male predominance (Cavaliere, 2019, p. 127; Engen & Hingorani, 2018, p. 1253; Kenagy & Vogt, 2013, pp. 430–431; Merguerian & Rowe, 2018, p. 1271; Sherman, 2015, p. 731; Vogt & Dell, 2015, p. 1694).

Clinical Presentation

- Infants born with prune belly syndrome are first noted to have wrinkled skin on the abdomen with the appearance of a "prune." The abdomen appears large and distended (Bradshaw, 2015, p. 618). The bladder is often noted to be enlarged or distended on physical exam associated with other urinary tract abnormalities (Bradshaw, 2015, pp. 617–618; Cavaliere, 2019, p. 127). Infant boys will exhibit undescended testes (Bradshaw, 2015, p. 617). Gastrointestinal (GI) abnormalities with obstruction and distention of the gut may also present (Bradshaw, 2015, p. 617; Cavaliere, 2019, p. 127).

Diagnosis

- Diagnosis is initially by observation. An ultrasound and/or VCUG can be used to evaluate the urinary tract, though there is some controversy about use of VCUG (Bates & Schwaderer, 2018, pp. 1278–1279; Bradshaw, 2015, p. 617). CT and nuclear scan are also possible methods of evaluating the urinary tract (Bradshaw, 2015, p. 618).

Complications

- Infants with prune belly syndrome may develop an enlargement of the bladder from the hydronephrosis and renal dysplasia, distension of the intestines from an obstruction, and renal failure (Bradshaw, 2015, p. 617; Cavaliere, 2019, p. 127)

Management

- Possible management plans depend on the extent of the abnormality and renal/respiratory symptoms. Management may include vesicostomy, self-catheterization, surgery on the abdominal wall or urinary tract, bilateral orchiopexy, and dialysis or renal transplant if needed (Bradshaw, 2015, p. 618; Kenagy & Vogt, 2013, pp. 430–431; Merguerian & Rowe, 2018, p. 1271; Vogt & Dell, 2015, p. 1694).

Outcomes

- If the infant has dysplastic kidneys, the infant may die in infancy. Many infants survive into adulthood after urinary tract and abdomen reconstruction and repair are completed (Bradshaw, 2015, p. 618; Merguerian & Rowe, 2018, p. 1271).

PATENT URACHUS

Definition and Etiology

- The urachus is a prenatal communication between the bladder and the umbilicus which usually regenerates but can remain patent after birth (Goodwin, 2019, p. 114; Ledbetter, Chabra, & Javid, 2018, pp. 1069–1070; Merguerian & Rowe, 2018, pp. 1267–1268).
- The cause of this defect is a failure of the normal closing of the urachal tube during fetal development (Blackburn, 2013, p. 372).

Clinical Presentation

- The appearance of urine or clear fluid from the umbilicus at birth or in the newborn period is one of the first signs of a patent urachus (Merguerian & Rowe, 2018, p. 1268). The umbilicus can appear "wet," and the wetness can cause a delay in cord separation from the stump for greater than 14 days (Cavaliere, 2019, p. 128; Merguerian & Rowe, 2018, p. 1268).

Diagnosis

- Confirmed diagnosis is made after analysis of fluid for urea and creatinine to confirm urine (Cavaliere, 2019, p. 128). Abdominal ultrasound may show the defect, but a VCUG is definitive (Bates & Schwaderer, 2018, pp. 1278–1279).

Complications

- Infants with patent urachus can develop an infection/UTI or excoriation of the skin after exposure to the urine (Cavaliere, 2019, p. 128).

Management

- Infants with a patent urachus are given supportive care. Surgical closure will occur after 1 year of age if spontaneous closure does not occur (Merguerian & Rowe, 2018, p. 1268).

Outcomes

- Most infants will have a good outcome with few if any complications (Ledbetter et al., 2018, pp. 1069–1070).

HYPOSPADIAS AND EPISPADIAS

Definition and Etiology

- These two defects occur when the urethral meatus is located on the ventral surface of the penis (hypospadias) or located on the dorsal surface of the penis (epispadias) rather than on the tip (Merguerian & Rowe, 2018, p. 1269).
- The most probable cause of abnormal urethral placement is due to a multifactorial mode of inheritance; therefore, related to a delay or arrest of the normal sequence of urethral development (Sherman, 2015, p. 732).

Incidence

- About one per 250 to 300 live male births. and may be increasing in the United States (Merguerian & Rowe, 2018, p. 1269; Sherman, 2015, p. 732)

Clinical Presentation

- The hypospadias is visually apparent on the underside of the penis, especially during voiding. The urinary stream comes from the underside of the penis with hypospadias and from the top with epispadias.

Diagnosis

- Observation or a physical exam is necessary for diagnosis by identifying the location of meatus or opening. Chordee often occurs with downward curving of penis. Incomplete formation of the prepuce often occurs with hypospadias, so the first indication of hypospadias could be what is sometimes called a "natural circumcision" on a male infant.
- Hypospadias was classified on the basis of the location of the meatus; however, this classification was not sufficient to encompass the complexity of this defect. A new scoring system called the GMS score (glans, meatus, shaft) has been used. This scale includes a scale of 1-4 for each component, with higher scores indicating unfavorable characteristics (Merguerian & Rowe, 2018, p. 1269).

Complications

- Chordee is an abnormal ventral curvature of the penile shaft and results in a deviation of stream during voiding (Merguerian & Rowe, 2018, p. 1269).

Management

- Infants with a hypospadias or epispadius should not be circumcised because the foreskin will be used for surgical repair and correction of the defect, which is usually completed between 6 and 18 months of age (Merguerian & Rowe, 2018, p. 1269; Remeithi & Wherritt, 2015, p. 1548).

Outcomes

- Hypospadias is usually repaired at 6-18 months of age. More severe cases will be delayed and repaired after the age of 1 year. Testosterone therapy may be given to increase phallic size if necessary (Merguerian & Rowe, 2018, p 1269)

EXSTROPHY OF THE BLADDER

Definition and Etiology

- Exstrophy of the bladder is defined as an exposed bladder through the lower anterior abdominal wall (Ledbetter et al., 2018, p. 1076; Ringer & Hansen, 2017, p. 959). The umbilicus can be displaced downward, and most are associated with epispadias and separation of the symphysis pubis (Ledbetter et al., 2018, p. 1076; Merguerian & Rowe, 2018, p. 1267; Vogt & Dell, 2015, pp. 1694–1695).
- Etiology is essentially unknown; but may be due to abnormal development of the cloacal membrane with rupture, and a possible genetic influence (Ledbetter et al., 2018, p. 1076; Merguerian & Rowe, 2018, pp. 1266–1267; Vogt & Dell, 2015, p. 1694).

Incidence

- Incidence of bladder exstrophy is about one in 10,000 to 60,000 live births, with a male predominance (Ledbetter et al., 2018, p. 1076)

Clinical Presentation

- Infants present with an external bladder (outside the lower abdominal wall), usually with epispadias (male) or bifid clitoris (female), anterior displacement of the anal opening, and may present with undescended testes, inguinal hernia, or umbilical hernia (Merguerian & Rowe, 2018, p. 1267; Vogt & Dell, 2015, pp. 1694–1695)

Diagnosis

- Is made by prenatal ultrasound or by observation after birth. An ultrasound and flat plate x-ray of the abdomen should be done to rule out any other urinary tract or bone anomalies (Ledbetter et al., 2018, p. 1076; Vogt & Dell, 2015, p. 1695).

Complications

- Infections, postop hydronephrosis, or anal incontinence may occur after surgery (Merguerian & Rowe, 2018, p. 1267). A malignancy of renal tissue may occur in childhood or adulthood.

Management

- Early management would include providing a cover to the exposed bladder with clear plastic or saline dressing to permit drainage but also to protect the bladder (Ledbetter et al., 2018, p. 1076; Merguerian & Rowe, 2018, p. 1267). Later management includes surgical closure, reconstruction of the bladder with antispasmodics, analgesics, and antibiotics (Merguerian & Rowe, 2018, p. 1267).

Outcomes

- Good bladder control is likely with proper management (Merguerian & Rowe, 2018, p. 1267).

TESTICULAR TORSION

Definition and Etiology

- A testicular torsion is when a testicle twists around the spermatic cord causing the blood flow to the testes to be cut off, resulting in necrosis (Cavaliere, 2015, p. 133).
- A testicular torsion is caused by an incomplete attachment of the testes allowing it to twist (Cavaliere, 2015, p. 133)

Incidence

- Most torsions of the testes occur prenatally rather than during the neonatal period, though they are diagnosed after birth (Cavaliere, 2015, p. 133; Ringer & Hansen, 2017, p. 961; Sherman, 2015, p. 732).

Clinical Presentation

- Infant with testicular torsion will present with swelling of testes in the scrotum and discoloration of the testes/scrotum; the scrotum appears bruised or "dusky" and bluish; and the testes will be painful to palpation if it is a recent strangulation; necrotic testes are not painful to palpation (Cavaliere, 2015, p. 133; Ringer & Hansen, 2017, p. 961).

Diagnosis

- Diagnosis of testicular torsion is by observation. Upon assessment, there is no cremasteric reflex noted and the testes tests negative to transillumination. The testis and blood flow may be seen by ultrasound (Merguerian & Rowe, 2018, p. 1271; Ringer & Hansen, 2017, p. 961).

Complications

- Most infants with testicular torsion noted will already have a loss of function of the testes and necrosis will occur (Merguerian & Rowe, 2018, p. 1271). Oligospermia is the main complication of testicular torsion (Ringer & Hansen, 2017, p. 962).

Management

- Emergent surgery for detorsion should occur within 4 to 6 hours and will include a contralateral orchiopexy to protect the nonaffected testes (Cavaliere, 2019, p. 133; Ringer & Hansen, 2017, p. 961; Sherman, 2015, p. 732).

Outcomes

- Use of testicular protheses can occur for cosmetic purposes (Ringer & Hansen, 2017, p. 962).

INGUINAL HERNIA

Definition and Etiology

- Failure of the proximal part of the processes vaginalis to close at birth ,producing a hernia sac (Cavaliere, 2019, p. 132; Ledbetter et al., 2018, p. 1077).

Incidence

- About 5% of infants under 1,500 g at birth and about 30% of infants under 1,000 g at birth (more frequent in males, premature infants, and small for gestational age (SGA) infants; Ledbetter et al., 2018, p. 1077; Ringer & Hansen, 2017, pp. 960–961).

Clinical Presentation

- An inguinal hernia will present as a swelling, lump, or bump in the inguinal area (groin) of female infants or in the scrotal sac(s) of male infants. Cryptorchidism may be present with the inguinal hernia (Cavaliere, 2019, pp. 132–133; Ledbetter et al., 2018, p. 1077).

Diagnosis

- Diagnosis is made by observation of the swelling/lump and by palpation of the herniated bowel or abdominal organs through the skin with the ability to manually reduce the herniation (Cavaliere, 2019, pp. 132–133; Ledbetter et al., 2018, p. 1077).

Complications

- Incarceration of the hernia (inability to manually reduce the hernia), ischemic injury, or a venous infection are serious complications (Cavaliere, 2019, p. 133; Ledbetter et al., 2018, p. 1077).

Management

- Treatment for unilateral or bilateral inguinal hernia is a herniorrhaphy, usually just prior to discharge in a premature infant (Cavaliere, 2019, p. 133; Ledbetter et al., 2018, p. 1077; Ringer & Hansen, 2017, pp. 960–961).

Outcomes

- Prognosis for full recovery is excellent. Recurrence risk is very small (Cavaliere, 2019, p. 133; Ledbetter et al., 2018, p. 1077; Ringer & Hansen, 2017, p. 961).

CRYPTORCHIDISM

Definition and Etiology

- Cryptorchidism is defined as undescended testicles. The testes (one or both) are not in the scrotal sac or scrotum.
- There are three possible causes of cryptorchidism: (a) endocrine dysfunction of the hypothalamic-pituitary-gonadal axis, (b) abnormal epididymal development without testicular descent into the scrotum, or (c) an anatomical abnormality preventing the descent of the testes into the scrotum (Merguerian & Rowe, 2018, p. 1268; Swartz & Chan, 2017, p. 939; Vogt & Dell, 2015, pp. 1549–1550).

Incidence

- The incidence of undescended testes is about 1% to 7% in full-term infants and up to as much as 45% in premature infants, with most being unilateral (about 70%; Merguerian & Rowe, 2018, p. 1268; Vogt & Dell, 2015, pp. 1549–1550). Most spontaneous descent occurs within six to ten weeks after birth, but usually by 6–9 months of age (Merguerian & Rowe, 2018, pp. 1268–1269).

Clinical Presentation

- Absence of testes in the scrotum
- Types of Undescended Testicles
  - Abdominal—testes are located inside the internal inguinal ring, therefore remaining in the abdomen.
  - Canalicular—testes located between the internal and external inguinal rings, remains within the canal
  - Ectopic—testes located between the abdominal cavity and the scrotum, but outside the inguinal canal
  - Retractile—testes are fully descended but move between the scrotum and the groin (Cavaliere, 2019, p. 131).
- The following syndromes have all been associated with undescended testes: Down, Klinefelter, Noonan, Prader-Willi, and fetal hydantoin syndrome, as well as other genetic, neurologic, or renal abnormalities (Swartz & Chan, 2017, p. 939).

Diagnosis

- Ultrasound and/or CT scan are both used for diagnosis as well as physical exam (Bates & Schwaderer, 2018, pp. 1278–1279).

Complications

- Testicular torsion, inguinal hernia, testicular cancer, and potential infertility have all been associated with persistent undescended testes (Merguerian & Rowe, 2018, p. 1268; Vogt & Dell, 2015, pp. 1549–1550).

Management

- Infants with undescended testes will usually have an orchiopexy between 6 and 24 months of age (Merguerian & Rowe, 2018, p. 1269; Swartz & Chan, 2017, p. 939; Vogt & Dell, 2015, pp. 1549–1550). Hormonal treatment with human chorionic gonadotropin can also be attempted (Merguerian & Rowe, 2018, p. 1269; Swartz & Chan, 2017, p. 939; Vogt & Dell, 2015, pp. 1549–1550).

Outcomes

- Fertility may be impaired, though the overall outcome is very good (Merguerian & Rowe, 2018, p. 1269; Swartz & Chan, 2017, p. 939; Vogt & Dell, 2015, pp. 1549–1550).

RENAL TUBULAR ACIDOSIS (RTA)

Definition and Etiology

- The kidneys excrete hydrogen (H^+) ion and reabsorb bicarbonate (HCO^-) ion to compensate for acidosis in the bloodstream. This disorder is the failure of the kidneys to respond and/or attempt to compensate for a metabolic acidosis (Sherman, 2015, p. 729).
- Types:
- There are four types of RTA:
  - **Type 1**—distal RTA is a defect in the ability to secrete the hydrogen ion.
  - **Type 2**—proximal RTA is a defect in the ability to reabsorb bicarbonate.
  - **Type 3**—a combination of types 1 and 2.
  - **Type 4**—hyperkalemic tubular type is due to a problem with aldosterone; either aldosterone deficiency or aldosterone resistance, which then results in high serum potassium levels (Richardson & Yonekawa, 2018, pp. 1305–1306; Samuels et al., 2017, pp. 398–399; Sherman, 2015, pp. 729–730; Vogt & Dell, 2015, p. 1697).

Clinical Presentation

- Infants with RTA will have signs of polyuria and weight loss despite adequate caloric intake (Richardson & Yonekawa, 2018, p. 1304).

Diagnosis

- Serum electrolytes with anion gap, blood gas for acidosis and bicarbonate level, and urine analysis for pH should be tested when the infant is acidotic (Richardson & Yonekawa,

2018, p. 1304). Infants with RTA will have a normal anion gap (Richardson & Yonekawa, 2018, p. 1304).

Management

- Treatment of infants with RTA is with sodium bicarbonate or Bicitra to correct the acidosis (Samuels et al., 2017, p. 399). Type 4 may require sodium supplementation and potassium restriction (Richardson & Yonekawa, 2018, p. 1306).

Outcomes

- Infants with Type 2 RTA may also have Fanconi anemia, and this needs to be explored (Richardson & Yonekawa, 2018, pp. 1304–1305).
- Treatment may cause a resolution of the symptoms and resolve the problem in some infants, but it depends on the cause of the tubular acidosis (see sections on renal dysplasia, obstruction, and hydronephrosis) (Samuels et al., 2017, p. 399).

NEPHROTOXICITY

Definition and Etiology

- Nephrotoxic drugs can damage the kidney of the newborn infant, either prenatally or after birth.
- Drugs that cross the placenta and may damage the kidney are the following:
  - Aminoglycosides
  - Heavy metals—lead and mercury
  - Alcohol intake by the mother can cause fetal alcohol syndrome (FAS) in the newborn infant and should be avoided or drastically limited. FAS can involve the kidney as well as other areas (Falck, Mooney, & Bearer, 2015, pp. 218–219).
  - Organic solvents (toluene)
  - Phthalates have produced hypospadias and cryptorchidism in rats (Askenazi et al., 2018, pp. 1285–1286; Falck et al., 2015, pp. 218–219, 222).
- Drugs given to the neonate may also damage the kidney. The following drugs are used to treat the infant in the NICU:
  - Aminoglycosides—direct tubular damage
  - Cephalosporins—direct tubular damage
  - Rifampin—direct tubular damage
  - Vancomycin—direct tubular damage
  - Indomethacin—decreased renal perfusion, direct tubular damage
  - Amphotericin B—direct tubular damage, decreased GFR
  - Acyclovir—tubular obstruction & decreased GFR
  - Radiocontrast agents—direct tubular damage
  - ACE inhibitors—decreased renal perfusion
  - Myoglobinuria—hemoglobinuria—direct tubular damage
  - Diuretics—decreased renal perfusion (Askenazi et al., 2018, pp. 1285–1286; Falck et al., 2015, pp. 218–219).

Incidence

- Recently evaluated cumulative nephrotoxic medication exposure of a cohort of 107 VLBW neonates. In this study, 87% of the cohort was exposed to at least one nephrotoxic medication, and on average these neonates were exposed to over 14 days of nephrotoxic medications (Askenazi, Selewski, Willig & Warady, 2018, p. 1286).

Clinical Presentation

- Nephrotoxicity may manifest clinically as nonoliguric renal failure, with a slow rise in serum creatinine and hypo-osmolar urine.
- Other alterations may include proteinuria and increasing in blood urea nitrogen (BUN) (Cadnapaphornchai, Schoebein, Woloschuk, Soranno & Hernandez, 2016, p. 698).

Management

- Aminoglycosides should be used with caution in an infant with pre-existing renal dysfuction
- Aminoglycoside toxicity is usually nonoliguric, therefore serial monitoring of serum creatinine values is necessary (Askenazi, Selewski, Willig & Warady, 2018, p. 1286)

CONCLUSION

This chapter has provided a brief review of the anatomy and physiology of the kidney, along with accompanying pathologies which may be congenital or develop during an infant's hospitalization. Guides for assessment of the infant with suspected renal dysfunction was reviewed as well as potential interventions from benign to invasive. The kidney is a vital organ which is essential to the infant's survival, so renal function must be considered when discussing any neonatal therapies.

REVIEW QUESTIONS

1. The fractional excretion of sodium (FENa) reflects the balance of sodium between:
   A. glomerular filtration and tubular reabsorption
   B. major and minor calyces and Bowman's capsule
   C. renal vein and the intraparenchymal pyramids

2. A medication which, if administered to the mother during pregnancy, can cause structural and/or functional anomalies of the fetal kidney is:
   A. dexamethasone (Decadron)
   B. indomethacin (Indocin)
   C. magnesium sulfate (MgSO$_4$)

3. An infant is born with a lack of abdominal wall muscles, hydronephrosis with a dilated bladder, and cryptorchidism. The most likely diagnosis is:
   A. Bardet–Biedl syndrome
   B. Churg–Strauss syndrome
   C. Eagle–Barrett syndrome

4. A genitourinary system abnormality that is considered a surgical emergency in the neonate is a/an:

    A. inguinal hernia

    B. patent urachus

    C. testicular torsion

5. A medication which can damage the neonate's kidney if given in high doses or over a prolonged period of time is:

    A. ampicillin (Omnipen)

    B. cefotaxime (Claforan)

    C. gentamicin (Garamycin)

REFERENCES

Askenazi, D., Selewski, D., Willig, L., & Warady, B. A. (2018). Acute kidney injury and chronic kidney disease. In C. A.Gleason & S. E. Juul (Eds.), *Avery's diseases of the newborn* (10th ed., pp. 1280–1300). Philadelphia, PA: Elsevier.

Bates, C. M., & Schwaderer, A. L. (2018). Clinical evaluation of renal and urinary tract disease. In C. A. Gleason & S. E. Juul (Eds.), *Avery's diseases of the newborn* (10th ed., pp. 1274–1323). Philadelphia, PA: Elsevier.

Blackburn, S. T. (2013). Renal system and fluid and electrolyte homeostasis. In *Maternal, fetal, and neonatal physiology: A clinical perspective* (4th ed., pp. 356–392). St. Louis, MO: Saunders

Bradshaw, W. (2015). Gastrointestinal disorders. In M. T. Verklan & M. Walden (Eds.), *Core curriculum for neonatal intensive care nursing* (5th ed., pp. 583–631). St. Louis, MO: Saunders Elsevier.

Cadnapaphornchai, M., Schoenbein, M., Woloschuk, R., Soranno, D., & Hernandez, J. (2016). Neonatal Nephrology. In S. Gardner, B. Carter, M. Hines, & J. Hernandez (Eds.). *Merenstein & Gardner's handbook of neonatal intensive care* (8th ed. pp. 689–726.e4).St. Louis, MO. Elsevier.

Cavaliere, T. (2019). Genitourinary assessment. In E. P. Tappero & M. E. Honeyfield (Eds.), *Physical assessment of the newborn—A comprehensive approach to the art of physical examination* (8th ed., pp. 121–138). New York, NY: Springer Publishing Company.

Diab, Y., & Luchtman-Jones, L. (2015). Hematologic and oncologic problems in the fetus and neonate. In R. J. Martin, A. A. Fanaroff, & M. C. Walsh, (Eds.) *Fanaroff and Martin's neonatal-perinatal medicine* (10th ed., pp. 1294–1343). Philadelphia, PA: Elsevier.

Doherty, E. G. (2017). Fluid and electrolyte management. In E. C. Eichenwald, A. R. Hansen, C. R. Martin, & A. R. Stark (Eds.), *Cloherty and Stark's manual of neonatal care* (8th ed., pp. 296–311). Philadelphia, PA: Wolters Kluwer.

Engen, R., & Hingorani, S. (2018). Developmental abnormalities of the kidneys. In C. A. Gleason & S. E. Juul (Eds.), *Avery's diseases of the newborn* (10th ed., pp. 1250–1259). Philadelphia, PA: Elsevier.

Falck, A. J., Mooney, S. M., & Bearer, C. F. (2015). Adverse exposures to the fetus. In R. J. Martin, A. A. Fanaroff, & M. C. Walsh, (Eds.) *Fanaroff and Martin's neonatal-perinatal medicine* (10th ed., pp. 211–226). Philadelphia, PA: Elsevier.

Goodwin, M. (2019). Abdominal assessment. In E. P. Tappero & M. E. Honeyfield (Eds.), *Physical assessment of the newborn—A comprehensive approach to the art of physical examination* (8th ed., pp. 111–120). New York, NY: Springer Publishing Company.

Kenagy, D. N., & Vogt, B. A. (2013). The kidney. In J. M. Fanaroff & A. A. Fanaroff (Eds.), *Klaus and Fanaroff's care of the high-risk neonate* (6th ed., pp. 410–431). Philadelphia, PA: Elsevier.

Ledbetter, D. J., Chabra, S., & Javid, P. J. (2018). Abdominal wall defects. In C. A. Gleason & S. E. Juul (Eds.), *Avery's diseases of the newborn* (10th ed., pp. 1068–1078). Philadelphia, PA: Elsevier.

Leonard, E. G., & Dobbs, K. (2015). Postnatal bacterial infections. In R. J. Martin, A. A. Fanaroff, & M. C. Walsh, (Eds.) *Fanaroff and Martin's neonatal-perinatal medicine* (10th ed., pp. 734–750). Philadelphia, PA: Elsevier.

Letterio, J., Ahuja, S. P., Petrosiute, A. (2013). Hematologic problems. In J. M. Fanaroff & A. A. Fanaroff (Eds.), *Klaus and Fanaroff's care of the high-risk neonate* (6th ed., pp. 432–475). Philadelphia, PA: Elsevier.

McAleer, I. (2018). Renal development. In C. A. Gleason & S. E. Juul (Eds.), *Avery's diseases of the newborn* (10th ed., pp. 1238–1249). Philadelphia, PA: Elsevier.

Merguerian, P. A., & Rowe, C. K. (2018). Developmental abnormalities of the genitourinary system. In C. A. Gleason & S. E. Juul (Eds.), *Avery's diseases of the newborn* (10th ed., pp. 1260–1273). Philadelphia, PA: Elsevier

Remeithi, S. A., & Wherritt, K. (2015). Disorders of sexual development. In R. J. Martin, A. A. Fanaroff, & M. C. Walsh, (Eds.) *Fanaroff and Martin's neonatal-perinatal medicine* (10th ed., pp. 1548–1550). Philadelphia, PA: Elsevier.

Richardson, K., & Yonekawa, K. (2018). Glomerulonephropathies and disorders of tubular function. In C. A. Gleason & S. E. Juul (Eds.), *Avery's diseases of the newborn* (10th ed., pp. 1301–1307). Philadelphia, PA: Elsevier.

Ringer, S. A., & Hansen, A. R. (2017). Surgical emergencies in the newborn. In E. C. Eichenwald, A. R. Hansen, C. R. Martin, & A. R. Stark (Eds.), *Cloherty and Stark's manual of neonatal care* (8th ed., pp. 942–966). Philadelphia, PA: Wolters Kluwer.

Samuels, J. A., Munoz, H., & Swinford, R. D. (2017). Neonatal kidney conditions. In E. C. Eichenwald, A. R. Hansen, C. R. Martin, & A. R. Stark (Eds.), *Cloherty and Stark's manual of neonatal care* (8th ed., pp. 366–400). Philadelphia, PA: Wolters Kluwer.

Sherman, J. (2015). Renal and genitourinary disorders. In M. T. Verklan & M. Walden (Eds.), *Core curriculum for neonatal intensive care nursing* (5th ed., pp. 719–733). St. Louis, MO: Saunders Elsevier.

Sparger, K. A., & Gupta, M. (2017). Neonatal thrombosis. In E. C. Eichenwald, A. R. Hansen, C. R. Martin, & A. R. Stark (Eds.), *Cloherty and Stark's manual of neonatal care* (8th ed., pp. 595–612). Philadelphia, PA: Wolters Kluwer

Swartz, J. M., & Chan, Y. M. (2017). Disorders of sexual development. In E. C. Eichenwald, A. R. Hansen, C. R. Martin, & A. R. Stark (Eds.), *Cloherty and Stark's manual of neonatal care* (8th ed., pp. 923–941). Philadelphia, PA: Wolters Kluwer.

Vogt, B. A., & Dell, K. M. (2015). The kidney and urinary tract of the neonate. In R. J. Martin, A. A. Fanaroff, & M. C. Walsh, (Eds.) *Fanaroff and Martin's neonatal-perinatal medicine* (10th ed., pp. 1676–1699). Philadelphia, PA: Elsevier.

Wang, P., Djahangirian, O., & Wehbi, E. (2018). Urinary tract infections and vesicoureteral reflux. In C. A. Gleason & S. E. Juul (Eds.), *Avery's diseases of the newborn* (10th ed., pp. 1308–1313). Philadelphia, PA: Elsevier.

20 THE ENDOCRINE/METABOLIC SYSTEM

Elena Bosque

INTRODUCTION

The goal of this chapter is to provide an overview of the problem in conceptual terms, and a general approach to care, which can be applied to cases that the NNP may encounter. The learner is encouraged to refer to the texts in the references for entire lists and explanations of all of the specific disorders.

The pathophysiology and treatment sections will be presented as metabolic and endocrine disorders. Metabolic disorders include those of carbohydrate, fat, and protein metabolism, problems of infants of diabetic mothers (IDM), and inborn errors of metabolism. Endocrine disorders include those of calcium, phosphorus, and magnesium metabolism, osteopenia, as well as thyroid, pituitary, and adrenal disorders, including disorders of sex development. There is some overlap among these categories because there is some overlap with these conditions. For example, problems of IDMs can be categorized as either or both a metabolic disorder, because of problems of carbohydrate metabolism, and an endocrine disorder, because of abnormal hormone production, with hyperinsulinism.

The NNP is expected to be able to identify typical clinical expressions of these disorders, to describe appropriate first-line interventions in collaboration with a neonatologist, to refer to a subspecialist, and to talk to parents about these problems. These activities involve anticipatory guidance of all team members to establish rigorous systems for obtaining, reporting, and responding to newborn screening results. Expected competencies include familiarity with characteristic signs and symptoms, communication with and integration of family members related to diagnosis and plan of care, and communication with subspecialists regarding inpatient and follow-up services (Merritt & Gallagher, 2018, p. 230).

OVERVIEW OF DISORDERS

- Metabolic or endocrine disorders of the newborn include problems known as inborn errors of metabolism and encompass both metabolic and biochemical genetic disease.
  - ○ Some of the expressions of metabolic disorders overlap with endocrine disorders, such as hypothyroidism and congenital adrenal hyperplasia (CAH).
  - ○ Most conditions involve gene mutation which causes an absent or defective enzyme, or over- or underproduction of hormones, with life-threatening

physiological or biochemical system regulation dysfunction (Cederbaum, 2018, p. 224; Divall & Merjaneh, 2018, p. 1324).

- Collectively, the incidence of metabolic or endocrine disorders is estimated to be approximately one per 1,000 to 2,000 live births. Newborn screening has identified disorders in one per 2,000 to 4,000 live births (El-Hattab & Sutton, 2017, p. 859; Nodine, Hastings-Tolsma, & Arruda, 2015, p. 14; Zinn, 2015, p. 1553).
  - ○ The most common disorders, such as phenylketonuria (PKU), occur approximately one per 10,000 to 15,000 live births (Nodine et al., 2015, p. 14; Zinn, 2015, p. 1553).
  - ○ Conversely, some disorders occur rarely, such as homocystinuria, which is diagnosed in approximately one per 1,800 to one per 900,000 live births (Merritt & Gallagher, 2018, p. 241).
- It is possible that the incidence of metabolic or endocrine disorders is underestimated if conditions are undetected. It is important to remember that multiple disorders of intermediary metabolism and energy metabolism are not detected through newborn screening. Intermediary metabolic disorders include aminoacidopathies, organic acidemias, and fatty acid oxidation disorders (Merritt & Gallagher, 2018, p. 230; Zinn, 2015, p. 1553)
- Many of these disorders are present during the neonatal period and are revealed as the protective effect of the maternal placenta ceases. Disorders, then, develop as acute, chronic, or progressive diseases, with potential life-threatening harm (Cederbaum, 2018, p. 224; Devaskar & Garg, 2015, p. 1434; Merritt & Gallagher, 2018, p. 230; Thomas, Lam, & Berry, 2018, p. 254).
  - ○ The normal transition from the maternal-fetal transport of nutrients to extrauterine homeostasis of the neonate may be disrupted by metabolic problems or dysfunction of regulatory systems (Devaskar & Garg, 2015, p. 1434; Divall & Merjaneh, p. 1325; Koves, Ness, Nip, & Salehi, 2018, p. 1333).
- Most neonates with metabolic or endocrine disorders are healthy at birth and present with nonspecific signs in hours or days after birth, and most are inherited in an autosomal recessive manner (El-Hattab & Sutton, 2017, pp. 858–859).
- If undiagnosed, many metabolic or endocrine disorders have profound negative consequences for the individual (El-Hattab & Sutton, 2017, p. 858; Swartz & Chan, 2018, p. 923; Wassner & Belfort, 2018, p. 892). In modern neonatology, with the standard use of the expanded newborn

screen, diagnosis and treatment usually occur early and before symptomatic presentation, and treatment can occur before the condition harms the individual (Cederbaum, 2018, p. 224; Merritt & Gallagher, 2018, p. 230; Zinn, 2015, p. 1553).

- Because some of the disorders present early, before the results of the newborn screen are known, or are not identified by the screen, it is important for healthcare providers to be able to identify clinical manifestations of these disorders, to provide initial care, and to recognize appropriate times to involve subspecialists (Cederbaum, 2018, p. 227; Merritt & Gallagher, 2018, p. 230; Zinn, 2015, p. 1608).
- Diagnosis of neonatal metabolic or endocrine problems is challenging for most clinicians. Many are intimidated because of the fear of making an incorrect diagnosis. Nonspecific presentations and individual rarity of diseases mean limited exposure for clinicians. Inherited metabolic or endocrine disorders will not be diagnosed unless specific investigations for that disorder are undertaken. It becomes important to understand basic pathophysiology, and to develop an approach to the investigation, upon presentation of symptoms (El-Hattab & Sutton, 2017, p. 859).

PHYSIOLOGY AND PATHOPHYSIOLOGY

Metabolic Disorders in the Neonate

DISORDERS OF CARBOHYDRATE METABOLISM

- Although the fetus is entirely dependent upon the mother for nutrients, it is hormonally independent. Maternal glucose is the major nutrient and the only source of fetal glucose. Fetal hormone responses are mediated by maternal supply of nutrients, even as maternal concentration fluctuates with pathology, as in the case of maternal diabetes.
  - ○ Substrates delivered to the human fetus for metabolism include glucose, fatty acids, amino acids, ketone bodies, glycerol, and other minor nutrients.
  - ○ Fetal hormones responsible for uptake of nutrients include insulin, glucagon, human chorionic somatomammotropin, and human growth hormone (Devaskar & Garg, 2015, pp. 1434–1435).
- At birth, when maternal supply of nutrients ceases, there is a surge of levels of epinephrine, norepinephrine, and glucagon in the neonate. This causes a fall in insulin level to mobilize glycogen and stimulate gluconeogenesis, resulting in a rise, initially, then a steady glucose production (Devaskar & Garg, 2015, p. 1436).
- In healthy full-term newborn infants, the plasma glucose concentration remains at a steady level of 40 to 80 mg/dL.
  - ○ Breastfed, small for gestational age, and premature infants may have lower steady-state glucose levels.
  - ○ Most investigators have defined hypoglycemia as plasma glucose level lower than 40 mg/dL, independent of gestational age or other factors (Devaskar & Garg, 2015, p. 1436).

HYPERINSULINEMIA

- Transient hyperinsulinism may result in neonatal hypoglycemia secondary to be an IDM, perinatal stress, or being small for gestational age.
- Hyperinsulinism which results in incalcitrant hypoglycemia is usually related to metabolic disorders associated

with genetic mutations, or tumors (Werny, Taplin, Bennett, & Pihoker, 2018, p. 1406).
  - ○ Diagnostic criteria for the diagnosis of hyperinsulinism is based upon a critical sample at the time of hypoglycemia, and includes:
    - ■ Insulin level >2 µIU/mL
    - ■ B-Hydroxybutyrate level <1.8 mmol/L
    - ■ Free fatty acid level <1.7 mmol/L
    - ■ Glucose rise ≥30 mg/dL after glucagon administration
    - ■ Insulin-like growth factor-binding protein 1 level ≤110 ng/mL (Werny et al., 2018, p. 1411).
  - ○ Normal insulin levels associated with transient hypoglycemia with may be caused by immaturity, increased metabolic expenditure, or maternal conditions.
  - ○ If hypoglycemia persists in the presence of normal insulin levels, this may be caused by endocrine disorders such as hypopituitarism or primary adrenal insufficiency or inborn errors of metabolism (see later sections; Werny et al., 2018, p. 1406).

HYPOGLYCEMIA

- Any alteration in either maternal metabolism or intrinsic metabolic problems of the neonate may cause hypoglycemia.
  - ○ Transient hypoglycemia, during the transition period after birth, may require brief surveillance and intervention, but resolves. It is usually the consequence of changes in the metabolic environment in utero, maternal drugs (e.g., tocolytics, diuretics, propranolol), or perinatally (Blackburn, 2012, p. 574; Devaskar & Garg, 2015, pp. 1438–1439).
  - ○ Persistent or recurrent hypoglycemia is a form which requires prolonged management, including high rates of glucose infusions for several hours, or potentially days, or pharmacologic intervention, such as use of diazoxide. Persistent hypoglycemia is the product of intrinsic metabolic problems of the infant, such as hyperinsulinism, congenital disorders, endocrine disorders, or inborn errors of metabolism (Devaskar & Garg, 2015, p. 1439; Werny et al., 2018, p. 1410).
- Defects of any of the enzymes in the carbohydrate metabolic pathways will result in pathogenesis of many organs, including the liver, kidney, brain, heart, intestine, ovaries, and skin.
  - ○ These disorders include galactosemia, glycogen storage diseases, and fructose-1-6-phosphatase deficiency.
  - ○ For example, infants with galactosemia often present with severe jaundice and coagulopathy, while infants with other disorders of carbohydrate metabolism may present with hypoglycemia, lactic acidosis, infection, or intestinal problems (Merritt & Gallagher, 2018, p. 236).
- Many of the disorders of carbohydrate metabolism are confirmed through newborn screening and genetic testing. Hyperinsulinemia will be diagnosed with measurement of glucose, insulin, cortisol, beta-hydroxybutyrate, and free fatty acid levels (Burris, 2017, p. 317). Treatment approaches vary per disorder, but may include dietary, medication, or vitamin management.

INFANTS OF DIABETIC MOTHERS

- The incidence of neonatal hypoglycemia in IDMs varies from 5% to 50%, with a lower incidence rate in infants of mothers with good glycemic control in pregnancy (Brown & Chang, 2019, p. 99).

○ The reported rates vary because of controversies and inconsistencies in the medical literature with definitions of hypoglycemia (Brown & Chang, 2018, p. 99).

- IDMs, who experience intermittent fetal hyperglycemia in response to maternal hypoglycemia, develop hypertrophic pancreatic islets and beta cells with increased fetal insulin secretion.
  ○ These fetuses and infants have high stores of glycogen and fat.
  ○ These fetuses and infants are at risk for numerous morbidities including congenital anomalies, heart failure, cardiac septal hypertrophy, surfactant deficiency, respiratory distress syndrome, persistent pulmonary hypertension, hyperbilirubinemia, hypoglycemia, hypocalcemia, hypomagnesemia, macrosomia, nerve injury related to birth trauma, renal vein thrombosis, small left colon, unexplained intrauterine demise, polycythemia, visceromegaly, neurosensory impairment, and predisposition to later-life obesity and diabetes (Brown & Chang, 2018, p. 99; Devaskar & Garg, 2015, p. 1440; Gorman, 2017, pp. 916–921).
- Neonatal hypoglycemia in IDMs is most likely due to hyperinsulinism. The fetus was hyperglycemic in relation to maternal hyperglycemia and responded with production of insulin.
  ○ Despite high energy stores, after birth, the amount of insulin production remains the same, with less neonatal glucose supply, so the neonate has hypoglycemia in the first few hours of life, which may persist for several days (Brown & Chang, 2018, p. 100; Werny et al., 2018, p. 1411).
- Symptoms may include sweating, pallor, tachycardia, tachypnea, tremor, "jittery", abnormal cry (weak or high-pitched), hypotonia, weak suck, lethargy, coma, seizure. Polycythemia is an associated feature related to increased erythropoiesis.
  ○ Not all infants with hypoglycemia, as defined in the medical literature, have symptoms or adverse effects (Brown & Chang, 2018, p. 99; Werny et al., 2018, p. 1405).
- Treatment of IDMs with hypoglycemia may include early feeding, frequent feeding, oral dextrose gel (40%), intravenous dextrose administration. Central venous catheter placement is recommended for dextrose concentration greater than 12.5%, with careful calculation of fluids and glucose index rate (mg/kg/min), then judicious weaning over first days or weeks of life (Burris, 2017, Fig. 24.1, p. 320; Werny et al., 2018, p. 1411).

DISORDERS OF FAT METABOLISM

- Lipids are necessary for retinal and neuronal development, including myelin sheath synthesis.
  ○ Essential fatty acids (EFAs) and linoleic acids are essential for brain, retinal, prostaglandin, thromboxane, and leukotrienes development.
  ○ Cholesterol is necessary for embryogenesis, cell membranes growth and function, bile acid synthesis, and steroid production.
  ○ The fetus is somewhat dependent on placental transfer of lipids, with some lipogenesis occurring in the fetal liver and other tissue (Blackburn, 2012, p. 577).
- The transition of the fetus to extra-uterine life includes lipid mobilization.
  ○ As with carbohydrates, an increase of catecholamines and glucagon, with a decrease in insulin levels and a

surge in thyroid hormones, promote fatty acid mobilization and glucagon production.
  ○ The newborn changes from glucose to fatty acid oxidative metabolism to conserve glucose for the brain.
  ○ Free fatty acid production is used by the heart and brain in the absence of glucose and results in ketone bodies (Blackburn, 2012, p. 578).
- Lipogenesis is dependent on cholesterol metabolism and substrate availability. Lipogenic precursors include glucose, lactate, and ketone bodies. During anaerobic metabolism, for example, during asphyxia, inefficient anaerobic glycolysis cannot meet energy requirements, resulting in precursors of gluconeogenesis, including lactate, pyruvate, and glycerol (Devaskar & Garg, 2015, p. 1437).
- Any disruption of enzyme activity in fatty acid metabolism will result in failure of oxidation within or transport of free fatty acids into the mitochondria.
  ○ This transport activity depends on carnitine.
  ○ These disorders lead to a deficit in energy production and can be life-threatening.
  ○ Infants with these disorders present after a few days of life, in a catabolic state, with breakdown of fatty acids from adipose tissue. This may occur before newborn screening results are known.
  ○ These infants may present with hypoglycemia, liver problems, cardiomyopathy, cardiac dysrhythmias, skeletal myopathy, and retinal degeneration (Merritt & Gallagher, 2018, p. 245).
- Diagnosis of many fatty acid oxidation disorders is made with plasma acylcarnitine levels, free carnitine levels, and genetic testing.
  ○ These disorders include long-chain acyl-CoA dehydrogenase deficiency (LCHADD), multiple acyl-CoA dehydrogenase deficiency (MADD), medium-chain acyl-CoA dehydrogenase deficiency (MCADD), short-chain acyl-CoA dehydrogenase deficiency (SCADD), and very long chain acyl-CoA dehydrogenase deficiency (VLCADD).
- Many of the devastating organ effects of these disorders may be avoided with early treatment. Some of these disorders require avoidance of dietary fat, so breastfeeding may be contraindicated.
- Treatment may include frequent feedings, avoidance of fasting, and diet, medication, or vitamin management (Merritt & Gallagher, 2018, p. 245).

DISORDERS OF PROTEIN METABOLISM

- Amino acids are necessary for protein synthesis and oxidative activities during organ development and tissue remodeling. Some amino acids are used for energy.
  ○ The fetus receives maternal amino acids via active transport across the placenta or produced by the placenta.
- After birth, the newborn is in a catabolic state relative to the anabolic state during fetal life. Serum amino acids are higher in newborns than later in life. The newborn infant has limited ability to synthesize amino acids, partly, due to limited liver enzyme function (Blackburn, 2012, p. 581).
- An infant with a disorder in protein metabolism may present with hypoglycemia, poor feeding, vomiting, odor, hypothermia, respiratory distress, hyperammonemia, azotemia, metabolic acidosis, ketosis, cholestasis, hepatosplenomegaly, lymphadenopathy, or hematologic problems.

○ These defects may lead to cirrhosis, renal dysfunction, cardiomyopathy, central nervous system abnormalities, developmental delay, or death.

○ Some of the amino acid metabolic disorders are associated with dysmorphic features but some are not (El-Hattab & Sutton, 2017, pp. 865–881; Zinn, 2015, pp. 1585–1591).

- The most common inborn error of amino acid metabolism is PKU, which affects approximately 1 in 12,000 live births (Sahai & Levy, 2018, p. 338).

  ○ It is an autosomal recessive disorder from deficiency of phenylalanine hydroxylase, required to convert phenylalanine to tyrosine.

  ○ PKU was the first disorder detected by the development of the newborn screen, in the 1960s.

  ○ Since tyrosine is elemental to the production of dopamine and other essential neurotransmitters, infants with this disorder experience developmental and intellectual disabilities, skin problems, and epilepsy (Merritt & Gallagher, 2018, pp. 241–242).

  ○ Treatment for PKU is life long dietary therapy.

- The diagnosis of amino acid metabolic disorders may be made, depending upon the disorder, by newborn screening, plasma, urine, and cerebral spinal fluid amino acid analysis, plasma acyl-carnitine analysis, urine organic acid analysis, chromatography, tandem mass spectrometry, in vitro cell studies of cultured skin fibroblasts, enzyme assay, or genetic testing.

  ○ Treatment for some of these disorders may include diet, vitamin supplementation, or liver transplantation; however, with some of these disorders, there is no known effective treatment (El-Hattab & Sutton, 2017, pp. 865–881; Zinn, 2015, pp. 1585–1591).

Inborn Errors of Metabolism

- Inborn errors of metabolism are also known as inherited metabolic disease (Zinn, 2015, p. 1553).

  ○ Enzyme proteins normally catalyze metabolic processes, and thousands of enzymes are required to perform critical biochemical reactions for processing or transport of amino acids, carbohydrates, or fatty acids.

  ○ The substance upon which the enzyme acts is the substrate.

- With absence or deficiency of these enzymes, the substrate molecules accumulate and may be converted to products that are not usually present. These alternative end products also interfere with normal metabolic processes. Finally, there is an inability to degrade end products.

  ○ Symptoms result from increased levels of normal substrate that become toxic, or lack of normal end products necessary for cellular function.

  ○ The toxic levels of metabolites or deficient cellular function can lead to decreased muscle tone, seizures, organ failure, blindness, deafness, mental retardation, and death (Cederbaum, 2018, p. 224; El-Hattab & Sutton, 2017, p. 858).

- Various strategies for conceptualization, classification, evaluation, and treatment of inborn errors of metabolism that present in the newborn period, or later, have been proposed (Cederbaum, 2018, p. 224; El-Hattab & Sutton, 2017, p. 859).

  ○ Inborn errors of metabolism are presented in this chapter as small-molecule disorders, lysosomal storage disorders, energy metabolism disorders, and heterogenous disorders.

  ○ In Table 20.1, classification groups, examples of metabolic problems, examples of some common specific disorders, and treatments are presented (Cederbaum, 2018, p. 224; El-Hattab & Sutton, 2017, p. 859).

Small Molecule Disorders

- The small molecule disorders include aminoacidopathies, including PKU, organic acidurias, urea cycle defects, and sugar intolerances, including galactosemia. They result from the accumulation of toxic compounds before the blockage in the metabolic pathway or process

  ○ The infant may be symptom-free initially; then demonstrate acute or progressive intoxication. The infant presents with increased drowsiness and poor feeding, after the metabolite accumulates, with stress, or when feeds are introduced.

  ○ Without intervention full decompensation will occur with acidosis, seizure, obtundation, coma, and death (Merritt & Gallagher, 2018, p. 231).

- Lysosomal storage diseases result from defective function of a catabolic hydrolase located in the lysosome that is responsible for metabolism of glycosaminoglycans and sphingolipids.

  ○ Other disorders in this category include a group of metabolic disorders that share dysfunction and defects of glycosylation, or cholesterol synthesis.

  ○ With most of these disorders, pathologic metabolites accumulate slowly with time and may not present in the newborn period. However, there are a few disorders of mucopolysaccharides and glycolipids which do present in neonates, including Pompe disease and Krabbe disease (Cederbaum & Berry, 2018, p. 226).

- Energy metabolism disorders are notable for insufficient generation of energy by the mitochondria. These include disorders such as fatty acid oxidation defects, disorders of ketogenesis, glycogen storage disease Type I, and disorders of gluconeogenesis (Cederbaum, 2018, p. 226).

  ○ Mitochondrial disorders and long-chain fatty acid oxidation defects can present with many symptoms, especially neurological or cardiac ones, but may also include disruptions of energy metabolism.

  ○ Infants may present at birth, or later, with hypoglycemia, lactic acidosis, or cardiac decompensation (Cederbaum, 2018, pp. 225–228; Merritt & Gallagher, 2018, p. 231; Thomas et al., 2018, pp. 253–255).

- Heterogenous disorders are very rare disorders resulting from absence or dysfunction of enzymes, which include carbohydrate-deficient glycoprotein disorders, lysosomal storage disease, peroxisomal disorders, disorders involving transport or receptor enzymes, or purine and pyrimidine disorders.

  ○ These complex molecules are key to embryogenesis, so infants with these disorders often present with dysmorphic features, which may be subtle at birth but become more pronounced as storage material accumulates (Thomas et al., 2018, pp. 253–255).

  ○ These disorders usually present in the extended neonatal period and may be diagnosed with enzyme assay or genetic sequencing testing.

TABLE 20.1 Example of Classification System for Neonatal Inborn Errors of Metabolism

Groups	Metabolic Problem	Disorder	Treatment
Small molecule disorders	Amino acids Organic acids Sugars	Includes aminoacidemias, for example, phenylketonuria, organic acidurias, urea cycle disorders, sugar intolerances, for example, galactosemia	Diet Extracorporeal procedures Drugs Vitamins
Lysosomal storage disorders	Lipids Glycoproteins Glycolipids Mucopolysaccharides Shingolipids	Include diseases with lysosomal, defects, for example, glycogen storage disease Type II (Pompe), Gaucher, Niemann–Pick type A or type B, Krabbe, Fabry disease, or mucopolysacchari-dosis	Mostly untreatable Some new or experimental enzyme, organ transplant, or gene therapy
Energy metabolism disorders	Inborn errors of intermediary metabolism that affect the cytoplasmic and mitochondrial energetic processes Oxidation disorders Fatty acid mobilization and metabolism disorders Glycogen storage diseases	Include: Cytoplasmic defects encompass those affecting glycolysis, glycogenosis, gluconeogenesis, hyperinsulinism (most treatable) Creatine (partly treatable) and pentose phosphate pathways (untreatable) Mitochondrial defects include respiratory chain disorders, and Krebs cycle and pyruvate oxidation defects (Mostly untreatable) Disorders of fatty acid oxidation and ketone bodies (treatable)	For some, dextrose, diet, supplements For others, no treatment
Heterogenous	Carbohydrate-deficient glycoprotein disorders Peroxisomal biogenesis disorders Cholesterol biosynthetic disorders Disorders of biogenic amines, folate, and pyridoxine Transport disorders Purine and pyrimidine metabolism disorders Receptor disorders	Include: Smith–Lemli–Opitz syndrome, melovalonic aciduria, folate deficiencies, Fanconi syndrome, Menkes disease, Zellweger syndrome, X-linked adrenoleukodystrophy, and so on	For some, nutritional, dietary, or vitamin supplements Medication Replacement therapy For others, no treatment

Sources: Data from Bacino, C. (2017). Genetic issues presenting in the nursery. In Eichenwald et al. (Eds.), *Cloherty and Stark's manual of neonatal care* (8th ed., pp. 117–130). Philadelphia, PA: Lippincott, Williams & Wilkins; Brown, Z., & Chang, J. (2018). Disorders of carbohydrate metabolism. In C. Gleason & S. Juul (Eds.), *Avery's disease of the newborn* (10th ed., pp. 1403–1416). Philadelphia, PA: Elsevier; Burris, H. (2017). Hypoglycemia and hyperglycemia. In Eichenwald et al. (Eds.), *Cloherty and Stark's manual of neonatal care* (8th ed., pp. 312–334). Philadelphia, PA: Lippincott, Williams & Wilkins; Cederbaum, S. (2018). Introduction to metabolic and biochemical genetic diseases. In C. Gleason & S. Juul (Eds.), *Avery's disease of the newborn* (10th ed., pp. 209–214). Philadelphia, PA: Elsevier; Cederbaum, S., & Berry, G. T. (2018). Inborn errors of carbohydrate, ammonia, amino acid, and organic acid metabolism. In C. Gleason & S. Juul (Eds.), *Avery's disease of the newborn* (10th ed., pp. 215–238). Philadelphia, PA: Elsevier; El-Hattab, A. W., & Sutton, V. R. (2017). Inborn errors of metabolism. In Eichenwald et al. (Eds.), *Cloherty and Stark's manual of neonatal care* (8th ed., pp. 858–891). Philadelphia, PA: Lippincott, Williams & Wilkins.

ENDOCRINE DISORDERS IN THE NEONATE

Disorders of Calcium, Phosphorus, and Magnesium Metabolism

- The majority of calcium, phosphorus, and magnesium stores can be found in the human skeleton, but also in the intracellular and extracellular spaces. These minerals are necessary for many biochemical reactions and cell functions in the body, including cardiovascular, nervous system, muscular, and homeostatic processes.
  - Bone minerals are important for ion transport across cell membranes, enzyme activity, intracellular regulation of metabolic pathways, hormone activity, coagulation activity, muscle contractility, and nerve conduction (Abrams & Tiosan, 2015, p. 1460; Blackburn, 2012, p. 589; Koves et al., 2018, p. 1333).

- During fetal life, these nutrients are transferred across the placenta. After birth, the supply of calcium is dependent upon enteral absorption through active and passive transport in the intestine with adequate vitamin D levels. For this reason, serum calcium levels normally decline after birth.
  - Calcium is excreted by the kidney. Nutrient intake from unfortified human milk has been calculated to be inadequate compared to fetal levels (Abrams & Tiosan, 2015, p. 1460; Blackburn, 2012, p. 589).
- Serum calcium represents less than 1% of whole-body calcium. Of this, about 50% of total serum calcium is in the ionized form and is the only physiologically active fraction. About 40% of total serum calcium is bound to proteins.
- Serum calcium is regulated by parathyroid hormone and 1,25-dihydroxyvitamin D (calcitriol), which increases serum calcium and by calcitonin, which decreases it.

○ Total serum calcium can be decreased by hypoalbuminemia.

○ Ionized calcium levels may be decreased by alkalosis as this increases albumin affinity for calcium.
  ▪ In the converse, acidosis decreases albumin binding and increases the ionized calcium.
  ▪ (Abrams & Tiosan, 2015, p. 1460; Blackburn, 2012, p. 590; Koves et al., 2018, p. 1333).

• Phosphorus accounts for about 10% to 15% of stores and is present in soft tissues and in extracellular fluid.
  ○ Phosphorus is absorbed in the intestine and reabsorbed and excreted by the kidney.
  ○ Absorption depends on dietary phosphorus as well as relative concentrations of calcium and phosphorus.
  ○ Deficiencies may result in muscle weakness, impaired leukocyte function, and abnormal bone metabolism (Abrams & Tiosan, 2015, p. 1463; Koves et al., 2018, p. 1334).

• Magnesium is stored in the skeleton at about 60%, and the remainder can be found in muscle, the nervous system, and organs with high metabolic rates.
  ○ Magnesium is absorbed in the intestine via both active and passive mechanisms. It is excreted and reabsorbed via the kidney to maintain homeostasis.
  ○ Magnesium is required for normal parathyroid secretory responses, protein synthesis, membrane integrity, nervous tissue, conduction, neuromuscular excitability, muscle contraction, hormone secretion, and intermediate metabolism.
  ○ One-third of serum magnesium is bound to albumin (Abrams & Tiosan, 2015, p. 1467; Koves et al., 2018, p. 1334).

• Homeostasis of all three elements, calcium, phosphorus, and magnesium require normal parathyroid hormone and calcitonin function as well as sufficient vitamin D levels.
  ○ The parathyroid glands secrete parathyroid hormone, which mobilizes calcium and phosphorus from bone and stimulates calcium reabsorption in the kidneys.
  ○ Calcitonin is synthesized by the thyroid in response to elevated serum calcium and lowers serum calcium and phosphorus secretions by inhibition of bone resorption and increased renal secretion.
  ○ Vitamin D is synthesized through the skin after sunshine exposure, or is absorbed from dietary sources in the intestine. It is transported to the liver, bound to protein, and metabolized in the kidney. Vitamin D maintains calcium and phosphorus balance through effects on the small intestine, through the synthesis of calcium-binding proteins, and on the kidney (Abrams & Tiosan, 2015, p. 1469; Koves et al., 2018, p. 1334).

Calcium, Magnesium, and Phosphate Imbalances

CALCIUM

• The definition of neonatal hypocalcemia varies with gestational age and birth weight but has been defined as a serum calcium level of less than 7 mg/dL or an ionized calcium less than 4 mg/dL (1 mmol/L (Abrams, 2017, p. 326). Definitions of normal values may also vary, slightly, depending upon the reference source.
  ○ In sick infants, it may be useful to measure the ionized calcium, which is the physiologically active portion.
  ○ Early hypocalcemia in the first 3 days of life commonly occurs with prematurity, asphyxia, in IDMs, and with intrauterine growth restriction (Koves et al., 2018, p. 1338).
  ○ Late neonatal hypocalcemia, after 3 to 5 days of life, may be associated with high phosphate load, maternal

vitamin D deficiency, congenital hypoparathyroidism including DiGeorge syndrome, maternal hyperparathyroidism, secondary to renal hypomagnesemia or renal tubular acidosis, abnormalities in vitamin D metabolism, and other rare causes (Koves et al., 2018, pp. 1338–1342).

• Signs of hypocalcemia are variable and may not correlate with calcium level, but may include jitteriness, poor feeding, vomiting, hematemesis, melena, hypotonia, apnea, tachycardia, prolonged cardiac QT interval, respiratory distress, high-pitched cry, hyperactivity, irritability, or seizures (Koves et al., 2018, p. 1338).

• Infants may not require treatment of hypocalcemia if stable and without symptoms.
  ○ Treatment during the acute stage may include a constant infusion of intravenous administration of calcium gluconate, if the calcium level is very low, or there are symptoms.
  ○ Risks of calcium infusion include bradyarrhythmias with rapid boluses, or subcutaneous tissue injury with infiltration.
  ○ Longer term treatment may include calcium supplementation, diet therapy, magnesium supplementation, or vitamin D treatment, depending upon the cause.

• Neonatal hypercalcemia has been defined as total serum calcium greater than 11.0 mg/dL or ionized calcium levels greater than 0.28 mmol/L (Koves et al., 2018, p. 1343).
  ○ Hypercalcemia may occur when there is a disruption in the interactive activities of parathyroid hormone, calcium-sensing receptors, calcitonin, and vitamin D in the intestine and kidney.
  ○ This may be caused by calcium-sensing receptor mutations with hyperparathyroidism, other forms of hyperparathyroidism, Williams syndrome, subcutaneous fat necrosis, iatrogenic excessive intake of calcium or vitamin D, iatrogenic decreased intake of phosphorus, or other rare causes (Koves et al., 2018, p. 1335).

• Hypercalcemia at low levels may be asymptomatic. Symptoms of hypercalcemia at high levels may include vomiting, respiratory distress, apnea, hypotonia, lethargy, polyuria, and seizures.
  ○ Treatment may include restriction of calcium and vitamin D, rehydration, or medication to treat acute effects, including calcitonin, loop diuretics and steroids (Koves et al., 2018, p. 1343).

MAGNESIUM

• Neonatal hypomagnesemia has been defined as serum magnesium level less than 1.6 mg/dL.
  ○ Neonatal hypomagnesemia is uncommon but may be associated with hypocalcemia or therapeutic cooling.
  ○ Symptoms may include apnea, poor tone, or seizures. Treatment of hypomagnesemia, with seizures, may include slow intravenous infusion of magnesium sulfate (Abrams, 2017, p. 333).

• Hypermagnesemia has been defined as serum magnesium level of greater than 3 mg/dL.
  ○ Hypermagnesemia is usually due to exogenous load that exceeds renal clearance.
  ○ Common causes include maternal magnesium therapy, administration of neonatal antacids, excessive magnesium in total parenteral nutrition, or medication errors (Abrams, 2017, p. 333; Koves et al., 2018, p. 1346).

○ Signs of hypermagnesemia include apnea, respiratory depression, lethargy, hypotonia, hyporeflexia, poor suck, decreased intestinal motility, delayed passage of meconium, hypotension, arrhythmias, coma, complete heart block, asystolic cardiac arrest.

○ Treatment is supportive until the magnesium is cleared by the kidney (Abrams, 2017, p. 333; Koves et al., 2018, p. 1346).

PHOSPHATE

• Normal term neonatal serum phosphate levels are 5.5 to 7.0 mg/dL, and may be higher than adult levels because of released stores, decreased or immature renal function, increased energy demand, and delayed feeding (Blackburn, 2012, p. 598).

○ Phosphorus, along with calcium, is necessary for bone mineralization, skeletal and skin growth, glucose metabolism, cardiovascular function, neuromuscular depolarization, immune system function, and hormone regulation.

○ Phosphorus is absorbed in the small intestine. Absorption and metabolism of phosphorus are under the influence of vitamin D and parathyroid hormone (Blackburn, 2012, pp. 589–590).

• Hypophosphatemia is rare, and usually related to parenteral or enteral nutritional causes or, rarely, renal causes. Symptoms would be related to hypercalcemia, including feeding intolerance, lethargy, irritability, hypertension, or seizures (Abrams, 2017, p. 328).

• Hyperphosphatemia is usually related to hypocalcemia, dietary excesses, or ordering error.

○ Infants with hyperphosphatemia may be asymptomatic, or with symptoms related to hypocalcemia such as apnea, jitteriness, increased tone, hyperreflexia, abnormalities of cardiac function, or seizures.

○ Treatment would include detection and correction of hypocalcemia, change in diet, or prevention of ordering errors (Abrams, 2017, p. 328).

METABOLIC BONE DISEASE

• Metabolic bone disease is defined as inadequate postnatal bone mineralization and is common among very low birth weight infants.

○ It is often called osteopenia or rickets of prematurity and is caused by deficiency of calcium and phosphorus due to poor mineral intake and absorption.

○ Less common causes include long-term fluid restriction, long-term total parenteral nutrition, furosemide therapy, or long-term steroid use (Abrams, 2017, p. 853; Koves et al., 2018, p. 1347).

○ This condition can lead to osteoporosis, with fractures, due to decreased bone mineral density, or rickets, which involves the growth plate.

• Rarely, metabolic bone disease may be associated with genetic disorders, including 1 alpha-hydroxylase deficiency or maternal vitamin D deficiency, Fanconi syndrome, or tumors.

○ Diagnosis may be made by laboratory analysis of mineral and hormone levels, rapid increase in alkaline phosphatase value, fracture seen per radiograph, or, rarely, with genetic testing.

○ Treatment includes diet management, diet fortification, mineral supplementation, vitamin therapy, passive physical activity, and surveillance (Abrams, 2017, p. 857; Wassner & Belfort, 2017, p. 892).

Disorders of the Thyroid

• Thyroid embryogenesis is complete by 10 to 12 weeks of gestation. At this time the fetal thyroid gland starts to concentrate iodine and secrete triiodothyronine (T3) and thyroxine (T4).

○ Thyrotropin/thyroid-stimulating hormone (TSH) secretion from the fetal pituitary gland increases, beginning mid-gestation.

○ Maternal TSH does not cross the placenta but maternal thyrotropin-releasing hormone (TRH) does cross.

○ After birth, there is a dramatic surge of TSH which peaks at 6 hours of life. In the preterm this surge is less marked (Chuang, Gutmark-little & Rose, 2015, p. 1498; Wassner & Belfort, 2017, p. 897).

• Thyroid hormone is essential for fetal brain development and for growth and metabolism regulation throughout childhood (Kim, Nandi-Munshi, & DiBlasi, 2018, p. 1388).

○ Thyrotropin/TSH is a pituitary hormone that stimulates the thyroid gland to secrete triiodothyronine (T3) and thyroxine (T4) into the circulation to regulate metabolism of thyroid-dependent tissues in the body.

○ Thyroid hormone is critical for normal growth and function, including the brain (Chuang et al., 2015, p. 1498).

• Control of thyroid hormone secretion is centered in the hypothalamic–pituitary–thyroid axis (HPA).

○ Thyroid hormones are iodinated amino acids.

○ Iodine is required by the thyroid gland and made available, when ingested or absorbed, via an active transport process that requires oxidative phosphorylation.

○ Thyrotropin is a glycoprotein that stimulates the thyroid to produce thyroxine (T4). Thyroxine (T4) is converted to triiodothyronine (T3), which is the active hormone that stimulates metabolism in most body tissue.

○ There are many intermediary hormones, antibodies, and other proteins that may affect normal thyroid function (Chuang et al., 2015, p. 1498)

HYPOTHYROIDISM

• Congenital hypothyroidism can be caused by primary hypothyroidism, including thyroid dysgenesis, inborn errors of thyroid hormone synthesis or secretion, mutations in the TSH receptor causing resistance, maternal ingestion of antithyroid drugs, or as a result of iodine deficiency (cretinism).

○ Congenital hypothyroidism may also be due to central congenital hypothyroidism, a genetic disorder either through inheritance or mutation.

○ This disorder has been attributed to difficult birth, birth injury, anoxia, growth or pituitary hormone deficiencies, and may be associated with any midline congenital defect (Chuang et al., 2015, pp. 1502–1504; Wassner & Belfort, 2017, pp. 901).

• Transient congenital hypothyroidism can be caused by anti-thyroid drugs, iodine excess or deficiency, transient hypothyroxinemia of prematurity, maternal TSH receptor-blocking antibodies, liver hemangiomas, and hypothyroxinemia associated with sick euthyroid syndrome (Wassner & Belfort, 2017, pp. 901–903). Most of these infants require treatment with thyroid hormone replacement but will not require lifelong treatment (Kim et al., 2018, p. 1398).

• Diagnosis of congenital hypothyroidism is made, most often, through the newborn screen, which permits early diagnosis and treatment, with optimal outcome.

○ Clinical signs of hypothyroidism include constipation, hypothermia, poor tone, lethargy, inactivity, respiratory distress, mottled skin, prolonged jaundice, poor feeding, large tongue, periorbital edema, large anterior and posterior fontanels, pallor, perioral cyanosis, poor or hoarse cry, lingual thyroid, or goiter.

○ If clinical signs of hypothyroidism are present, thyroid function studies should be performed, even if newborn screening results are negative.

○ Radiographic studies of bone maturation, radiograph or echocardiogram to evaluate for cardiomegaly, or ultrasound of the thyroid may be considered.

○ Other tests that should be considered may include cortisol and growth hormone levels and imaging of the hypothalamus and pituitary, to rule out pituitary-hypothalamic defects.

- Treatment of hypothyroidism includes thyroid hormone replacement therapy and proper nutrition and vitamin support. Congenital hypothyroidism is one of the most preventable causes of intellectual disability (Chuang et al., 2015, pp. 1505–1509; Wassner & Belfort, 2017, pp. 897–906).

HYPERTHYROIDISM
- Neonatal hyperthyroidism is uncommon and, usually, transient.
  ○ Most infants with hyperthyroidism are born to mothers with Graves' disease and results from transplacental transfer of stimulating TSH-receptor antibodies (TRAb) from mother to newborn. About 1% to 5% of infants born to mothers with Graves' disease have neonatal hyperthyroidism.
  ○ Rarely, infants have permanent hyperthyroidism from an autosomal dominant trait resulting in activating mutation of the TSH receptor (Chuang et al., 2015, pp. 1505–1509; Wassner & Belfort, 2017, pp. 897–906).
- Signs of hyperthyroidism and neonatal thyrotoxicosis include prematurity, intrauterine growth restriction, irritability, excessive movement, tremor, flushing of cheeks, hyperthermia, sweating, increased appetite, weight loss or poor growth, supraventricular tachycardia, arrhythmia, goiter, exophthalmos, lymphadenopathy, hepatosplenomegaly, craniosynostosis, thrombocytopenia, hypoprothrombinemia, and coagulopathy.
  ○ Treatment includes anti-thyroid drugs. Supportive care may include a beta-blocker, such as propranolol to treat tachycardia or steroids.
  ○ Death may occur if the condition is not treated. If condition is caused by genetic defect, and permanent, thyroid gland removal or ablation may be considered (Chuang et al., 2015, pp. 1511; Wassner & Belfort, 2017, pp. 907–908).

Disorders of the Pituitary

- Deficiencies of cortisol or growth hormone can cause neonatal hypoglycemia, in the context of hypopituitarism, with adrenocorticotropic hormone (ACTH) and growth hormone deficiency (Werny et al., 2018, p. 1406).
  ○ Hypopituitarism, and altered functioning of the hypothalamic–pituitary–thyroid axis, is often associated with midline, facial, cranial, or intracranial defects.
  ○ Septo-optic dysplasia is often associated with pituitary hormone deficiencies.
  ○ Clinical signs of hypopituitarism include hypoglycemia related to growth and ACTH deficiencies, polyuria

from antidiuretic hormone deficiency, microphallus in boys from gonatotropin hormone deficiency, nystagmus, and hypothyroidism.
  ○ Diagnosis is made with endocrine studies after other causes of symptoms are ruled out.
  ○ Treatment may include corticosteroids and thyroid, sex, or growth hormone replacement (Chuang et al., 2015, p. 1498, 1504).

Disorders of the adrenal

- Normal adrenal function is essential for fetal and extra-uterine growth and homeostasis. Adrenal disorders can be life-threatening.
- The major adrenal hormones are cortisol and aldosterone, regulated in response to corticotropin-releasing hormone (CRH) from the hypothalamus and adrenocorticotropic hormone (ACTH) from the pituitary gland (Blackburn, 2012, p. 630).
  ○ Glucocorticoids, primarily cortisol, are metabolized in the zona fasciculata, and are responsible for regulation of fluid and electrolyte balance, glucose stability, regulation of blood pressure, response to stress, and response to inflammation with immune suppression.
  ○ Mineralocorticoids are produced in the zona glomerulosa, which regulate fluid and electrolyte balance.
    ■ Epinephrine and norepinephrine, which have both glucocorticoid and mineralocorticoid properties, are produced in the adrenal medulla and are also involved in stress responses and cardiovascular function
  ○ Androgens are produced in the zona reticularis and in the gonads. Androgens are important for sexual differentiation (Blackburn, 2012, p. 630).
- Disorders of the adrenal glands may include Cushing syndrome (too much cortisol secondary to tumor), Addison's disease (primary adrenal insufficiency), hyperaldosteronism, pheochromocytoma or paraganglioma (primary tumors), or adrenal problems secondary to pituitary tumors, but these rarely present in the neonate.

CONGENITAL ADRENAL HYPERPLASIA
- CAH comprises a group of disorders in which there is an inherited defect in one of the enzymes required for the adrenocortical synthesis of cortisol from cholesterol. This leads to impaired cortisol production and elevated ACTH levels.
  ○ The clinical problems are caused by impaired synthesis of glucocorticoids, mineralocorticoids, or gonadal sex steroids, and overproduction of precursor steroids or their side products (Remeithi & Wherrett, 2015, p. 1542; Swartz & Chan, 2017, p. 923).
- CAH is a fairly common disorder, with a worldwide incidence of one per 16,000 births, and is included in newborn screening.
  ○ This problem involves problems with both adrenal function and sex development (Swartz & Chan, 2017, p. 934).
- The most common cause of CAH is 21-hydroxylase enzyme deficiency, accounting for more than 95% of all cases.
  ○ The most common forms of CAH include the simple virilizing form, with increased secretion of androgens before the enzyme block.
  ○ In the female fetus, this leads to varying degrees of male differentiation of the external genitalia, but internal sex organs develop normally. In the male fetus, the effect of increased androgens in insignificant and penile enlargement is, usually, not recognizable as such. Both female and males may have increased pigmentation of

genitalia (Remeithi & Wherrett, 2015, p. 1543; Swartz & Chan, 2017, p. 934).

- Severe deficiency of the 21-hydroxylase enzyme with impairments of cortisol and aldosterone synthesis results in the salt-wasting form of CAH.
  - Hypo-aldosteronism causes renal sodium wasting with depletion of total-body sodium content and impaired ability to secrete potassium and hydrogen ions via the kidney. This may lead to hyponatremia, hyperkalemia, or metabolic acidosis.
  - Hypocortisolemia causes impairment of cardiovascular, metabolic, and other system functions, including the renin-angiotensin axis, which results in hypoglycemia and shock (Remeithi & Wherrett, 2015, p. 1543; Swartz & Chan, 2017, p. 934).
- Diagnosis of CAH is made via the newborn screen in most cases.
  - The most common disorder of sex development with presentation in the newborn period is a 46, XX female with CAH. Females with the salt-losing form of CAH may present with complete masculinization of the external genitalia, and some are incorrectly identified as male.
    - Infants born with ambiguous genitalia, non-palpable testes, or severe hyponatremia should be evaluated for adrenal disorders (Fechner, 2018, p. 1351; Swartz & Chan, 2017, p. 934).
    - Although most disorders of sex development involve a virilized infant with 46 XX karyotypes, and caused by CAH, it is important to understand the differential diagnoses, clinical assessment, appropriate referral, and parental support for all possible presentations (Shnorhavorian & Fechner, 2018, pp. 1365–1366). Males usually receive medical attention when they develop a salt-losing crisis caused by adrenal insufficiency (Fechner, 2018, p. 1356).
- When CAH is suspected, diagnosis may be facilitated by readily available algorithms, as well as referral to pediatric subspecialists.
  - General concepts include performance of a complete physical exam with thorough documentation of symmetry, presence, and description of external genitalia, appropriate laboratory and genetic analysis, and imaging of internal gonads (Fechner, 2018, pp. 1356–1357).
- The goal of treatment of CAH is to normalize ACTH secretion, and provide replacement or correction of cortisol, aldosterone, or gonadal sex steroid deficiencies.
  - Treatment of salt-wasting CAH may include glucocorticoid (cortisol) and mineralocorticoid replacement, sodium replacement, hydration, other supportive care, and surveillance.
  - These infants may require cortisol stress doses with any illness, surgery, or trauma (Fechner, 2018, pp. 1356–1357).

ADDITIONAL DISORDERS OF SEX DEVELOPMENT

- This heterogenous group of disorders is associated with developmental, genetic or endocrine causes and includes the findings of ambiguous genitalia, cryptorchidism, hypospadias, microphallus, clitoromegaly, asymmetry of genitalia, and discordance of external genitalia with prenatal karyotype.
  - Because internal genital anatomy, karyotype, and sex assignment cannot be determined from external

appearance, a rapid and thorough evaluation is required, including a suspicion of CAH, which would necessitate urgent treatment (Swartz & Chan, 2017, p. 923, 930).

- The differential diagnosis for ambiguous genitalia includes categories of problems that include causes of 46, XX virilized female, 46, XY undervirilized male, gonadal differentiation and chromosomal disorders, and syndromes associated with ambiguous genitalia (Shnorhavorian & Fechner, 2018, p., 1366).
- General considerations in the approach to assessment and care of the newborn with ambiguous genitalia include initial history collection and physical exam, including notation of genitalia asymmetry, gonadal size, position, and descent, and description of associated anomalies.
  - Laboratory testing may include genetic testing, 17-hydroxyprogesterone before newborn screen results are available, pertinent adrenal precursors, hormones and chemistries, imaging of gonads and other pertinent structures, and possibly, biopsies (Shnorhavorian & Fechner, 2018, p. 1365; Swartz & Chan, 2017, pp. 923–932).
  - Referrals to appropriate subspecialists may include neonatologist, pediatric surgeon, pediatric endocrinologist, pediatric urologist, geneticist, and child psychologist (Shnorhavorian & Fechner, 2018, p. 1365; Swartz & Chan, 2017, p. 941).
- Care of the family should include open and honest discussion of available assessment and test results, avoidance of premature sex assignment until a collaborative decision is made by the multidisciplinary team and parents after thorough evaluation, and psychological support.
  - Until sex assignment is made, gender-specific names, pronouns, and other references should be avoided (Shnorhavorian & Fechner, 2018, p. 1365; Swartz & Chan, 2017, p. 924).
  - The main goal of sex assignment is to attempt to match the child's future gender identity (Swartz & Chan, 2017, p. 923).

ASSESSMENT AND TREATMENT OF METABOLIC AND ENDOCRINE DISORDERS

The NNP Role in Evaluation

- The NNP may not be able to identify the specific disorder, but he or she should be able to describe and document a complete history, physical, and first-line laboratory and radiographic evaluation. Any infant who presents with hypoglycemia, acidosis, lethargy, temperature instability, or neurological abnormalities should be considered to possibly have a metabolic or endocrine disorder if there is concern that this infant's condition does not fit the pattern of sepsis or hypoxia (Blackburn, 2012, p. 582; Cederbaum, 2018, p. 226; El-Hattab & Sutton, 2017, p. 859; Wassner & Belfort, 2017, p. 893, 903).
- Because the care of the infant with suspected metabolic and endocrine disorders can feel overwhelming, it is helpful to emphasize the priorities and interventions of the NNP, within the scope of practice granted by state licensure. All of these efforts will involve collaboration with the neonatologist.

○ These priorities include identification of abnormal symptoms, evaluation, stabilization, communication with parents, notification of colleagues and consultants, consideration of need for transport, and discharge planning.

○ A guide to the approach to care of infants with metabolic or endocrine disorders is presented in Table 20.2.

Clinical Presentation

• Generally, newborn infants with metabolic or endocrine disorders have relatively non specific types of presenting symptoms. The most common presenting symptoms include dysmorphic features (sometimes), hypoglycemia, poor feeding, vomiting, poor growth, jaundice, organomegaly, acidosis, cardiomyopathy, respiratory distress, lethargy, apnea, hypotonia, hypothermia, cyanosis, seizures, encephalopathy, obtundation, coma, and sudden death.

○ Since some of these symptoms may be caused by some common neonatal problem such as breastfeeding difficulty, jaundice, benign cardiac murmur, or infection, then it becomes clear why a consistent, thorough, differential, and systematic approach is necessary for the assessment of all infants (Blackburn, 2012, p. 582; Cederbaum, 2018, p. 226; El-Hattab & Sutton, 2017, p. 859; Werny et al., 2018, p. 1405; Zinn, 2015, pp. 1554, 1568).

Perinatal History

• Parents and family members should be asked about a history of neonatal death or sudden, unexplained death of any infant or child within the family, as well as any incidences of mental retardation, developmental delay, or heart problems.

• It is helpful to remember that X-linked conditions have male predominance, but females may have milder forms, so it may be important to listen, carefully, to how mild abnormalities are described, especially of female relatives.

• Parents should be asked if they are related at all, as autosomal recessive disorders are more likely to occur with parental consanguinity.

• Although pregnancy history may be available in the medical record, parents should still be questioned since information may be lacking or prenatal care may have been received elsewhere without transfer of records.

○ Infants with metabolic or endocrine disorders are, often, born to mothers with normal pregnancies. However, in some cases, the pregnancies may have had associated severe hyperemesis, liver dysfunction, fatty liver of pregnancy, or HELLP (including hemolysis, elevated liver enzymes, and low platelet count) syndrome.

○ Fetal ultrasound results may have revealed congenital malformations associated with genetic metabolic disorders (Bacino, 2017, pp. 118–122; El-Hattab & Sutton, 2018, pp. 859–861)

Systematic Physical Examination

• In this chapter, only the organs or systems most commonly affected by metabolic or endocrine disorders, which may be identified during a physical exam, are presented.

• The physical exam should be performed with a consistent, thorough approach of all organs or systems to identify all abnormalities to assist in the evaluation and care of the infant.

• It is important to start with a general assessment of the infant for evaluation of phenotype, and activity as there may or may not be phenotype abnormalities with specific metabolic or endocrine disorders, but a thorough evaluation may reveal physical dysmorphology that is present with some disorders (Cederbaum, 2018, p. 226).

• it is also important to initiate a neurological evaluation of the infant at rest in terms of position, tone, and activity before the infant is disturbed.

• It is possible to have confounding problems as in the case, for example, of an infant with a metabolic disorder, who, also, has respiratory distress because of meconium aspiration syndrome.

• A more complete description of presenting signs of metabolic and endocrine disorders in infants is presented in Table 20.2 (Cederbaum, 2018, p. 226; Devaskar & Garg, 2015, p. 1440; Thomas et al., 2018, pp. 256–259; Zinn, 2015, pp. 1585–1591).

TABLE 20.2 Presenting Signs of Metabolic and Endocrine Disorders in Infants

Organ System Mainly Involved	Presenting Signs	Metabolic/Endocrine Disorder
Neurologic	Encephalopathy High-pitched cry Jitteriness Lethargy Hypotonia Abnormal movements Coma	Hypoglycemia, hypo/hypercalcemia, hypomagnesemia Amino acid disorders Organic acidemias Respiratory chain defects Urea cycle defects
	Seizures	Neurotransmitter disorders
	Seizures + Microcephaly	3-phosphoglycerate dehydrogenase Glucose transporter type 1 deficiency

Organ System Mainly Involved	Presenting Signs	Metabolic/Endocrine Disorder
Eye	Cataracts	Galactosemia Carbohydrate defects Lysosomal storage disease Peroxisomal disorders Respiratory chain defects
	Cherry spots	Sphingolipidoses
	Retinopathies	Congenital disorders of glycolysation Lysosomal storage disorders Peroxisomal disorders
	Abnormal movements or gaze	Mitochondrial cytopathies or Gaucher disease
Hepatic	Liver failure	Galactosemia Hereditary fructose intolerance Tyrosinemia type I Phosphomannoisomerase
	Jaundice, cholestasis	Galactosemia Long-chain 3-hydroxy-acyl-CoA dehydrogenase deficiency Bile acid synthesis defects Cerebrotendinous xanthomatosis
	Hepatosplenomegaly	Congenital erythropoietic porphyria
Cardiac	Cardiomyopathy Arrhythmias	Fatty acid oxidation defects Glycogen storage diseases Lysosomal storage diseases Respiratory chain defects
Endocrine	Hepatosplenomegaly –Metabolic acidosis –Hypoglycemia	Amino acid defects Bile acid biosynthetic defects Carbohydrate defects Congenital disorders of glycosylation Fatty acid oxidation defects Peroxisomal disorders Respiratory chain defects Organic acidemias
	–Severe hypoglycemia –Ambiguous genitalia	Congenital hyperinsulinism Congenital adrenal hyperplasia
	Cardiac involvement	Fatty acid oxidation defects Carnitine uptake defect
Gastrointestinal/hepatic	–Poor feeding –Jaundice –Hepatomegaly, splenomegaly –Vomiting –Diarrhea, rarely	Bile acid biosynthetic defects Carbohydrate defects Congenital glycosylation disorders Fatty acid beta-oxidation disorders Lysosomal storage disorders Organic acidemias Respiratory chain defects Glycogen storage diseases
Hair/skin/skeletal anomalies	–Increased skin pigmentation –Fair hair and skin –Brittle, coarse hair –Alopecia –Rash –Unusual odor –Fractures	Amino acid disorders Organic acidemias Menkes disease Phenylketonuria Osteopenia of prematurity

(continued)

TABLE 20.2 Presenting Signs of Metabolic and Endocrine Disorders in Infants *(cont.)*

Organ System Mainly Involved	Presenting Signs	Metabolic/Endocrine Disorder
Hematologic anomalies	–Neutropenia –Thrombocytopenia –Anemia –Pancytopenia	Organic acidemias Respiratory chain defects

Sources: Data from Bacino, C. (2017). Genetic issues presenting in the nursery. In Eichenwald et al. (Eds.), *Cloherty and Stark's manual of neonatal care* (8th ed., pp. 117–130). Philadelphia, PA: Lippincott, Williams & Wilkins; Brown, Z., & Chang, J. (2018). Disorders of carbohydrate metabolism. In C. Gleason & S. Juul (Eds.), *Avery's disease of the newborn* (10th ed., pp. 1403–1416). Philadelphia, PA: Elsevier; Burris, H. (2017). Hypoglycemia and hyperglycemia. In Eichenwald et al. (Eds.), *Cloherty and Stark's manual of neonatal care* (8th ed., pp. 312–334). Philadelphia, PA: Lippincott, Williams & Wilkins; Cederbaum, S., & Berry, G. T. (2018). Inborn errors of carbohydrate, ammonia, amino acid, and organic acid metabolism. In C. Gleason & S. Juul (Eds.), *Avery's disease of the newborn* (10th ed., pp. 215–238). Philadelphia, PA: Elsevier; El-Hattab, A. W., & Sutton, V. R. (2017). Inborn errors of metabolism. In Eichenwald et al. (Eds.), *Cloherty and Stark's manual of neonatal care* (8th ed., pp. 858–891). Philadelphia, PA: Lippincott, Williams & Wilkins.

- An eye examination may reveal, or suggest, galactosemia, sphingolipids, mitochondrial cytopathies, Kearns–Sayre syndrome, and other metabolic or endocrine disorders.
  - Infants with these conditions may present with cataracts, cherry spots, retinopathies, or abnormal gaze.
  - It is possible to miss some of these anomalies during the initial eye exam, without dilation of the pupils, so if a metabolic or endocrine disorder is suspected, a referral to a pediatric ophthalmologist is appropriate (Cederbaum, 2018, p. 227; Thomas et al., 2018, p. 256).
- Infants may present with respiratory distress, including tachypnea (Cederbaum, 2018, p. 226).
- A cardiac exam should be performed in any infant with suspected metabolic disorder. However, for some disorders, the cardiac problem, when accompanied by hemodynamic instability, is the presenting symptom.
  - The symptoms of metabolic or endocrine disorders with cardiac involvement may include cardiac murmur, arrhythmia, cardiomyopathy with signs of failure, or hemodynamic decompensation.
  - There may be significant cardiac problems and symptoms with mitochondrial disorders, for example, mitochondrial respiratory chain disorders, or glycogen storage disease, for example, Pompe disease. (Blackburn, 2012, p. 650; Cederbaum, 2018, p. 228; Thomas et al., 2018, p. 257, 258)
- The abdomen should be evaluated for distension, associated with vomiting or diarrhea, may be assessed for many of the intoxication disorders.
  - Liver, or spleen, involvement is common to many metabolic or endocrine disorders.
  - Signs of liver failure may be seen with disorders such as galactosemia and tyrosinemia.
  - Hepatosplenomegaly may be seen with congenital erythropoietic porphyria or lysosomal storage diseases, for example, Gaucher disease (Cederbaum, 2018, p. 227; Thomas et al., 2018, pp. 257–258).
- Genitalia should be assessed for appropriateness for gestational age and for any abnormalities.
  - Abnormalities such as ambiguous genitalia in a female may be associated with endocrine disorders such as CAH.
  - Other abnormalities may be related to other sex development disorders (Blackburn, 2012, p. 651; Thomas et al., 2018, p. 259)

- Extremities should be assessed for bone fracture by inspection or radiological determination that may be associated with osteopenia of prematurity, also called metabolic bone disease or rickets of prematurity (Abrams & Tiosano, 2015, p. 1485).
  - Subcutaneous fat necrosis, associated with birth trauma, may be associated with hypercalcemia later, as calcification resolves (Abrams & Tiosano, 2015, p. 1481; Thomas et al., 2018, pp. 256–259)
- Abnormal neurologic signs may present in many infants with metabolic or endocrine disorders.
  - Sometimes these are subtle and ubiquitous signs, such as "poor feeding." However, infants may present with progressive or significant neurological symptoms.
  - Infants with either metabolic or endocrine disorders, such as hypoglycemia, may present with irritability, high-pitched cry, apnea, jitteriness, tremors, feeding difficulty, lethargy, stupor, seizures, hypothermia, sweating, or hypotonia (Abrams & Tiosano, 2015, p. 1474, 1484; Devaskar & Gar, 2015, p. 1437; El-Hattab & Sutton, 2017, pp. 860–861; Thomas et al., 2018, pp. 256–259)
  - With many of the acidemia disorders, and lysosomal storage, as well as heterogenous disorders, the infant will present with neurological signs, including hypotonia, seizures, obtundation, and may progress to coma. They may also have accompanying abnormal, distinctive odors of urine, breath, saliva, or sweat (El-Hattab & Sutton, 2017, pp. 860–861; Kim et al., 2018, p. 1393; Thomas et al., 2018, pp. 257–258).
    - Abnormal odor may be an important diagnostic feature of some disorders, such as PKU, which presents with a stale, mousy, barn-like smell, or tyrosinemia, which presents with a rancid smell, like sulfur (El-Hattab & Sutton, 2017, p. 863).

First-Line Investigations

- If metabolic or endocrine disorders are suspected, the goal is to promote cardiopulmonary and metabolic stability and to obtain some basic measures that are routinely available, before more specialized investigation. Even if the NNP is uncertain about ordering some of these first-line studies before discussion with a neonatologist, much may be revealed by, at least, blood sugar levels and arterial blood gas tests, as well as some other commonly ordered metabolic tests (see Table 20.3) (El-Hattab & Sutton, 2017, pp. 864–865).

- ○ First-line investigations of blood often include blood glucose levels, arterial pH, carbon dioxide, bicarbonate, and base deficit, complete blood count, serum lactate, ammonia, amino acids, liver function studies, and clotting studies.
- ○ First-line investigations of urine include ketones, organic acids (including orotic acid), reducing substances (if suspecting galactosemia), and amino acids.
- • If any of the physical examination findings or laboratory test results are abnormal, or if the clinician is concerned despite normal results, then this may be the appropriate time to ask for a consult from a pediatric subspecialist. Depending on the case and stability of the infant, it may be appropriate to request a consult from a pediatric endocrinologist, geneticist, neurologist, cardiologist, gastroenterologist, infectious disease specialist, dermatologist, and so on. Depending on the suspected disorder, further

testing will be performed (Cederbaum, 2018, p. 226; El-Hattab & Sutton, 2017, pp. 860–891; (Swartz & Chan, 929–940; Wassner & Belfort, 2017, 898–909).

NEWBORN SCREENING

- • Newborn screening is a successful public health program that began, in 1963, with drops of blood on filter paper, and a process of bacterial inhibition assay to detect PKU, a preventable cause of mental retardation. In the following years, more screening tests were developed to detect a few more conditions. As conditions were identified, treatment and follow-up recommendations were established (Sahai & Levy, 2018, p. 332).
- • In the 1990s, with the application of tandem mass spectrometry, many metabolic and hematological disorders could be detected, and the list of conditions was broadened.
  - ○ Examples of some of the disorders that can be detected include endocrine disorders, hemoglobinopathies, immunodeficiencies, and cystic fibrosis, as well as PKU and

TABLE 20.3 Screening Tests of Metabolic or Endocrine Disorders That Should Be Considered by the NNP Before Further Investigations

Test	Reason	Clinical Importance: Abnormalities may be Associated with Disorders
Glucose—metabolic or endocrine disorders should be suspected in any infant with prolonged, persistent hypoglycemia	Normal, low, or high	Small molecule disorders: glucose with poor feeding, obtundation Energy metabolism disorders: normal Lysosomal storage disorders: may be normal Endocrine: hypoglycemia, TSH, T3, T4
Arterial blood gas	To determine metabolic acidosis	Small molecule disorders: pH, carbon dioxide (CO_2) with coma and respiratory failure, or CO_2 with hyperventilation. Energy metabolism disorders: pH with lactic acidosis, base deficit, carbon dioxide with alkalosis Lysosomal storage disorders: may be normal
Electrolytes/minerals	Especially serum bicarbonate, to determine metabolic acidosis To determine anion gap with acidosis	Small molecule disorders: abnormal electrolytes with vomiting and acidosis Energy metabolism disorders: bicarbonate, abnormal with acidosis Lysosomal storage disorders: may be normal Endocrine: sodium, potassium, calcium magnesemia, alkaline phosphatase
Liver function studies with bilirubin, coagulopathy studies	To determine liver involvement and jaundice	Small molecule disorders: liver function tests Energy metabolism disorders: liver function tests Lysosomal storage disorders: bilirubin or normal
Ammonia	May be elevated	Small molecule disorders: may be elevated Energy metabolism disorders: may be elevated Lysosomal storage disorders: may be elevated or normal
Lactate	May be elevated	Small molecule disorders: lactate Energy metabolism disorders: lactate Lysosomal storage disorders: may be normal
Urinary ketones	To determine if present, which is abnormal	Small molecule disorders: ketones Energy metabolism disorders: normal or ketones Lysosomal storage disorders: may be normal

TSH, thyroid-stimulating hormone.

Sources: Data from Bacino, C. (2017). Genetic issues presenting in the nursery. In Eichenwald et al. (Eds.), *Cloherty and Stark's manual of neonatal care* (8th ed., pp. 117–130). Philadelphia, PA: Lippincott, Williams & Wilkins; Brown, Z., & Chang, J. (2018). Disorders of carbohydrate metabolism. In C. Gleason & S. Juul (Eds.), *Avery's disease of the newborn* (10th ed., pp. 1403–1416). Philadelphia, PA: Elsevier; Burris, H. (2017). Hypoglycemia and hyperglycemia. In Eichenwald et al. (Eds.), *Cloherty and Stark's manual of neonatal care* (8th ed., pp. 312–334). Philadelphia, PA: Lippincott, Williams & Wilkins; Cederbaum, S., & Berry, G. T. (2018). Inborn errors of carbohydrate, ammonia, amino acid, and organic acid metabolism. In C. Gleason & S. Juul (Eds.), *Avery's disease of the newborn* (10th ed., pp. 215–238). Philadelphia, PA: Elsevier; El-Hattab, A. W., & Sutton, V. R. (2017). Inborn errors of metabolism. In Eichenwald et al. (Eds.), *Cloherty and Stark's manual of neonatal care* (8th ed., pp. 858–891). Philadelphia, PA: Lippincott, Williams & Wilkins.

other inborn errors of metabolism (Blackburn, 2012, p. 652; Sahai & Levy, 2018, p. 332).

- Presently in the United States, the newborn screening programs are mandated and more than 60 conditions are included, although specific tests done will vary state to state. In some states, parents are allowed to refuse screening.
  - ○ The goal is to screen all infants and provide the necessary follow-up evaluation and intervention to prevent death or disability. However, some experts question if there exists clear scientific evidence of long-term benefit of screening and treatment. Controversies exist among experts in different countries about the benefits and risks of certain therapies, especially with disparate availability of resources, and about which disorders should be included in the screen (Sahai & Levy, 2018, pp. 344–346).
- The concept of "newborn screening" has been broadened to include other technologies such as hearing screening, with automated auditory brainstem response (ABR) to screen for hearing loss, and critical congenital heart disease (CHD) screening, with pulse oximetry (Sahai & Levy, 2018, p. 332).
- In the future, it may be possible to perform a genetic and mutational scan across the whole genome of the fetus, in a noninvasive manner, by analyzing cell-free fetal DNA in maternal blood as early as the fifth week of gestational age. This technology and approach remains controversial because of methodological, ethical, and political issues.

Second-Line Investigations

- Second-line investigations are usually performed as a result of the consultants' recommendations and may include urine, cerebral spinal fluid, or serum samples for metabolites or markers, such as urine succinylacetone, cerebral spinal fluid glycine, serum acylcarnitines, and other markers or metabolites. Chromosomes and other specific genetic studies may also be requested.
- Organ or organelle-specific investigations may include studies such as long-chain fatty acids, transferrin isoelectric focusing, and peroxisomal function tests. Skin, muscle, liver biopsies may be performed at this time, if possible and appropriate, or during postmortem studies.
- Specific imaging may include tandem mass spectrometry as well as other radiographic or ultrasound studies.
- Depending on the resources at the facility where the infant was born or evaluated, sometimes the infant must be transported to a regional pediatric medical center for some of these tests.
- For the second-line investigations, it is important to determine, with the collaborative team, an appropriate medical order to prevent excessive exsanguination and handling.
  - ○ It is also important to contact the laboratory personnel in the facility to determine if the tests are analyzed at that facility or must be sent out, to plan for optimum collection and processing of the samples.
  - ○ To accomplish this goal, one must establish proper timing (e.g., not before long weekend if sample needs to be sent to another lab), confirm proper tubes, proper handling (e.g., does sample need to be placed on ice), and notice to the lab technologists when these tests are to be sent so that they are processed immediately (Cederbaum, 2018, p. 226; El-Hattab & Sutton, 2017, pp. 860–891; Kim et al., 2018, p. 1395; Swartz & Chan, 2017, pp. 929–940; Wassner & Belfort, 2017, pp. 898–909).

Treatment Goals

ACUTE MANAGEMENT

- The goals of acute management of metabolic or endocrine problems are to stop further de-compensation and buildup of toxic metabolites and support with appropriate nutrient, substrate, enzyme, or hormone. This may be accomplished through:
  - ○ Reducing or eliminating any food or drug that cannot be metabolized properly
  - ○ Replacing missing or inactive enzymes or other chemicals if possible
  - ○ Removing toxic products of metabolism that accumulate due to the metabolic disorder (El-Hattab & Sutton, 2017, pp. 866–868; Swartz & Chan, 2017, p. 936, 940; Wassner & Belfort, 2017, p. 905)
- If the infant's oral feedings are stopped at the time of evaluation, 10% dextrose with electrolytes should be administered, or high glucose rate of infusion if hypoglycemic.
  - ○ The exception to this strategy would occur if congenital lactic acidosis or mitochondrial disorders were suspected, since higher carbohydrates exacerbate acidosis. In that situation, 5% dextrose with electrolytes should be administered
  - ○ If the infant is hyperglycemic, then insulin should be considered rather than decrease the dextrose infusion index.
  - ○ If fat oxidation defects are excluded from the evaluation, then provide lipids (Cederbaum, 2018, p. 229; El-Hattab & Sutton, 2017, pp. 866–868).
- For disorders of calcium, phosphorus, and magnesium, intravenous correction or adjustment should occur while laboratory investigation is pending.
- Treatment of rare conditions involving toxicities may include parenteral rehydration, diuretics, corticosteroids, antacids, and enemas (Abrams & Tiosano, 2015, pp. 1474–1479).
- Electrolytes should be monitored because of intravenous fluid therapy and underlying conditions.
  - ○ Potassium levels should be monitored if acidotic, since potassium falls as acidosis is corrected.
  - ○ Both sodium and potassium should be ordered if certain endocrine disorders are suspected which alter electrolyte balance.
- With certain disorders, it may be necessary to remove or divert toxic metabolites. All of these interventions can be determined in collaboration with the neonatologist and appropriate subspecialist consultants (Cederbaum, 2018, p. 229; El-Hattab & Sutton, 2017, p. 858, 861, 868; Koves et al., 2018, p. 1343; Thomas et al., 2018, pp. 258–25)

LONG-TERM MANAGEMENT

- Lifelong treatment may include diet management, provision of a deficient substance, or vitamin therapy such as vitamin B12, biotin, riboflavin, thiamine, pyridoxine, or folate.
- Supportive therapy includes early intervention, education, family, genetic counseling, and continued follow-up with the pediatrician and appropriate pediatric subspecialists, depending on the case.
- Some of the treatments for metabolic or endocrine disorders are listed in Table 20.4 (El-Hattab & Sutton, 2017, p. 868; Koves et al., 2018, pp. 1342–1346; Merritt & Gallagher, 2018, p. 232; Thomas et al., 2018, pp. 263–272)

TABLE 20.4 NNP Guide for Approach to Care of Infant With Suspected Metabolic or Endocrine Disorder

Priority	Intervention
Proper *identification* of abnormal symptoms	Complete physical assessment and documentation of abnormalities Obtain family, maternal, pregnancy, and labor and delivery histories
Initial *evaluation*	*Obtain first-line investigatory lab tests, but, at least, obtain arterial blood gas sample and blood sugar level.* Obtain other tests as indicated (laboratory, radiological, pulse oximetry, echocardiogram)
Initial stabilization	Provide basic stabilization per Neonatal Resuscitation Program guidelines and systems approach to problems. Treat acid base imbalances. If metabolic disorder is suspected, consider nothing per mouth and intravenous dextrose infusion. Do not transfuse without consultation with at least the neonatologist, since genetic studies may be required before transfusion.
Communicate with parents initially	Provide honest description of what is observed as abnormal findings. Do not offer a diagnosis, unless it is confirmed. Reassure parents that further tests will be performed, infant will be supported, and specialists are available if needed. *Remember, you are not expected to be a subspecialist, but are expected to support the infant and obtain resources to benefit the infant.*
Proper *notification* of colleagues	Notify the neonatologist per institutional and practice expectations.
Consider *need for transport*	Based on the stability of the infant and resources in this institution, consider need for transport to regional children's hospital with subspecialist support at this time.
Further evaluation	Consider the remainder of first-line investigation studies, if not already obtained.
Consideration of *need for subspecialist* consult	If symptoms persist or worsen and diagnosis unclear, consider subspecialist consultation request. The type of consultation depends on the case presentation and systems involved.
Support recommendations of consultant	Based on discussion with team, as recommended by consultants, order further second-line diagnostic tests Provide supportive interventions per recommendations.
Family conference	Once a diagnosis or plan for diagnostic tests is made, conduct an interdisciplinary family conference to answer all questions, provide information regarding possible differential diagnoses, and identify goals of hospitalization, for example, cardiorespiratory stability, feeding (oral, nasogastric, etc.), and discharge to home or eventual transport. If necessary, discuss the need for transport to regional children's hospital.
Plan for *functional goals*	Identify appropriate plan for functional goals for this infant. Communicate plan to entire team (neonatology, nursing, support staff). Refer to social worker for support.
Discharge planning	Identify pediatrician comfortable to follow infant with this disorder. Plan for support, if appropriate; for example, home oxygen, home support for tube feedings. Support nurses to write specific discharge teaching plan. Plan for discharge medications, metabolites, vitamins, and diet, and allow time to obtain necessary supplements before discharge. Avoid discharge on weekend or holiday unless all necessary items are obtained.
Make appropriate *referrals and follow-up* appointments	*If able to be discharged from your institution without transport to regional children's hospital, then:* Make pediatrician follow-up appointment. Complete referral documentation for sub specialist out-patient clinic referrals. If appropriate, complete paperwork to obtain special formulas through government-funded programs. If necessary, make first appointments at sub specialist clinics. If diagnosis is known, refer parents to appropriate support groups.

Sources: Data from Bacino, C. (2017). Genetic issues presenting in the nursery. In Eichenwald et al. (Eds.), *Cloherty and Stark's manual of neonatal care* (8th ed., pp. 117–130). Philadelphia, PA: Lippincott, Williams & Wilkins; Brown, Z., & Chang, J. (2018). Disorders of carbohydrate metabolism. In C. Gleason & S. Juul (Eds.), *Avery's disease of the newborn* (10th ed., pp. 1403–1416). Philadelphia, PA: Elsevier; Burris, H. (2017). Hypoglycemia and hyperglycemia. In Eichenwald et al. (Eds.), *Cloherty and Stark's manual of neonatal care* (8th ed., pp. 312–334). Philadelphia, PA: Lippincott, Williams & Wilkins; Cederbaum, S., & Berry, G. T. (2018). Inborn errors of carbohydrate, ammonia, amino acid, and organic acid metabolism. In C. Gleason & S. Juul (Eds.), *Avery's disease of the newborn* (10th ed., pp. 215–238). Philadelphia, PA: Elsevier; El-Hattab, A. W., & Sutton, V. R. (2017). Inborn errors of metabolism. In Eichenwald et al. (Eds.), *Cloherty and Stark's manual of neonatal care* (8th ed., pp. 858–891). Philadelphia, PA: Lippincott, Williams & Wilkins.

CONCLUSION

The evaluation and treatment of metabolic and endocrine disorders can be daunting for the care provider because of nonspecific, rare presentations and complexities of the disorders. An overview of metabolic or endocrine disorders has been presented, including a strategy for evaluation and treatment, to guide the NNP. This approach includes a thorough assessment, first-line investigation, second-line investigation, short- and long-term management options, referrals, discharge planning, and follow-up. The key concepts presented emphasize that an infant may have subtle symptoms of metabolic or endocrine problems that may be in common or co-exist with other problems. If a thorough systems approach is applied, and referrals to consultants are made at appropriate times, then one does not need to feel intimidated by these problems. The goal is, as with all other neonatal problems, to support the infant and family with the goal of discharge to home with the necessary support, follow-up care, and referrals.

REVIEW QUESTIONS

1. Gene mutation which causes an absent or defective enzyme, or over- or underproduction of hormones, with life-threatening physiological or biochemical system regulation dysfunction are termed:
   A. antigen–antibody disorders
   B. endocrine/metabolic disorders
   C. hepatobiliary regulation disorders

2. Phenylketonuria (PKU) is the most common inborn error of amino acid metabolism and is treated with:
   A. avoidance of legumes
   B. dietary therapy
   C. oral medications

3. The NNP is caring for a term newborn who was transferred from the postpartum unit with vomiting, poor feeding, lethargy, and petechiae. The infant had been breastfeeding well, and voiding and stooling for 2 days prior to transfer. The most recent laboratory findings are notable for hyperbilirubinemia, coagulopathy, and blood culture positive for *Escherichia coli*. Lactate levels were normal. The most likely cause is:
   A. galactosemia
   B. hyperammonemia
   C. phenylketonuria

4. A possible symptom of a metabolic/endocrine disorder is unresponsive, intractable:
   A. diarrhea
   B. fevers
   C. hypoglycemia

5. After feedings have been established in a neonate who had an initial normal examination, a common presenting symptom of an organic acidemia metabolic disorder is:
   A. drowsiness
   B. hypertonia
   C. seizures

REFERENCES

Abrams, S. A. (2017). Abnormalities of serum calcium and magnesium. In E. Eichenwald, A. Hansen, C. Marin, & A. Stark (Eds.), *Cloherty and Stark's manual of neonatal care* (8th ed., pp. 296–311). Philadelphia, PA: Wolters Kluwer.

Abrams, S., & Tiosano, D. (2015). Disorders of calcium phosphorus, and magnesium metabolism in the neonate. In R. J. Martin, A. A. Fanaroff, & M. C. Walsh (Eds.), *Fanaroff and Martin's neonatal-perinatal medicine: Diseases of the fetus and infant* (10th ed., pp. 1460–1489). Philadelphia, PA: Elsevier.

Bacino, C. (2017). Genetic issues presenting in the nursery. In E. Eichenwald, A. Hansen, C. R. Martin, & A. Start (Eds.), *Cloherty and Stark's manual of neonatal care* (8th ed., pp. 117–130). Philadelphia, PA: Lippincott, Williams & Wilkins.

Blackburn, S. (2012). *Maternal, fetal, & neonatal physiology: A clinical perspective* (4th ed., pp. 560–588). Maryland Heights, MO: Elsevier.

Brown, Z., & Chang, J. (2018). Disorders of carbohydrate metabolism. In C. Gleason & S. Juul (Eds.), *Avery's disease of the newborn* (10th ed., pp. 1403–1416). Philadelphia, PA: Elsevier.

Burris, H. (2017). Hypoglycemia and hyperglycemia. In E. Eichenwald, A. Hansen, C. R. Martin, & A. Start (Eds.), *Cloherty and Stark's manual of neonatal care* (8th ed., pp. 312–334). Philadelphia, PA: Lippincott, Williams & Wilkins.

Cederbaum, S. (2018). Introduction to metabolic and biochemical genetic diseases. In C. Gleason & S. Juul (Eds.), *Avery's disease of the newborn* (10th ed., pp. 209–214). Philadelphia, PA: Elsevier.

Cederbaum, S., & Berry, G. T. (2018). Inborn errors of carbohydrate, ammonia, amino acid, and organic acid metabolism. In C. Gleason & S. Juul (Eds.), *Avery's disease of the newborn* (10th ed., pp. 215–238). Philadelphia, PA: Elsevier.

Chuang, J., Gutmark-Little, I., & Rose, S. R. (2015). Thyroid disorders in the neonate. In R. J. Martin, A. A. Fanaroff, & M. C. Walsh. (Eds.), *Neonatal-perinatal medicine: Diseases of the fetus and infant* (pp. 1490–1515). Philadelphia, PA: Elsevier Mosby.

Devaskar, S. U., & Garg, M. (2015). Disorders of carbohydrate metabolism. In R. J. Martin, A. A. Fanaroff, & M. C. Walsh (Eds.), *Neonatal-perinatal medicine: Diseases of the fetus and infant*. Philadelphia, PA: Elsevier Mosby.

Divall, S. A., & Megjaneh, L. (2018). Developmental endocrinology. In C. Gleason & S. Juul (Eds.), *Avery's disease of the newborn* (10th ed., pp. 1224–1332). Philadelphia, PA: Elsevier.

El-Hattab, A. W., & Sutton, V. R. (2017). Inborn errors of metabolism. In E. Eichenwald, A. Hansen, C. R. Martin, & A. Start (Eds.), *Cloherty and Stark's manual of neonatal care* (8th ed., pp. 858–891). Philadelphia, PA: Lippincott, Williams & Wilkins.

Fechner, P. Y. (2018). Disorders of the adrenal gland. In C. Gleason & S. Juul (Eds.), *Avery's disease of the newborn* (10th ed., pp. 1351–1364). Philadelphia, PA: Elsevier.

Gorman, T. (2017). Neonatal effects of maternal diabetes. In E. Eichenwald, A. Hansen, C. R. Martin, & A. Start (Eds.), *Cloherty and Stark's manual of neonatal care* (8th ed., pp. 910–922). Philadelphia, PA: Lippincott, Williams & Wilkins.

Kim, G., Nandi-Munshi, D., & Diblasi, C. C. (2018). Disorders of the thyroid gland. In C. Gleason & S. Juul (Eds.), *Avery's disease of the newborn* (10th ed., pp. 1388–1402). Philadelphia, PA: Elsevier.

Koves, I. H., Ness, K. D., Nip, A. S., & Salehi, P. (2018). Disorders of calcium and phosphorus metabolism. In C. Gleason & S. Juul (Eds.), *Avery's disease of the newborn* (10th ed., pp. 1333–1350). Philadelphia, PA: Elsevier.

Merritt, J. L., & Gallagher, R. C. (2018). Inborn errors of carbohydrate, ammonia, amino acid, and organic acid metabolism. In C. Gleason & S. Juul (Eds.), *Avery's disease of the newborn* (10th ed., pp. 230–252). Philadelphia, PA: Elsevier.

Nodine, P. A., Hastings-Tolsma, P. A., & Arruda, J. (2015). Prenatal environment: Effect on neonatal outcome. In S. Gardner, B. S. Carter, M. E. Hines, & J. A. Hernandez (Eds.), *Merenstein & Gardner's handbook of neonatal intensive care* (8th ed., pp. 11–31). St. Louis, MO: Elsevier.

Remeithi, S. A., & Wherrett, D. K. (2015). Disorders of sex development. In R. J. Martin A. A. Fanaroff, & M. C. Walsh. (Eds.), *Neonatal-perinatal medicine: Diseases of the fetus and infant* (10th ed., pp. 1516–1552). St. Louis, MO: Elsevier.

Sahai, I., & Levy, H. L. (2018). Newborn screening. In C. Gleason & S. Juul (Eds.), *Avery's disease of the newborn* (10th ed., pp. 332–346). Philadelphia, PA: Elsevier.

Shnorhavorian, M., & Fechner, P. Y. (2018). Disorders of sexual differentiation. In C. Gleason & S. Juul (Eds.), *Avery's disease of the newborn* (10th ed., pp. 1365–1387). Philadelphia, PA: Elsevier.

Swartz, J. M., & Chan, Y. (2017). Disorders of sex development. In E. Eichenwald, A. Hansen, C. R. Martin, & A. Start (Eds.), *Cloherty & Stark's manual of neonatal care* (8th ed., pp. 922–941). Philadelphia, PA: Lippincott, Williams & Wilkins.

Thomas, J. A., Lam, C., & Berry, G. T. (2018). Lysosomal storage, peroxisomal, and glycosylation disorders and Smith-Lemli-Optiz presenting in the neonate. In C. Gleason & S. Juul (Eds.), *Avery's disease of the newborn* (10th ed., pp. 253–272). Philadelphia, PA: Elsevier.

Wassner, A. J., & Belfort, M. B. (2017). Thyroid disorders. In E. Eichenwald, A. Hansen, C. R. Martin, & A. Start (Eds.), *Cloherty & Stark's manual of neonatal care* (8th ed., pp. 892–909). Philadelphia, PA: Lippincott, Williams & Wilkins.

Werny, D., Taplin, C., Bennett, J. T., & Pihoker, C. (2018). Disorders of carbohydrate metabolism. In C. Gleason & S. Juul (Eds.), *Avery's disease of the newborn* (10th ed., pp. 1403–1416). Philadelphia, PA: Elsevier.

Zinn, A. B. (2015). Inborn errors of metabolism. In R. J. Martin, A. A. Faranoff, & M. C. Walsh (Eds.) *Neonatal-perinatal medicine: Diseases of the fetus and infant* (10th ed., p. 1553). St. Louis, MO: Elsevier Mosby.

THE HEMATOPOIETIC SYSTEM

Denise Kirsten
Kelly Sulo
Amy Koehn

INTRODUCTION

The neonatal hematologic system is a complex interaction between multiple organ systems to support growth and function of blood cells within the serous fluids of the body. This chapter covers the basics of hematopoiesis and alterations which affect blood cells' volume, content, and efficiency. Anemias, platelet disorders, and coagulopathies are covered, and then discussion moves to maternal-fetal ABO and Rh compatibilities. Neonatal hyperbilirubinemia, which can result from one or the other of these is covered, as is common management of types of hyperbilirubinemia. Finally, the bases of transfusion medicine are covered as interventions when physiological systems cannot maintain hemostasis.

FETAL HEMATOPOIETIC DEVELOPMENT

- Hematopoiesis is responsible for the formation, production, and maintenance of blood cells. It is the process of pluripotent, stem cells delineation into different blood cells. Hematopoiesis begins in the yolk sac as early as 2 weeks' gestation and results in red blood cells (RBCs) and macrophages, implying that the other types blood cells are not critical during early embryonic development.
  - Hematopoietic stem cells originate from the mesoderm and are found in organs such as the yolk sac, liver, and bone marrow. The liver becomes the main source of hematopoiesis by 6 weeks' gestation and remains the major site of hematopoiesis until the 16th week of gestation (Blackburn, 2013a, p. 229; Diab & Luchtman-Jones, 2015, p. 1294; Diehl-Jones & Fraser, 2015, p. 662; Juul & Christensen, 2018, p. 1113, 1116).
- By 24 weeks' gestation, the bone marrow becomes the primary site of hematopoiesis. From late gestation to the end of the first postnatal year, RBCs gradually shift from the production of fetal hemoglobin (HgF) to the production of adult hemoglobin (HgA); (Diab & Luchtman-Jones, 2015, p. 1294; Juul & Christensen, 2018, p. 1116).
  - Figure 21.1 describes stem cell differentiation.

Erythropoiesis

- Fetal erythropoiesis, the process of RBC production, is controlled in the fetus by the protein erythropoietin (EPO). EPO is the primary growth factor that stimulates the growth and development of erythrocytes and is regulated by mechanisms in the fetal liver and kidney that sense hypoxia-based oxygen concentration of tissue and oxygen saturation of hemoglobin (Diab & Luchtman-Jones, 2015, p. 1297; Diehl-Jones & Fraser, 2015, p. 663; Juul & Christensen, 2018, p. 1114).

- The bone marrow becomes the primary site for erythropoiesis from 22 weeks' gestation and continues postnatally (Diehl-Jones & Fraser, 2015, p. 662; Juul & Christensen, 2018, p. 1116).
  - Once the bone marrow becomes the primary site of RBC production, extramedullary erythropoiesis can occur during periods or hemolysis, common with congenital infections. Extramedullary sites include the liver, spleen, adrenal glands, pancreas, thyroid, endocardium, testes, uterus, brain, or skin.
  - When extramedullary erythropoiesis occurs in the skin, the characteristic "blueberry muffin rash" associated with congenital cytomegalovirus (CMV) infection can be seen (Blackburn, 2013a, p. 229).
- After delivery, EPO is produced in the kidneys. As RBCs mature they become very dependent on EPO (Diehl-Jones & Fraser, 2015, p. 663).
  - The EPO concentration in the neonate decreases rapidly in response to the relatively hyperoxic extrauterine environment.
  - EPO levels reach their nadir by 1 month of life in normal, term newborns. Then EPO levels increase to their peak at 2 months of life, then gradually decline to adult levels (Diab & Luchtman-Jones, 2015).
- EPO levels will again increase in response to anemia and in the presence of decreased availability of oxygen to the tissues. Other situations in which EPO levels increase include Down syndrome or intrauterine growth restriction, as well as infants born to mothers with diabetes or pregnancy-induced hypertension. EPO levels decrease after transfusion of packed RBCs (Diehl-Jones & Fraser, 2015, p. 663).

Hemoglobin Synthesis

- The primary purpose of mature RBCs is to carry oxygen to the body's tissues as well as to maintain adequate adenosine triphosphate (ATP) stores, to produce substances that act as antioxidants and to produce 2,3-diphosphoglycerate (2,3 DPG), which modifies the oxygen affinity of hemoglobin (Blackburn, 2013a, p. 231; Diab & Luchtman-Jones, 2015, p. 1304).
- Hemoglobin is the most common protein in RBCs. Each hemoglobin molecule has four globin chains, two alpha chains, and two beta chains. The synthesis of fetal hemoglobin begins around the 14th day of embryonic development. The transition from production of fetal hemoglobin to adult hemoglobin begins near term or at the end of fetal life.

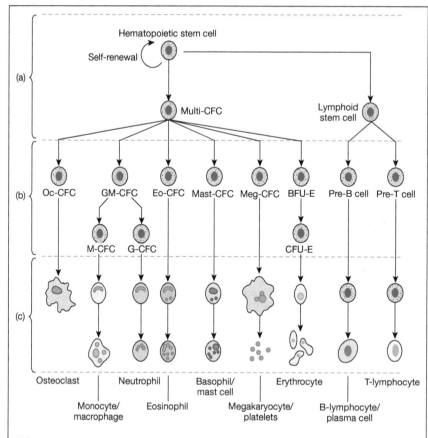

FIGURE 21.1 Stem cell differentiation (A) stem cells, (B) committed progenitors, and (C) mature cells

Source: Adapted from Diab, Y., & Luchtman-Jones. (2015). Hematologic and oncologic problems in the fetus and neonate. In R. Martin, A. Fanaroff, & M. Walsh (Eds.), *Fanaroff and Martin's neonatal-perinatal medicine: Diseases of the fetus and infant* (10th ed., pp. 1294–1343). Philadelphia, PA: Elsevier.

○ RBCs contain approximately 70% to 90% of fetal hemoglobin at birth. A delay in this transition can occur in certain situations, including maternal hypoxia or fetal growth restriction and in infants of diabetic mothers (Blackburn, 2013a, p. 231; Diab & Luchtman-Jones, 2015, p. 1296; Diehl-Jones & Fraser, 2015, p. 663).

- The reticulocyte count can be a useful measure of erythrocyte production. High reticulocyte levels reflect active erythropoiesis, while low values indicate reduced levels of erythropoiesis. Immediately after delivery, reticulocyte values tend to be higher in preterm infants when compared to term newborns (Juul & Christensen, 2018, p. 1117).

ANEMIA

- Anemia is defined as a hemoglobin level two standard deviations below the mean for age, or when the hemoglobin, hematocrit, or RBC count is below the fifth percentile lower reference level for gestational and postnatal age (Diab & Luchtman-Jones, 2015, p. 1300; Juul & Christensen, 2018, p. 1152).

- Hematocrit values increase immediately after delivery and then decline during the first week of life. In the absence of any stress and while in the bone marrow, reticulocytes mature in approximately 1 to 2 days and then another day in the circulation before maturing into erythrocytes.

- The average life span of the RBC is related and proportional to the gestational age of the infant, with an average of 35 to 50 days among premature infants and 60 to 70 days in term infants. This is in contrast to adults, who have an average RBC life span of 100 to 120 days (Juul & Christensen, 2018, p. 1156; Kaplan, Wong, Sibley, & Stevenson, 2015, p. 1299).

Physiologic Anemia

DEFINITION AND PATHOPHYSIOLOGY

- In utero, a low fetal PaO_2 stimulates EPO production, resulting in erythropoiesis. The relatively hyperoxic extrauterine environment results in suppression of EPO production from approximately 2 days of life until 6 to 8 weeks of life. The result is an expected decline in hemoglobin levels over the first 2 to 3 months of life, with a nadir at 6 to 12 weeks of life. Physiologic anemia is the expected, asymptomatic decline in erythropoiesis seen in term and preterm infants following birth as a result of postnatal EPO suppression (Blackburn, 2013a, p. 242).

- The decline in hemoglobin, and thus oxygen-carrying capacity, is offset by the gradual right shift of the oxygen–hemoglobin dissociation curve.
  - A right shift of the oxygen-hemoglobin dissociation curve increases oxygen availability to the tissue (see Figure 21.2). Eventually, a continued decline in hemoglobin levels results in a decrease in oxygen delivery to the tissue, stimulating EPO production.
  - By 10 to 12 weeks of life, EPO levels in infants are similar to those of adults. By 4 to 6 months of life, physiologic anemia has resolved, and normal levels of hemoglobin are once again present (Blackburn, 2013a, p. 243).

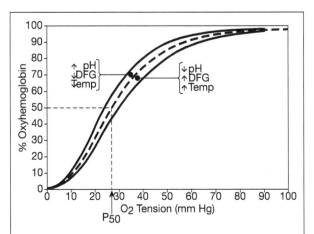

FIGURE 21.2 Oxygen-hemoglobin dissociation curve

Source: Reproduced with permission from Diab, Y., & Luchtman-Jones. (2015). Hematologic and oncologic problems in the fetus and neonate. In R. Martin, A. Fanaroff, & M. Walsh (Eds.), *Fanaroff and Martin's neonatal-perinatal medicine: Diseases of the fetus and infant* (10th ed., pp. 1294–1343). Philadelphia, PA: Elsevier.

- Once hemoglobin synthesis restarts following the physiologic nadir, iron stored from the reticuloendothelial system is released. Term infants have sufficient iron stores to last for approximately 6 to 12 weeks; subsequently, without adequate iron availability (approximately 1 mg/kg/day), hemoglobin production will decrease (Blackburn, 2013a, p. 243).
  - Infants who have received an exchange transfusion or multiple RBC transfusions may experience a later hemoglobin nadir. Blood used in transfusions results in increased HgA in these neonates and thus in increased oxygen availability to tissue, resulting in suppression of EPO production.
  - Infants with hemolysis due to isoimmunization may experience a late, severe anemia due to the continued presence of maternal antibodies that cause continued hemolysis (Blackburn, 2013a, p. 243).

RISK FACTORS

- The physiologic anemia of infancy can be exaggerated in the sick or premature infant by frequent blood sampling: the smaller the infant, the proportionally greater the volume of blood that is withdrawn for laboratory testing (Diab & Luchtman-Jones, 2015, p. 1315)
- Infants with hemolytic disorders due to isoimmunizations may experience a late and often severe anemia that is not physiologic, but the result of continued hemolysis (Blackburn, 2013a, p. 243).
- The normal hemoglobin decrease after birth is often not seen in infants with cyanotic heart disease who maintain higher EPO levels because of their low PaO_2 levels and thus higher hemoglobin levels (Blackburn, 2013a, p. 243).

CLINICAL PRESENTATION

- Physiologic anemia is usually well tolerated without any clinical indications (Blackburn, 2013a, p. 242).
  - The method to determine hematocrit can significantly affect the value. Capillary hematocrit measurements are highly subject to variations in blood flow, which may produce an artificially high hematocrit value. Prewarming does minimize the artifactual increase in the sample. There may be as much as a 20% difference between the value obtained from a capillary sample and the hematocrit value obtained from a central (venous or arterial) sample (Manco-Johnson, McKinney, Knapp-Clevenger, & Hernandez, 2016, p. 480).
- In extremely low birth weigh (ELBW) infants whose nadir falls below 7 g/dL, this can be associated with pallor, tachypnea, tachycardia, poor feeding, and poor weight gain. Other causes of blood loss and suppression of erythropoiesis in the ill neonate can contribute to more severe and earlier anemia (Diab & Luchtman-Jones, 2015, p. 1315).

MANAGEMENT

- Physiologically lower levels of EPO in neonates provided the rationale for the pharmacologic use of recombinant human EPO (r-HuEPO) to treat symptomatic anemia or as prophylactic therapy to reduce the volume and risks of blood transfusions (Blackburn, 2013a, p. 243; Diehl-Jones & Fraser, 2015, p. 684).
  - Supplementation of between 1 mg/kg per day and 10 mg/kg per day elemental iron has been used to lessen the risk of iron deficiency (Diab & Luchtman-Jones, 2015, p. 1315).
- Therapy with r-HuEPO and iron stimulates erythropoiesis and increases reticulocyte counts (Diehl-Jones & Fraser, 2015, p. 684).

OUTCOMES

- Two approaches to EPO therapy have been systematically reviewed in neonates:
  - The early approach, defined by the use of r-HuEPO before day 8 of life, has been shown to reduce (but not eliminate) RBC transfusions and donor exposures, but did not impact morbidity and mortality measures.
  - The later use of r-HuEPO (on day 8 of life or after) resulted in a reduction in the number of blood transfusions, but not the total volume of blood, per infant, so that meaningful clinical outcomes were not affected by the use of r-HuEPO (Diab & Luchtman-Jones, 2015, p. 1315).

Anemia of Prematurity

DEFINITION AND PATHOPHYSIOLOGY
- Because preterm infants have more fetal hemoglobin and the lifespan of fetal hemoglobin is shorter than the lifespan of adult hemoglobin, physiologic anemia of preterm neonates occurs earlier and is more pronounced (Martin & Fanaroff, p. 1307). This normocytic normochromic anemia is characterized by low EPO levels (Blackburn, 2013a, p. 243).
- Preterm infants, especially those born prior to 32 gestational weeks, experience a lower nadir and lower hemoglobin levels for a longer period of time.
  - For these preterm infants, hemoglobin levels may reach the lowest point by about 4 to 6 weeks of life and remain low for 3 to 6 months of life. The more preterm the infant, the lower the nadir (Blackburn, 2013a, p. 243).
- Once RBC production resumes, iron stores are quickly depleted by 2 to 3 months of life (Blackburn, 2013a, p. 244). As a result, adequate iron intake is necessary for continued erythropoiesis.

RISK FACTORS
- Rates of decline and nadir are inversely proportional to gestational age (Diehl-Jones & Fraser, 2015, p. 671).
- Low birth weight (LBW) infants are at high risk for late-onset anemia of prematurity due to the low endogenous production of EPO and frequent laboratory sampling (Diehl-Jones & Fraser, 2015, p. 671; Manco-Johnson et al., 2016, p. 491).
- The precipitous drop in hematocrit may be intensive in sick infants who have repeated blood draws. Additionally, preterm infants do not readily increase serum EPO levels in the presence of hypoxia (Blackburn, 2013a, p. 243).

CLINICAL PRESENTATION
- Infants with anemia of prematurity may be symptomatic or asymptomatic. Symptoms of anemia include the following: tachycardia, tachypnea, poor feeding or fatigue with feeding, poor weight gain, pallor, increased lactate levels, increased oxygen requirement, or apnea and bradycardia (Blackburn, 2013a, p. 244; Diab & Luchtman-Jones, 2015, p. 1297; Diehl-Jones & Fraser, 2015, p. 671).
- If levels drop below a tolerable point, the infant may display decreased activity, poor growth, tachypnea, and tachycardia (Manco-Johnson et al., 2016, p. 483).

MANAGEMENT
- Small, premature infants often undergo transfusions because they are critically ill and have the highest blood sampling loss in relation to their weight (Manco-Johnson et al., 2016, p. 491). More than 90% of very low birth weight (VLBW) infants weighing less than 1,000 grams or less at birth receive at least one RBCs (red blood cells) transfusion during their hospital course. There is no standardized guideline for transfusing with RBCs (red blood cells) and practices vary among units (Blackburn, 2013a, p. 243, Kaplan et al., 2018, p. 1181).
- The goal of transfusion for infants with anemia of prematurity is to restore or maintain oxygen delivery without increasing oxygen consumption (Blackburn, 2013a, p. 244).
  - The appropriate time to transfuse an infant is an area of controversy since there are no clinical signs which are consistently useful or predictive alone or when in a group (Blackburn, 2013a, p. 244). Advantages of transfusion must be weighed against risks and in consideration of gestational, postnatal age, intravascular volume, and coexisting cardiac, pulmonary, or vascular conditions (Diehl-Jones & Fraser, 2015, p. 673).
  - Potential complications of red cell blood transfusions may include:
    - Acute hemolytic transfusion reactions—These types of reactions usually occur secondary to an incompatibility of the donor's RBCs with antibodies in the infant's plasma.
  - Volume overload—This condition may occur with large-volume transfusions, greater than 20 mL/kg. Infants with chronic anemia are more vulnerable to volume overload from transfusions. Congestive heart failure and pulmonary edema are consequences of fluid volume overload (Sloan, 2017, p. 580; Patel & Josephson, 2018, p. 1183).
- Research has demonstrated successful use of r-HuEPO to decrease the severity of anemia of prematurity and lessen the use of blood transfusions in smaller, premature infants (Manco-Johnson et al., 2016, p. 483).
- The American Academy of Pediatrics (AAP) recommends 2 to 4 mg/kg/day of elemental iron for preterm infants; however, higher doses for prevention of iron deficiency may be associated with improved outcomes (Manco-Johnson et al., 2016, p. 483)

OUTCOMES
- The use of restrictive transfusion guidelines appears to have similar results in terms of numbers of transfusion as use of r-HuEPO. Concerns have been raised that transfusion guidelines are too restrictive and may increase the risk of neurologic injury and altered outcomes (Blackburn, 2013a, p. 244).
- Iron deficiency with or without accompanying anemia has been associated with cognitive and behavioral deficits (Manco-Johnson et al., 2016, p. 483).
- Rate of common morbidities such as chronic lung disease, necrotizing enterocolitis (NEC), and intraventricular hemorrhage were found to be similar in control and experimental (r-HuEPO) groups (Blackburn, 2013a, p. 244).

Polycythemia

DEFINITION AND PATHOPHYSIOLOGY
- Polycythemia is defined as a peripheral venous hemoglobin and hematocrit more than two standard deviations above the mean. This is equivalent to a venous hematocrit of 65% or greater or a hemoglobin of 22 mg/dL or greater (Blackburn, 2013a, p. 244; Diab & Luchtman-Jones, 2015, p. 1317; Diehl-Jones & Fraser, 2015, p. 680; Mancho-Johnson et al., p. 492; O'Reilly, 2017, p. 624).
  - Hematocrit values vary greatly based on several factors, including sample site with some capillary hematocrits higher than 20% that of venous samples (Diab & Luchtman-Jones, 2015, p. 1317; O'Reilly, 2017, p. 624).
  - Capillary sampling can be used as a screening test, but a central venous sample should be analyzed to confirm polycythemia (Manco-Johnson et al., 2016, p. 492).
- Box 21.1 summarizes potential causes of polycythemia.

BOX 21.1 Causes of polycythemia

Causes or Etiologic Factors
- Placental transfusion
  - Holding the infant below the mother at delivery
  - Maternal-to-fetal transfusion
  - Twin-to-twin transfusion
- Placental insufficiency
  - Small-for-gestational age
  - Intrauterine growth restriction
  - Maternal hypertension syndromes, such as preeclampsia and renal disease
  - Maternal diabetes
  - Maternal smoking
  - Cyanotic heart disease or pulmonary disease in the mother
  - Post term infants or large-for-gestational-age infants
  - High-altitude pregnancies
- Fetal factors
  - Trisomy 13, 18, and 21
  - Hyperthyroidism
  - Neonatal thyrotoxicosis
  - Congenital adrenal hyperplasia
  - Beckwith–Wiedemann syndrome
- Other conditions
  - Certain maternal medications, such as propranolol
  - Neonatal dehydration
  - Sepsis

Sources: Data from Blackburn, S. (2018). *Maternal, fetal, and neonatal physiology: A clinical perspective* (5th ed., p. 244). Maryland Heights, MO: Elsevier; Diab, Y., & Luchtman-Jones. (2015). Hematologic and oncologic problems in the fetus and neonate. In R. Martin, A. Fanaroff, & M. Walsh (Eds.), *Fanaroff and Martin's neonatal-perinatal medicine: Diseases of the fetus and infant* (10th ed., pp. 1294–1343). Philadelphia, PA: Elsevier; Manco-Johnson, M., McKinney, C., Knapp-Clevenger, R., & Hernandez, J. (2016). Neonatal hyperbilirubinemia. In S. Gardner, B. Carter, M. Hines, & J. Hernandez (Eds.), *Merenstein & Gardner's handbook of neonatal intensive care* (8th ed., pp. 470–510). St. Louis, MO: Elsevier; O'Reilly, D. (2017). Polycythemia. In E. Eichenwald, A. Hansen, C. Martin, & A. Stark (Eds.), *Cloherty and Stark's manual of neonatal care* (8th ed., pp. 624–629). Philadelphia, PA: Wolters Kluwer.

DELAYED CORD CLAMPING

- Delayed clamping of the umbilical cord by 30 to 90 seconds has been reported as a successful variation of autologous transfusion. Two recent randomized clinical trials have disproven the concern regarding delayed cord clamping leading to polycythemia. There was no increased incidence of polycythemia or hyperbilirubinemia (Diab & Luchtman-Jones, 2015, p. 1299; Fasano, Said, & Luban, 2015, p. 1352; Manco-Johnson et al., 2016, p. 492).

HYPERVISCOSITY

- It is important to recognize that polycythemia is not synonymous with hyperviscosity and that not every neonate with polycythemia also has hyperviscosity (Christensen, 2018, p. 1176). The viscosity of blood increases linearly with hematocrit up to 60% then increases exponentially. Viscosity cannot easily be measured directly, so hematocrit is often used as a surrogate for viscosity (Manco-Johnson et al., 2016, p. 492).
  - Viscosity is the property of a liquid to resist changes in shape; for example, honey is more viscous than water.
  - When whole blood viscosity testing is not convenient, hyperviscosity can be inferred when a neonate with polycythemia has signs of hyperviscosity (Christensen, 2018, p. 1176).

- Blood viscosity increases with hematocrits greater than 65% or when venous hemoglobin is greater than 22 g/dL. Hyperviscosity leads to reduction of blood flow to the organs (Diehl-Jones & Fraser, 2015, p. 680)

RISK FACTORS
- Polycythemia is estimated to occur anywhere from 1% to 5% of term infants. The incidence is increased in infants who are growth restricted, small-for-gestational age, or post term (Diab & Luchtman-Jones, 2015, p. 1317; O'Reilly, 2017, p. 572)
- Identification of maternal–fetal risk factors such as insulin-dependent diabetes, hypertension and heart disease, cigarette smoking, and living at high altitude. Fetal risk factors including intrauterine growth restriction and delayed cord clamping (Manco-Johnson et al., 2016, p. 493).

CLINICAL PRESENTATIONS
- Most polycythemic infants have no symptoms, particularly if the polycythemia becomes apparent only on routine neonatal screening. Infants are often asymptomatic. Symptoms tend to appear at or after 2 hours of life when the hematocrit is at its highest value. In some infants, especially those with excessive extracellular fluid losses, symptoms may not be apparent until day of life 2 or 3. Symptoms are typically transient (Christensen, 2018, p. 1176; Diab & Luchtman-Jones, 2015, p. 1317).
- Symptoms, when present, are usually attributable to hyperviscosity and poor tissue perfusion characterized by impaired circulation occurring from an increased resistance to blood flow, or to associated metabolic abnormalities, such as hypoglycemia and hypocalcemia (Christensen, 2018, p. 1176; Diab & Luchtman-Jones, 2015, p. 1317; Manco-Johnson et al., 2016, p. 492).
- The clinical manifestations associated with polycythemia and hyperviscosity are common to many neonatal conditions and may include:
  - Central nervous abnormalities, such as lethargy or irritability, jitteriness, hypotonia, apnea, seizures, and cerebral venous thrombosis
  - Respiratory distress, including tachypnea, pulmonary edema, and pulmonary hemorrhage, and persistent pulmonary hypertension of the newborn. There may be prominent vascular markings on chest radiograph
  - Cardiac compromise, including cyanosis, tachycardia, congestive heart failure, heart murmur, cardiomegaly, and elevated pulmonary vascular resistance
  - Renal manifestations, such as renal vein thrombosis, hematuria, and proteinuria
  - Gastrointestinal signs including behaviors associated with poor feeding, such as poor nippling and emesis, decreased bowel sounds, abdominal distention. The increased RBC load also contributes to hyperbilirubinemia (Diab & Luchtman-Jones, 2015, p. 1317; Manco-Johnson et al., 2016, p. 492; O'Reilly, 2017, pp. 572–574).

MANAGEMENT
- The management of polycythemia should be based on the presence of clinical manifestations that are consistent with hyperviscosity and not laboratory values alone (Manco-Johnson et al., 2016, p. 493).
- Asymptomatic infants with a hematocrit between 60% and 70% can be managed by increasing the total fluid intake

and repeating the hematocrit 4 to 6 hours later (O'Reilly, 2017, p. 672).

- ○ Supportive care, which includes insertion of a peripheral intravenous catheter (PIC) and initiation of intravenous (IV) fluids and initiation of phototherapy to treat hyperbilirubinemia (Manco-Johnson et al., 2016, p. 493).
- ○ A normal saline bolus of 10 mL/kg can be given for asymptomatic infants whose hematocrit is greater than 70% or in infants who demonstrate clinical manifestations of polycythemia with a hematocrit between 65% and 70% (Diehl-Jones & Fraser, 2015, p. 680; Manco-Johnson et al., 2016, p. 494).
- Symptomatic infants may require a partial exchange transfusion to dilute the circulating blood volume and improve perfusion to vulnerable areas. Blood is removed from the infant via the umbilical cord and replaced (also through the cord) with normal saline. The total volume exchanged is usually 15 to 20 mL/kg of body weight; however, this will depend on the infant's body weight (O'Reilly, 2017, pp. 627–628).

OUTCOMES

- Hyperviscosity syndrome is associated with development of vascular thrombosis (renal cerebral, mesenteric), neurologic sequalae, fine motor abnormalities, and speech delays (Diehl-Jones & Fraser, 2015, p. 680).
- The long-term neurologic outcomes in infants with asymptomatic polycythemia and/or hyperviscosity remain controversial (O'Reilly, 2017, p. 628). A partial exchange transfusion has not shown to improve neurodevelopmental outcomes in infants with asymptomatic polycythemia (Diab & Luchtman-Jones, 2015, p. 1318; O'Reilly, 2017, p. 628).
- Newborns with a diagnosis of hyperviscosity are at greater risk for adverse neurologic outcomes. The presence of adverse neurologic outcomes may be related to the underlying risk factors as opposed to polycythemia alone (Diehl-Jones & Fraser, 2015, p. 680; Manco-Johnson et al., 2016, p. 493).

NEONATAL PLATELET DISORDERS

Thrombocytosis

DEFINITION AND PATHOPHYSIOLOGY

- Primary (essential) thrombocytosis is extremely rare in infants and children and is often caused by monoclonal antibodies or other etiology which can lead to an uncontrollable production of platelets (Deschmann & Sola-Visner, 2018, p. 1141).
- Secondary (reactive) thrombocytosis tends to occur more often in infants and neonates (Deschmann & Sola-Visner, 2018, p. 1141). Following the interruption of platelet consumption by thrombus, after successful anticoagulation, infant may manifest thrombocytosis from increased bone marrow production (Manco-Johnson et al., 2016, p. 505).

RISK FACTORS

- The most common causes of reactive thrombocytosis in neonates and children are infections, tissue damage (surgeries, trauma, burns), and anemia (frequently, iron deficiency). Reactive thrombocytosis has also been described in association with medications (i.e., corticosteroids), maternal exposure to methadone or psychopharmaceutical drugs,

and metabolic diseases, myopathies, or neurofibromatosis (Deschmann & Sola-Visner, 2018, p. 1141).

CLINICAL PRESENTATION

- Based on severity, thrombocytosis has been traditionally classified as
  - ○ mild (platelet counts between 500 and $700 \times 10^9/L$)
  - ○ moderate ($700–900 \times 10^9/L$)
  - ○ severe ($900–1000 \times 10^9/L$)
  - ○ extreme thrombocytosis (platelet counts $> 1000 \times 10^9/L$ (Deschmann & Sola-Visner, 2018, p. 1141)

MANAGEMENT

- Reactive thrombocytosis usually does not lead to thromboembolic or hemorrhagic complications, and for that reason therapy with anticoagulants or platelet function inhibitors (i.e., aspirin) is usually not indicated in asymptomatic children. Individually tailored thrombosis prophylaxis should be considered only in neonates with additional thrombotic risk factors, such as maternal antiphospholipid syndrome or cardiac malformation (Deschmann & Sola-Visner, 2018, p. 1141).

OUTCOMES

- No long-term complications from thrombocytosis have been studied (Deschmann & Sola-Visner, 2018, p. 1141).

Thrombocytopenia

DEFINITION AND PATHOPHYSIOLOGY

- Platelets are small, nonnucleated cells which are derived from megakaryocytes in the bone marrow. After release into the bloodstream, they will circulate for 7 to 10 days before being removed by the spleen. They are hypoactive in the first few days after birth, which protects the infant against thrombosis but may increase risk of bleeding (Diehl-Jones & Fraser, 2015, p. 666).
- Thrombocytopenia is a general term to reflect a decreased number of platelets in the infant's blood (Manco-Johnson et al., 2016, p. 498). Traditionally defined as a platelet count of less than $150 \times 10^9/L$ (Diab & Luchtman-Jones, 2015, p. 1328). A normal platelet count in healthy newborn infants regardless of gestational age is 150,000 to 450,000 (Blackburn, 2013a, p. 236; Letterio, Ahuja, & Petrosiute, 2013, p. 457)
- Neonatal thrombocytopenia is the most common acquired disease hematologic condition in the infant, occurring in approximately 1% to 5% of healthy term infants at birth and up to 35% of critically ill neonates (Deschmann, Saxonhouse, & Sola-Visner, 2017, p. 631; Diab & Luchtman-Jones, 2015, p. 1328; Diehl-Jones & Fraser, 2015, p. 677; Letterio et al., 2013, p. 457).
  - ○ In infants admitted to the NICU and those that are critically ill, the incidence of thrombocytopenia increases to 22% to 35% (Diehl-Jones & Fraser, 2015, p. 677; Letterio et al., 2013, p. 457).

RISK FACTORS

- Infants predisposed to thrombocytopenia include those who are exposed to maternal antibodies or whose fetal platelets contain an antigen lacking in the mother. Congenital or acquired infections may cause thrombocytopenia. Infants born with hemangiomas such as Kasabach–Merritt syndrome will demonstrate thrombocytopenia, as will some infants born with Trisomy 13 or 18 (Diehl-Jones & Fraser, 2015, pp. 677–678).

CLINICAL PRESENTATION

- Patients with platelet function disorders present with bleeding signs including mucocutaneous bleeding (nose, mouth, gastrointestinal tract, genitourinary tract) and bruising. The extent, location, and nature of the bruises are generally related to birth trauma and invasive procedures (e.g., IV starts, heel sticks, or endotracheal suctioning; Deschmann & Sola-Visner, 2018, p. 1150). They also show platelet-type bleeding such as petechiae, purpura, and epistaxis. If delivered vaginally, the infant will have a cephalohematoma (Diehl-Jones & Fraser, 2015, p. 678)
- When evaluating a thrombocytopenic neonate, the first step to narrow the differential diagnosis is to classify the thrombocytopenia as either early onset (within the first 72 hours of life) or late onset (after 72 hours of life) and to determine whether the infant is clinically ill or well (Deschmann et al., 2017, p. 631; Deschmann & Sola-Visner, 2018, p. 1141).

EARLY ONSET

- The most frequent cause of early-onset thrombocytopenia in a well-appearing neonate is placental insufficiency, seen in infants born to mothers with pregnancy-induced hypertension/preeclampsia and in those with intrauterine growth restriction. The thrombocytopenia is usually mild to moderate and resolves within 72 hours (Deschmann & Sola-Visner, 2018, pp. 1141–1142).
  - ○ *Severe* early-onset thrombocytopenia in an otherwise healthy infant should trigger suspicion for an immune-mediated thrombocytopenia, either autoimmune (if the mother is also thrombocytopenic) or alloimmune (if the mother has a normal platelet count) (Deschmann & Sola-Visner, 2018, p. 1142).

IMMUNE THROMBOCYTOPENIA

- Immune thrombocytopenia occurs because of the passive transfer of antibodies from the maternal to the fetal circulation. There are two distinct types of immune-mediated thrombocytopenia:
  - ○ *Neonatal alloimmune thrombocytopenia (NAIT)*, in which the antibody is produced in the mother against a specific human platelet antigen (HPA) present in the fetus but absent in the mother (Deschmann et al., 2017, p. 835; Deschmann & Sola-Visner, 2018, p. 1144; Diab & Luchtman-Jones, 2015, p. 1328).
  - ○ *Autoimmune thrombocytopenia* should be considered in any neonate who has early-onset thrombocytopenia and a maternal history of either immune thrombocytopenic purpura (ITP) or an autoimmune disease. Neonatal thrombocytopenia secondary to maternal ITP may last for weeks to months (unlike NAIT, which usually resolves within 2 weeks) and requires long-term monitoring (Deschmann et al.,2017, p. 837; Deschmann & Sola-Visner, 2018, p. 1145; Diab & Luchtman-Jones, 2015, p. 1329).

LATE ONSET

- The most common causes of thrombocytopenia of any severity presenting after 72 hours of life are sepsis

(bacterial or fungal) and NEC. Thrombocytopenia can be the first presenting sign of these processes and can precede clinical deterioration. If bacterial/fungal sepsis and NEC are ruled out, viral infections such as herpes simplex virus (HSV), CMV, or enterovirus should be considered.
  - ○ Other less common causes of late-onset thrombocytopenia include inborn errors of metabolism and Fanconi anemia (rare); (Deschmann et al., 2017, p. 633; Deschmann & Sola-Visner, 2018, p. 1143).

MANAGEMENT

- Random donor platelet transfusions are now considered the first line of therapy for infants with suspected NAIT (Deschmann & Sola-Visner, 2018, p. 1144) although it rarely results in sustained increase due to antibody destruction (Diehl-Jones & Fraser, 2015, p. 679).
  - ○ If able, obtain HPA testing on the infant, and in the absence of neonatal HPA, the use of maternal platelets is recommended (Diehl-Jones & Fraser, 2015, p. 679).
- First-line therapy for autoimmune thrombocytopenia is IV immunoglobin Ig (IVIG) with the addition of random donor platelets for infants with active bleeding (Deschmann et al., 2017, p. 636; Deschmann & Sola-Visner, 2018, p. 1145).
- Management of late-onset thrombocytopenia includes treatment appropriate to the suspected etiology (i.e., antibiotics, supportive respiratory and cardiovascular care, bowel rest in case of NEC, and surgery in case of surgical NEC). The platelet count usually improves in 1 to 2 weeks, although in some infants the thrombocytopenia persists for several weeks for unclear reasons (Deschmann & Sola-Visner, 2018, p. 1143; Diehl-Jones & Fraser, 2015, p. 679).

OUTCOMES

- The outcomes for patients with thrombocytopenia are variable and depend on the specific disorders (Deschmann & Sola-Visner, 2018, p. 1147; Diehl-Jones & Fraser, 2015, p. 680).

COAGULOPATHIES

Vitamin K Deficiency

DEFINITION AND PATHOPHYSIOLOGY

- Newborns are deficient in all vitamin K dependent factors: II, VII, IX, X (Blackburn, 2013a, p. 239). In the absence of vitamin K, these proteins are dysfunctional and are released into the circulation informs knows as proteins induced by vitamin K absence (PIVKA); (Diab & Luchtman-Jones, 2015, p. 1334). Previously termed 'hemorrhagic disease of the newborn," the newer term ,"vitamin K-dependent bleeding (VKDB)" is thought to more accurately describe the link between vitamin K deficiency and spontaneous bleeding (Croteau, 2017, p. 586; Diehl-Jones & Fraser, 2015, p. 673; Manco-Johnson et al., 2016, p. 496; Saxonhouse, 2018, p. 1125).
- The etiology of vitamin K dependent factor deficiency is twofold:
  - ○ Vitamin K is poorly transferred through the placenta to the fetus during pregnancy.
  - ○ The newborn intestine lacks colonization of bacteria normally responsible for producing vitamin K (Blackburn, 2013a, pp. 239–241; Diab & Luchtman-Jones, 2015,

p. 1334; Diehl-Jones & Fraser, 2015, p. 674; Saxonhouse, 2018, p. 1125).

RISK FACTORS

- Risk factors are related to three forms of VKDB:
  - Early onset (within 24 hours)—can occur in infants of mothers who are taking certain anticonvulsants (e.g., phenytoin) and vitamin K antagonists such as warfarin (Coumadin).
  - Classic onset (2–6 days)—Classical VKDB occurs because of a physiologic deficiency in vitamin K at birth combined with a sole breast milk diet or inadequate feeding (Saxonhouse, 2018, p. 1125).
  - Late onset (2–12 weeks of age)—occurs in infants who did not receive vitamin K at birth and are receiving an inadequate dose (e.g., breastfeeding) or in infants with hepatobiliary disease (Croteau, 2017, p. 594; Diehl-Jones & Fraser, 2015, p. 674; Manco-Johnson et al., 2016, p. 501).

CLINICAL PRESENTATION

- In general, oozing, which may be localized or diffuse. Frequently gastrointestinal (hematemesis, melena) or from puncture sites, the umbilical cord, or post-circumcision. There may also be diffuse ecchymosis and/or petechiae (Diehl-Jones & Fraser, 2015, p. 674).
- Laboratory assessment showed elevated prothrombin time (PT) and partial thromboplastin time (PTT), low levels of vitamin K-dependent clotting factors, and PIVKA levels are high (Croteau, 2017, p. 591; Diehl-Jones & Fraser, 2015, p. 674; Saxonhouse, 2018, p. 1125).

MANAGEMENT

- Prophylactic vitamin K (phytonadione) intramuscular (IM) injection at the time of delivery
- If VKDB occurs, transfusions of blood products (RBCs, fresh frozen plasma) and repeated doses of vitamin K may be indicated (Croteau, 2017, p. 592; Diab & Luchtman-Jones, 2015, p. 1335; Diehl-Jones & Fraser, 2015, p. 675).

OUTCOMES

- Prophylactic therapy has mostly eliminated VKDB (Diehl-Jones & Fraser, 2015, p. 675). When IM vitamin K prophylaxis is provided, the incidence of late VKDB decreases to 0.24 to 3.2 per 100,000 live births (Saxonhouse, 2018, p. 1125).

Disseminated Intravascular Coagulation (DIC)

DEFINITION AND PATHOPHYSIOLOGY

- DIC is a complex process that is characterized by systemic activation of coagulation and fibrinolysis, consumption of platelets and coagulation factors, and generation of fibrin clots that can lead to ischemic organ damage or failure (Diab & Luchtman-Jones, 2015, p. 1335; Saxonhouse, 2018, p. 1125).
  - This dysregulation of the coagulation and inflammatory systems results in massive thrombin generation with widespread fibrin deposition and consumption of coagulation proteins and platelets, ultimately leading to multiorgan damage (Saxonhouse, 2018, p. 1125).
- In DIC, activation of blood clotting proteins is initiated by tissue factor from bacterial products (endotoxin) or inflammation. The activation of clotting proteins leads to a hypercoagulable state and thromboses form, especially in

the small vessels of the liver, spleen, brain, lungs, kidneys, and adrenal glands. The bone marrow releases platelets; however, the system which regulates coagulation is immature and the ability to neutralize activated clotting proteins is quickly overwhelmed. This results in deficient of platelets and clotting factors and is called consumptive coagulopathy (Manco-Johnson et al., 2016, p. 500; Diehl-Jones & Fraser, 2015, p. 675).

RISK FACTORS

- It is important to remember that *DIC always occurs as a secondary event*, and can be triggered by a variety of pathologic conditions (Diab & Luchtman-Jones, 2015, p. 1335) These include birth asphyxia, respiratory distress syndrome, meconium aspiration syndrome, infection, NEC, hypothermia, severe placental insufficiency, and thrombosis (Saxonhouse, 2018, p. 1125).
- Neonatal precipitating factors include infection (bacterial, viral, fungal); conditions causing hypoxia, acidosis, and shock; severe Rh incompatibility; and tissue injury (traumatic birth, or NEC); (Diehl-Jones & Fraser, 2015, p. 675).

CLINICAL PRESENTATION

- The cardinal manifestations of overt DIC are caused by excessive bleeding and microvascular thrombosis. Hemorrhagic symptoms include petechiae and bruising, oozing from venipuncture sites, bleeding from traumatic and surgical wounds, and, in severe cases, bleeding involving internal organs, and organ and tissue ischemia. Microvascular thrombosis causes potential ischemia and necrosis of any organ, particularly the kidney. Organ failure can result in the end stage (Diab & Luchtman-Jones, 2015, p. 1335; Diehl-Jones & Fraser, 2015, p. 676).
- The diagnosis of DIC, particularly in the early stages, can be problematic because there is no single laboratory test that can establish or rule out DIC. Hence, the diagnosis is often made on the basis of an appropriate clinical suspicion supported by laboratory evidence of procoagulant and fibrinolytic system activation coupled with anticoagulant consumption and diffuse clinical bleeding.
  - Laboratory abnormalities seen in DIC include thrombocytopenia, elevated fibrin degradation products (FDP) or D-dimers, prolonged PT, prolonged aPTT, prolonged thrombin clotting time, and a low fibrinogen (Diab & Luchtman-Jones, 2015, p. 1335; Diehl-Jones & Fraser, 2015, p. 676).

MANAGEMENT

- The most important aspect of treatment for DIC is to treat the underlying disorder (Croteau, 2017, p. 593; Saxonhouse, 2018, pp. 1125–1126). Successful treatment of DIC relies largely on reversal of the underlying condition and supporting adequate blood flow and oxygen delivery (Diab & Luchtman-Jones, 2015, p. 1335; Diehl-Jones & Fraser, 2015, p. 676).
- The focus of acute management in the neonate is to support adequate hemostasis to reduce the risk of spontaneous hemorrhage. This is usually achieved with platelet transfusions, fresh frozen plasma (FFP), or cryoprecipitate (Croteau, 2017, p. 593; Diehl-Jones & Fraser, 2015, p. 677; Saxonhouse, 2018, pp. 1125–1126).
  - Blood component transfusions (platelets, fresh frozen plasma, and cryoprecipitate) are an important part of supportive treatment in DIC. In cases of DIC in which thrombosis predominates, such as arterial or venous

thromboembolism or severe purpura fulminans, therapeutic anticoagulation with unfractionated heparin may be considered (Diab & Luchtman-Jones, 2015; p. 1335; Diehl-Jones & Fraser, 2015, p. 676).

OUTCOMES

- Outcomes are related to the prognosis of the underlying disease and the severity of DIC (Diehl-Jones & Fraser, 2015, p. 677).

IMMUNE-MEDIATED HEMOLYTIC DISEASE

- Immune-mediated disorders are the most common cause of hemolysis in neonates and should be suspected when there is:
  - ○ a heterospecific mother–infant pair where the infant expresses a red cell antigen(s) foreign to the mother,
  - ○ the presence of a maternal antibody directed to the infant RBC antigen, and
  - ○ a positive direct Coombs test in the neonate indicating maternal antibody bound to the infant RBC (Watchko, 2018, p. 1201).

Rh Disease

DEFINITION AND PATHOPHYSIOLOGY

- The basis of alloimmune hemolytic anemia is transfer of maternal antibody against fetal RBC antigens inherited from the father and absent in the mother. In the developed world, most cases of alloimmune hemolytic disease of the fetus and newborn are now the result of maternal antibodies to ABO, Kell, Duffy, Kidd, and MNS antigens and other Rh antigens, particularly c and E (Christensen, 2018, pp. 1165–1167).
  - ○ Several Rh antigens are recognized, each of which is detected by specific antibodies. The most clinically relevant of the membrane Rh proteins to neonatal hemolytic disease is the D antigen since the D antigen is most commonly implicated in maternal–fetal incompatibility (Blackburn, 2013b, p. 470). The D antigen may produce maternal sensitization with a fetomaternal hemorrhage as small as 0.1 mL (Kaplan et al., 2015, p. 1361).
  - ○ Rh-positive RBCs are those that possess the D antigen. A lowercase *d* is used to denote the absence of the D antigen, or Rh-negative status (Christensen, 2018, p. 1167).
- The hallmark of isoimmunization is a positive direct antiglobulin test (DAT) (also known as the Coombs test). This is indicative of maternally produced antibody that has traversed the placenta and is now found within the fetus.
  - ○ The test is termed *direct* if the antiglobulin is adhered to the RBCs.
  - ○ An *indirect* test refers to the antibody being detected in the serum (Kaplan et al., 2015, p. 1630).
- Rh isoimmunization is of particular concern because the D antigen is strongly expressed in large amounts early in gestation. Additionally, the D antigen stimulates production of maternal IgG and memory cells in the mother. Following exposure to the D antigen on the fetal RBCs, the mother's immune system responds by forming anti-D immunoglobulin G (IgG) antibodies. The IgG then crosses the placenta and adheres to fetal RBCs containing the D antigen. The subsequent antigen-antibody interaction leads to hemolysis and anemia (Kaplan et al., 2015, p. 1631).

- ○ Isoimmune hemolytic disease, hemolytic disease of the newborn, and erythroblastosis fetalis are synonymous with the disorder by which maternal IgG antibodies cross into the fetal circulation (Blackburn, 2013b, p. 470).
- Rh hemolytic disease is rare during the first pregnancy involving an Rh-positive fetus, but the risk increases with each subsequent pregnancy. This is because small volumes of fetal RBCs enter the maternal circulation throughout gestation, although the major fetomaternal bleeding responsible for sensitization occurs during delivery. Once sensitization has occurred, reexposure to Rh(D) RBCs in subsequent pregnancies leads to an exaggerated response, with an increase in the maternal anti-D titer.
- Rh-negative mothers are unlikely to have anti-D antibodies unless they have been exposed to D antigen in a previous pregnancy or have received a mismatched blood transfusion (Blackburn, 2013b, p. 472). Significant hemolysis occurring in the first pregnancy indicates previous maternal exposure to Rh-positive RBCs. On occasion the sensitization is a consequence of an earlier transfusion in which Rh-positive RBCs were administered by mistake or in which some other blood component (e.g., platelets) containing Rh(D) RBCs was transfused. Even a tiny amount of Rh-positive fetal blood is enough to cause anti-D antibody formation and memory cell production in the mother (Blackburn, 2013b, p. 472, Kaplan et al., 2015, p. 1631).

MANAGEMENT

- Management requires first the identification of those fetuses at risk. An increase in the maternal anti-D titer in a previously sensitized Rh-negative woman is a good serologic measure of a fetus in potential jeopardy. A history of neonatal hemolytic disease resulting from anti-D antibodies suggests that the current fetus also may be at risk (Christensen, 2018, p. 1168).
- Rh immune globulin (RhIG) (RhoGAM) is a concentrated form of anti-D antibodies, given to Rh-negative women at various points antepartum and postpartum in order to prevent hemolytic disease of the newborn. RhIG works by destroying fetal Rh-positive RBCs in the maternal circulation before the D antigen is recognized by the maternal circulation so that antibodies and memory cells are not made.
  - ○ RhIg is administered at 28 weeks' gestation prophylactically, within 72 hours of delivery of an Rh-positive newborn, or after any other event that may increase the risk of maternal fetal blood mixing, including after an abortion, amniocentesis, or with significant bleeding during pregnancy (Blackburn, 2013b, p. 472; Christensen, 2018, p. 1168).
- It is important to note that Rh-D-positive infants delivered to Rh-D-negative women during the first isoimmunized pregnancy (conversion from negative to positive maternal antibody titer in that pregnancy) are at an approximately 20% risk of developing hemolytic disease of the newborn. An infant born of a pregnancy during which maternal antibody conversion occurs will by definition carry the foreign antigen and may have a positive direct Coombs test. Such infants are at risk of hemolytic diseases, and should be monitored closely for severe hyperbilirubinemia with serial serum total bilirubin (TSB) measurements and not discharged early from the birth hospital as they will likely require treatment, including the possibility of an exchange transfusion (Watchko, 2018, p. 1201).

ABO Incompatibility

DEFINITION AND PATHOPHYSIOLOGY

- With the reduction of the incidence of Rh isoimmunization by immune prophylaxis, DAT-positive ABO incompatibility is now the single most prominent cause of immune hemolytic disease in the neonate (Kaplan et al., 2015, p. 1631).
  - Although ABO incompatibility is much more common that Rh disease, it is less severe than Rh incompatibility. Mechanisms responsible for Rh isoimmunization, such as previous exposure and immunization, are not needed with ABO incompatibility because the mother has naturally occurring antibodies to fetal ABO antigens (Blackburn, 2013b, p. 472).
- ABO incompatibility occurs most frequently when a type O mother is pregnant with a baby with A blood type. By ABO blood group heterospecificity, we refer to the situation in which a blood group A or B baby is born to a group O mother, a setup occurring in about 12% of pregnancies (Christensen, 2018, p. 1168; Kaplan et al., 2015, p. 1631).
- In mothers with type A or type B blood, naturally occurring anti-B and anti-A isoantibodies are typically IgM antibodies and consequently do not cross the placenta to affect fetal RBCs. In contrast, the anti-A and anti-B alloantibodies present in mothers with type O blood typically also include IgG antibodies that can cross the placenta and affect the fetal erythrocytes. For this reason, ABO hemolytic disease of the fetus and newborn is largely limited to type O mothers carrying type A or type B fetuses (Christensen, 2018, p. 1168).
  - About one-third of blood group A or B neonates born to a blood group O mother will have a positive direct Coombs test (Kaplan et al., 2015, p. 1632).

MANAGEMENT

- It is essential to closely observe any newborn born to a blood group O mother and to perform a TcB or TB measurement at the first appearance of jaundice. Routine blood group and DAT determination on umbilical cord blood is an option, which may allow for additional risk determination (Kaplan et al., 2015, p. 1632).
- ABO hemolytic disease is often detected within the first 12 to 24 hours of life ("icterus praecox") (Watchko, 2018, p. 1203).
- In most cases, pallor and jaundice are minimal. Hepatosplenomegaly is uncommon. Laboratory features include evidence of minimal to moderate hyperbilirubinemia and, occasionally, some degree of anemia. The DAT is sometimes negative (Christensen, 2018, p. 1168).
- Symptomatic ABO hemolytic should be considered in infants who develop marked jaundice in the context of ABO incompatibility that is generally accompanied by a positive direct Coombs test and prominent microspherocytosis on red cell smear (Watchko, 2018, p. 1202).
  - In suspected cases of ABO incompatibility, it is essential to exclude other antibodies and other nonimmune causes of hemolysis such as glucose 6-phosphate dehydrogenase (G6PD) deficiency or hereditary spherocytosis.
- Severe cases are generally treated effectively with phototherapy, occasionally with an exchange transfusion in which group O Rh-compatible RBCs is used. Additional follow-up at 2 to 3 weeks of age to check for anemia in these infants is essential (Christensen, 2018, p. 1169)

NEONATAL JAUNDICE AND LIVER DISEASE

Biliary Atresia (BA)

DEFINITION AND PATHOPHYSIOLOGY

- BA is a condition in infants that is characterized by inflammation and fibrosis of the bile ducts. The hepatic biliary ducts become scarred and as the disease progresses, there is complete obliteration of the bile ducts. As the bile builds up in the liver, damage to this organ occurs.
  - Biliary atresia is one of the more common causes of chronic liver disease in infants with an incidence of approximately 0.5 to 3.2 per 10,000 live births. This reported incidence varies based on geographic location and ethnicity (Kaplan et al., 2015, p. 1660; Lane, Chisholm, & Murray, 2018, p. 1100).

RISK FACTORS

- BA is characterized by the anatomy of extrahepatic biliary obstruction. Two clinical phenotypes exist:
  - "Classical" BA, which is not associated with extrahepatic congenital anomalies
  - "BA with splenic malformation," which presents with other congenital anomalies such as situs inversus, polysplenia or asplenia, vascular and cardiac malformations, and intestinal malrotation

CLINICAL PRESENTATION

- Infants with BA typically present between 2 and 5 weeks of life with symptoms including:
  - Acholic stools which can appear after the onset of jaundice
  - Cholestatic or prolonged jaundice. The cholestatic jaundice may not be recognized as new; this highlights the importance of evaluating any prolonged or new jaundice in infants.
  - Ascites may present later in the disease course.
  - Inadequate weight gain related to malabsorption that occurs secondary to chronic inflammation and cholestasis (Lane et al., 2018, p. 1100)

MANAGEMENT

- Expedient differentiation of BA from other causes of neonatal cholestasis is critical, as surgical intervention before 2 months of age has been shown to improve surgical success and outcome (Lane et al., 2018, p. 1100). The immediate goal for surgical correction is the reestablishment of bile drainage, which is now achieved in most neonates when operated on before 3 months of age (Kaplan et al., 2015, p. 1665).
- BA may be suspected based on the clinical manifestations. The following is part of the workup to confirm a diagnosis of biliary atresia:
  - Conjugated hyperbilirubinemia, which is often between 2 and 7 mg/dL
  - Total serum bilirubin levels ,which may be between 5 and 12 mg/dL
  - Elevated alanine aminotransferase (ALT), ALP, and GGT

- Abdominal ultrasound (US) should be performed if BA is present, and US will demonstrate absence of the gallbladder or a fibrotic remnant of the extrahepatic bile duct. There may also be the "triangle cord sign," which is a triangular or tubular echogenic cord of fibrous tissue that represents the biliary remnant (Lane et al., 2018, p. 1100).
- Hepatobiliary iminodiacetic acid (HIDA) scan. In infants with biliary atresia, there is a lack of excretion into the bowel of the radioactive tracer that is injected into the infant. Oral phenobarbital can be administered at 5 mg/kg/day to the infant for 5 days prior to the procedure to enhance sensitivity of the scan (Lane et al., 2018, p. 1100).
- Once a diagnosis is confirmed, surgery is done with a Kasai hepatic portoentereostomy, which attempts to restore the normal flow of the bile. This may prevent or delay progression of the disease as well as worsening of fibrosis and development of end-stage liver disease (Lane et al., 2018, p. 1101).
  - ○ The Kasai hepatic portoenterostomy is a surgical procedure that excises the bile duct that is obstructed with creation of an anastomosis. An anastomosis is created with a jejunal limb of a Roux-en-Y with the liver at the porta hepatis, the latter the area of the liver where the

bile duct is located outside of the liver (extrahepatic); (Juul & Christensen, 2018, p. 1101).

OUTCOMES
- Without rapid intervention, the natural history of BA is uniform fatality by 2 years of age (Lane et al., 2018, p. 1101). Unrelieved by surgery, the defect inevitably leads to death from biliary cirrhosis in the first 2 to 3 years of life (Kaplan et al., 2015, p. 1661).
- Even with surgery intervention with the Kasai portoenterostomy, many infants tend to go on to develop cirrhosis and portal hypertension with the need for a liver transplant (Lane et al., 2018, p. 1101; Kaplan et al., 2015, p. 1665).

HYPERBILIRUBINEMIA

Normal Physiology

- In order to understand bilirubin pathology, an understanding of the natural physiology is necessary.
- Physiology. The pathway of bilirubin synthesis, transport, and metabolism is summarized in Figure 21.3

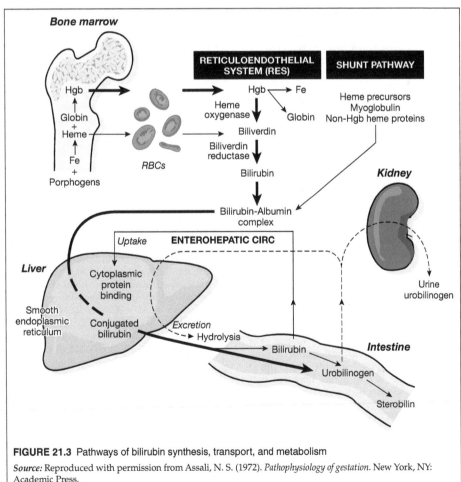

FIGURE 21.3 Pathways of bilirubin synthesis, transport, and metabolism

Source: Reproduced with permission from Assali, N. S. (1972). *Pathophysiology of gestation.* New York, NY: Academic Press.

Bilirubin Production

- Bilirubin production in the newborn is as high as 8 to 10 mg/kg/24 hour which, when compared to adults, is 2 to 2.5 times faster (Blackburn, 2013c, p. 610; Kamath-Rayne, Thilo, Deacon, & Hernandez, 2016, p. 511; Kaplan et al., 2015, p. 1620; Maisels & Watchko, 2018, p. 313).
- A majority of bilirubin (75%–85%) production occurs from the breakdown of hemoglobin from RBCs or ineffective erythropoiesis, a process that is accelerated in infants (Blackburn, 2013c, p. 611; Kamath-Rayne et al., p. 511; Maisels & Watchko, 2018, 2013, p. 310).
  - Each gram of hemoglobin produces 35 mg of bilirubin (Maisels & Watchko, 2018, 2013, p. 310).
- The remaining 15% to 25% of bilirubin is derived from the breakdown of other forms of heme in the body. This form of hemoglobin includes heme in the liver, such as in cytochromes and in muscle myoglobin. Ineffective erythropoiesis in the bone marrow also contributes to the production of bilirubin (Kamath-Rayne et al., 2015, p. 511; Maisels & Watchko, 2018, 2013, p. 310).
- Bilirubin metabolism occurs in the reticuloendothelial system, primarily in the liver and spleen as old or abnormal RBCs are removed from the circulation. The breakdown of RBCs is a normal process that destroys red cells that are aging, immature, or malformed (Kamath-Rayne et al., 2016, p. 511; Kaplan et al., 2015, p. 1620).
  - The enzyme heme oxygenase acts on heme to produce biliverdin. Biliverdin reductase will then convert biliverdin into bilirubin (Kamath-Rayne et al., 2016, p. 511).

TRANSPORT OF BILIRUBIN
- Once converted to bilirubin by biliverdin reductase, the unconjugated bilirubin is released into the bloodstream (Kamath-Rayne et al., 2016, p. 511).
- Once in the bloodstream, bilirubin must be bound to a carrier for transport to the liver. Albumin is this carrier which rapidly and tightly binds with bilirubin (Kaplan et al., 2015, p. 1621).
  - Each molecule of adult albumin is able to bind with at least two molecules of bilirubin with the first molecule being more tightly bound than the second (Kaplan et al., 2015, p. 1621).
- Infants have a reduced capacity to bind albumin with bilirubin when compared to adults and older children secondary to reduced concentrations of albumin (Kaplan et al., 2015, p. 1621).

HEPATIC UPTAKE OF BILIRUBIN
- Prior to entering the cells in the liver, bilirubin is removed from albumin. Bilirubin is then transported into the hepatocyte by intracellular carrier proteins. Once in the liver, unconjugated bilirubin is bound to glutathione-S-transferase A, or also known as ligandin or with B-ligandin (Y protein). To a lesser degree, unconjugated bilirubin may also bind with Z protein, another hepatic carrier (Kamath-Rayne et al., 2016, p. 512; Kaplan et al., 2015, p. 1621; Maisels & Watchko, 2018, 2013, p. 312).

CONJUGATION OF BILIRUBIN
- Conversion of unconjugated bilirubin to a more polar, water-soluble substance must occur in order for bilirubin to be excreted in bile. Conjugated occurs within the smooth endoplasmic reticulum of the liver cell (Kamath-Rayne et al., 2016, p. 512; Kaplan et al., 2015, p. 1622).

- In the liver, conjugation of bilirubin occurs by another enzyme, *uridine diphosphate glucuronosyl transferase* (UGT-1A1) which leads to the formation of water-soluble compounds called bilirubin glucuronides (Kamath-Rayne et al., 2016, p. 512; Kaplan et al., 2015, p. 1622; Maisels & Watchko, 2018, 2013, p. 312).

EXCRETION OF BILIRUBIN
- Conjugated bilirubin can now be actively secreted in the bile and into the small intestine (Kamath-Rayne et al., 2016, p. 512; Maisels & Watchko, 2018, 2013, p. 312).

ENTEROHEPATIC ABSORPTION OF BILIRUBIN
- Enterohepatic circulation is the reabsorption and recycling of the unconjugated form of bilirubin back into the circulation (Kamath-Rayne et al., 2016, p. 512).
- Enterohepatic reabsorption of bilirubin that is excreted into the intestine is enhanced in infants. This increases their risk for hyperbilirubinemia (Watchko, 2018, p. 1204).
- Conjugated bilirubin can be spontaneously or enzymatically converted back to unconjugated bilirubin. Typically, the more unstable forms of conjugated bilirubin are reverted back to unconjugated bilirubin, such as the mono- and diglucuronides of bilirubin (Kaplan et al., 2015, p. 1623; Watchko, 2018, p. 1204).
- Reverted unconjugated bilirubin can now readily cross the intestinal mucosa and contribute to the circulating pool of unconjugated bilirubin through the enterohepatic circulation (Kaplan et al., 2015, p. 1623; Watchko, 2018, p. 1204).
- Additional factors that play a role in enterohepatic circulation include a mildly alkaline pH of the duodenum and jejunum and a lack of intestinal flora, the latter which reduces bilirubin to urobilinogen. High concentrations of bilirubin are also found in meconium (Kaplan et al., 2015, p. 1623; Watchko, 2018, p. 1204).

Factors That Affect Bilirubin Levels

- Delayed passage of meconium—Meconium contains a substantial amount of bilirubin (Kamath-Rayne et al., 2016, p. 517).
- A reduction in UGT activity
- Albumin levels—An increase in the amount of albumin limits the amount of unbound, unconjugated bilirubin that is available to cross the blood–brain barrier to cause neuronal damage (Kamath-Rayne et al., 2016, p. 512).
- Decreased life span of the RBC—The life span of the RBC is shorter at 70 to 90 days in newborns (Kamath-Rayne et al., 2016, p. 511).
- An accelerated breakdown of RBCs produces more bilirubin production in newborns (Kamath-Rayne et al., 2016, p. 511).
- Diminished hepatic uptake of bilirubin—may be related to inadequate perfusion of the sinusoids in the liver or a deficiency of the carrier proteins Y and Z (Kamath-Rayne et al., 2016, p. 517).

Unconjugated (Indirect) Nonpathologic "Physiologic" Hyperbilirubinemia

DEFINITION AND PATHOPHYSIOLOGY
- Bilirubin is a weak acid that is not water-soluble or easily excreted from the body. In order to be excreted from

the body it must be conjugated to glucuronic acid (Kaplan et al., 2015, p. 1618).

- A majority of fetal bilirubin is in the unconjugated form, which can be found in amniotic fluid as early as 12 weeks' gestation. The fetus begins producing bile acids and pigments early in pregnancy, a majority of which is biliverdin and bilirubin (Blackburn, 2013c, p. 608).
  - Bilirubin levels in the amniotic fluid usually rise followed by a plateau between 16 and 25 weeks before decreasing and disappearing by 36 weeks' gestation (Blackburn, 2013c, p. 610).
- Bile acids and bilirubin levels are low in the fetus related to enzymes and transport systems that encourage the removal of these potentially harmful substances (Blackburn, 2013c, p. 610).
  - Bilirubin in the unconjugated state occurs for many reasons, including liver and intestinal immaturity. The ductus venous also shunts some placental blood away from the liver, thereby decreasing blood flow to this organ. Additionally, bilirubin is recirculated by the enterohepatic shunt. All of these processes allow bilirubin to remain in the unconjugated form (Blackburn, 2013c, p. 608).
- There is evidence to suggest that bilirubin may not only be toxic but beneficial as well in infants. Unconjugated bilirubin has the ability to diffuse into any cell and might be helpful in times of stress, and at lower levels bilirubin acts as an antioxidant. As an antioxidant, bilirubin limits cellular damage by binding to the membrane to prevent peroxidation and scavenging of reactive oxygen species (Blackburn, 2013c, p. 610; Kaplan et al., 2015, p. 1620).
- Unconjugated hyperbilirubinemia is the most common condition in the neonatal period that requires evaluation and treatment; however, for a majority of newborns it is a benign condition without clinical significance (Blackburn, 2013c, p. 611; Kamath-Rayne et al., 2016, p. 511; Watchko, 2018, p. 1198).
  - It is the most common reason for readmission to the hospital during the first week of life (Blackburn, 2013c, p. 611; Kamath-Rayne et al., 2016, p. 511; Watchko, 2018, p. 1198).
- There is no consistent definition for hyperbilirubinemia of the neonate (Blackburn, 2013c, p. 614). Jaundice is a self-limiting process with bilirubin levels typically returning to normal, defined as less than 1 mg/dL by 12 days of life (Dragoo, 2017, p. 255).
- Physiologic jaundice occurs in approximately 85% of infants during the first several days after delivery. Almost all term infants will have a bilirubin level greater than 2 mg/dL during the first week of life (Blackburn, 2013c, p. 593). Approximately 60% to 80% of normal newborns will appear jaundiced during the first week of life (Kamath-Rayne et al., 2016, p. 511).
  - In a minority of healthy infants, approximately 6%, bilirubin levels increase to 12 mg/dL while about 3% of healthy newborns will have bilirubin levels that exceed 15 mg/dL (Dragoo, 2017, p. 255).
- Occurs in term infants and is characterized by progressive increase in total bilirubin concentration and peaks between 3 and 4 days of life in White and African American infants. This is followed by a rapid decline in bilirubin levels to approximately 3 mg/dL by the fifth day of life in White and African American infants and by the seventh day on Asian American infants (Kamath-Rayne et al., 2016, p. 514; Kaplan et al., p. 1626).

- Physiologic jaundice in premature infants tends to be more severe when compared to term neonates with peak total bilirubin concentrations in larger preterm newborn that may reach 10 to 12 mg/dL by the fifth day of life (Kaplan et al., 2015, p. 1627).

RISK FACTORS

- Some infants are at greater risk for hyperbilirubinemia when compared to other neonates. Risk factors for hyperbilirubinemia can be divided into three categories, and are listed in Box 21.2. Highlights of these risks include:
  - Previous sibling with jaundice treated with phototherapy
  - Late-preterm gestation
  - Exclusive breast milk feeding
  - African American ethnicity
  - East Asian ethnicity
  - Jaundice within the first 24 hours of life
  - Intracranial hemorrhage or other trauma (Kaplan et al., 2015, p. 1628; Watchko, 2018, p. 1206)

BOX 21.2 **Risk factors for hyperbilirubinemia in the newborn**

Risk Factors for Hyperbilirubinemia in Newborns
Major risk factors
- A serum or transcutaneous bilirubin level in the high-risk zone prior to discharge
- Jaundice observed within the first 24 hours of life
- Blood group incompatibility with positive direct antiglobulin test, other known hemolytic disease (such as G6PD deficiency)
- Late preterm infant of 35 to 36 weeks' gestation
- Previous sibling who received phototherapy
- Cephalohematoma or significant bruising
- Exclusive breastfeeding, especially if breastfeeding is not going well and weight loss is excessive
- East Asian race

Minor risk factors
- A serum or transcutaneous bilirubin level in the high intermediate risk zone prior to discharge
- Gestational age of 37 to 38 weeks
- Jaundice observed prior to discharge
- Previous sibling who received phototherapy
- Macrosomic infant of a diabetic mother
- Maternal age greater than 25 years
- Male gender

Decreased risk
- A serum or transcutaneous bilirubin level in the low-risk zone prior to discharge
- Gestational age greater than 41 weeks
- Exclusive breastfeeding
- African American race
- Discharge after 72 hours of age

Source: Data from Kamath-Rayne, B., Thilo, E., Deacon, J., & Hernandez, J. (2016). Neonatal hyerbilirubemia. In S. Gardner, B. Carter, M. Hines, & J. Hernandez (Eds.), *Merenstein & Gardner's handbook of neonatal intensive care* (8th ed., pp. 511–536). St. Louis, MO: Elsevier.)

Clinical Presentation

VISUAL INSPECTION

- When serum bilirubin levels are elevated, jaundice becomes visible in the skin (Watchko, 2018, p. 1208). Jaundice does not become visible in infants until levels exceed 5.0 to 7.0 mg/dL (Dragoo, 2017, p. 263; Kaplan et al., 2015, p. 1625; Watchko, 2018, p. 1208).
- Visual inspection for jaundice should be performed in a well-lit room with natural lighting or daylight at least every 8 hours when hyperbilirubinemia is suspected.
- Jaundice initially becomes apparent on the face and progresses in a cephalocaudal fashion; therefore, assessment for jaundice includes blanching the skin with pressure using the fingers on the forehead, sternum, or knee to reveal the underlying color or tone (Dragoo, 2017, p. 263; Watchko, 2018, p. 1208).
  - ○ Inspecting the skin of the infant is helpful in identifying jaundice, but is not an accurate method to determine bilirubin levels. Because accuracy of identifying jaundice varies with clinician experience and neonatal skin differences, it is very important to obtain bilirubin levels for all newborns who appear jaundiced with either a serum or transcutaneous bilirubin measurement (Dragoo, 2017, p. 263; Watchko, 2018, p. 1208).

BILIRUBIN MEASUREMENT

- Bilirubin levels can be measured within the blood sera or through the skin using a transcutaneous device.
  - ○ Serum measurement is most commonly obtained from heel puncture. This is the most accurate method to determine a bilirubin level, but is also the most painful as obtaining the blood sample is painful for the infant. The total serum bilirubin is the most recommended method on which to make clinical decisions (Dragoo, 2017, p. 263; Kamath-Rayne et al., 2016, p. 524).
  - ○ Transcutaneous bilirubinometry (TcB) is a noninvasive method that uses reflectance photometry or transcutaneous colorimetry as a way to estimate the bilirubin level.. Several studies have demonstrated that using a handheld TcB device can accurately determine TSB levels in term and late–preterm infants of different ethnic groups to within 2 to 3 mg/dL when the TSB is less than 15 mg/dL.
    - One limitation of using the TcB device is that it often underestimates the bilirubin level when total serum levels are greater than 15 mg/dL. The recommendation is that all bilirubin levels greater than 15 and above the 75th percentile be confirmed with serum bilirubin levels (Dragoo, 2017, p. 263; Kaplan et al., 2015, p. 1646).
- All bilirubin level concentrations must be interpreted based on the infant's age in hours. Using the nomogram developed by Bhutani and colleagues for infants greater than 35 weeks' gestation, the newborn's TSB should be plotted and interpreted based on age in hours to determine the risk for hyperbilirubinemia and need for additional testing. Once plotted, the nomogram suggests whether the infant is at high, intermediate, or low risk for requiring further intervention for hyperbilirubinemia, based on total serum bilirubin concentration (Dragoo, 2017, p. 264; Kamath-Rayne et al., 2016, p. 521; Maisels & Watchko, 2018, 2013, p. 329).

Management

PHOTOTHERAPY

- Phototherapy was initially introduced in 1958. It is the most common and effective form of therapy to treat unconjugated hyperbilirubinemia. Phototherapy is the mainstay of treatment for indirect hyperbilirubinemia (Blackburn, 2013c, p. 618; Kamath-Rayne, Thilo, Deacon, & Hernandez, 2016, p. 525; Kaplan et al., 2015, p. 1647).
- The use of phototherapy reduces the rise of the total bilirubin concentration, regardless of gestational age, the presence or absence of hemolysis and the degree of skin pigmentation (Kaplan et al., 2015, p. 1647).
- The widespread use of phototherapy to treat hyperbilirubinemia has greatly reduced the need for exchange transfusions in infants. Additionally, the incidence of kernicterus and long-term neurobehavioral performance in children is greatly decreased in infants treated with phototherapy. There has been no documentation of adverse long-term outcomes in infants who received phototherapy in the neonatal period (Kaplan et al., 2015, p. 1647; Merenstein & Gardner, 2016, p. 525).

MECHANISM OF ACTION

- Phototherapy works by creating a photochemical reaction that transforms the unconjugated bilirubin in the capillaries and interstitial spaces of the skin and subcutaneous tissue into photoisomers that can be excreted from the body in the bile and urine without conjugation (Blackburn, 2013c, p. 618; Merenstein & Gardner, p. 526; Dragoo, 2017, p. 265).
- During phototherapy, bilirubin absorbs the light so that photochemical reactions occur. These photochemical reactions, photoisomerization and photooxidization, facilitate changing the structure and shape of bilirubin and converting it to photoproducts that can be excreted from the body in bile and urine without conjugation (Blackburn, 2013c, p. 600; Maisels & Watchko, 2013, p. 337; Merenstein & Gardner, p. 526).
  - ○ Photoisomerization, which is responsible for more than 80% of the bilirubin that is eliminated with the use of phototherapy, converts indirect bilirubin that is poorly soluble into a water-soluble reversible configurational or an irreversible structural photoisomer. The photoisomers can then be excreted into the bile without conjugation (Blackburn, 2013c, p. 600; Kaplan et al., 2015, p. 1648).
- Lumirubin is the major pathway through which bilirubin is eliminated with phototherapy use. It is a stable, nonreversible structural photoisomer that does not require conjugation and is formed slowly but is excreted very rapidly in both bile and to a lesser extent in urine with a serum half-life of 2 hours.
  - ○ The production of lumirubin is dose dependent with the amount of irradiance (Blackburn, 2013c, p. 600; Kaplan et al., 2015, pp. 1648–1649; Merenstein & Gardner, p. 527).
  - ○ The photoisomers are unlikely to cross the blood–brain barrier because they are polar and need transporters in order to reach neurons. For this reason, they do not enter the brain to cause kernicterus (Blackburn, 2013c, p. 600).
- The breakdown of bilirubin in the presence of phototherapy occurs primarily in the superficial capillaries and in the

intestinal spaces (Blackburn, 2013c, p. 600). Configurational isomers are formed very rapidly but are excreted very slowly in bile. They have a serum half-life of 12 to 21 hours. After 6 to 12 hours of phototherapy, approximately 20% of the total serum bilirubin has been converted to configurational isomers. Because these isomers are unstable and the process reversible, they may be reverted back to unconjugated bilirubin in the intestines and recirculated by way of enterohepatic shunting (Blackburn, 2013c, p. 600; Kaplan et al., 2015, p. 1648; Merenstein & Gardner, p. 526).

TYPES OF PHOTOTHERAPY

- Special blue fluorescent lights are the most effective available for phototherapy because they deliver light in the blue–green spectrum and have more irradiance at 450 nm. They provide maximal absorption and adequate skin penetration (Blackburn, 2013c, p. 621; Kaplan et al., 2015, p. 1649).
  - There are many types of fluorescent lights, including daylight, white, and blue lamps. Although widely used, these types of lights are less effective than special blue fluorescent tubes, which provide significantly more irradiance in the blue spectrum.
  - High-pressure mercury vapor halide lamps provide adequate output in the blue range, but they cannot be brought close to the infant to increase the irradiance without risk of thermal injury. Additionally, the amount of surface covered by many halogen lamps is small with a reduced spectral power (Klaus & Fanaroff, p. 338).
- Fiberoptic blankets use a tungsten–halogen lamp as the light source for use as a spotlight. This type of system is a convenient way of delivering phototherapy above and below the infant simultaneously. They generate little heat and provide higher irradiance when compared to fluorescent lights. Because they are small, they cover only a small surface area, which significantly reduces the achieved spectral power. For this reason, they are rarely effective when used alone in term infants (Klaus & Fanaroff, p. 339).
- Another method of delivering phototherapy is with the use of blue light-emitting diodes (LEDs), which allows a higher level of irradiance to be delivered to the infant with minimal generation of heat. An LED unit is a low weight, low-voltage, low-power device that has shown to be an effective and safe alternative to other modes of phototherapy. They are available as either overhead or underneath device (Kaplan et al., 2015, p. 1651; Klaus & Fanaroff, p. 339).

INDICATIONS FOR PHOTOTHERAPY

- The AAP issued comprehensive guidelines for the initiation of phototherapy in infants 35 weeks or greater. The guidelines are based on limited evidence and the levels for initiation of treatment are estimates.
  - Additional online applications, such as the BiliTool, has been endorsed and recommended by the AAP to aid in the decision-making process regarding the treatment of jaundice in infants (Kaplan et al., 2015, pp. 1651–1652; Snell & Gardner, p. 265).
- There is no single serum bilirubin level at which phototherapy should be initiated. Instead, each infant needs to be evaluated individually with consideration to the bilirubin level and the infant's level of risk for hyperbilirubinemia (Kaplan et al., 2015, pp. 1651–1652; Snell & Gardner, 2016, p. 265).

- When discontinuing phototherapy, the level must be considered in combination with the overall clinical presentation and risk factors of the infant. A rebound bilirubin level should be obtained for at least 24 hours in infants less than 37 weeks, have a positive DAT and those treated at or before 72 hours of age. A rebound total serum bilirubin level of 1 to 2 mg/dl or more can occur after phototherapy has been discontinued (Kaplan et al., 2015, p. 1652; Snell & Gardner, p. 266; Merenstein & Gardner, p. 530).
- The guidelines by the AAP do not apply to premature infants born less than 35 weeks' gestation.

FACTORS THAT IMPACT THE EFFICACY OF PHOTOTHERAPY

- There are many factors that influence the efficacy of phototherapy, including variations among light sources, the spectrum of light that is delivered, the intensity of the energy output or irradiance, peak wavelength of the light that is delivered, the surface area of exposed skin to the light, and the transmission of the light through the infant's skin (Blackburn, 2013c, p. 619).

BODY SURFACE AREA

- The amount of body surface exposed to phototherapy light also determines effectiveness of therapy. Under ideal circumstances, the infant should be naked when under phototherapy. However, a diaper is often in place and folded back to expose as much surface area as possible (Kaplan et al., 2015, p. 1650).
- The use of several phototherapy lamps positioned around the infant or a combination of a phototherapy mattress with overhead lights can increase the intensity and effectiveness of therapy (Blackburn, 2013c, p. 618; Kaplan et al., 2015, p. 1650).
- Using a reflective surface, such as a white sheet, around the incubator or open crib can encourage more light to be transmitted to the skin, especially onto relatively underexposed areas, thus increasing the light irradiance (Blackburn, 2013c, p. 618; Kaplan et al., 2015, p. 1650).

COMPLICATIONS

- Although complications associated with the use of phototherapy are rare, several may occur. There have been no studies suggesting that there is an increase in mortality or morbidity with the use of phototherapy (Kaplan et al., 2015, pp. 1653–1654). Some complications may include the following:
  - Intestinal hypermotility—Stools may be more loose and diarrhea-looking in appearance. Infants may more frequent stools (Kaplan et al., 2015, p. 1653; Snell & Gardner, p. 267).
  - Temperature instability—Phototherapy may potentially cause an increase in body and environmental temperature.
  - Increased insensible water losses—With the use of phototherapy, increased insensible and intestinal water losses can occur and need to be taken into consideration with fluid management. The overall fluid intake may need to be increased by as much as 25% above the estimated fluid needs without phototherapy. The use of fiberoptic phototherapy seems to result in insensible water losses that are lower and therefore less need for an increase in the maintenance fluids (Blackburn, 2013c, p. 601; Kaplan et al., 2015, p. 1653; Snell & Gardner, p. 267).

○ Retinal degeneration—This condition can occur after several days using phototherapy. For this reason, the eyes must be covered with adequate layers to protect against the possibility of damage. The use of fiberoptic phototherapy does not eliminate the need to protect the infant's eyes (Kaplan et al., 2015, p. 1653).

○ Bronze baby syndrome—Bronze baby syndrome is characterized by a brown–black (bronze) color appearance of the serum, urine, and skin that appears several hours or more after initiation of phototherapy lights, especially if the serum conjugated bilirubin is elevated. A majority of reported infants with this condition have recovered without sequelae (Blackburn, 2013c, p. 602; Kaplan et al., 2015, p. 1653).

○ Psychobehavioral issues—include a lack of sensory experiences, behavioral and activity changes, and alterations in state organization and biologic rhythms. Parenteral stress has also been documented with the use of phototherapy. Maternal separation with the potential for interference with parental bonding may occur (Blackburn, 2013c, p. 618; Snell & Gardner, p. 267).

BREASTMILK JAUNDICE

Definition and Pathophysiology

- Breastmilk jaundice differs from physiologic jaundice because in the former, bilirubin levels begin to rise during the second week of life when physiological jaundice is beginning to improve (Dragoo, 2017, p. 262).
- Breastmilk jaundice is often a benign condition that occurs during the first weeks of life in newborns receiving mother's own milk (MOM). These infants have exaggerated unconjugated bilirubin levels that can persist through the end of the first week of life. They are three times more likely to have a TSB level greater than 12 mg/dL, with levels reaching as high as 25 to 30 mg/dL (Dragoo, 2017, p. 262).
  - ○ Breastmilk jaundice typically may be prolonged, occurring after the first 3 to 5 days of life and persisting into the third week of life or beyond. Peak bilirubin levels tend to occur at 4 weeks of life and last up to 12 weeks of age (Dragoo, 2017, p. 262; Kamath-Rayne et al., 2016, p. 519; Kaplan et al., 2015, p. 1637).
- Infants with breastmilk jaundice are well appearing. They appear healthy with normal weight gain, stooling patterns, and urine output. The physical examination on these infants is normal. There is no evidence of hemolysis in infants with breastfeeding-associated jaundice (Kamath-Rayne et al., 2016, p. 519; Kaplan et al., 2015, p. 1637).
- Breastmilk jaundice typically resolves without the need for intervention (Kamath-Rayne et al., 2016, p. 519).

PHASES OF BREASTMILK JAUNDICE

- Breastmilk jaundice can occur in two forms or phases. Breastfeeding-associated jaundice that occurs early is the more common form, while late breastmilk jaundice is less prevalent. These phases can overlap and may not be distinguishable from one another (Blackburn, 2013c, p. 615l; Kaplan et al., 2015, p. 1637).

PHASE ONE

- The phase historically associated with breastfeeding-associated jaundice. A major factor that increases the risk for breastfeeding-associated jaundice is increased enterohepatic shunting. Increased enterohepatic shunting occurs in infants exclusively breastfeeding because these infants have a reduced fluid and caloric intake and less frequent feedings and stooling patterns. In the presence of decreased caloric intake, there is an increase in the breakdown of fat, which is needed for energy (Blackburn, 2013c, p. 615).
  - ○ Additionally, infants who are fed breastmilk produce lower weight stools and their stool output is initially lower when compared to newborns fed formula. The stools of breast-fed infants contain less bilirubin than formula-fed neonates This occurs because more conjugated direct bilirubin is switched back to indirect bilirubin by β-glucuronidase, which has a greater affinity in breast fed infants (Blackburn, 2013c, p. 615).

PHASE TWO

- Breastmilk jaundice that occurs during phase two occurs later and is characterized by increasing bilirubin levels after 3 to 5 days of life with peak levels of 5 to 10 mg/dL by 2 weeks of life. These levels eventually decrease to more normal levels over the next 3 to 12 weeks of life (Blackburn, 2013c, p. 615; Kaplan et al., 2015, p. 1637).
  - ○ This phase of jaundice is thought to be related to the properties of breast milk that interferes with normal conjugation and excretion (Blackburn, 2013c, p. 615; Kaplan et al., 2015, p. 1637).

Risk Factors

- Decreased fluid and/or poor caloric intake due to delay in lactation or lactation failure)
- Large amount of weight loss. Infants who lose more than 7% of their birth weight are at greater risk for significant dehydration and subsequent jaundice.
- Delayed passage of meconium
- The type of number of bacteria in the intestine of breastfed infants
- Breastfeeding failure jaundice—the intricates of breastfeeding (poor technique, cracked nipples, fatigue) may be difficult, especially with first-time mothers (Dragoo, 2017, p. 262; Watchko, 2018, p. 1206).

Clinical Presentation

- Usually, other than jaundice, the neonates appear healthy, and no abnormal findings are noted (Kaplan et al., 2015, p. 1638).

Management

- Jaundice occurring in breastfed infants can be minimized by preventive measures. Frequent feeding with breastmilk, as often as eight or nine times within a 24-hour period during the first 3 days of life, is encouraged. Frequent feeding stimulates intestinal activity and the passage of meconium, allowing for less availability of bilirubin for enzymes to convert back to the indirect form. It also reduces the risk of enterohepatic shunting and facilities stimulation of breastmilk production. Continued and frequent breastmilk feedings also increase intestinal motility and can act as a laxative to encourage the passage of meconium. This removes conjugated bilirubin from the small intestinal, thereby decreasing the tendency that this bilirubin will be deconjugated and recirculated by the enterohepatic shunt (Blackburn, 2013c, p. 616; Stark & Bhutani, 2017, p. 340).

- Replacing breastmilk with formula may be warranted at a bilirubin level greater than 25 mg/dL even while undergoing intensive phototherapy. Also consider formula if the infant's weight loss from birth is greater than 12% or if there is clinical evidence of dehydration (Blackburn, 2013c, p. 616).
  - If interruption of breastfeeding is indicated, emotional support should be provided to the mother. The mother should also be provided with a breast pump to allow expression of breast milk (Blackburn, 2013c, p. 616; Stark & Bhutani, 2017, p. 340).

Outcomes

- Although not recommended unless hyperbilirubinemia levels reach levels that might be of danger to the infant, interruption of nursing and substitution with formula feeding for 1 to 3 days usually causes a prompt decline of the bilirubin level to about half or less of the original level. On resumption of nursing, the bilirubin level does not usually increase substantially (Kaplan et al., 2015, p. 1638).

KERNICTERUS

Definition and Pathophysiology

- The term kernicterus is derived from bilirubin staining of the "kern" or nuclear region of the brain. Kernicterus is an irreversible condition causing devastating injury to the brain. Also known as chronic bilirubin encephalopathy (CBE); (Watchko, 2018, p. 1208).
- CBE defines the permanent clinical sequelae of bilirubin toxicity that become evident in the first year of life. Sequelae are distinguished by remarkably selective involvement of the globus pallidus, subthalamic nucleus, sectors of the hippocampus, the reticular portion of the substantia nigra, the red nuclei, dentate nuclei and Purkinje cells of the cerebellum, and select brainstem nuclei (Watchko, 2018, p. 1209).
- The blood–brain barrier is normally intact and with tight junctions between the endothelial cells of the cerebral blood vessels. These junctions are permeable to lipid-soluble substances and impermeable to water-soluble substances, proteins, and other large molecules.
  - Unconjugated bilirubin is fat-soluble. Under normal conditions, the blood–brain barrier is impermeable to bilirubin that is bound to albumin. However, when this barrier becomes damaged, reversible alterations or "openings" occur, which allows the entry of albumin-bound bilirubin into the brain. There may also be an increased movement of unbound bilirubin across a blood–brain barrier that is damaged (Blackburn, 2013c, p. 622; Kamath-Rayne et al., 2016, p. 328; Kaplan et al., 2015, p. 1640).
- It not exactly known how bilirubin exerts its toxic effects in the brain. It is thought that bilirubin enters the brain through several different mechanisms.
  - Bilirubin can enter the brain when there is a significant increase in the amount of unbound bilirubin in the bloodstream. In the presence of an increased amount of unbound bilirubin, the normal buffering capacity of the blood and tissues becomes overwhelmed and bilirubin enters the brain.
  - Alterations in the bilirubin-binding capacity of albumin and other proteins can lead to increased levels of unconjugated bilirubin the blood stream. Even when bound to albumin, bilirubin can enter the brain when the blood–brain barrier is disrupted. Disruption of the blood–brain barrier increases permeability of the central nervous system to bilirubin (Blackburn, 2013c, p. 622; Kamath-Rayne et al., 2016, p. 328; Kaplan et al., 2015, p. 1640).
- Conditions that can potentially damage the blood–brain barrier include infection, dehydration, severe respiratory acidosis, hypoxemia, or other injury (Blackburn, 2013c, p. 622). Additionally, ability of bilirubin to bind to albumin is decreased in sick term and preterm infants and the serum albumin concentration lower in this population. These factors can increase the risk for kernicterus at lower serum bilirubin levels in the sick term or preterm infant when compared to the term newborn (Kaplan et al., 2015, p. 1642).
- Other areas of the brain at risk for bilirubin toxicity include the hippocampal cortex, subthalamic nuclei, and cerebellum. The cerebral cortex is generally spared and not affected by elevated levels of unconjugated bilirubin (Blackburn, 2013c, p. 622; Kaplan et al., 2015, p. 1640).
- The incidence of kernicterus varies among countries as well as between industrialized countries and those with developing medical systems. It is estimated that kernicterus occurs between 0.4 and 2 per 100,000 children (Kaplan et al., 2015, p. 1639). CBE as a consequence for infants born in developing countries is a serious *endemic* problem; for example, in Nigeria approximately 3% of neonatal hospital admissions evidence bilirubin encephalopathy (Watchko, 2018, p. 1209)

Risk Factors

- A diagnosis of kernicterus tends to occur more often in infants born term or late preterm (Blackburn, 2013c, p. 604). The most important determinants of brain injury caused by hyperbilirubinemia are the concentration of unconjugated bilirubin and free (unbound) bilirubin (Kamath-Rayne et al., 2016, p. 520).
- Although rare in preterm infants, it can occur in this population because of an immature central nervous system and clinical conditions that potentiate bilirubin neurotoxicity (Blackburn, 2013c, p. 604).
- Additional risk factors for kernicterus, especially at lower bilirubin levels, include prematurity, respiratory distress syndrome, G6PD deficiency, hypoxia, asphyxia, hypercapnia, and acidosis (Blackburn, 2013c, p. 622).

Clinical Manifestations

- Symptoms of bilirubin toxicity do not become clinically apparent until serum bilirubin levels are elevated for several hours. The infant passes through several stages of bilirubin encephalopathy, characterized by abnormal clinical symptoms that are progressive in severity.

○ The initial phase of acute bilirubin encephalopathy, which is reversible in its early stages, is characterized by symptoms of poor sucking, progressive lethargy, vomiting, temperature instability, and hypotonia.

○ If left untreated, pathology advances to the intermediate stage. Infants may demonstrate alternating hypotonia and hypertonia of the extensor muscles and a high-pitched cry. Hypertonia is characterized by backward arching of the neck (retrocollis) and a high-pitched cry.

○ Symptoms of advanced kernicterus include ataxia, opisthotonos, choreoathetoid movements (rapid, highly complex, involuntary, spasmodic movements), extrapyramidal disturbances, auditory abnormalities with sensorineural hearing loss, and oculomotor paresis. At this stage, permanent damage to the brain has occurred (Blackburn, 2013c, p. 604; Kaplan et al., 2015, p. 1640; Watchko, 2018, p. 1209).

OUTCOMES

- The central nervous system sequelae reflect the regional topography of bilirubin-induced neuronal damage. These include the extrapyramidal movement disorders of dystonia and/or choreoathetosis, hearing loss caused by auditory neuropathy spectrum disorders, and the eye movement abnormality of paresis of upward gaze (Watchko, 2018, p. 1209).

- Although there is overwhelming evidence to suggest that infants with advanced clinical manifestations of CBE have permanent central nervous damage, recent studies have challenged this notion. There are a few reports in the literature that some infants who present with advanced symptoms of CBE may have no neurologic sequelae if treated aggressively (Watchko, 2018, p. 1210).

CONCLUSION

An understanding of the neonatal hematopoietic system and process of erythropoiesis is important to the evaluation of and decision for intervention in the neonate. The role and importance of red cells, platelets, and coagulation factors cannot be overstated, and the NNP must recognize the pathophysiology involved in order to intervene appropriately. Recognition and appropriate management of infants at risk for hyperbilirubinemia will prevent long-term sequalae. Overall the hematologic system is vital to the continued healthy growth and development of the neonate.

REVIEW QUESTIONS

1. The process which is responsible for the formation, production, and maintenance of pluripotent stem cells as they delineate into segregated blood cells is:
   A. erythropoiesis
   B. hematopoiesis
   C. monopoiesis

2. When assessing a neonate with polycythemia, the NNP understands that the infant will also:
   A. be at high risk for hyperviscosity
   B. have confirmed hyperviscosity
   C. require treatment of hyperviscosity

3. In order to effectively remove bilirubin from the body's system, an enzyme is necessary to covert the heme from red blood cells into:
   A. biliflavo
   B. bilipurpura
   C. biliverdin

4. The NNP correctly interprets a positive, indirect Coombs test to mean a maternal antibody is found in the infant's:
   A. blood sera
   B. progenitor cells
   C. red blood cells

5. Prior to beginning phototherapy, the NNP considers an infant's individual:
   A. current bilirubin level and the level of risk
   B. blood type compared to the mother's type
   C. hours of age and anticipated rate of rise

REFERENCES

Assali, N. S. (1972). *Pathophysiology of gestation.* New York, NY: Academic Press.

Blackburn, S. (2013a). Hematologic and hemostatic systems. In S. Blackburn (Ed.), *Maternal, fetal, & neonatal physiology: A clinical perspective* (4th ed., pp. 216–251). Maryland Heights, MO: Elsevier.

Blackburn, S. (2013b). Immune system and host defense mechanisms. In S. Blackburn (Ed.), *Maternal, fetal, & neonatal physiology: A clinical perspective* (4th ed., pp. 443–483). Maryland Heights, MO: Elsevier.

Blackburn, S. (2013c). Bilirubin metabolism. In S. Blackburn (Ed.), *Maternal, fetal, & neonatal physiology: A clinical perspective* (4th ed., pp. 607–626). Maryland Heights, MO: Elsevier.

Christensen, R. (2018). Neonatal erythrocyte disorders. In C. Gleason & S. Juul (Eds.), *Avery's diseases of the newborn* (10th ed., pp. 1152–1179). Philadelphia, PA: Elsevier.

Croteau, S. (2017). Bleeding. In E. Eichenwald, A. Hansen, C. Martin, & A. Stark (Eds.), *Cloherty and Stark's manual of neonatal care* (8th ed., pp. 586–594). Philadelphia, PA: Wolters Kluwer.

Deschmann, E., Saxonhouse, M., & Sola-Visner, M. (2017). Thrombocytopenia. In E. Eichenwald, A. Hansen, C. Martin, & A. Stark (Eds.), *Cloherty and Stark's manual of neonatal care* (8th ed., pp. 630–640). Philadelphia, PA: Wolters Kluwer.

Deschmann, E., & Sola-Visner, M. (2018). Neonatal platelet disorders. In C. Gleason & S. Juul (Eds.), *Avery's diseases of the newborn* (10th ed., pp. 1139–1151). Philadelphia, PA: Elsevier.

Diab, Y., & Luchtman-Jones. (2015). Hematologic and oncologic problems in the fetus and neonate. In R. Martin, A. Fanaroff, & M. Walsh (Eds.), *Fanaroff and Martin's neonatal-perinatal medicine: Diseases of the fetus and infant* (10th ed., pp. 1294–1343). Philadelphia, PA: Elsevier.

Diehl-Jones, W., & Fraser, D. (2015). Hematologic disorders. In T. Verklan & M. Walden (Eds.), *Core curriculum for neonatal intensive care nursing* (5th ed., pp. 662–686). St. Louis, MO: Elsevier.

Dragoo, S. (2017). Hyperbilirubinemia of the newborn born after 35 weeks' gestation. In B. J. Snell & S. Gardner (Eds.), *Care of the well newborn* (pp. 253–271). Burlington, MA: Jones & Barlett.

Fasano, R., Said, M., & Luban, N. (2015). Blood component therapy in martin. In R. Fanaroff & M. Walsh (Eds.), *Fanaroff and Martin's neonatal-perinatal medicine: Diseases of the fetus and infant* (10th ed., pp. 1344–1361). Philadelphia, PA: Elsevier.

Juul, S., & Christensen, R. (2018). Developmental hematology. In C. Gleason & S. Juul (Eds.), *Avery's diseases of the newborn* (10th ed., pp. 1113–1120). Philadelphia, PA: Elsevier.

Kamath-Rayne, B., Thilo, E., Deacon, J., & Hernandez, J. (2016). Neonatal hyperbilirubinemia. In S. Gardner, B. Carter, M. Hines, & J. Hernandez (Eds.), *Merenstein & Gardner's handbook of neonatal intensive care* (8th ed., pp. 511–536). St. Louis, MO: Elsevier.

Kaplan, M., Wong, R., Sibley, E., & Stevenson, D. (2015). Neonatal jaundice and liver disease. In R. Martin, A. Fanaroff, & M. Walsh (Eds.), *Fanaroff and Martin's neonatal-perinatal medicine: Diseases of the fetus and infant* (10th ed., pp. 1618–1673). Philadelphia, PA: Elsevier.

Lane, E., Chisholm, K., & Murray, K. (2018). Disorders of the liver. In C. Gleason & S. Juul (Eds.), *Avery's diseases of the newborn* (10th ed., pp. 1098–1112.e1). Philadelphia, PA: Elsevier.

Letterio, J., Ahuja, S., & Petrosiute, A. (2013). Hematologic problems. In A. Fanaroff & J. Fanaroff (Eds.), *Klaus and Fanroff's care of the high-risk neonate* (6th ed., pp. 432–475). Cleveland, OH: Elsevier.

Maisels, J., & Watchko, J. (2013). Neonatal hyperbilirubinemia. In A. Fanaroff & J. Fanaroff (Eds.), *Klaus and Fanroff's care of the high-risk neonate* (6th ed., pp. 310–344). Cleveland, OH: Elsevier.

Manco-Johnson, M., McKinney, C., Knapp-Clevenger, R., & Hernandez, J. (2016). Neonatal hyperbilirubinemia. In S. Gardner, B. Carter, M. Hines, & J. Hernandez (Eds.), *Merenstein & Gardner's handbook of neonatal intensive care* (8th ed., pp. 470–510). St. Louis, MO: Elsevier.

O'Reilly, D. (2017). Polycythemia. In E. Eichenwald, A. Hansen, C. Martin, & A. Stark (Eds.), *Cloherty and Stark's manual of neonatal care* (8th ed., pp. 624–629). Philadelphia, PA: Wolters Kluwer.

Patel, R., & Josephson, C. (2018). Neonatal transfusion. In C. Gleason & S. Juul (Eds.), *Avery's diseases of the newborn* (10th ed., pp. 1180–1186.e3). Philadelphia, PA: Elsevier.

Saxonhouse, M. (2018). Neonatal bleeding and thrombotic disorders. In C. Gleason & S. Juul (Eds.), *Avery's diseases of the newborn* (10th ed., pp. 1121–1138.e4). Philadelphia, PA: Elsevier.

Sloan, S. (2017). Blood products used in the newborn. In E. Eichenwald, A. Hansen, C. Martin, & A. Stark (Eds.), *Cloherty and Stark's manual of neonatal care* (8th ed., pp. 576–585). Philadelphia, PA: Wolters Kluwer.

Stark, A., & Bhutani, V. (2017). Neonatal hyperbilirubinemia. In E. Eichenwald, A. Hansen, C. Martin, & A. Stark (Eds.), *Cloherty and Stark's manual of neonatal care* (8th ed., pp. 335–352). Philadelphia, PA: Wolters Kluwer.

Watchko, J. (2018). Neonatal indirect hyperbilirubinemia and kernicterus. In C. Gleason & S. Juul (Eds.), *Avery's diseases of the newborn* (10th ed., pp. 1198–1218). Philadelphia, PA: Elsevier.

22 NEONATAL INFECTIOUS DISEASES

Debra Armbruster
Valerie Marburger
Jenni Etheridge

INTRODUCTION

Of any age group, newborns and infants are at the highest risk of infection-induced morbidity and mortality. The unique functions of fetal, neonatal, and maternal immunity reflect adaptation to developmental challenges, such as preservation of fetal well-being as an allogeneic graft versus adequate immunologic protection in the extrauterine environment. There are differences in immunologic responsiveness between newborns and adults, which are highly regulated ontogenic differences that facilitate transitions between distinct age-specific challenges (Weitkamp, Lewis, & Levy, 2018, p. 453).

This chapter provides a basic review of developmental immunity and infections of concern in the neonatal period. Overall risk factors, incidence, and organisms, as well as treatment recommendations, will be discussed. Pharmacology related to the treatment of sepsis is reviewed in a separate chapter (Chapter 13).

IMMUNE SYSTEM DEVELOPMENTAL IMMUNITY

- In general, the immunological system is comprised of two major defense mechanisms: innate-nonspecific immune response and acquired-specific immune response. Defense mechanisms that operate effectively without prior exposure to a microorganism or its antigens are *innate-nonspecific immune responses*. This includes physical barriers—skin and mucous membranes—and chemical barriers—gastric acid and digestive enzymes (Benjamin, Mezu-Ndubuisi & Maheshwari, 2015, p. 696).
- An *acquired-specific immune response* describes the development of a protective response to a specific foreign antigen that has been processed and presented by the innate immune system, and establishment of an immunologic memory of responses. It includes cell-mediated (T-lymphocyte) and humoral (B lymphocyte and immunoglobulin; Blackburn, 2013, pp. 446–447).

Innate Immunity

POLYMORPHONUCLEAR NEUTROPHILS (PMNS)

- Polymorphonuclear neutrophils (PMNs), monocytes, and macrophages include the major phagocytic cell types that function to ingest and kill bacteria and other microorganisms. Natural killer (NK) cells kill invading pathogens by non phagocytic mechanisms. These cell types eliminate pathogens from the host more efficiently when the pathogens are opsonized, or coated, by complement components and other soluble proteins of the innate immune system. Equally, non phagocytic methods such as lysis of infected cells by NK cells, PMNs, and monocytes are augmented in the presence of specific antibody to the target organism (Benjamin, Mezu-Ndubuisi, & Maheshwari, 2015, p. 697).
- Progenitor cells that are committed to maturation along the granulocyte or macrophage cell lineages (granulocyte–macrophage colony-forming units) are detectable in the human liver between 6 and 12 weeks. Human fetal blood has detectable granulocyte–macrophage colony-forming units from 12 weeks' gestation to term. Cells committed to phagocyte maturation are seen in the human fetal liver by 6 weeks and the peripheral fetal blood by 15 weeks' gestation (Weitkamp, Lewis, & Levy, 2018, p. 462). In the human fetus, granulocytopoiesis takes place almost exclusively in the bone marrow (Benjamin et al., 2015, p. 697).
- Mature PMNs are first identified in the fetal bone marrow at approximately 14 weeks of gestation. By 22 to 23 weeks' gestation the circulating PMN count has increased but remains lower than in term infants. By mid-gestation fetus and preterm infant, the neutrophil storage pool (NSP) is very small and can be readily exhausted during sepsis. The neutrophil proliferating pool (NPP) is also small. PMNs of term and preterm infants are limited in chemotactic, phagocytic, and microbicidal activities. Circulating PMNs increase dramatically at birth, peak at 12 to 24 hours, and decline slowly by 72 hours to remain stable during the rest of the neonatal period.
- The PMN is qualitatively and quantitatively the most effective killing phagocyte of the host defense. The influx of mononuclear phagocytes to sites of inflammation is delayed and attenuated in newborns. This defect is most likely related to the impaired chemotactic activity by the peripheral blood monocytes of these infants. Phagocytosis and microbicidal activity seem equivalent to the level displayed by mononuclear phagocytes of adults (Benjamin et al., 2015, pp. 703–704).
- When searching for the cause of neutropenia (<1,500 PMNs/mm³) in infants, a strong suspicion of infection is warranted, although maternal preeclampsia, premature birth, birth depression, intravascular hemorrhage, and hemolytic disease may result in low peripheral PMN counts (Benjamin, Mezu-Ndubuisi, & Maheshwari, 2015, p. 698).

MONOCYTES

- The first monocytes in circulation are not seen until about the fifth month of gestation, and remain uncommon until bone marrow becomes the predominant site of hematopoiesis.
- In neonates, monocytosis has been associated with lower birth weight and gestational age (GA), multiple transfusions, albumin infusions, and theophylline therapy.

- The ability of fetal monocytes to kill a variety of pathogens, including *Staphylococcus aureus, Staphylococcus epidermidis, Escherichia coli,* and *Candida albicans,* appears to be equivalent to that of adults.
- Impaired migration in response to chemoattractants may be a primary factor in the delayed influx of monocytes at inflammatory sites during the neonatal period.
- Impaired monocyte function in neonates may be partially responsible for poorer cytokine responses of neonatal T-cells.
- Generally, mononuclear phagocyte recruitment and accumulation lag behind the brisk PMN influx by 6 to 12 hours, but the former process persists for several days.

MACROPHAGES
- Resident macrophages are often the first phagocytic cells of the innate immune system to encounter invading pathogens. These cells serve important host defense functions through phagocytosis and also as sentinel cells that regulate local inflammatory responses by producing various cytokines and chemokines.
- During resolution of inflammation, the macrophage populations switch from a pro-inflammatory to an anti-inflammatory phenotype (Benjamin, Mezu-Ndubuisi & Maheshwari, 2015, p. 703).
- Newborn monocytes, macrophages, and dendritic cells (DCs) demonstrate a reduced chemotaxis and phagocytosis, as well as anti-inflammatory cytokine production (Weitkamp, Lewis, & Levy, 2018, p. 462).

NATURAL KILLER CELLS
- NK cells are relatively normal in number in the neonatal period, but surface membrane expression of certain antigens is altered compared with adult NK cells. NK cell cytolytic activity against target cells in vitro is diminished during the neonatal period. The role of NK cell immaturity in contributing to the increased susceptibility of newborns to viral infection remains unknown (Benjamin, Mezu-Ndubuisi & Maheshwari, 2015, p. 704).
- NK progenitor cells have been identified in the fetal thymus, bone marrow, and liver as early as 6 weeks' gestation. In the human neonate, the NK cell population is immature, but expresses decreased cytolytic activity (Weitkamp, Lewis, & Levy, 2018, pp. 460–461).
- Table 22.1 lists, compares, and contrasts the innate and adaptive immune systems.

THE COMPLEMENT SYSTEM
- Its major function is to facilitate the neutralization of foreign substances either in the circulation or on mucous membranes (Benjamin et al., 2015, p. 704).
- Complement proteins are synthesized early in gestation.
- *The classic pathway* of complement activation requires the presence of specific antibodies against a particular antigen and the formation of immune complexes.
  - Newborns have a limited spectrum of antibody transmitted across the placenta; they receive immunoglobulin G (IgG), no immunoglobulin M (IgM), and little antibody to the entire range of Gram-negative bacteria.
  - The classic pathway has relatively little value at and shortly after birth.
  - Therefore, it follows that in the absence of specific antibody, activation of the biologically active fragments and complexes of the complement system through the

alternative or lectin pathways becomes an extremely important defense mechanism for neonates during the first encounter with bacteria.
- In contrast, *the alternative pathway* may be activated by bacterial or mammalian cell surfaces in the absences of specific antibodies.
  - Activation of the alternative pathway or lectin pathway enables opsonization of invading organisms without specific Ig immunoglobulin recognition.
  - For preterm infants or those without organism-specific maternal IgG, alternative or lectin pathways activation provides a critical mechanism for engaging complement effector functions (Weitkamp et al., 2018, p. 453).
  - Proteins in the lectin pathways are also lower in neonates compared with adults and are decreased in preterm compared to term infants.
    - Defects in the complement system, and the alternative pathway in particular, likely play a role in susceptibility to infection, especially in preterm infants.
  - The components of the classic and alternative complement systems and their functional activity in full-term neonates are generally lower than in normal adults.
  - Serum alternative complement component values reach adult levels by 6 to 18 months.
  - In most neonates, functional deficiencies in these pathways, in conjunction with impaired functioning PMNs, are likely clinically relevant (as suggested by lower levels of manose-binding lectins (MBL) and ficolin lectins in neonates with culture-proven sepsis; Benjamin et al., 2015, p. 706).

NEONATAL COMPLEMENT SYSTEM FUNCTION
- Newborn infants have an increased susceptibility to infection because of various host defense impairments that exist during the neonatal period.
- A network of regulatory glycoproteins and phospholipids that mediate the interactions between cells control the responses.
- These cytokines and chemokines are responsible for the generation of the immune response and differentiation of a wide variety of immune and nonimmune cells.
- The infant's ability to generate the right balance of pro-inflammatory and anti-inflammatory cytokines when challenged with an infectious agent allows recovery from the encounter with minimal residua.
  - Circulating concentrations of fibronectin are decreased in the neonatal period and are directly correlated with GA (lower GA = lower levels).
  - Even lower plasma concentrations are measured in infants who are ill.
- Plasma fibronectin increases phagocyte function in vitro.
  - The role of fibronectin in host immune defense in neonates remains uncertain, but in vitro data suggest a potential role as an enhancer of phagocyte function.
  - Antigen-presenting cells (APCs) of the innate immune system (e.g., macrophages, NK cells, neutrophils, mucosal epithelial cells, endothelial cells, and DCs) play pivotal roles in the initiation of an inflammatory response to invading pathogens.
  - Activated, macrophages synthesize and secrete a cascade of proinflammatory cytokines, chemokines, and mediators. Some of these cytokines activate neutrophils to release proteases and free radicals that have the capacity to damage endothelium and promote capillary leak.

TABLE 22.1 Comparison of Innate and Acquired Immunity

	Innate Immunity	Adaptive Immunity
Function	Includes inflammation, lysis of an antigen cell membrane, and phagocytosis. Activation of adaptive immune response.	Development of a protective response to a specific foreign antigen that has been processed and presented by the innate immune system, and establishment of an immunologic memory of responses.
Mechanism of response	First line of defense following exposure to antigen. No long-term memory with repeat exposures producing same response.	Includes both humoral-mediated and antibody-mediated (B-lymphocytes) responses Cell-mediated (T-lymphocytes) Long-term memory with repeat exposures producing heightened response.
Key characteristics	Involves nonspecific inborn responses to foreign antigen activated the first time an antigen is encountered. Important characteristics: 1. Prior exposure is not required 2. Repeated exposures to an antigen will not alter response 3. Ability to recognize molecular patterns shared by groups	Six characteristics: 1. Specificity—ability to respond to distinct antigen or part of an antigen 2. Diversity—ability to respond to wide variety of antigens 3. Memory—repeated exposures to an antigen elicit more vigorous responses 4. Specialization—optimizing immune responses against different antigens 5. Self-limiting—ability to return to homeostasis 6. Nonreactive to self-defend foreign antigens while not harming the human's own cells
Effector cells	Polymorphonuclear neutrophils, macrophages, monocytes, mast cells, and natural killer cells. TLRs—on cell surfaces, responsible for recognizing molecular patterns of microbials. Endothelial cells, circulating factors—complement and acute phase proteins—CRP and cytokines and chemokines (secreted by macrophages; mediate the innate immune response)	T-lymphocytes, B-lymphocytes APCs: dendritic cells, monocytes, macrophages Effector cells: mononuclear phagocytes
Activation	TLRs sense molecular patterns of pathogens; induce expression of cytokines and chemokines to activate defensive cells. Pattern recognition receptors on cell surfaces, intracellular vesicles, and cytoplasm recognize damaging molecular patterns (cytokines, intracellular proteins, substances released from damaged cells, and pathogen associated with molecular patterns). Pathogens bind to TLR and other receptors on monocytes, macrophages, initiate a complement cascade with release of prostaglandin. Transcription factor NK-κB is released, which stimulates synthesis and release of both proinflammatory (IL-1B, IL-6, TNF-) and anti-inflammatory (IL-1, IL-10) cytokines.	Primary antibody response: activation, proliferation, and differentiation of naive B-lymphocytes into antibody secreting cells or memory cells. Secondary antibody response: memory B-lymphocytes that are activated to produce increasing amounts of antibodies. *Cell-mediated response* by T-lymphocytes 1. Presentation of antigen by histocompatibility glycoprotein complexes (MCHs) on surface of APC or B-lymphocyte. 2. Cell associated antigen recognition by naive T cells. 3. Activation of T cells to produce cytokines. 4. T-cell proliferation and clonal expansion. 5. Differentiation of naive T cells into effector or memory cells. 6. Inhibition of response by suppressor or regulatory T cells when control or elimination foreign antigen complete.

APCs, antigen-presenting cells; CRP, C-reactive protein; IL, interleukin; MCH, major histocompatibility complexes; NK-kB, natural killer kappa B; TLR, toll-like receptors; TNF-α, tumor necrosis factor alpha.

Source: Data from Blackburn, S. T. (2013). *Maternal, fetal, & neonatal physiology: A clinical perspective* (4th ed.), Philadelphia, PA: Elsevier.

- The proinflammatory cascade is interrupted by the initiation of counter-regulatory mechanisms.
  - The concentration of anti-inflammatory substances (e.g., interleukin (IL)-1ra and soluble receptors) increases substantially with time and has been termed the *compensatory anti-inflammatory response syndrome.*
  - This is a response of the host to limit the toxicity of pro-inflammatory substances (Benjamin et al., 2015, p. 712).

Neonatal-Acquired Immunity Function

- The ability to mount cell-mediated or antibody-mediated immune responses to specific antigens is acquired sequentially during the course of embryonic development.
  - Early in gestation, fetuses can respond to certain antigens, whereas other antigens elicit antibody production or cell-mediated immune responses only after birth.
- Fetuses and newborns do not respond to some antigens (e.g., pneumococcal polysaccharide), and the antibody

responses to other antigens (e.g., rubella, cytomegalovirus [CMV], *Toxoplasma*] are predominately of the IgM type.

- T lymphocytes are less experienced in neonates and tend to suppress rather than stimulate B-cell differentiation.
- B cells of newborns differentiate predominantly into IgM-secreting plasma cells, whereas activated adult B cells produce IgG- and IgA-secreting plasma cells.
  - This adult pattern of differentiation develops over the first year of life.
- Along with quantitative differences, neonatal T cells are also functionally distinct from adult cells. This deficiency in T-cell subsets may contribute to the increased susceptibility to infections in the preterm infant.
  - Cord blood T cells have reduced ability to proliferate and synthesize cytokines such as Il-2, interferon gamma (IFN-*y*), Il-4, and granulocyte–macrophage colony-stimulating factor (GM-CSF). Both CD4+ and CD8+ lymphocytes decrease with GA and are lower at birth in preterm compared to term infants. (Benjamin et al., 2015, p. 717)
- Neonatal T cells are impaired in producing a robust Th1 response and produce less INF-*y* and TNF under conditions of physiologic stimulation, including in response to the multi-chain T cell receptor/CD3 complex (TCR-CD3) stimulation, although, adult-level cytokine production can be elicited in human neonatal T cells by increasing the magnitude of Th-1 promoting costimulatory signals. (Benjamin et al, 2015, p. 719).
  - However, neonatal cytotoxic T lymphocytes are capable of generating long-lasting memory effectors against several viral infections, including CMV (and Rous sarcoma virus).
  - Qualitative differences in neonatal T cells and APCs compared with adult cells might contribute to these deficient T-cells-mediated responses of neonates (Benjamin et al., 2015, p. 725).

Passive Immunity

- Maternal transfer of IgG antibodies across the placenta provides a newborn with a measure of immune protection.
- Both protective and potentially damaging maternal antibodies cross the placenta. Maternal IgG antibodies are the only ones to cross in significant amounts. Maternal antibody has multiple functions in the fetus and neonate, including passive immunity against pathogens, epigenetic inheritance of immunologic memory, immunological imprinting, suppression of immunoglobulin E (IgE) responsiveness, and suppression of tumor development.
- Fetal levels of IgG are low until 20 to 22 weeks' gestation, when passive and active transfer of IgG across the placenta increases. All four IgG subclasses cross, although IgG$_1$ and IgG$_3$ subclasses predominate and are transferred more efficiently. Active transfer allows for movement of IgG to the fetus even when maternal levels are low. IgG$_1$ is the primary immunoglobulin before 28 weeks. IgG$_3$ crosses later and does not reach maternal levels until after 32 to 33 weeks' gestation. In most infants, IgG levels near term are higher than maternal levels.
  - Depending on the maternal antibody complement, the newborn may have passive immunity against tetanus, diphtheria, polio, measles, mumps, group B streptococcus (GBS), *E. coli*, hepatitis B virus (HBV), *Salmonella enterica*, and others (Blackburn, 2013, p. 454).

- Antibodies to viral agents, diphtheria, and tetanus antitoxins, which are usually of the IgG class, are efficiently transported across the placenta and attain protective levels in the fetus.
- However, antibodies to agents that evoke primarily immunoglobulin A (IgA) or IgM antibody responses are poorly transported across the placenta, thereby leaving the neonate unprotected against those organisms.
- Infants are not protected against agents to which the mother has not made significant amounts of antibody (Benjamin et al., 2015, p. 727).
- Most viruses and many bacteria are capable of being transferred across the placenta, although relatively few are actually transferred. Immune factors that prevent maternal rejection of the fetus also protect the placenta from infectious agents (Blackburn, 2013, p. 454).
  - The organisms that most commonly cross the maternal-placental barrier are *Listeria monocytogenes*, *Treponema pallium*, HIV, paravirus B19, rubella, *Toxoplasmosis gondii*, and CMV.
  - Amniotic fluid also protects the fetus through antibacterial and other substances found in maternal milk, including transferrin, beta-lysin, peroxidase, fatty acids, IgG and IgA immunoglobulins, and lysozyme (Blackburn, 2013, p. 455).

NEONATAL SEPSIS

- Epidemiologically, neonatal sepsis is divided into the following categories: early-onset sepsis (EOS), late-onset sepsis (LOS), and very LOS. The age of onset of sepsis reflects the likely mode of acquisition, microbiologic features, mortality rate, and presentation of infection (Baley & Leonard, 2013, p. 346; Leonard & Dobbs, 2015, p. 734).
- Sources of infection in a newborn can be divided into three categories: transplacental acquisition, perinatal acquisition, and hospital acquisition (Pammi, Brand, & Weismann, 2016, p. 537; Wilson & Tyner, 2015, p. 697).
  - An infection occurs when a susceptible host comes in contact with a potentially pathogenic organism. And when the encountered organism proliferates and overcomes the host defenses, infection results (Pammi et al., 2016, p. 537).
- Sepsis is a common cause of death in infants born <1,500 g (Baley & Leonard, 2013, p. 347). Failure to identify early signs of sepsis contribute to morbidity, mortality, and increased healthcare costs (Wilson & Tyner, 2015, p. 689).
- Table 22.2 compares EOS and LOS

Risk Factors for Neonatal Sepsis

- Newborns are extremely susceptible to infection. The immature immune system of the neonate is characterized by immature activation and function of the immune system responses that make newborns more susceptible to infections with a frequency and an intensity greater than any other period of life (Baley & Leonard, 2013, p. 346; Leonard & Dobbs, 2015, p. 734; Wilson & Tyner, 2015, p. 689).
  - This susceptibility stems from maternal risk factors, obstetrical complications, the postnatal environment, and the immature host defenses of the newborn (Baley & Leonard, 2013, p. 346).
  - The main goal is to prevent infection in the fetus and the newborn (Baley, & Leonard, 2013, p. 346).

TABLE 22.2 Comparisons of Early-Onset Sepsis and Late-Onset Sepsis

	Early-Onset Sepsis	Late-Onset Sepsis
Definition	Commonly occurs before 72 hours of life, and 90% of infants are symptomatic by 24 hours of age. Horizontal acquisition during birth.	Commonly occurs after the first week of life (7 days), but may occur as early as 3 days. Described as community-acquired infection (CAI) or hospital-acquired infection (HAI). Vertical acquisition from infant's environment. Infants colonized with pathogenic bacteria ubiquitous to their physical environment—including flora of caregivers.
Risk Factors	Maternal factors: Premature rupture of membranes, prolonged rupture of membranes (>18 hours), chorio-amnionitis, fever (>100.4 F) GBS status, and maternal UTI. Neonatal factors: Prematurity, gestational age, and low BW.	Neonatal factors: Prematurity inversely related to gestational age, low BW. Need for NICU devices: Intubation, mechanical ventilation, OG/NG tube insertion, central lines (CLABSI, most common HAI). Need for high-risk medications: Broad-spectrum antibiotics (increase bacterial colonization), parenteral nutrition, antacids, H_2 blockers, proton pump inhibitors.
Presentation	Clinical signs and symptoms are variable and nonspecific. Common signs include: Respiratory distress (most common), hemodynamic instability with poor perfusion or shock, and temperature instability. May present as fulminant onset of respiratory symptoms—due to pneumonia, shock, or poor perfusion resulting in a systemic, multiorgan disease. Clinical signs and symptoms may reflect noninfectious etiologies.	Presentation may be slow and progressive or fulminant. Common signs: Poor feeding, temperature instability, and lethargy. Focal disease common: UTI, osteoarthritis, or soft tissue infection. Meningitis is common. GBS LOS is more often complicated by meningitis (primarily caused by polysaccharide serotype strains).
Etiology	Most commonly acquired before delivery via vertical transmission either through ascending amniotic fluid infection or through acquisition of bacterial flora from the mother's ano-genital tract during vaginal delivery, and reflects maternal genitourinary and gastrointestinal colonization.	Most commonly acquired from infants postnatal environment. Prematurity is most significant factor; invasive procedures performed on a neonate (intubation, catheterization, and surgery) increase the risk of bacterial infection. CLABSIs prominent concern in NICU setting. VAP second most common HAI in NICU; associated with aspiration of secretions, colonization, and use of contaminated equipment.
Incidence	Incidence in the United States estimated to be 0.98 per 1,000 live births overall. Birthweight <1,500 g 10.96 per 1,000 live births. Birthweight 1,500–2,500 g 1.38 per 1,000 live births. Universal antenatal screening for GBS colonization with antibiotic prophylaxis for women colonized with GBS has significantly reduced the rate of early-onset GBS sepsis. Increases in non-GBS EOS and ampicillin-resistant EOS are reported among VLBW infants.	Incidence 0.27 cases per 1,000 live births (2013 data). Approximately 50% of cases occur in infants born <37 weeks. Rates of LOS are most common in LBW infants, and are inversely associated with birthweight. IAP has no impact on LOS GBS.
Microorganisms	Most common: Group B streptococcus, *E. coli* and Listeria monocytogenes. Less common: *Staphylococcus aureus*, viridans group Streptococci, Enterococci, group A Streptococci, Listeria monocytogenes, Haemophili, other Gram-negative Klebsiella, Enterobacter, Citrobacter, Acinetobacter, and Pseudomonas. Fungal species can cause EOS primarily in preterm infants. Since IAP began, predominance of Gram-negative organisms has been noted in infants weighing less than 1,500 g at birth.	Gram-positive organisms predominate in LOS in VLBW and premature infants, coagulase negative staphylococcus (CONS), and *S. aureus*, as well as invasive candidiasis. Approximately 50% of LOS cases are caused by CONS. Gram-negative organisms account for about one-third of LOS cases in VLBW infants. GBS and *E. coli* are common organisms—*E. coli* is frequent cause of urosepsis in young infants. Common community LOS organisms include: GBS, *E. coli*, or Klebsiella, and less common organisms include: *Streptococcus pneumonia* and *Neisseria meningitides*. Very LOS disease includes GBS, Gram-negative bacilli, and Streptococcus pneumonia

(*continued*)

Table 22.2 Comparisons Of Early-Onset Sepsis And Late-Onset Sepsis *(Cont.)*

	Early-Onset Sepsis	Late-Onset Sepsis
Evaluation	Blood culture, CBC, and LP (urine unlikely to yield results in EOS)	Blood culture, CBC, LP, and urine culture
Treatment	The most appropriate regime is ampicillin and gentimicin. (The use of broad spectrum antibiotics is associated with increased antibiotic resistance and fungicemia.) Antibiotic regimes should cover GBS, Gram-negative bacilli, and L.monocytogenes.	Empiric therapy usually consists of vancomycin and an aminoglycoside, providing coverage for coagulase-negative Staphylococci, *S. aureus*, and Gram-negative organisms. The antibiotic therapy in LOS and very LOS onset disease are not definitively in favor of any one regimen. Naficillin appropriate coverage for MSSA. Vancomycin is first-line coverage for MRSA. Consider empiric antifungal coverage for invasive candidiasis. Local variation in microbiology of LOS is important in considering empiric antibiotic therapy. The regime for an infant admitted from the community should include coverage for GBS, *E. coli*, and *S. pneumoniae*.
Mortality Morbidity	Mortality may be as high as 30% to 50%. GBS—38% to 45%, and *E. coli* 24% to 29%. Mortality rate for early preterm infants is as high as 30% to 54%. Mortality rates are inversely proportional to gestational age.	Mortality is lower than EOS but may still be 20% to 40%. Mortality from GBS LOS is low at 1% and 5% in term and preterm infants, respectively. The sequelae in survivors of GBS meningitis can be severe.

BW, birthweight; CBC, complete blood count; CLABSI, central line blood-stream infection; EOS, early-onset sepsis; GBS, group B streptococcus; IAP, intrapartum antibiotic prophylaxis; LOS, late-onset sepsis; LP, lumbar puncture; MRSA, Methicillin-resistant *S. aureus*; MSSA, methicillin-susceptible *S. aureus*; UTI, urinary tract infection; VAP, ventilator associated-pneumonia; VLBW, very low birthweight.

Sources: Data from Baley, J. E., & Leonard, E. G. (2013). Infections in the neonate. In A. Fanaroff & A. Fanaroff (Eds.), *Klaus and Fanaroff's care of the high-risk neonate* (6th ed., pp. 346–367). Cleveland, OH: Elsevier; Leonard, E. G., & Dobbs, K. (2015). Postnatal bacterial infections. In R. Martin, A. Fanaroff, & M. Walsh (Eds.), *Fanaroff and Martin's neonatal-perinatal medicine: Diseases of the fetus and infant* (10th ed., pp. 737–741). Philadelphia, PA: Elsevier; Pammi, M., Brand, M. C., & Weismann, L. (2016). Infection in the neonate. In S. Gardner, B. Carter, M. Hines, & J. Hernandez (Eds.), *Merenstein & Gardner's handbook of neonatal intensive care* (8th ed., pp. 537–562). St. Louis, MO: Elsevier; Puopolo, K. M. (2017). Bacterial and fungal infections. In Eichenwald et al. (Eds.), *Cloherty and Stark's manual of neonatal care* (8th ed., pp. 641–650, 691–718). Philadelphia, PA: Wolters Kluwer.

Maternal Risk Factors

ANTEPARTUM

- Inadequate prenatal care, inadequate nutrition, low socioeconomic status, recurrent abortion, substance abuse, history of maternal sexually transmitted diseases (STDs), maternal urinary tract infections (UTIs), and premature rupture of membranes (PROM).

INTRAPARTUM

- PROM (>12–18 hours) prior to labor/delivery, GBS colonization, chorioamnionitis, uterine tenderness, purulent amniotic fluid, foul-smelling amniotic fluid, maternal fever (>101F), prolonged or difficult labor, premature birth, maternal UTI, invasive intrapartum procedures (internal fetal monitoring), elevated maternal heart rate (HR; >100 bpm), and elevated fetal HR (>180 bpm).

Neonatal Risk Factors

- Prematurity, low birth weight (LBW), difficult birth, birth asphyxia, meconium staining, resuscitation, low Apgar score (<6 at 5 min), congenital anomalies, breach of skin integrity, and multiple births.

ENVIRONMENTAL

- Hospital admission, length of stay; invasive procedures: peripheral intravenous catheter (PIV), intubation, umbilical venous/arterial catheters (UVC/UAC), central venous catheters (CVC),

peripherally inserted central catheters (PICCs), chest tubes (CTs), and other surgical interventions; use of broad-spectrum antibiotics; and use of humidification systems in ventilation and incubators (Wilson & Tyner, 2015, p. 690).

Incidence of Neonatal Sepsis

- The incidence of neonatal sepsis ranges from one to eight cases per 1,000 live births (whereas meningitis may occur in one of every six septic infants; Baley & Leonard, 2013, p. 346), although the incidence is twice as high among moderately premature infants compared to term infants and highest among very low birth weight (VLBW; <1,500 g) infants with recent reports ranging from 10 to 15 cases per 1,000 VLBW births (Puopolo, 2017, p. 685).
  - The most important risk factors for neonatal sepsis are prematurity and low BW and incidence is inversely proportional to gestational age (GA) or birth weight (BW).
- Other risk factors include compromised immune function, exposure to invasive procedures, hypoxia, metabolic acidosis, hypothermia, and low socioeconomic status, all of which are factors associated with prematurity and low BW (Baley & Leonard, 2013, p. 346–347).
- Neonatal sepsis is twice as common in Black infants than White infants (Baley & Leonard, 2013, p. 347). African American preterm neonates account for 5.14 cases per 1,000 births, with a fatality rate of 24.4% (Wilson & Tyner, 2015, p. 694). African American preterm infants remain at considerably greater risk than do White preterm infants and both Black and White term infants (Pammi et al., 2016, p. 537).

- Males have higher incidence, but not a higher risk.
- Sepsis is more common in firstborn twins.
- Infants with a diagnosis of galactosemia are more likely to become infected with gram-negative organisms, particularly *E. coli* (Baley & Leonard, 2013, p. 347).

Clinical Signs and Symptoms

- Detection of neonatal sepsis requires a high index of suspicion as clinical signs may be nonspecific and nonlocalizing (Leonard & Dobbs, 2015, p. 735; Pammi et al., 2016, p. 537; Wilson & Tyner, 2015, p. 690).
  - Familiarity with epidemiology risk factors is crucial to determining the threshold index of suspicion because most neonates are asymptomatic without correlation with positive cultures.
  - Lethargy or poor feeding may be the only symptoms initially, although the most common clinical sign is respiratory distress (Leonard & Dobbs, 2015, p. 735; Wilson & Tyner, 2015, p. 690).
  - Other less specific signs of sepsis include irritability, lethargy, temperature instability, poor perfusion, and hypotension, but disseminated intravascular coagulation (DIC) with purpura and petechiae can occur in more severe septic shock. However, lethargy, irritability, and seizures can all occur secondary to electrolyte or metabolic disturbances, including endocrinologically (Puopolo, 2017, p. 685).
- Metabolic manifestations may include hyperglycemia or hypoglycemia, acidosis, and jaundice.
- Noninfectious etiologies that may mimic neonatal sepsis include transient tachypnea of the newborn (TTNB), pulmonary hypertension, cardiogenic pulmonary edema, surfactant deficiency, noninfectious metabolic acidosis, and meconium aspiration syndrome (MAS; Leonard & Dobbs, 2015, p. 735).

Diagnosis

- Definitive diagnosis is the isolation of an organism from a sterile body site, such as blood, cerebrospinal fluid (CSF), or urine (Baley & Leonard, 2013, p. 347; Leonard & Dobbs, 2015, p. 735; Wilson & Tyner, 2015, p. 694).
- Blood culture volume should be at least 1 mL for improved recovery, particularly in low colony count bacteremia (Leonard & Dobbs, 2015, p. 735; Wilson & Tyner, 2015, p.694).
  - A blood culture may be falsely negative if mother received antibiotics or if infant has been exposed to multiple courses of antibiotics.
- A lumbar puncture (LP) should be considered in any infant with suspected sepsis (Baley & Leonard, 2013, p. 347; Leonard & Dobbs, 2015, p. 735).
  - There is a poor correlation between the results of neonatal blood cultures and CSF cultures (underscores the need for LP); however, an LP may be deferred in unstable infants (Leonard & Dobbs, 2015, p. 735).
  - Meningitis rate as high as 23% in infants with bacteremia (Baley & Leonard, 2013, p. 347; Leonard & Dobbs, 2015, p. 735; Wilson & Tyner, 2015, p. 694).
  - A study among VLBW infants with meningitis showed that one-third had corresponding negative blood cultures; therefore, a failure to perform an LP may result in a missed diagnosis (Baley & Leonard, 2013, p. 346; Leonard & Dobbs, 2015, p. 736).

- 92% of cultures are positive by 24 hours.
  - Contaminates usually take a longer time to grow (>2–3 days), although if infant is symptomatic, infection should be presumed.
  - If positive culture is obtained from blood, CSF, or urine, a follow-up culture should be obtained to document sterility.
  - Gram-positive bacteria can be detected after up to 36 hours of antimicrobial therapy, and some Gram-negative organisms can be detected for several days in CSF (Wilson & Tyner, 2015, p. 695).

Indirect Markers of Sepsis

- Indirect indices of infection include the following: white blood cells (WBC), absolute neutrophil count (ANC), C-reactive protein (CRP), procalcitonin level, and various cytokines; none are specific or sensitive enough to confirm or exclude sepsis (Baley & Leonard, 2013, p. 347).
  - These indices can be used to help identify infected infants and guide decisions on antimicrobial therapy (Leonard & Dobbs, 2015, p. 736).
- Other nonspecific laboratory abnormalities that may accompany neonatal sepsis include hyperglycemia, hypoglycemia, and unexplained metabolic acidosis (Pammi et al., 2016, p. 537).

WHITE BLOOD CELLS

- There is a roller coaster shape of the WBC and ANC and immature to total neutrophil ratio (I/T) curves in the first 72 hours of life (Puopolo, 2017, p. 689).
  - It is recommended to wait for 6 to 12 hours after birth for WBC evaluation as later counts are more likely to be abnormal and reflect an inflammatory response of the neonate compared to those obtained at birth (Leonard & Dobbs, 2015, p. 736).
  - Optimal interpretation of WBC data to predict EOS should account for the natural rise and fall in WBC during this period.
- The WBC and ANC are most predictive of infection when these values are low (WBC <5,000 and ANC <1,000).
  - Calculation of ANC:

$$\% \text{ WBCs} \times \left(\% \text{ Immature neutrophils} + \% \text{ Mature neutrophils}\right) \times 0.01$$

  - The immature to total I/T is most informative if measured between 1 to 4 hours after birth.
  - Calculation of I/T:

$$\frac{\% \text{ Bands} + \% \text{ Immature forms}}{\% \text{ Mature} + \% \text{ Bands} + \% \text{ Immature forms}}$$

- The I/T is best used for negative predictive value: If I/T is normal; likelihood infection is absent with 99% predictive value (Wilson & Tyner, 2015, p. 692).
- The combination of low ANC and elevated I/T ratio is the most predictive combination of WBC indices for EOS (Puopolo, 2017, p. 689).
- The WBC and its components may be of more value in the VLBW infant and/or in the evaluation of LOS infection, especially if interpreted in relation to values obtained prior to the concern for infection (Puopolo, 2017, p. 689).
- Studies have shown that leukopenia and high percentage of immature to total WBCs are associated with EOS. LOS

has been associated with both low and high WBC, high ANC and high percentage of immature to total WBCs (Leonard & Dobbs, 2015, p. 736).

C-Reactive Protein

- CRP is a nonspecific marker of inflammation. It is one of the most rapidly responsive acute-phase proteins, with increases of 100- to 1,000-fold (in adults) in the serum concentration detectable during an infection. CRP is produced by both the fetus and the newborn. In surveys of infants with proven infections, an elevation of CRP serum concentration has been observed in 50% to 100% of patients (Benjamin et al., 2015, p. 697).
    - An elevated CRP may be found in bacterial sepsis and meningitis (Puopolo, 2017, p. 693).
    - Elevated cord blood CRP levels are associated with chorioamnionitis with prolonged rupture of membranes (ROMs; Wilson & Tyner, 2015, p. 693).
- CRP levels increase within 6 to 8 hours and peak after 24 hours. CRP sensitivity is lowest early, and sensitivity increases with serial values 24 to 48 hours after onset of symptoms. Serial levels may be useful for identifying infants who do not have a bacterial infection or in monitoring response to treatment for infected infants (Leonard & Dobbs, 2015, p. 736).
- A single determination of CRP at birth lacks both sensitivity and specificity for infection, although serial CRP determinations at the time of blood culture, 12 to 24 hours and 48 hours later, have been used to manage infants at risk for LOS (Puopolo, 2017, p. 693), and can be helpful in exclusion of serious infection (Wilson & Tyner, 2015, p. 693).
    - Serial CRP patterns have been found to be useful to follow resolution of infection and guide antibiotic therapy (Pammi et al., 2016, p. 537; Puopolo, 2017, p. 693).

Procalcitonin

- Procalcitonin is an acute-phase reactant that is elevated in response to bacterial toxins.
- Procalcitonin concentrations peak 12 hours after infection (physiologic increase 24 hours after birth). Increases can be seen in noninfectious causes, such as respiratory distress syndrome (RDS).
    - Procalcitonin appears to have better sensitivity but less specificity than CRP for identifying neonatal sepsis. The most important information guiding clinical decisions continues to be a patient's overall clinical status and culture data (Leonard & Dobbs, 2015, p. 736).

Treatment Recommendations

- Once a pathogen is identified, therapy should be tailored to the species and antimicrobial susceptibilities.
- Duration of therapy determined by the site of infection and patient's clinical response (Leonard & Dobbs, 2015, p. 736).
- The most appropriate and least toxic antibiotic or antibiotic combination should be continued for an appropriate period by a suitable route.
- Antibiotics are not the entire solution to treating the infected newborn—meticulous attention to the treatment of associated conditions (shock, hypoxemia, thermal abnormalities, electrolyte or acid–base imbalance, inadequate nutrition, anemia, or presence of pus or foreign bodies) is as important as choosing an antibiotic (Pammi et al., 2016, p. 537).
    - Supportive treatments for sepsis include mechanical ventilation, exogenous surfactant therapy for pneumonia and RDS, volume and pressor support for hypotension, sodium bicarbonate for metabolic acidosis, and anticonvulsants for seizures.
    - Adjunct therapies for neonatal sepsis including double-volume exchange transfusions and granulocyte infusions, intravenous immunoglobulin G (IVIG) have been studied with variable results (Puopolo., 2017, p. 686).

Sepsis Prevention Strategies

- Intrapartum antibiotic prophylaxis (IAP) has been highly effective in reducing GBS EOS, although there has been no direct effect on LOS GBS (Leonard & Dobbs, 2015, p. 737).
- Table 22.3 offers recommended maternal IAP.
- Preventative efforts to reduce the risk of LOS focus on infection control/hand hygiene, proper management of CVCs, appropriate use of antibiotics, limited use of H-2 blockers, and proton pump inhibitors (Leonard & Dobbs, 2015, p. 737; Pammi et al., 2016, p. 537; Wilson & Tyner, 2015, p. 715).
- A systematic and multidisciplinary approach to reducing central line bloodstream infections (CLABSIs) should be included in the infection-control policies of every NICU.
- Prevention of healthcare-associated infection.
    - Two-tiered approach recommended by the Centers for Disease Control and Prevention (CDC):
        - Standard precautions—use with all patients; universal precautions.
        - Transmission-based precautions.
    - Hand hygiene (Pammi et al., 2016, p. 537; Wilson & Tyner, 2015, p. 715).

TABLE 22.3 Recommended Maternal Intrapartum Antibiotic Prophylaxis

Prophylaxis	No Prophylaxis
Women with positive GBS culture results Women with history of GBS bacteremia during current pregnancy Women with a history of previous infant with invasive GBS disease Pregnant women in preterm labor, if ≥37 weeks, unknown GBS status, IAP recommended if fever ≥100.5°F occurs, or ROM >18 hours prior to delivery	Women with intact membranes and planned casarean delivery Women with negative GBS prenatal culture results

GBS, group B streptococcus; IAP, intrapartum antibiotic prophylaxis; ROM, rupture of membranes

Sources: Data from Leonard, E. G., & Dobbs, K. (2015). Postnatal bacterial infections. In R. Martin, A. Fanaroff, & M. Walsh (Eds.), *Fanaroff and Martin's neonatal-perinatal medicine: Diseases of the fetus and infant* (10th ed., pp. 737–741). Philadelphia, PA: Elsevier; Puopolo, K. M. (2017). Bacterial and fungal infections. In Eichenwald et al. (Eds.), *Cloherty and Stark's manual of neonatal care* (8th ed., pp. 641–650, 691–718). Philadelphia, PA: Wolters Kluwer.

SEPTIC SHOCK AND SYSTEMIC INFLAMMATORY RESPONSE SYNDROME (SIRS)

Septic Shock

- Shock is defined as a state of cellular energy failure resulting from an inability of tissue oxygen delivery to satisfy tissue oxygen demand. When the tissue oxygen demand cannot be met, the organs begin to fail and without corrective measures will progress to irreversible damage, end-organ failure, and death (Noori, Azhibekov, Lee, & Seri, 2018, p. 741).
- Septic or distributive shock is a type of shock where there is profound sepsis resulting in insufficient perfusion, oxygenation, and delivery of nutrients to satisfy tissue requirements, resulting in cellular dysfunction and ultimately cell destruction (Wilson & Tyner, 2015, p. 691).
- There are three phases of shock: the compensated phase, the uncompensated phase, and the irreversible phase.
  - During the *compensated* phase, blood flow to nonvital organs is sacrificed in order to continue to perfuse vital organs such as the brain and heart. This is accomplished with vasoconstriction to the former and vasodilation to the latter. During this phase blood pressure is maintained in the normal range but HR increases. Additionally, signs of nonvital organ compromise begin to appear along with evidence of overall poor perfusion. If untreated or inadequately treated the infant will progress to uncompensated shock.
  - In *uncompensated* shock, perfusion to the vital organs can no longer be maintained and blood pressure falls. Cardiac output and systemic perfusion decrease and lactic acidosis develops.
  - Without correction and treatment, the infant progresses to *irreversible shock*, where permanent damage to organ systems occur and death is imminent without reversal of the infant's condition (Noori et al., 2018, p. 749).
- Limited data are available on the exact hemodynamics of neonatal septic shock. Two patterns have been identified in older patients, warm and cold shock; with cold shock being well described in neonates.
  - Cold shock is characterized by increased vascular tone, low systemic blood flow, and eventually falling blood pressure.
  - Warm shock, which is characterized by loss of vascular tone, increased systemic blood flow, and low blood pressure, is more difficult to clinically recognize. Recent studies have described high cardiac output, low systemic vascular resistance, and increased left ventricular output consistent with neonatal warm shock.
    - The mediators of neonatal warm septic shock remain unclear; but if similarity to the adult pathogenesis is assumed, the dysregulated cytokine release and the upregulated nitric oxide production combined with the deficiency of vasopressin production could have relevance to vasopressor-resistant hypotension in preterm infants (Noori et al., 2018, p. 754).
- Rapid identification and treatment are paramount in preventing the progression of septic shock and death. Clinical presentation includes:
  - Tachycardia or bradycardia
  - Respiratory distress progressing to respiratory insufficiency and failure
  - Persistent pulmonary hypertension (PPHN) with decreased oxygenation
  - Poor perfusion
  - Hypotension with resulting decreased urinary output, organ dysfunction, and ileus
  - Metabolic acidosis and other electrolyte disorders
  - Coagulopathy, oozing, or bleeding that can progress to DIC
  - Edema due to capillary leak
  - Myocardial complications, arrhythmias, and eventually cardiac arrest (Wilson & Tyner, 2015, p. 691)
- Treatment of septic shock is centered around supporting body systems and function with a goal of restoring adequate tissue perfusion to improve outcomes. This includes:
  - Adequate respiratory support
  - Treatment of hypovolemia with normal saline, lactated Ringer's, or blood productions
  - Infant may need any combination of red blood cells (RBCs), platelets, fresh frozen plasma and/or cryoprecipitate to treat blood loss and DIC.
  - Electrolyte imbalances and metabolic acidosis need to be corrected while providing adequate nutrition and euglycemia.
  - Inotropic agents, typically dopamine, epinephrine, or hydrocortisone, may be required to support blood pressure.
  - The underlying infection must be treated with tailored antimicrobial therapy.
  - Close watch must be kept on cardiac function and arrhythmias with echocardiograms and electrocardiograms.
  - Extracorporeal membrane oxygenation (ECMO) can be considered for infants greater than 34 weeks not responding to the treatments listed above (Wilson & Tyner, 2015, p. 696–697).

Systemic Inflammatory Response Syndrome

- SIRS of the neonate is a state of physiologic dysregulation that is associated with deviations in laboratory values and vital signs (Wilson & Tyner, 2015, p. 695).
- SIRS is poorly understood and presumed to be caused by infection, although numerous noninfective etiologies exist that mimic a septic presentation.
  - In the presence of a negative culture, the differential diagnosis includes viral infections, cardiopulmonary disease, intraventricular hemorrhage, seizures, subgaleal or intracranial hemorrhage, opiate withdrawal, necrotizing enterocolitis (NEC), malrotation, bowel obstruction, metabolic disorders, and inborn errors of metabolism.
- It is difficult to define in term and preterm infants due to significant variations in "normal" vital sign values. Based on guidelines adapted by the International Pediatric Sepsis Consensus Conference, an infant must have two of the following, one of which must be an abnormal temperature or leukocyte count, to qualify for a diagnosis of SIRS:
  - Core temperature abnormality: defined as greater than 38.5°C (101.3°F) or less than 36°C (96.8°F)
  - Tachycardia: defined as a mean HR greater than 2 standard deviations (SDs) above normal for age without the presences of external or painful stimuli or chronic medications, for a half-hour to 4-hour time frame

○ Bradycardia: defined as an HR less than the 10th percentile for age without external stimulus, β-blocker medications, or heart disease, for a half-hour to 4-hour time frame
○ Respiratory rate: greater than 2 SDs above normal for age or mechanical ventilation requirement due to acute decompensation unrelated to anesthesia or neuromuscular disease
○ Leukocyte count: elevated or depressed for gestation or greater than 10% immature neutrophils
○ Sepsis: proven or suspected, caused by a pathogen or clinical syndrome with a high likelihood of infection
  ■ Positive evidence of infection includes abnormalities in examination, imaging, or laboratory tests. Examples of this include abdominal perforation, petechiae, purpura, chest radiograph demonstrating pneumonia, or the presence of WBCs in normally sterile fluid.
○ Diagnosis of SIRS is accomplished with culture and sensitivities. Antimicrobial therapy depending on prevalent organisms, age of onset of symptoms, and environmental setting is the standard treatment. If culture results are negative antibiotics may be discontinued after 48 to 72 hours but are usually continued for 5 to 7 days at the discretion of the clinician (Wilson & Tyner, 2015, p. 696).

MENINGITIS

- Meningitis is defined as the isolation of a pathogen in the CSF and can occur independently or as a sequela of bacteremia (Wilson & Tyner, 2015, pp. 698–699). The incidence of bacterial meningitis is less than one per 1,000 live births but occurs more often in preterm and LBW infants, and in anywhere from 15% to 38% of bacteremic infants (Baley & Leonard, 2013, p. 346; Pammi et al., 2016, p. 553; Wilson & Tyner, 2015, p. 694 & 698).
- Meningitis can manifest in EOS or LOS with either vertical or horizontal transmission. EOS is vertically transmitted from the maternal genital tract and occurs within the first week of life, while LOS can be either vertically transmitted from maternal flora or horizontally transmitted from colonized caregivers (Leonard & Dobbs, 2015, p. 737; Wilson & Tyner, 2015, p. 698).
  ○ Within the first week of life, GBS or *E. coli* cause 70% of cases with an additional 5% due to *L. monocytogenes*. After the first week of life coagulase-negative staphylococci are the most common isolates (Ferrieri & Wallen, 2018, p. 563).
  ○ Other less common causative organisms include *Klebsiella, Enterobacter, Citrobacter, Serratia,* and *Candida* (Hostetter & Gleason, 2018, p. 583; Leonard & Dobbs, 2015, p. 737).
- The clinical presentation of meningitis is difficult to distinguish from sepsis. Non-neurologic symptoms include temperature instability, poor feeding, respiratory distress, apnea, and diarrhea. Neurologic signs include irritability, lethargy, poor tone, seizures, and, later, a full or bulging fontanelle. Seizures are more common in Gram-negative meningitis and are usually focal (Ferrieri & Wallen, 2018, pp. 564–565; Leonard & Dobbs, 2015, p. 737; Wilson & Tyner, 2015, pp. 698–699).
- Diagnosis of meningitis requires a full septic workup and must include an LP for CSF cell count, glucose, protein,

Gram stain, and culture. The WBC count and protein levels in the CSF can be difficult to interpret as they vary with gestational and postnatal age (Ferrieri & Wallen, 2018, pp. 564–565; Leonard & Dobbs, 2015, p. 737; Puopolo, 2017, p. 691).
  ○ Generally, CSF glucose will be low and WBC and protein levels high, although up to 10% of infants have normal CSF analysis, leaving culture and Gram stain as the gold standard (Ferrieri & Wallen, 2018, p. 564; Wilson & Tyner, 2015, p. 699).
- Treatment of meningitis requires a tailored antibiotic regimen with repeat CSF cultures to verify sterility. Gram-positive organisms will usually clear within 24 to 48 hours, but Gram-negative organisms may persist.
  ○ Infants are frequently very ill and require supportive therapy with any combination of mechanical ventilation, complex fluid management, vasopressor support, and cardiopulmonary monitoring. Length of treatment depends on the organism and the quickness of CSF clearance; usually 2 weeks after sterilization of Gram positive bacteria and 3 weeks after clearance of Gram-negative organisms (Ferrieri & Wallen, 2018, p. 564; Wilson & Tyner, 2015, p. 700).
- Overall mortality of Gram-positive disease is about 10%, increasing to 40% to 80% when the organism is Gram-negative (Wilson & Tyner, 2015, p. 698).
  ○ The mortality for the two most common causes of meningitis, GBS and *E. coli*, are 30% and 20% to 60% respectively (Ferrieri & Wallen, 2015, p. 564).
  ○ Of the survivors, 40% to 50% have some evidence of neurologic damage due to complications from hydrocephalus, multicystic encephalomalacia, porencephaly, white matter atrophy, abscesses, subdural effusions, and ventriculitis, manifesting as developmental delays, late-onset seizures, cerebral palsy, hearing loss and blindness (Ferrieri & Wallen, 2015, p. 565; Wilson & Tyner, 2015, p. 700).

OSTEOMYELITIS

- Osteomyelitis is an infection of the bone that is uncommon and difficult to diagnose in neonates due to the delayed onset of symptoms. Neonates are susceptible in part because of immature immune responses resulting in vulnerability to organisms not ordinarily virulent (White, Bouchard, & Goldberg, 2018, p. 1448). The most common sites of infection are femur, humerus, tibia, radius, and maxilla (Puopolo, 2017, p. 718).
- There are three causative mechanisms associated with osteomyelitis: bacteremia or hematogenous spread; direct inoculation from a puncture wound; and a contiguous spread from an adjacent infection. The most common of these is hematogenous spread, with the metaphysis as the most common site (Gilmore & Thompson, 2015, p. 1784).
- The structure and circulation of bone during the neonatal period predisposes infants to infection.
  ○ Unlike older children and adults, in the first 12 to 18 months of life the epiphysis and metaphysis are not separated by a formed physis; consequently, their blood supply is linked.
  ○ The epiphyseal and metaphyseal blood flow are connected because the barrier created by the formed physis (growth plate) has yet to completely develop.

This allows bacteria and infection to spread from one to the other and to cross and touch the physeal area. This contact with the forming physis may account for the increased incidence of growth plate damage seen with neonatal osteomyelitis when compared to childhood osteomyelitis (Gilmore & Thompson, 2015, p. 1784).

○ Additionally, blood vessels enter the bone centrally and ascend to the metaphysis, making a 180-degree turn when they reach the physis and emptying into the venous sinusoids. The 180-degree turn creates an area of sluggish blood flow where bacteria can become trapped and proliferate (Gilmore & Thompson, 2015, p. 1784; Leonard & Dobbs, 2015, p. 740).

- The most common organism responsible for osteomyelitis is *S. aureus* with Methicillin-resistant *S. aureus* (MRSA) being particularly destructive. Other common offenders include GBS and *E. coli*, with some cases caused by *Neisseria gonorrhoeae*, candida, other enteric Gram-negative bacteria, and group A streptococcus (Gilmore & Thompson, 2015, p. 1748; Leonard & Dobbs, 2015, p. 740; Puopolo, 2017, p. 718)

- The signs and symptoms of osteomyelitis are subtle, vary with age, and can mimic sepsis, with severity of presentation directly correlated to the health of the infant prior to infection (Gilmore & Thompson, 2015, p. 1785; Leonard & Dobbs, 2015, p. 740).

○ In term, previously healthy neonates' symptoms usually occur around 2 to 4 weeks of life with limited spontaneous movement and pseudoparalysis of the involved extremity, local tenderness, erythema, swelling, and increased warmth. Term infants are less ill, afebrile or run a lower grade fever, and have less leukocytosis and erythrocyte sedimentation rate (ESR) elevation (Gilmore & Thompson, 2015, p. 1785; White et al., 2018, p. 1448).

○ Premature neonates in the NICU commonly present with systemic illness and require prolonged hospitalization. Infants most at risk are those with a history of multiple peripheral and central vascular catheters and repetitive percutaneous arterial blood sampling. Forty percent of these infants have multiple areas of involvement with swelling (White et al., 2018, p. 1448).

- Evaluation of osteomyelitis should initially mimic a septic work up with blood, CSF, and urine cultures along with the culture of any purulent skin lesions (Puopolo, 2017, p. 718). Radiographic testing along with ultrasound and bone aspiration can aid diagnosis. MRI and nuclear scintigraphy may be used. Fluid collection from bone aspirations is positive 70% of the time and blood cultures are positive 50% to 60% of the time (Gilmore & Thompson, 2015, p. 1785; Leonard & Dobbs, 2015, p. 740). It is unusual to have a fever, elevated ESR, or leukocytosis, although CRP is a reliable indicator (White et al., 2018, p. 1448).

○ Ultrasound is the preferred method of diagnosis and evaluation as it detects joint effusions, deep edema, and subperiosteal and soft tissue fluid collection, and can guide aspiration (Gilmore & Thompson, 2015, pp. 1785–1786; White et al., 2018, pp. 1448–1449).

○ Early radiographs may be normal, with soft tissue swelling presenting by 3 days and bone changes at 7 to 10 days. More advanced films will show deep edema;

joint effusion, separation, and dislocation; and even bone destruction (Gilmore & Thompson, 2015, p. 1785; Leonard & Dobbs, 2015, p. 740; White et al., 2018, pp. 1448–1449).

○ MRI and nuclear scintigraphy are both highly sensitive and can be considered. Scintigraphy is useful for identifying multifocal involvement, while MRI provides accurate regional information on both the soft tissue and bones and is highly sensitive in identifying early infection. Unfortunately, both require sedation of the infant and therefore require the balancing of risks versus benefit (White et al., 2018, pp. 1448–1449).

○ Fluid collection in the soft tissue and bone should be aspirated and sent for culture and Gram stain. Aspiration should be done over the point of maximal swelling, bone tenderness, and fluctuation (Gilmore & Thompson, 2015, p. 1785).

- Treatment of uncomplicated osteomyelitis requires antimicrobial therapy for 3 to 6 weeks. If there is abscess formation in the bone or soft tissue or septic arthritis, then surgical drainage and debridement are required followed by immobilization of the affected limb. If the infant is unresponsive to the initial treatment of an isolated infection, suspect that an abscess has formed (Gilmore & Thompson, 2015, p. 1449; White et al., 2018, p. 1449).

- Due to the previously described physiology of neonatal bone, osteomyelitis can lead to epiphyseal and physeal damage, chronic infection and joint infection, or septic arthritis, with septic arthritis occurring in 76% of neonates. Damage to the physis and articular cartilage can cause growth disturbances, limb shortening, angular deformity, physeal closure, loss of motion, and precocious arthritis (Gilmore & Thompson, 2015, p. 1784; White et al., 2018, p. 1449).

- Table 22.4 lists suggested duration of antibiotic therapy based on location.

TABLE 22.4 Duration of Antibiotic Therapy

Location of Disease	Recommended Treatment Time Frame
Bacteremia with a focus	7–10 days
Meningitis	14–21 days
Septic arthritis	14–21 days (up to 4 weeks)
Osteomyelitis	4–6 weeks
Endocarditis or ventriculitis	Up to 4 weeks

Sources: Data from Baley, J. E., & Leonard, E. G. (2013). Infections in the neonate. In A. Fanaroff & A. Fanaroff (Eds.), *Klaus and Fanaroff's care of the high-risk neonate* (6th ed., pp. 346–367). Cleveland, OH: Elsevier; Leonard, E. G., & Dobbs, K. (2015). Postnatal bacterial infections. In R. Martin, A. Fanaroff, & M. Walsh (Eds.), *Fanaroff and Martin's neonatal-perinatal medicine: Diseases of the fetus and infant* (10th ed., pp. 737–741). Philadelphia, PA: Elsevier; Puopolo, K. M. (2017). Bacterial and fungal infections. In Eichenwald et al. (Eds.), *Cloherty and Stark's manual of neonatal care* (8th ed., pp. 641–650, 691–718). Philadelphia, PA: Wolters Kluwer.

BACTERIAL CAUSES OF SEPSIS

Enterococcus

- *Enterococcus faecalis* and *Enterococcus faecium* are responsible for specifically LOS and infections associated with indwelling central line catheters (Puopolo, 2017, p. 702). These organisms resemble coagulase-negative *staphylococcus* (CONS) organisms in their ability to produce a biofilm and slime and adhere to catheter surfaces (Puopolo, 2017, p. 702).
- Approximately 3% of NICU bloodstream infections are attributable to these bacteria (Srinivasan & Evans, 2018, p. 574), but *Enterococcus* spp. can also be associated with meningitis, UTIs, and NEC, but with low overall mortality (Puopolo, 2017, p. 702).
    - Gram-positive organisms such as enterococcus, CONS, *S. aureus*, *L. monocytogens*, and beta hemolytic streptococci contribute to 4% of cases of meningitis, with an approximate mortality rate of 10% (Wilson & Tyner, 2015, p. 698).
    - As a Gram-positive coccus, enterococcus is the third most common organism responsible for UTIs in the neonate, causing 10% to 16% of infections (Wang, Djahangirian, & Wehbi, 2018, p. 1309).
- Enterococci are one of the common fecal organisms found in preterm infants, along with Enterobacteriaceae, *E. coli*, staphylococci, streptococci, *Clostridium* species, and *Bacteroides* species. The colonization of these pathogenic bacteria last longer in preterm infants than in term infants, and this abnormal colonization of the preterm gut is thought to contribute to the pathogenesis of NEC (McElory, Frey, Torres, & Maheshwari, 2018, pp. 1064–1065).

Vancomycin-Resistant Enterococci (VRE)

- Widespread use of antibiotics has caused a mutation of the enterococcus virus leading to the development of VRE (Srinivasan & Evans, 2018, p. 574). VRE has been seen in some NICUs and is difficult to treat (Puopolo, 2017, p. 703). Treatment for VRE should be discussed and decided on in consultation with infectious disease experts and will also require infection control measures such as isolation, barrier precautions, and cohorting of patients (Puopolo, 2017, p. 703; Srinivasan & Evans, 2018, p. 574).

Escherichia Coli

- *E. coli* are aerobic Gram-negative rods that are found universally in human intestinal tract, human vagina, and urinary tract (Puopolo, p. 697, 2017). It is the organism most commonly implicated in neonatal UTI (LOS; Pammi et al., 2016, p. 537).
    - With implementation of IAP for GBS, an increasing proportion of cases of EOS are caused by Gram-negative organisms. Controversy is whether IAP is responsible for increased incidence of Gram-negative, and in particular ampicillin-resistant Gram-negative organisms.
- EOS *E. coli* infections, particularly those complicated with meningitis, are primarily due to strains with the K1-type polysaccharide capsule. Strains with complete LPS and K1 capsule have been shown to specifically evade both complement-mediated bacteriolysis and neutrophil-mediated killing (Puopolo, 2017, p. 697). There is usually little protective maternal antibody of K1 strain available to infant.

Group B Streptococcal

- GBS or *Streptococcus agalactiae* are Gram-positive diplococcus encapsulated bacterium and have been the principal GBS pathogen for over 50 years (Wilson & Tyner, 2015, p. 702).
- GBS is the most common cause of vertically transmitted neonatal sepsis (Baley & Leonard, 2013, p. 348).
    - Factors for GBS can be modified by IAP at least 4 hours prior to delivery (Puopolo, 2017, p. 685).
    - Primary mode of transmission is following rupture of membranes (ROM) and during passage through the birth canal. High genital inoculum at delivery increases the likelihood of transmission and the consequential rate of EOGBS (Baley & Leonard, 2013, p. 348).
- The bacteria are subtyped into 10 distinct serotypes. Most neonatal GBS diseases in the United States are currently caused by types Ia, Ib, II, III, and V GBS, although type III GBS is associated with the development of meningitis and is a common cause of LOS (Puopolo, 2017, p. 693) followed by subtypes 1a and V.
- Virulence has been associated with a polysaccharide capsule, although surface-localized GBS proteins may also be factors (Ferrieri & Wallen, 2018, p. 556).
- GBS disease accounts for 95% of EOS, and more than 90% of LOS in neonates in the United States today (Wilson & Tyner, 2015, p. 702).
    - Neonatal GBS infection is acquired in utero or during passage through the birth canal (Puopolo, 2017, p. 693) and is the most common cause of vertically transmitted neonatal sepsis in the United States today (Baley & Leonard, 2013, p. 348; Leonard & Dobbs, 2015, p. 742).
    - Nearly 50% of infants who pass through colonized birth canal become colonized; however, only 1% to 2% will develop invasive disease (Wilson & Tyner, 2015, p. 703).
    - Documented maternal colonization of GBS is the strongest predictor for GBS EOS (Puopolo, 2017, p. 693).
- GBS or *Streptococcus agalactiae* are a significant cause of maternal bacteriuria and endometritis and a major cause of serious bacterial infection in infants up to 3 months of age (Baley & Leonard, 2013, p. 348).
    - Maternal factors predictive of GBS disease include documented maternal GBS colonization, intrapartum fever (>38°C) and other signs of chorioamnionitis, and prolonged ROM (>18 hours). Primary risk factor is intrapartum maternal colonization of genitourinary or gastrointestinal tract-disease acquired vertically, during passage through the birth canal (Leonard & Dobbs, 2015, p. 742).
    - Neonatal risk factors include prematurity (<37 weeks' gestation) and LBW (<2,500 g; Puopolo, 2017, p. 685).
        - Lack of maternally derived, protective capsular polysaccharide-specific antibody is associated with the development of GBS invasive disease (Ferriere & Wallen, 2018, p. 556; Puopolo, 2017, p. 694).
- Table 22.5 lists maternal and neonatal risk factors of GBS.

INCIDENCE

- Maternal IAP has reduced neonatal EOS GBS disease by 80%, from 1.7 cases per 10,000 live births to 0.28 cases per

TABLE 22.5 Maternal and Neonatal Risk Factors of Group B Streptococcus (GBS)

Maternal	Neonatal
GBS colonization Intrapartum fever (>100.4°F) Chorioamnionitis Premature rupture of membranes Prolonged rupture of membranes (>18 hours) GBS bacteremia	Prematurity (<37 weeks' gestation) Low birthweight (<2,500 g) (Vaginal birth[b])

Sources: Data from Baley, J. E., & Leonard, E. G. (2013). Infections in the neonate. In A. Fanaroff & A. Fanaroff (Eds.), *Klaus and Fanaroff's care of the high-risk neonate* (6th ed., pp. 346–367). Cleveland, OH: Elsevier; Leonard, E. G., & Dobbs, K. (2015). Postnatal bacterial infections. In R. Martin, A. Fanaroff, & M. Walsh (Eds.), *Fanaroff and Martin's neonatal-perinatal medicine: Diseases of the fetus and infant* (10th ed., pp. 737–741). Philadelphia, PA: Elsevier; Puopolo, K. M. (2017). Bacterial and fungal infections. In Eichenwald et al. (Eds.), *Cloherty and Stark's manual of neonatal care* (8th ed., pp. 641–650, 691–718). Philadelphia, PA: Wolters Kluwer; Wilson, D. J., & Tyner, C. I. (2015). Infectious diseases in the neonate. In T. Verklan & M. Walden (Eds.), *Core curriculum for neonatal intensive care nursing* (5th ed., pp. 689–718). St. Louis, MO: Elsevier.

1,000 live births, per 2010 CDC data (Leonard & Dobbs, 2015, p. 743; Puopolo, 2017, p. 694). However, despite the implementation of IAP, GBS remains the leading cause of EOS in term infants (Puopolo, 2017, p. 694).

○ Neither maternal IAP nor neonatal antibiotic administration prevents the development of primary onset GBS disease infection ≥7 days of life (LOS GBS disease; Leonard & Dobbs, 2015, p. 743; Puopolo, 2017, p. 695).

• Infants whose mothers received IAP are less likely to have sepsis, need assisted mechanical ventilation, or have documented GBS bacteremia (Wilson & Tyner, 2015, p. 703).

• Neonatal GBS EOS without a focus accounts for approximately 80% to 85% of cases, however the overall incidence of GBS EOS has fallen to 0.24 cases per 1,000 births.

○ Fifty percent of the cases of GBS LOS are attributed to vertical transmission at birth or horizontal transmission in household or community settings (Wilson & Tyner, 2015, p. 703).

○ One-quarter of all GBS EOS occurs among infants >37 weeks—most GBS EOS occurs in culture-negative antepartum screens, although culture surveillance remains standard (Puopolo, 2017, p. 695).

○ Black infants are at a higher risk for GBS EOS disease by nearly three times White infants (Puopolo, 2017, p. 694; Wilson & Tyner, 2015, p. 703), as well as, infants born to mothers who are less than 20 years of age, although the exact etiology is unclear (Puopolo, 2017, p. 694).

MATERNAL EVALUATION

• The 2010 CDC guidelines for maternal surveillance of GBS includes rectal and vaginal screening at 35 to 37 weeks' gestation for all women, except those with bacteremia during the current pregnancy and those with a history of

previous infant with GBS invasive disease, as these women should receive IAP regardless of GBS culture results.

○ *Adequate IAP* includes administration of penicillin, ampicillin, or cefazolin at least 4 hours prior to delivery (Puopolo, 2017, pp. 695–696).

○ If GBS IAP was indicated *but inadequate*, limited diagnostic evaluation only if other risk factors for EOS are present, such as GA < 37 weeks and/or ROM >18 hours (Puopolo, 2017, p. 696).

○ Pregnant women in preterm labor with *unknown GBS status*: If ≥37 weeks, IAP is recommended if maternal fever ≥100.5°F occurs or ROM >18 hours prior to delivery.

○ Cesarean section delivery with intact membranes does not require antibiotic treatment (Leonard & Dobbs, 2015, p. 742).

○ Table 22.6 describes the evaluation of an infant for GBS disease.

TREATMENT

• Although to date no studies have shown an association between penicillin and ampicillin IAP and the emergence of antibiotic resistance in other bacteria, this risk remains a concern (Baley & Leonard, 2013, p. 348).

○ Thirty percent of GBS isolates are resistant to erythromycin, while 20% are resistant to clindamycin (Leonard & Dobbs, 2015, p. 743).

• Penicillin remains preferred agent (Wilson & Tyner, p. 703, 2015) and is the narrowest spectrum agent (Baley & Leonard, 2013, p. 348), with ampicillin acceptable alternative. Other acceptable alternatives include 1st+2nd cephalosporin and vancomycin (Leonard & Dobbs, 2015, p. 743).

• Recurrent GBS infections are infrequent (1%–6%).

• Mortality from GBS disease is highest in preterm infants or LBW infants.

TABLE 22.6 Evaluation of Infant for Group B Streptococcus (GBS) Disease

Asymptomatic infant	Symptomatic infant
If signs/symptoms of maternal chorioamnionitis present: Limited evaluation recommended and includes: CBC with differential Blood cultures Empiric antibiotic therapy • Inadequate IAP (<4 hours prior to delivery)	Full diagnostic evaluation includes: CBC with differential Blood culture Lumbar puncture including CSF culture Chest radiograph Empiric antibiotic therapy

CBC, complete blood count; CSF, cerebrospinal fluid; IAP, intrapartum antibiotic prophylaxis.

Source: Data from Puopolo, K. M. (2017). Bacterial and fungal infections. In Eichenwald et al. (Eds.), *Cloherty and Stark's manual of neonatal care* (8th ed., pp. 641–650, 691–718). Philadelphia, PA: Wolters Kluwer.

KLEBSIELLA SPECIES (SPP.)

- Gram-negative organisms such as *Klebsiella* spp and *E. coli* are leading causes of LOS and nosocomial infections (Puopolo, 2017, p. 699) and are important causes of bloodstream infections, meningitis, and pneumonia. These bacteria are responsible for 15% of NICU infections and are associated with up to a 3.5-fold higher risk of death as opposed to Gram-positive bacteria (Srinivasan & Evans, 2018, p. 574).
- With the introduction of intrapartum prophylaxis of GBS, Gram-negative enteric bacteria-like *Klebsiella* are increasingly responsible for EOS in term and preterm infants (Baley & Leonard, 2013, p. 346; Puopolo, 2017, p. 693). *Klebsiella* is a common cause of early-onset neonatal pneumonia and can result in lung injury, abscess formation, empyema, and pneumatoceles (Leonard & Dobbs, 2015, p. 738).
- *Klebsiella* can also be the offending organism in UTIs and omphalitis (Leonard & Dobbs, 2015, p. 739 & p. 741).
  - ○ Neonatal UTIs are commonly caused by Gram-negative rods, with *E. coli* (40%–72%) and *Klebsiella* species (7%–40%) responsible for over 80% of cases. In addition, *Klebsiella pneumonia* has a higher incidence in neonates with vesicular urethral reflux (VUR) presenting with a UTI compared with those without VUR (Wang et al., 2018, pp. 1309–1310).
  - ○ Omphalitis is a bacterial infection of the umbilical stump that presents around day 3 of life. It is commonly caused by *S. aureus*, *S. epidermidis*, *Streptococcus* spp, *E. coli*, *Clostridium difficile*, *Klebsiella*, and *Pseudomonas* (Boos & Sidbury, 2018, p. 1497).

Pseudomonas spp

- Pseudomonas is noted as a cause of EOS and LOS, specifically bloodstream infections, meningitis, omphalitis, UTIs, and pneumonia. In preterm infants, *Pseudomonas*, along with other Gram-negative enteric bacteria, are a leading cause of EOS (Puopolo, 2017, p. 693). Of particular interest is the species *Pseudomonas aeruginosa*, which can be quite wide-reaching and virulent (Boos & Sidbury, 2018; Leonard & Dobbs, 2015; Puopolo, 2017; Srinivasan & Evans, 2018; Wilson & Tyner, 2015). According to the National Institute of Child Health and Human Development, Gram-negative LOS is associated with an overall 40% mortality rate (Puopolo, 2017, p. 703).
- *Pseudomonas* thrives in moist environments, such as respiratory equipment, and can lead to colonization of the respiratory tract (Srinivasan & Evans, 2018, p. 571). *P. aeruginosa* pneumonia can cause pneumatoceles (Wilson & Tyner, 2015, p. 701).
- *P. aeruginosa* is particularly virulent in LBW babies, with a mortality rate as high as 76%. This is due to its bacterial factors: a lipopolysaccharide outer membrane (endotoxin), mucoid capsule, adhesins, invasins, and toxins, specifically exotoxin A.
  - ○ Nosocomial acquisition and IV antibiotic exposure lead to overcolonization of this bacteria in the preterm gut. This is due in part to *Pseudomonas*' resistance to most common antibiotics. A severe illness during or after prolonged exposure to common antibiotics should trigger suspicion for *Pseudomonas*-induced LOS (Puopolo, 2017, p. 703).
  - ○ Of Gram-negative bacteria *P. aeruginosa* is a less common cause of meningitis, an infection of the central nervous system (Wilson & Tyner, 2015, p. 698). *P. aeruginosa* can cause a rare and devastating form of bacterial

conjunctivitis, requiring IV antibiotics (Puopolo, 2017, p. 716).
- *Pseudomonas* causes LOS, and nosocomial infections, specifically bloodstream infections, meningitis, and pneumonia. In these instances, it is frequently resistant to ß-lactamase antibiotics (Leonard & Dobbs, 2015, p. 737; Srinivasan & Evans, 2018, p. 574). *Pseudomonas* is particularly virulent among the enteric bacteria, causing death in 42% to 75% of infected neonates (Srinivasan & Evans, 2018, p. 574).
- As opposed to simple UTIs commonly caused by *E. coli* and *Klebsiella*, UTIs that are associated with VUR have distinctly different bacterial etiology, including *P. aeruginosa* (Wang et al., 2018, p. 1309).
  - ○ *Pseudomonas* can cause omphalitis, an infection of the umbilical stump (Boos & Sidbury, 2018, p. 1497).

Coagulase-Negative Staphylococci (CONS or CNS)

- This describes a heterogeneous group of Gram-positive organisms with structure similar to *S. aureus*. These bacteria lack protein A and have different cell wall components (Puopolo, 2017, pp. 700–701). CONS is a facultative anaerobic Gram-positive organism frequently found in respiratory tract and on skin (Leonard & Dobbs, 2015, p. 743).
- *S. epidermidis* is the most common species of CONS recovered from human skin and mucous membranes (Baley & Leonard, 2013, p. 349; Leonard & Dobbs, 2015, p. 743) and is the primary cause of NICU disease (Baley & Leonard, 2013, pp. 348–349; Puopolo, 2017, p. 701).
  - ○ Most infants are colonized within the first week of life from passage through the birth canal and repeated exposure from colonized caregivers (Baley & Leonard, 2013, p. 349).
  - ○ Neonates most common source of LOS, but does not commonly occur in first 72 hours (Leonard & Dobbs, 2015, p. 743).
  - ○ Bloodstream infections caused by CONS are much more prevalent than bacteremia caused by *S. aureus* (Baley & Leonard, 2013, p. 350) and are most commonly associated with umbilical or central venous lines (Leonard & Dobbs, 2015, p. 743).
    - Believed to first colonize central catheter surfaces, polysaccharide surface adhesion (PSA) adheres to catheter surfaces biofilm and slime production inhibit host defenses to eliminate organisms (Puopolo, 2017, p. 701).
- Infants may present with systemic instability, temporary cessation of enteral feeding, escalated respiratory support, and is associated with prolonged hospitalizations and poorer neurodevelopmental outcomes. Typically, infants present without localizing signs, such as fever, new-onset respiratory distress, or deterioration in respiratory status (Puopolo, 2017, p. 701).
  - ○ Other common nonspecific signs include apnea, bradycardia, poikilothermia, poor perfusion, poor feeding, irritability, and lethargy (Baley & Leonard, 2013, p. 349), as well as, pneumonia, conjunctivitis, and skin and soft tissue infections (SSTIs; Leonard & Dobbs, 2015, p. 743).
- Indolent disease is more common than fulminant disease, and mortality is generally under 15%. However, CONS are a major source of morbidity leading to increased antibiotic exposure, length of stay, and hospital costs (Baley & Leonard, 2013, p. 349).

○ Rarely fatal, and rarely causes meningitis or site-specific disease (Puopolo, 2017, p. 701).

○ Neonatal infection may be associated with maternal infection: mastitis, cellulitis, or cesarean section wound infection (Leonard & Dobbs, 2015, p. 743).

Staphylococcus aureus

• *S. aureus* is an encapsulated Gram-positive organism that may result in multiple adhesions, produce virulence-associated enzymes, and/or release toxins to cause a wide range of systemic dysfunctions, including bacteremia, meningitis, cellulitis, omphalitis, osteomyelitis, and arthritis (Puopolo, 2017, pp. 701–702).

• *S. aureus* differs from CONS by the production of coagulase and the presence of protein A, which is a component of the cell wall that contributes to virulence by binding to a portion of the IgG antibody and blocks the body's ability to break down the bacteria (Puopolo, 2017, pp. 701–702), however *S. aureus* is identical to CONS under light microscopy (Baley & Leonard, 2013, p. 350).

○ It is normal skin flora, which can cause a much wider and potentially more invasive disease than CONS through production of numerous toxins, enzymes, and binding proteins that facilitate its ability to establish possible life-threatening pyogenic infection (Baley & Leonard, p. 350, 2013).

• Symptoms of *S. aureus* disease begin after the first week of life (Leonard & Dobbs, 2015, p. 743).

• Frequently complicated with focal site infections: soft tissue, bone/joint infections, and marked by persistent bacteremia despite antibiotic administration (Puopolo, 2017, pp. 701–702)

○ Joint infections often require open reduction—may lead to joint destruction and permanent disability (Baley & Leonard, 2013, p. 350; Puopolo, 2017, pp. 701–702).

○ Small-inoculum colonization or infection can cause catastrophic, toxin-mediated disease—that is, scalded skin syndrome or toxic shock (Baley & Leonard, 2013, p. 350).

• LOS caused by *S. aureus* can result in significant morbidity (Puopolo, 2017, pp. 701–702).

TREATMENT OF *S. AUREUS*

• Most resistant to penicillin, semisynthetic penicillins, and gentamicin

○ Empiric therapy commonly includes vancomycin (Puopolo, 2017, p. 701) or nafcillin (Leonard & Dobbs, 2015, p. 743).

○ Commonly treatment of CONS often requires vancomycin, as more than 80% of strains acquired in the hospital are resistant to beta-lactam antibiotics (Baley & Leonard, 2013, p. 349).

• Nafcillin is appropriate for methicillin-susceptible *S. aureus* (MSSA; Leonard & Dobbs, 2015, p. 743; Puopolo, pp. 701–702, 2017); however, vancomycin is the preferred treatment for MRSA in neonates (Leonard & Dobbs, 2015, p. 743).

• Clindamycin or linezolid—can be used as alternative to vancomycin; however, it should be noted that clindamycin is bacteriostatic, not bactericidal, and should not be used for bacteremia or severe infection (Leonard & Dobbs, 2015, p. 743).

○ More than 50% of CONS are resistant to clindamycin, trimethoprim–sulfamethoxazole, gentamicin, and ciprofloxacin and others isolated from hospital patients show varying rates of antibiotic resistance to tetracyclines, chloramphenicol, rifampin, and newer generation of quinolone antibiotics.

• Some CONS show resistance to vancomycin (VRSA), but these species are susceptible to the newer agents for Gram-positive organisms: linezolid, quinupristin-dalfopristin, and daptomycin. There is little pharmacokinetic data and clinical experience with these agents in neonates, therefore consult specialty MD with experience in infectious diseases.

• Most effective treatment includes systemic antibiotic and removal of foreign body, but if the device cannot be removed, consult an infectious disease specialist to determine best antimicrobial agents and duration of therapy treatment combination (Baley & Leonard, 2013, p. 350).

• Empiric treatment for *Staphylococcus* skin and soft tissue infections (SSTIs) includes vancomycin, clindamycin, and linezolid.

○ Localized pustulosis and omphalitis without associated cellulitis or systemic symptoms can be treated with topical antibiotics, that is, mupirocin.

○ Cellulitis may be treated with oral or parenteral antibiotics (Leonard & Dobbs, 2015, p. 743).

Alternative Treatment Options

• Infants who clinically improve and have a negative blood culture or CSF culture can be switched to oral therapy. Infants with systemic symptoms (especially, preterm infants and LBW infants) should be treated with parenteral antibiotics.

○ Oral therapy options: cephalexin, clindamycin, and amoxicillin clavulanate with a total duration of treatment for 7 to 14 days.

○ There is little evidence for the treatment of healthy, full-term newborns with mild, localized *S. aureus* skin infections (Leonard & Dobbs, 2015, p. 743).

Methicillin Resistant Staphylococcus Aureus (MRSA)

• MRSA isolates categorized as hospital associated (HA-MRSA) or community associated (CA-MRSA) and can be rapidly spread in NICU by nosocomial transmission on hands of caregivers (Puopolo, 2017, p. 702).

○ Drug resistant *S. aureus* (MRSA) is a problem for all ages (Leonard & Dobbs, 2015, p. 743) and is increasingly a recognized pathogen in NICU.

○ During the last two decades, MRSA has shown increasing resistance to beta-lactamase antibiotics, all penicillins, penicillin-beta-lactamase inhibitor combination drugs, cephalosporins, and carbapenems, and most hospital-acquired strains are resistant to clindamycin (Baley & Leonard, 2013, p. 350).

○ Community MRSA has developed an additional virulence factor which has a significant increase in pyogenic infection by MRSA (Baley & Leonard, p. 350, 2013; Puopolo, 2017, p. 702), and may present in previously healthy neonates as pustulosis, cellulitis, skin abscess, or mastitis with invasive disease and bacteremia, UTI, pneumonia, or musculoskeletal infections (Leonard & Dobbs, 2015, p. 743).

• Infection of MRSA can be complicated with deep tissue involvement and persistent bacteremia that may require surgical debridement for resolution.

- MRSA infections require treatment with vancomycin (Baley & Leonard, p. 350, 2013; Leonard & Dobbs, 2015, p. 743; Puopolo, 2017, p. 702).
  - ○ Routine surveillance, cohorting, and isolation of colonized infants may be required to prevent spread and persistence of organism (Puopolo, 2017, p. 702).
  - ○ Drugs with activity against MRSA include tetracycline and trimethoprim sulfamethoxazole, but these are typically avoided in neonates.
  - ○ Consultation with an infectious disease specialist is recommended when the treatment of MRSA in a neonate is complicated (Baley & Leonard, 2013, p. 351).
  - ○ Rifampin can be used as adjunctive therapy for persistent MRSA infection, but not as single agent. Consultation with an infectious disease specialist is recommended for persistent MRSA infection (Puopolo, 2017, p. 702).

VIRAL INFECTIONS

The following section will review neonatal viral infections. Overall risk factors, incidence, and organisms, as well as treatment recommendations, will be discussed.

Cytomegalovirus

- CMV is a member of the herpes virus family (Permar, 2017, p. 642).
- Hallmark of the virus is the histologic presence of large cells with generous amounts of cytoplasm (cytomegaly) and "inclusion-bearing" cells in both the nucleus and cytoplasm (Permar, 2017, p. 642; Schleis & Marsh, 2018, p. 494).
- Infection with the virus results in lifelong disease (Permar, 2017, p. 642).

INCIDENCE

- The incidence of CMV is 0.5% to 2% of live births, or about 40,000 infants born in the United States (Schleis & Marsh, 2018, p. 494).
  - ○ Most common cause of congenital infection in the United States. Infants are at high risk for brain damage and birth defects (Permar, 2017, p. 644).
- In the United States, the seropositivity rate in women is 50% to 85%, whereas in undeveloped countries, the seropositivity rate in women is as high as 90% (Baley & Leonard, 2013, pp. 353–354).

EPIDEMIOLOGY

- The virus may be found in body fluids of saliva, urine, blood and blood products, breastmilk, and genital fluids (cervical and seminal secretions; Permar, 2017, p. 644; Wilson & Tyner, 2014, p. 708)
- Transmitted horizontally and vertically.
  - ○ Horizontal transmission results from by person-to-person contact with virus-containing secretions.
- If fresh donor milk is indicated, only use breastmilk from CMV seronegative women. Horizontal transmission can be decreased through pasteurization of breastmilk.
- For blood/blood product transfusions, use only CMV-negative blood products.

- ○ CMV transmission through blood products can be minimized or eliminated by freezing the RBCs in glycerol before administration or by a specified filtration process (Wilson & Tyner, 2014, p. 708).
- Good handwashing techniques and wearing gloves when handling body fluids can reduce the spread of CMV infection (Pammi et al., 2016, p. 539).

RISK FACTORS

- Single, unmarried women of non-White race; immunocompromised individuals, including neonates; infected breastmilk exposure in the premature neonate and/or transfused with unscreened blood products (Permar, 2017, p. 646; Schleis & Marsh, 2018, pp. 495–498)

PRESENTATION AND EVALUATION

- Peripartum or intrapartum infections do not commonly present with clinical illness unless infant is immunocompromised, that is, preterm neonate. Eighty-five percent of infants born with CMV are asymptomatic at birth but may present with disabilities later in childhood. Most severe sequelae are associated with a primary or acute infection during the first trimester of pregnancy (Permar, 2017, p. 644; Wilson & Tyner, 2013, p. 708).
- Testing using polymerase chain reaction (PCR) can be done on blood, urine, or saliva by viral isolation in tissue culture from the infant's urine or saliva, and by spin-enhanced urine culture (Baley & Leonard, 2013; Greenberg, Narendran, Schibler, Warner, & Haberman, 2014, p. 1236; Wilson & Tyner, 2014, p. 708).
  - ○ Testing of CMV should be completed within 2 weeks after birth to differentiate congenital infection from perinatal or postnatal infection.
  - ○ Testing completed after 3 weeks of age may represent a perinatal infection (Schleis & Marsh, 2018, p. 497).
  - ○ Table 22.7 presents clinical findings of congenital CMV infection

TREATMENT AND OUTCOMES

- Ganciclovir is the antiviral of choice for congenital CMV infection with proven CNS involvement.
- If the infection is acquired peripartum or postnatally, ganciclovir is not recommended due to the potential toxic side effects (Greenberg et al., 2014, p. 1236; Wilson & Tyner, 2014, p. 708).
- Primary CMV infection during the first trimester of pregnancy carries the greatest risk of neonatal congenital infection and the highest (as high as 30%) mortality rate (Baley & Leonard, 2013, p. 355).
- Only 10% to 15% of neonates with congenital CMV will have symptomatic CMV infection.
  - ○ 90% of infants with congenital CMV are asymptomatic at birth, however, may have sensorineural hearing loss (SNHL) later in childhood.
- Term infants who contract CMV during the peripartum or postnatal period are usually asymptomatic.
- Preterm or immunocompromised who contract CMV during the peripartum or postnatal period may develop systemic CMV disease (Permar, 2017, p. 645).
- Figure 22.1 identifies outcomes of CMV-exposed neonates.

TABLE 22.7 Clinical Findings of Congenital Cytomegalovirus (CMV) Infection

Timing of presentation	Clinical findings
Prenatal signs of CMV infection	• Fetal growth restriction • Cerebral periventricular echogenicity or calcifications • Cerebral ventriculomegaly • Microcephaly • Polymicrogyria • Cerebellar hypoplasia • Hyperechogenic fetal bowel • Hepatosplenomegaly • Amniotic fluid abnormalities • Ascites and/or pleural effusions • Placental enlargement
Symptoms present at birth: 1. Fulminant infection (congenital symptomatic CMV infection) 2. Nonlife-threatening infection	• Intrauterine growth restriction • Hepatosplenomegaly with jaundice, abnormal LFTs • Thrombocytopenia with or without purpura • Severe central nervous system involvement (50%–90% of symptomatic newborns) • Neurologic complications (microcephaly, intracerebral calcifications, chorioretinitis) • Hemolytic anemia • Pneumonitis • IUGR • Microcephaly • Cranial calcifications • Sensorineural hearing loss
Asymptomatic at birth: Late or subclinical disease	• Infancy to the first 2 years of life • Developmental abnormalities • Hearing loss • Seizures • Mental retardation • Motor spasticity • Acquired microcephaly • Visual impairment

IUGR, intrauterine growth restriction; LFT, liver function tests.

Source: Data from Permar, S. R. (2017). Bacterial and fungal infections. In Eichenwald et al. (Eds.), *Cloherty and Stark's manual of neonatal care* (8th ed., pp. 641–650). Philadelphia, PA: Wolters Kluwer.

Enterovirus

INCIDENCE

• Human enteroviruses (HEV) are single-stranded RNA viruses and belong to one of the two genera in the Picornaviridae family (Permar, 2017, p. 67; Schleis & Marsh, 2018, p. 508). They are the most commonly diagnosed viruses in the NICU (Pammi et al., 2016, p. 544).

• HEVs are classified into four major groups: coxsackievirus group A, coxsackievirus group B, echovirus, and polio virus.

  ○ Most congenital enteroviruses are caused by coxsackie B and echoviruses, with 70% caused by echovirus 11 (Permar, 2017, p. 677).

• Infections can occur throughout the year in tropical climates, but are more common between July and November in temperate climates (Permar, 2017, p. 677; Wilson & Tyner, 2015, p. 710).

  ○ Enteroviruses are also responsible for a large portion of febrile infants under 2 months of age who are readmitted to hospitals, and the cause for neonatal aseptic meningitis (Schleis & Marsh, 2018, p. 508).

EPIDEMIOLOGY

• In the general population, transmission of HEV is primarily through fecal-oral or respiratory routes. Perinatally, the virus can spread in utero transplacentally (Permar, 2017, p. 677); intrapartum through contact with maternal blood, fecal material, or vaginal or cervical secretions (Schleis & Marsh, 2018, p. 508); and postpartum, HEV may be spread through breastfeeding (Wilson & Tyner, 2015, p. 544).

RISK FACTORS

• Risk factors for severe infection in the neonate include prematurity, early onset of disease (less than 7 days of age) and a maternal history of illness with a high white count (15,000/mm³ or greater) and low hemoglobin (less than 10.7 g/dL; Pammi et al., 2016, p. 544).

PRESENTATION AND EVALUATION

• Infants exposed to maternal HEV infection in utero are often asymptomatic at birth; however, 50% will develop generalized symptoms such as fever, coryza, poor feeding, and vomiting within five days after birth (Permar, 2017, p. 677; Schleis & Marsh, 2018, p. 509).

• A mother who presents with a febrile illness and negative cultures may have an enteroviral infection, although most enterovirus infections are asymptomatic (Pammi et al., 2016, p. 544) and, therefore, there may be no clinical history of symptoms.

  ○ Mothers infected prior to term are at risk of preterm delivery (Schleis & Marsh, 2018, p. 509).

• Most infants are asymptomatic. Clinical symptoms may manifest during the first 2 weeks of life, which may be mild to severe multiorgan involvement and include rash, aseptic meningitis, hepatitis, pneumonia (Permar, 2017, p. 677; Schleis & Marsh, 2018, p. 509).

  ○ Other symptoms that have been documented in HEV are respiratory symptoms, including (bronchiolitis and pneumonia) pulmonary edema and hemorrhage, hand–foot and mouth disease, meningitis, encephalitis, paralysis, vomiting, diarrhea, hepatitis, acute hemorrhagic conjunctivitis, myocarditis, sepsis, and coagulopathy (Wilson & Tyner, 2015, p. 711).

  ○ There may be an association between sudden infant death syndrome (SIDS) and viral infections with enterovirus as the most common isolate (Schleis & Marsh, 2018, p. 508).

• A neonate commonly presents with one of three major clinical entities: meningoencephalitis, myocarditis, or a sepsis-like presentation. A septic-like presentation has the highest mortality (Permar, 2017, p. 677).

• HEV is rare in neonates; however, if there is an outbreak of similar symptoms in the NICU and there is an increased incidence in the general population, the practitioner should be suspicious of enteroviral infection (Schleis & Marsh, 2018, p. 508).

• Evaluation includes a thorough history of recent viral illness of all family members, complete physical exam, and to differentiate viral sepsis from bacterial sepsis (Permar, 2017, p. 677).

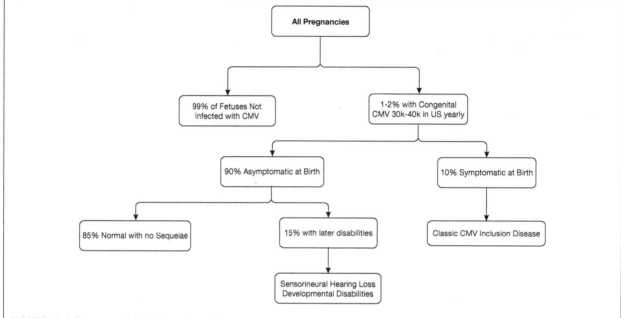

FIGURE 22.1 Outcomes of CMV-exposed neonates

Sources: Baley, J. E., & Leonard, E. G. (2013). Infections in the neonate. In A. Fanaroff & A. Fanaroff (Eds.), *Klaus and Fanaroff's care of the high-risk neonate* (6th ed., pp. 346–367). Cleveland, OH: Elsevier; Greenberg, J. M., Narendran, V., Schibler, K. R., Warner, B. B., & Haberman, B. E. (2014). Neonatal morbidities of prenatal and perinatal origin. In R. Resnik, R. K. Creasy, J. D. Iams, C. J. Lockwood, T. Moore, & M. F. Greene (Eds.), *Creasy & Resnik's maternal-fetal medicine principles and practice* (7th ed., pp. 1215–1239.e7). St. Louis, MO: Elsevier; Permar, S. R. (2017). Bacterial and fungal infections. In Eichenwald et al. (Eds.), *Cloherty and Stark's manual of neonatal care* (8th ed., pp. 641–650). Philadelphia, PA: Wolters Kluwer; Wilson, D. J., & Tyner, C. I. (2015). Infectious diseases in the neonate. In T. Verklan & M. Walden (Eds.), *Core curriculum for neonatal intensive care nursing* (5th ed., pp. 689–718). St. Louis, MO: Elsevier.

○ Cultures are the gold standard, however may take up to a week or longer (Schleis & Marsh, 2018, p. 509). Viral infection evaluation requires cultures from rectal swab, nasopharyngeal swab, blood, and urine.

- Reverse transcription PCR (RT-PCR) assay for HEV can be obtained from nasopharyngeal swab, blood, urine, or CSF (Wilson & Tyner, 2015, p. 711).
  ○ RT-PCR is the most sensitive and specific for CSF (Schleis & Marsh, 2018, p. 509).

TREATMENT AND OUTCOMES
- For most cases of enterovirus, supportive care is adequate. For those infants with severe, life-threatening disease, high-dose immune globulin has been found to be beneficial (Permar, 2017, p. 678)
- There are no approved antiviral agents; however, the antiviral drug pleconaril is under investigation in the use of enteroviral infection (Pammi et al., 2016, p. 544; Wilson & Tyner, 2015, p. 711).
- If a pregnant woman is suspected of having an enteroviral infection, it would be prudent to delay delivery until the acute infection is over, thus allowing transplacental passage of maternal antibodies that will decrease the severity of an infection in the neonate (Permar, 2017, p. 678).
- Broad spectrum antibiotics and acyclovir are recommended until bacterial cultures and herpes simplex virus (HSV) cultures are negative. Other therapies for treatment of infants with severe HEV infection include eomycin (administered prophylactically to reduce intestinal flora; Permar, 2017, p. 678) and pleconaril (Schleis & Marsh, 2018, p. 510).

- Outcomes in terms of mortality and long-term morbidity are directly proportional to the severity of the disease and, therefore, neonates who present with more severe clinical disease tend to have greater long-term morbidities (Wilson & Tyner, 2105, p. 711).
  ○ High mortality rates are associated with the combination of severe hepatitis, coagulopathy, and myocarditis. Additionally, the presence of DIC has a poor prognosis (Schleis & Marsh, 2018, p. 510).
  ○ Most infants with congenital or neonatal HEV infection recover completely without morbidities (Schleis & Martin, 2018, p. 510).
  ○ If central nervous system (CNS) infection is present there is a small incidence of intellectual impairment.

Hepatitis B Virus

INCIDENCE
- It is a DNA virus and one of the most common causes of acute and chronic hepatitis worldwide.
- HBV has a spherical structure with a double shell: HBV concentrates in the hepatic parenchymal cells and circulates in the blood (Schleis & Marsh, 2018, p. 513).
  ○ The outer surface lipoprotein layer (HBsAg) and inner core nucleocapsid layer (HBcAg). A regulatory X protein and viral polymerase soluble antigen (HBeAg) are also present (Greenberg et al., 2014, pp. 1236–1237; Permar, 2017, pp. 668–672).
  ○ HBV may remain in blood for days to years (Schleis & Marsh, 2018, p. 513).

EPIDEMIOLOGY

- Transmission is by the following mechanisms (Permar, 2017, p. 669; Schleis & Martin, 2018, pp. 514–515):
  - Transplacental—either during pregnancy or at the time of delivery secondary to placental leaks. Rarely do the viral antigens cross the placenta.
    - Occurrence more likely if mother is HBeAg-positive.
  - Natal transmission—by exposure during labor and delivery to HBV in amniotic fluid, vaginal secretions, or maternal blood.
  - Postnatal transmission may be by fecal–oral spread, blood transfusion, or other means (Greenberg et al., 2014, pp. 1236–1237; Permar, 2017, pp. 668–672; Schleis & Marsh, 2018, p. 513; Wilson & Tyner, 2014, p. 710).
  - Age at the time of acute infection is the primary determinant of risk of progression to chronic Hepatitis B infection:
    - For neonates born to mothers who are HBsAg-positive and HBeAg-positive, the risk of acquiring HBV is higher than if HBsAg-positive alone. HBsAg has been found in breastmilk of HBsAg-positive mothers, but transmission not documented. With use of appropriate immunoprophylaxis breastfeeding is safe (Greenberg et al., 2014, pp. 1236–1237; Schleis & Marsh, 2018, p. 514; Wilson & Tyner, 2014, p. 710).

RISK FACTORS

- The virus is highly transmissible via contact with blood and/or body fluids or infected individuals (Permar, 2017, pp. 668–672).
  - Mother with HBsAg, especially with HBeAg present; especially if born in endemic areas such as Alaskan natives and Pacific Islanders, or native of China, Southeast Asia, the majority of Africa, and parts of the Middle East
  - Persons with high-risk behavior, for example: IV drug use, multiple sex partners, close contacts with HBV-infected persons, persons receiving multiple blood products or blood product transfusions, and healthcare workers (Permar, 2017, pp. 668–672).

PRESENTATION AND EVALUATION

- Neonates with an HBV infection are usually asymptomatic at birth due to the long incubation period of the virus (Pammi et al., 2016, pp. 547–548; Wilson & Tyner, 2014, p. 710). Without appropriate immunoprophylaxis a percentage will become HBsAg-positive within 4 to 12 weeks. When they become HBsAg-positive it places them at risk for becoming chronically infected and therefore at risk of having chronic hepatitis, cirrhosis, or hepatocellular carcinoma as an adult (Pammi et al., 2016, pp. 547–548; Schleis & Marsh, 2018, p. 513; Wilson & Tyner, 2014, p. 710).
- Without immunoprophylaxis, clinical findings between 2 and 6 months of age may include:
  - Jaundice, hepatomegaly, and mild prolonged enzyme level elevations as well as development of antibodies, followed by either recovery or chronic active hepatitis. Rarely, fulminant hepatitis is seen and can be fatal.
  - Fever
  - Anorexia (Schleis & Marsh, 2018, p. 51; Wilson & Tyner, 2014, p. 710)
- The diagnosis of HBV is made by specific serologies with the detection of viral antigens and antibodies as described below:

- Hepatitis B surface antigen (HBsAg) is a protein on the surface of the HBV, usually found 1 to 2 months after exposure and lasts a variable period of time. Any patient positive with HBsAg is potentially infectious.
- Hepatitis B surface antibody (Anti-HBs or HBsAb) appears after resolution of infection or immunization and indicates immunity.
- Hepatitis B core antigen (HBcAg) assists in differentiating between natural immunity from disease and immunity from vaccination.
- Hepatitis B core antibody (Anti-HBc or HBcAb) is present with all HBV infections and lasts for an indefinite period of time.
- IgM antibody to hepatitis B core antigen (Anti-HBc IgM) appears early in infection, is detectable for 4 to 6 months after infection, and is a good marker for acute or recent infection.
- Hepatitis B e antigen (HBeAg) is present in both acute and chronic infections and correlates with viral replication and high infectivity.
- Hepatitis B e antibody (Anti-HBeAg or HBeAb) develops with resolution of viral replication and indicates resolving infection (Permar, 2017, pp. 668–672).
- Hepatitis B DNA (HBV DNA) is measured by PCR and the concentration correlates with amount of virus present.
- Table 22.8 outlines interpretation of hepatitis B serologies.

TABLE 22.8 Interpretation of Hepatitis B Serologies

HBsAg **anti-HBc** **anti-HBs**	Negative Negative Negative	Susceptible
HBsAg **anti-HBc** **anti-HBs**	Negative Positive Positive	Immune due to natural infection
HBsAg **anti-HBc** **anti-HBs**	Negative Negative Positive	Immune due to hepatitis B vaccination
HBsAg **anti-HBc** **IgM anti-HBc** **anti-HBs**	Positive Positive Positive Negative	Acutely infected
HBsAg **anti-HBc** **IgM anti-HBc** **anti-HBs**	Positive Positive Negative Negative	Chronically infected
HBsAg **anti-HBc** **anti-HBs**	Negative Positive Negative	Interpretation unclear; four possibilities: 1. Resolved infection (most common) 2. False-positive anti-HBc, thus susceptible 3. "Low-level" chronic infection 4. Resolving acute infection

Source: Adapted from A Comprehensive Immunization Strategy to Eliminate Transmission of Hepatitis B Virus Infection in the United States: Recommendations of the Advisory Committee on Immunization Practices. Part I: Immunization of Infants, Children, and Adolescents. MMWR 2005;54 (No. RR-16).

- An HBV DNA PCR may assist in confirming the diagnosis but also to assess the viral load and monitor the response to therapy.
- Baseline and follow-up of the infant's liver function, including aspartate aminotransferase (AST), alanine transaminase (ALT), and bilirubin levels, should be done (Schleis & Marsh, 2018, p. 513)

TREATMENT AND OUTCOMES
- There are two types of products available for hepatitis B immunoprophylaxis (Greenberg et al., 2014, pp. 1236–1237):
  - Hepatitis B immune globulin (HBIG) provides short-term protection from 3 to 6 months, indicated in post-exposure circumstance.
  - Hepatitis B vaccine is used for preexposure and postexposure protection and provides long-term protection. The vaccine is safe and effective.
- Oral antiviral agents are available for adults and older children, but currently there is no specific therapy for infants (Permar, 2017, pp. 668–672).
- A four-pronged approach is used for prevention in the United States:
  - 1. Universal immunization of all infants beginning at birth (Wilson & Tyner, 2014, p. 710).
    - Premature infants can have HBV delayed 30 to 60 days if mom is seronegative.
    - By 1 month of age, medically stable preterm infants should be immunized, regardless of initial birthweight or GA (Greenberg et al., 2014, pp. 1236–1237).
  - 2. Prevention of perinatal infection through routine screening of all pregnant women and appropriate immunoprophylaxis of infants born to HBsAg-positive women (or whose status is unknown).
  - 3. Routine immunization of children and adolescents who have not been immunized previously.
  - 4. Immunization of nonimmunized adults at increased risk of infection (Schleis & Marsh, 2018, p. 513).
  - Neonatal therapy is based on maternal status:
    - Infants born to HBsAg-positive mothers:
      - Should receive both active and passive immunization within 12 hours of birth.
      - Should be followed up with Hepatitis B serologies at 9 and 12 months of age.
    - Therapy for infants born to mother with unknown maternal HBV status:
      - The mother's status should be checked immediately.
      - The infants should receive the first dose of the HBV within 12 hours of birth. And HBIG should be given prior to 1 week of age, if maternal status remains unknown (Schleis & Marsh, 2018, p. 513).
- Age at the time of acute infection is the principal factor in the risk of progression to chronic HBV infection.
  - More than 90% of infants with perinatal infection develop chronic HBV.
  - Between 25% and 50% of children infected at 1 to 5 years of age develop chronic HBV.
  - 2% to 6% of older children or adults develop chronic HBV infection.
- Perinatally infected infants have a 90% risk of progressing to chronic infection.
  - 15% to 25% of those will die of HBV-related complications later in life (Schleis & Marsh, 2018, p. 513).

- Chronic HBV causes cirrhosis and hepatic carcinoma, of which cirrhosis is the primary cause of Hepatitis B mortality (Permar, 2017, pp. 668–672; Schleis & Marsh, 2018, p. 513).
  - Five percent to 10% of infants born to HbeAg-positive mothers, regardless of appropriate immunoprophylaxis, progress to become chronic HBV carriers (Schleis & Marsh, 2018, p. 513).
  - If a neonate progresses to fulminant hepatitis disease, the mortality is around 67% (Wilson & Tyner, 2014, p. 710).

Herpes Simplex Virus

INCIDENCE
- HSV is a double-stranded DNA virus with the ability to enter a latent state and produce a lifelong infection. It consists of a viral DNA core surrounded by a protein capsid, which is surrounded by an envelope of proteins. There are two distinct types: HSV-1 and HSV-2. Both types induce congenital infections that are clinically identical (Baley & Leonard, 2015, p. 356; Permar, 2017, p. 650).
- In the past clinicians concluded that HSV-1 affected the person above the waist (face and skin) and that HSV-2 involved the area below the waist (genitals). It is now accepted that both viruses can affect any of the body and the neonate, although 75% of congenital HSV is due to HSV-1 (Schleis & Marsh, 2018, p. 485; Wilson & Tyner, 2015, p. 708).

EPIDEMIOLOGY
- Congenital transmission of HSV to the fetus is greatest if mother has a primary infection at or near the time of delivery. During the first trimester the transmission rate is less than 2%, whereas near the end of pregnancy it rises to 25% to 60%.
- Most mothers of severely affected infants have no known history of HSV or lesion present at the time of delivery (Greenberg et al., 2014, p. 1237), therefore a negative maternal history should not deter the practitioner from evaluating the infant with HSV symptoms (Schleis & Marsh, 2018, p. 485).
- HSV recurrence can lead to person-to-person transmission, including maternal-fetal and maternal-infant, but the maternal-fetal transmission rate is low (Schleis & Marsh, 2018, p. 485). If a woman has a recurrent infection, the fetus may have received some immunity to HSV and therefore exposure is less problematic (Greenberg et al., 2014, p. 1237).
  - Neonatal infection can occur through a contact with the hands or mouth of a care provider or from breast lesions during breastfeeding (Schleis & Marsh, 2018, pp. 485–491; Wilson & Tyner, 2015, pp. 708–710).
- Prevention is key in decreasing the mortality and morbidity in neonates and infants (Pammi et al., 2016, p. 548; Permar, 2017, p. 654). Pregnancy strategies include:
  - If mother negative HSV, avoid sex with HSV-seropositive partner in the third trimester.
  - If mother has a primary HSV infection, treat with oral or IV acyclovir for 10 days and consider delivery by cesarean section.
  - Mothers with HSV infections need to use strict handwashing techniques before touching the infants and wear gowns to cover active lesions. If oral lesions are

present in a mother or other caregiver, they should wear a mask. Breastfeeding is permissible if there are no breast lesions (Pammi et al., 2016, p. 549; Wilson & Tyner, 2015, p. 709).
  ○ The exception to covering the lesion is, if herpetic whitlow present (finger lesions), caregivers should not be providing direct patient care without gloves (Baley & Leonard, 2015, p. 357).

RISK FACTORS
- Women who are sexually active, of lower socioeconomic status, and are in proximity to others with HSV type 1 or type 2 with oral or skin lesions. Risks to the infant increase, especially in a primary infection, near the end of pregnancy. Risk of transmission is present if the mother has vesicles on breast.

PRESENTATION AND EVALUATION
- Table 22.9 outlines the category of HSV in correlation with presentation, evaluation, and suggested treatment.

TREATMENT AND OUTCOMES
- Treatment with IV acyclovir has decreased the mortality rate of disseminated disease and neurologic sequelae of surviving infants. Infants with CNS disease have a higher mortality rate (Schleis & Marsh, 2018, pp. 487–489).
- Prognosis depends on both the viral antigen type and the location of the infection, with poor prognostic indicators including prematurity, coma, DIC, pneumonitis, and seizures at the onset of therapy (Baley & Leonard, 2015, p. 359).

HIV

INCIDENCE
- HIV is a cytopathic ribonucleic acid (RNA) virus of the lentivirus genus, which belongs to the retroviridae family (Baley & Leonard, 2015, p. 359; Wilson & Tyner, 2015, p. 713).
- HIV results in a lifelong infection and may progress to AIDS. Supportive therapies are available for AIDS, but there is no cure (Permar, 2017, p. 641).
- There are two types of HIV viruses: HIV-1 and HIV-2.
  ○ HIV-1 is the most prevalent in the United States and is the most pathogenetic of the two types.
  ○ HIV-1 enters immune system, especially the CD4+ T-lymphocytes, where it incorporates itself through RNA to the host's DNA and becomes a part of the genome, where it replicates (Permar, 2017, p. 641).
  ○ HIV-2 is mostly found in West Africa and is a milder virus (Wilson & Tyner, p. 713).

EPIDEMIOLOGY
- HIV is transmitted by three primary modes: sexual contact, parenteral inoculation, and pre/perinatal transfer (Permar, 2017, p. 661). HIV is found in blood, semen, vaginal secretions, and breastmilk (Pammi et al., 2016, p. 538).
- The rate of transmission of HIV from is highest in the late third trimester or at delivery. If untreated, the infant's transmission rate has been estimated to be between 15% and 40%. Infection risk increases with ROMs and assistive techniques (Permar, 2017, p. 661).

  ○ Other factors that increase maternal–neonatal transmission are low maternal CD4+ counts, maternal IV drug use, no antiviral treatment during pregnancy, premature birth, and breastfeeding.

RISK FACTORS
- Either parent having multiple sex partners—especially among high-risk groups such as persons with a history of exchanging sex for money, both heterosexual and homosexual.
- Diagnosis of others sexually transmitted infections (STIs)
- IV drug users, including those who may be incarcerated.
- Persons who require multiple blood transfusions and blood products, including hemophiliacs and/or spouses of hemophiliacs (Permar, 2017, p. 661; Schleis & Marsh, 2018, p. 521).

PRESENTATION AND EVALUATION
- Infants are generally asymptomatic at birth.
  ○ Early symptoms could be missed since they are nonspecific and consistent with other more common viruses (Schleis & Marsh, 2018, p. 521). Infants who are infected in utero may present with growth restriction, hepatosplenomegaly, and/or recurrent *Candidiasis*.
- Most neonates with untreated HIV infection present with acute illness during the first 2 to 4 weeks of life. Infants may present with any of the following symptoms, which may develop, persist, or recur during the first year of life:
  ○ Unexplained fevers, opportunistic infections (viral and bacterial)
  ○ Chronic diarrhea, failure to thrive
  ○ Generalized lymphadenopathy, hepatosplenomegaly, parotitis, hepatitis, nephropathy, and cardiomyopathy
  ○ Recurrent oral and diaper candidiasis
  ○ Lymphoid interstitial pneumonitis
  ○ Cardiac abnormalities (pericardial disease, myocardial dysfunction, dysrhythmias)
  ○ Encephalopathy, neurologic disease that is either delayed or progressive (Baley & Leonard, 2015, p. 360; Permar, 2017, p. 664; Wilson & Tyner, 2015, p. 713)
- HIV antibody tests can be performed on samples of serum/plasma, whole blood, or oral fluid; antigen/antibody tests can be performed only on serum or plasma.
- Immunoassays are used widely as the initial test for serum HIV antibody or for p24 antigen (see subsequently) and HIV antibody. Serologic assays that are cleared by the Food and Drug Administration (FDA) for the diagnosis of HIV include:
  ○ Nucleic acid amplification assays. Plasma HIV, DNA, or RNA assays have been used to diagnose HIV infection. Currently, there is one HIV-1 qualitative RNA assay cleared by the FDA as a diagnostic test. The DNA PCR assays can detect one to 10 DNA copies of proviral DNA in peripheral.
  ○ Antigen detection. Detection of the p24 antigen (including immune complex–dissociated) is less sensitive than the HIV proviral DNA PCR assay or culture. False-positive test results occur in samples obtained from infants younger than 1 month.
  ○ HIV-2 detection. Most HIV immunoassays currently approved by FDA, including third-generation assays, detect but do not differentiate between HIV-1 and HIV-2 antibodies.

TABLE 22.9 Herpes Simplex Virus (HSV) Presentation, Evaluation, and Suggested Treatment

Category of HSV	Presentation	Diagnostics/Evaluation	Treatment
Asymptomatic infants born to mothers with suspected or proven primary infection with active lesions at delivery	Asymptomatic	Thorough physical assessment CBC Surface cultures at 24 hours of age Blood DNA PCR for HSV	Dependent on maternal history and infant virology testing Pending diagnostic results may treat with IV acyclovir versus routine follow-up
Localized skin, eyes, and mouth (SEM) disease	Symptoms present by 7-14 days of life Skin lesions (in <30%) Lesions localized to mouth and eyes	Culture of vesicular fluid, blood (CSF culture yield is less than 50%) Surface cultures from mouth, nasopharynx, conjunctiva, and anus after 24 hours from birth and after initial bath Direct fluorescent antibody (DFA) test Enzyme immunoassay antigen detection (EIA) Tzanck test on the skin at the base of the vesicle The evaluation should include ophthalmologic examination, brain imaging, EEG, and audiologic testing.	Oral acyclovir is not adequate therapy. Recommendation includes 14 days of IV acyclovir therapy Ocular antiviral therapy with: 3% vidarabine, 1% trifluridine, or 0.1% iododeoxyuridine Adequate hydration to prevent nephrotoxicity
Localized CNS disease (encephalitis)	Symptoms present by 14 to 21 days of life May have skin lesions Lethargic, irritable, and tremors Meningoencephalitis Seizures Microcephaly	The indicated diagnostic tests stated above plus: HSV PCR of CSF Culture of CSF (culture CSF yields less than 50%)	IV acyclovir as oral therapy is not adequate. 21 days of IV acyclovir therapy Obtain a CSF PCR at the end of treatment; if positive continue treatment. Adequate hydration to prevent nephrotoxicity If ocular lesions present: Ocular antiviral therapy with: 3% vidarabine, 1% trifluridine, or 0.1% iododeoxyuridine
Disseminated disease	Initially, asymptomatic Skin lesions (in <30%) Present at 7 to 14 days of life CNS involvement Fever/temperature instability Pneumonia Severe liver dysfunction Abnormal CSF findings Seizures Profound sepsis with septic shock Microcephaly		

CBC, complete blood count; CSF, cerebrospinal fluid; CNS, central nervous system; HSV, herpes simplex virus; IV, intravenous; PCR, polymerase chain reaction.

Sources: Data from Baley, J. E., & Leonard, E. G. (2013). Infections in the neonate. In A. Fanaroff & A. Fanaroff (Eds.), *Klaus and Fanaroff's care of the high-risk neonate* (6th ed., pp. 346–367). Cleveland, OH: Elsevier; Greenberg, J. M., Narendran, V., Schibler, K. R., Warner, B. B., & Haberman, B. E. (2014). Neonatal morbidities of prenatal and perinatal origin. In R. Resnik, R. K. Creasy, J. D. Iams, C. J. Lockwood, T. Moore, & M. F. Greene (Eds.), *Creasy & Resnik's maternal-fetal medicine principles and practice* (7th ed., pp. 1215–1239.e7). St. Louis, MO: Elsevier; Pammi, M., Brand, M. C., & Weismann, L. (2016). Infection in the neonate. In S. Gardner, B. Carter, M. Hines, & J. Hernandez (Eds.), *Merenstein & gardner's handbook of neonatal intensive care* (8th ed., pp. 537–562). St. Louis, MO: Elsevier; Schleis, M. R., & Marsh, K. J. (2018). Viral infections of the fetus and newborn. In C. Gleason & S. Juul (Eds.), *Avery's diseases of the newborn* (10th ed., pp. 482–526.e18). Philadelphia, PA: Elsevier; Wilson, D. J., & Tyner, C. I. (2015). Infectious diseases in the neonate. In T. Verklan & M. Walden (Eds.), *Core curriculum for neonatal intensive care nursing* (5th ed., pp. 689–718). St. Louis, MO: Elsevier.

○ Therefore, FDA-approved HIV-1/HIV-2 antibody differentiation assays should be used in lieu of the Western blot to identify antibodies and distinguish HIV-1 from HIV-2 (American Academy of Pediatrics, 2018a, pp. 463–465).

- Transplacental transfer of maternal antibodies occurs in all deliveries, therefore, do not use antibody-based assays (ELISA or Western Blot) to diagnose neonatal HIV.
- Do not use cord blood as there may be maternal blood present (Greenberg et al., 2015, p. 1237).

TREATMENT AND OUTCOMES
- HIV-infected pregnant women should receive combined antiretroviral therapy (cART) regimens, both for treatment of infection and for prevention of mother-to-child transmission (MTCT). The goal during pregnancy is virologic suppression.
- Because HIV recommendations and therapies change over time, consultation with an infectious disease specialist is recommended when managing neonatal HIV. The most recent recommendations can also be found online through the CDC or NIH websites.
- Combination antiretroviral therapy (cART) is indicated for HIV-infected neonatal patients should be provided as soon as the HIV diagnosis is confirmed. The principle objective of therapy is suppression of viral replication, to preserve immune function, and reduce associated morbidities.
- Due to unproven ability of prophylaxis to completely protective against MTCT of HIV, in countries where safe alternative sources are available, such as the United States, HIV-infected women should be counseled not to breastfeed their infants or to donate to human milk banks.
  - ○ If a mother still chooses to breastfeed, it is vital that an appropriate plan of management be developed, including encouraging prolonged use of ARVs in both the mother and infant while breastfeeding.
- Caregivers should remain vigilant for the risk of opportunistic infections such as pneumonia. The HIV-positive infant should receive all recommended childhood immunizations.

- With the prevention and treatment protocols and subsequent interruption of vertical transmission, the number of infected children has been greatly reduced. HIV infection in untreated infants has a mortality rate of 20% by 4 years of age as the virus spreads more rapidly in infants and children due to their immature immune and organ systems (Wilson & Tyner, 2015, p. 713).
  - ○ Without the appropriate treatment infants would progress quickly to having HIV-related complications, including AIDS, pneumocystis jiroveci pneumonia, and other bacterial and viral opportunistic infections (Baley & Leonard, 2015, p. 360).
- Table 22.10 describes the plan of care for maternal HIV in correlation with neonatal treatment and monitoring.
- Table 22.11 outlines a suggested plan of care for an infant who tests positive for HIV.

Respiratory Syncytial Virus (RSV)

INCIDENCE
- The majority of infants infected with RSV experience upper respiratory tract symptoms, but 20% to 30% will go on to develop lower respiratory tract disease.
  - ○ 1% to 3% of these will be hospitalized because of RSV lower respiratory tract disease. Most hospitalization occurs between 30 and 60 days of age.
- Fewer than 125 deaths of infants less than 2 years of age are associated with RSV infection in the United States yearly, and 40% of those deaths occur secondary to a primary diagnosis of RSV (American Academy of Pediatrics, 2018b, pp. 682–683).

TABLE 22.10 Plan of Care for Maternal HIV

Scenario	Maternal treatment/monitoring	Neonatal treatment/monitoring

Mom HIV-1-positive with no HAART or HIV RNA load greater than 1,000 copies/ml	Mom to continue cART during and after pregnancy:
	–Includes a minimum of three antiretroviral treatments regardless of CD4 count or viral load
	–IV zidovudine 3 hours prior to delivery or ASAP
	• Monitoring:
	  ○ Viral resistance testing
	  ○ HIV RNA PCR for viral load
	• Delivery:
	  ○ Plan for c/s delivery at 38 weeks
	  ○ Avoid artificial rupture of membranes, invasive fetal monitoring, and use of forceps or vacuum-assisted delivery as these will increase the risk of maternal-child transmission.
		Therapy:
		–vART started within 6 to 12 hours of birth for the first 4 to 6 weeks
		–No breastfeeding
		Evaluation:
		–HIV DNA PCR at 0 to 2 days, 6 weeks, and 3 months
		–Baseline CBC and differential (at risk for anemia)
		–Additional confirmatory testing includes HIV, RNA PCR, HIV viral resistance, CD4 counts

Mom HIV-positive with HAART and HIV RNA load less than 1,000 copies/ml or unknown HIV RNA load	Mom to continue cART during and after pregnancy -Including a minimum of three antiretroviral treatments regardless of CD4 count or viral load IV zidovudine not indicated Individualize decision for cesarean section	Therapy: –ART for the first 4 to 6 weeks Monitoring: –HIV DNA PCR at 0 to 2 days, 6 weeks, and 3 months No breastfeeding

ART, antiretroviral therapy; CBC, complete blood count; HAART, Highly active antiretroviral therapy; PCR, polymerase chain reaction.

Sources: Data from Baley, J. E., & Leonard, E. G. (2013). Infections in the neonate. In A. Fanaroff & A. Fanaroff (Eds.), *Klaus and Fanaroff's care of the high-risk neonate* (6th ed., pp. 346–367). Cleveland, OH: Elsevier; Pammi, M., Brand, M. C., & Weismann, L. (2016). Infection in the neonate. In S. Gardner, B. Carter, M. Hines, & J. Hernandez (Eds.), *Merenstein & Gardner's handbook of neonatal intensive care* (8th ed., pp. 537–562). St. Louis, MO: Elsevier; Schleis, M. R., & Marsh, K. J. (2018). Viral infections of the fetus and newborn. In C. Gleason & S. Juul (Eds.), *Avery's diseases of the newborn* (10th ed., pp. 482–526.e18). Philadelphia, PA: Elsevier.

TABLE 22.11 Plan of Care for HIV-Positive Neonate

Monitoring	Treatment
–HIV DNA PCR at 0 to 2 days, 6 weeks, and 3 months of age –HIV phenotypic and genotypic resistance testing –Monitor for AIDS –Monitor for pneumocystis jiroveci pneumonia (PCP) prophylaxis (TMP/SMX for 1 year) –Screening: audiology, dental, neurodevelopmental, ophthalmology, TB –Other viral serologies as indicated –Chest x-ray (CXR) –Brain imaging –Consultation with a pediatric HIV specialist	–ZDV given between 6 and 12 hours of birth –Nevirapine × three doses in first week of life –Once the neonate/infant is confirmed HIV-positive, a multidrug antiretroviral therapy is initiated and a specialists should be consulted. –Zodovudine is only approved HIV drug for premature infants. –Term infants regime: zidovudine, lamivudine, emtricitabine, and stavudine –After 14 days of age there are more antiretroviral drugs that can be added to the term neonate's therapy, such as didanosine, ritonavir-boosted lopinovir, and nevirapine (Schleis & Marsh, 2018, p. 525).

ZDV, zidovudine.

Sources: Data from Baley, J. E., & Leonard, E. G. (2013). Infections in the neonate. In A. Fanaroff & A. Fanaroff (Eds.), *Klaus and Fanaroff's care of the high-risk neonate* (6th ed., pp. 346–367). Cleveland, OH: Elsevier; Pammi, M., Brand, M. C., & Weismann, L. (2016). Infection in the neonate. In S. Gardner, B. Carter, M. Hines, & J. Hernandez (Eds.), *Merenstein & Gardner's handbook of neonatal intensive care* (8th ed., pp. 537–562). St. Louis, MO: Elsevier; Schleis, M. R., & Marsh, K. J. (2018). Viral infections of the fetus and newborn. In C. Gleason & S. Juul (Eds.), *Avery's diseases of the newborn* (10th ed., pp. 482–526.e18). Philadelphia, PA: Elsevier.

EPIDEMIOLOGY
- Respiratory syncytial virus (RSV) is an RNA virus of the Paramyxovirus with two major strains: group A and group B. The virus replicates in the nasopharynx and spreads to the small bronchiolar epithelium (Permar, 2017, p. 681; Wilson & Tyner, 2015, p. 707).
  - Humans are the only source of infection and the transmission is through respiratory droplets or fomites.
  - The incubation period is 2 to 8 days and viral shedding may take from 3 days to weeks (Permar, 2017, p. 681; Wilson & Tyner, 2015, p. 707).
- RSV is a virus found globally and one of the most common diseases in early childhood. Most children are affected during their first 2 years of life.
  - There is no lifelong immunity.
- In the NICU, RSV is a common nosocomial infection. Most commonly, RSV is spread by via hands of healthcare workers or family members.
- Community epidemics occur most commonly November through March, but can vary in warmer climates (Wilson & Tyner, 2015, p. 707).

RISK FACTORS
- Infants less than 6 months of age, especially those born prematurely and developed lung disease
- Infants <2 years of age with heart disease
- Infants who were the product of multiple-birth pregnancies
- Infants with school-aged siblings or those who attend day care
- Neonates less than 1 month of age and formula fed
- Male infants and male or female infants who are immunocompromised
- Regular exposure to secondhand smoke or air pollution and/or family history of asthma (Schleis & Marsh, 2018, p. 519)

PRESENTATION AND EVALUATION
- RSV is the most common cause of bronchiolitis and pneumonia in infants (Wilson & Tyner, 201, p. 707).
- Symptoms of RSV may be nonspecific, such as rhinorrhea and general malaise. Other symptoms that manifest include:
  - Inflamed mucous membranes with cough, dyspnea, wheezing, and congestion, any of which may be accompanied by cyanosis. Work of breathing may lead to apnea, especially new-onset disease (Wilson & Tyner, 2015, p. 707).
  - Audible rales and rhonchi on physical examination
  - Lethargy, irritability, poor feeding (Schleis & Marsh, 2018, p. 519)
- Neonates and infants who present with respiratory infections require a thorough clinical evaluation.
  - Rapid diagnosis is made by PCR or immunofluorescent antigen testing of respiratory secretions (95% sensitivity with good specificity).
  - Respiratory viral cultures (results not until 3–5 days) (Permar, 2017, p. 681)

TREATMENT AND OUTCOMES
- The best treatment is prevention of the disease.
- RSV is a common respiratory virus, which is benign in the healthy term infant or young child and requires minimal intervention.
- High-risk populations are more commonly at risk for severe disease course and accompanying complications.
  - Isolation precautions are necessary if the infant/child requires hospitalization.
  - Supportive care with hydration, supplemental oxygen, nebulized bronchodilators, and mechanical ventilation as needed (Wilson & Tyner, 2015, p. 707).
- Palivizumab (Synagis) and ribavirin are available but should be considered on a case-by-case basis (Permar, 2017, p. 682; Schleis & Marsh, 2018, p. 519; Wilson & Tyner, 2015, p. 707)
- Passive immunization: palivizumab (Synagis) provides passive immunity and should be given monthly to high-risk infants during RSV season:
  - Infants born before 32 weeks' gestation with chronic lung disease during their first year of life or second year if additional qualifiers are met.
  - Infants born <29 weeks' gestation without chronic lung disease during their first year of life

○ Children ≤24 months of age with hemodynamically significant acyanotic congenital heart disease
○ Infants with anatomic pulmonary abnormalities of the airway or neuromuscular disorder during their first year of life
○ Severely immunocompromised infants (such as SCID) up to 24 months of age
■ Infants with symptomatic cystic fibrosis (Permar, 2017, p. 681)

- Most infants have a complete recovery with no long-term complications; however, there are approximately 400 deaths of children in the United States annually due to RSV.
- There is an increase in mortality rates for premature infants, infants with complex congenital heart disease, those with pulmonary hypertension or bronchopulmonary dysplasia, or immunodeficiencies (Wilson & Tyner, 2015, p. 707).

Varicella–zoster virus (VZV)

INCIDENCE
- Prior to introduction of routine immunization, an average of 100 to 125 people died of chickenpox in the United States each year.
- The incidence of the congenital varicella syndrome among infants born to mothers who experience varicella during pregnancy is approximately 2% when infection occurs between 8 and 20 weeks of gestation. Rarely, cases of congenital varicella syndrome have been reported in infants of women infected after 20 weeks of pregnancy.
  ○ Varicella infection has a high fatality rate in infants when the mother develops varicella from 5 days before to 2 days after delivery, because there is inadequate time for the development and transfer of maternal antibody across the placenta.
  ○ When varicella develops in a mother more than 5 days before delivery and GA is 28 weeks or more, the severity of disease in the newborn infant is modified by transplacental transfer of VZV-specific maternal immunoglobulin (Ig) G antibody (American Academy of Pediatrics, 2018c, p. 869).

EPIDEMIOLOGY
- VZV is a member of the Herpesviridae family (Wilson & Tyner, 2015, p. 712), which affects neurons and can lie dormant to reactivate at a later time.
- Primary varicella infection is *chickenpox*, whereas reactivation of a latent virus is *zoster* or *shingles* (Schleis & Marsh, 2012, p. 491).
- Individuals are contagious 1 to 2 days before onset of lesions and until all lesions are crusted (Schleis & Marsh, 2012, p. 493; Wilson & Tyner, 2015, p. 712).
- Maternal infection during the first or second trimester can be devastating to the fetus, resulting in limb, skin, CNS abnormalities and death (Wilson & Tyner, 2015, p. 712). Transmission during the first two trimesters of pregnancy (less than 20 weeks) holds an increased the risk of teratogenic effects to a fetus (congenital viral syndrome [CVS]). Maternal infection in the third trimester is not associated with CVS (Schleis & Marsh, 2012, p. 492).

Transmission occurs through direct contact with individuals that have vesicular lesions or respiratory tract secretions.
○ Transmission in the pregnant woman is transplacentally or ascending through the birth canal.
○ Theoretical risk of transmission via breastfeeding, while mother is contagious (Wilson & Tyner, 2015, p. 712)

RISK FACTORS
- Varicella is much more contagious than is herpes zoster.
- Skin lesions appear to be the major source of transmissible VZV. Person-to-person transmission occurs either from direct contact with VZV lesions from varicella or herpes zoster or from airborne spread.
- VZV infection in a household member usually results in infection of almost all susceptible people in that household. Children who acquire their infection at home (secondary family cases) often have multiple skin lesions. Healthcare-associated transmission is well-documented in pediatric units.
- Patients are contagious from 1 to 2 days before onset of the rash until all lesions have crusted (American Academy of Pediatrics, 2018c, pp. 870–871).

PRESENTATION AND EVALUATION
- Diagnosis via PCR assay of vesicular fluid, scab, saliva, or buccal swabs, and via tissue culture of vesicles, CSF, or biopsy (Wilson & Tyner, 2015, p. 712).
  ○ PCR has low yield in congenital viral infection compared to acquired infection (Schleis & Marsh, 2012, p. 493).

TREATMENT AND OUTCOMES
- Full-term healthy infants who acquire varicella postnatally only require routine supportive care.
- Acyclovir is recommended when:
  ○ A full-term infant acquires a congenital infection (Permar, 2017, p. 674)
  ○ An infection becomes systemic, even in a full-term healthy infant (Schleis & Marsh, 2012, p. 493)
- Varicella immune globulin (VariZIG) should be administered when:
  ○ A neonate is exposed to a maternal infection between 5 days prior to and 2 days after delivery
  ○ Immunoprophylaxis should be given within 96 hours of exposure.
  ○ IVIG may be given when VariZIG is not available (Permar, 2017, p. 674).
- Infants treated with immunoglobulins need to be in respiratory isolation for 28 days following treatment. Women who are not immune should not receive varicella vaccine during pregnancy or 1 to 3 months prior to becoming pregnant and should avoid exposure to infected persons.
- Varicella immunization is recommended for all nonimmune women as part of prepregnancy and postpartum care (Wilson & Tyner, 2015, p. 712).
- Table 22.12 summarizes the stages of varicella exposure, clinical findings, and suggested therapies.

TABLE 22.12 Congenital Varicella Exposure, Clinical Findings, and Treatment

Stage	Exposure to VZV	Clinical findings	Treatment
Fetal varicella syndrome (FVS)	In utero transmission Mother exposed during the first half of pregnancy	1. Skin lesions may scar with skin loss 2. Profound neurologic impairment: Microcephaly, seizures, encephalitis, cortical atrophy, cerebral calcifications 3. Ocular abnormalities: microphthalmia, chorioretinitis, and/or cataracts 4. Limb hypoplasia and other skeletal defects 5. Prematurity and intrauterine growth restriction (IUGR) 6. Mortality rate 30% during first months of life 7. Survivors may have profound mental retardation and major neurologic disabilities.	Supportive care Acyclovir therapy may be beneficial to prevent progressive complications No isolation indicated
Congenital (early neonatal) syndrome (CVS)	Active maternal VZV in the last 3 weeks of pregnancy or within the first few days postpartum Transmitted transplacentally or via ascending infection through the birth canal	1. Active VZV begins in the neonate before delivery or within 10 to 12 days, after birth. 2. Variable presentation 3. A centripetal rash 4. A generalized pruritic, vesicular rash 5. Low-grade fever 6. Potential superinfection of skin lesions 7. Pneumonia 8. Thrombocytopenia 9. occurs rarely: 10. Glomerulonephritis, hepatitis, and arthritis 11. Prognosis is good if maternal infection occurs more than 5 days prior to delivery 12. Infant mortality increases with maternal infection within 5 days to 2 days after delivery. 13. Latent infection may occur. 14. Infection after vaccination may also occur.	Administer varicella–zoster immune globulin (VZIG or VariZIG) within 96 hours of exposure. If VZIG not available, then administer IVIG. Provide supportive care. Requires strict respiratory isolation for 28 days Acyclovir may be prescribed as adjunct therapy. Antibiotics may be prescribed for secondary skin infections, prn.
Postnatal chickenpox	Not transmitted transplacentally.	Presents between 12 and 28 days of life May see a typical chickenpox rash: erythematous macular rash to vesicular rash occurring in multiple stages	If acquired postnatally, disease is usually mild.

VZV, varicella–zoster virus.

Sources: Data from Permar, S. R. (2017). Bacterial and fungal infections. In Eichenwald et al. (Eds.), *Cloherty and Stark's manual of neonatal care* (8th ed., pp. 641–650). Philadelphia, PA: Wolters Kluwer; Schleis, M. R., & Marsh, K. J. (2018). Viral infections of the fetus and newborn. In C. Gleason & S. Juul (Eds.), *Avery's diseases of the newborn* (10th ed., pp. 482–526.e18). Philadelphia, PA: Elsevier; Wilson, D. J., & Tyner, C. I. (2015). Infectious diseases in the neonate. In T. Verklan & M. Walden (Eds.), *Core curriculum for neonatal intensive care nursing* (5th ed., pp. 689–718). St. Louis, MO: Elsevier.

OTHER INFECTIONS AFFECTING NEONATES

The following section reviews chlamydia, gonorrhea, syphilis, and toxoplasmosis, which that may cause other infections in neonates. Organisms involved, incidence, risk factors, and treatment recommendations are discussed.

Chlamydia

- *Chlamydia trachomatis* is an obligate intracellular organism that can cause ophthalmia neonatorum and pneumonia in the infant and neonate (Leonard & Dobbs, 2015, p. 738).
  - ○ Infants born to infected mothers have a 50% chance of acquiring an infection primarily transmitted through infected genital secretions, although transmission through intact membranes has been reported in infants delivered by cesarean section.
  - ○ *C. trachomatis* is the leading cause of ophthalmia neonatorum in the United States due to its prevalence in the population (Baley & Leonard, 2013, p. 362; Puopolo, 2017, p. 716). Infected infants have a 25% to 50% chance of developing conjunctivitis and a 5% to 20% chance of developing pneumonia (Baley & Leonard, 2013, p. 362).
- Usual presentation of symptoms occurs between 5 and 14 days of life with a spectrum ranging from mild eyelid edema to mucopurulent discharge with significant swelling and redness (Leonard & Dobbs, 2013, p. 741).
- The infection is diagnosed with culture and sensitivity and the culture must contain epithelial cells due to the intracellular nature of the organism (Baley & Leonard, 2013, p. 362). If positive, infants should also be evaluated for pneumonia (Puopolo, 2017, p. 716).
  - ○ Systemic treatment along with follow-up retesting are necessary, with up to 20% of infants requiring a second course of therapy (Baley & Leonard, 2013, p. 363; Leonard & Dobbs, 2015, p. 741; Puopolo, 2017, p. 716).
  - ○ If untreated, symptoms of the infection can last up to one year and result in conjunctival scarring, micropannus formation, and, less frequently, corneal scarring (Baley & Leonard, 2013, p. 362; Leonard & Dobbs, 2015, p. 741; Puopolo, 2017, p. 716).
- *C. trachomatis* can cause pneumonia in the presence or absence of conjunctivitis, with approximately 50% of pneumonia cases having a conjunctival history (Leonard & Dobbs, 2015, p. 741).
  - ○ *C. trachomatis* pneumonia usually presents between 2 and 4 weeks of life but can present as early as week 1 through the first 4 months of life (Baley & Leonard, 2013, p. 363; Leonard & Dobbs, 2015, pp. 738, 741; Wilson & Tyner, 2015, p. 701).
- Symptoms usually include a persistent staccato cough, tachypnea, and nasal congestion without a fever (Baley & Leonard, 2013, p. 363; Leonard & Dobbs, 2015, p. 741).
- Diagnoses are largely clinical, but chest radiographs usually show bilateral interstitial infiltrates with hyperinflation. Some infected infants will have a positive nasopharyngeal swab although a negative swab does not exclude the disease. *C. trachomatis* IgM titers do elevate, with a 1:32 or greater titer being diagnostic.
- As with *C. Trachomatis* conjunctivitis, systemic treatment and rescreening are required with pneumonia (Baley & Leonard, 2013, p. 363).

Gonorrhea

- The most common manifestation of *N. gonorrhoeae* in neonates is ophthalmia neonatorum with rare dissemination to bacteremia, osteomyelitis, septic arthritis, and meningitis. In the United States, most systemically infected infants do not have ocular disease due to universal prophylaxis at birth (Baley & Leonard, 2013, pp. 361–362).
  - ○ Infection of mucosal surfaces can occur along with scalp abscesses when fetal electrode monitoring is used (Leonard & Dobbs, 2015, p. 741; Puopolo, 2018; p. 716).
- Ophthalmia neonatorum or bacterial conjunctivitis typically presents within 1 to 5 days of life with profuse and purulent drainage, bilateral eyelid edema, and chemosis. Without treatment it can progress to clouding and damage of the cornea and pan-ophthalmitis (Baley & Leonard, 2013, p. 361; Leonard & Dobbs, 2015, p. 741; Puopolo, 2018, pp. 715–716).
- An infant born to a mother with a known gonococcal infection should be evaluated for other STDs and hospitalized for treatment and testing for invasive disease (Puopolo, 2017, pp. 715–716). Like *C. trachomatis*, systemic treatment is required for gonococcal conjunctivitis (Leonard & Dobbs, 2015, p. 741).

Syphilis

- Congenital syphilis (CS) infection is caused by the *Treponema pallidum* organism, a hematogenous and sexually transmitted corkscrew shaped spirochete (Baley & Leonard, 2013, p. 364; Heresi, 2017, p. 729; Michaels, Sanches, & Lin, 2018, p. 532).
- Syphilis is the common neonatal infection worldwide (Michaels et al., 2018, p. 532).
- The CDC recommends syphilis testing for all pregnant women.
  - ○ No newborn should be discharged from the hospital without documented results of maternal serologic testing (Greenberg et al., 2014, p. 1239; Heresi, 2017, p. 730; Michaels et al., 2018, p. 532).
- Can infect the fetus at any time during gestation with an increase in the risk as the pregnancy progresses (Heresi, 2017, p. 728). Transmitted to the fetus transplacentally in utero or during delivery via contact with a maternal genital lesion (Michaels et al., 2018, p. 533).
  - ○ Vertical transmission is highest during a recent maternal infection (Heresi, 2017, p. 728) in either the primary and secondary stages of syphilis (Michaels et al., 2018, p. 533).
- For the untreated mother, primary or secondary stage of syphilis has a transmission rate of nearly 100%, and decreases to between 10% and 30% during the latent stages (Heresi, 2017, p. 533).
- Infants with "snuffles" are rarely seen in today's nurseries, but if noted are highly contagious. The skin lesions or pemphigus sypiliticus are vesicles or bullous lesions unique to infants.
  - ○ Lesions are highly contagious after rupture (Baley & Leonard, 2013, p. 364).
- Risk factors include women with poor or no prenatal care, and Black women are at the highest risk (Michaels et al., 2018, p. 532); also, those who lack syphilis screening or are noncompliant serologic positive mothers. Maternal history of drug use, especially cocaine, also increases risk (Heresi, 2017, p. 730)

- Maternal data, a thorough infant exam, and appropriate laboratory testing are essential (Heresi, 2017, p. 729). Symptoms are difficult to differentiate from other neonatal infections.
  - ○ The placenta and umbilical cord should be examined as this can aid in the diagnosis (Michaels et al., 2018, p. 533).
- Table 22.13 identifies the classifications for evaluating infants for CS.
- More than 50% of infants with CS will be asymptomatic at birth (Baley & Leonard, 2013, p. 364).
  - ○ In contrast, infants may present with multisystem organ involvement.
  - ○ Symptoms of early-onset syphilis may develop in the first 2 years of life and late-onset syphilis after 2 years of life.
- Evaluation includes maternal history, physical examination, and laboratory testing (Greenberg et al., 2014, p. 1239).

The laboratory testing for an infant should be identical to maternal testing for comparison (Baley & Leonard, 2013, p. 365).

- Table 22.14 lists clinical findings of CS in the neonatal period.
- Laboratory tests are grouped into two distinctive categories; nonspecific nontreponemal antibody (NTA) tests and specific treponemal antibody (STA) tests (Heresi, 2017, pp. 730–731).
  - ○ Pregnant women should be screened at the first prenatal visit and at delivery (Heresi, 2017, p. 730).
  - ○ If the NTA test of the infant a four-fold increase over the mother's NTA test, the infant has an active infection and an STA test should follow (Greenberg et al., 2014, p. 1239).
- Table 22.15 lists laboratory testing for *T. pallidum*

TABLE 22.13 Classifications for Evaluating Infants for Congenital Syphilis

Presentation	Findings	Recommended Neonate Evaluation	Recommended Treatment
1. Proven or highly probable disease	1. Abnormal physical exam consistent with congenital syphilis 2. NTA fourfold maternal result 3. Positive darkfield test or PCR of lesions or body fluids	• CSF for VDRL, cell count, protein • CBC w/differential and platelets • Long-bone radiographs • Chest radiograph • Liver function tests • Neuroimaging • Ophthalmologic exam • Auditory brainstem response	1. Aqueous crystalline penicillin G 50,000 units/kg/dose intravenous (IV) every 12 hours the 1st 7 days of life then every 8 hours for 3 more days **or** 2. Penicillin G procaine 50,000 units/kg/dose IM once daily for 10 days
3. Possible congenital syphilis	1. Normal physical exam 2. NTA less than or equal to 4-fold maternal result and *one* of the following: ○ Mother not treated, inadequately treated or no record of treatment. ○ Mother treated less than 4 weeks prior to delivery.	• CSF for VDRL, cell count, protein • CBC w/differential and platelets • Long-bone radiographs	1. Aqueous crystalline penicillin G 50,000 units/kg/dose IV every 12 hours the first 7 days of life then every 8 hours for 3 more days **or** 2. Penicillin G procaine 50,000 units/kg/dose once daily for 10 days **or** (if evaluation completely normal) 3. Penicillin G benzathine 50,000 units/kg/dose IM X 1 dose
4. Congenital syphilis less likely	1. Normal physical exam 2. NTA less than or equal to fourfold maternal result and *both* of the following are true: ○ Mother was treated appropriately greater than 4 weeks before delivery ○ No evidence of maternal reinfection or relapse	No further evaluation	
3. Congenital syphilis unlikely	Normal physical exam • NTA less than or equal to 4-fold higher than maternal result and *both* of the following: • Mother was treated appropriately prior to pregnancy • Maternal NTA low and stable before and during pregnancy and at delivery	No further evaluation	

CBC, complete blood count; CSF, cerebrospinal fluid; NTA, nontreponemal antibody; VDRL, Venereal Disease Research Laboratory.

Source: Reproduced, with permission from Heresi, G. (2017). Syphilis. In Eichenwald et al. (Eds.), *Cloherty and Stark's manual of neonatal care* (8th ed., pp. 788–737). Philadelphia, PA: Wolters Kluwer.

TABLE 22.14 Clinical Findings of Congenital Syphilis in the Neonatal Period

Most common:
Hepatitis
Hepatomegaly with or without splenomegaly
Radiographic bone changes (periostitis, osteochondritis)
Rash involving the palms and soles
Oval and maculopapular rash that becomes copper-colored with desquamation
Condylomata lata
Mucocutaneous lesions
Jaundice, both direct and indirect hyperbilirubinemia
Bone marrow failure, anemia, and/or thrombocytopenia with petechiae or purpura

Less common to rare:
Lymphadenopathy
Pemphigus syphiliticus
Respiratory distress due to pneumonia or pneumonitis
Myocarditis
Meningitis or other central nervous symptom findings (leptomeningitis, cranial nerve palsies, cerebral infarction, seizures, hypopituitarism)
Nephrotic syndrome
Rhinitis (snuffles)
Pseudoparalysis of an extremity, pseudoparalysis of Parrot Fever
Small for gestational age
Nonimmune hydrops

Sources: Data from Baley, J. E., & Leonard, E. G. (2013). Infections in the neonate. In A. Fanaroff & A. Fanaroff (Eds.), *Klaus and Fanaroff's care of the high-risk neonate* (6th ed., pp. 346–367). Cleveland, OH: Elsevier; Heresi, G. (2017). Syphilis. In Eichenwald et al. (Eds.), *Cloherty and Stark's manual of neonatal care* (8th ed., pp. 788–737). Philadelphia, PA: Wolters Kluwer; Michaels, M. G., Sanchez, P., & Lin, L. (2018). Congenital toxoplasmosis, syphilis, malaria, and tuberculosis. In C. Gleason & S. Juul (Eds.), *Avery's diseases of the newborn* (10th ed., pp. 527–552.e6). Philadelphia, PA: Elsevier; Pammi, M., Brand, M. C., & Weismann, L. (2016). Infection in the neonate. In S. Gardner, B. Carter, M. Hines, & J. Hernandez (Eds.), *Merenstein & Gardner's handbook of neonatal intensive care* (8th ed., pp. 537–562). St. Louis, MO: Elsevier.

- CS can be prevented when maternal infection is detected and treated during pregnancy (Heresi, 2017, p. 735; Michaels et al., 2018, p. 535).
  - ○ Infants should be treated for CS when proven or probable disease suspected (Greenberg et al., pp. 1238–1249; Pammi et al., 2016, p. 541).
  - ○ Aqueous penicillin G is the only acceptable antimicrobial treatment for syphilis in both the mother and the infant. Erythromycin is not an appropriate treatment for syphilis (Pammi et al., 2016, p. 541).
- Undiscovered or untreated infections may result in stillbirth, preterm birth, congenital anomalies, long-term neurologic impairment, and fetal or neonatal death (Heresi, 2017, p. 728)
  - ○ Manifestations of untreated CS may develop after 2 years of age whether or not the baby had clinical symptoms during infancy.
  - ○ Long-term complications include impairments of the bones, CNS, eyes, joints, and teeth (Greenberg et al., p. 1238; Michaels et al., 2018, p. 531).

Toxoplasmosis

- Toxoplasmosis is caused by *T. gondii*, an intracellular parasitic protozoan (Wilson & Tyner, 2014, p. 705) that is found most places in nature (Michaels et al., 2018, p. 527).

- The incidence of congenital toxoplasmosis in the United States is estimated between 500 and 5.000 infants each year (Holzmann-Pazgal, 2017, p. 720).
- Risk factors include lower socioeconomic status, lower levels of education, and having at least three or more kittens.
  - ○ Cats are the host where *T. gondii* is shed by oocysts in the cat's intestinal tract. The oocysts enter the cat's feces and are left in the soil.
- Risk is higher in those who work with raw meats. Additional food risk factors are eating undercooked or raw meats, including oysters and clams.
  - ○ Intermediate hosts include all warm-blooded animals (sheep, cattle, and pigs) and humans.
  - ○ Infective tissue cysts accumulate in the organs, particularly the brain, eye, and skeletal muscle, of these animals and can remain in the muscle (Holzmann-Pazgal, 2017, p. 721; Michaels et al., 2018, p. 528).
- High risk of transmission when consuming unwashed raw fruits and vegetables, drinking unpasteurized goat's milk, or water from an untreated well (Michaels et al., 2018, p. 527)
- Table 22.16 lists toxoplasmosis infection transmission rates.
- Toxoplasmosis has very similar clinical characteristics to other viral infections (Michaels et al., 2018, p. 528). There are four recognized patterns of presentation for congenital toxoplasmosis (Holzmann-Pazgal, 2017, p. 720):
  - ○ **Subclinical/asymptomatic infection**—Most infants fall into this category (79%–90%) and do not have clinical symptoms at birth. If untreated, a large population will later demonstrate visual and CNS deficits, including hearing impairment, learning disabilities, or mental retardation several months to years later.
  - ○ **Neonatal symptomatic disease**—signs of congenital disease at birth include maculopapular rash, lymphadenopathy, hepatosplenomegaly, jaundice, petechiae, and thrombocytopenia.
  - ○ **Delayed onset**—This is most often seen in premature infants and usually occurs within the first 3 months of age. It can behave like neonatal symptomatic disease.
  - ○ **Sequelae or relapse in infancy through adolescence of a previously untreated infection**—chorioretinitis develops in up to 85% of adolescents/young adults with previously untreated congenital infection.
- Table 22.17 offers a summation of clinical symptoms of congenital toxoplasmosis.
- A congenital toxoplasmosis infection results when a maternal primary infection during pregnancy spreads to the placenta and fetus. A reactivated infection does not predispose the infant to infection.
  - ○ The severity of the infection is greater in the first trimester, but the transmission rate is lower (Holzmann-Pazgal, 2017, p. 721; Michaels et al., 2018, p. 528).
- Postnatal transmission can occur from blood product or bone marrow transfusion via a seropositive donor with a latent infection.
  - ○ There is no documentation of transmission through breastfeeding.
- Prevention of congenital toxoplasmosis is through avoidance of high-risk behaviors. If exposed to cats:
  - ○ Avoid changing cat litter, or change cat litter daily because the oocysts are not infective during first 1 to 2 days after passage.
  - ○ Keep cats indoors and feed them commercially prepared foods rather than undercooked meats or rodents (Michaels et al., 2018, p. 531).

TABLE 22.15 Laboratory Testing for *T. pallidum*

Diagnostic Test Category	Specific Diagnostic Test	Testing Information
Nonspecific nontreponemal antibody (NTA) tests	Venereal Disease Research Laboratory (VDRL)	A screening tool Allows quantitative monitoring Follow serially to evaluate therapy effectiveness. A normal result in either test equates to a negative result. Any positive test should be followed with a (STA) test. VDRL is the test to use on CSF fluid (not RPR).
	Rapid Plasma Reagin (RPR)	
Specific treponemal antibody (STA) tests Not used for quantitative findings	Fluorescent treponemal antibody absorption (FTA-ABS)	Verify presence of the antibody, indicating current or past infection. If positive, remains positive, always May be used for testing CSF
	Microhemagglutination test for antibodies to *T. pallidum* (MHA-TP)	
	T. pallidum enzyme immunoassay (TP-EIA)	Used for screening in some institutions (instead of NTA)
	T. pallidum-specific IgM immunoblot testing in the newborn (TP-Pa)	High sensitivity (Not commercially available)
Direct identification of *T. pallidum*	Microscopic dark field examination and	May be used to detect spirochetes and their antigens
	Direct fluorescent antibody staining	
	PCR	Can detect spirochete DNA (Not commercially available)

CSF, cerebrospinal fluid; NTA, nontreponemal antibody; PCR, polymerase chain reaction.

Source: Reproduced with permission from Heresi, G. (2017). Syphilis. In Eichenwald et al. (Eds.), *Cloherty and Stark's manual of neonatal care* (8th ed., pp. 788–737). Philadelphia, PA: Wolters Kluwer.

TABLE 22.16 Toxoplasmosis Infection Transmission Rates

	1st Trimester	2nd Trimester	3rd Trimester
Fetal infection rates increase as gestation increases	6%–17%	25%–40%	60%–72%
Severity of fetal disease decreases as gestation increases	40% severe fetal disease Plus 35% stillbirth or perinatal death		Most have a subclinical infection

Sources: Data from Holzmann-Pazgal, G. (2017). Congenital toxoplasmosis. In Eichenwald et al. (Eds.), *Cloherty and Stark's manual of neonatal care* (8th ed., pp. 720–727). Philadelphia, PA: Wolters Kluwer; Michaels, M. G., Sanchez, P., & Lin, L. (2018). Congenital toxoplasmosis, syphilis, malaria, and tuberculosis. In C. Gleason & S. Juul (Eds.), *Avery's diseases of the newborn* (10th ed., pp. 527–552.e6). Philadelphia, PA: Elsevier.

- Many congenital infections are asymptomatic at birth.
- Treatment for diagnosed toxoplasmosis is long term and requires antiparasitics for no less than 1 year. Most common antiparasitics include pyrimethamine, sulfadiazine, and folinic acid.
- The pregnant mother with known toxoplasmosis infection and in the neonate with a confirmed or probable diagnosis is treated with the same medications. Treatment of infants with toxoplasmosis infections can reduce the risk of SNHL and visual and neurodevelopmental morbidities (Michaels et al., 2018, p. 530).
  - If there is ophthalmic or CNS involvement, or if the mother is HIV positive, additional therapy with a corticosteroid may improve long-term outcomes (Michaels et al., 2018, p. 530; Pammi et al., 2016, p. 543).
- Congenital infection with *T. gondii* has a mortality rate as high as 12%. Morbidities may include ophthalmologic, neurodevelopmental, and audiologic impairments, including mental retardation, seizures, spasticity and palsies, and deafness, which may occur in subclinical infection (Michaels et al., 2018, pp. 529–531).

TABLE 22.17 Clinical Symptoms of Congenital Toxoplasmosis

Prenatal Presentation on Ultrasound	Postnatal Presentation	
	One-third present with generalized symptoms	Two-thirds present mostly with CNS symptoms, which is the hallmark of congenital *T. gondii* infection
• Intracranial hyperechogenic foci • Ventricular dilation • Anemia • Hydrops • Ascites • Brain, splenic, and hepatic calcifications • Hepatosplenomegaly	• IUGR • Temperature instability • Hepatosplenomegaly • Jaundice • Pneumonitis • Generalized lymphadenopathy • Maculopapular rash • Petechiae • Chorioretinitis • Anemia • Thrombocytopenia • Eosinophilia • Abnormal CSF • Diarrhea	Classic triad of congenital toxoplasmosis 1. Chorioretinitis 2. Diffuse Intracranial calcifications 3. Obstructive hydrocephalus Other CNS symptoms: • Pleocytosis (elevated WBC in CSF) • Elevated protein count in CSF • Microcephaly • Hyper/hypothermia related to hypothalamic involvement • Seizures • Direct hyperbilirubinemia • Meningoencephalitis

CSF, cerebrospinal fluid; IUGR, intrauterine growth restriction; WBC, white blood cell.

Sources: Data from Holzmann-Pazgal, G. (2017). Congenital toxoplasmosis. In Eichenwald et al. (Eds.), *Cloherty and Stark's manual of neonatal care* (8th ed., pp. 720–727). Philadelphia, PA: Wolters Kluwer; Michaels, M. G., Sanchez, P., & Lin, L. (2018). Congenital toxoplasmosis, syphilis, malaria, and tuberculosis. In C. Gleason & S. Juul (Eds.), *Avery's diseases of the newborn* (10th ed., pp. 527–552.e6). Philadelphia, PA: Elsevier; Pammi, M., Brand, M. C., & Weismann, L. (2016). Infection in the neonate. In S. Gardner, B. Carter, M. Hines, & J. Hernandez (Eds.), *Merenstein & Gardner's* handbook of neonatal intensive care (8th ed., pp. 537–562). St. Louis, MO: Elsevier.

CONCLUSION

Throughout pregnancy the fetus is protected to an extent by the chorioamniotic membranes, the placenta, and various anti-microbial factors in the amniotic fluid that are poorly understood. Even with these protections, congenital bacterial and viral infections may occur and have long-term impact on the neonate's growth and development. Understanding the implications of an immature immune system and the common bacterial and viral risks facing the neonate will allow the NNP to make clinically appropriate decisions in the evaluation and treatment of neonatal infections.

REVIEW QUESTIONS

1. A 16-day-old neonate presents with poor feeding and lethargy. What type of evaluation is warranted?
   A. complete blood count (CBC), C-reactive protein (CRP), and blood culture
   B. CBC, blood cultures, and lumbar puncture (LP)
   C. CBC, blood cultures, urine culture, and LP

2. Neonatal sepsis has varying presentations, which may include:
   A. epidemiological risk factors
   B. nonspecific and nonlocalized signs
   C. specific and localized signs

3. Which of the following supports a proactive preventative approach to hospital-acquired infections (HAIs)?
   A. hand hygiene, proper management of central venous catheters, appropriate use of antibiotics, and limited use of H-2 blockers and proton pump inhibitors

   B. hand hygiene, central line dressing changes every 3 days, limited use of antibiotics, and antibiotic prophylaxis for every NICU admission
   C. hand hygiene, limited use of antibiotics, antibiotic prophylaxis for central lines, and limited use of H-2 blockers and proton pump inhibitors

4. A neonate presents at birth with low birth weight, jaundice, and hepatosplenomegaly. The maternal history is negative other than a mononucleosis-like illness during the pregnancy. The NNP knows that further diagnostic testing should include:
   A. both treponemal and non-tremponemal tests
   B. head ultrasound, eye exam, and hearing screen
   C. polymerase reaction on nasopharyngeal secretions

5. A neonate presents at 7 days of age with a fever, and during the physical examination the NNP notes a cluster of vesicles on the scalp over the occipital region. The NNP reviews mother's history and does not find any history of herpes lesions. The NNP decides the risk of the infant having HSV is:
   A. somewhat likely, although it could be a rash
   B. negative without a positive maternal history
   C. highly possible, based on exam and timing

REFERENCES

American Academy of Pediatrics. (2018). Human immunodeficiency virus infection. In D. Kimberlin, M. Brady, M. Jackson, & S. Long (Eds.), *Red book: 2018 Report of the committee on infectious diseases* (31st ed., pp. 459–475). Itasca, IL: American Academy of Pediatrics.

American Academy of Pediatrics. (2018b). Respiratory syncytial virus. In D. Kimberlin, M. Brady, M. Jackson, & S. Long (Eds.), *Red book: 2018 Report of the committee on infectious diseases* (31st ed., pp. 682–691). Itasca, IL: Author.

American Academy of Pediatrics. (2018c). Varicella-zoster virus infection. In D. Kimberlin, M. Brady, M. Jackson, & S. Long (Eds.), *Red book: 2018 Report of the committee on infectious diseases* (31st ed., pp. 869–882). Itasca, IL: Author.

Baley, J. E., & Leonard, E. G. (2013). Infections in the neonate. In A. Fanaroff & A. Fanaroff (Eds.), *Klaus and Fanaroff's care of the high-risk neonate* (6th ed., pp. 346–367). Cleveland, OH: Elsevier.

Benjamin, J. T., Mezu-Ndubuisi, O. J., & Maheshwari, A. (2015). Developmental immunology. In R. Martin, A. Fanaroff, & M. Walsh (Eds.), *Fanaroff and Martin's neonatal-perinatal medicine: Diseases of the fetus and infant* (10th ed., pp. 737–741). Philadelphia, PA: Elsevier.

Blackburn, S. T. (2013). *Maternal, fetal, & neonatal physiology: A clinical perspective* (4th ed.). Philadelphia, PA: Elsevier.

Boos, M. D., & Sidbury, R. (2018). Infections of the skin. In C. Gleason & S. Juul (Eds.), *Avery's diseases of the newborn* (10th ed., p. 1495–1502.e2). Philadelphia, PA: Elsevier.

Ferrieri, P., & Wallen, L. (2018). Newborn sepsis and meningitis. In C. Gleason & S. Juul (Eds.), *Avery's diseases of the newborn* (10th ed., pp. 546–565). Philadelphia, PA: Elsevier.

Gilmore, A., & Thompson, G. H. (2015). Bone and joint infections in neonates. In R. Martin, A. Fanaroff, & M. Walsh (Eds.), *Fanaroff and Martin's neonatal-perinatal medicine: Diseases of the fetus and infant* (10th ed., pp. 1784–1786). Philadelphia, PA: Elsevier.

Greenberg, J. M., Narendran, V., Schibler, K. R., Warner, B. B., & Haberman, B. E. (2014). Neonatal morbidities of prenatal and perinatal origin. In R. Resnik, R. K. Creasy, J. D. Iams, C. J. Lockwood, T. Moore, & M. F. Greene (Eds.), *Creasy & Resnik's maternal-fetal medicine principles and practice* (7th ed., pp. 1215–1239.e7). St. Louis, MO: Elsevier.

Heresi, G. (2017). Syphilis. In E. Eichenwald, A. Hansen, C. Martin, & A. Stark (Eds.), *Cloherty and Stark's manual of neonatal care* (8th ed., pp. 788–737). Philadelphia, PA: Wolters Kluwer.

Holzmann-Pazgal, G. (2017). Congenital toxoplasmosis. In E. Eichenwald, A. Hansen, C. Martin, & A. Stark (Eds.), *Cloherty and Stark's manual of neonatal care* (8th ed., pp. 720–727). Philadelphia, PA: Wolters Kluwer.

Hostetter, M. & Gleason, C. (2018). Fungal infections in the neonatal intensive care unit. In C. Gleason & S. Juul (Eds.), *Avery's diseases of the newborn* (10th ed., pp. 581–585.e2). Philadelphia, PA: Elsevier.

Leonard, E. G., & Dobbs, K. (2015). Postnatal bacterial infections. In R. Martin, A. Fanaroff, & M. Walsh (Eds.), *Fanaroff and Martin's neonatal-perinatal medicine: Diseases of the fetus and infant* (10th ed., pp. 734–750). Philadelphia, PA: Elsevier.

McElory, S. J., Frey, M. R., Torres, B. A., & Maheshwari, A. (2018). Innate and mucosal immunity in the developing gastrointestinal tract. In C. Gleason & S. Juul (Eds.), *Avery's diseases of the newborn* (10th ed., pp. 1064–1065). Philadelphia, PA: Elsevier.

Michaels, M. G., Sanchez, P., & Lin, L. (2018). Congenital toxoplasmosis, syphilis, malaria, and tuberculosis. In C. Gleason & S. Juul (Eds.), *Avery's diseases of the newborn* (10th ed., pp. 527–552.e6). Philadelphia, PA: Elsevier.

Noori, S., Azhibekov, T., Lee, B., & Seri, I. (2018). Cardiovascular compromise in the newborn. In C. Gleason & S. Juul (Eds.), *Avery's diseases of the newborn* (10th ed., pp. 741–754). Philadelphia, PA: Elsevier.

Pammi, M., Brand, M. C., & Weismann, L. (2016). Infection in the neonate. In S. Gardner, B. Carter, M. Hines, & J. Hernandez (Eds.), *Merenstein & Gardner's handbook of neonatal intensive care* (8th ed., pp. 537–562). St. Louis, MO: Elsevier.

Permar, S. R. (2017). Bacterial and fungal infections. In E. Eichenwald, A. Hansen, C. Martin, & A. Stark (Eds.), *Cloherty and Stark's manual of neonatal care* (8th ed., pp. 641–650). Philadelphia, PA: Wolters Kluwer.

Puopolo, K. M. (2017). Bacterial and fungal infections. In E. Eichenwald, A. Hansen, C. Martin, & A. Stark (Eds.), *Cloherty and Stark's manual of neonatal care* (8th ed., pp. 684–719). Philadelphia, PA: Wolters Kluwer.

Schleis, M. R., & Marsh, K. J. (2018). Viral infections of the fetus and newborn. In C. Gleason & S. Juul (Eds.), *Avery's diseases of the newborn* (10th ed., pp. 482–526.e18). Philadelphia, PA: Elsevier.

Srinivasan, L., & Evans, J. R. (2018). Health care-associated infections. In C. Gleason & S. Juul (Eds.), *Avery's diseases of the newborn* (10th ed., pp. 571–574). Philadelphia, PA: Elsevier.

Wang, P., Djahangirian, O., & Wehbi, E. (2018). Urinary tract infections and vesicoureteral reflux. In C. Gleason & S. Juul (Eds.), *Avery's diseases of the newborn* (10th ed., pp. 1309–1310). Philadelphia, PA: Elsevier.

Weitkamp, J. H., Lewis, D. B., & Levy, O. (2018). Immunology of the fetus and newborn. In C. Gleason & S. Juul (Eds.), *Avery's diseases of the newborn* (10th ed., pp. 453–481, 1448–1449). Philadelphia, PA: Elsevier.

White, K. K., Bouchard, M., & Goldberg, M. J. (2018). Common neonatal orthopedic conditions. In C. Gleason & S. Juul (Eds.), *Avery's diseases of the newborn* (10th ed., pp. 1448–1449). Philadelphia, PA: Elsevier.

Wilson, D. J., & Tyner, C. I. (2015). Infectious diseases in the neonate. In T. Verklan & M. Walden (Eds.), *Core curriculum for neonatal intensive care nursing* (5th ed., pp. 689–718). St. Louis, MO: Elsevier.

Christi Olsen

INTRODUCTION

Complete understanding of the development and abnormalities throughout the musculoskeletal system is crucial to prompt diagnosis and treatment of abnormalities and congenital syndromes.

MUSCULOSKELETAL DEVELOPMENT

Embryologic Development

- The embryologic development of the musculoskeletal system stems from both the mesoderm and the neural crest, as the musculoskeletal system requires both functional tissue and innervation to function properly (Liu & Thompson, 2015, p. 1777).
- Development and differentiation of both the mesoderm and neural crest being in weeks 3 to 4.
  - ○ The innervation of the musculoskeletal system rises from the notochord, a tubular column of cells formed cephalocaudally on the long axis of the embryo (Liu & Thompson, 2015, p. 1777).
- The extremities develop from the limb buds beginning in week 4 and continue in a proximal–distal pattern until week 8.
  - ○ During this time, cells forming connective tissue differentiate from the mesoderm into three segments:
    - Dermatomes, which become the skin
    - Myotomes, which become muscle cells
    - Sclerotomes, which become cartilage and bone
- Differentiation of the spinal cord begins week in fourth week of embryologic development, beginning with somites which create mesodermal tissue that migrates dorsally and anterolaterally to give rise to the trunk structures and limbs (Liu & Thompson, 2015, pp. 1776–1777).
- Teratogens and genetic abnormalities in the embryologic period affecting the musculoskeletal system result in malformations of the extremities and spine.
  - ○ Teratogens include irradiation, industrial chemicals, therapeutic drugs, and maternal infections such as rubella, congenital syphilis, cytomegalic inclusion disease, and congenital herpes (Heresi, 2017, p. 729; Liu & Thompson, 2015, p. 1777).
  - ○ Genetic disorders are classified as either Mendelian, chromosomal, or multifactorial (see Genetics for definition of inheritance patterns; Liu & Thompson, 2015, p. 1777).

Fetal Development

- After the embryologic foundation is laid, skeletal development continues throughout gestation, the postnatal period, and through the end of adolescence (Liu & Thompson, 2015, p. 1777).
  - ○ Primary skeletal ossification centers are present in the long bones near the end of the first trimester, and growth occurs from the ends of the long bones (i.e., humerus, radius, ulna, metacarpals, phalanges, femur, tibia, fibula, metatarsals) (Liu & Thompson, 2015, p. 1777).
- In utero fetal movement and "kicking" strengthen and develop muscular system. Muscle cells (myocytes) continue to differentiate and mature, with full maturation present at 38 weeks' post-menstrual age. Myocytes grow primarily by hypertrophy with little myogenesis occurring after birth (Blackburn, 2013, p. 510; Liu & Thompson, 2015, p. 1776; Tappero, 2016, p. 139).
- Muscle tone develops in a caudocephalad and distal–proximal patterns and active tone develops prior to passive tone (Blackburn, 2013, p. 510).

CONGENITAL SYNDROMES AFFECTING THE MUSCULOSKELETAL SYSTEM

Apert Syndrome

DEFINITION

- Characterized by craniosynostosis involving the coronal sutures and wide anterior fontanelle and metopic suture, micrognathia or maxillary hypoplasia, hypertelorism with downward slanting palpebral fissures, symmetric syndactyly of hands and feet (Robinson & Cohen, 2015, pp. 984–985)

INCIDENCE AND ETIOLOGY

- Occurs in approximately one in 55,000 births, and is typically described as a sporadic mutation involving FGFR2 gene (Robinson & Cohen, 2015, p. 984).

PRESENTATION

- Congenital craniosynostosis of the coronal sutures, wide anterior fontanelle and metopic suture, micrognathia, short beaked nose, and symmetric syndactyly of hands and feet (Robinson & Cohen, 2015, p. 984)
  - ○ May present in respiratory distress due to small, beaked nose (Robinson & Cohen, 2015, p. 984).
- Ventriculomegaly, which typically does not progress but may precipitate hydrocephalus

INTERVENTION AND OUTCOMES

- Routine management of respiratory distress (Robinson & Cohen, 2015, p. 985)
- Consider cranial ultrasound and neurosurgical consult if ventriculomegaly is present. Ventriculomegaly and/

or hydrocephalus does not appear to affect intellectual functions (Robinson & Cohen, 2015, p. 985).

Crouzon

DEFINITION
- Crouzon syndrome is characterized by craniosynostosis not usually present at birth, bulging and wide set eyes due to shallow eye sockets, micrognathia, fusion of cervical vertebrae, and ankylosis of elbows that become more emphasized as the infant grows (Robinson & Cohen, 2015, p. 984).

INCIDENCE AND ETIOLOGY
- Approximately 50% of Crouzon cases are familial; the other half of cases have been linked to mutations of the FGFR2 gene.
- The incidence of Crouzon is approximately one in 25,000 live births.

PRESENTATION
- Presentation includes craniosynostosis not usually present at birth, bulging and wide set eyes due to shallow eye sockets, micrognathia, beaked nose, small nasopharynx, fusion of cervical vertebrae, ankylosis of elbows that become more emphasized as the infant grows.
  - ○ May present in respiratory distress initially, due to malformed nasal structures.
- Subluxation of the eyes may occur.
- Hydrocephalus may occur (Robinson & Cohen, 2015, p. 984).

INTERVENTION AND OUTCOMES
- Routine management of respiratory distress
- Consider cranial ultrasound and neurosurgical consult if ventriculomegaly is present, although hydrocephalus does not appear to affect intellectual functions.
- Ophthalmology follow-up may be indicated if exophthalmos is severe (Robinson & Cohen, 2015, p. 984).

Congenital Myotonic Dystrophy

DEFINITION
- Congenital myotonic dystrophy (CMD) is a genetic disorder characterized by muscular dystrophy and hypotonia (Bass, Lotze, & Miller, 2015, p. 958).

INCIDENCE AND ETIOLOGY
- Congenital myotonic dystrophy is an autosomal dominant disease that affects one in 3,500 live births, and is caused by genetic mutations of chromosome 19q13.3. It is typically inherited from the mother, who is also affected but typically to a lesser degree (Bass et al., 2015, p. 958).

PRESENTATION
- Prenatal history of polyhydramnios and decreased fetal movement is common. In addition, mothers may experience prolonged labor due to poor uterine contractions related to their own myotonic dystrophy (Bass et al., 2015, p. 958).
- Infants may require resuscitation at birth secondary to poor respiratory quality due to muscular weakness and pulmonary immaturity and may succumb to complications such

as hypoxic-ischemic encephalopathy (Bass et al., 2015, p. 958).
- CMD ranges in severity, but presents as respiratory distress accompanied by profound generalized hypotonia, diminished or absent deep tendon reflexes, and facial diplegia with ptosis (Bass et al., 2015, p. 958).
- Generalized hypotonia with weak suck-swallow may lead to feeding aspiration (Bass et al., 2015, p. 958).

INTERVENTION AND OUTCOMES
- Upon suspicion of CMD, clinical and electromyographic exams of the mother should be performed as well as genetic studies, including molecular genetic analysis (Bass et al., 2015, p. 958).
- Routine management of respiratory distress depending on degree of severity
- Infant may require ancillary services such as physical, occupational, and speech therapies.
- Mortality of neonates with CMD is high, despite intensive care. Mortality is increased in infants requiring mechanical ventilation for greater than 30 days.
  - ○ Of infants who survive without comorbidities of prematurity, such as cerebral palsy, most walk by age 3. However, significant learning disabilities develop with maturation (Bass et al., 2015, p. 959).

ABNORMALITIES OF THE EXTREMITIES

Syndactyly

DEFINITION
- Syndactyly—fusion of digits, which is likely a normal variant but can be associated with genetic syndromes (see Box 23.1; Son-Hing & Thompson, 2015, p. 1790; Tappero, 2016, p. 162).

INCIDENCE AND ETIOLOGY
- Syndactyly occurs in one in 2,000 to 3,000 live births, is more common in males than females, and occurs more frequently in White infants than infants of African descent

---

BOX 23.1 Congenital syndromes associated with syndactyly and polydactyly

> Syndactyly
>   Apert syndrome
>   Streeter's dysplasia
>
> Polydactyly
>   Trisomy 13
>   Trisomy 21
>   Meckel–Gruber syndrome
>   Other skeletal malformations in White infants with postaxial polydactyly

Sources: Data from Son-Hing, J., & Thompson, G. (2015). Congenital abnormalities of the upper and lower extremities and spine. In R. Martin, A. Fanaroff, & M. Walsh (Eds.), *Fanaroff and Martin's neonatal–perinatal medicine: Diseases of the fetus and infant* (10th ed., pp. 1789–1808). Philadelphia, PA: Elsevier; Tappero, E. (2016). Musculoskeletal system assessment. In E. P. Tappero & M. E. Honeyfield (Eds.), *Physical assessment of the newborn* (5th ed., pp. 139–166). New York, NY: Springer Publishing Company.

(Son-Hing & Thompson, 2015, p. 1790; Tappero, 2016, p. 162).

- Most cases (approximately 80%) are spontaneous without genetic transmission (Son-Hing & Thompson, 2015, p. 1790; Tappero, 2016, p. 162).
- Syndactyly is the most common congenital abnormalities involving the upper extremities and is a result of failure of separation during the fifth to eighth week of gestation (Son-Hing & Thompson, 2015, p. 1790).
- May be an incidental, familial finding, or associated with several congenital syndromes (Son-Hing & Thompson, 2015, p. 1790).

PRESENTATION

- Severity of syndactyly ranges from mild webbing to complete fusion with bone structure involvement. May be present on fingers, toes, or both (Son-Hing & Thompson, 2015, p. 1790; Tappero, 2016, p. 162).

INTERVENTION AND OUTCOMES

- Intervention of syndactyly is not routine but may be requested by parents, and treatment depends on the severity of the webbing, bony structure, and vascular involvement (Son-Hing & Thompson, 2015, p. 1790).
  - When encountered, consultation with pediatric orthopedic and plastic surgery is recommended to determine course of treatment for function and cosmetic appearance (Tappero, 2016, p. 162).
  - Near-equal-length digits typically do not need separation until 2 to 3 years of age (Son-Hing & Thompson, 2015, p. 1791; Tappero, 2016, p. 162).
- Syndactyly of toes does not affect function (Tappero, 2016, p. 162).
- Syndactyly of unequal lengths, that is, thumb and index finger fused, can cause tethering and deformity of longer digit. Earlier intervention is recommended (Son-Hing & Thompson, 2015, p. 1791; Tappero, 2016, p. 162).

Polydactyly

DEFINITION

- Polydactyly is a duplication of digits, and is most commonly an incidental, familial finding but may also be associated with several congenital syndromes (Kasser, 2017, p. 846; Son-Hing & Thompson, 2015, p. 1791; Tappero, 2016, p. 162).

INCIDENCE AND ETIOLOGY

- Polydactyly also occurs commonly; approximately one in 300 African American live births and one in 3,000 White live births.
  - Radial polydactyly rates are similar in African American and White infants. Ulnar polydactyly is more common in African American infants and associated anomalies are **not** usually present.
  - In White infants, ulnar polydactyly is less common and often **is** associated with other skeletal anomalies, that is, syndactyly, coalescence of carpal bones, radioulnar synostosis, tibia and fibula hypoplasia and/or aplasia, hemivertebrae, and dwarfism (Son-Hing & Thompson, 2015, p. 1791; Tappero, 2016, p. 163).

PRESENTATION

- Presence of extra digits on the radial or ulnar aspect of the hand or the medial or lateral aspect of the foot. May be present unilaterally or bilaterally (Son-Hing & Thompson, 2015, p. 1791; Tappero, 2016, p. 163)
- Severity ranges from bulbous formation to complete skeletal and vascular formation of the digit (Kasser, 2017, p. 846; Son-Hing & Thompson, 2015, p. 1791; Tappero, 2016, p. 163).

INTERVENTION AND OUTCOMES

- Treatment may or may not be necessary and outcome depends on severity of defect and presence of associated syndromes. Decisions to treat also depend on the degree of development of the digit; some less severe tags can be tied off, whereas some digits with bony structures and complete vasculature may require more complex surgical intervention. Surgical intervention is usually completed between 6 and 18 months of age (Son-Hing & Thompson, 2015, p. 1791; Tappero, 2016, p. 163).
- Ligation of extra radial digits should not be routinely performed by the NNP due to risk of incomplete arterial ligation, resulting in subsequent venous congestion and pain. Instead ,consultation with a pediatric hand specialist should be completed (Kasser, 2017, p. 846; Tappero, 2016, p. 163).

Developmental Dysplasia of the Hip

DEFINITION

- Developmental dysplasia of the hip (DDH) is the presence of a dislocatable femoral head from the acetabulum present at birth, which may be unilateral or bilateral and ranges in severity from hip laxity to complete, irreducible dislocation (Son-Hing & Thompson, 2015, p. 1796; Sterk, 2015, p. 783; Tappero, 2016, p. 157).
- DDH is classified as typical when the infant has normal neurologic findings, or it may be classified as teratogenic when the infant has other neuromuscular abnormalities (Son-Hing & Thompson, 2015, p. 1796).

INCIDENCE AND ETIOLOGY

- DDH of ranging severity occurs in 11.5 per 1,000 live births and frank dislocations occurs in two per 1,000 live births in the United States. It occurs more commonly in females than males, and in Native American and Eastern European ethnicities (Son-Hing & Thompson, 2015, p. 1796; Sterk, 2015, p. 783; Tappero, 2016, p. 157).
- Typical DDH is a multifactorial condition involving genetic predisposition, physiology, and mechanical factors. See Box 23.2 for risk factors for DDH.
- The most common risk factors resulting in DDH are first born and breech presentation. Breech position results in extreme flexion and decreased motion causing increased instability (Son-Hing & Thompson, 2015, p. 1796; Sterk, 2015, p. 783; Tappero, 2016, p. 157).

PRESENTATION

- DDH diagnosis is highly suspected when Barlow and Ortolani tests are positive, asymmetric thigh and gluteal skin folds, uneven knee levels (Allis or Galeazzi sign), and the absence of normal knee flexion contractures (Son-Hing & Thompson, 2015, p. 1796; Sterk, 2015, p. 783; Tappero, 2016, p. 157).

BOX 23.2 Risk factors for developmental dysplasia of the hip

Genetic Factors
  Family history of DDH
  Inherited ligamentous laxity

Physiologic Factors
  Female
  Maternal estrogen and other hormones related to pelvic
    relaxation during labor

Mechanical Factors
  Primigravida
  Breech presentation
  Postnatal positioning including adduction and extension of
    lower extremities

Sources: Data from Sterk, L. (2015). Congenital anomalies. In M. T. Verlan & M. Walden (Eds.), *Core curriculum for neonatal intensive care nursing* (5th ed., pp. 767–794). Maryland Heights, MO: Elsevier/Saunders; Son-Hing, J., & Thompson, G. (2015). Congenital abnormalities of the upper and lower extremities and spine. In R. Martin, A. Fanaroff, & M. Walsh (Eds.), *Fanaroff and Martin's neonatal–perinatal medicine: Diseases of the fetus and infant* (10th ed., pp. 1789–1808). Philadelphia, PA: Elsevier; Tappero, E. (2016). Musculoskeletal system assessment. In E. P. Tappero & M. E. Honeyfield (Eds.), *Physical assessment of the newborn* (5th ed., pp. 139–166). New York, NY: Springer Publishing Company.

INTERVENTION AND OUTCOMES
- Interventions include accurate and early diagnosis, use of Pavlik harness, and orthopedic referral. If spontaneous reduction or recurrent dislocation occurs, surgical closed reduction may be necessary (Kasser, 2017, p. 847; Tappero, 2016, p. 157; White, Bouchard, & Goldberg, 2018, p. 1351).
- Imaging includes hip ultrasound ,and radiographs may be performed to confirm diagnosis.
- Decreased motion results in decreased stimulation and growth of the acetabulum cartilage (Son-Hing & Thompson, 2015, p. 1796).

Talipes Equinovarus (Club Foot)

DEFINITION
- Talipes equinovarus (TE) is characterized as adduction of forefoot, pronounced varus, foot and toes in downward pointing position, equinus position, and atrophy of the affected lower extremity. TE may be unilateral or bilateral (Kasser, 2017, p. 851; Son-Hing & Thompson, 2015, p. 1802; Tappero, 2016, pp. 160–116, 226; White et al., 2018, p. 1354).

INCIDENCE AND ETIOLOGY
- Most common neonatal foot abnormalities occurring in one to two in 1,000 live births (Son-Hing & Thompson, 2015, p. 1802; Tappero, 2016, p. 160).
- Three classifications: congenital, teratologic, and positional
  - Congenital TE is generally an isolated abnormality and the etiology is unknown; however, there is thought to be a familial component.
  - Teratologic TE is associated with neuromuscular disorders such as myelodysplasia or arthrogryposis.
  - Positional TE occurs in utero when a normal foot has been held in the equinovarus position (Kasser, 2017, p. 851; Son-Hing & Thompson, 2015, p. 1802; Tappero, 2016, pp. 160–116, 226; White et al., 2018, p. 1354).

PRESENTATION
- When manipulated, the foot is unable to be passively positioned midline; this differentiates club foot from metatarsus adductus (Kasser, 2017, p. 851; Son-Hing & Thompson, 2015, p. 1802; Tappero, 2016, pp. 160–116, 226; White et al., 2018, p. 1354).

INTERVENTION AND OUTCOMES
- Intervention includes range of motion exercises to be started in the nursery, followed by pediatric orthopedic and physical therapy referrals.
  - The Ponseti method of positioning and serial casting is the common form of treatment; occasionally surgical intervention is necessary for severe deformities or when nonoperative treatments are unsuccessful.
- Successful treatment using nonoperative methods has been achieved when treatment begins prior to 1 year of age. Nonoperative treatment is a lengthy process that can take several years to fully correct TE (Kasser, 2017, p. 851; Son-Hing & Thompson, 2015, p. 1802; Tappero, 2016, pp. 160–116, 226; White et al., 2018, p. 1354).

Metatarsus Adductus

DEFINITION
- Metatarsus adductus is the medial positioning of the forefoot without pathologic structural changes to the metatarsals.

INCIDENCE AND ETIOLOGY
- Metatarsus adductus is the most common foot anomaly in neonates.
  - Approximately 10% of children with metatarsus adductus have DDH.
- Etiology is unclear; however, it is suspected that intrauterine positioning is a contributing factor (Son-Hing & Thompson, 2015, p. 1800).

PRESENTATION
- Presentation includes adduction of the forefoot with occasional supination. Infant will have normal ankle dorsiflexion and plantar flexion.
- The degree of flexibility of the foot determines severity of malformation; however, the foot should be able to be positioned midline (Kasser, 2017, p. 850; Son-Hing & Thompson, 2015, p. 1800; White et al., 2018, p. 1443).

INTERVENTION AND OUTCOMES
- Typically corrects without intervention by age 3. Imaging is unnecessary initially, but weight-bearing radiographs may be necessary to diagnosis rigid versus moderate deformities.
- Intervention includes parental reassurance and routine pediatric follow-up (Kasser, 2017, p. 850; Son-Hing & Thompson, 2015, p. 1800; White et al., 2018, p. 1443).

SKELETAL DYSPLASIA

Achondroplasia

DEFINITION
- Achondroplasia is a form of dwarfism, characterized by frontal bossing and shortened lower limbs (Son-Hing & Thompson, 2015, p. 1803; Tappero, 2016, p. 263).

INCIDENCE AND ETIOLOGY

- It is estimated that achondroplasia occurs one in 15,000 to one in 40,000 live births. However, it is more common for the parents of achondroplastic patients to be of normal stature (Son-Hing & Thompson, 2015, p. 1803; Tappero, 2016, p. 263).
- Achondroplasia is cause by a mutation in the gene that controls fibroblast growth factor receptor 3 (FGFB3), causing disturbances in bone growth in early development. In achondroplasiam, the mutations of FGFB3 cause an overproduction of the protein responsible for converting cartilage to bone. This occurs in an autosomal dominant inheritance pattern (Son-Hing & Thompson, 2015, p. 1803; Tappero, 2016, p. 263).

PRESENTATION

- Characteristics include frontal bossing, flattened nasal bridge, shortened arms and thighs, and average torso length with protruding abdomen. Knees and hands may be hyperextendable. Hands may be short and broad with widely spaced long and ring fingers, forming a "trident hand." There is generally some degree of genu varum. Mild to moderate hypotonia is also common in newborns (Son-Hing & Thompson, 2015, p. 1803; Tappero, 2016, p. 263).

INTERVENTION AND OUTCOMES

- The infant should receive routine care unless other concerns are noted, and if so, then consultation with neurology, genetics, and orthopedics should be considered (Son-Hing & Thompson, 2015, p. 1803; Tappero, 2016, p. 263).
- Homozygous achondroplasia is a lethal defect due to respiratory insufficiency related to rib cage hypoplasia (Son-Hing & Thompson, 2015, p. 1803).
- Infants with heterozygous achondroplasia have a normal life expectancy. However, these children are at high risk for motor milestone delays as well as middle ear infections and unresolving genu varum (Son-Hing & Thompson, 2015, p. 1803; Tappero, 2016, p. 263).

Arthrogryposis Multiplex Congenita

DEFINITION

- Arthrogryposis multiplex congenita (AMC) is a syndrome classified by the presence of multiple joint contractures present at birth (Bennett & Meier, 2019, p. 231; Son-Hing & Thompson, 2015, p. 1804).

INCIDENCE/ETIOLOGY

- AMC occurs in approximately one in 8,000 live births and the cause is attributed to intrinsic and extrinsic factors (Son-Hing & Thompson, 2015, p. 1804).
  - Intrinsic factors include neurologic, muscular, and joint problems, with neurologic problems being most common.
  - Extrinsic factors include fetal crowding or intrauterine constraint.

PRESENTATION

- Infants present with multiple contractures, fixed or limited mobility limb extensions, and joint dislocations at birth (Bennett & Meier, 2019, p. 231; Son-Hing & Thompson, 2015, p. 1804).

INTERVENTION AND OUTCOMES

- The infant should be evaluated for the degree of contracture and the presence of scoliosis, which may include radiographs (Son-Hing & Thompson, 2015, p. 1804).
- Given the cause of AMC, referral to pediatric neurology and orthopedics should be considered, and neonates may require physical therapy and serial casting to correct club foot and other contractures (Son-Hing & Thompson, 2015, p. 1804).
- Outcomes depend on the cause of AMC and severity of contractures. In some cases, surgical interventions are necessary to aid in range of motion, but this is not typically done in the neonatal period (Son-Hing & Thompson, 2015, p. 1804).

SPINAL ABNORMALITIES

Congenital Scoliosis and Kyphosis

DEFINITION

- Congenital scoliosis is a lateral curvature of the spine resulting from an embryologic failure of spinal formation or segmentation.
- Congenital kyphosis is the failure of formation of all or part of the vertebral body with preservation of the posterior elements as well as the failure of anterior segmentation of the spine (Kasser, 2017, p. 847; Son-Hing & Thompson, 2015, p. 1793; Tappero, 2016, p. 153; White et al., 2018, p. 1358).

INCIDENCE AND ETIOLOGY

- Congenital spinal deformities, including scoliosis, kyphosis, or a combination of the two, occurs in 0.5 to one in 1,000 live births. Neither are inherited or chromosomal, but typically result from and embryologic failure of formation or segmentation of the vertebrae. Congenital scoliosis is more common in females than males, and may be accompanied by cardiac or genitourinary anomalies (Kasser, 2017, p. 847; Son-Hing & Thompson, 2015, p. 1793; Tappero, 2016, p. 153; White et al., 2018, p. 1446).
- Congenital spinal anomalies can occur in Klippel-Feil and VACTERL/VATER syndromes.

PRESENTATION

- Both scoliosis and kyphosis may be difficult to detect at birth; however, early detection is critical to prevent severe deformities and maintain neurologic function (Kasser, 2017, p. 847; Son-Hing & Thompson, 2015, p. 1793; Tappero, 2016, p. 153; White et al., 2018, p. 1446).

INTERVENTION AND OUTCOMES

- Evaluation includes radiographic evaluation of spine, echocardiogram, renal ultrasound, and orthopedic follow-up.
- Outcomes depend on the severity and location of the deformity as well as the presence of multiple anomalies at multiple levels such as hemivertebrae. Progressive kyphosis in the thoracic region can result in paraplegia (Kasser, 2017, p. 847; Son-Hing & Thompson, 2015, p. 1793; Tappero, 2016, p. 153; White et al., 2018, p. 1358).

Sacral Agenesis

DEFINITION

- The complete absence of the sacrum; with lower lumbar spine involvement, it is termed lumbosacral agenesis (Son-Hing & Thompson, 2015, p. 1794).

INCIDENCE AND ETIOLOGY

- Sacral agenesis is a rare disorder, occurring in one in 25,000 live births. Etiology is unknown; however, it tends to be associated with maternal diabetes (Son-Hing & Thompson, 2015, p. 1794).

PRESENTATION

- Presentation is variable, but in most severe forms includes a small pelvis, pterygia (webbing) of the hips and knees, and bilateral foot deformities.
- Spinopelvic instability may be present.
- Neurologic exam tends to show no motor function below the last complete vertebrae; however, innervation and sensation may be present (Son-Hing & Thompson, 2015, p. 1794).

INTERVENTIONS AND OUTCOMES

- Observation is appropriate for patients with partial agenesis and stable spinopelvic exam. Depending on degree of agenesis, ambulation may be possible with proper orthopedic consultation and orthotic use (Son-Hing & Thompson, 2015, p. 1794).
- Orthopedic and neurosurgical consultation should be included in the plan of care in case patients with complete agenesis or unstable spinopelvic exam require spinal fusion during childhood.
  - Spinal fusion can enhance sitting balance and improve upper extremity function (Son-Hing & Thompson, 2015, p. 1794).

MUSCULOSKELETAL BIRTH INJURIES

Fractures

CLAVICULAR FRACTURES

- Clavicle fractures are one of the most common birth injuries, and associated with shoulder dystocia and difficult delivery.
- Intervention includes pinning the sleeve of the infants' shirt to the front as a means to immobilize the extremity for 7 to 10 days (Abdulhayoglu, 2017, pp. 64–73; Son-Hing & Thompson, 2015, p. 1779; Tappero, 2016, p. 145; White et al., 2018, p. 1359).

HUMERAL FRACTURES

- Humeral fractures are second to clavicle fractures and are also associated with difficult delivery.
- Intervention includes immobilization via plaster splint or elastic bandage.

FEMORAL FRACTURES

- Femoral fractures are less common and associated with breech delivery.
- Intervention includes immobilization via simple plaster splint or Pavlik harness.
  - Splinting may be discontinued when callus formation is evident on radiograph (Abdulhayoglu, 2017, pp. 64–73; Son-Hing & Thompson, 2015, p. 1779; Tappero, 2016, p. 145; White et al., 2018, p. 1359).

Brachial Plexus Injuries

ERB'S PALSY

- Caused by injury to the fifth and sixth cervical nerve roots
- Defining characteristics of the affected arm include adducted, internally rotated, and extended at the elbow with flexion of the wrist with an intact grasp, as known as the "waiter's tip" position. The infant may have normal grasp with absent Moro reflex.
- Intervention includes gentle handling of affected arm and gentle passive range of motion to prevent contractures of the shoulder, elbow, forearm, and hand.
- Outcomes depend on nerve root involvement; most infants achieve functional improvement by 3 months of age. If improvement is not seen by 3 months, surgical intervention may be necessary (Abdulhayoglu, 2017, p. 71; Tappero, 2016, pp. 155–156; White et al., 2018, p. 1359).

KLUMPKE'S PALSY

- Caused by injury to the eighth cervical and first thoracic nerve roots
- Defining characteristics include upper arm mobility with complete lower arm paralysis with absent grasp. This is a less common birth injury compared to Erb's palsy.
- Intervention includes gentle handling of affected arm and gentle passive range of motion to prevent contractures of the shoulder, elbow, forearm, and hand (Abdulhayoglu, 2017, p. 71; Manguten et al., 2015, p. 419; Tappero, 2016, pp. 155–156; White et al., 2018, p. 1359).

TORTICOLLIS

- Caused by injury to the sternocleidomastoid (SCM) muscle, likely due to intrauterine positioning or birth trauma
- Defining characteristics include firm, immobile circumscribed mass on SCM present at birth to 14 days of age, tilting of the head toward the affected side with inability to passively move to neutral position.
- Intervention includes early physical therapy, if torticollis persists greater than four years, possible surgical interventions may be necessary.
  - If undiagnosed, torticollis may go unnoticed until plagiocephaly is evident (Kasser, 2015, p. 68; Son-Hing, 2015, pp. 423 and 1781, p. 423; Tappero, 2016, p. 153; White et al., 2018, p. 1353).

CONCLUSION

The musculoskeletal development spans from infancy through adolescence. A thorough understanding of fetal and neonatal musculoskeletal development and associated pathologies is vital to provide quick and accurate diagnosis a variety of birth related injuries, anomalies, and associated genetic disorders.

REVIEW QUESTIONS

1. The NNP performs an admission assessment on a 41-week infant who was delivered via cesarean section for breech presentation, and notes uneven gluteal folds. The correct next step for the NNP's assessment is to:
   A. Defer further examination and continue to monitor.
   B. Order an ultrasound examination of the hips.
   C. Perform the Barlow and Ortolani maneuvers.

2. On an initial exam, the NNP discovers the infant exhibits a lateral curvature of the spine and bilateral radial polydactyly. A radiograph of the chest revealed poorly formed

spinal vertebral bodies, leading the NNP to become concerned the infant has congenital:

A. arthrogryposis multiplex.

B. caudo-sacral agenesis.

C. scoliosis or kyphosis.

3. An infant is found to have complete syndactyly of the first and second digit on one hand. Parental education should focus on the fact that syndactyly is a:

A. disfigurement requiring surgical correction.

B. hallmark of several genetic syndromes.

C. normal variant and no special care is necessary.

4. The NNP attends the delivery of a small-for-gestational-age, 38 weeks' gestational-age infant. The prenatal history is significant for oligohydramnios and maternal bicornate uterus. The NNP notes on the initial exam the left foot is adducted and pointed downward and cannot be positioned midline, and correctly documents the finding in the chart as a:

A. metatarsus abduction.

B. talipes equinovarus.

C. varus adductus.

5. The most common neonatal fracture site is the:

A. clavicle.

B. femur.

C. humerus.

REFERENCES

Abdulhayoglu, E. (2017) Birth trauma. In E. Eichenwald, A. Hansen, C. Martin, & A. Stark (Eds.), *Cloherty and Stark's manual of neonatal care* (8th ed., pp. 64–75). Philadelphia, PA: Wolters Kluwer.

Bass, N., Lotze, T., & Miller, G. (2015). Hypotonia and neuromuscular disease in the neonate. In R. Martin, A. Fanaroff, & M. Walsh (Eds.), *Fanaroff and Martin's neonatal-perinatal medicine: Diseases of the fetus and infant* (10th ed., pp. 950–962). Philadelphia, PA: Elsevier.

Bennet, M., & Meier, S. (2019). Assessment of the dysmorphic infant. In E. P. Tappero & M. E. Honeyfield (Eds.), *Physical assessment of the newborn* (5th ed., pp. 219–237). New York, NY: Springer Publishing Company.

Blackburn, S. (2013). *Maternal, fetal, & neonatal physiology: A clinical perspective* (4th ed.). Maryland Heights, MO: Elsevier/Saunders.

Heresi, G. (2017) Syphilis. In E. Eichenwald, A. Hansen, C. Martin, & A. Stark (Eds.), *Cloherty and Stark's manual of neonatal care* (8th ed., pp. 728–737). Philadelphia, PA: Wolters Kluwer.

Kasser, J. (2017). Orthopedic problems. In E. Eichenwald, A. Hansen, C. Martin, & A. Stark (Eds.), *Cloherty and Stark's manual of neonatal care* (8th ed., pp. 845–852). Philadelphia, PA: Wolters Kluwer.

Liu, R., & Thompson, G. (2015). Musculoskeletal disorders in neonates. In R. Martin, A. Fanaroff, & M. Walsh (Eds.), *Fanaroff and Martin's neonatal–perinatal medicine: Diseases of the fetus and infant* (10th ed., pp. 1776–1783). Philadelphia, PA: Elsevier.

Robinson, S., & Cohen, A. (2015). Disorders of head shape and size. In R. Martin, A. Fanaroff, & M. Walsh (Eds.), *Fanaroff and Martin's neonatal–perinatal medicine: Diseases of the fetus and infant* (10th ed., pp. 964–987). Philadelphia, PA: Elsevier.

Son-Hing, J., & Thompson, G. (2015). Congenital abnormalities of the upper and lower extremities and spine. In R. Martin, A. Fanaroff, & M. Walsh (Eds.), *Fanaroff and Martin's neonatal-perinatal medicine: Diseases of the fetus and infant* (10th ed., pp. 1789–1808). Philadelphia, PA: Elsevier.

Sterk, L. (2015). Congenital anomalies. In M. T. Verlan & M. Walden (Eds.), *Core curriculum for neonatal intensive care nursing* (5th ed., pp. 767–794). Maryland Heights, MO: Elsevier/Saunders.

Tappero, E. (2016). Musculoskeletal system assessment. In E. P. Tappero & M. E. Honeyfield (Eds.), *Physical assessment of the newborn* (5th ed., pp. 139–166). New York, NY: Springer Publishing Company.

White, K., Bouchard, M., & Goldberg, M. (2018). Common neonatal orthopedic conditions. In C. Gleason & S. Juul (Eds.), *Avery's diseases of the newborn* (10th ed., pp. 1438–1449.e3). Philadelphia, PA: Elsevier.

24 INTEGUMENTARY SYSTEM

Rebecca Chuffo Davila

INTRODUCTION

Neonatal nurse practitioners need to be familiar with newborn skin development, skin care, and common skin disorders of the integumentary system. The skin is the largest organ in the body and is responsible for many functions, including protection, metabolic functions, sensation, and thermoregulation. Understanding of skin variations can alert the practitioner to a benign versus a life-threatening disease process. This chapter addresses general skin development, reviews newborn skin care, and reviews common skin disorders in neonates.

GENERAL SKIN DEVELOPMENT AND CARE

- The skin is comprised of three layers: the epidermis, the dermis, and the subcutaneous layer (Lund & Durand, 2016, p. 464).
  - The *epidermis* consists of an outer stratum corneum, stratum granulosum, and the stratum germinativum, which consists of the stratum spinosum, and the stratum basale. The basal layer contains the melanocytes and keratinocytes. Keratinocytes are the major cells of the epidermis.
  - The *dermis* lies beneath the epidermis. It is formed from fibrous protein, collagen, and elastin fibers that are woven together. The dermis contains nerves and blood vessels and carries sensations from the skin to the brain.
  - A *subcutaneous layer* is composed of fatty connective tissue that provides insulation and caloric storage (Blackburn, 2013, p. 489).

General Skin Development

EMBRYOLOGIC DEVELOPMENT

- The *epidermis* develops around 5 to 8 weeks' gestation. By 30 to 40 days, two layers can be identified: the inner basal layer and the outer periderm. The inner basal layer develops into the true epidermis.
  - The periderm is an embryonic layer that is gone by the second half of gestation. It is protective for the embryo and fetus and forms part of the vernix caseosa, and acts as a nutrient interface between the embryo and the amniotic fluid (Blackburn, 2013, p. 490).
  - By 60 days the epidermis now has 3 layers—the basal layer (where melanocytes are found), an intermediate layer, and the superficial periderm.
- The *dermis* lies beneath the epidermis and is comprised of connective tissue, nerves, blood vessels, and lymphatic vessels. It also contains mast cells, histiocytes, and neutrophils (Blackburn, 2013, p. 494). The dermis provides mechanical strength, protection, and elasticity to skin (Lund & Durand, 2016, p. 467).

- The intermediate layer of the integumentary system becomes more complex by the end of the fourth month, when the epidermis has stratified (Blackburn, 2013, p. 493; Lund & Durand, 2016, p. 464).

EPIDERMAL APPENDAGES

- Glands, the hair, and the nails are considered epidermal appendages.
  - Glands consist of sebaceous, eccrine, apocrine, and mammary.
    - Sebaceous glands are formed from epidermal cells around 4 weeks' gestation and are complete around 8 to 16 weeks. They are only found where hair grows.
    - Eccrine and apocrine are two types of sweat glands located within the dermal layer.
    - Mammary glands are adapted sweat glands seen at 4 weeks of gestation.
  - Hair originates in the dermis and projects up through the epidermis. Hairs are first seen at 10 to 12 weeks. The hair that appears along the embryo's body is called lanugo.
  - Fingernails and toenails develop as thickenings in the epidermal layer appearing around the 10th week (Lund & Durand, 2016, p. 464).

Differences in Full and Preterm Infant Skin

- In full and preterm infants, the skin is an organ that comprises at least 13% of the total body weight in contrast to only 3% of body weight in adults.
- The term infant has fewer problems with thermoregulation and fluid and electrolyte management, and are able to use calories for growth (Lund & Durand, 2016, p. 464, 467).
- Preterm infants have many more issues related to electrolyte disturbances and fluid shifts. Their skin is very thin and fragile and may be gelatinous due to the underdeveloped stratum corneum (Lund & Durand, 2016, p. 467).
  - The extremely low birth weight infant (ELBW) can have water losses 10 times higher than term infants (Lund & Durand, 2016, p. 467).
- Preterm infants are unable to manage thermoregulation and need a heat source to keep them normothermic.
- Though both term and preterm infants are at risk for developing infections, preterm infants are at higher risk due to fewer layers of stratum corneum for protection (Lund & Durand, 2016, p. 466).

General Skin Care

- Understanding the physiology of skin development is important in the understanding of how to care for the skin of term and preterm infants. The next section will discuss skin care for both the term and preterm neonates.

Bathing

- Immersion bathing for stable term and preterm infants have been shown to be beneficial. Such baths can be more soothing and less stressful. However, bathing can alter the skin pH, so baths should be done every 4 days or less (Lund & Durand, 2016, p. 469).
  - ○ Baths should be delayed in the term infant until he or she is physiologically stable.
  - ○ Term infants should be bathed infrequently with water or mild soaps which have a neutral pH (Witt, 2015, p. 797).

Umbilical Cord Care

- Sterile cutting of the cord at delivery, drying of the cord, and keeping the cord free of urine and feces is helpful in preventing umbilical infections (Lund & Durand, 2016, p. 472; Witt, 2015, p. 798).
  - ○ Intravenous (IV) antibiotics should be given if there is suspected omphalitis (Lund & Durand, 2016, p. 472).

Emollients

- Maintaining the hydration of the stratum corneum is essential for intact skin and normal barrier function (Lund & Durand, 2016, p. 470).
  - ○ If emollients are used, they should be free of dyes and perfumes. They should be single-patient-use tubes or jars and not shared among infants (Lund & Durand, 2016, p. 470).

Skin Disinfectants

- Skin decontamination is necessary prior to procedures in the NICU. Which and when to use a disinfectant is a common issue in the NICU.
  - ○ Povidone-iodine is widely used.
  - ○ Whichever skin disinfectant is used, it should be completely removed from the infant's skin once the procedure is finished (Lund & Durand, 2016, p. 470).

Adhesive Removal

- There is risk of damage to the skin in all the infants we care for in the NICU. There should be minimization in use of adhesives, solvents, and bonding agents (Hoath & Narendran, 2015, p. 1703).
- Damage that can occur from adhesive removal include epidermal stripping, tearing of the skin, maceration, tension blisters, chemical irritation, sensitization, and folliculitis (Lund & Durand, 2016, p. 472).
- Hydrocolloid barriers may be helpful in securing tubes and lines to the skin. They can aid in preventing permanent damage and scarring of the skin (Lund & Durand, 2016, p. 472).
- Silicone tapes are very gentle to the skin, but do not adhere well to plastics. They should not be used when securing critical, life-sustaining tubes and appliances (Lund & Durand, 2016, p. 473).

Treatment for Skin Excoriations

- Topicals antimicrobial creams such as bacitracin (Bacitin), mupirocin (Bactroban), or a combination of bacitracin and polymyxin B (Polysporin) should be used sparingly.

- Seeking help and guidance from a wound/ostomy nurse can be very beneficial (Lund & Durand, 2016, p. 474).

INTRAVENOUS EXTRAVASATIONS

- Once the extravasation is identified, the IV should be removed and the extremity involved should be elevated.
- The use of heat or cold is not recommended because the tissue is susceptible to extended injury from these extreme temperatures.
- Hyaluronidase can be helpful to prevent tissue necrosis if given within 1 hour of the extravasation.
- Phentolamine should be used in the event of extravasation by a vasoconstrictive drug such as dopamine (Lund & Durand, 2016, p. 475).

Risk Factors for Skin Injury

- Gestational age <32 weeks
- Edema
- Use of paralytic agents and vasopressors
- Multiple tubes and lines
- Numerous monitors
- Surgical wounds
- Ostomies
- Technologies that limit movement—high frequency oscillator ventilation (HFOV), extracorporeal membrane oxygenation (ECMO) (Lund & Durand, 2016, p. 474)

SKIN DISORDERS

Definitions Used to Describe Skin Lesions/Disorders

- Macule—pigmented, flat spot that is visible but not palpable. If >1 cm in diameter may be referred to as a patch.
- Papule—a solid, elevated, palpable lesion with distinct borders and <1 cm in diameter
- Plaque—a solid, elevated, palpable lesion with distinct borders that is >1 cm in diameter
- Nodule—a solid lesion that is elevated with depth and up to 2 cm in size
- Tumor—a solid lesion that is elevated with depth and greater than 2 cm in size
- Vesicle—an elevated lesion or blister filled with serous fluid less than 1 cm in diameter
- Bulla—a fluid filled lesion larger than 1 cm
- Pustule—a vesicle filled with cloudy or purulent fluid
- Petechiae—subepidermal hemorrhages and are pinpoint in size. They do not blanch with pressure.
- Ecchymosis—a large area of subepidermal hemorrhage
- Wheal—area of edema in the upper dermis, creating a palpable, slightly raised lesion
- Ulcer—erosion of skin with damage of the epidermis into the dermis. This will leave a scar after healing (Witt, 2015, p. 799).

Hemangiomas

INCIDENCE

- Infantile hemangiomas (IHs) are the most common skin anomaly of infancy (Gupta & Sidbury, 2018, p. 1511).

ETIOLOGY/RISK FACTORS

- Risk factors for developing IHs include prematurity, multiple gestation, preeclampsia, placental abnormalities, advanced maternal age, and in vitro fertilization (Gupta & Sidbury, 2018, p. 1511). It is hypothesized that formation of IHs is linked to hypoxia (Gupta & Sidbury, 2018, p. 1512).

FINDINGS/ASSESSMENT
- Hemangiomas are clinically heterogeneous.
- Solitary cutaneous lesion
- Superficial hemangiomas are located in the upper dermis and present as elevated, bright red, well-demarcated papules or plaques, which sometimes are referred to as "strawberry hemangiomas" (Gupta & Sidbury, 2018, p. 1512).

TREATMENT
- Hemangiomas that require immediate attention are those that are in the airway and those involved in the hepatic and parotid areas (Gupta & Sidbury, 2018, p. 1518). Treatment therapies include topicals such as timolol maleate and systemic agents such as propranolol; other treatments include prednisone/rednisolone, interferon alpha, and vincristine. Laser therapy and surgical excision have also been used (Gupta & Sidbury, 2018, p. 1519).

OUTCOMES
- Most IHs (80%) have completed their growth by 3 months of age and 90% regress by 4 years of age (Gupta & Sidbury, 2018, p. 1512). Up to 40% can cause permanent skin changes, including disfigurement (Gupta & Sidbury, 2018, p. 1519). Complications include ulceration; those located around the eyes could cause visual impairment and those around the ears could cause hearing deficits (Gupta & Sidbury, 2018, p. 1518).

HYPERPIGMENTATION
- Café au ait macules are well-demarcated oval or round light-brown macules or patches that differ in size. Six or more of these macules measuring 0.5 cm or greater in diameter should alert the practitioner to the possible diagnosis of neurofibromatosis Type 1 (NF 1) (Gupta & Sidbury, 2018, p. 1527).

HYPOPIGMENTATION
- Ash-leaf macules are small, oval areas of hypopigmentation. They are one of the few congenital markers for infants with tuberous sclerosis (TS) (Gupta & Sidbury, 2018, p. 1526).
  - TS is a hereditary disorder characterized by cutaneous and central nervous system (CNS) tumors resulting in seizures, developmental delays, and behavioral problems (Witt, 2018, p. 52).

Subcutaneous Fat Necrosis

INCIDENCE
- More common in term newborns

ETIOLOGY/RISK FACTORS
- Subcutaneous fat necrosis is a skin lesion caused secondary by some form of intrauterine or perinatal trauma (Witt, 2018, pp. 52–53).
- Reported in some infants undergoing therapeutic hypothermia (Witt, 2018, p. 53)

FINDINGS/ASSESSMENT
- Subcutaneous nodule or nodules that are hard, nonpitting, and sharply circumscribed

- May be red or purplish in color (Witt, 2018, p. 53)
- The lesions are located in areas with fat pads, such as buttocks, thighs, arms, face, and shoulders.

TREATMENT
- Nodules may grow slightly larger over several days, but then resolve on their own after several weeks to months (Khorsand & Sidbury, 2018, p. 1509; Witt, 2018, p. 53).
- Calcification can occur and be associated with hypercalcemia (Khorsand & Sidbury, 2018, p. 1509).

OUTCOMES
- Hypercalcemia may occur up to 6 months after presentation of the initial nodule.
- Serum calcium levels should be monitored.
- Intervention with fluids, calcium-wasting diuretics, and glucocorticoids may be necessary (Witt, 2018, p. 53).

Epidermolysis Bullosa

INCIDENCE
- The exact prevalence of epidermolysis bullosa (EB) is unknown, but it is estimated to affect one in 30,000 to 50,000 people.

ETIOLOGY/RISK FACTORS
- EB is a group of inherited diseases that are characterized by blistering lesions.
- There are both autosomal dominant and recessive forms of this disease (Witt, 2015, p. 809).
- The dermal–epidermal junction is critical for skin integrity. EB is a disorder of the dermal–epidermal junction (Blackburn, 2013, pp. 493–494).

FINDINGS/ASSESSMENT
- Blister lesions occur on the skin and mucous membranes.
- Simple lesions are bullae that heal without scarring; dystrophic lesions may cause scarring and infection that could lead to death, and EB lethalis is the most severe form. Treatment is mostly supportive (Witt, 2015, p. 809).
- Blisters may be readily elicited by gentle rubbing (known as Nikolsky sign).
- The initial diagnosis of EB is a clinical one. Other disorders that cause blistering (i.e., infections) should be excluded.

TREATMENT
- There is no effective treatment for EB.
- Treatment aims are preventing trauma to skin, providing wound-healing dressings, maximizing nutrition, and preventing secondary infections.

OUTCOMES
- Repeated episodes of blistering, infection, and scar formation can lead to severe deformities, loss of hair, scarring of the mucosa, multi-organ dysfunction, and impaired physical and sexual development.

Collodion Baby

INCIDENCE
- Rare

ETIOLOGY/RISK FACTORS
- This term describes an appearance rather than a disease.
- Many will have some form of ichthyosis.
- May represent a phenotypic expression of several genotypes

FINDINGS/ASSESSMENT
- Cellophane-like membrane that is very taut and can distort facial features and digits
- Often are premature
- Fissuring and peeling begin shortly after birth.

TREATMENT
- Treatment consists of sterile olive oil or mineral oil several times a day, careful handling, and prevention of infection (Witt, 2015, p. 809).

OUTCOMES
- Since these infants have an abnormal epidermal barrier, the practitioner needs to follow closely for complications such as dehydration, electrolyte imbalance, temperature instability, and infection.
- Complete shedding of the collodion membrane may take several weeks.

Ichthyosis

INCIDENCE
- Rare disorder; X-linked ichthyosis is the most common form of ichthyosis in the newborn period, affecting approximately one in 2,500 male babies.

ETIOLOGY/RISK FACTORS
- Ichthyosis is caused by excessive production of stratum corneum cells or faulty appropriate shedding of the stratum corneum.
- The term ichthyosis derives from the similarity of the skin condition to the scales of a fish.

FINDINGS/ASSESSMENT
- The four types of ichthyosis:
  o Ichthyosis Vulgaris
    ■ Ichthyosis vulgaris is an autosomal dominant disorder and usually appears after 3 months of age. It presents as fine white scales and excessively dry skin. It is the most common and most benign of the four types (Witt, 2015, p. 809).
  o X-Linked Ichthyosis
    ■ X-linked ichthyosis appears at birth or during the first year of life. There are large thick, brown scales over the entire body excluding the palms and soles. This form only occurs in males (Witt, 2015, p. 810).
  o Lamellar Ichthyosis
    ■ Lamellar ichthyosis is an autosomal recessive disorder that is manifested at birth as bright red erythema and desquamation. Some of these infants may resemble collodion babies. Scales are large, flat, and coarse. They may have eversion of lips and eyelids (Witt, 2015, p. 810).
  o Bullous Ichthyosis
    ■ Bullous ichthyosis is an autosomal dominate disorder characterized by recurrent bullous lesions. There is excessive dryness and peeling. Infection caused by *Staphylococcus aureus* is a concern (Witt, 2015, p. 810).

TREATMENT
- Family history and skin biopsy are necessary to determine the subtype of ichthyosis.
- Treatment of infection if arises
- Reduce dryness of the skin and protect skin from infection.

OUTCOMES
- Prevention of infection is key as there is no definitive cure.

HARLEQUIN FETUS
- Previously had been considered to be a severe form of ichthyosis, but may be a rare autosomal disease. These infants have hard, thick, gray or yellow scales that cause severe deformities. The condition is usually lethal (Witt, 2015, p. 810).

NORMAL SKIN FINDINGS AND VARIATIONS

Milia

- Is common in up to 40% to 50% of newborns
- They present as tiny, white, monomorphic papules with a smooth surface.
- Commonly seen on the forehead, cheeks, and chin
- They are tiny inclusion cysts that form in the epidermis.
- No treatment is necessary and they will resolve spontaneously over several months (Khorsand & Sidbury, 2018, p. 1505).

Miliaria

- Miliaria is a benign rash due to obstruction of the eccrine ducts occurring in the first 1 to 2 weeks of life with rapid resolution within days.
- There are three types of known miliaria: miliaria crystallina, miliaria rubra, and miliaria profunda.
  o Miliaria Crystallina—eccrine ducts within or below the stratum corneum are blocked, and this causes small, clear vesicles that can be wiped away.
  o Miliaria Rubra—blockage of the eccrine duct at the level of the epidermis. This is thought to be related to overheating.
  o Miliaria Profunda—blockage of the eccrine ducts at or below the dermal–epidermal junction. It resembles a papular eruption that is rarely seen in newborns (Khorsand & Sidbury, 2018, p. 1505).

Hyperpigmented Macule (Dermal Melanocytosis) (Previously Mongolian Spot)

- This common skin finding is seen mainly in infants of African American, Asian, and Hispanic descent.
- Seen mostly on the buttocks and lower back
- It is caused by excessive number of dermal melanocytes.
- The characteristic "bluish-gray" color is due to the Tyndall effect, which is light reflection off the dermal-based melanocytes.
- They fade over time and approximately 42% disappear by 1 year of age (Khorsand & Sidbury, 2018, p. 1510).

Erythema Toxicum

- Erythema toxicum neonatorum is a benign, inflammatory condition in the newborn period.
- It presents in the first 1 to 3 days of life.

- It is most commonly seen on the trunk.
- If examined microscopically, would reveal a large number of *eosinophils*.
- No treatment is required (Khorsand & Sidbury, 2018, p. 1503).

Transient Neonatal Pustular Melanosis

- More commonly seen in African American infants.
- A distinctive eruption that consists of three types of lesions: first stage—superficial vesiculopustules, second stage—collarettes of scale or scale crust, third stage—scale or scale crust surrounding the hyperpigmented macule.
- If examined would reveal a predominance of *neutrophils*.
- The residual hyperpigmentation may take months to resolve (Khorsand & Sidbury, 2018, p. 1504).
- No therapy is required as this skin condition is benign and transient.

Petechiae/Purpura

- Petechiae are pinpoint, flat, round, red spots under the skin surface caused by intradermal hemorrhage. They will not blanch when compressed.
- Can commonly be seen right after birth, especially on the presenting part (Witt, 2015, p. 799)
  - If the infant is delivered vaginally following a rapid labor, presented in a vertex position, or had a tight nuchal cord, petechiae may be present (Verklan, 2015, p. 63).
- Petechiae may be benign or an indication of severe platelet malfunction; further evaluation should be done if the infant is symptomatic (e.g., prolonged bleeding from heel sticks; Diab & Luchtman-Jones, 2015, p. 1328).

Ecchymosis

- Ecchymosis is a hemorrhagic blotching due to pooling of blood under the skin or mucous membrane. It also does not blanch with pressure (Witt, 2015, p. 799).
- Ecchymosis in newborns most commonly is caused by birth, in particular if assistive devices are used, such as mid-forceps or vacuum extraction (Mangurten, Puppala, & Prazad, 2015, p. 411). Fetuses, especially large ones, who are delivered vaginally in breech position may demonstrate ecchymosis from birth. The ecchymosis is transient and will fade away in a few days (Cavaliere, 2018, p. 124).
  - Presence of a large cephalohematoma or extensive ecchymosis places the infant at higher risk of hyperbilirubinemia (Pappas & Robey, 2015, p. 442).
- May also be concerning for a primary hematologic disease (Diab & Luchtman-Jones, 2015, p. 1327)

Accessory Tragus (Preauricular Tags)

- Accessory tragi are a relatively common congenital malformation of the external ear.
- They are present at birth and can be multiple and/or bilateral.
- Association between deafness and renal abnormalities are controversial.
- Removal by tying off of the tragi should not be done and could lead to complications (Gupta & Sidbury, 2018, p. 1534).

Capillary Malformation: Port-Wine Stain

- A port-wine stain is a flat, pink or reddish-purple lesion.
- A lesion on the face may follow a pattern similar to that of the trigeminal nerve and may be associated with the diagnosis of Sturge-Weber syndrome (SWS).
- Infants with SWS can have seizures, hemiparesis, developmental delays, and ophthalmologic abnormalities—most commonly glaucoma (Gupta & Sidbury, 2018, p. 1523; Witt, 2016, p. 54).

CONCLUSION

Knowing the physiology of skin development and careful physical assessment of the newborn skin is of utmost importance for NNPs. Thorough examination and understanding of the skin allows insight into the health and well-being of the newborn. Being able to distinguish between benign and life-threatening skin conditions is imperative.

REVIEW QUESTIONS

1. The NNP is caring for a newly born preterm infant born at 30 weeks' gestation who weighs 1,200 g. The intervention most appropriate to promote skin integrity is the use of:
   A. alcohol routinely to remove adhesives
   B. immersion bathing done every 4 days
   C. soap and water during daily bathing

2. An infant is noted to have a small strawberry hemangioma located on the scalp, and the NNP counsels the family based on the knowledge that:
   A. Increasing size will occur before regression.
   B. Prophylactic oral antibiotic therapy is needed.
   C. Surgical removal is necessary at 6 months of age.

3. A full-term neonate is diagnosed with epidermolysis bullosa (EB). When planning care for this infant, the primary complication which should be anticipated is the occurrence of:
   A. electrographic seizures
   B. indirect hyperbilirubinemia
   C. secondary infections

4. The NNP is called to talk to parents of an approximately 38-hour-old term infant. The parents are concerned about tiny white papules on the infant's forehead, cheeks, and chin. The NNP responds based on the knowledge that:
   A. Erythema toxicum results from eosinophilia.
   B. Milia are common and need no intervention.
   C. Pustular melanosis will resolve in a few months.

5. When noting the presence of an ear tag on a newborn infant, the parents should be counseled as to the:
   A. necessity of surgery to remove it at a later date.
   B. potential for the infant to develop hearing losses.
   C. relatively common occurrence of this anomaly.

REFERENCES

Blackburn, S. (2013). The integumentary system. In S. Blackburn (Ed.), *Maternal, fetal, and neonatal physiology* (4th ed., pp. 484–408). St. Louis, MO: Elsevier.

Cavaliere, T. (2018). Genitourinary assessment. In E. P. Tappero & M. E. Honeyfield (Eds.), *Physical assessment of the newborn* (6th ed., pp. 121–137). New York, NY: Springer Publishing Company.

Diab, Y., & Luchtman-Jones, L. (2015). Hematologic and oncologic problems in the fetus and neonate. In R. Martin, A. Fanaroff, & M. Walsh (Eds.), *Fanaroff and Martin's neonatal–perinatal medicine: Diseases of the fetus and infant* (10th ed., pp. 1294–1343). Philadelphia, PA: Elsevier.

Gupta, D., & Sidbury, R. (2018). Cutaneous congenital defects. In C. Gleason & S. Juul (Eds.), *Avery's diseases of the newborn* (10th ed., pp. 1511–1535.e4). Philadelphia, PA: Elsevier.

Hoath, S., & Varendran, V. (2015). The skin of the neonate. In R. Martin, A. Fanaroff, & M. Walsh (Eds.), *Fanaroff and Martin's neonatal–perinatal medicine: Diseases of the fetus and infant* (10th ed., pp. 1702–1732). Philadelphwia, PA: Elsevier.

Khorsand, K., & Sidbury, R. (2018). Common newborn dermatoses. In C. Gleason & S. Juul (Eds.), *Avery's diseases of the newborn* (10th ed., pp. 1503–1510.e1). Philadelphia, PA: Elsevier.

Lund, C., & Durand, D. (2016). Skin and skin care. In S. Gardner, B. Carter, M. Hines, & J. Hernandez (Eds.), *Merenstein & Gardner's handbook of neonatal intensive care* (8th ed., pp. 464–478.e3). St. Louis, MO: Elsevier.

Mangurten, H., Puppala, B., & Prazad, P. (2015). Birth injuries. In R. Martin, A. Fanaroff, & M. Walsh (Eds.), *Fanaroff and Martin's neonatal–perinatal medicine: Diseases of the fetus and infant* (10th ed., pp. 407–435). Philadelphia, PA: Elsevier.

Pappas, B., & Robey, D. (2015). Care of the late preterm infant. In T. Verklan & M. Walden (Eds.) *Core curriculum for neonatal intensive care nursing* (5th ed., pp. 439–446). St. Louis, MO: Elsevier.

Verklan, T. (2015). Adaptation to extrauterine life. In T. Verklan & M. Walden (Eds.) *Core curriculum for neonatal intensive care nursing* (5th ed., pp. 58–76). St. Louis, MO: Elsevier.

Witt, C. (2015). Neonatal dermatology. In T. Verklan & M. Walden (Eds.), *Core curriculum for neonatal intensive care nursing* (5th ed., pp. 795–812). St. Louis, MO: Elsevier.

Witt, C. (2018). Skin assessment. In E. P. Tappero & M. E. Honeyfield (Eds.), *Physical assessment of the newborn* (6th ed., pp. 45–59). New York, NY: Springer Publishing Company.

25 EYES, EARS, NOSE, MOUTH, AND THROAT

Christi Olsen
Yvette Pugh

INTRODUCTION

Complete understanding of the development and pathology of the structures of the eyes, ears, nose, mouth, and throat is crucial to providing prompt and accurate evaluation and treatment of potentially life-threatening or debilitating disease processes. Craniofacial malformations affect multiple systems and can have an impact on breathing, vision, swallowing, and hearing, which in some cases can be life-threatening.

THE EYES

- The initial weeks of an infant's life are critical in terms of the visual development in the brain, and clinicians are on the front line when it comes to identifying potential vision problems.
- It is important for clinicians to recognize the signs and symptoms of eye disease or disorders early. Prompt intervention can prevent loss of vision, identify systemic illnesses, or can be life-saving. The clinician must first know what is normal in order to identify abnormalities.

Embryology

- Optic evagination occurs during the first trimester at 24 days of embryonic development during which early somites and the optic cup is formed at 30 days.
- Lens development occurs between 34 and 44 days of embryonic development.
  - Lens invagination occurs at 34 days.
  - At 38 days, the lens is detached and the pigmentation of the retina occurs.
  - At 44 days, lens fibers are formed as migration of the retinal cells occurs and the hyaloid vessels are formed.
  - The eyelids are formed at 55 days. At 70 days, the iris and ciliary body form, and the eyelids fuse (Blackburn, 2013, p. 74).
  - Pupillary light reaction is present at 28 to 30 weeks' gestation, and lid closure in response to bright light occurs at 30 weeks' gestation (Blackburn, 2013, p. 74; Őrge & Grigorian, 2015, p. 1735).
  - Vestibular (doll's eye) rotations are well-developed at 34 weeks' gestation (Őrge & Grigorian, 2015, p. 1735).
  - Visual fixation and conjugate horizontal gaze are well-developed and present at birth.
  - Visual milestones from 30 weeks' gestation to 6 months of age is summed in Table 25.1.

Postnatal Visual Progression

- Pupillary light reaction is well-developed by 1 month.
- Color vision is present at 2 months and reaches adult level by 6 months (Őrge & Grigorian, 2015, p. 1735).
- The infant can coordinate vision at 3 to 5 months (Blackburn, 2013, p. 74).

TABLE 25.1 Visual Milestones Up To 6 Months Corrected Gestational Age

Age	Visual Milestone Present
30 weeks' gestation	Pupillary response to light present Lid closure in response to bright light
34 weeks' gestation	Well-developed vestibular rotation (doll's eye reflex)
Full-term birth	Visual fixation present Well-developed conjugate horizontal gaze Well-developed optokinetic nystagmus Eyeball development 70% of adult diameter Cornea development 80% of adult diameter
1 month	Well-developed pupillary response to light
2 months	Well-developed fixation Color vision present Well-developed conjugate vertical gaze Blink response to visual threat (present 2–5 months)
3 months	Visual following is well-developed
4 months	Well-developed accommodation Stable ocular alignment Differentiation of fovea complete
6 months	Visual evoked potential acuity at adult level Color vision at adult level Stereopsis developed Fusional convergence well-developed Iris pigmentation well-developed

Sources: Data from Blackburn, S. (2013). The prenatal period and placental physiology. In S. Blackburn (Ed.), *Maternal, fetal, & neonatal physiology: A clinical perspective* (4th ed., pp. 61–114). Maryland Heights, MO: Elsevier; Őrge, F., & Grigorian, F. (2015). Examination and common problems of the neonatal eye. In R. Martin, A. Fanaroff, & M. Walsh (Eds.), *Fanaroff and Martin's neonatal–perinatal medicine: Diseases of the fetus and infant* (10th ed., pp. 1734–1766). Philadelphia, PA: Elsevier.

- The iris is immature at birth, and the color tends to be gray or blue. The iris may become darker as the pigmented layer of the iris stroma becomes more fully developed. Pigmentation of the iris occurs by 6 months of age (Blackburn, 2013, p. 74; Campomanes & Binenbaum, 2018, p. 1538).
- The eyeball is 70% of adult diameter at birth and 95% of adult diameter at 3 years (Örge & Grigorian, 2015, p. 1735).
- Maximal vision is reached by 5 years (Blackburn, 2013, p. 74).

Examination of the Eye

- A thorough examination of the eyes can yield a great deal of valuable information pertaining to intrauterine infection, congenital abnormalities, trauma, and genetic disorders. Screening eye examinations are done during the newborn physical exam and during routine well-baby visits. Additional exams for retinopathy of prematurity (ROP) are performed at more frequent intervals based on risk factors.
- The screening eye examination begins with a careful history, noting family history of eye disease. It is also important to note maternal diseases, medications, or drugs taken during pregnancy, and conditions that occurred during pregnancy, labor, and delivery,; for example, a difficult delivery with forceps can result in direct ocular trauma (Örge & Grigorian, 2015, p. 1734).
- The eye exam is best done prior to insertion of eye prophylaxis (see section "Eye Prophylaxis") and when the infant is in the quiet alert state or is aroused to wakefulness with manipulation (Boucher, Marvicsin, & Gardner, 2017, p. 113; Fraser & Diehl-Jones, 2015, p. 815; Vargo, 2014, p. 605).
- The eyes should be checked both by inspection and with an ophthalmoscope (Lissauer, 2015, p. 394). By following a simple examination framework, I-ARM (inspection, acuity, red reflex, and motility), the clinician can identify abnormalities or asymmetries in the structure or function of the eye (Campomanes & Binenbaum, 2018, p. 1536).
- The screening eye examination should include an evaluation of visual function, preferably one eye at a time. Visual function in infants less than 4 to 6 weeks of age is assessed by withdrawal or blinking to light or pupil constriction to light (Örge & Grigorian, 2015, p. 1734). At this time, the pupils should be observed for being equal, round, and reactive to light (Boucher et al., 2017, p. 113).
- Red reflex testing using an ophthalmoscope is a mandatory element of all newborn and well-baby physical examinations (Campomanes & Binenbaum, 2018, p. 1537). The light from the ophthalmoscope should be directed at the pupil from approximately 6 inches away to elicit the red reflex (Johnson, 2016, p. 72). The red reflex normally appears as homogeneous and bright red-orange (Fraser & Diehl-Jones, 2015, p. 815).
  - The red reflex test is vital for early detection of vision and potentially life-threatening conditions such as a congenital cataract, glaucoma, retinoblastoma, retinal abnormalities, systemic diseases with ocular manifestations, and high refractive errors (Campomanes & Binenbaum, 2018, p. 1540; Johnson, 2016, p. 72).
  - A positive red reflex is indicative of an intact lens and retina and may appear milky white, rather than red, in darker-skinned infants (Boucher et al., 2017, p. 113, p. 119).
  - If a red reflex cannot be seen, the pupils can be dilated with cyclomydril eye drops. If a clear and equal red reflex is still not seen, the baby should be referred to an ophthalmologist (Örge & Grigorian, 2015, p. 1738).

Eye Prophylaxis

- Neonatal eye prophylaxis is the practice of instilling eye drops or an antibiotic ointment in the neonate's eyes to protect against maternal infections, such as *Neisseria gonorrheae* or *Chlamydia trachomatis*.
- A sterile ophthalmic ointment containing 0.5% erythromycin ointment, 1% tetracycline ointment, or an ophthalmic solution of 2.5% povidone–iodine is used for prophylaxis of ophthalmia neonatorum due to *N. gonorrhoeae* while erythromycin or tetracycline is used for prophylaxis against *C. trachomatis* (Campomanes & Binenbaum, 2018, p. 1545; Örge & Grigorian, 2015, p. 1762; Vargo, 2014, p. 604; Verklan, 2015, p. 64).
  - Gentamicin ointment should be avoided, as it is associated with periocular ulcerative dermatitis when used on the newborn eye (Campomanes & Binenbaum, 2018, p. 1545).
- A 1- to 2-inch ribbon of medication, if an ointment is used, is instilled into the conjunctival sac before 1 hour of age but may be delayed until after the first breastfeeding (Verklan, 2015, p. 64).

Cataracts

DEFINITION

- A cataract is defined any opacity or abnormality within the structure of the lens.
  - The lens is a biconvex, transparent capsule that refracts light and helps images focus on the retina. It is preserved in capsules (anterior and posterior) and has a nuclear core and surrounding cortical portion (Campomanes & Binenbaum, 2018, p. 1542; Fraser & Diehl-Jones, 2015, p. 818; Örge & Grigorian, 2015, p. 1749).
  - Normally, the light from an object passes directly through the lens to a focal point on the retina, producing a sharp image. Cataracts result in a degraded image or no image at all (Fraser & Diehl-Jones, 2015, p. 818).

INCIDENCE AND ETIOLOGY

- The incidence of congenital cataract is approximately two in 10,000 live births (Campomanes & Binenbaum, 2018, p. 1542). Cataracts are responsible for 10% blindness worldwide (Örge & Grigorian, 2015, p. 1749).
  - Infants with isolated unilateral cataracts often do not have a family history and rarely have associated systemic disorders (Campomanes & Binenbaum, 2018, p. 1543).
- There are several causes of cataracts, including heredity, maternal infections, and congenital rubella. See Table 25.2 for a summation of possible etiologies of cataracts, including percentages of some of the etiologies.

PRESENTATION

- Normally, when light is directed at the pupils, they appear black to the naked eye of the examiner, but cataracts present as white pupils (leukocoria) that can be dense, milky white opacities in the lens.

TABLE 25.2 Cataract Classification and Possible Etiologies

Classification of Cataracts	Possible Etiology
Hereditary (30%)	Most common mode of inheritance—autosomal dominant
Metabolic and endocrine disorders	Galactosemia, Fabry disease, hemolytic jaundice, neonatal hypoglycemia, diabetes mellitus, hypoparathyroidism
Traumatic/iatrogenic	Birth trauma, blunt trauma, perforating injuries, high-voltage electric shock, battered child syndrome
Idiopathic (30%)	Developmental variation; not associated with other abnormalities
Secondary	Maternal infection, inflammation, steroid use
Congenital rubella	Present in 30% of newborn infants with congenital rubella syndrome
Other congenital infections	Toxoplasmosis, CMV infection, herpes simplex, varicella
Chromosomal abnormalities	Down syndrome, trisomy 13, Turner syndrome
Renal disorders	Lowe, Alport, Hallermann–Streiff–François syndromes
Skeletal and connective tissue disorders	Smith–Lemli–Opitz, Marfan, Conradi, and Weill–Marchesani syndromes
Clinical syndromes	Crouzon syndrome, Pierre Robin syndrome

CMV, cytomegalovirus.

Sources: Data from Campomanes, A. G., & Binenbaum, G. (2018). Eye and vision disorders. In C. Gleason & S. Juul (Eds.), *Avery's diseases of the newborn* (10th ed., pp. 1536–1557). Philadelphia, PA: Elsevier; Fraser, D., & Diehl-Jones, W. (2015). Ophthalmologic and auditory disorders. In Verklan et al. (Eds.), *Core curriculum for neonatal intensive care nursing* (pp. 813–831). St. Louis, MO: Saunders, Elsevier; Örge, F., & Grigorian, F. (2015). Examination and common problems of the neonatal eye. In R. Martin, A. Fanaroff, & M. Walsh (Eds.), *Fanaroff and Martin's neonatal–perinatal medicine: Diseases of the fetus and infant* (10th ed., pp. 1734–1766). Philadelphia, PA: Elsevier.

○ Dense central opacities greater than 3 mm are considered visually significant.

○ Should consider other diseases of the eye that may produce a white pupil (e.g., retinoblastoma).

- Rapid, searching eye movements are known as nystagmus. It should be noted that limited horizontal nystagmus elicited with rotational movements is a normal variant until 3 to 4 months of age. However, spontaneous horizontal, vertical, torsional, or persistent nystagmus (occurring greater than 4 months of age) is considered pathologic and warrants further intervention.

○ The presence of nystagmus before surgery is a marker for poor visual prognosis (Campomanes & Binenbaum, 2018, p. 1542; Fraser & Diehl-Jones, 2015, p. 818; Johnson, 2019, p. 72).

INTERVENTION AND OUTCOMES

- Interventions should target the cause of cataracts; therefore the following evaluations should be considered: TORCH (toxoplasmosis, other, ruebella, cytomegalovirus, herpes virus) titers (including syphilis), urine tests for reducing substance (galactosemia), plasma urea, electrolyte and urine amino acid levels (Lowe syndrome), quantitative amino acid levels and red blood cell enzyme levels (galactokinase, galactose-1-phosphate uridyltransferase), complete blood count and ferritin, blood glucose, calcium, and phosphate levels, genetic consultation, chromosome analysis and next-generation sequencing (focused on the 115 cataract-causing genes known to date), and ocular examination of parents and siblings.

- Children with a family history of infantile or juvenile cataracts should be examined early by a pediatric ophthalmologist, and infants with cataracts may undergo selective diagnostic evaluation, especially if the infant has bilateral cataracts.

- Congenital cataracts are the main treatable cause of visual impairment in infancy and should be surgically removed within 6 to 8 weeks of birth. Aphakic (without a lens) glaucoma is one of the most common sight-threatening complications of cataract surgery in infants (Campomanes & Binenbaum, 2018, p. 1542–1543; Fraser & Diehl-Jones, 2015, p. 818).

- Cataracts lead to varying degrees of visual impairment, from blurred vision to blindness, depending on the location and extent of the opacity. In neonates, cataracts may be transient, disappearing spontaneously within a few weeks (Campomanes & Binenbaum, 2018, p. 1539; Fraser & Diehl-Jones, 2015, p. 818).

○ Useful vision can be restored if the surgery is completed within the first 6 weeks after birth. Beyond this time, visual restoration becomes progressively more difficult because of irreversible deprivation amblyopia (Campomanes & Binenbaum, 2018, p. 1542).

○ Visual prognosis depends not only on the extent of cataracts, age at removal, surgical outcome, and rapid optical correction, but also on the nature of other associated anomalies of the eye or syndromes (Fraser & Diehl-Jones, 2015, p. 819).

- Intensive visual rehabilitation strategies must be implemented, and if the infant is left aphakic (without a lens), optical correction is achieved with special contact lenses or glasses.

○ Critical intervention involves adherence to the use of contact lenses and glasses; and, in the case of monocular cataracts, aggressive amblyopia treatment by penalizing (patching) of the sound eye is critical and directly affects the child's ultimate visual outcome (Campomanes & Binenbaum, 2018, p. 1542).

Coloboma

DEFINITION

- Ocular coloboma: a congenital anatomic defect or cleft that results from failure of the optic fissure to close during embryogenesis. The result is an area of missing tissue in the eye, most commonly, in the inferonasal quadrant (Campomanes & Binenbaum, 2018, p. 1544; Õrge & Grigorian, 2015, p. 1749; Tappero & Honeyfield, 2016, p. 267).

IRIS COLOBOMA

- The iris coloboma is one of the most common congenital abnormalities of the eye (Õrge & Grigorian, 2015, p. 1748). The iris coloboma is a malformation that is sometimes seen as a key-shaped pupil (Tappero & Honeyfield, 2016, p. 267).

EYELID COLOBOMA

- Eyelid colobomas are partial-thickness or complete defects that can range from a small notching of the lid borders to involvement of the entire length of the lid (Õrge & Grigorian, 2015, p. 1741).

INCIDENCE AND ETIOLOGY

- Depending on the population studied, its incidence ranges from 0.5 to 7.5 per 10,000 births and accounts for 3% to 11% of blind children worldwide and can be isolated, associated with a chromosomal abnormality, or can be syndromic.
- Colobomas occur in the inferonasal quadrant, where the embryonic fissure closes. Typical iris colobomas result from an abnormal closure of the embryonic fissure. Because of this, iris colobomas also may be associated with a coloboma of the ciliary body, fundus, or optic nerve and can affect the eyelid, lens, macula, optic nerve, or uvea.
  ○ The cause of lid colobomas is often unknown unless associated with a craniofacial syndrome. Isolated eyelid colobomas could possibly arise from the localized failure of adhesion of the lid folds resulting in a lag of growth, or from mechanical effects of amniotic bands.
- There are numerous ocular abnormalities and systemic findings associated with colobomas, including more than 200 syndromes such as CHARGE syndrome, 22q11 deletion, and Treacher Collins, Walker–Warburg, Aicardi, and Goldenhar (eyelid coloboma) syndromes (Campomanes & Binenbaum, 2018, p. 1544; Õrge & Grigorian, 2015, p. 1748).

PRESENTATION

- An iris coloboma appears as an irregular "keyhole," or "cat's-eye" pupil. A chorioretinal or optic nerve head coloboma will appear as an abnormal red reflex or leukocoria. The affected eye may be microphthalmic.
- Most eyelid colobomas occur in the medial aspect of the upper lid. When the lower lid is involved, the defect is more often in the lateral aspects. Atypical iris colobomas occur away from the inferonasal quadrant (Campomanes & Binenbaum, 2018, p. 1544; Õrge & Grigorian, 2015, p. 1741, 1749).

INTERVENTION AND OUTCOMES

- The systemic diagnostic testing in patients with apparently isolated bilateral or unilateral uveal coloboma should include a kidney ultrasound examination, audiometry, spine radiographs, and possibly an echocardiogram and neuroimaging.
  ○ When an iris coloboma is detected, it is always wise to evaluate the fundus for a pathologic condition.
- When the lid defect prevents adequate lid closure and allows exposure of the cornea, early surgical correction is often required when the coloboma is greater than one third of the eyelid margin.
- When the optic nerve or central macula is involved in the coloboma, visual difficulty occurs (Campomanes & Binenbaum, 2018, p. 1544; Õrge & Grigorian, 2015, pp. 1741, 1749).
  ○ Atypical colobomas, which vary from a small notch in the pupil to the absence of an entire segment of the iris, are not usually associated with visual difficulties (Õrge & Grigorian, 2015, p. 1749).
- With retinal and optic nerve colobomas, there is a long term, variable risk of complicating retinal detachment or choroidal neovascularization (Campomanes & Binenbaum, 2018, p. 1544).

Glaucoma

DEFINITION

- Glaucoma is an optic neuropathy usually associated with raised intraocular pressure (IOP); (Campomanes & Binenbaum, 2018, p. 1544).

INCIDENCE AND ETIOLOGY

- Congenital glaucoma can occur as a primary disease or secondary to numerous other ocular conditions or systemic syndromes, such as aniridia, congenital rubella, Hallermann–Streiff syndrome, Lowe syndrome, Axenfeld or Rieger syndrome, Sturge-Weber syndrome, and neurofibromatosis.
  ○ One cause of congenital glaucoma is inadequate drainage of aqueous fluid that leads to increased pressure in the eye, resulting in damage of the optic nerve (Campomanes & Binenbaum, 2018, pp. 1538, 1544; Õrge & Grigorian, 2015, p. 1748).

PRESENTATION

- Symptoms of congenital glaucoma can be apparent at birth or weeks to months later and include tearing, light sensitivity, blepharospasm (blinking), Haab striae (tears in the Descemet membrane, seen as lines in the red reflex), or lack of a red reflex. Congenital glaucoma is uncommon but can have devastating effects, so it is an important disease to consider (Campomanes & Binenbaum, 2018, p. 1544; Õrge & Grigorian, 2015, p. 1748; Vargo, 2014, p. 604).
- With acute glaucoma, high IOP is painful enough to manifest as crying, irritability, grimacing, poor feeding, or emesis in an infant. Tearing may be sign of glaucoma, not just of a blocked tear duct.

○ If the IOP is high enough for any prolonged period, irreversible optic nerve damage can ensue, with permanent vision loss (Campomanes & Binenbaum, 2018, p. 1538, 1549; Őrge & Grigorian, 2015, p. 1745).

- Cloudy corneas may be present in the premature baby for up to 7 days and the term baby for up to 48 hours of life. A persistently hazy cornea beyond these times may be suggestive of birth trauma or glaucoma (Őrge & Grigorian, 2015, p. 1747).
  ○ Cloudy corneas represent glaucoma until proven otherwise and require prompt ophthalmologic evaluation even if buphthalmos is not present (Walker, 2018, p. 303).
- As the disease progresses, the increased IOP produces stretching of the eye, creating a cloudy cornea, and corneal and eye enlargement (buphthalmos), progressive myopia (nearsightedness), and loss of vision (Campomanes & Binenbaum, 2018, p. 1544; Őrge & Grigorian, 2015, p. 1748).
  ○ Most newborn infants have a corneal diameter of about 9 to 10 mm. If this measurement exceeds 12 mm, congenital glaucoma must be considered, especially if corneal haze, tearing, and photophobia are present (Őrge & Grigorian, 2015, p. 1747).

INTERVENTION AND OUTCOMES
- Treatment is surgical in most cases, and medical management is used only for temporizing the condition or better visualization for various surgical procedures.
  ○ Congenital glaucoma is a surgical disease that requires prompt intervention, frequently in the neonatal period.
- The prognosis depends on the age of onset, time to diagnosis, and associated ocular and systemic conditions. Vision loss from glaucoma is typically irreversible. Should consider genetic testing to rule out associated syndromes (Campomanes & Binenbaum, 2018, p. 1544; Őrge & Grigorian, 2015, p. 1748).

Retinopathy of Prematurity

DEFINITION
- ROP is a disease of the developing retinal vasculature of premature infants. It first became a significant cause of blindness in children in the 1950s due to increased survival of premature infants mainly because of the use of supplemental oxygen (Campomanes & Binenbaum, 2018, p. 1550; Sun, Hellstrom, & Smith, 2015, p. 1767).

INCIDENCE AND ETIOLOGY
- The overall incidence of ROP of any severity was reported to be 66%; moderately severe ROP, 18%; and severe ROP, 6% (Fraser & Diehl-Jones, 2015, p. 823; Sun et al., 2015, p. 1767).
  ○ The incidence of ROP decreases with increasing gestational age and occurs in most babies with birth weights less than 1,500 g (very low birth weight [VLBW]), with an even greater proportion of babies developing ROP in the less than 1,000 g birth-weight category (extremely low birth weight [ELBW]; Campomanes & Binenbaum, 2018, p. 1552; Sun et al., 2015, p. 1768; Fraser & Diehl-Jones, 2015, p. 823).
  ○ In most cases, ROP develops at 31 to 33 weeks' postmenstrual age (Campomanes & Binenbaum, 2018, p. 1552; Fraser & Diehl-Jones, 2015, p. 822).

- The human retina is avascular until 16 weeks of gestation, after which a capillary network begins to grow, starting at the optic nerve and branching outward toward the ora serrata (edge of the retina). The nasal periphery is vascularized by about 32 weeks of gestation, but the process is not complete in the more distant temporal periphery until 40 to 44 weeks (Fraser & Diehl-Jones, 2015, p. 822).
  ○ Lower gestational age and birth weight are the main risk factors of ROP given that at lower gestational ages, retinal development is less complete (Campomanes & Binenbaum, 2018, p. 1552; Fraser & Diehl-Jones, 2015, p. 823; Sun et al., 2015, p. 1767).
- Relative hyperoxia, aggravated by exogenous oxygen supplementation, damages existing retinal blood vessels, and inhibits retinal secretion of vascular endothelial growth factor (VEGF), a hypoxia-induced vasoactive molecule responsible for normal and pathologic blood vessel development and growth in the body. ROP develops because of poor retinal vascularization resulting in retinal hypoxia and pathologic neovascularization (Campomanes & Binenbaum, 2018, p. 1552; Sun et al., 2015, p. 1769).
  ○ After the initial insult, vessel growth may proceed without ROP, or growth may remain arrested, and the vessels pile up within the retina forming a ridge that might become very thick. If the new vasculature develops abnormally, these capillaries may extend into the vitreous body and/or over the surface of the retina (where they do not belong), and leakage of fluid from these weak, abnormally growing blood vessels may occur.
  ○ Blood and fluid leakage into various parts of the eye can result in scar formation and traction on the retina; visual acuity may be affected depending on the extent to which the macula is pulled out of position (Fraser & Diehl-Jones, 2015, p. 823).
- Other risk factors for ROP are slow postnatal weight gain, low insulin-like growth factor-1 (IGF-1), hyperglycemia and insulin use, hyper/hypocapnia, sepsis, and other prematurity-related morbidities (Campomanes & Binenbaum, 2018, p. 1550, p. 1552; Fraser & Diehl-Jones, 2015, p. 823; Sun et al., 2015, pp. 1768–1769).

CLASSIFICATION
- The standardized approach for describing ROP, developed by the International Committee for the Classification of Retinopathy of Prematurity (2005) takes into account four components: anterior–posterior location of the retinopathy (zone), severity (stage), extent of the disease at the circumference of the vascularized retina (in clock hours), and the presence or absence of plus disease (Campomanes & Binenbaum, 2018, p. 1551; Fraser & Diehl-Jones, 2015, pp. 823–824; Sun et al., 2015, p. 1769).
- The ROP status of an eye is determined by the highest stage and the lowest zone observed, along with noting the presence or absence of plus disease.
  ○ Plus disease is defined as engorged and tortuous vessels of the posterior pole and is indicative of a more serious form of ROP (Campomanes & Binenbaum, 2018, p. 1551).
- See Table 25.3 for the classification of ROP.

TABLE 25.3 Classification of ROP

Stage (severity)	Stage Description	Zone (Anterior–Posterior Location of the Retinopathy)	Zone Description
Stage 0	- Mildest form of ROP - Immature retinal vasculature	Zone 1	- Zone 1 is the most labile - The center of zone 1 is the optic nerve - Most severe retinopathy occurs in zone I or posterior zone II
Stage 1	- Mildly abnormal blood vessel growth - A fine, thin line of demarcation between the vascular and avascular region is present	Zone 2	- Zone 2 is a circle surrounding the zone 1 circle with the nasal ora serrata as its nasal border - Most retinopathy occurs in zone 2
Stage 2	- Moderately abnormal blood vessel growth - Ridge at the junction between vascularized and avascular retina	Zone 3	- Zone 3 is the crescent that the circle of zone 2 does not encompass temporally - Aggressive disease rarely is seen in this zone - ROP with an onset in zone 3 has a good prognosis
Stage 3	- Severely abnormal blood vessel growth - Growth of vessels into the vitreous	x	x
Stage 4	- Partial retinal detachment	x	x
Stage 5	- Total retinal detachment	x	x
Plus disease	- Blood vessels of the retina have become enlarged and twisted, indicating a worsening of the disease	x	x

Sources: Data from Campomanes, A. G., & Binenbaum, G. (2018). Eye and vision disorders. In C. Gleason & S. Juul (Eds.), *Avery's diseases of the newborn* (10th ed., pp. 1536–1557). Philadelphia, PA: Elsevier; Fraser, D., & Diehl-Jones, W. (2015). Ophthalmologic and auditory disorders. In Verklan et al. (Eds.), *Core curriculum for neonatal intensive care nursing* (pp. 813–831). St. Louis, MO: Saunders, Elsevier; Sun, Y., Hellstrom, A., & Smith, L. (2015). Retinopathy of prematurity. In R. Martin, A. Fanaroff, & M. Walsh (Eds.), *Fanaroff and Martin's neonatal–perinatal medicine: Diseases of the fetus and infant* (10th ed., pp. 1767–1774). Philadelphia, PA: Elsevier. See Figure 25.1 for the clock hours and zones of the retina.

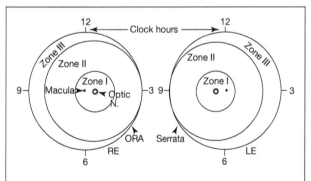

FIGURE 25.1 Clock hours and zones of ROP

Source: Image used with permission from Campomanes, A. G., & Binenbaum, G. (2018). Eye and vision disorders. In C. Gleason & S. Juul (Eds.), *Avery's diseases of the newborn* (10th ed., p. 1551). Philadelphia, PA: Elsevier.

ROP EXAM

- It is critical for clinicians to identify the at-risk baby so that timely examinations can be performed to decrease the likelihood of or prevent blindness. In the United States, the recommended guidelines for detection of serious ROP indicate that diagnostic examinations should be performed on:
  - Infants with birth weights less than 1,500 g or of 30 weeks' gestation, along with babies in the 1,501 to 2,000 g birth-weight group thought to be at high risk
  - The first exam should occur 4 to 6 weeks after birth (approximately 31–33 weeks of postconceptional age; Campomanes & Binenbaum, 2018, p. 1553; Fraser & Diehl-Jones, 2015, p. 824; Sun et al., 2015, p. 1772).
- Infants who are found to have areas of retinal immaturity on initial examination should have repeated examinations every other week, then every 2 to 3 weeks until vascularization has reached the ora serrata (Campomanes & Binenbaum, 2018, p. 1553; Fraser & Diehl-Jones, 2015, p. 824; Sun et al., 2015, p. 1772).
- If ROP is present during the initial examination, the infant should be examined weekly or every other week, depending on the severity of clinical findings (Campomanes & Binenbaum, 2018, p. 1553; Fraser & Diehl-Jones, 2015, p. 824).

PREPARATION FOR THE ROP EXAM

- Preparation for the ROP examination includes dilating the eyes with sympathomimetic drugs (e.g., phenylephrine) and anticholinergic drugs (e.g., tropicamide, cyclopentolate, atropine) (Campomanes & Binenbaum, 2018, p. 1537).

- Phenylephrine is a sympathetic mydriatic (pupil dilator) agent, and the 2.5% solution is considered safe in the pediatric population (Taketomo, Hodding & Kraus, 2018, p. 1615).
- Anticholinergic drugs cause dilation by inhibiting the parasympathetic constrictor muscle and bringing about cycloplegia (paralysis of the ciliary muscle of the eye) (Taketomo et al., 2018, p. 532).
  - ○ Cyclomydril (cyclopentolate and phenylephrine) is the preferred agent for use in neonates and infants because lower concentrations of both drugs provide optimal dilation while minimizing the systemic side effects of a higher concentration of each drug used alone (Campomanes & Binenbaum, 2018, p. 1537; Taketomo et al., 2018, p. 532).
    - ■ Potential side effects of these drugs include increased heart rate, elevated blood pressure, cardiac arrhythmias, feeding intolerance, slowed gastric emptying, urticaria, contact dermatitis, and seizures. Premature infants are susceptible to bradycardic and apneic events with cyclopentolate and are pain response reactions and not a direct effect of the drugs.
  - ○ Adverse effects can be of greater concern in preterm infants since they weigh less and usually require multiple doses to achieve adequate dilation, as well as many children with dark irises (Campomanes & Binenbaum, 2018, p. 1537).

INTERVENTIONS FOR ROP
- Laser photoablation therapy for ROP is recommended for infants with the following classifications:
  - ○ Zone II: Plus disease with stage 2 or 3 ROP
  - ○ Zone I: Plus disease with stage 1 or 2 ROP
  - ○ Zone I: Stage 3 ROP (Campomanes & Binenbaum, 2018, p. 1554; Fraser & Diehl-Jones, 2015, p. 825; Sun et al., 2015, p. 1771)
- Another treatment option that is in the experimental stages is anti-VEGF therapy. Anti-VEGF agents are being considered more frequently as a first-line treatment alternative, especially for eyes with zone I ROP, because laser photoablation is relatively ineffective in decreasing retinal detachment in those cases (Campomanes & Binenbaum, 2018, p. 1554; Fraser & Diehl-Jones, 2015, p. 826).
  - ○ Bevacizumab (Avastin) is a monoclonal antibody that inhibits angiogenesis and is administered as an intraocular injection and suppresses the development of blood vessels in the retina.

OUTCOMES FROM ROP
- Ninety percent (or more) of cases of acute ROP resolve spontaneously, with little or no loss of vision. Timely treatment has been shown to decrease the risk of blinding complications of ROP by 50% (Fraser & Diehl-Jones, 2015, p. 826).
- ROP located in the most immature zone I has the worst prognosis (Fraser & Diehl-Jones, 2015, p. 826; Sun et al., 2015, pp. 1769–1770).
- ROP with an onset in zone 2, or a slower evolution of the disorder, more often leads to complete resolution.
- ROP with an onset in zone 3 has a good prognosis for full recovery (Sun et al., 2015, p. 1770).

- Blindness or severe visual impairment commonly results from progression of the retinopathy to retinal detachment or severe distortion of the posterior retina (Campomanes & Binenbaum, 2018, p. 1552; Fraser & Diehl-Jones, 2015, p. 823).

Strabismus

DEFINITION
- Strabismus is the appearance of crossed eyes often seen in newborns because of weak eye musculature and lack of coordination (Tappero & Honeyfield, 2016, p. 285; Vargo, 2014, p. 604).

INCIDENCE AND ETIOLOGY
- Strabismus is more common in preterm infants, especially those with a history of ROP, intracranial hemorrhage, or white matter injury (Stewart, Hernandez, & Duncan, 2017, p. 195).
- Strabismus results from muscular incoordination and gives the appearance of crossed eyes (Johnson, 2019, p. 72). Transient deviations (neonatal ocular misalignments) occur very commonly in the first month of life in visually normal infants, and at this age it is not possible to distinguish those infants who will progress to develop pathologic strabismus from those who will develop normal binocular vision (Campomanes & Binenbaum, 2018, p. 1540).
- Conjugate horizontal gaze (movement of both eyes with the visual axes parallel) should be evident in the newborn, and vertical conjugate gaze develops by 2 months of age (Őrge & Grigorian, 2015, p. 1739).

PRESENTATION
- The most common form of strabismus is esotropia (crossed eyes), but exotropia (wall-eye) and hypertropia (vertical misalignment of the eyes where one eye is higher than the other) also occur (Stewart et al., 2017, p. 195).
- Pseudostrabismus due to a flat nasal bridge usually resolves within a year and can be differentiated from strabismus by the presence of symmetrical corneal light reflexes (Johnson, 2016, p. 73).
- Strabismus may also produce abnormal or asymmetric red reflexes. An additional observation is the position of the light reflex on the corneal surface. Asymmetric positioning of this reflex can indicate misalignment of the eyes (strabismus) (Campomanes & Binenbaum, 2018, p. 1542).

INTERVENTIONS AND OUTCOMES
- Premature and low birth weight infants are at increased risk of developing strabismus and other amblyogenic conditions throughout their childhood. Any constant strabismus beyond the age of 4 months requires further evaluation.
  - ○ This is especially important as, in some cases, strabismus can also be the first sign of serious ocular or systemic disorders (Campomanes & Binenbaum, 2018, p. 1542). Infants with strabismus require a fundus exam to exclude retinoblastoma (Őrge & Grigorian, 2015, p. 1756).
- Strabismus may be treated with eye patching, atropine drops, and corrective lenses. Surgical intervention may be necessary depending of the cause (Stewart et al., 2017, p. 195).

- Premature infants have a higher incidence of myopia, amblyopia, and strabismus in childhood. Careful follow-up of all children born prematurely is advisable to ensure early detection of these ocular conditions (Őrge & Grigorian, 2015, p. 1740).

Conjunctivitis

DEFINITION
- Neonatal conjunctivitis (ophthalmia neonatorum) is an inflammatory reaction resulting from invasion of the conjunctivae by pathologic organisms (Campomanes & Binenbaum, 2018, p. 1545; Fraser & Diehl-Jones, 2015, p. 816; Őrge & Grigorian, 2015, p. 1762).

INCIDENCE AND ETIOLOGY
- Conjunctivitis caused by bacterial and viral infections is typically acquired from the mother as the child passes through the birth canal, but it can occur after cesarean section (Őrge & Grigorian, 2015, p. 1762).
  - The incidence of neonatal conjunctivitis has decreased dramatically since the introduction of prophylaxis in 1881, but still blinds thousands of babies annually worldwide (Campomanes & Binenbaum, 2018, p. 1545).
  - Chlamydial conjunctivitis is the most common cause of neonatal conjunctivitis, and the rates are higher when there is absent prenatal care (Fraser & Diehl-Jones, 2015, p. 817; Őrge & Grigorian, 2015, p. 1762).
  - About 20% to 50% of babies born vaginally to mothers with a *C. trachomatis* infection of the cervix will develop conjunctivitis, and 10% to 20% develop pneumonia (Fraser & Diehl-Jones, 2015, p. 817).
- See Table 25.4 for the causes and treatment of conjunctivitis.

PRESENTATION
- The infant with mucopurulent discharge must be distinguished from the infant who exhibits only excessive tearing and a relatively white eye, which is most likely nasolacrimal duct obstruction; but the possibility of congenital glaucoma must always be ruled out (Campomanes & Binenbaum, 2018, p. 1546; Őrge & Grigorian, 2015, p. 1745).

INTERVENTIONS AND OUTCOMES
- Since the timing of the onset of conjunctivitis is not a reliable diagnostic clue, and because significant overlap exists among the different etiologic agents, conjunctival cultures and conjunctival scraping for Gram and Giemsa staining are mandatory and should be performed without delay (Campomanes & Binenbaum, 2018, p. 1545; Őrge & Grigorian, 2015, p. 1762).
- Infants with gonococcal conjunctivitis are at risk of having corneal ulceration, perforation, and subsequent visual impairment. Systemic complications involving the blood, joints, or central nervous system (CNS) may occur in a small number of infants (Fraser & Diehl-Jones, 2015, p. 817).
- Chlamydial infections are spread through the nasolacrimal duct system and can lead to Chlamydia-related pneumonia (Fraser & Diehl-Jones, 2015, p. 817).

TABLE 25.4 Causes and Treatment of Conjunctivitis

Type	Causative Factor	Onset	Presentation	Treatment
Chemical	Instillation of silver nitrate or other antibiotic prophylaxis	1–2 days	- Low amount of purulence - No organisms on Gram stain - Usually resolves in 1–2 days	None
Bacterial	*Neisseria gonorrhea*	3–4 days	Bilateral, hyperacute purulent conjunctivitis, marked lid edema, copious discharge	Ceftriaxone 25–50 mg/kg daily Intravenously Topical irrigation Topical antibiotics useful only if corneal ulcer present
	Chlamydia trachomatis - Most common cause of conjunctivitis in the neonatal period - Can lead to Chlamydia-related pneumonia if left untreated	5–7 days	Mild mucopurulent, nonfollicular conjunctivitis, lid edema, pseudomembrane formation	Erythromycin, 12.5 mg/kg orally every 6 hours for 2 weeks or azithromycin suspension, 20 mg/kg orally daily for 3 days
	Staphylococcus aureus, Streptococcus, and other bacteria	5–14 days	Nosocomial mucoid discharge, conjunctival hyperemia, and swelling	Broad-spectrum topical antibiotic (e.g., polymyxin B–trimethoprim, one drop every 4 hours for 7 days)
Viral	Herpes simplex virus	6–14 days	Unilateral or bilateral conjunctivitis, serous discharge, associated lid vesicles	Acyclovir, 60 mg/kg per day in three divided doses for 2 weeks (3 weeks if CNS or disseminated disease) plus topical drops (1% trifluridine, 0.1% iododeoxyuridine, or 3% vidarabine)

CNS, central nervous system.

Sources: Data from Campomanes, A. G., & Binenbaum, G. (2018). Eye and vision disorders. In C. Gleason & S. Juul (Eds.), *Avery's diseases of the newborn* (10th ed., pp. 1536–1557). Philadelphia, PA: Elsevier; Fraser, D., & Diehl-Jones, W. (2015). Ophthalmologic and auditory disorders. In Verklan et al. (Eds.), *Core curriculum for neonatal intensive care nursing* (pp. 813–831). St. Louis, MO: Saunders, Elsevier; Őrge, F., & Grigorian, F. (2015). Examination and common problems of the neonatal eye. In R. Martin, A. Fanaroff, & M. Walsh (Eds.), *Fanaroff and Martin's neonatal–perinatal medicine: Diseases of the fetus and infant* (10th ed., pp. 1734–1766). Philadelphia, PA: Elsevier.

- Neonatal herpes infection is most often acquired during passage through the birth canal and can cause typical herpetic eye disease such as blepharoconjunctivitis, keratitis, iritis, or chorioretinitis (Őrge & Grigorian, 2015, p. 1763).

THE NOSE

Embryology

- Olfactory placodes, nasal swellings, choana, and primitive palate develop and olfactory evagination occurs at 34 to 44 days of gestation (Blackburn, 2013, p. 74).
- Lacrimal apparatus consists of structures that produce tears (lacrimal glands) and structures responsible for drainage of tears (upper and lower puncta, canaliculi, lacrimal sac, and nasolacrimal duct; Fraser & Diehl-Jones, 2015, p. 817; Őrge & Grigorian, 2015, p. 1745).
- Lacrimal duct becomes fully patent at about 4 to 6 months (Vargo, 2014, p. 604).
- Term and preterm newborn infants have the capacity to secrete tears as a reflex to irritants, but usually do not secrete emotional tears until 2 to 3 months of age (Fraser & Diehl-Jones, 2015, p. 817).

Nasolacrimal Duct Obstruction

DEFINITION

- Obstruction or stenosis of the nasolacrimal duct (dacrostenosis; Campomanes & Binenbaum, 2018, p. 1538; Őrge & Grigorian, 2015, p. 1745)

INCIDENCE AND ETIOLOGY

- The duct is blocked at birth in 5% to 10% of newborns, resulting in epiphora (excessive tearing) and discharge in an otherwise white and quiet eye; 90% of such blockages clear by 1 year of age.
- Congenital nasolacrimal duct obstruction is usually caused by an imperforate membrane at the distal end of the nasolacrimal duct (Fraser & Diehl-Jones, 2015, p. 817). Nasolacrimal duct obstruction is an ophthalmic manifestation of Goldenhar syndrome (Campomanes & Binenbaum, 2018, pp. 1538, 1555; Őrge & Grigorian, 2015, p. 1745).

PRESENTATION

- Nasolacrimal duct obstruction presents with epiphora (excess tearing) and usually does not occur until after the first 3 weeks of life when the major portion of the lacrimal gland has become functional (Őrge & Grigorian, 2015, p. 1745).
- Nasolacrimal duct obstruction also presents with crusting or matting of the eyelashes, the spilling of tears over the lower lid and cheek, and absence of conjunctival infection (Fraser & Diehl-Jones, 2015, p. 817).
  - Chronic obstruction may lead to secondary infection in the lacrimal sac may occur, a condition known as dacryocystitis (Campomanes & Binenbaum, 2018, p. 1546; Őrge & Grigorian, 2015, p. 1745).
  - Dacryocystocele is formed when a proximal and a distal obstruction coexist in the lacrimal sac, and the lacrimal sac becomes distended.

- Manifested as a bluish, nontender mass just inferior and medial to the canthus causing bulging of the mucosa at the lower end of the nasolacrimal duct and can significantly compromise the airway (Campomanes & Binenbaum, 2018, p. 1547)

INTERVENTIONS AND OUTCOMES

- Simple nasolacrimal duct obstruction (NLDO) usually requires conservative management. This consists of digital massage downward from the lacrimal sac over the nasolacrimal duct on the side of the nose. The massage empties the sac, reducing the opportunity for bacterial growth. Dacrocystocele should be ruled out by inspection of the nasal passage (Campomanes & Binenbaum, 2018, pp. 1546–1547).
- Once confirmed, prompt intervention with oral antibiotics is recommended to prevent infection of the dacryocystocele, which can occur in up to two-thirds of these patients, and surgical treatment with a nasolacrimal probing should be considered within the next 2 to 4 days (Őrge & Grigorian, 2015, p. 1745).
  - Topical broad-spectrum antibiotic drops or ointment, such as Bacitracin Zinc and polymyxin B sulfate ophthalmic ointment or drops, can be used if there is conjunctival infection and discharge.
- Dacrocystitis, if not treated, can have potentially serious consequences in a neonate, including meningitis and septicemia (Campomanes & Binenbaum, 2018, pp. 1546–1548).

Choanal Atresia

DEFINITION

- Choanal atresia is a membranous or bony obstruction in the nasal passage and may be bilateral or unilateral (Gardner & Hernandez, 2016, p. 94).

INCIDENCE AND ETIOLOGY

- Choanal atresia occurs in approximately one in 7,000 live births, with associated anomalies present in 20% to 50% of infants with choanal atresia (Otteson & Arnold, 2015, p. 1147).
- Choanal atresia is a feature of CHARGE syndrome (Bennett & Meier, 2016, p. 233).

PRESENTATION

- Choanal atria presents with noisy breathing, cyanosis that resolves during crying, and apnea of the quiet infant (Benjamin & Furdon, 2015, p. 129; Gardner & Hernandez, 2016, p. 94; Walker, 2018, p. 304).
- As infants are preferential nose breathers for the first 4 to 6 weeks of life, symptoms of bilateral choanal atresia can be severe and depends on the severity of the lesion (Otteson & Arnold, 2015, p. 1147).
- Bilateral choanal atresia, as in other conditions with severe airway obstruction or swallowing dysfunction, polyhydramnios is commonly present prenatally (Evans, Hing, & Cunningham, 2018, p. 1433).

INTERVENTIONS AND OUTCOMES

- Passage of a thin (6-French) catheter through both nostrils to evaluate the newborn for potential choanal atresia (Otteson & Arnold, 2015, p. 1147; Walker, 2018, p. 291)

○ An oral airway should be placed if bilateral choanal atresia is suspected. This can stabilize the airway by bypassing the choanal obstruction. Once the airway has been secured, a confirmatory CT scan of the nasal passages can be obtained.

- If the oral airway does not allow adequate air entry, endotracheal intubation may be required. In consultation with a pediatric otolaryngologist, transnasal stents may be placed to keep the nasal passages patent in choanal stenosis (and postoperatively after choanal atresia repair).
  ○ Left untreated, the newborn with bilateral choanal atresia can asphyxiate and die (Evans et al., 2018, p. 1433–1434).
- Definitive therapy includes opening a hole through the bony plate with the use of a laser (Ringer & Hansen, 2017, p. 951).
- Bottle feeding or breastfeeding is contraindicated in an infant with choanal atresia, and the infant should be gavage-fed instead (Verklan, 2015, p. 66).

Deviated Septum

DEFINITION

- A deviated septum is a dislocation of the cartilaginous part of the septum from the vomerine groove and columella and is a cause of nasal obstruction (Benjamin & Furdon, 2015, pp. 129–130; Mangurten, Puppala, & Prazed, 2015, p. 414).

INCIDENCE AND ETIOLOGY

- A deviated septum is the most frequent neonatal nasal injury that can result from intrauterine factors such as a uterine tumor, persistent pressure on the nose by fetal small parts, or during delivery from pressure on the nose by the symphysis pubis, sacral promontory, or perineum.
  ○ Asymmetries of the nose caused by in utero compression are common and need to be distinguished from true septal deviation. (Benjamin & Furdon, 2015, p. 130; Johnson, 2016, p. 73; Mangurten et al., 2015, p. 414; Walker, 2018, p. 302)

PRESENTATION

- The neonate is an obligate nose breather and presents with respiratory distress if there is a blockage (Benjamin & Furdon, 2015, p. 129).

INTERVENTION AND OUTCOMES

- To differentiate nasal asymmetry from septal deviation, gently compress naris on side of asymmetrical naris. A dislocated septum remains angled at base. In the nasal asymmetry, no nasal deviation occurs with compression.
- Consult otolaryngologist for septal dislocation; reduction of a dislocated septum should be done within a 7 to 10 days of birth for the best outcome because lacrimal bones unite quickly (Benjamin & Furdon, 2015, p. 130; Mangurten et al., 2015, p. 415; Walker, 2018, p. 302).
  ○ If surgery is required, the provider should provide an oral airway to relieve respiratory distress (Mangurten et al., 2015, p. 415).

- Fractures of the septal cartilage also may be reduced by manual remolding, but most are associated with hematomas that should be promptly incised and drained.
- Prompt fracture reduction and fixation provides rapid healing without complications. Inadequate, missed, or delayed identification and treatment may lead to subsequent developmental deformities (Mangurten et al., 2015, p. 415).

THE EARS

Embryology

- The structures of the ear begin to form at 9 weeks' gestation and continue until 32 weeks' gestation. The cartilage continues to mature until 40 weeks' gestation and is used as a criteria for gestational assessment (Bajaj & Gross, 2015, p. 137; Trotter, 2015, p. 33).
- Hearing begins to develop in utero and continues to approximately 9 months of age (Lehtonon, 2017, p. 1003).

Preauricular Tags and Sinuses

DEFINITION

- Preauricular tags are minor malformations of skin generally found on the anterior tragus.
- Preauricular sinuses is an indentation on the anterior tragus that may be blind or communicate with the inner ear or brain (Douma, Casey, & Greene, 2017, p. 976; Johnson, 2019, p. 68).

INCIDENCE AND ETIOLOGY

- Preauricular and auricular skin tags occur rarely, in approximately 0.23% of newborns. Auricular sinuses occur even less often, in approximately 0.12% of newborns (Parikh & Mitchell, 2015, p. 440).
- Preauricular tags are thought to be embryologic remnants of the first brachial arch or cleft.
- Preauricular tags are likely benign but warrant investigation as they may be familial or associated with syndromes (CHARGE), hearing loss or deafness, renal anomalies, brachial arch anomalies, and oral clefts (Johnson, 2019, p. 68; Lissauer, 2015, p. 395).

PRESENTATION

- Upon inspection preauricular tags or sinuses are evident (Benjamin & Furdon, 2015, p. 131; Lissauer, 2015, pp. 394–395).

INTERVENTION AND OUTCOMES

- When single or bilateral preauricular tags are present with other abnormalities or risk factors, a renal ultrasound is indicated (Benjamin & Furdon, 2015, p. 131; Lissauer, 2015, pp. 394–395).
  ○ No surgical intervention is required in cases of preauricular tags. Parents may desire cosmetic removal and should be referred to a plastic surgeon.
- Preauricular sinuses are usually benign. Surgical removal may be necessary as the child gets older due to recurrent infection. Increased risk of deafness and renal anomalies (Benjamin & Furdon, 2015, p. 131; Douma et al., 2017, p. 976).

- Isolated preauricular tags and sinuses are generally benign. In the presence of associated anomalies or risk factors, further evaluation is warranted (Johnson, 2019, p. 68; Lissauer, 2015, pp. 394).
- Routine hearing screening should occur due to associations with congenital hearing loss (Lissauer, 2015, pp. 394–395).

Malformation and Deformities of the Ear

DEFINITION
- Normal ear position occurs when the attachment of the ear is above the horizontal plane from the inner to outer canthus. If the ear attachment falls below this plane, the ear is considered "low set" (Johnson, 2019, p. 68; Lissauer, 2015, pp. 394).
  - *Malformation* of the ear occurs when the anatomic structures of the ear are not formed correctly due to a primary defect in tissue formation.
  - *Deformation* of the ear is a result of external, mechanical forces acting on normal ear structures (Parikh & Mitchell, 2015, 436).

Incidence and Etiology

MALFORMATIONS
- Microtia is a disorganized, dysplastic, or dysmorphic external ear which may be unilateral or bilateral. Ears may appear low set. Microtia is associated with other malformations and abnormalities of the middle ear (Benjamin & Furdon, 2015, p. 130; Walker, 2018, p. 302).
- Low set, posteriorly rotated, or poorly formed ears may be associated with chromosomal abnormalities and syndromes (Johnson, 2019, pp. 69–70).

DEFORMATIONS
- Deformation of the ear may occur due to in utero positioning or prematurity and may be associated with auditory atresia and conductive hearing loss (Lissauer, 2015, p. 395).
- Incidence regarding congenital malformations and deformations of the ear are not identified.

PRESENTATION
- Normal ear placement is considered to be above the imaginary line drawn from the inner to outer canthus of the eye toward the ear. If the insertion of the ear is lower than this point, the ear is considered low set. Both ears should be examined for insertion and rotation as one ear may be posteriorly rotated and appear low set, while the other ear appears in normal position (Bennett & Meier, 2019, p. 221; Johnson, 2019, p. 69; Lissaur, 2015, p. 394).
- Posterior rotation occurs when the ear deviates more than 10° from the vertical axis (Bennett & Meier, 2019, p. 221).

INTERVENTIONS AND OUTCOMES
- Microtia or posteriorly rotated or low-set ears should alert the provider to conduct further testing such as hearing screening and possible genetic testing. Microtia may indicate middle ear abnormalities, while posterior rotation and low-set ear insertions are associated with several genetic syndromes (Benjamin & Furdon, 2015, p. 129; Bennett & Meier, 2019, p. 221).

Congenital Hearing Loss

DEFINITION
- Hearing loss is one of the most common major abnormalities present at birth; universal hearing screening is recommended with appropriate follow-up intervention by 6 months of age (Johnson, 2019, pp. 69–70; Vohr, 2015, p. 993).

INCIDENCE AND ETIOLOGY
- Approximately 50% of congenital hearing loss is hereditary. Genetic hearing loss is more likely to be nonsyndromic, autosomal recessive (30% syndromic and 70% nonsyndromic). Over 400 syndromes have association with congenital hearing loss (Vohr, 2015, p. 993).
- See Box 25.1 for risk factors for hearing loss.

BOX 25.1 Risk Factors for Congenital Hearing Loss

- Caregiver concerns regarding hearing, speech, language, or developmental delay
- Family history of permanent hearing loss
- NICU admission for greater than 5 days, including and of the following regardless of length of stay:
  - Extracorporeal membrane oxygenation
  - Assisted ventilation
  - Exposure to ototoxic medications or loop diuretics
  - Hyperbilirubinemia requiring exchange transfusion
  - Intrauterine TORCH infection
  - Craniofacial abnormalities involving the ear structures and temporal
  - White forelock, associated with sensorineural or permanent conductive hearing loss
  - Syndromes such as neurofibromatosis, osteopetrosis, and Usher syndrome, associated with progressive hearing loss
  - Neurodegenerative disorders, i.e., Hunter syndrome, or sensory motor neuropathies such as Friedreich ataxia or Charcot-Marie-Tooth disease
  - Postnatal bacterial or viral infection confirmed with culture, including meningitis
  - Head trauma requiring hospitalization
  - Chemotherapy

Source: Data from Vohr, B. (2015). Hearing loss in the newborn. In R. Martin, A. Fanaroff, & M. Walsh (Eds.), *Fanaroff and Martin's neonatal–perinatal medicine: Diseases of the fetus and infant* (10th ed., pp. 993–1000). Philadelphia, PA: Elsevier.

PRESENTATION
- Symptoms of hearing loss may be difficult to assess in the neonatal period due to responsivity. However, the infant should startle, cry, or respond to loud noises and should alert to voices (Johnson, 2015, p. 70).

INTERVENTIONS AND OUTCOMES
- Universal hearing screening is recommended for all infants in the United States. Two of the common physiologic tests performed prior to hospital discharge are the otoacoustic emissions (OAEs) and auditory brainstem response (ABR); (Johnson, 2019, p. 68; Stewart et al., 2017, p. 996, Vohr, 2015, p. 993).
  - OAE and ABR do not require active response, therefore they can be performed while the infant sleeps. Both OAE and ABR testing methods detect sensorineural and conducting hearing loss. However, false-positive

fail screenings can occur due to middle ear dysfunction, presence of fluid or debris (transient conductive hearing loss), or noise interference (Stewart, 2017, p. 996; Vohr, 2015, pp. 993–995).

- Failed hearing screening should be referred to a pediatric audiologist for further diagnostic testing, including CT or MRI, genetic counseling, and pediatric ophthalmology (Stewart et al., 2017, p. 997).
- Providers should aim to identify infants with congenital hearing loss and enroll qualified infants into early intervention services by 3 months of age to optimize speech and language development (Stewart et al., 2017, p. 998, Vohr, 2015, p. 995).
- Outcomes depend greatly on severity of hearing loss, time of diagnosis and treatment initiation as well as presence of syndromes or comorbidities. Earlier identification and treatment leads to better achievement of age-appropriate speech and language milestones.
  - Fitting of hearing aids by age 6 months has shown improved speech outcomes (Stewart et al., 2017, p. 998).

Birth Injury of Ear

DEFINITION
- Any impairment of the structure or function due to adverse influences that occur at birth (Abdulhayoglu, 2017, p. 64).

INCIDENCE AND ETIOLOGY
- Birth injuries of the ear are usually caused by misplaced or slipping forceps application during delivery, with bruising, lacerations, abrasions, and hematomas the most common types of injuries (Abdulhayoglu, 2017, p. 68; Mangurten et al., 2015, p. 417).

PRESENTATION
- Careful inspection of the ear structures should yield any evidence of ear trauma. Particular care should be taken following forceps-assisted deliveries, as this is the most common cause of ear trauma (Abdulhayoglu, 2017, p. 68; Mangurten et al., 2015, p. 417).

INTERVENTION AND OUTCOMES
- Hematomas should be drained to prevent "cauliflower ear." Infant may need follow-up with otolaryngologist if temporal bone and cartilage are involved (Abdulhayoglu, 2017, p. 68; Mangurten et al., 2015, p. 417).
- Severe lacerations may require consultation from a plastic surgeon depending on severity.

MOUTH AND THROAT

Embryology

- The mouth and throat structures develop between weeks 5 and 9 of gestation, with fusion of the lip and primary palate occurring in week 7 (Bajaj & Gross, 2015, p. 137; Blackburn, 2013, pp. 69–79; Evans et al., 2012, p. 1333).

Cleft Lip and/or Palate

DEFINITION
- Cleft lip generally occurs at the lateral aspect, along one of the philtral ridges or along the midline.
- Cleft palate can occur on any area of the hard or soft palate.

INCIDENCE AND ETIOLOGY
- The causes of orofacial clefting are usually nonsyndromic and unknown in 75% of infants with cleft lip with or without cleft palate and 50% of infants with isolated cleft palate. The prevalence of cleft lip and palate is approximately 0.8 per 1,000 births (Evans et al., 2012, p. 1331; Lissauer, 2015, p. 392). See Table 25.4 for syndromes with potential oral anomalies.
- As an isolated anomaly, cleft palate is rarely associated with genetic anomalies. Midline cleft lip is associated with holoprosencephaly, where U-shaped clefts are associated with Pierre-Robin sequence (Evans et al., 2012, p. 1331; Parikh & Mitchell, 2015, p. 447).

PRESENTATION
- Palpation of the hard and soft palate should be completed with exam in order to identify submucosal or posterior clefts (Johnson, 2019, p. 74; Lissauer, 2015, p. 395).
- Location, shape, and degree of cleft should be noted, as this information will guide the need for further genetic evaluation.

INTERVENTION AND OUTCOMES
- Presence of atypical cleft lip and or plate, for example, midline cleft lip, U-shaped or V-shaped cleft palate, and any additional anomalies, should lead the provider to complete genetic testing and genetic counseling referrals.
- Cleft lip/palate is not an automatic ICU admission. A multidisciplinary approach to management and early intervention follow-up is recommended. Nutritionist consult should be considered as cleft lip and palate infants may have higher caloric requirements and are at higher risk for failure to thrive.
  - Parents should be taught to feed the infant safely using a specialized bottle. Breastfeeding may pose a challenge due to inability to create adequate suction, especially in cases of cleft palate. Proper feeding technique is important to reduce potential aspiration and subsequent airway inflammation.
- Surgical intervention occurs around 6 months of age for cleft lip and 9 to 12 months of age for cleft lip and palate, to optimize speech and language development.
- Outcomes vary depending on type and location and any associated syndromes. Early diagnosis and repair will lead to optimized speech and language development (Evans et al., 2012, pp. 1335, 1337).

Laryngeal Clefts

DEFINITION
- Cleft of the airway structures, which may include the larynx, trachea, and/or esophagus.

INCIDENCE AND ETIOLOGY

- Laryngeal clefts are a result of the failure of posterior cricoid lamina fusion. Laryngeal clefts are not typically associated with cleft palate (Evans et al., 2012, p. 1334; Otteson & Arnold, 2015, p. 1154).

PRESENTATION

- Infant with laryngeal clefts may present with stridor, respiratory distress, dysphagia, or feeding difficulties, including aspiration (Evans et al., 2012, p. 1334; Otteson & Arnold, 2015, p. 1154).

INTERVENTION AND OUTCOMES

- Definitive diagnostic testing for laryngeal cleft is microlarygoscopy under general anesthesia. Early diagnosis is key to reduce lung inflammation and injury (Evans et al., 2012, p. 1334; Ringer & Hansen, 2017, p. 951)
- A chest x-ray should be obtained to evaluate airway and lung fields for aspiration. The primary concern is for aspiration of secretions and feeds.
  - Thickened feedings may be sufficient in mild cases; however, if aspiration or distress with feedings persists or cleft is severe, gastrostomy tube placement may be necessary to prevent aspiration (Otteson & Arnold, 2015, p. 1154).
- Surgical treatment may initially require tracheostomy to allow growth and insure airway patency (Evans et al., 2012, p. 1334).

Micrognathia and Retrognathia

DEFINITION

- Micrognathia is an excessively small jaw.
- Retrognathia refers to the position of the jaw, being set further back. Infants may have a combination of micrognathia and retrognathia (Evans et al., 2012, p. 1331; Parikh & Mitchell, 2015, p. 448).

INCIDENCE AND ETIOLOGY

- Incidence of isolated micrognathia and retrognathia are difficult to discern due to association with genetic syndromes. However, estimates the prevalence of Pierre Robin sequence range from 1:8,500 to 1:20,000 live births.
- Micrognathia is present in several syndromes, most commonly Pierre Robin sequence, Strickler syndrome, and Treacher Collins syndrome (Evans et al., 2012, p. 1331, 1345; Parikh & Mitchell, 2015, p. 448).

PRESENTATION

- Micrognathia and retrognathia are evident on exam of the infant's facies. Macroglossia (large, protruding tongue) may be exaggerated as the oral cavity is not large enough for the tongue (Johnson, 2019, p. 74; Parikh & Mitchell, 2015, p. 448).
  - Presence of respiratory distress with accompanying jaw deformity requires prompt intervention (Evans et al., 2012, p. 1332).

INTERVENTION AND OUTCOMES

- Systematic examination of oral cavity should be performed when micrognathia and retrognathia are present (Benjamin & Furdon, 2015, p. 130; Johnson, 2019, p. 74).

- Initial airway stabilization including prone positioning, nasopharyngeal, or endotracheal airway. Nasopharyngeal airway is preferred as it is the least invasive treatment (Evans et al., 2012, p. 1332, Pappas & Robey, 2015, p. 90).
- Factors that determine treatment plan include presence of additional airway anomalies or presence of musculoskeletal or neurologic syndromes or skeletal dysplasia,s which may contribute to degree of airway obstruction.
- As the infant grows, subsequent growth of the mandible may occur and alleviate airway obstruction. Multidisciplinary approach should include consultations include otolaryngology and nutrition.
- Surgical treatments differ by facility and provider but may include mandibular distraction with osteogenesis, tongue-lip adhesion, or tracheostomy (Evans et al., 2012, p. 1332; Ringer & Hansen, 2017, p. 951)

Macroglossia

DEFINITION

- Macroglossia is the presence of a large tongue, which does not allow for complete closure of the mouth (Johnson, 2019, p. 74).

INCIDENCE AND ETIOLOGY

- Incidence of macroglossia is unknown, however, it is commonly seen in genetic disorders such as Beckwith-Wiedemann syndrome and Down syndrome. It may also be associated with hypothyroidism and mucopolysaccharidosis (Bennett & Meier, 2019, p. 222; Johnson, 2019, p. 74).

PRESENTATION

- Macroglossia is a large protruding tongue, which hinders the mouth from closing. Care should be taken when examining an infant with presumed macroglossia, as micrognathia may be the cause of the protruding tongue.
- The tongue may obstruct the airway or make feeding difficult (Johnson, 2019, p. 74).

INTERVENTIONS AND OUTCOMES

- Testing should be completed to determine the cause of the macroglossia, which may include genetic and metabolic testing.
- Interventions regarding airway obstruction and feeding difficulties are necessary if these issues arise and compromise the infant.
- Outcomes of macroglossia depend on the root cause and outpatient support. Infants with Beckwith–Wiedemann and Down syndrome may need outpatient services, such as physical, occupational, and speech therapies to achieve optimum functioning.
- Table 25.5 describes syndromes and potential associated oral anomalies.

AIRWAY OBSTRUCTIONS

Laryngeal Webs

DEFINITION

- Membranous tissue most commonly covering the glottis to the anterior vocal process (Otteson & Arnold, 2015, p. 1153)

TABLE 25.5 Syndromes and Potential Associated Oral Anomalies

Syndromes	Associated Oral Obstructions
Pierre Robin sequence	Micrognathia, retrognathia, U-shaped bilateral cleft, glossoptosis
Treacher Collins syndrome	Micrognathia with glossoptosis
Crouzon syndrome	Retrognathia
Trisomy 21	Glossoptosis (downward placement or retraction of the tongue)
Trisomy 18	Microstomia (abnormally small mouth opening)
Cornelia de Lange syndrome, fetal alcohol syndrome	Thin upper lip, flattened philtrum
Beckwith-Wiedemann syndrome, hypothyroidism, mucopolysaccoridosis	Macroglossia, macrostomia (abnormally wide mouth)
Holoprosencephaly	Midline cleft lip or palate

Sources: Data from Evans, K. N., Hing, A. V., & Cunningham, M. L. (2018). Craniofacial malformations. In C. Gleason & S. Juul (Eds.), *Avery's diseases of the newborn* (10th ed., pp. 1417–1437). Philadelphia, PA: Elsevier; Johnson, P. (2016). Head, eyes, ears, nose, mouth, and neck assessment. In E. Tappero & M. E. Honeyfield (Eds.), *Physical assessment of the newborn* (5th ed., pp. 61–78). New York, NY: Springer Publishing Company; Parikh, A. S., & Mitchell, A. (2015). Congenital anomalies. In R. Martin, A. Fanaroff, & M. Walsh (Eds.), *Fanaroff and Martin's neonatal–perinatal medicine: Diseases of the fetus and infant* (10th ed., pp. 436–457). Philadelphia, PA: Elsevier.

INCIDENCE AND ETIOLOGY
- Due to error in recanalization of the laryngeal inlet at 10 weeks' gestation. Thickness of this tissue varies (Otteson & Arnold, 2015, p. 1153).

PRESENTATION
- Infants may not be symptomatic at birth and depending on thickness of the web, infant may present several weeks after birth with biphasic stridor. Cry may be soft or nonexistent (Otteson & Arnold, 2015, p. 1153).
  - When severe webbing is present at birth and causes severe respiratory distress, perforation with stiff endotracheal tube is necessary (Ringer & Hansen, 2017, p. 951).

INTERVENTION AND OUTCOMES
- Biphasic increases as age and activity level increases. Laryngeal webs should be evaluated endoscopically when presentation of such symptoms occurs at 4 to 6 weeks of age.
- Diagnosis and treatment of thin webs is done endoscopically using carbon dioxide laser. Thicker webs may require tracheostomy and external stent placement. In either case, referral to otolaryngologist is necessary (Otteson & Arnold, 2015, p. 1153).

Laryngomalacia

DEFINITION
- Laryngomalacia is classified as a congenital flaccid larynx (Otteson & Arnold, 2015, p. 1153).

INCIDENCE AND ETIOLOGY
- Laryngomalacial comprises approximately 60% of all pediatric laryngeal problems and is the most common cause of stridor. Etiology of laryngomalacia is unknown, but it is commonly thought to be caused by neurologic immaturity of respiratory and digestive tracts (Otteson & Arnold, 2015, p. 1551).

PRESENTATION
- Characterized as inspiratory stridor, generally presenting at 2 to 4 weeks of age, but stridor may be present at birth. Gastroesophageal reflex is commonly present with laryngomalacia (Otteson & Arnold, 2015, p. 1151).

INTERVENTION AND OUTCOMES
- When not associated with cyanotic events, fiberoptic nasolaryngoscopy is performed to confirm diagnosis.
- Management includes prone positioning to decrease supraglottic collapse, surgical intervention may be needed if infant presents as failure-to-thrive. Agitation may worsen degree of stridor. Direct laryngoscopy via rigid bronchoscopy may be warranted in atypical cases to evaluate for secondary obstructive lesion.
- Infants with laryngomalacia typically improve by 8 to 12 months of age and symptoms typically resolve with minimal intervention by 2 years of age.
- Observation, education, and reassurance of caregivers is the primary therapy for laryngomalacia (Otteson & Arnold, 2015, p. 1151).

Congenital Subglottic Stenosis

DEFINITION
- Congenital subglottic stenosis is defined as subglottic diameter <4 mm at birth in at term infant, generally a result of a malformed cricoid ring or excessive thickening of subglottic tissue (Otteson & Arnold, 2015, p. 1153).

INCIDENCE AND ETIOLOGY
- Congenital subglottic stenosis results from an abnormally shaped (elliptical) cricoid ring or thickened subglottic tissue. Many mild cases are undetected until 2 to 3 years of age (Otteson & Arnold, 2015, p. 1153).

PRESENTATION

- Presents as biphasic stridor and/or coup-like cough with the absence of systemic signs of infection. Infants usually have normal cry, but tend to have respiratory distress with feeding, including tachypnea (Otteson & Arnold, 2015, p. 1153).

INTERVENTION AND OUTCOMES

- Endoscopic evaluation should be performed to diagnose subglottic narrowing (Otteson & Arnold, 2015, p. 1153).

In most cases of congenital subglottic stenosis, treatment depends on the severity of the narrowing. Infants should be referred to otolaryngology for possible cricoid split or tracheostomy in severe cases (Otteson & Arnold, 2015, p. 1153).

Intubation Trauma

DEFINITION

- Iatrogenic injury of the airway following endotracheal intubation and may include granuloma formation, subglottic stenosis, subglottic cysts, or arytenoid dislocation with vocal cord fixation (Otteson & Arnold, 2015, p. 1153).

INCIDENCE AND ETIOLOGY

- Iatrogenic subglottic stenosis related to endotracheal intubation risk factors included prematurity, Down syndrome, and long-term intubations (Otteson & Arnold, 2015, p. 1154).

PRESENTATION

- Progressive hoarseness following extubation may indicate granuloma or subglottic cyst formation.
- Persistent stridor may indicate iatrogenic subglottic stenosis (Otteson & Arnold, 2015, p. 1155).

INTERVENTIONS AND OUTCOMES

- Precautionary steps should be taken to reduce intubation trauma and associated injuries (see Box 25.2; Otteson & Arnold, 2015, p. 1154).

BOX 25.2 Interventions to Reduce Incidence of Intubation-Related Airway Injuries

- Use smaller diameter, uncuffed endotracheal tubes. Tight tubes increase risk of upper-airway injury.
- Aggressively treat systemic infection.
- Sedate as necessary to minimize patient movement, thereby preventing subglottic and exposed cartilage abrasions and accidental extubation requiring further manipulation.
- Consider tracheostomy if prolonged intubation is anticipated.
- Extubate under ideal conditions. In the difficult airway, high-dose systemic steroids for 24–48 hours before and after may aid extubation.
- Use of inhaled/racemic epinephrine immediately following extubation may reduce airway edema.

Sources: Data from Otteson, T. D., & Arnold, J. E. (2015). Upper airway lesions in the neonate. In R. Martin, A. Fanaroff, & M. Walsh (Eds.). *Fanaroff and Martin's neonatal–perinatal medicine: Diseases of the fetus and infant* (10th ed., pp. 1147–1156). Philadelphia, PA; Said, M. M., & Rais-Bahrami, K. (2013). Endotracheal intubation. In M. G. MacDonald, J. Ramasethu, & K. Rais-Bahrami (Eds.), *Atlas of procedures in neonatology* (5th ed., pp. 236–249). Philadelphia, PA: Lippincott Williams & Wilkins.

- Treatment depends on the severity of the stenosis. Tracheostomy or tracheal reconstruction using rib cartilage may be necessary in severe cases.
- In cases of laryngeal granulomas or subglottic cyst, removal via microlaryngoscopy generally relieves symptoms (Otteson & Arnold, 2015, p. 1154).
- Box 25.2 suggests means to reduce incidence of intubation-related airway injuries.

CONCLUSION

Thorough assessment and understanding of the anatomy and pathology of the eyes, ears, nose, and mouth allows the practitioner to provide accurate diagnosis and implement the appropriate interventions necessary to decrease comorbidities associated with prematurity and genetic abnormalities.

REVIEW QUESTIONS

1. The NNP explains the etiology of retinopathy of prematurity (ROP) to an infant's mother based on the knowledge that ROP develops because of:
   A. scar formation and traction placed on the retina
   B. poor retinal vascularization and resultant hypoxia
   C. vitreous neovascularization of the retinal surface

2. An infant is transferred to the NICU due to suspected upper-airway obstruction. The infant is reported to not sleep more than a few minutes at a time, becomes cyanotic and then wakes crying, and the cyanosis resolves. Extreme upper-airway "noise" is audible when the infant takes a pacifier. The NNP begins the evaluation with the differential diagnosis of:
   A. choanal atresia
   B. deviated septum
   C. nasolacrimal sheath

3. To establish normal ear placement, the NNP imagines a line drawn from the ear to the:
   A. external antihelix
   B. inner concha
   C. outer canthus

4. The NNP is called to evaluate a newly born infant with a cleft lip/palate that was unknown before birth. The infant has no other obvious anomalies and is pink and crying with good tone. The mother asks if the infant will have to be transferred to the NICU, and the NNP bases the response on the knowledge that an NICU admission:
   A. can occur if the otolaryngologist requests that for the infant
   B. is mandatory for all infants until surgical correction occurs
   C. will be necessary only if the infant cannot safely orally feed

5. Macroglossia is most commonly associated with:
   A. Beckwith–Wiedemann syndrome
   B. Cru du Chat syndrome
   C. VATER/VACTERL association

REFERENCES

Abdulhayoglu, E. (2017). Birth trauma. In E. Eichenwald, A. N. Hansen, C. Martin, & A. Stark (Eds.), *Cloherty and Stark's manual of neonatal care* (8th ed., pp. 64–75). Philadelphia, PA: Elsevier.

Bajaj, K., & Gross, S. J. (2015). Genetic aspects of perinatal disease and prenatal diagnosis. In R. Martin, A. Fanaroff, & M. Walsh (Eds.). *Fanaroff and Martin's neonatal–perinatal medicine: Diseases of the fetus and infant* (10th ed., pp. 130–146). Philadelphia, PA: Elsevier.

Benjamin, K., & Furdon, S. A. (2015). Physical assessment. In M. T. Verklan & M. Walden (Eds.), *Core curriculum for neonatal intensive care nursing* (pp. 110–145). St. Louis, MO: Saunders, Elsevier.

Bennett, M., & Meier, S. (2016). Assessment of the dysmorphic infant. In E. Tappero & M. H. Honeyfield (Eds.), *Physical assessment of the newborn* (5th ed., pp. 221–238). New York, NY: Springer Publishing Company.

Blackburn, S. (2013). The prenatal period and placental physiology. In S. Blackburn (Ed.), *Maternal, fetal, & neonatal physiology: A clinical perspective* (4th ed., pp. 61–114). Maryland Heights, MO: Elsevier.

Boucher, N., Marvicsin, D., & Gardner, S. (2017). Physical examination, interventions, and referrals. In B. Snell & S. Gardner (Eds.), *Care of the well newborn* (pp. 101–134). Burlington, VT: Jones & Bartlett.

Campomanes, A. G., & Binenbaum, G. (2018). Eye and vision disorders. In C. Gleason & S. Juul (Eds.), *Avery's diseases of the newborn* (10th ed., pp. 1536–1557). Philadelphia, PA: Elsevier.

Douma, C. E., Casey, D., & Greene, A. K. (2017). Skin care. In E. Eichenwald, A. N. Hansen, C. Martin, & A. Stark (Eds.), *Cloherty and Stark's manual of neonatal care* (8th ed., pp. 967–977). Philadelphia, PA: Elsevier.

Evans, K. N., Hing, A. V., & Cunningham, M. L. (2018). Craniofacial malformations. In C. Gleason & S. Juul (Eds.), *Avery's diseases of the newborn* (10th ed., pp. 1417–1437). Philadelphia, PA: Elsevier.

Fraser, D., & Diehl-Jones, W. (2015). Ophthalmologic and auditory disorders. In M. T. Verklan & M. Walden (Eds.), *Core curriculum for neonatal intensive care nursing* (pp. 813–831). St. Louis, MO: Saunders, Elsevier.

Gardner, S., & Hernandez, J. (2016). Initial nursery care. In S. Gardner, B. Carter, M. Hines, & J. Hernandez (Eds.), *Merenstein & Gardner's handbook of neonatal intensive care* (pp. 71–104). St. Louis, MO: Elsevier.

Johnson, P. (2016). Head, eyes, ears, nose, mouth, and neck assessment. In E. Tappero & M. E. Honeyfield (Eds.), *Physical assessment of the newborn* (5th ed., pp. 61–78). New York, NY: Springer Publishing Company.

Lissauer, T. (2015). Physical examination of the newborn. In R. Martin, A. Fanaroff, & M. Walsh (Eds.), *Fanaroff and Martin's neonatal–perinatal medicine: Diseases of the fetus and infant* (10th ed., pp. 391–406). Philadelphia, PA: Elsevier.

Mangurten, H., Puppala, B., & Prazed, P. (2015). Physical examination of the newborn. In R. Martin, A. Fanaroff, & M. Walsh (Eds.), *Fanaroff and Martin's neonatal–perinatal medicine: Diseases of the fetus and infant* (10th ed., pp. 407–435). Philadelphia, PA: Elsevier.

Őrge, F., & Grigorian, F. (2015). Examination and common problems of the neonatal eye. In R. Martin, A. Fanaroff, & M. Walsh (Eds.), *Fanaroff and Martin's neonatal–perinatal medicine: Diseases of the fetus and infant* (10th ed., pp. 1734–1766). Philadelphia, PA: Elsevier.

Otteson, T. D., & Arnold, J. E. (2015). Upper airway lesions in the neonate. In R. Martin, A. Fanaroff, & M. Walsh (Eds.). *Fanaroff and Martin's neonatal–perinatal medicine: Diseases of the fetus and infant* (10th ed., pp. 1147–1156). Philadelphia, PA: Elsevier.

Pappas, B. E., & Robey, D. L. (2015). Neonatal delivery room resuscitation. In M. T. Verklan & M. Walden (Eds.), *Core curriculum for neonatal intensive care nursing* (pp. 80–94). St. Louis, MO: Saunders, Elsevier., Philadelphia, PA: Elsevier.

Parikh, A. S., & Mitchell, A. (2015). Congenital anomalies. In R. Martin, A. Fanaroff, & M. Walsh (Eds.), *Fanaroff and Martin's neonatal–perinatal medicine: Diseases of the fetus and infant* (10th ed., pp. 436–457). Philadelphia, PA: Elsevier.

Ringer, S., & Hansen, A. (2017). Surgical emergencies in the newborn. In E. Eichenwald, A. N. Hansen, C. Martin, & A. Stark (Eds.), *Cloherty and Stark's manual of neonatal care* (8th ed., pp. 942–966). Philadelphia, PA: Elsevier.

Said, M. M., & Rais-Bahrami, K. (2013). Endotracheal intubation. In M. G. MacDonald, J. Ramasethu, & K. Rais-Bahrami (Eds.), *Atlas of procedures in neonatology* (5th ed., pp. 236–249). Philadelphia, PA: Lippincott Williams & Wilkins.

Stewart, J. R., Bentley, J., & Knorr, A. (2017). Hearing loss in neonatal intensive care graduates. In E. Eichenwald, A. N. Hansen, C. Martin, & A. Stark (Eds.), *Cloherty and Stark's manual of neonatal care* (8th ed., pp. 993–999). Philadelphia, PA: Elsevier.

Sun, Y., Hellstrom, A., & Smith, L. (2015). Retinopathy of prematurity. In R. Martin, A. Fanaroff, & M. Walsh (Eds.), *Fanaroff and Martin's neonatal–perinatal medicine: Diseases of the fetus and infant* (10th ed., pp. 1767–1774). Philadelphia, PA: Elsevier.

Taketomo, C., Hodding, J., & Kraus, D. (Eds.). (2018). *Lexicomp pediatric & neonatal dosage handbook* (25th ed.). Hudson, OH: Wolters Kluwer.

Tappero, E., & Honeyfield, M. E. (2016). Glossary of terms. In E. Tappero & M. E. Honeyfield (5th ed.). *Physical assessment of the newborn* (pp. 263–288). New York, NY: Springer Publishing Company.

Trotter, C.W. (2015). Gestational age assessment. In Tappero, E. P. & Honeyfield, M. E. (eds.), *Physical assessment of the newborn* (5th ed., pp. 23–43). New York, NY: Springer Publishing Company.

Vargo, L. (2014). Newborn physical assessment. In K. R Simpson & P. A. Creehan (eds.), *AWHONN's perinatal nursing* (4th ed., pp. 600–606). Philadelphia, PA: Lippincott Williams & Wilkins.

Verklan, M. T. (2015). Adaptation to extrauterine life. In M. T. Verklan & M. Walden (Eds.), *Core curriculum for neonatal intensive care nursing* (pp. 58–76). St. Louis, MO: Saunders, Elsevier.

Vohr, B. (2015). Hearing loss in the newborn. In R. Martin, A. Fanaroff, & M. Walsh (Eds.), *Fanaroff and Martin's neonatal–perinatal medicine: Diseases of the fetus and infant* (10th ed., pp. 993–1000). Philadelphia, PA: Elsevier.

Walker, V. (2018). Newborn evaluation. In C. Gleason & S. Juul (10th ed.), *Avery's diseases of the newborn* (pp. 289–311). Philadelphia, PA: Elsevier.

26 INTRAUTERINE DRUG EXPOSURE

Amy Koehn
Lisa R. Jasin

INTRODUCTION

Substance use in pregnancy is a preventable public health and social problem (Nocon, 2013, p. 217). Prevalence rates for perinatal substance use are difficult to determine due to underreporting, unreliable drug use survey and detection methods, and societal attitudes (Wallen & Gleason, 2018, p. 126). However, available data identify that pregnant women use illicit drugs at almost half the rate of the general population. During pregnancy, 16.3% of pregnant women report tobacco use and 10.8% report alcohol use (Prasad & Jones, 2019, p. 1243). Nearly 5.9% of pregnant women use illicit drugs (Sullivan, 2016, p. 564). In the 30 days prior, one in 10 pregnant women reported consuming alcohol and one in 10 pregnant women reported binge drinking (Reis & Jnah, 2017, p. 51). It is estimated that 400,000 to 440,000 neonates annually are affected by intrauterine exposure to alcohol or illicit drugs (Sullivan, 2016, p. 565).

SUBSTANCE USE DISORDER

- It is important for the NNP to be aware of and have a basic knowledge of the psychology and physiology of dependence. It is necessary in order to be able to work successfully with the parents, caregivers, and other family members of our infants.
- Psychological dependence, or addiction, is now replaced by the term "substance use disorder (SUD)" (Nocon, 2013, p. 218). SUD refers to the compulsive use of drugs despite negative consequences. Cravings and continued use can be triggered by cues derived from the environment that are associated with previous drug use (Luscher, 2015, p. 552). The American Society of Addiction Medicine (ASAM) describes five characteristics (the ABCs) in its definition of addiction:
  - Inability to consistently **A**bstain
  - Impairment in **B**ehavioral control
  - **C**raving, or increased "hunger" for drugs or rewarding experiences
  - **D**iminished recognition of significant problems with one's behaviors and interpersonal relationships
  - A dysfunctional **E**motional response (Nocon, 2013, p. 220)
- In 2011, the National Survey on Drug Use and Health (NSDUH) found marijuana to be the most commonly used illegal drug for Americans age 12 and older in the previous 30 days, followed by cocaine, hallucinogens,inhalants, methamphetamine, and heroin. The NSDUH estimated 6.1 million Americans 12 and older used prescription drugs without a medical indication in the previous 30 days (Hudak, 2015, p. 682).

- Polysubstance use, including alcohol, tobacco, and other drugs, has become more common (Sullivan, 2016, p. 564). The most frequently used substances in pregnancy are alcohol, tobacco, marijuana, cocaine, opioids, and amphetamines, with alcohol and nicotine causing more damage to the fetus than all the other drugs combined (Nocon, 2013, p. 224).
- Drug use is less likely by pregnant women in the third trimester. This may indicate pregnancy is a motivator to treatment for SUD (Patrick, 2017, p. 141).

Dependence

- Pregnant woman may be physically dependent and/or psychologically addicted to a substance. Recently, physical dependence has been termed "dependence." Physical dependence may occur with multiple classes of nonpsychoactive drugs such as sympathomimetic vasoconstrictors and bronchodilators as well as psychoactive drugs. While each drug causes different acute effects, all cause feelings of euphoria and reward. With repeated use, tolerance occurs, requiring escalation of dosing for maintenance (Luscher, 2015, p. 552).

Classification of Substances

- The initial molecular and cellular targets must be identified in order to understand the long-term changes induced by drugs of abuse. Much research has revealed the mesolimbic dopamine system as the prime target of addictive drugs. This system originates in a tiny structure at the tip of the brainstem, the ventral tegmental area (VTA), which projects to the nucleus accumbens, the amygdala, the hippocampus, and the prefrontal cortex. These projection neurons are dopamine-producing neurons, and when they begin to fire in large bursts, excessive amounts of dopamine are released.
  - Disproportionate amounts of dopamine reinforce the reward-processing centers of the brain, enough to elicit rapid adaptive behavior changes as the good feelings of reward and satisfaction become associated with the additive drug (Luscher, 2015, p. 556).
- All addictive drugs increase dopamine concentration in the mesolimbic projections. Each addictive drug has a specific molecular target that engages distinct cellular mechanisms to activate the mesolimbic system:
  - G_{io} protein-couples receptors (e.g., opioids, cannabinoids, and hallucinogens)
  - Ionotropic receptors or ion channels (e.g., nicotine, alcohol, benzodiazepines, and some inhalants)
  - Dopamine transmitters (e.g., cocaine, amphetamines, and ecstasy; Luscher, 2015, p. 558)

Maternal Screening and Treatment

- Identification of perinatal substance use is accomplished by obtaining a thorough and accurate history of risk factors for maternal substance use (Table 26.1), self-reported use, neonatal history and presentation, and toxicology screens that support maternal substance use (urine screens) or neonatal exposure (urine, meconium, umbilical cord samples; Wallman, 2018, p. 256).
- The American Congress of Obstetricians and Gynecologists (ACOG) and the American Medical Association endorse universal screening (Nocon, 2013, p. 218; Prasad & Jones, 2019, p. 1245).
  - ○ Every pregnant patient is asked about substance use at the first visit and in each trimester (universal screening; Nocon, 2013, p. 240) using screening, brief intervention, and referral to treatment (SBIRT; Hudak, 2015, p. 683).
- Brief intervention should include available community resources for education and treatment. These brief interventions may influence women using substances during pregnancy (Prasad & Jones, 2019, p. 1243).

SUBSTANCE USE SCREENING INSTRUMENTS

SBIRT procedures should be performed periodically for each pregnant woman. Pregnancy is a motivator for long-term recovery. SBIRT results in increased effectiveness in treating alcohol addiction in pregnancy, increased compliance with prenatal visits, and reduction in preterm labor and birth (Nocon, 2013, p. 221–222).

- The substance use screening tools, questions, and scoring are contained in Table 26.2.
- Even with these actions, screening that targets risk factors for substance use does not identify all women who need intervention (Prasad & Jones, 2019, p. 1243).
  - ○ Shame and stigma are associated with SUD and may contribute to delay in diagnosis and treatment (Hudak, 2015, p. 683; Nocon, 2013, p. 222; Wallen & Gleason, 2018, p. 127).
  - ○ Pregnant women experience increased stigma due to potential fetal harm, which calls maternal fitness into question. Questions of maternal fitness may lead to punitive measures such as criminalizing drug use while pregnant (Hudak, 2015, p. 683; Wallen & Gleason, 2018, p. 127).

  - ○ A nonjudgmental approach to SUD is critical (Hudak, 2015, p. 683), as well as identification and treatment of psychiatric comorbidities (Table 26.2; Nocon, 2013, p. 223).

BIOCHEMICAL SCREENING

- In the prenatal and perinatal period, biochemical screening is used to test for drug exposure including nicotine. Specimens such as hair (Patrick, 2017, p. 143; Sherman, 2015, p. 48), cord blood, human milk, and amniotic fluid may be tested (Wallman, 2018, pp. 256–257). However, ACOG does not support biochemical screening as the method of detecting substance use in pregnancy. If biochemical testing is performed, maternal consent should be obtained (Prasad & Jones, 2019, p. 1244).
- Urine is the most commonly used substance tested as it is easy to collect. Urine testing may detect threshold levels of drug metabolites only for several days after use (Patrick, 2017, p. 143; Sherman, 2015, p. 48).
  - ○ Urine testing can be used for testing for substance use as well as evidence of compliance (Nocon, 2013, p. 241).
  - ○ Positive results may occur with use of prescribed drugs or secondhand exposure and should be confirmed with mass spectrometry or gas chromatography (Hudak, 2015, p. 683).
    - Positive urine drug screen results may deter pregnant women from seeking prenatal care due to legal consequences (Nocon, 2013, p. 240).
  - ○ False negative can occur even with significant drug exposure (Hudak, 2015, p. 683; Patrick, 2017, p. 143; Sherman, 2015, p. 48; Wallman, 2018, p. 256–257).
- Table 26.3 shows complications of pregnancy and potential outcomes of pregnancy influenced by substance use.

TREATMENT

- Pharmacologic treatment may alleviate withdrawal syndrome, in particular after use of opioids and use of nicotine. The most common treatment for withdrawal is to slowly taper long-acting opioids. Another treatment approved for opioids and nicotine is substitution of a legally available agonist that acts at the same receptor as the misused drug (Luscher, 2015, p. 564).

TABLE 26.1 Maternal Screening for Substance Use

Risk Factors for Perinatal Substance Use Disorder	Comorbid Psychiatric Disorders Common in Women
Limited, inadequate, or no prenatal care Exposure to violence Unresolved trauma Perinatal depression Poor nutrition Sexually transmitted maternal diseases Premature onset of labor Abruptio placentae Intrauterine growth restriction Congenital malformations Significant mental illness	Bipolar disorders Panic disorder PTSD Bulimia Depression

Sources: Data from Nocon, J. (2013). Substance use disorders. In D. Mattison (Ed.), *Clinical pharmacology during pregnancy* (p. 223). San Diego, CA: Elsevier; Wallman, C. (2018). Assessment of the newborn with antenatal exposure to drugs. In E. P. Tappero & M. E. Honeyfield (Eds.), *Physical assessment of the newborn* (6th ed., p. 256). New York, NY: Springer Publishing.

TABLE 26.2 Substance Use Screening Instruments

Instrument		Scoring
The CAGE-AID	– C: Have you ever felt that you ought to **Cut** down on your drinking or drug use? – A: Have people **Annoyed** you by criticizing your drinking and drug use? – G: Have you ever felt bad or **Guilty** about your drinking or drug use? – E: Have you ever had a drink or used drugs first thing in the morning to steady your nerves or to get rid of a hangover (**Eye** opener)?	One or more yes answers indicates intervention needed
CRAFFT	During the past 12 months: – Have you ever ridden in a **Car** driven by someone (including yourself) who was high or had been using alcohol or drugs? – Did you ever use alcohol or drugs to **Relax**, feel better about yourself, or fit in? – Did you ever use alcohol or drugs while you were by yourself, or **Alone**? – Did you ever **Forget** things you did while using alcohol or drugs? – Did your **Family** or friends ever tell you that you should cut down on your drinking or drug use? – Have you ever gotten in **Trouble** while you were using drugs or alcohol?	Two or more yes answers indicates need for further assessment.
4 P's Plus	– Did your **PARENTS** have trouble with alcohol or drugs? – Do any of your **PEERS** have a problem with alcohol or drugs? – Does your **PARTNER** have a problem with alcohol or drugs? – Have you ever drunk beer, wine, or liquor to excess in the **PAST**? – Have you smoked any cigarettes, used any alcohol, or any drug at any time in this **PREGNANCY**? – Did you ever drink beer, wine, or liquor in the month before you knew you were pregnant? – How many cigarettes did you smoke in the month before you knew you were pregnant? – How many beers, how much wine, and how much liquor did you drink in the month before you knew you were pregnant?	Positive alcohol or tobacco in the month prior to pregnancy indicates need for assessment. If positive screen, all women should be given educational materials and have follow-up monitoring.

T-ACE	T: **Tolerance:** "How many drinks does it take you to feel high?"
	   More than 2 drinks is a positive response—score 2 points.
	A: **Annoyed:** "Have people annoyed you by criticizing your drinking?"
	   Yes—score 1 point.
	C: **Cut down:** "Have you ever felt you ought to cut down on your drinking?"
	   Yes—score 1 point.
	E: **Eye Opener:** "Have you ever had a drink first thing in the morning to steady your nerves or get rid of a hangover?"
	   Yes—score 1 point.
		A score of 2 or more indicates potential prenatal risk for substance use.

Sources: Data from Hudak, M. (2015). Infants with antenatal exposure to drugs. In R. Martin, A. Fanaroff, & M. Walsh (Eds.), *Fanaroff and Martin's neonatal–perinatal medicine: Diseases of the fetus and infant* (10th ed., p. 683). Philadelphia, PA: Elsevier; Nocon, J. (2013). Substance use disorders. In D. Mattison (Ed.), *Clinical pharmacology during pregnancy* (pp. 243–244). San Diego, CA: Elsevier; Patrick, S. (2017). Maternal drug use, infant exposure, and neonatal abstinence syndrome. In E. Eichenwald, A. Hansen, C. Martin, & A. Stark (Eds.), *Cloherty and Stark's manual of neonatal care* (8th ed., p. 142). Philadelphia, PA: Wolters Kluwer; Prasad, M., & Jones, H (2019) Substance abuse in pregnancy. In R. Resnik, C. Lockwood, T. Moore, M. Greene, J. Copel, & R. Silver (Eds.), *Creasy and Resnik's maternal–fetal medicine: Principles and practice* (8th ed., p. 1244). Philadelphia, PA: Elsevier; Sullivan, C. (2016). Substance abuse in pregnancy. In S. Mattson & J. Smith (Eds.), *Core curriculum for maternal-newborn nursing* (5th ed., p. 574). St. Louis, MO: Elsevier.

TABLE 26.3 Drug Use and Pregnancy

May Compromise Outcomes of Pregnancy With Drug Use	Obstetric Complications of Drug Use
Anemia Bacteremia Cardiac disease Cellulitis Depression Diabetes Edema Hepatitis B and C TB Hypertension Phlebitis STIs Urinary tract infections Vitamin deficiencies	Abruptio placenta Placenta previa Intrauterine death Spontaneous abortion Premature labor and delivery PROM IUGR Polyhydramnios

IUGR, intrauterine growth restriction; PROM, premature rupture of membranes; STIs, sexually transmitted infections; TB, tuberculosis.

Source: Reproduced with permission from Sullivan, C. (2016). Substance abuse in pregnancy. In S. Mattson & J. Smith (Eds.), *Core curriculum for maternal-newborn nursing* (5th ed., p. 565). St. Louis, MO: Elsevier.

TABLE 26.4 Fetal Effects of Substance Use

Direct Effects	Indirect Effects
Embryonic (early) phase of gestation – Teratogenic effects Fetal period (after major structural development) – Abnormal growth – Abnormal maturation – Alterations in neurotransmitters – Alterations in neural receptors – Alterations in brain organization	Vasoconstriction of uterine/placental vessels – Placental insufficiency – Altered nutrition to the fetus Altered maternal health behaviors – Altered nutrition to the fetus

Sources: Data from Hudak, M. (2015). Infants with antenatal exposure to drugs. In R. Martin, A. Fanaroff, & M. Walsh (Eds.), *Fanaroff and Martin's neonatal–perinatal medicine: Diseases of the fetus and infant* (10th ed., p. 682). Philadelphia, PA: Elsevier; Reis, P., & Jnah, A. (2017). Perinatal history: Influences on newborn outcome. In B. Snell & S. Gardner (Eds.), *Care of the well newborn* (p. 51). Burlington, MA: Jones & Bartlett Learning; Sherman, J. (2015). Perinatal substance abuse. In T. Verklan & M. Walden (Eds.), *Core curriculum for neonatal intensive care nursing* (5th ed., p. 54). St. Louis, MO: Elsevier; Wallman, C. (2018). Assessment of the newborn with antenatal exposure to drugs. In E. P. Tappero & M. E. Honeyfield (Eds.), *Physical assessment of the newborn* (6th ed., p. 257). New York, NY: Springer Publishing.

INTRAUTERINE EFFECTS OF PERINATAL SUBSTANCE EXPOSURE

- Prenatal exposure to alcohol, tobacco, and illicit drugs has the potential to cause significant harm to the fetus and neonate. Effects may persist into childhood (Sherman, 2015, p. 43).
  - All drugs associated with SUD have low-molecular weight and are lipid soluble, thus they all cross the placenta and cause direct effects on the fetus (Weiner & Finnegan, 2016, p. 200).
  - Drugs taken orally may have a decreased ability to cross the placenta; intravenous (IV) drugs may cross the placenta readily.
  - The use of IV drugs increases exposure of both the mother and fetus to HIV and hepatitis (Sullivan, 2016, pp. 564–565).
- Table 26.4 details the direct and indirect effects of substance use on the embryo and fetus.
- Intrauterine exposure to drugs is associated with fetal distress, fetal demise, lower Apgar scores, and withdrawal in the newborn (Smith & Carley, 2014, p. 680). Symptoms of drug withdrawal are similar to sepsis, hypoglycemia, and central nervous system (CNS) disorders in the newborn (Sullivan, 2016, p. 565).

Neonatal Screening

- Testing for in utero substance exposure is often based on risk factors; however, using only risk factors fails to identify all substance-exposed neonates (Hudak, 2015, p. 682). Box 26.1 details risk factors associated with maternal SUD.
  - Due to liberal state laws, a pediatrician can legally order urine and meconium tests on a newborn without parental consent if a mother refuses a urine drug screen. The refusal to be tested provides a reasonable basis for suspicion of substance use (Nocon, 2013, p. 241).
- Urine and meconium can be used testing for substance exposure in utero. Meconium is more accurate, but is more expensive. Meconium is generally not used for prevalence testing (Nocon, 2013, p. 240).

URINE
- Easy to collect and reflects drug exposure in the days prior to delivery (Nocon, 2013, p. 241).

MECONIUM
- Two to three grams of stool is necessary for testing; therefore the collection of multiple samples is highly recommended. (Patrick, 2017, p. 143; Sherman, 2015, p. 48).
- Drug use during the second and third trimesters can be detected through the testing of meconium (Patrick, 2017, p. 143; Sherman, 2015, p. 48; Prasad & Jones, 2019, p. 1244; Weiner & Finnegan, 2016, p. 209).

UMBILICAL CORD
- 6-inch segment required for testing and results are returned more rapidly than meconium.
- Appears to be as reliable as meconium (Sherman, 2015, p. 48); however, collection and storage may require increased resources (Patrick, 2017, p. 143).

BOX 26.1 Maternal risk factors indicating need for newborn testing for intrauterine substance exposure

- Self-report of alcohol or drug use
- Inadequate or no prenatal care
- Sexually transmitted disease
- Premature labor
- Abruptio placentae
- Intrauterine growth restriction
- Congenital malformations
- Signs of neonatal withdrawal

Source: Reproduced with permission from Hudak, M. (2015). Infants with antenatal exposure to drugs. In R. Martin, A. Fanaroff, & M. Walsh (Eds.), *Fanaroff and Martin's neonatal–perinatal medicine: Diseases of the fetus and infant* (10th ed., p. 682). Philadelphia, PA: Elsevier.

Outcomes

- Substance exposure in utero may have long-term effects on behavior, learning, school performance, and emotional stability.
- Environmental factors may also contribute to these effects. Infants exposed to illicit drugs, alcohol, and tobacco demonstrate fewer behaviors that encourage bonding. They are also at risk for physical, sexual, and emotional abuse; neglect; and developmental delay (Sherman, 2015, p. 55).
  - Initially, substance-using mothers and their infants may have difficulty with bonding behaviors. Mothers who are substance users have significantly less positive affect and greater detachment when evaluated with their infant.
  - Parents of drug-exposed infants may need assistance recognizing infant cues necessary for caregiving and infant symptoms that signal problems (Weiner & Finnegan, 2016, p. 217).

Prevention

- Preconception education of women of childbearing age, families, and physicians is key to prevention of drug effects on the fetus and newborn. Early education about drug effects on a fetus and newborn that begins at home and is reinforced in elementary and middle school is optimal. Teenagers who become pregnant are more likely to engage in substance use than their nonpregnant peers (Hudak, 2015, p. 682).

COMMON SUBSTANCES USE IN PREGNANCY

Tobacco/Nicotine

- Nicotine, including traditional and electronic cigarettes, smokeless tobacco, and nicotine replacement patches, is the substance most frequently used in pregnancy. Nicotine has the most adverse effect on perinatal outcomes, in particular preterm birth (Wallen & Gleason, 2018, p. 131).

Prevalence

- Prevalence is difficult to determine secondary to failure to self-report. In 2016, the percentage of pregnant women from ages 15 to 44 who used cigarettes was 10.1% (decreased from 13.6% in 2015) (Sullivan, 2016, p. 570; Wallman, 2018, p. 255). Among pregnant women 15 to 17 years of age, the rate of cigarette smoking was 22.7% versus 13.4% in nonpregnant women of the same age group (Sherman, 2015, p. 45).
  - Smoking among opioid-dependent women is common, at almost 90%. Data reveal 24% to 50% of pregnant women do not disclose smoking status when questioned (Prasad & Jones, 2019, p. 1245).

Pharmacology

- The addictive properties of nicotine arise from dopaminergic effects on the brain. Cotinine is the metabolite of nicotine that is measured in a urine drug screen. Nicotine rapidly reaches peak levels in the bloodstream and enters the brain, where peak levels are reached within 10 seconds after inhalations. Immediately after nicotine exposure, the adrenal glands are stimulated and epinephrine is released, causing an increase in blood pressure, respiration, and heart rate (Prasad & Jones, 2019, p. 1245).
  - Cotinine levels consistent with smoking can be seen in women exposed to secondhand smoke (Prasad & Jones, 2019, p. 1245; Sullivan, 2016, p. 570).
- Cigarette smoke contains approximately 4,000 compounds, including cyanide, carbon monoxide, and many toxic hydrocarbons, which affect oxygen transport in the placenta and can cause adverse effects on the fetus (Nocon, 2013, p. 226; Wallen & Gleason, 2018, p. 131). Nicotine crosses the placenta with levels in the fetal blood and amniotic fluid significantly exceeding maternal levels (Wallen & Gleason, 2018, p. 131).

Screening

- Screening measures in use include the Tobacco Screening Measure. The pregnant woman is asked:
- "Have you ever smoked cigarettes or used other tobacco products?"
  - If "yes," further probing accomplished by, "Have you ever smoked or used an in the past 30 days?"
  - If "yes,": "On average, how many cigarettes do you smoke (or times do you use) per day?" yields more information.
  - Finally, If "yes,": "How long have you been smoking (using) at that rate?"

Fetal Effects

- Nicotine affects umbilical blood flow and fetal cerebral artery blood flow, and potentiates the effects of the smoke (Nocon, 2013, p. 226). It is possible that vasospasm secondary to smoking leads to decreased intervillous perfusion, hypoxia, and decreased nourishment to the fetus (Sherman, 2015, p. 4; Prasad & Jones, 2019, p. 1245; Wallen & Gleason, 2018, p. 131). Carbon monoxide is slow to clear from fetal circulation and a left shift of the oxyhemoglobin dissociation curve occurs (Prasad & Jones, 2019, p. 1245).
  - Low birth weight is dose dependent, with the more smoking during pregnancy the lower the birth weight (Sullivan, 2016, p. 571). One study suggested each pack of cigarettes smoked per day caused a reduction in relative fetal weight of 5% (Wallman, 2018, p. 257).
- Smoking may also lead to chromosomal instability secondary to genotoxicity (Box 26.2). The most common translocation or deletion was in the 11q23 region. This region is implicated in hematologic malignancies. An association with childhood cancers has been suggested (Prasad & Jones, 2019, p. 1246).

Neonatal Effects

- Maternal genotype appears to have an impact on the risk of low birth weight (LBW) and pulmonary function in children of smokers (Prasad & Jones, 2019, p. 1246). Serum erythropoietin levels are higher in tobacco smoke–exposed infants at delivery, a finding that is presumed to reflect fetal hypoxia (Wallen & Gleason, 2018, p. 131).

BOX 26.2 Effects of nicotine

- Maternal
  - Placental pathology
  - Ectopic pregnancies
  - Spontaneous abortion
- Fetal
  - Intrauterine growth restriction
  - Fetal hypoxia
  - Cleft lip or palate
  - Urinary tract malformations
  - Cardiac malformations
  - Limb reductions defects
  - Talipes
  - Craniosynostoses
- Neonatal
  - Small for gestational age
  - Low birth weight
  - Jitteriness
  - Hypertonicity
  - Altered respiratory function
  - Increased respiratory infections
  - Sudden infant death syndrome
- Childhood
  - Impulsivity
  - Attention deficit hyperactivity disorder
  - Altered learning and memory function
  - Lower IQ scores
  - Auditory processing dysfunction
  - Anxiety/depression
  - Reduced lung function/asthma

Sources: Data from Blackburn, S. (2013). *Maternal, fetal, & neonatal physiology: A clinical perspective* (4th ed., p. 207). Maryland Heights, MO: Elsevier; Prasad, M., & Jones, H (2019) Substance abuse in pregnancy. In R. Resnik, C. Lockwood, T. Moore, M. Greene, J. Copel, & R. Silver (Eds.), *Creasy and Resnik's maternal-fetal medicine: Principles and practice* (8th ed., p. 1246). Philadelphia, PA: Elsevier; Sherman, J. (2015). Perinatal substance abuse. In T. Verklan & M. Walden (Eds.), *Core curriculum for neonatal intensive care nursing* (5th ed., p. 54). St. Louis, MO: Elsevier; Smith, J. R., & Carley, A. (2014). Common neonatal complications. In K. Simpson & P. Creehan (Eds.), *Perinatal nursing* (4th ed., p. 681). St. Louis, MO: Lippincott Williams & Wilkins; Sullivan, C. (2016). Substance abuse in pregnancy. In S. Mattson & J. Smith (Eds.), *Core curriculum for maternal-newborn nursing* (5th ed., p. 571). St. Louis, MO: Elsevier; Wallman, C. (2018). Assessment of the newborn with antenatal exposure to drugs. In E. P. Tappero & M. E. Honeyfield (Eds.), *Physical assessment of the newborn* (6th ed., p. 131, 257). New York, NY: Springer Publishing.

Breastfeeding

- Nicotine is found in breastmilk in 1.5 to 3 times greater than in maternal blood plasma. Smoking is not an absolute contraindication to breastfeeding according to the American Academy of Pediatrics (AAP; Prasad & Jones, 2019, p. 1245), but is associated with an increased incidence of infant respiratory allergy and sudden infant death syndrome (SIDS). Smoking may also decrease milk supply and lead to poor neonatal weight gain (Sherman, 2015, p. 55).
- Smoking and bottle feeding has a greater negative effect on an infant than smoking and breastfeeding due to the effects on bonding and the lack of maternal nutrients passed through the milk. Babies of mothers who smoke may sleep less and have more ear and respiratory infections (Sullivan, 2016, p. 571).

Childhood Effects

- Potential long-term effects of prenatal exposure to nicotine have been identified. Box 26.3 lists childhood effects of fetal nicotine exposure.

BOX 26.3 Fetal impacts of prenatal cocaine exposure

Fetal hypoxia
Congenital heart defects (first trimester use)
Reduction in growth (length, weight, head circumference)
Preterm labor
Low birth weight
Microcephaly

Sources: Data from Hudak, M. (2015). Infants with antenatal exposure to drugs. In R. Martin, A. Fanaroff, & M. Walsh (Eds.), *Fanaroff and Martin's neonatal-perinatal medicine: Diseases of the fetus and infant* (10th ed., p. 691). Philadelphia, PA: Elsevier; Nocon, J. (2013). Substance use disorders. In D. Mattison (Ed.), *Clinical pharmacology during pregnancy* (p. 236). San Diego, CA: Elsevier; Sherman, J. (2015). Perinatal substance abuse. In T. Verklan & M. Walden (Eds.), *Core curriculum for neonatal intensive care nursing* (5th ed., p. 43). St. Louis, MO: Elsevier; Sullivan, C. (2016). Substance abuse in pregnancy. In S. Mattson & J. Smith (Eds.), *Core curriculum for maternal-newborn nursing* (5th ed., pp. 565–566). St. Louis, MO: Elsevier; Wallman, C. (2018). Assessment of the newborn with antenatal exposure to drugs. In E. P. Tappero & M. E. Honeyfield (Eds.), *Physical assessment of the newborn* (6th ed., pp. 257–258). New York, NY: Springer Publishing; Weiner, S., & Finnegan, L. (2016). Drug withdrawal in the neonate. In S. Gardner, B. Carter, M. Hines, & J. Hernandez (Eds.), *Merenstein & Gardner's handbook of neonatal intensive care* (8th ed., p. 202). St. Louis, MO: Elsevier.

Treatment

- Women who are most likely to quit have done so by their first prenatal visit, while women who have not quit by the first prenatal visit are likely to continue smoking throughout pregnancy without effective intervention. A Cochrane Review suggested that interventions geared toward smoking cessation have the potential to decrease LBW and preterm births (Nocon, 2013, p. 226; Prasad & Jones, 2019, p. 1246).
- The U.S. Department of Health and Human Services made three recommendations:
  - Offer psychosocial interventions that exceeds minimal advice to quit.
  - Offer interventions throughout pregnancy.
  - Offer pharmacotherapy (nicotine replacement or bupropion) (Prasad & Jones, 2019, p. 1246).
- Pharmacologic therapy for nicotine use focuses on detoxification and abstinence support. Nicotine replacement treatment (NRT) helps prevent relapse and removes the effects of the smoke on the fetus. The patient must be advised not to smoke while using NRT because the combined dose of nicotine substantially increases fetal exposure (Nocon, 2013, p. 226).

ALCOHOL

Prevalence

- Alcohol is one of the most misused substances during pregnancy (Sherman, 2015, p. 44; Weiner & Finnegan, 2016,

p. 202) and the most common teratogen to which the fetus is exposed. Alcohol exposure in utero is the leading cause of preventable birth defects in the United States (Sullivan, 2016, pp. 572–573).

- Some data suggest that 20% to 30% of women drink at some time during pregnancy (Sherman, 2015, p. 44). Among pregnant women aged 15 to 44 years, 10.8% reported current alcohol use, 3.7% reported binge drinking, and 1% reported heavy drinking. Binge drinking in the first trimester of pregnancy was reported by 10.1% of women 15 to 44 (Prasad & Jones, 2019, p. 1247) and has been reported as high as 11.9% of pregnant women (Sullivan, 2016, p. 564, 573).
- The highest use of alcohol use in pregnancy is not determined by socioeconomic status. In some states, alcohol use in pregnancy was highest in women older than 35, non-Hispanic women, women with more than a high school education, and women with higher degrees (Prasad & Jones, 2019, p. 1247).

Pharmacology

- Ethanol, the alcohol contained in alcoholic beverages, is absorbed via the digestive tract and into body fat and the bloodstream. Alcohol is metabolized to acetaldehyde by alcohol dehydrogenase, primarily in the liver. Acetaldehyde is short-lived but can cause significant tissue damage, particularly in the liver where most alcohol is metabolized (Wallen & Gleason, 2018, p. 128).
  - Pregnant women clear alcohol more slowly than nonpregnant women when consuming the same amount of alcohol, likely related to hormonal alterations in alcohol metabolizing enzymes (Wallen & Gleason, 2018, p. 128).
- Ethanol enhances the effects of the inhibitory neurotransmitter γ-aminobutyric acid and lessens the effect of the excitatory neurotransmitter glutamate. Ethanol acts as a CNS depressant or sedative (Wallen & Gleason, 2018, p. 127). Alcohol acts as an antagonist at the N-methyl-D-aspartate (NMDA) receptors and as a facilitator at the gamma-amino-butyrate agonist (GABA) receptors. Dopamine is released in response to alcohol use and provides reinforcement of alcohol use (Prasad & Jones, 2019, p. 1247).

Screening

- Unless a pregnant woman is obviously intoxicated, biochemical screening is not endorsed (Prasad & Jones, 2019, p. 1248). Instruments are available for screening for alcohol use in pregnancy. The simplest and easiest tool for alcohol screening is the CAGE questionnaire (Prasad & Jones, 2019, p. 1247). T-ACE is another questionnaire in use. The T-ACE questions address Tolerance, Annoyance, the need to Cut down and the use of Eye-openers (Prasad & Jones, 2019, p. 1247). Table 26.2 has examples of screening instruments for alcohol use.

Fetal Effects

- Alcohol is a known teratogen and the AAP's Committee on Substance Abuse strongly affirmed there is no known

safe level for use in pregnancy (Nocon, 2013, p. 225; Prasad & Jones, 2019, p. 1248; Reis & Jnah, 2017, p. 51). Alcohol at any stage of pregnancy can affect the brain or other areas of development (Blackburn, 2013, p. 207).

- Ethanol easily crosses the placenta and is present in amniotic fluid well after the mother's level is metabolized to zero (Nocon, 2013, p. 224; Sherman, 2015, p. 47). Alcohol damage can occur early in pregnancy before a woman realizes she is pregnant. Fetal toxicity is dose related with greatest risk occurring early in the first trimester (Nocon, 2013, p. 225).
- The rate of stillbirth was increased across all categories of maternal alcohol use. The rate of death from otherwise unexplained stillbirth ranged from 1.37 cases per 100 women drinking less than one drink per week to 8.83 cases per 1,000 women drinking five or more drinks per week (Prasad & Jones, 2019, p. 1248). Healthcare professionals should counsel all women not to drink any alcohol while pregnant (Weiner & Finnegan, 2016, p. 202).
- There is a dose-related risk with increased risk of fetal alcohol spectrum disorders (FASDs) with heavy or binge drinking (Reis & Jnah, 2017, p. 51; Sherman, 2015, p. 44). Even small amounts of alcohol, less than one-half drink per day while pregnant, has resulted in harmful outcomes for the infant (Weiner & Finnegan, 2016, p. 202).
- Even high consumption of alcohol does not always result in birth of a child with fetal alcohol syndrome (FASDs). Adverse effects of alcohol are related to:
  - Gestational age at exposure and the individual susceptibility of the fetus
  - Amount and pattern of alcohol consumed
  - Maternal metabolism and peak blood alcohol levels
  - Risk factors that increase susceptibility to FAS include advanced maternal age, being of non-White race, and socioeconomic status (Wallen & Gleason, 2018, p. 129).

Neonatal Effects

- Decreased birth weight and impact on the fetus correlated with exposure in any trimester (Prasad & Jones, 2019, p. 1248; Wallman, 2018, p. 257). Dysmorphia and growth disturbance were increased in women with first trimester alcohol use. Birth weight was more significantly affected by second-trimester exposure (Prasad & Jones, 2019, p. 1248). FAS is estimated to occur in 0.2 to 1.5 of 1,000 births (Sullivan, 2016, p. 574; Wallman, 2018, p. 255).
- The most common preventable causes of developmental delay are FAS and FASDs, both of which are the result of neuronal damage by alcohol ingestion while pregnant (Nocon, 2013, p. 224; Reis & Jnah, 2017, p. 51). Physical characteristics may be noted in the neonate; behavioral problems and learning deficits may be identified after the neonatal period. Collectively, the findings are referred to as FASDs and the newborn with FAS may have craniofacial deformities, growth problems, and CNS abnormalities (Wallman, 2018, p. 257). Table 26.5 details the disorders associated with alcohol use in pregnancy.

TABLE 26.5 Disorders Associated With Alcohol Use in Pregnancy

FASD	FAS
• ARBDs • ARND • FAS	• Maternal drinking during pregnancy • Fetal growth problems • Facial dysmorphia (smooth philtrum, midface hypoplasia, broad flat nasal bridge, thin vermilion border, short palpebral fissures) • Central nervous system abnormalities (dysgenesis of the corpus callosum, cerebellar hypoplasia) • Less frequently described: skeletal anomalies, abnormal hand creases, and ophthalmologic, renal, and cardiac anomalies • Cognitive abnormalities; delayed brain development • Signs of neurologic impairment, including lifelong behavioral and psychosocial dysfunction

ARBDs, alcohol-related birth defects; ARND, alcohol-related neurodevelopmental disorder; FAS, fetal alcohol syndrome; FASD, fetal alcohol spectrum disorder.

Sources: Data from Barron, 2014, p. 103; Prasad, M., & Jones, H. (2019). Substance abuse in pregnancy. In R. Resnik, C. Lockwood, T. Moore, M. Greene, J. Copel, & R. Silver (Eds.), *Creasy and Resnik's maternal-fetal medicine: Principles and practice* (8th ed., p. 1248). Philadelphia, PA: Elsevier; Wallen, L., & Gleason, C. (2018). Prenatal drug exposure. In C. Gleason & S. Juul (Eds.), *Avery's diseases of the newborn* (10th ed., p. 129). Philadelphia, PA: Elsevier; Wallman, C. (2018). Assessment of the newborn with antenatal exposure to drugs. In E. P. Tappero & M. E. Honeyfield (Eds.), *Physical assessment of the newborn* (6th ed., p. 257). New York, NY: Springer Publishing; Weiner, S., & Finnegan, L. (2016). Drug withdrawal in the neonate. In S. Gardner, B. Carter, M. Hines, & J. Hernandez (Eds.), *Merenstein & Gardner's handbook of neonatal intensive care* (8th ed., p. 202). St. Louis, MO: Elsevier.

Breastfeeding

• The AAP advises pregnant and lactating women to abstain from alcohol. Women who drink while breastfeeding should be advised to have no more than one drink and to wait at least 2 hours before breastfeeding (Prasad & Jones, 2019, p. 1248).

• Alcohol is concentrated in breastmilk and can decrease milk production by decreasing the response of prolactin to infant breastfeeding (Prasad & Jones, 2019, p. 1248; Sherman, 2015, p. 54). Alcohol has negative effects on infant motor development (Sherman, 2015, p. 54).

Childhood Effects/FASD

• FASD, the term for the range of effects that may results from prenatal alcohol exposure, is among the most common identifiable causes of developmental delay and intellectual disability, with an average IQ of 67 (Nocon, 2013, p. 225; Reis, & Jnah, 2017, p. 51; Sullivan, 2016, p. 573; Weiner & Finnegan, 2016, p. 202). FASD is not a diagnostic term. It refers to specific conditions, such as FAS, alcohol-related neurodevelopmental disorder (ARND), and alcohol-related birth defects (ARBD; Sullivan, 2016, p. 573; Weiner & Finnegan, 2016, p. 202).

• It is difficult to obtain exact data on the number of infants exposed to alcohol in utero who subsequently develop FAS or FASD; it is estimated that potentially two to five of every 100 schoolchildren exhibit characteristics of FASD (Sullivan, 2016, p. 574; Wallman, 2018, p. 255). FAS is diagnosed based on history and physical findings. No laboratory tests are available to determine the extent of fetal alcohol exposure (Wallen & Gleason, 2018, p. 129).

• The Institute of Medicine has proposed a new term—ARND—for FAS. ARND includes structural CNS and cognitive abnormalities in children with confirmed fetal exposure to alcohol. A diagnosis of ARND does not require the presence of facial or other physical abnormalities (Sullivan, 2016, p. 573–574; Wallen & Gleason, 2018, p. 129). Table 26.5 details the disorders associated with alcohol use in pregnancy.

Treatment (Maternal)

• In most cases, the risk of alcohol use far outweighs the risk of treatment with medication. Treatment is based on detoxification and abstinence (Nocon, 2013, p. 225). Disulfiram is used to maintain abstinence. Disulfiram inhibits aldehyde dehydrogenase production. Use of alcohol while taking disulfiram leads to accumulation of acetaldehyde and to symptoms including facial flushing, tachycardia, hypotension, nausea, and vomiting. This negative reinforcement may not be well tolerated by the pregnant alcoholic in recovery (Nocon, 2013, p. 226)

MARIJUANA/TETRAHYDROCANNABINOL

Prevalence

• Marijuana is the most common illicit drug implicated in SUD (Hudak, 2015, p. 682; Nocon, 2013, p. 235; Prasad & Jones, 2019, p. 1249; Wallman, 2018, p. 255). Marijuana is commonly coupled with other exposures (Prasad & Jones, 2019, p. 1249). In 2011 there were 18.1 million past-month users (Sullivan, 2016, p. 567). Marijuana use during pregnancy continues to rise in correlation with the legalization of marijuana for both medical and recreational use in some states (Wallman, 2018, p. 258).

Pharmacology

• The active substance in marijuana is delta-9-tetrahydrocannabinol (THC; Nocon, 2013, p. 235; Wallman, 2018, p. 258). It is derived from the plant *Cannabis sativa*. Its lipophilic structure allows it to accumulate in fatty tissue and remains for days before it is metabolized in the liver. Inhalation of marijuana smoke is held in the lungs for long periods and results in higher levels of carboxyhemoglobin (Nocon, 2013, p. 235).

• THC content is 10% to 15%. Metabolites of THC are found in the urine for 1 to 3 days after a single use and up to 30 days if chronic use (Hudak, 2015, p. 684; Prasad & Jones, 2019, p. 1249). THC readily crosses the blood–brain barrier (Prasad & Jones, 2019, p. 1249) and the placenta (Hudak, 2015, p. 684; Wallman, 2018, p. 258).

Screening

- THC is the most common substance found in urine drug screens (Nocon, 2013, p. 235). Marijuana exposure can be detected in the mother's and the infant's hair (Weiner & Finnegan, 2016, p. 203).

Fetal Effects

- Marijuana extract and THC have been studied in many animal models and no pattern of malformation has emerged as uniquely associated with marijuana exposure (Hudak, 2015, p. 684; Prasad & Jones, 2019, p. 1249).
- Research in the literature is conflicting, with some studies finding no independent effect on the fetus and others finding decreased fetal growth restriction, prematurity, and stillbirth (Hudak, 2015, p. 684; Nocon, 2013, p. 236; Wallman, 2018, p. 258). Marijuana remains in the body tissues of chronic users for as long as 30 days and can result in prolonged fetal exposure (Hudak, 2015, p. 684).

Neonatal Effects

- In a large longitudinal study, rates of preterm birth, NICU admission, and perinatal mortality were not increased among users. But sustained weekly use was linked to a trend toward decreased birth weight (Prasad & Jones, 2019, p. 1250).
- Babies may display altered neurobehaviors including response to visual stimuli, increased tremulousness, and a high-pitched cry (Sullivan, 2016, p. 567; Weiner & Finnegan, 2016, p. 203), prolonged startle response, or altered sleep (Prasad & Jones, 2019, p. 1250) There is an association between newborns exposed to marijuana prenatally and decreased executive skills, including poor impulse control, visual memory, and attention deficit (Wallman, 2018, p. 258)

Breastfeeding

- Breastfeeding while using marijuana should be avoided. THC, the active metabolite of marijuana, is concentrated in breastmilk compared with maternal blood plasma levels (Prasad & Jones, 2019, p. 1249).

Childhood Effects

- No independent effect of prenatal marijuana exposure on childhood growth through adolescence has been found. Multiple studies have revealed issues with executive function, difficulty organizing, and integrating specific cognitive and output processes with difficulties in reading and spelling (Hudak, 2015, p. 684; Prasad & Jones, 2019, p. 1250; Sherman, 2015, p. 54; Weiner & Finnegan, 2016, p. 203). No effect on IQ or language has been found (Hudak, 2015, p. 684). Prenatal exposure to marijuana has been associated with increased marijuana use by age 14 (Nocon, 2013, p. 236).

Treatment

- No effective pharmacologic agent is available for the treatment of marijuana dependence (Prasad & Jones, 2019, p. 1250). Treatment of marijuana use is achieved with cognitive behavioral methods and motivational enhancement. Smoking cessation programs are effective. Most patients respond to "coercive therapy" which means the parent is informed if the baby tests positive for THC in the meconium, child protective services will investigate (Nocon, 2013, p. 236).

COCAINE

Prevalence

- The 2010 National Survey on Drug Abuse and Health found that 1.5 million Americans were current cocaine abusers (Prasad & Jones, 2019, p. 1252).

Pharmacology

- Cocaine is a highly addictive lipophilic alkaloid extracted from the plant *Erythroxylum coca* leaves. Rapid tolerance develops and is the basis for a rapid addictive process. It causes blockade of the myocardial fast sodium channels and results in prolongation of the QRS complex and dysrhythmia. Blockade of dopamine reuptake centrally produces a profound euphoria that is responsible for the high addictive potential. The norepinephrine release related to euphoria augments the norepinephrine reuptake mechanism and contributes further to vasoconstriction and pursuit of the pleasure response (Hudak, 2015, p. 690; Nocon, 2013, p. 236; Prasad & Jones, 2019, p. 1253; Sullivan, 2016, p. 566; Wallman, 2018, p. 257).
- Cocaine readily crosses the placenta by simple diffusion (Hudak, 2015, p. 690; Wallman, 2018, p. 257; Weiner & Finnegan, 2016, p. 201). This occurs because of its high lipid solubility, low molecular weight, and low ionization at physiologic pH.
  - ○ There is a low level of plasma esterases in the fetus and cocaine accumulates secondary to the relatively low pH of fetal blood (Weiner & Finnegan, 2016, p. 201).
- Cocaine is metabolized by plasma and hepatic cholinesterases with renal clearance of the inactive compounds produced. Plasma cholinesterase activity is decreased in pregnant women, fetuses, and infants which increases the half-life of cocaine (Hudak, 2015, p. 690).

Screening

- Cocaine is hydrolyzed to benzoylecgonine, which appears in the urine. Meconium drug screens have a high sensitivity for detecting cocaine use (Nocon, 2013, p. 236). Cocaine may be detected in neonatal urine for up to 7 days after delivery (Hudak, 2015, p. 691; Sherman, 2015, p. 50).

Fetal Effects

- Cocaine is lipid soluble and readily crosses the placenta and enters the fetal brain (Blackburn, 2013, p. 208; Prasad & Jones, 2019, p. 1253; Sherman, 2015, pp. 43; Sullivan, 2016, pp. 565–566). Cocaine causes significant vasoconstriction and decreases blood flow to the placenta and uterus. This decreases oxygen delivery to the fetus (Hudak, 2015, p. 690; Smith & Carley, 2014, p. 681; Weiner & Finnegan, 2016, p. 202).
- The vasoconstrictive properties of cocaine can have a wide range of fetal effects. Box 26.3 details the fetal associations

with prenatal cocaine exposure. Vasoconstriction related to cocaine use has been correlated with placental abruption, intestinal atresia, and necrotizing enterocolitis in a small series of term and preterm newborns (Wallman, 2018, p. 257–258). Cocaine users have an increased risk of giving birth to an infant with urinary tract defects (Prasad & Jones, 2019, p. 1253).

- Acute cocaine use in the third trimester can result in preterm labor, abruptio placenta, increased incidence of premature rupture of membranes, increased meconium staining, precipitous delivery, prematurity, and LBW (Hudak, 2015, p. 690; Sullivan, 2016, p. 566).

Neonatal Effects

- Cocaine crosses the placenta easily. Cocaine use in pregnancy is associated with preterm birth, small for gestational age (SGA) infants, younger gestational age at birth, and reduced birth weight. Infants who were exposed to tobacco and cocaine or marijuana had less alert responsiveness (Prasad & Jones, 2019, p. 1253). Infants with prenatal exposure to cocaine were significantly more likely to require medical support or resuscitation (Weiner & Finnegan, 2016, p. 202).
- The half-life of cocaine is longer in the fetus and neonate than the adult, thus cocaine may be present in the neonate for several days after birth (Blackburn, 2013, p. 208). Neurobehavioral abnormalities in infants with in utero cocaine exposure are often seen on day of life 2 or 3 (Hudak, 2015, p. 691; Sherman, 2015, p. 50; Sullivan, 2016, p. 565).
- Neonates exposed to cocaine are often irritable and tremulous, have a high-pitched cry and excessive sucking, and are difficult to console (Sherman, 2015, p. 50). These neurobehaviors may reflect the effect of the drug as opposed to withdrawal (Blackburn, 2013, p. 208; Hudak, 2015, p. 691).
- Newborns may also present with tachycardia, arrhythmias, hypertension, vasoconstriction, diaphoresis, and mild tremors when cocaine is present in the bloodstream as a result of maternal use (Wallman, 2018, p. 257). When cocaine use occurs shortly before delivery, there is an association with transient neonatal ventricular tachycardia (Hudak, 2015, p. 690).

Breastfeeding

- Breastfeeding is contraindicated during cocaine use (Prasad & Jones, 2019, p. 1253), due to being excreted into breastmilk (Hudak, 2015, p. 690; Wallman, 2018, p. 257). Cocaine may be found in breastmilk up to 36 hours after it is used (Blackburn, 2013, p. 208).

Childhood Effects

- Prenatal cocaine exposure was associated with an increased risk of specific cognitive impairments (visual spatial skills, general knowledge, and arithmetic skills; Prasad & Jones, 2019, p. 1254). Children exposed to cocaine in utero have self-reported attention processing deficits, increased symptoms of attention deficit hyperactivity disorder, and oppositional defiance disorder (Sherman, 2015, p. 54). Large prospective studies have shown relatively subtle cocaine-associated deficits that are dose dependent. Subtle effects may have a financial impact on schools due

to increased numbers of children requiring special services (Hudak, 2015, p. 691).

- The home environment was the most important independent predictor of outcome, suggesting the potential to compensate for in utero drug exposure (Prasad & Jones, 2019, p. 1254).

Treatment

- Pharmacologic treatment of cocaine use includes topiramate, an anticonvulsant, and baclofen, a GABA B receptor agonist that blocks the brain reward system (Nocon, 2013, pp. 236–237). Therapy for cocaine addiction is psychosocial treatment (Prasad & Jones, 2019, p. 1254), which is based on cognitive behavioral methods, motivational enhancement, and the "coercive approach" (Nocon, 2013, p. 237).

METHAMPHETAMINE

Prevalence

- In the National Survey on Drug Abuse in 2010, methamphetamine exposure decreased; however, despite the trend, methamphetamine use remains a significant problem in some areas (Prasad & Jones, 2019, p. 1254).

Pharmacology

- Methamphetamine blocks the reuptake of adrenergic neurotransmitters. Methamphetamine is a sympathomimetic agent that induces euphoria and increases alertness and self-confidence because it produces a massive efflux of dopamine in the CNS (Hudak, 2015, p. 692). Methamphetamine may be identified in urine drug screens and remains detectable for up to 3 days (Prasad & Jones, 2019, p. 1254; Sullivan, 2016, p. 567).

Screening

- There are no well-validated measures that accurately detect stimulant use. Detection depends on accurate self-report (Prasad & Jones, 2019, p. 1254).

Fetal Effects

- Methamphetamine readily passes through the placenta and the blood–brain barrier and stimulates the CNS. The mechanism of action may be an interaction with and alteration of neurotransmitter systems as well as alterations in brain morphogenesis (Sherman, 2015, p. 47).
- Prenatal amphetamine exposure has been shown in some early research to lead to congenital brain lesions, including hemorrhage, infarction, or cavitary lesions (Weiner & Finnegan, 2016, p. 202). Case reports demonstrate, but do not confirm, cardiovascular, gastrointestinal, and CNS abnormalities; facial clefts; and limb reduction defects with increased risk of malformation (Prasad & Jones, 2019, p. 1255).
- Due to vasoconstrictive properties, methamphetamine exposure during pregnancy increases the risk of preterm birth, LBW, and SGA infants (Hudak, 2015, p. 692; Prasad & Jones, 2019, p. 1255). Further effects on the fetus may include growth restriction, abruption, and withdrawal symptoms (Nocon, 2013, p. 237).

Neonatal Effects

- Neonatal effects mimic those of cocaine. In the neonatal period, neurologic abnormalities including decreased arousal, poor state control, difficulty with habituation, tremors, hyperactive neonatal reflexes, abnormal cry, increased stress, drowsiness, poor feeding, and seizures have been reported (Weiner & Finnegan, 2016, p. 203). Symptoms may alternate between lethargy and irritability, poor sucking patterns, and sleep disturbances (Weiner & Finnegan, 2016, p. 209). Use of methamphetamines may be toxic to the fetal brain and may increase the risk of SIDS (Weiner & Finnegan, 2016, p. 203).

Breastfeeding

- Breastfeeding is not recommended for women with ongoing methamphetamine use due to concentration in the breastmilk that is 2.8 to 7.5 times higher than that in maternal plasma (Prasad & Jones, 2019, p. 1255). High doses of methamphetamine in breastmilk have been associated with fetal levels in the infant (Nocon, 2013, p. 237). The high levels of methamphetamine in breastmilk may produce an acute neurotoxic syndrome with hypertonia, tremors, apnea, and seizures (Weiner & Finnegan, 2016, p. 203).

Child Effects

- Long-term effects of methamphetamine revealed delays in cognitive skills and growth (Nocon, 2013, p. 237). Long-term adverse neurotoxic effects of in utero methamphetamine exposure on behavior, cognitive skills, and physical dexterity have been reported (Hudak, 2015, p. 692; Sullivan, 2016, p. 568).

Treatment

- There is no pharmacologic treatment for methamphetamine use. Management is psychosocial (Prasad & Jones, 2019, p. 1255) with cognitive behavioral therapy and motivational enhancement as the primary mode of treatment (Nocon, 2013, p. 237).

BENZODIAZEPINES

Prevalence

- Benzodiazepines are among the most frequently prescribed medications for pregnant women. Diazepam (Valium), alprazolam (Xanax), lorazepam (Ativan), clonazepam (Klonopin), and chlordiazepoxide (Librium) are the most common drugs. Diazepam (Valium) is the only benzodiazepine for which there is sufficient research among pregnant women (Prasad & Jones, 2019, p. 1255).

Pharmacology

- Benzodiazepines affect the neuroinhibitory neurotransmitter GABA and appear to act on the limbic, thalamic, and hypothalamic level of the CNS to produce sedative and hypnotic effects, reduction of anxiety, anticonvulsant effects, and skeletal relaxation (Nocon, 2013, p. 235; Prasad & Jones, 2019, p. 1255).

Screening

- There are no well-validated brief measures to identify benzodiazepine use. Detection relies on self-report (Prasad & Jones, 2019, p. 1255).

Fetal Effects

- Diazepam (Valium) is transferred across the placenta and accumulates in the fetal circulation at about one to three times the level in maternal blood (Prasad & Jones, 2019, p. 1255).

Neonatal Effects

- Infants with extended exposure in utero to diazepam (Valium) have exhibited a neonatal abstinence syndrome (NAS) resembling that shown with opioid withdrawal. The onset of benzodiazepine-associated NAS may occur at up to 12 days for diazepam (Valium; Sherman, 2015, p. 51), and up to 2 to 3 weeks after birth, complicating diagnosis and treatment of the problem (Hudak, 2015, p. 690; Prasad & Jones, 2019, p. 1255). Benzodiazepines with longer half-lives are associated with more severe signs and length of withdrawal symptoms. Symptoms may include hypertonia, hypotonia, excessive or poor suck, and vomiting (Hudak, 2015, p. 690).
  - If an infant has severe signs, these infants are usually treated with phenobarbital. Outpatient weaning of phenobarbital (Luminal) has been reported to require weeks to months (Hudak, 2015, p. 690; Prasad & Jones, 2019, p. 1255).

Breastfeeding

- There is a paucity of research to guide recommendations for breastfeeding by mothers using benzodiazepines. Diazepam (Valium) and its metabolites have been found in breastmilk and infant blood (Prasad & Jones, 2019, p. 1255).

Childhood Effects

- The effects of in utero exposure to benzodiazepines are similar to those of opioids. It has been difficult to differentiate the relative contributions of the drug from those of the child's social environment (Prasad & Jones, 2019, p. 1255).

Treatment

- Treatment of benzodiazepine addiction is difficult because the drug is associated with poor psychological functioning and a reduced effect of other interventions for illicit drug use. Successful withdrawal from benzodiazepines is likely to occur only when the taper from benzodiazepine dose is slow and gradual and in the context of extensive psychological counseling and support (Prasad & Jones, 2019, p. 1255).

OPIOIDS

Prevalence

- The United States is experiencing an epidemic of addiction to prescribed controlled substances, often originally administered for the management of chronic pain. More than 116 million Americans receive pharmacologic treatment for chronic pain (Reis, & Jnah, 2017, p. 51). Opioid use among pregnant women increased six times from 2000 to 2009 and continues to increase. Women of 25 to 34 years are most likely to misuse prescription painkillers. The NSDUH in 2013 found that pregnant females ages 15 to 17 account for 14.6% of illicit drug users (Reis, & Jnah, 2017, p. 52). From 2000 to 2009, addiction to prescription painkillers by pregnant women caused cases of NAS to rise by almost 300% (Weiner & Finnegan, 2016, p. 199).

- Pregnant women are uniquely vulnerable to opiate use for many reasons. Opiates are exceedingly addictive and are often obtained by trading sex for drugs. Heroin use in particular is strongly associated with the behaviors of a male partner. Chronic heroin use is estimated to effect 810,000 to 1 million Americans (Prasad & Jones, 2019, p. 1250).

Pharmacology

- Opioids are alkaloids derived from the opium poppy and include all opiates plus the semisynthetics, which are derived from the alkaloids: hydrocodone (Hycodan), oxycodone (Oxycontin), and heroin, plus the synthetics: methadone (Dolophine), fentanyl (Duragesic), nalbuphine (Nubian), and buprenorphine (Subutex). The terms opiates and opioids are often used interchangeably (Hudak, 2015, p. 684; Nocon, 2013, p. 226; Weiner & Finnegan, 2016, p. 199).
  ○ Opiates/opioids are small molecular weight and variably lipophilic compounds that cross both blood–brain and placental barriers. Opiates can be inhaled injected, snorted, swallowed, or used subcutaneously.
- Opiates exert their effect by binding to the mu and kappa receptors in the limbic and limbic-related areas in the brain. Binding of the opiate receptors sends a signal to dopamine terminals to release dopamine. Opioids also acutely inhibit the release of noradrenaline at synaptic terminals. Activated mu receptors produce analgesia, euphoria, miosis, and reinforcement of the reward behavior. Activated kappa receptors produce the subjective sensation of dysphoria, spinal analgesia, sedation, and psychomimetic.
  ○ Opiates are highly addictive (Hudak, 2015, p. 684; Nocon, 2013, p. 227; Prasad & Jones, 2019, p. 1250); 70% of opiate users relapse within 6 weeks of nonmedication rehabilitation efforts (Prasad & Jones, 2019, p. 1250).

Screening

- There are no well validated screening measures for opioid dependence. A brief interview may uncover opioid abuse. Biologic testing, with the patient's consent, may be warranted (Prasad & Jones, 2019, p. 1251). A urine drug screen may be negative if a patient is in withdrawal. Morphine (MS Contin) is excreted within 72 hours and withdrawal occurs in 3 to 6 days (Nocon, 2013, pp. 227–228).

Fetal Effects

- Opioid use in pregnancy is associated with intrauterine growth restriction, LBW, placental abruption, preterm labor and birth, fetal death, and in utero passage of meconium (Reis, & Jnah, 2017, p. 53; Sullivan, 2016, p. 565). Animal studies have shown decreased brain growth and cell development (Sherman, 2015, p. 47). Human and animal studies have shown a direct effect on fetal growth with opioid exposure in pregnancy (Weiner & Finnegan, 2016, p. 201).

Neonatal Effects

- Common adverse outcomes include preterm delivery, LBW, and perinatal mortality. Other adverse outcomes are attributed to drug-seeking behaviors, concomitant smoking, and inadequate nutrition (Prasad & Jones, 2019, p. 1251). An increase in the frequency of SIDS has been noted.
- NAS is the most common effect on the neonate. Between 2000 and 2009, the rate of newborns diagnosed with NAS increased from 1.2 to 3.4 per 1,000 births (Sherman, 2015, p. 47). Signs of withdrawal can occur up to 6 days of life (Sullivan, 2016, p. 565).
- NAS is a risk for all opiate-exposed infants (Prasad & Jones, 2019, p. 1251). NAS most often occurs with a mean onset of treatable symptoms at 48 to 72 hours of life and average withdrawal lasting 28 or more days. No studies found a dose–response relationship with maternal use of methadone (Dolophine) and NAS (Reis, & Jnah, 2017, p. 54).

Breastfeeding

- Breastfeeding is not recommended for women who are abusing opioids (Patrick, 2017, p. 155; Prasad & Jones, 2019, p. 1251).
- Women who are compliant in opioid agonist treatment with methadone (Dolophine) or buprenorphine (Subutex) should be encouraged to breastfeed because drug concentrations in breastmilk are low (Hudak, 2015, p. 687; Patrick, 2017, p. 149; Prasad & Jones, 2019, p. 1251; Sherman, 2015, p. 54). Mothers should be encouraged to continue breastfeeding as long as the infant continues to gain weight (Hudak, 2015, p. 687; Patrick, 2017, p. 149).
  ○ Methadone (Dolophine) is on the approved category for women who are breastfeeding (Sherman, 2015, p. 55). The relative dose for the infant is approximately 1.9% to 6.5% via breastmilk. Buprenorphine (Subutex) appears in breastmilk approximately two hours after maternal ingestion (Weiner & Finnegan, 2016, p. 216).
- Infants who breastfeed have a reduction in neonatal abstinence symptoms when mother is on methadone (Dolophine) (Reis, & Jnah, 2017, p. 54; Sherman, 2015, p. 55; Weiner & Finnegan, 2016, p. 216). Infants who were breastfed required pharmacologic treatment 23.1% of the time compared to 30% need for pharmacologic care for infants who were not breastfed (Weiner & Finnegan, 2016, p. 216). Breastfed infants who were exposed to methadone (Dolophine) and buprenorphine (Subutex) required pharmacologic treatment for a shorter period of time than infants who did not breastfeed (Weiner & Finnegan, 2016, p. 216).

Childhood Effects

- Research suggests that school-age children who were exposed to heroin in utero experience developmental delay and may exhibit aggressiveness, hyperactivity, and disinhibition. Variations in parental care may modify expression of the effects of in utero drug exposure (Prasad & Jones, 2019, p. 1251). Hyperactivity and short attention span have been noted in toddlers prenatally exposed to opiates. Older exposed children have demonstrated memory and perceptual problems (Sherman, 2015, p. 54).

TREATMENT (MATERNAL)

- Opioid detoxification and abstinence during pregnancy is not recommended due to the risk of abruption, preterm labor, fetal distress, and fetal loss (Hudak, 2015, pp. 684–685; Nocon, 2013, p. 227). Detoxification in pregnancy has a relapse rate of more than 50% (Hudak, 2015, p. 685; Prasad & Jones, 2019, p. 1251). Inpatient detoxification may be the only alternative to illicit drug use if the mother does not have access to a supervised opioid maintenance program (Hudak, 2015, p. 684–685).
- The goal of treatment in pregnancy is maintenance (Hudak, 2015, p. 684–685; Nocon 2013, p. 227) and to provide a dosage of medication-assisted treatment that prevents drug cravings and illicit use and does not create euphoria (Hudak, 2015, p. 685; Prasad & Jones, 2019, p. 1251).

METHADONE (DOLOPHINE)

- Methadone (Dolophine) is a full mu agonist and a weak NMDA receptor agonist (Hudak, 2015, p. 685; Sherman, 2015, p. 45; Sullivan 2016, p. 51). It exerts secondary effects by acting as an NMDA receptor antagonist to block the actions of glutamate, the primary excitatory neurotransmitter in the CNS (Hudak, 2015, p. 684). It is well-absorbed orally and exhibits a mean half-life of approximately 1 day (vs. only 15 to 30 minutes for heroin) to produce a sustained effect (Hudak, 2015, p. 684). It is excreted in 4 to 5 days and withdrawal occurs in 10 to 20 days (Nocon, 2013, pp. 227–228).
- Benefits of methadone (Dolophine) treatment with dosing that sustains opioid concentrations in the mother and fetus include decreased high-risk behaviors, reduced incarceration, decreased spread of infectious disease (Prasad & Jones, 2019, p. 1252), decreased opioid craving, and prevention of fetal stress (Hudak, 2015, p. 685; Sherman, 2015, p. 51). Methadone (Dolophine) treatment of SUD is associated with decreased maternal complications, decreased prematurity, and improved birth weight (Sherman, 2015, p. 45; Sullivan, 2016, p. 567).

BUPRENORPHINE (SUBUTEX)

- Buprenorphine (Subutex) alone or combined with naloxone (Suboxone) has been used as a primary treatment for heroin addiction and as a replacement for methadone (Dolophine; Sherman, 2015, p. 51). Buprenorphine (Subutex) is a partial mu agonist and has a very high affinity for the mu opioid receptor (Hudak, 2015, p. 685; Prasad & Jones, 2019, p. 1252), and treatment can be accomplished on an outpatient basis and does not require a daily visit to a maintenance program (Sullivan, 2016, p. 567).
  - ○ One study demonstrated a shorter length of stay for infant treatment for NAS, lower doses of morphine (MS Contin) needed for NAS treatment, and shorter duration of treatment as outcomes of maternal treatment with buprenorphine (Subutex; Hudak, 2015, p. 685; Prasad & Jones, 2019, p. 1252; Sherman, 2015, p. 45).

NEONATAL ABSTINENCE SYNDROME

Incidence

- The collection of symptoms that are associated with withdrawal are called NAS. In the neonate exposed to opioids in utero, 55% to 94% will develop signs of withdrawal (Hudak, 2015, p. 685). The rate of NAS is 3.9 per 100 hospital births in the United States, with approximately 4 million births annually (Weiner & Finnegan, 2016, p. 199). From 2004 to 2013, the rate of NICU admissions for NAS increased from seven per 1,000 admissions to 27 cases per 1,000 admissions (Wallman, 2018, p. 255). Depending on the population, setting, and hospital, the rate of NAS ranges from 3% to 50% (Smith & Carley, 2014, p. 680).
  - ○ Infants with NAS have a 19% higher likelihood to have LBW, and a 13-day longer length of stay than an infant without NAS (Weiner & Finnegan, 2016, p. 199). From 2004 to 2013, the median length of stay of an infant with NAS increased from 13 to 19 days (Wallman, 2018, p. 255).
- The increase in infants diagnosed with NAS correlates directly with the increase in maternal opioid use in pregnancy (Hudak, 2015, p. 685; Wallman, 2018, p. 255). Studies demonstrate inconsistent results when evaluating the relationship between the mother's dose of methadone (Dolophine) and NAS severity; approximately 50% of studies find a relationship and 50% find no relationship (Weiner & Finnegan, 2016, p. 206).

Pathophysiology

- A neonate can develop a passive dependence secondary to exposure in utero to opiates or opioids used to treat chronic pain, misused by the mother, or for treatment of SUD. A neonate can also develop an iatrogenic dependence due to opioids used for analgesia and sedation after birth. Opiates and opioids that result in dependence include heroin, methadone (Dolophine), morphine (MS Contin), buprenorphine (Subutex), fentanyl (Duragesic), and other narcotic analgesics (Weiner & Finnegan, 2016, p. 200, 204).
- Opioid withdrawal is complicated in the newborn due to complex maternal–fetal–placental pharmacokinetics as well as the immaturity of the fetus and newborn neurologic system (Wallman, 2018, p. 259). The absence of opioids after birth causes an increase in norepinephrine production that causes most of the clinical symptoms in NAS (Wallman, 2018, p. 259).
  - ○ Because opioid receptors are located in the CNS and gastrointestinal (GI) tract (Sherman, 2015, p. 51; Wallman, 2018, p. 259), NAS causes CNS irritability, GI system dysfunction in addition to autonomic nervous system overactivity (Sherman, 2015, p. 51; Smith & Carley, 2014, p. 681).
- The collection of symptoms associated with withdrawal from a dependency-producing substance are called NAS (Hudak, 2015, p. 685; Smith & Carley, 2014, p. 681). The most severe withdrawal symptoms occur with exposure to opioids, though other drugs can also trigger symptoms (Smith & Carley, 2014, p. 681).
- Withdrawal in the newborn is physiologic and is not an addiction. Neonates should not be referred to as "addicts," because the practice of addiction involves active, drug-seeking behaviors (Wallman, 2018, p. 259).

Screening

- Amniotic fluid, cord blood, breastmilk, and newborn urine and meconium can be tested for morphine (MS Contin), a metabolite of heroin known as 6-AM, and methadone (Dolophine), as well as buprenorphine (Subutex) and its metabolites (Weiner & Finnegan, 2016, p. 200).

Clinical Features

- During in utero exposure to addictive substances, the fetus undergoes a biochemical adaptation. At delivery, supply of the substance is discontinued, but newborn metabolism and clearance continues. Withdrawal occurs when critically low levels of the substance in the neonatal system are reached (Weiner & Finnegan, 2016, p. 206).
- The timing of onset of withdrawal symptoms is dependent on multiple factors, including timing of most recent exposure, type of opioid exposure, dose of exposure, and level of neurologic maturity in the newborn (Wallman, 2018, p. 259; Weiner & Finnegan, 2016, p. 201, 205). The closer to delivery a mother takes a drug, the more severe the symptoms and the greater the delay in onset (Weiner & Finnegan, 2016, p. 206).
- Most infants exposed to opioids appear physically and behaviorally normal at birth. The presentation of symptoms often begins within 24 to 72 hours of birth (Hudak, 2015, p. 686; Sherman, 2015, p. 51; Smith & Corley, 2014, p. 681; Weiner & Finnegan, 2016, p. 201).
  - ○ Withdrawal from heroin, which has a short half-life, usually begins within 24 hours of birth.
  - ○ Withdrawal from treatment medications, which have a longer half-life, occurs at 48 to 72 hours after birth.
    - ■ Methadone (Dolophine) withdrawal, which is stored in the fetal lung, liver, and spleen, typically begins at 24 to 72 hours of life.
    - ■ Buprenorphine (Subutex) withdrawal symptoms peak at 40 hours and are most severe at 70 hours of age (Hudak, 2015, p. 686; Sherman, 2015, p. 51; Weiner & Finnegan, 2016, p. 205).
  - ○ Symptoms of withdrawal may present as late as 7 to 14 days after birth (Hudak, 2015, p. 686; Smith & Carley, 2014, p. 681; Weiner & Finnegan, 2016, p. 207).
- The most common symptoms of NAS primarily occur in the CNS, GI system, and autonomic nervous system (Hudak, 2015, p. 686; Sherman, 2015, p. 51; Weiner & Finnegan, 2016, p. 207). Table 26.6 details the symptoms of NAS.
  - ○ Tremors are typically mild and progress from occurring only with stimulation to occurring spontaneously.

Disturbed and undisturbed tremors, hyperactive Moro reflex, excess irritability, and failure to thrive are more frequent in infants exposed to methadone (Dolophine) in utero. Nasal stuffiness, sneezing, and loose stools are more commonly seen in infants exposed to buprenorphine (Subutex) in utero (Hudak, 2015, p. 686; Weiner & Finnegan, 2016, pp. 207–208).
  - ○ In 2% to 11% of infants, seizures may occur in acute withdrawal. These seizures have an unknown etiology and unknown long-term significance. In the absence of seizure activity, abnormal electroencephalograms have been noted in more than 30% of infants exposed to opiates in utero (Hudak, 2015, p. 686).
- Symptoms usually resolve within 2 weeks, but some mild signs persist for up to 6 months (Hudak, 2015, p. 686; Smith & Carley, 2014, p. 681). The severity of NAS does not correlate well with the dose or duration of in utero substance exposure, but is affected by the drug or drugs used (Smith & Carley, 2014, p. 681). Perceived severity of NAS may be affected by infant's hunger and environmental stimuli (Hudak, 2015, p. 686).

PREMATURE INFANTS AND NAS
- Lower gestational age is correlated with lower risk of withdrawal. This may be due to decreased length and dose of exposure and neurologic immaturity that limits the ability of the premature infant to exhibit signs of withdrawal (Hudak, 2015, p. 686; Wallman, 2018, p. 259). Compared to term infants whose mothers were treated with methadone (Dolophine), infants born at less than 35 weeks' gestational age had significantly lower total and CNS abstinence scores (Hudak, 2015, p. 686).

Assessment of Withdrawal

- Objective and ongoing scoring of symptoms of NAS can assist the clinician with decision-making (Hudak, 2015, p. 687). Multiple tools exist for assistance with discrete scoring for NAS. These include the Finnegan Neonatal Abstinence Scoring System, Neonatal Drug Withdrawal Scoring System (the Lipsitz Tool), Neonatal Withdrawal Inventory, Neonatal Narcotic Withdrawal

TABLE 26.6 Symptoms of Neonatal Abstinence Syndrome

CNS Symptoms	GI Symptoms	Autonomic Symptoms
Tremors (disturbed and undisturbed) Jitteriness Hyperactive Moro reflex Myoclonic jerks Seizures Irritability Poor sleep pattern Excessive/high pitched crying Tachypnea Tachycardia Skin excoriation Facial and body excoriation secondary to excessive irritation and movements	Poor feeding Poor weight gain Hyperphagia (excessive desire to eat) Emesis Diarrhea Perianal excoriation secondary to GI disturbance	Sneezing Yawning Mottling Hiccups Nasal stuffiness Fever Sweating

Sources: Data from Hudak, M. (2015). Infants with antenatal exposure to drugs. In R. Martin, A. Fanaroff, & M. Walsh (Eds.), *Fanaroff and Martin's neonatal–perinatal medicine: Diseases of the fetus and infant* (10th ed., p. 686). Philadelphia, PA: Elsevier; Sherman, J. (2015). Perinatal substance abuse. In T. Verklan & M. Walden (Eds.), *Core curriculum for neonatal intensive care nursing* (5th ed., p. 51). St. Louis, MO: Elsevier; Wallman, C. (2018). Assessment of the newborn with antenatal exposure to drugs. In E. P. Tappero & M. E. Honeyfield (Eds.), *Physical assessment of the newborn* (6th ed., pp. 259–260). New York, NY: Springer Publishing; Weiner, S., & Finnegan, L. (2016). Drug withdrawal in the neonate. In S. Gardner, B. Carter, M. Hines, & J. Hernandez (Eds.), *Merenstein & Gardner's handbook of neonatal intensive care* (8th ed., pp. 204, 207–208). St. Louis, MO: Elsevier.

Index, MOTHER NAS Scale, and Neonatal Network Neurobehavioral Scale (Wallman, 2018, p. 260).

- The Finnegan Neonatal Abstinence Scoring System is the tool used most frequently for scoring for neonatal withdrawal in the United States (Hudak, 2015, p. 687; Wallman, 2018, p. 260; Weiner & Finnegan, 2016, p. 210). The Finnegan scoring tool has been studied for validity and reliability (Wallman, 2018, p. 260).
    - ○ The Finnegan scoring tool uses 21 individual items with a weighted score based on severity. The total score is determined by adding the individual scores together during an assigned scoring interval (Hudak, 2015, p. 687; Patrick, 2017, p. 148; Weiner & Finnegan, 2016, p. 209).
    - ○ A score of 7 or less on day of life 2 is in the 95th percentile for infants not exposed to opioids. Any score of 8 or higher is highly suggestive of exposure to opioids in utero (Sherman, 2015, p. 51).
- The Lipsitz Tool was recommended in the 1998 AAP statement on neonatal drug withdrawal (Weiner & Finnegan, 2016, p. 210). The Lipsitz Tool is a simple to use and has good sensitivity to identify clinically important withdrawal (Hudak, 2015, p. 687).
- Regardless of the choice of scoring tool, one of the most important factors to effective utilization is training and ongoing education for the staff and providers who implement the tool; poor interrater consistency may lead to ineffective medical management (Wallman, 2018, p. 260).

Nonpharmacologic Treatment

- Supportive care of withdrawal symptoms can increase the newborn's ability to regulate his or her neurobehavior, improve neuromotor control, and promote maternal/infant dyad bonding (Smith & Carley, 2014, p. 682). Box 26.4 details nonpharmacologic supportive-care strategies for the infant with NAS. The goal of care and treatment is to ensure the infant is able to eat and sleep to ensure adequate weight gain and socialization skills (Hudak, 2015, p. 687).
    - ○ Regardless of nonpharmacologic or pharmacologic treatment needs, the infant with severe signs of withdrawal may require increased calories to achieve growth due to increased metabolic rate, emesis, and loose stools. Infants with NAS may require 150 to 250 cal/kg/day to achieve growth.
    - ○ The infant with severe NAS needs careful observation for fever, dehydration, and weight loss. Stabilization with gavage feeding, IV fluids, and electrolytes may be required (Hudak, 2015, p. 687; Sherman, 2015, p. 53).

Pharmacologic Treatment

- The goal of medication to treat NAS is to relieve severe signs and symptoms and prevent complications such as fever, weight loss, and seizures if nonpharmacologic care is not able to manage the symptoms. The reduction of symptoms is the only clear benefit of drug therapy (Hudak, 2015, p. 688; Sherman, 2015, p. 53). Treatment with drugs may disrupt maternal/infant bonding, as well as guarantees prolongation of hospitalization and increased drug exposure (Hudak, 2015, p. 688).
- Ideal drug treatment uses a protocol to drive drug titration and control symptoms (Sherman, 2015, p. 53). The literature does not identify an optimal drug or regimen for NAS treatment (Hudak, 2015, p. 689). Methadone (Dolophine), morphine (MS Contin), and buprenorphine (Subutex)

have been used to relieve the symptoms of NAS (Weiner & Finnegan, 2016, p. 200).

Opioids

- An opioid is the primary drug for opioid withdrawal symptoms associated with in utero exposure to opiates. Methadone (Dolophine) and morphine (MS Contin) are the drugs of first choice. Both drugs bind to opioid receptors in the CNS, causing inhibition of ascending pain pathways and altering the perception and response to pain. Methadone (Dolophine) has a long half-life and provides a steadier level with the benefit of administration at less frequent intervals. It is a full mu agonist and has approximately 90% oral bioavailability (Sherman, 2015, p. 53; Taketomo, Hodding, & Kraus, 2018, pp. 1400–1408, 1321).
- Buprenorphine (Subutex) is a partial mu agonist and kappa agonist, has a higher receptor affinity and a longer duration of action than methadone (Dolophine), and has approximately 50% oral bioavailability (Weiner & Finnegan, 2016, p. 205). It is rapidly absorbed sublingually and use in treatment revealed a shorter length of stay when compared to morphine (MS Contin; Sherman, 2015, p. 53).

BOX 26.4 Nonpharmacologic strategies for the infant with NAS

Rocking
Minimize environmental stimulation (light and noise)
Swaddle
Minimize unnecessary handling
Pacifier for excessive sucking (nonnutritive)
Diaper changing frequently
Soft sheets or sheepskin (decrease excoriation)
Mittens over hands (prevent scratching)
Small/frequent demand feedings
Increased calorie feedings

Sources: Data from Hudak, M. (2015). Infants with antenatal exposure to drugs. In R. Martin, A. Fanaroff, & M. Walsh (Eds.), *Fanaroff and Martin's neonatal–perinatal medicine: Diseases of the fetus and infant* (10th ed., p. 687). Philadelphia, PA: Elsevier; Sherman, J. (2015). Perinatal substance abuse. In T. Verklan & M. Walden (Eds.), *Core curriculum for neonatal intensive care nursing* (5th ed., pp. 43–57). St. Louis, MO: Elsevier; Smith, J. R., & Carley, A. (2014). Common neonatal complications. In K. Simpson & P. Creehan (Eds.), *Perinatal nursing* (4th ed., p. 682). St. Louis, MO: Lippincott Williams & Wilkins; Weiner, S., & Finnegan, L. (2016). Drug withdrawal in the neonate. In S. Gardner, B. Carter, M. Hines, & J. Hernandez (Eds.), *Merenstein & Gardner's handbook of neonatal intensive care* (8th ed., p. 212). St. Louis, MO: Elsevier.

ADJUNCT THERAPIES
PHENOBARBITAL (LUMINAL)

- If symptoms of NAS are not controlled despite higher ranges of opioid administration, in utero exposure to other nonopioid drugs should be suspected. This is an indication for a secondary drug therapy for the treatment of NAS, typically from another drug class (Hudak, 2015, p. 689). Phenobarbital (Luminal), a sedative–hypnotic, has been used as a primary treatment medication for NAS, but is also used as an adjunct therapy when symptoms are not resolved with the initial maximum opioid therapy (Hudak, 2015, p. 689; Sherman, 2015, p. 53). Phenobarbital is a long acting barbiturate with sedative, hypnotic, and anticonvulsant properties. It depresses the sensory cortex, decreases motor function, and produces drowsiness. Adjunct treatment with phenobarbital (Luminal) may allow weaning of the primary opioid, but outpatient therapy with phenobarbital (Luminal) may be prolonged as it is weaned (Hudak, 2015, p. 689; Taketomo et al., 2018, p. 1606–1608).

DIAZEPAM (VALIUM)

- Diazepam (Valium) is not recommended as a first-line treatment drug due a documented lack of efficacy and its adverse effects on the swallow reflex (Sherman, 2015, p. 53).

CLONIDINE (CATAPRES)

- Clonidine (Catapres) stimulates alpha-adrenergic receptor agonist in the brain stem, thus activating an inhibitory neuron that results in reduced sympathetic outflow from the CNS and palliation of symptoms of excess autonomic activity via a negative feedback mechanism (Taketomo et al., 2018, p. 491). It decreases symptoms such as tachycardia, diaphoresis, restlessness, and diarrhea. Clonidine (Catapres) has been used in combination with an opioid to treat withdrawal with limited case series in newborns (Hudak, 2015, p. 689; Patrick, 2017, p. 149).

Weaning

- When an infant is stable on a dose that is effective, weaning should begin and proceed slowly.
  - Weaning regimens vary, with some titrated by Finnegan scores with a frequent wean or increase based on individual scores. Other regimens wean by 10% to 20% of the total (or initial) dose every other day based on mild signs of withdrawal, weight gain, and ability to sleep (Hudak, 2015, p. 689).
  - One example of weaning uses average daily scores and begins to wean with average scores of less than 8 without a single score greater than or equal to 14.
    - Morphine (MS Contin) weans by dose and not interval. The morphine (MS Contin) is weaned first by 10% of the maximum dose every 48 hours as long as the average score remains less than 8 until 25% of the maximum dose is reached.
    - Once the baby is stable (scores less than 8) on 25% of the maximum dose for 48 hours, the morphine (MS Contin) is discontinued.
    - Scoring continues for 48 to 72 hours after the final dose is given. If scores are greater than or equal to 8 after morphine (MS Contin) is off, one rescue dose is considered and then the previous dose level is restarted (Patrick, 2017, p. 148).

Discharge

- An infant with NAS is two and one half times more likely to be readmitted to the hospital within 30 days of discharge than an uncomplicated term infant (Patrick, 2017, p. 155). Signs of NAS can continue for 6 months; therefore, parents and caregivers should be thoroughly educated about infant behaviors following treatment for NAS. In particular infants may be more irritable and less cuddly, and have tremors and increased tone (Weiner & Finnegan, 2016, p. 217).
- Parents should spend extended periods of observed time caring for and interacting with their infant during the hospitalization, which allows the nurse to observe parental interaction with the infant (Smith & Carley, 2014, p. 684). Parents of these infants may need guidance in recognizing behaviors necessitating caregiving and education on substances that

BOX 26.5 Parent teaching in caring for an infant with intrauterine opioid exposure

Some Symptoms May Persist for 2 to 6 Months

- Infants exposed to narcotics in utero are more irritable, less cuddly, and tremulous, and have increased tone: Parent(s) may interpret these behaviors as signs of rejection; infant may not want to be held or cuddled as other babies.
- Less responsive to visual stimulation
- Less likely to maintain a quiet-alert state: Let parent know symptoms are time limited.
- Poor feeding habits: Continues to regurgitate yet shows vigorous sucking of fists or pacifier. Constant sucking and exaggerated rooting reflex may lead to overfeeding the infant.
- Continuation of loose stools: Important to stress good diaper hygiene to prevent infection from excoriated skin.
- Infants easily disturbed by sounds: Parent may decrease stimuli in house.
- Sweats more than other newborns: Dress infant appropriately to avoid overheating.
- High-pitched cry: Not easily consoled; parents need someone to share infant care and give them some rest from an irritable infant to prevent neglect or abuse.
- Hypertonia
- Less eye-to-eye contact, which decreases social interaction

Source: Reproduced with permission from Weiner, S., & Finnegan, L. (2016). Drug withdrawal in the neonate. In S. Gardner, B. Carter, M. Hines, & J. Hernandez (Eds.), *Merenstein & Gardner's handbook of neonatal intensive care* (8th ed., pp. 199–217.e3). St. Louis, MO: Elsevier.

should not be used around infants as they are detrimental to the health of the baby (e.g., tobacco; Weiner & Finnegan, 2016, p. 217). Box 26.5 outlines some possible teaching needs of parents with infants after intrauterine drug exposure.

After Discharge

- Drug use may remain a factor after families are discharged; therefore, they should be followed after discharge by available community services. The pediatrician follow-up should occur within a few days after discharge, additional, home nurse visits, child protective services may become involved if necessary. A referral to early intervention services and other community services may be applicable (Patrick, 2017, p. 155; Smith & Carley, 2014, p. 684). Ideally, infant care would occur in conjunction with maternal care (Patrick, 2017, p. 155).
- SUD does not occur in isolation. Behaviors associated with substance dependence or addiction lead to adverse pregnancy outcomes. Contributing to the development and maintenance of substance use among pregnant women, these factors independently place the family, infant, and child at risk for poor developmental outcomes:
  - Maternal and neonatal/child malnutrition and/or dehydration
  - Impoverished housing
  - Polysubstance use and/or psychiatric comorbidity
  - Exposure to violence and/or physical abuse (Prasad & Jones, 2019, p. 1256)
- When substance-using mothers and their infants were assessed for pattern of interaction, both mothers and

newborns demonstrated poor performance on a measure of social engagement. Mothers demonstrated significantly less positive affect and greater detachment, and the infants presented fewer behaviors promoting social involvement (Weiner & Finnegan, 2016, p. 217). This has wide-reaching implications for bonding and future parent–child interactions. Staff should do what they can to encourage parent–infant contact and interaction while the child is hospitalized in order to maximize feelings of parenthood and lay the foundation for their future interactions.

CONCLUSION

While the NNP will manage primarily the neonate who has experienced intrauterine substance exposure, the import of treating the whole family cannot be overstated. The NNP must have an appreciation for the toll that SUD takes on the adults of the family as well. Regardless of the medication or protocol used in a specific institution, the overall goals remain the same: to decrease the infant's dependence on the substance by balancing the need for treatment with the desire not to extend the infant's hospital stay. The NNP, as part of the entire neonatology staff, has a duty to promote family integrity and prepare the infant and family to function successfully post-discharge.

REVIEW QUESTIONS

1. A mother of a newborn is involved in a therapy program and taking buprenorphine (Subutex) for substance use disorder. She asks the NNP about the option to breastfeed the infant, and the NNP answers based on the knowledge that breastfeeding is:
   A. contraindicated due to the crossing of medication into the breast milk
   B. recommended as long as the mother remains compliant with treatment
   C. vital to forming maternal-infant bond and reducing the risk of child abuse

2. The NNP is called to an emergency cesarean delivery of a term infant after the mother was involved in a car accident. The infant's physical exam reveals shortened palpebral fissures, a thin upper lip, and a smooth philtrum, which indicates to the NNP that the mother may abuse:
   A. alcohol
   B. cocaine
   C. tobacco

3. The NNP is called to assess a 46-hours-old term newborn with a history of intrauterine opioid exposure. Finnegan scores were 4 to 6 but is now increased to an 8. Upon exam, the infant is rooting vigorously and scratching his cheeks, has disturbed tremors with increased tone, is crying inconsolably, and is having loose watery stools. The NNP bases the decision to begin medication therapy based on:
   A. clinical symptoms
   B. finnegan scores
   C. hours of postnatal age

4. An infant who completed 5 days of observation following intrauterine opioid exposure is preparing for discharge. The infant did not require medication during hospitalization. The NNP knows to include in discharge teaching that withdrawal symptoms:
   A. are no longer a risk to the infant's health
   B. may still appear as late at 7 to 14 days
   C. will occur if the infant receives morphine

5. A key to preventing the effects of substance misuse on the fetus and neonate is:
   A. intrauterine detoxification
   B. legalizing prenatal abuse
   C. preconception education

REFERENCES

Blackburn, S. (2013). *Maternal, fetal, & neonatal physiology: A clinical perspective* (4th ed., pp. 183–215). Maryland Heights, MO: Elsevier.

Hudak, M. (2015). Infants with antenatal exposure to drugs. In R. Martin, A. Fanaroff, & M. Walsh (Eds.), *Fanaroff and Martin's neonatal–perinatal medicine: Diseases of the fetus and infant* (10th ed., pp. 682–694). Philadelphia, PA: Elsevier.

Luscher, C. (2015). Drugs of abuse. In B. Katzung, M. Weitz, & P. Boyle (Eds.), *Basic & clinical pharmacology* (13th ed., pp. 552–566). New York, NY: McGraw-Hill Education.

Nocon, J. (2013). Substance use disorders. In D. Mattison (Ed.), *Clinical pharmacology during pregnancy* (pp. 217–256). San Diego, CA: Elsevier.

Patrick, S. (2017). Maternal drug use, infant exposure, and neonatal abstinence syndrome. In E. Eichenwald, A. Hansen, C. Martin, & A. Stark (Eds.), *Cloherty and Stark's manual of neonatal care* (8th ed., pp. 141–157). Philadelphia, PA: Wolters Kluwer.

Prasad, M., & Jones, H (2019) Substance abuse in pregnancy. In R. Resnik, C. Lockwood, T. Moore, M. Greene, J. Copel, & R. Silver (Eds.), *Creasy and Resnik's maternal–fetal medicine: Principles and practice* (8th ed., pp. 1243–1257.e3). Philadelphia, PA: Elsevier.

Reis, P., & Jnah, A. (2017). Perinatal history: Influences on newborn outcome. In B. Snell & S. Gardner (Eds.), *Care of the well newborn* (pp. 69–100). Burlington, MA: Jones & Bartlett Learning.

Sherman, J. (2015). Perinatal substance abuse. In T. Verklan & M. Walden (Eds.), *Core curriculum for neonatal intensive care nursing* (5th ed., pp. 43–57). St. Louis, MO: Elsevier.

Smith, J. R., & Carley, A. (2014). Common neonatal complications. In K. Simpson & P. Creehan (Eds.), *Perinatal nursing* (4th ed., pp. 662–698). St. Louis, MO: Lippincott Williams & Wilkins.

Sullivan, C. (2016). Substance abuse in pregnancy. In S. Mattson & J. Smith (Eds.), *Core curriculum for maternal-newborn nursing* (5th ed., pp. 564–579). St. Louis, MO: Elsevier.

Taketomo, C., Hodding, J., & Kraus, D. (2018). *Lexicomp pediatric & neonatal dosage handbook* (25th ed.). Hudson, OH: Wolters Kluwer.

Wallen, L., & Gleason, C. (2018). Prenatal drug exposure. In C. Gleason & S. Juul (Eds.), *Avery's diseases of the newborn* (10th ed., pp. 126–144.e4). Philadelphia, PA: Elsevier.

Wallman, C. (2018). Assessment of the newborn with antenatal exposure to drugs. In E. P. Tappero & M. E. Honeyfield (Eds.), *Physical assessment of the newborn* (6th ed., pp. 255–262). New York, NY: Springer Publishing Company.

Weiner, S., & Finnegan, L. (2016). Drug withdrawal in the neonate. In S. Gardner, B. Carter, M. Hines, & J. Hernandez (Eds.), *Merenstein & Gardner's handbook of Neonatal intensive care* (8th ed., pp. 199–217.e3). St. Louis, MO: Elsevier.

EVIDENCE-BASED PRACTICE

Patricia E. Thomas

INTRODUCTION

This chapter provides an overview and history of evidence-based practice (EBP) in healthcare. The relationship between EBP and research is described. The process of EBP is outlined and resources for developing EBP projects are provided. Quality improvement is then described with strategies for improving the quality of care for newborns.

Definition and Evolution of EBP

- The process of EBP is the utilization of the best available evidence for care with the integration of nursing expertise and consideration of the individual needs and values of each patient (Polit & Beck, 2018, p. 21; Thomas, 2015, p. 840). In the medical literature, EBP may be referred to as evidence-based medicine (Walsh & Higgins, 2013, p. 1).
- Many factors have contributed to the growth of EBP among healthcare providers. Although there has been growth in the availability of research via database searches, healthcare systems are not always prepared to utilize evidence from research appropriately. The research evidence may be underused, overused, or misused. EBP provides a systematic way to evaluate the available evidence for practice within each individual healthcare system (Pantoja & Hines, 2016). With reimbursement increasingly tied to patient safety initiatives, nursing leaders have come to recognize the importance of organized efforts to improve patient outcomes. EBP is one strategy that can promote consistent quality of care in healthcare organizations (Thomas, 2015, p. 832).
- With their nursing expertise and educational preparation, nurse practitioners are in an excellent position to lead and participate in EBP projects.
  - Graduate nursing programs incorporate the Essentials for MSN Education from the American Association of Colleges of Nursing (AACN) into their curricula. MSN Essential IV is Translating and Integrating Knowledge into Practice (Thomas, 2015, p. 834).
  - AACN DNP Essential III is Clinical Scholarship and Analytical Methods, which includes developing guidelines for EBP (Thomas, 2015, p. 834).

Relationship Between Research and EBP

- Research is the generation of new knowledge. This new knowledge can be used to guide EBP. The EBP process includes taking knowledge gleaned from research and incorporating nursing expertise and patient values to establish best practices (Thomas, 2015, p. 840).

Research Utilization

- All nurses are consumers of research in their practice. Research utilization occurs when nurses identify a problem in the patients in their care and then search for research evidence for solutions. This is the first step toward reducing the gap between research and practice (Thomas, 2015, pp. 832–833).

Levels of Evidence

- One of the challenging aspects of selecting research that is appropriate for use as evidence lies in determining the quality of the research. Although sources vary in their designation of specific levels for each type of study, all reflect the strength of evidence found in meta-analyses of randomized-controlled trials (RCT) such as those published in the Cochrane Database of Systematic Reviews.
- The levels presented in Table 27.1 enable consumers of research to compare the strength of different types of evidence (Polit & Beck, 2018, pp. 23–34; Thomas, 2015, p. 840).

Resources for EBP

- Preappraised sources of evidence are readily available for clinicians to use, including systematic reviews and clinical practice guidelines (Polit & Beck, 2018, p. 25).
  - Systematic reviews are critical appraisals of existing research data using clear criteria. Reviewers who are

TABLE 27.1 Levels of Evidence

Level	Evidence Type
I	Meta-analysis and/or systematic review of RCT
II	Single RCT
III	Quasi-experiment (nonrandomized)
IV	Non experimental study (case-control, cohort, correlational)
V	Systematic reviews of descriptive studies or qualitative studies
VI	Single qualitative study or cross-section study (survey)
VII	Expert opinion, case reports, committee reports

RCT, randomized-controlled trials.

Sources: Data from Polit, D. F., & Beck, C. T. (2018). *Essentials of nursing research: Appraising evidence for nursing practice* (9th ed.). Philadelphia, PA: Wolters Kluwer; Thomas, K. A. (2015). Foundations of neonatal research. In M. T. Verklan & M. Walden (Eds.), *Core curriculum for neonatal intensive care nursing* (6th ed., pp. 832–842). St. Louis, MO: Elsevier Saunders.

transparent in sharing the details of their analysis and ultimate conclusions support the quality of the finished review (Lingappan & Suresh, 2016, p. 45e). Systematic reviews are rich sources of evidence, which can be found in the Cochrane Database of Systematic Reviews as well as in professional journals (Polit & Beck, 2018, p. 25). The international Cochrane Collaboration was formed in 1993 in Oxford, U.K., and is a collection of independent evidence that can be used by providers to inform practice (Polit & Beck, 2018, pp. 21–22).

○ Clinical practice guidelines are another source of pre-appraised evidence. Examples of neonatal clinical practice guidelines are those for skin care, pain management, and peripherally inserted central catheters developed by the National Association of Neonatal Nursing (Smith & Donze, 2015, p. 358).

- For those looking to improve care within their own healthcare system, frameworks exist to guide in the design and implementation of EBP projects. One of the most popular EBP models is the Iowa model of EBP to promote quality care. Others include the Advancing Research and Clinical Practice Through Close Collaboration (ARCC) model, the Johns Hopkins nursing EBP model, and the Promoting Action on Research implementation in Health Services (PARiHS) model (Polit & Beck, 2018, pp. 27–28).

The Process of EBP

- The process of EBP begins when a clinician identifies a question in her clinical practice. The clinician then searches for available evidence in the literature that could solve the clinical problem. Once the available research on the topic has been retrieved, the clinician appraises and synthesizes the evidence to determine which potential solutions are in line with her prior experience and relevant to her practice site. Prior to utilizing the new intervention, the clinician will consider its appropriateness to the individual patient based on the patient and family's beliefs and values. After initiating the new intervention, the clinician will then evaluate its effectiveness (Polit & Beck, 2018, p. 29).

Posing the Question

- Once a clinician has identified an issue in her clinical practice for which there may be solutions within the current body of research, the clinician must formulate the question in a way that will yield results from a literature search.
- The essential elements of the PIO question must identify the patient population (P), intervention (I), and outcome (O) of interest (Polit & Beck, 2018, p. 30).
- An alternate intervention of interest may be included as the comparison (C) treatment, which will result in a PICO question (Polit & Becka, 2018, p. 30).
- Another component which can be added to the PICO question includes that of time frame (T) of the proposed intervention, resulting in a PICOT question (Polit & Beck, 2018, p. 30).
  ○ Examples of PIO, PICO, and PICOT questions:
    ▪ An example of a **PIO** question that an NNP might ask is, "Will adding clindamycin to ampicillin in a VLBW infant with stage 2 necrotizing enterocolitis reduce mortality prior to hospital discharge?" In this example, the patient population (P) is very low

birth weight (VLBW) infants with stage 2 necrotizing enterocolitis. The intervention (I) is the addition of clindamycin. The outcome (O) is reduced mortality.

▪ An example of a **PICO** question is, "Are premature babies who receive Curosurf® less likely to develop bronchopulmonary dysplasia than those who receive Infasurf®?" In this example, the patient population (P) is premature babies. The intervention (I) is Curosurf®. The comparison (C) is Infasurf® and the outcome (O) is bronchopulmonary dysplasia.

▪ An example of a **PICOT** question is, "Do term newborns who are given glucose gel prior to a heel stick have lower pain scores on the NIPS than babies who are only swaddled?" The patient population (P) in this example is term babies. The intervention (I) is glucose gel with a comparison (C) of swaddling. The timing (T) of the intervention is prior to heel stick and the outcome (O) is pain score on the Neonatal Infant Pain Scale (NIPS).

Searching for Evidence

- The plethora of available evidence means that the search for relevant evidence can be the most time-consuming part of the EBP process. In order to narrow the search to one that will yield the highest quality results, Walsh and Higgins (2013) recommend starting with the Cochrane Collaboration database and then searching Google Scholar (p. 2). Additional individual research studies published in professional journals can then be found from searching medical databases such as PubMed (Walsh & Higgins, 2013, p. 2). Lingappan and Suresh (2016) recommend using the "Clinical Queries" feature in PubMed to focus the search (p. 41e).

Appraising the Evidence

- One strategy to ensure the quality of the evidence used in the EBP process is to use preappraised evidence such as that found in systematic reviews and meta-analyses, which can be found in the Cochrane Database of Systematic Reviews and clinical practice guidelines (Polit & Beck, 2018, p. 25). When evaluating individual sources of evidence, the level of the evidence can be determined from Table 27.1. For single studies, RCT provides the strongest evidence for practice as randomization of patients to treatment groups is the best way to assess the effect of the treatment (Walsh & Higgins, 2013, p. 3).

Integrating Evidence in EBP

- Once the practitioner identifies relevant evidence in the literature to answer the PIO, PICO, or PICOT question, the next step is to integrate those findings into the individual's setting and experience. Each practitioner views evidence for practice through the lens of his or her own clinical experience. In addition, the practitioner has knowledge of the clinical setting which must be considered when utilizing research findings for practice. The process of EBP must include consideration of patient values and preferences, as well (Polit & Beck, 2018, p. 33).

Implementing Evidence and Evaluating Outcomes

- After completing the steps outlined above, the practitioner is ready to make the evidence-based decision for the patients' care. The final step in the process is evaluation. The question must be asked, Did the action that was made based on the EBP process improve the patient outcome as expected? It can be challenging to answer that question as an individual, and that is why some EBP questions are better answered within a group, such as the organization in which care is provided (Polit & Beck, 2018, p. 34).

Promoting EBP Within Organizations

- While the essential steps of the EBP process are the same for groups and individuals, there are factors that should be considered when engaging in a group or organizational EBP project. The trigger for an EBP project within an organization may evolve from staff's concern over an issue they are seeing in practice or may be generated from the discovery of a new clinical practice guideline or recommendation from a national organization (Polit & Beck, 2018, p. 34).
- For EBP projects within an organization, Polit and Beck (2018) recommend that a model of EBP, such as the Iowa model, be used to ensure that a proper site-specific assessment is made prior to the project and that strategies are developed to ensure staff support with the proposed practice change (pp. 34–35). Also, training of staff on the new intervention and an evaluation plan are crucial to the success of an organizational EBP project (Polit & Beck, 2018, p. 35).

Quality Improvement

- Medical and nursing providers of healthcare must work together to ensure the quality and safety of their patients through the process of continuous quality improvement. Hospital performance on quality indicators is increasingly important as results are being shared publicly and with accrediting organizations. Patient outcomes vary in NICUs across the world (Profit, Lee, Gould, & Horbar, 2015, p. 59). Quality-of-care issues may include the overuse, underuse, and/or misuse of interventions (Profit et al., 2015, p. 60). The systematic use of quality improvement can be used to improve the quality and safety of the care delivered to babies in the NICU (Profit et al., 2015, p. 59).

Assessing and Monitoring the Quality of Care

- The choice of quality indicators to be monitored depends upon the individual NICU's priorities, practice patterns, and resources including access to databases on patient outcomes. Clinicians utilize outcome data on quality indicators from databases such as the Vermont Oxford Network or the Pediatrix neonatal database to benchmark their own unit's performance. Common quality improvement (QI) indicators of interest involve patient safety, such as medication errors and nosocomial infection rates (Suresh & Ragahavan, 2016, p. 50e).

Team Approach

- Unlike EBP, which can be used by any individual practitioner, QI requires a team approach. A core group of clinicians dedicated to each QI project is necessary. In addition to the work of the QI process, these individuals are responsible for garnering the collaboration of their professional peers in the NICU as well as ensuring the cooperation of those who are involved in the babies' care (Suresh & Ragahavan, 2016, p. 51e).

Identifying Aims

- The first step of any QI project is to determine the aim, or focus, of the project. The team should identify patient problems in their individual unit that could be viewed as an opportunity for improvement (Suresh & Ragahavan, 2016, p. 51e). The aim should be phrased in a way that it is "specific, measureable, achievable, realistic, and time-bound" (Suresh & Ragahavan, 2016, p. 51e). Examples of patient outcomes that are often of interest to NICU QI teams include bronchopulmonary dysplasia, intraventricular hemorrhage, and retinopathy of prematurity (Suresh & Ragahavan, 2016, p. 51e).

Measurement

- Effective QI projects rely on measurement of outcomes. The QI process begins with measurement of the outcome of interest prior to initiation of any changes to establish a baseline. This baseline can be compared with benchmark data retrieved from a neonatal database to determine priorities for the individual NICU. The Vermont Oxford Network was developed by neonatologists in the late 1980s to improve the safety of care for newborns (Palma & Tarczy-Hornoch, 2018). The next step involves process mapping where the steps of a care intervention are broken down to determine which factors may be affecting the patient outcome of interest. Next, members of the team search for available evidence on interventions which could improve the outcome of interest in their patients (Suresh & Ragahavan, 2016, pp. 51e–52e).

PDSA Cycles

- Once the desired change in practice has been identified and implemented, clinicians can use a plan-do-study-act (PDSA) cycle to test the change. The intervention is planned (plan), is implemented in practice (do), outcome data are collected (study), and outcome data are evaluated to determine what changes (if any) should be made (act) at that point (Suresh & Ragahavan, 2016, pp. 52e–53e).

Overcoming Barriers

- With the focus on quality improvement from accrediting bodies, it is essential for every NICU to embody the culture of continuous QI. While this culture must include all levels of caregivers, the commitment of leadership to continuous quality improvement (CQI) is essential to the success of any QI project. Potential barriers to a specific project can be identified by leaders and QI committee members by meetings with caregivers on all shifts to hear any concerns and to note their recommendations for the project (Suresh & Ragahavan, 2016, p. 54e).

CONCLUSION

EBP is the integration of the best available research for practice into patient care with consideration of the patients' values and clinicians' experience. The process begins with the identification of important clinical questions. Then PIO questions are formulated and relevant evidence is evaluated for use. Models exist to help formulate and implement EBP projects within organizations.

Quality improvement is the process by which clinicians identify possible measures to improve the quality of care for patients. Many QI initiatives have a focus on patient safety. PDSA cycles can be used to implement and monitor the effectiveness of quality initiatives.

REVIEW QUESTIONS

1. Evidence-based practice (EBP) is informed by research with the integration of provider expertise and:
   A. patient beliefs and values
   B. patient educational preparation
   C. provider educational preparation

2. A new NNP graduate volunteers to participate in an evidence-based practice (EBP) project in the NICU. The leader of the EBP team asks what expertise the NNP could lend to the project. Which of the following would be the best response?
   A. I was a research assistant in an animal lab during graduate school.
   B. My graduate nursing program included a course in translating research into practice.
   C. My manager requires that all NNPs participate in unit committees.

3. Key differences between research and evidence-based practice (EBP) include:
   A. the originality of results
   B. systematic approach
   C. values in management

REFERENCES

Lingappan, K., & Suresh, G. K. (2016). Evidence-based respiratory care. In J. P. Goldsmith, E. Karotkin, G. Suresh, & M. Kessler (Eds.), *Assisted ventilation of the neonate: An evidence-based approach to newborn respiratory care* (6th ed., pp. 41e–48e). Philadelphia, PA: Elsevier Saunders.

Palma, J. P., & Tarczy-Hornoch, P. (2018). Biomedical informatics in neonatology. In C. A. Gleason & S. E. Juul (Eds.), *Avery's diseases of the newborn* (10th ed., pp. 11–19). Philadelphia, PA: Elsevier.

Pantoja, A. F., & Hines, M. E. (2016). Evidence-based clinical practice. In S. L. Gardner, B. S. Carter, M. Enzman Hines, & J. A. Hernandez (Eds.), *Merenstein & Gardner's handbook of neonatal intensive care* (8th ed.). St. Louis, MO: Elsevier.

Polit, D. F., & Beck, C. T. (2018). *Essentials of nursing research: Appraising evidence for nursing practice* (9th ed.). Philadelphia, PA: Wolters Kluwer.

Profit, J., Lee, H. C., Gould, J. B., & Horbar, J. D. (2015). Evaluating and improving the quality and safety of neonatal intensive care. In R. J. Martin, A. A. Fanaroff, & M. C. Walsh (Eds.), *Fanaroff and Martin's neonatal–perinatal medicine: Disease of the fetus and infant* (10th ed., Vol. 1, pp. 59–88). Philadelphia, PA: Elsevier Saunders.

Smith, J. R., & Donze, A. (2015). Patient safety. In M. T. Verklan & M. Walden (Eds.), *Core curriculum for neonatal intensive care nursing* (5th ed., pp. 348–372). St. Louis, MO: Elsevier Saunders.

Suresh, G. K., & Raghavan, A. (2016). Quality and safety in respiratory care. In J. P. Goldsmith, E. Karotkin, G. Suresh, & M. Kessler (Eds.), *Assisted ventilation of the neonate: An evidence-based approach to newborn respiratory care* (6th ed., pp. 49e–55e). Philadelphia, PA: Elsevier Saunders.

Thomas, K. A. (2015). Foundations of neonatal research. In M. T. Verklan & M. Walden (Eds.), *Core curriculum for neonatal intensive care nursing* (6th ed., pp. 832–842). St. Louis, MO: Elsevier Saunders.

Walsh, M. C., & Higgins, R. D. (2013). Evidence-based medicine and the role of networks in generating evidence. In A. A. Fanaroff & J. M. Fanaroff (Eds.), *Klaus & Fanaroff's care of the high-risk neonate* (6th ed., pp. 1–9). Philadelphia, PA: Elsevier Saunders.

28 LEGAL, ETHICAL, AND COMMUNICATION ISSUES

Rebecca Chuffo Davila

INTRODUCTION

Professional, ethical, and legal issues are important concepts for all NNPs. Knowing and understanding key concepts related to ethics and the law will only enhance the NNP's practice. This chapter explores ethical theories and frameworks as they relate to nursing. Key legal concepts such as tort law, malpractice, and liability will be addressed. Other topics will include the consent process, the importance of accurate documentation, and privacy rights. Finally, the topic of staffing and safety issues related to NNP practice will be reviewed.

PROFESSIONAL ISSUES

Ethical Theories

Three ethical theories that are commonly referenced in bioethics are *Kantianism, Utilitarianism, and Liberal Individualism* (Sudia-Robinson, 2015, p. 845).
- Kantianism, or deontology, is an obligation-based theory from the 1700s. This theory requires that individuals act with a sense of obligation. This theory, however, lacks direction in what to do if there are conflicting obligations.
- Utilitarianism focuses on the maximization of the goodness of an act. The decision-maker has to identify the greatest good while balancing the interests of all affected. This theory was also from the 1700s and its application to present day NICUs may not be relevant.
- Liberal Individualism addresses the rights, both positive and negative, that individuals in our society possess. A positive right requires someone to do something for another individual in need. A negative right keeps individuals from being directly harmed by others (Sudia-Robinson, 2015, pp. 845–846).

Ethical Decision-Making Frameworks

- The NNP's ability to respond to ethical dilemmas may be influenced by four factors as described by Guido (2014):
  - The nurse's perception of his or her level of influence within the healthcare setting
  - Level of clinical expertise and competence
  - Degree of ethical concern
  - Past experience with ethics education
- Ethical decision-making frameworks can help guide one in resolving ethical dilemmas. Various models for ethical decision-making typically have five to 14 ordered steps that begin with fully comprehending the ethical dilemmas and conclude with the evaluation of the implemented decision (Guido, 2014, p. 44).
- The **MORAL** model may be one of the easier models to use for NNPs at the bedside. This model includes the following steps:
  - **M**assage the dilemma. Identify and define the issues. Consider the opinions of the major stakeholders as well as their value system.
  - **O**utline the options. Examine all options fully, including the less realistic and the conflicting ones. Identify all the pros and cons. This stage is to evaluate options and not to make the final decision.
  - **R**esolve the dilemma. Review the issues and options, applying basic ethical principles to each option.
  - **A**ct by applying the chosen option. This step requires actual implementation.
  - **L**ook back and evaluate the entire process. Ensure that all involved are able to follow through on the final option. If they cannot, then a second decision may be necessary and the whole process should begin again (Guido, 2014, p. 44).

Ethical Foundations of Healthcare and Nursing Practice

- Ethics: From the Greek word *ethos*, meaning "custom" or "character"; established by Socrates. The Socratic discipline deals with what is good or bad and with moral duty and obligation (Stephenson, 2016, p. 662).

PROFESSIONAL CODE OF ETHICS
- The professional code of ethics enumerates standards of integrity, professionalism, and ethical norms for members of a given discipline (Guido, 2014, p. 43).
  - *Bioethics* is a subdivision of ethics to determine the most morally desirable course of action in healthcare when there are conflicting values inherent in varying treatment options (Stephenson, 2016, p. 662).
  - *Metaethics* is the division of ethics where professional ethicists or philosophers attempt to analyze reasons behind the ethical principles (Stephenson, 2016, p. 663).
  - *Descriptive ethics* is where sociologists, anthropologists, psychologists, historians, and others describe or attempt to explain moral behaviors and why humans are moral (Stephenson, 2016, p. 663).
  - *Normative ethics* are moral standards based on the fundamental principle that determines right or wrong (Stephenson, 2016, p. 664).

○ *Consequentialism or goal outcomes ethics* explains that the rightness or wrongness of an act depends on its utility, usefulness, or outcome. Right consists of actions that have good consequences, and wrong consists of actions that have bad consequences (Stephenson, 2016, p. 665).

○ *Principle-based ethics* attempts to identify the fundamental principles that form the foundation of ethical deliberation (Swaney, English, & Carter, 2016, p. 927).

○ *Virtue ethics* is based in character and therefore identifies moral aspects rather than the applied principles (Swaney et al., 2016, p. 927).

○ *Narrative ethics* uses the narrative of the story itself as the method of clinical reasoning (Swaney et al., 2016, p. 927).

- Related principles guiding healthcare and nursing practice:
  ○ Social contract theory holds that individual moral behavior, moral responsibility, and accountability are influenced by social context, social structures, and public policy issues (Stephenson, 2016, p. 665).
  ○ Duty and obligation involves a duty to follow universally accepted rules of what is right and wrong (Stephenson, 2016, p. 664).
  ○ Principles of autonomy, beneficence, nonmaleficence, and justice are summarized in Table 28.1 (Stephenson, 2016, p. 664).

- Ethics in nursing are utilized as foundational professional knowledge and ongoing teaching and learning.

- On the national level, the American Nurses Association (ANA) first published a code for nurses in 1950, most recently revised in 2001. The Code of Ethics for Nurses with Interpretive Statements has nine provisions regarding the professional practice of nursing, and serves the following purposes: It gives direction for those entering the nursing profession about their ethical accountability, sets a nursing standard for ethical practice, and informs the consumer about nursing's ethical standards (Guido, 2014, p. 43). The concepts of caring and nursing are intertwined. The "Five 'C's' of Caring" are Compassion, Conscience, Competence, Commitment, and Confidence (Stephenson, 2016, pp. 666–667).
  ○ For the NICU nurse, primary professional guidance is provided through the ANA Code of Ethics for Nurses with Interpretive Statements (Sudia-Robinson, 2015, p. 884); the ANA Position Statements on Ethics and Human Rights.

- Neonatal nurses utilize the ethical guidance as established by professional nursing organizations, such as the ANA Code of Ethics (2015) and the National Association of Neonatal Nurses (NANN, 1999) Position Statement on NICU Nurse Involvement in Ethical Decisions. These key documents provide the foundation for ethical practice in the NICU (Sudia-Robinson, 2015, p. 884).

- The NICU NNP plays a critical role in both direct care of the neonate and support for the parents. Parents will need help coping and understanding all the intricacies of the NICU. They will also need support to learn how to care for their infant (Sudia-Robinson, 2015, p. 847). NNPs, along with other members of the healthcare team, have an obligation to keep the parents thoroughly informed of the infant's condition and honestly outline the risks and benefits of that care (Sudia-Robinson, 2015, p. 847).

NNPs' Professional Regulation and Practice

- Credentials are the practitioner's proof of qualifications. Nursing credentials are those of licensure and certification. NNPs, like all other advanced practice registered nurses (APRNs), require licensure and certification (Guido, 2014, p. 200).

- The legal description of the NNPs scope of practice according to state law is important for the following reasons:
  ○ To establish the NNP as a professional entity and allow NNPs to perform at their level of education and training. By doing so, the NNP avoids any charges of practicing medicine without a license; however, it will allow for reimbursement for physician services, when provided by an NNP. Accountability for both benefits and harm to patients is placed squarely on the NNP.
  ○ Each state has its own set of nurse practice acts. Some states are more restrictive than others when it comes to APRNs. However, with more autonomy of practice also comes increased responsibility. Advance practice providers have a legal responsibility to their patients.

- A *Standard of Care* is the minimum criteria by which proficiency is defined in the clinical arena. There are five basic types of evidence that are used to establish the legal standard of care. Those include:

TABLE 28.1 Four Key Principles Needed to Examine Ethical Issues

Beneficence	This ethical principle is derived from the Hippocratic Oath, which states a duty to help others and to balance good and harm. Some people, however, may have difficulty in deciding what is "good" for others.
Nonmaleficence	This ethical principle is also derived from the Hippocratic Oath. It is an obligation to "first do no harm." A person must avoid intentional harm. The key aspect of this principle is the intent of the healthcare provider's actions.
Respect autonomy	Autonomy addresses personal freedom. There are four important concepts of autonomy: liberty, self-determination, independence, and agency. Liberty is the freedom to choose without coercion. Self-determination is the ability to access information and then act upon it with the understanding of that information. Independence is the ability to act, reason, and decide for oneself. And agency is the power to be in command and responsible for one's actions.
Justice	This ethical principle is derived from Aristotle. It is the obligation to treat individuals equally or comparably and to distribute benefits and burdens equally throughout society.

Sources: Data from Guido, G. W. (2014). *Legal and ethical issues in nursing* (6th ed., pp. 35–38). Upper Saddle River, NJ: Pearson Education; Stephenson, C. (2016). Ethics. In S. Mattson & J. Smith (Eds.), *Core curriculum for maternal-newborn nursing* (5th ed., pp. 664–665). St. Louis, MO: Elsevier; Sudia-Robinson, T. (2015) Ethical issues. In T. Verklan, & M. Walden, (Eds.), *Core curriculum for neonatal intensive care nursing* (5th ed., pp. 845–855). St. Louis, MO: Elsevier.

- State and federal regulations
- Institutional policies
- Procedures and protocols
- Testimony from expert witnesses
- Standards of professional organizations and current professional literature (Verklan, 2015, p. 851)
- State and federal regulations establish NNPs' care and scope of practice (Verklan, 2015, p. 851). Hospital policies, procedures, and protocols are very important to acknowledge and outline the standard of care for that particular institution. Standards are also outlined by NNPs' various professional organizations. It is very important for practitioners to utilize the most up-to-date evidence and keep current with practice guidelines.
- Professional decision-making should be based on standards of care and ethical concepts of duty, beneficence, and nonmaleficence (Stephenson, 2016, p. 670). Treatment goals for NICU infants should include contribution by both healthcare professionals and parents, respecting parental autonomy so that there is a common plan.

LEGAL ISSUES

- Though each state has its own practice act, some things ring true for any state in which NNPs practice. With increasing scope of practice, autonomy, and authority, there is an increase risk in greater exposure to liability situations. APRNs are held to a higher standard than RNs when it comes to legal liability. All NNPs should be familiar with legal terms and precedence.

Torts

- Tort law is the most commonly seen classification of law in healthcare settings. A tort is a civil wrong committed against a person or the person's property. Tort law is based in fault and applicable to situations where a professional either failed to meet his or her responsibility or performed the act below the allowable standard of care. Torts are civil wrongs based on personal transgressions rather than contracts (Guido, 2014, p. 69).

Negligence and Malpractice

- *Negligence* is a general term that denotes conduct lacking in due care and equates with carelessness. A person commits negligence when deviating from actions a reasonable person would use in a particular set of circumstances. The reverse is also true, in that negligence may also denote a person acting in a manner that the reasonable and prudent person would **not** act (Guido, 2014, p. 69).
  - To clarify, a *mistake in judgment* is not evidence of negligence if the nurse possesses reasonable and ordinary skills akin to professional colleagues. The nurse will not be guilty of negligence even if the decision made subsequently proves incorrect (Verklan, 2015, p. 853).
- *Malpractice*, or *professional negligence*, is a more specific term that addresses a professional standard of care. Malpractice has routinely been defined by the courts as any professional misconduct, or unreasonable lack of skill or fidelity, in professional duties which then resulted in injury, unnecessary suffering, or death to the injured party. There must be a clear precedent of ignorance, carelessness, want

of proper professional skill, disregard of established rules and principles, neglect, or a malicious or criminal intent.
  - In a more modern definition, malpractice is the failure of a professional person to act in accordance with the prevailing professional standards or failure to foresee consequences that a professional person, having the necessary skills and education, should foresee (Guido, 2014, p. 69; Verklan, 2015, p. 853).
  - To be liable for malpractice, the tortfeasor (person committing the civil wrong) must be a professional such as a nurse, NPP, or physician (Guido, 2014, p. 69).

ELEMENTS OF MALPRACTICE OR NEGLIGENCE

- To be successful in a court case involving malpractice or negligence, the plaintiff (injured party) must prove the following four elements in a malpractice case; a malpractice suit cannot be won if all four elements are not present (Verklan, 2015, p. 854):
  - A duty was owed to the patient.
    - An individual is under a legal duty to act as an ordinary, prudent, reasonable person would act given the same set of circumstances, including taking precautions against risk of injury to other persons (Guido, 2014, p. 70).
  - There was a breach of that duty.
  - Harm or damage occurred to the patient.
  - Breach of the duty resulted in harm (proximal cause):
    - This involves showing a deviation from the standard of care owed the patient—that is, something was done that should not have been done or nothing was done when it should have been done (Guido, 2014, p. 70; Verklan, 2015, p. 853).

AVOIDING MALPRACTICE CLAIMS

- NNPs should practice without fear of legal ramifications. Common sense and understanding of patients and their families is important. Being empathetic and genuine are traits that are desirable in the medical profession (Box 28.1). NNPs are rarely sued, but do need to be aware of malpractice law and follow a few basic recommendations:
  - Always be honest and respectful with patients and their families.
  - Know relevant law and legal doctrine. (Just saying "I didn't know" is not a defense!)
  - Be a lifelong learner.
  - Join and support your professional organizations.
  - Know and understand that many malpractice claims occur from lack of knowledge of patient education and discharge planning issues (Guido, 2014, pp. 83–84).

Examples of other legal pitfalls to avoid are summarized in Box 28.2.

BOX 28.1 What NNPs can do to avoid negligent torts

- Treat patients and their families with dignity and respect.
- Use your education knowledge.
- First line of duty is to the patient.
- Be current and up-to-date on your skills and education.
- Document
- Ensure that parental education is thorough prior to discharging the infant home.

(continued)

Liability

- Nurses and NNPs are recognized as professionals who are responsible and accountable for the care they give to their patients (Verklan, 2015, p. 853). If the nurse/NNP is liable to the patient because of negligent conduct, that nurse/NNP can be held legally responsible for the harm incurred by the patient. APRNs are held to a higher standard than a registered nurse due to the necessary training and education that is necessary to become an NNP. The standard of care expected of the APRN is the degree of care expected of any reasonable and prudent APRN who practices in the same specialty (Verklan, 2015, p. 858).
- The most common areas in which APRNs have incurred liability are the following:
  - Conduct exceeding their scope of expertise, resulting in damages
  - Conduct exceeding physician-delegated authority, resulting in damages
  - Practicing independently in a state that mandates a sponsoring physician
  - Failure of referral
  - Failure to correctly diagnose (Verklan, 2015, p. 853)
- The costs of liability when a neonate is involved are high for three reasons: (1) the costs of healthcare for a damaged infant with a normal life expectancy are high, (2) there is a longer statute of limitations for minors, and (3) sympathy toward the family (Verklan, 2015, p. 854).
- Essentially four types of damages may be compensated:
  - General damages are inherent to the injury itself.
  - Special damages account for all losses and expenses incurred as a result of the injury.
  - Emotional damages may be compensated if there is apparent physical harm as well.
  - Punitive or exemplary damages may be awarded if there is malicious, willful, or wanton misconduct (Guido, 2014, p. 76).

Consent

- Consent has two key components:
  - The prevention of a battery (nonconsensual touching)
  - The person's right to control what is done to his or her body (Guido, 2014, p. 118)
- In getting consent for procedures and consent for research studies, one must be sure that the patient or the patient's legal representative understands fully and does not feel coerced in any way (Polit & Beck, 2018, p. 83).
  - *Informed consent* is the voluntary authorization by a patient or the patient's legal representative to do something to the patient. The key to true and valid consent is patient (or legal representative) comprehension (Guido, 2014, p. 118).
  - *Expressed consent* is consent given by direct words, written or oral (Guido, 2014, p. 119). *Implied consent* refers to the patient's conduct or what may be perceived in an emergency situation. For emergency consent, the patient must not able to make their wishes known and a delay in providing care could have devastating outcomes that may lead to death (Guido, 2014, p. 119).
- To satisfy the definition of informed consent, the consent needs to be authorized by someone who has the legal capacity for giving such consent. In most cases this is the patient or the patient's legal representative.
  - The person giving the consent must fully comprehend the procedure to be done and who will be doing it; the risks involved; expected or desired outcomes; any complications or side effects; and alternative therapies, including none at all (Guido, 2014, p. 129).
  - Our society has designated parents as the patient's legal representative, with rights to make decisions about their children; however, there are a variety of reasons why a social worker or a state-appointed guardian may be designated the patient's legal representative (Stephenson, 2016, p. 669; Verklan, 2015, p. 862).
- The right of consent also involves the right of refusal. For *informed refusal*, the patient or the patient's legal representative have to fully understand what the consequences are to them (or their child) by their refusal of treatment or diagnostic tests (Guido, 2014, p. 118).
- Courts recognize the following four exceptions to the need for informed consent in circumstances in which consent is required:
  - *Emergency situations*, as these give rise to implied consent
  - *Therapeutic privileges* describes the situation where caregivers are allowed to withhold information based on the emotional stability of the recipient and that could potentially cause significant harm to the recipient.
  - *Patient waiver* is used when the patient or the patient's legal representative does not wish to know about the potential complications or risks. This is the only situation in which the patient or the patient's legal representative may initiate a consent waver; medical personnel are not allowed to initiate the conversation.
  - *Prior patient knowledge* waiver is in effect when the procedure has been explained to the patient or the patient's

legal representative with a previous procedure. The consent process does not need to be repeated (Guido, 2014, p. 121–122).

- The physician or the NNP has the responsibility of obtaining informed consent on procedures for which they are responsible (Verklan, 2015, p. 862).
- Professionals have an ethical and legal obligation to inform parents with facts regarding care of their neonate. The NNP and/or physician should update parents on their infant's diagnosis, and what interventions are available given the infant's overall condition. Being truthful regarding outcomes, risks, and benefits of certain procedures is imperative (Stephenson, 2016, p. 670).

Documentation

- The most important purpose of documentation is communication (Guido, 2014, p. 154).
- Documentation is a professional responsibility. Medical records are used by attorneys to provide evidence in legal proceedings.
  - For proper documentation, all entries must be signed with name and proper credentials. Proper documentation also includes avoiding inappropriate comments, making corrections to charting appropriately, documenting events accurately and concisely, and documenting objectively and promptly (Verklan, 2015, pp. 859–861).
- Effective documentation includes an entry for every observation in clear and objective language that is factual and realistic. Chart only your observations, chart refusal of care, and chart all patient education.
  - Never alter the medical record at someone else's request.
  - Use of standardized checklists, daily notes, and procedure notes may help in preventing liability (Guido, 2014, pp. 154–168).

Confidentiality/Right to Privacy

NNPs have the duty to maintain and protect patients' and their families' confidentiality of their medical records. The right to privacy should always be maintained (Polit and Beck, 2018, p. 82).

HIPAA and PHI

- In August 1996, President Bill Clinton signed the Health Insurance Portability and Accountability Act (HIPAA) into law (Public law 104–191; Guido, 2014, p. 177). This act provides for:
- The portability of healthcare coverage through the streamlining of the transfer of patient information between insurers and providers
- An antifraud and abuse program
- Tax incentives toward the acquisition of health insurance and accelerated benefits
- The establishment of the federal government as a national healthcare regulator (Guido, 2014, p. 177)
- HIPAA also protects patients' protected health information (PHI). Information such as name, phone number, Social Security number, and other unique identifiers are PHI. One should only know pertinent information that is needed to care for your patient. Violations of HIPAA could result in termination and loss of license (Guido, 2014, pp. 177–179).

STAFFING AND SAFETY ISSUES

- The National Association of Neonatal Nurse Practitioners (NANNP) acknowledges the limited evidence upon which to recommend specific patient-to-NNP ratios or caseload ranges for workload management. NNP workload must take into account the clinical setting, patient acuity, resources, census, team workload distribution, flexibility in role expectation, shift length, and competence level (NANN, 2013, p. 4).
- The following guidelines have been established by NANN and the NANNP council. NANNP and its members are committed to providing safe, ethical, and professionally accountable care. Position statements have been developed that address the issues of NNP workload and on shift length and fatigue. The NNP workload should:
  - Consider the NNPs level of competence and experience.
  - Be consistent with the body of evidence related to fatigue and its impact on safety and quality (NANN, 2015, p. 2).
  - Evaluate the level of patient acuity and other functional responsibilities that may occupy the attention and concentration of the NNP (NANN, 2013, p. 2).
- Determinations of site-specific workloads should be supported through outcomes monitoring, including and amount and length of time spent on:
  - Reviewing delivery room resuscitation documentation and adherence to the neonatal resuscitation program and/or average amount of time spent per delivery
  - Documentation and/or billing/charges
  - Discharge management, parental satisfaction with NNPs, and/or customer complaints, including grievances
  - Reviewing adverse events
- NNP workload cannot only include the hands-on patient care in the delivery room and/or at the bedside. Workloads must also take into consideration time for the NNP to fully participate in personal and professional development of leadership, process improvement, clinical practice, consultation, research, education, and advocacy (NANN, 2013, p. 7).
- The NNP shift length and prevention of fatigue should include education related to recognition and management of fatigue and system management.
  - Workplace fatigue remains a critical issue in healthcare. NNPs are accountable for ensuring they are fit to care for their patients and their families. NNPs are encouraged to create responsible staffing patterns and work models in their institutions that would promote decrease in fatigue and foster patient and personal safety (NANN, 2015, p. 9).
- NNPs in practice may be called on to precept NNP students. Students are required to complete 600 hours of clinical time in the NICU with preceptors who are, at a minimum, master's prepared and nationally certified with a minimum of 1-year full-time-equivalent employment at the clinical site. These requirements ensure that the preceptor at a given site has the clinical expertise and the familiarity with the site to provide the best supervision of the NNP student (NANN, 2013, p. 12).
  - The preceptor-to-student ratio should not exceed 1:2, and the preceptors for other clinical experiences (i.e., antenatal, intrapartum, and primary care) must have the clinical expertise necessary to provide safe guidance

and education for the NNP student. Preceptors must be oriented to NNP program requirements and expectations for the supervision and evaluation of the NNP student. Preceptors must also be evaluated annually for the purpose of ensuring quality of the NNP students' learning experiences and overall relationship with student learners (NANN, 2017, p. 13).

CONCLUSION

The understanding of ethical and legal issues is critical for all NNPs. As NNPs, we cannot practice fully unless we have knowledge of these key concepts. NNPs who have proper training and education should not have to practice in fear of legal ramifications; but having an understanding of the law and ways to prevent negligence and malpractice are so very important. Understanding ethical concepts will not only help in your practice day to day, but will guide you through many tough situations personally and professionally.

REVIEW QUESTIONS

1. The prevention of battery and the person's right to control what is done to their body are the components of:
   A. confidentiality
   B. consent
   C. malpractice

2. The four elements that must be proven to win a malpractice case are: a duty owed, breach of that duty, harm or damage, and:
   A. absent documentation
   B. negativity of intent
   C. proximal cause

3. The NNP understands the importance of treating all patients and their families equally, and by doing this is practicing the ethical principle of:
   A. beneficence
   B. justice
   C. respect

REFERENCES

American Nurses Association. (2015). *Code of ethics for nurses with interpretive statements*. Silver Spring, MD: nursingbooks.org. Retrieved from https://www.nursingworld.org/practice-policy/nursing-excellence/ethics/code-of-ethics-for-nurses/coe-view-only/

Guido, G. W. (2014). *Legal and ethical issues in nursing* (6th ed., pp. 42–53). Upper Saddle River, NJ: Pearson Education.

National Association of Neonatal Nurses. (1999). *Position statement #3015: NICU nurse involvement in ethical decisions*. Retrieved from http://nann.org/uploads/About/PositionPDFS/1.4.12_Nurse%20Involvment%20in%20Ethical%20Decisions.pdf

National Association of Neonatal Nurses. (2013). *Neonatal nurse practitioner workforce* [Position Statement #3058]. Retrieved from http://nann.org/uploads/About/PositionPDFS/NNP_Workforce_Position_Statement_01.22.13_FINAL.pdf

National Association of Neonatal Nurses. (2015). *The effect of staff nurses' shift length and fatigue on patient safety and nurses' health* [Position Statement #3066]. Retrieved from http://nann.org/uploads/About/PositionPDFS/1.4.1_Effect%20of%20Staff%20Nurses%20Shift%20Length%20and%20Fatigue%20on%20Patient%20Safety%20and%20Nurses%20Health.pdf

Polit, D., & Beck, C. (Eds.). (2018). *Essentials of nursing research: Appraising evidence for nursing practice* (9th ed., pp. 77–91). Philadelphia, PA: Wolters Kluwer.

Stephenson, C. (2016). Ethics. In S. Mattson & J. Smith (Eds.), *Core curriculum for maternal-newborn nursing* (5th ed., pp. 662–681). St. Louis, MO: Elsevier.

Sudia-Robinson, T. (2015) Ethical issues. In T. Verklan, & M. Walden, (Eds.), *Core curriculum for neonatal intensive care nursing* (5th ed., pp. 843–848). St. Louis, MO: Elsevier.

Swaney, J., English, N., & Carter, B. (2016) Ethics, values, and palliative care in neonatal intensive care. In S. Gardner, B. Carter, M. Hines, & J. Hernandez (Eds.), *Merenstein & Gardner's handbook of neonatal intensive care* (8th ed. pp. 924–945.e3). St. Louis, MO: Elsevier.

Verklan, M. T. (2015). Legal issues. In T. Verklan, & M. Walden (Eds.), *Core curriculum for neonatal intensive care nursing* (5th ed., pp. 849–865). St. Louis, MO: Elsevier.

29 PATIENT SAFETY

Terri Schneider-Biehl
Amy Koehn

INTRODUCTION

Since 1999, patient safety has become a national priority. That year, the Institute of Medicine of the National Academy of Sciences issued two landmark reports that set a challenge to all levels of healthcare professionals to improve the safety and quality of care for all patients and families. Medically fragile NICU patients are at a great risk for medical errors that lead to adverse events due to the fast-paced and complex environment. In the NICU, care is around the clock, with multiple team members and many handoffs, high-technology equipment, weight-based medication, and neonates who have limited physiologic capacity to defend against adverse events; and, they are nonverbal, which adds to the risk of medical errors. There are many agencies and resources available to assist with identifying risk and applying quality-improvement processes to help prevent errors.

KEY CONCEPTS IN PATIENT SAFETY

Quality in Healthcare

- The National Academy of Medicine, formerly known as the Institute of Medicine (IOM), defines *healthcare quality* as the degree to which individual and population health services promote desired health outcomes (quality principles), are in line with current professional knowledge (professional practitioner skill), and meet the expectations of the marketplace (Suresh & Raghavan, 2017, p. 49; Tyler & Napoli, 2019, p. 670).
- Patient safety is defined by the National Academy of Medicine as the prevention of harm to patients by placing emphasis on the system in which that care is delivered. Safety is the foundation on which all other aspects of quality are built (Tyler & Napoli, 2019, p. 670).
  - The standard framework for quality of care was proposed by Donabedian in the 1960s and is still the foundation today. The Donabedian Triad focuses on system structure, processes, and outcomes (Suresh & Raghavan, 2017, p. 49).
- A culture of safety involves understanding the limitations of human abilities, anticipating and planning for the unexpected, and actively modeling a nonpunitive learning environment. This comprehensive approach, using human factors science, can improve system processes and structure (Smith & Donze, 2015, p. 350).
- Identifying and eliminating sources of patient harm or potential harm are critical for the delivery of safe and quality care in nursing and all other healthcare disciplines (Smith & Donze, 2015, p. 348).

COMPONENTS OF HIGH-QUALITY CARE

- As defined by the IOM committee, there are six concrete components of high-quality care:
  - Safe—the patient is not injured by any care or procedure.
  - Effective—the desired outcome is produced.
  - Patient-centered—care is provided with respect and awareness of the individuality of the patient.
  - Timely—care is provided at the right time without delays.
  - Efficient—care is organized and performed with minimum waste in time, effort, or supplies.
  - Equitable—there is impartiality in care provision (Suresh & Raghavan, 2017, pp. 49–50; Tyler & Napoli, 2019, p. 670).

ORGANIZATIONAL APPROACHES TO DEVELOPING AND SUSTAINING A CULTURE OF SAFETY

- In 1999, the concepts, theories, and attributes of high-reliability organizations (HROs) was applied to clinical practice. HROs share similar characteristics, such as a preoccupation with failure, a reluctance to simplify interpretations, a sensitivity to operations, commitment to resilience, and deference to expertise (Simpson, 2014, p. 3; Suresh & Raghavan, 2017, p. 59). HROs operate highly complex and hazardous technological systems essentially without mistakes over long periods of time.
- Organizational approaches used in developing and sustaining a culture of safety include both technological and nontechnological improvements:
  - Nontechnological improvements:
    - *Five rights*—right patient, right drug, right dose, right route, and right time
    - *Forcing functions* guide the user to the next appropriate action/decision.
    - *Medication reconciliation processes* create the most accurate list of medications a patient is taking.
    - *Read backs* require the repetition of a message one has received in order to acknowledge its correctness.
    - *Time outs* are a preprocedure pause that allows all members involved to identify the correct patient and procedure.
    - *Executive walk arounds* occur when healthcare leaders visit each unit/department to show the organization prioritizes patient safety and to learn from the healthcare team about near misses, errors, or challenges to patient safety.
    - *Storytelling* is intended to open dialogue among healthcare providers, who may be able to prevent similar occurrences.
    - *Safety briefings* allow information to be shared among staff both to increase safety awareness among staff and to cement the principles of a culture of safety into the daily routine (Smith & Donze, 2015, p. 350).

○ Technological improvements:
  ■ Health information technology (HIT) has proven effective in reducing human errors in industries such as aviation and banking. HIT systems enable a more reliable, effective means of communication between and across healthcare settings and improve accessibility to patient information at the time of care (Tyler & Napoli, 2019, p. 678).
    • Technology eliminates duplicate work, improves caregivers' decision-making through automated menus, places evidence-based clinical guidelines within easy access, and removes the dangers of illegible handwriting.
    • Some technologies that improve medication administration are electronic medical records (EMR), computerized provider order entry (CPOE), bar coding medications, smart infusion pumps, and automated dispensing units (ADUs; Smith & Donze, 2015, pp. 355–357).
    • If the HIT is not wellintegrated into the workflow of the organization, it may become more dangerous than valuable. HIT may also be costly to acquire, implement, train staff on, and "go live" over time. Culture barriers may also exist which challenge the implementation of a new or different HIT (Tyler & Napoli, 2019, p. 678).

Creating a Culture of Safety

• A culture of safety uses a comprehensive approach based on human factors science to improve system processes and structures in a nonpunitive environment.
  ○ Traditional practice is for organizations to respond to errors by naming and blaming individuals. This is known as a *person-centered approach*.
  ○ A *systems approach* recognizes the complexity of a system and that most errors are based in flawed systems in which the individuals work (Smith & Donze, 2015, p. 350).
    ■ Potential for errors within systems are generally related to either:
      – *Active failures*, which are unsafe acts committed by person or persons who are in direct contact with the patient or system
      – *Latent conditions*, which are flaws within the system caused by failures in design (Tyler & Napoli, 2019, p. 682)
  ○ A *just culture* recognizes that individuals should not be held responsible for system failures and that even the most competent professionals can be prone to errors (Smith & Donze, 2015, pp. 350–351).

SAFETY BEHAVIORS
• All members involved in patient care need to engage in the culture of safety, including hospital administrators, all healthcare team members, and families. Safety is the number one priority and takes precedence over institution and provider convenience, production issues, and costs. Safety guides all unit operations and clinical actions. Safety is created through accountability based on standardization, simplification, and clarity, as supported by the principles of safety science (Simpson, 2014, pp. 2–3; Smith & Donze, 2015, p. 350; Suresh & Raghavan, 2017, p. 54).

• Safety behaviors should be promoted throughout the organizational culture, and means to incorporate safety behaviors should be viewed as a positive intervention rather than punitive action. Examples of these actions are:
  ○ Cross checking—involves confirmation of information from two separate sources to verify the accuracy.
  ○ Speaking up for safety—involves the use of key phrases that focus on the system concern and not an individual.
  ○ Coaching—modeling the safety behaviors and encouraging their use by others (Tyler & Napoli, 2019, p. 683)
• Systemwide approaches that may both initiate and continue conversations about safety concerns may include safety huddles, daily check-ins, executive rounds, and performance management concepts (Tyler & Napoli, 2019, p. 675).
• Transparency and full disclosure are also important concepts in the development and maintenance of a culture of safety. Transparency is a process in which errors are fully disclosed to the patients and/or the families, including details before, during, and after the error.
  ○ All healthcare providers find these to be very difficult conversations, although research routinely supports the expressed desire of the patient/family to be informed of an error. Literature reviews also confirm providers are less likely to be sued if an error is fully disclosed in a timely manner rather than hidden from the patient/family (Smith & Donze, 2015, p. 360).

SAFETY SYSTEM PROCESSES
• There are multiple strategies an organization may choose to employ to enhance patient safety. Although none have been subjected to a rigorous randomized controlled trial, evidence indicates these techniques are useful in maximize a safety culture.
  ○ Outside expert review—removes the biases which may be in place when a system is examined by someone deep within it (Pettker & Grobman, 2019, p. 843). There exists a risk of "normalization of deviance," defined as a degradation of professional, behavioral, and technical standards that occurs over time and increases probability of a major accident or harm (Simpson, 2014, p. 2).
  ○ Bundles, guidelines, and protocols provide a common foundation for healthcare providers to use in approaching patient care and help to maintain standards and practice patterns in order for the staff to provide consistent care.
    ■ Bundles are sets of evidence-based interventions grouped together under a care target that aim to be implemented together or in part. Bundles include checklists, guidelines, protocols, and educational materials necessary to facilitate the implementation of the practices (Pettker & Grobman, 2019, p. 844). When implemented collectively, the use of a bundle and its components reliably results in significantly better patient outcomes than when individually applied (Tyler & Napoli, 2019, p. 684).
    ■ Guidelines and protocols should be based on evidence, when available, or expert opinion. However, even if based only on consensus and expert opinion, they will provide consistency among caregivers necessary for smooth workflow and safe practices (Pettker & Grobman, 2019, p. 844).
  ○ Checklists
    ■ These have been improving safety since the 1930s in aviation, for the first flight tests of the B-17 bomber

(aka the "flying fortress"). The plane was considered too much for one man to fly; therefore, pilots introduced a system of checklists to streamline the processes of takeoff, flight, and landing.

- Checklists are a cognitive tool that uses two strategies to reduce potential errors. The first goal of a checklist is to implement evidence-based and best-practice strategies in a systematic fashion, making their use routine and universal. Second, checklists aim to improve the function of a team by creating a shared set of standards and goals (Pettker & Grobman, 2019, p. 845; Profit, Lee, Gould, & Horbar, 2015, p. 68, 84; Simpson, 2014, p. 24).
- The use of a checklist in conjunction with real-time surveillance is useful in identifying pitfalls in care practices that are particularly prone to error, such as mislabeled medications, absent patient identifiers, or failure to follow hand hygiene practices. Errors in these practices cross many parts of the healthcare processes and may have systemwide implications (Simpson, 2014, p. 24; Smith & Donze, 2015, p. 360).

DESIGNING SAFE PROCESSES

- *Plan-do-study-act (PDSA)* cycles are part of the Institute for Healthcare Improvement (IHI) Model for Improvement. Each PDSA cycle is a test of a hypothesis of how a specific change will affect the system, and can accelerate quality improvement (Profit et al., 2015, p. 66). This method implements small and frequent changes that are analyzed for effectiveness before being introduced on a larger scale (Tyler & Napoli, 2019, p. 680). By doing a series of PDSA cycles and thus learning from each effort at improvement, the team can achieve lasting improvements in the way they provide patient care and in patient outcomes (Suresh & Raghavan, 2017, pp. 52–53).
- *Lean methodology* was derived from the production system of Toyota and works through targeting the needs and aims of the customer. Minimization of waste is the focus, and processes that are deemed to be of no value are discontinued. The definition of "value" is widely discussed (Tyler & Napoli, 2019, p. 679).
- *Six Sigma* reflects the measure of standard deviations or known variance and the degree to which almost perfect production can occur (Tyler & Napoli, 2019, p. 678). If there are six standard deviations between the process mean and the nearest specification limit, only 3.4 out of 1 million outputs will fail to meet specifications (Profit et al., 2015, p. 63). These metrics drive the system to reduce error and eliminate defects from processes in the delivery of care (Smith & Donze, 2015, p. 361).
- *Root cause analysis* (RCA) is a structured method to analyze adverse events retrospectively through a specific protocol based on the belief that the system, not individual, is the likely root cause of most errors. Analysis is labor intensive and involves the formation of a multidisciplinary team that retrospectively investigates the sentinel events using chart reviews, interviews, and field observations to reconstruct the timeline of events that led to the undesirable outcome, and to identify common underlying factors. The Joint Commission, which is responsible for accreditation of hospitals and hospital organizations, now requires RCA be performed in response to all sentinel events (Profit et al., 2015, p. 66; Simpson, 2014, p. 28; Tyler & Napoli, 2019, p. 679).

MEASURING SAFETY PROCESSES

- Safety events are generally classified in four ways:
  - Near misses—these errors are detected before they reach the patient, usually through skillful nursing assessment and intervention.
  - Precursor events—these errors reach the patient but result in no detectable or only minimal harm.
  - Serious safety issues—any error that reaches the patient and results in moderate to severe harm, including death. May also be called a "sentinel" event (Simpson, 2014, p. 27).
    - It has been suggested that for every serious safety issue, there are potentially tens of precursor safety events and hundreds of near misses. Reporting these less-severe errors may prevent the occurrence of a serious safety issue (Tyler & Napoli, 2019, p. 673, 682).
  - "Never" events—errors that are unambiguous (clearly identifiable and measurable), serious (usually resulting in death), and considered universally preventable (Simpson, 2014, p. 29).
- Benchmarking
  - Benchmarking in healthcare is defined as collaborative and continual measurement of key results of work processes against those who are considered to have "'best demonstrated practices." Using benchmarking allows organizations to routinely measure services, practices, costs, and products against an established standard.
    - Internal benchmarks are used to identify best practices within an organization over time.
    - External benchmarks require a comparison of an organization with other organizations, with the intent to identify new ideas, methods, products, or services (Tyler & Napoli, 2019, p. 674).

TEAMWORK AND COMMUNICATION

- A healthy work environment is critical to promoting patient safety (Simpson, 2014, p. 4), and the work environment is enhanced through effective communication and teamwork from all disciplines. These will create and sustain a culture of safety (Smith & Donze, 2015, p. 351).
- The Joint Commission records that more than two-thirds of serious safety issues were caused primarily by breakdown in communication (Smith & Donze, 2015, p. 351). Other data cite the root cause of an error as poor communication (72%), with 55% of cases involving an organizational culture that prevented effective teamwork and communication (Pettker & Grobman, 2019, p. 843).

Methods to Improve Communication

- Respectful communication is highly valued and rewarded. Team members in HROs do not wait until there is an adverse outcome to evaluate operations and practices. Evaluation is ongoing through use of established measurement processes (Simpson, 2014, p. 3).
- Crew Resource Management (CRM)
  - Each team member is empowered within his or her role and responsibilities to alert on safety concerns. In fact, assertions of safety concerns are not only encouraged, it is promoted as an expectation and part of the role of team member (Smith & Donze, 2015, p. 353; Tyler & Napoli, 2019, p. 671).

- Team Strategies and Tools to Enhance Performance and Patient Safety (TeamSTEPPS)
  - A three-step process developed by the Agency for Healthcare Research and Quality (AHRQ) founded on four core competencies: leadership, situation monitoring, mutual support, and communication. TeamSTEPPS is designed to provide hospitals a systematic approach to integrating teamwork into everyday practices of healthcare workers to improve quality, safety, and efficiency of care (Tyler & Napoli, 2019, pp. 671–672).
- Situation, Background, Assessment, and Recommendation (SBAR)
  - A tool used to help prevent omission of information through standardization of presentation. Also used to ensure consistency in methods of communication between team members during critical time periods such as shift change, team reports, and patient transfers (Simpson, 2014, p. 21; Smith & Donze, 2015, p. 353).
- Communication among team members must flow freely regardless of their authority gradient. Patient care decision-making should be shared among all members of the healthcare team (Smith & Donze, 2015, p. 352).
  - Respectful, collegial interactions between nurses and physicians and with patients are the bedrock of the unit culture. The *different but equal* contribution of nurses to clinical outcomes should be recognized and valued.
  - Aggressive or disruptive behavior (e.g., throwing items, intimidation, angry outbursts, making demeaning comments to team members and/or patients, or using profanity) should not be tolerated within the system, regardless of with whom the provider is involved. Competent clinical practice is a basic expectation and cannot be substituted for irresponsible, inappropriate, dysfunctional, or abusive behavior (Simpson, 2014, p. 6).
- Examples of other structured communication processes are summarized in Table 29.1.

Simulation

- Simulation used to provide skills on low-frequency, high-severity events or of an actual event that has previously occurred or could potentially occur. The IOM encourages the use of simulation as a means to encourage teamwork and communication and thereby improve patient safety (Pettker & Grobman, 2019, p. 848; Smith & Donze, 2015, p. 352).
  - Healthcare providers tend to be trained as individuals even though they function almost exclusively as teams, and patient safety programs that promote team training and functioning need to be adopted.
  - Debriefing after a simulation provides the opportunity for teams to critique performances and learn lessons as to how, when, and where errors happened and could be prevented in a real-life situation.
  - Simulation in conjunction with debriefing is an effective method that allows team members to become aware of their role in error occurrence and/or prevention (Smith & Donze, 2015, pp. 352–353).
- Skills training for healthcare professions involving simulation-based training focuses on communication skills, include speaking up, performing check-ins, and closing the loop.
- There is now good evidence that simulation and debriefing improve self-confidence, knowledge, and operational performance in simulated settings. Emerging evidence supports that simulation and debriefing can improve performance in clinical settings and can result in safer patient outcomes (Smith & Donze, 2015, p. 361).

ERRORS IN THE NICU

- NICU data have demonstrated that 47% of errors were medication related, 11% were related to patient misidentification, 7% were from delay or errors in diagnosis, and 14% involved errors in the administration or methods of using a treatment (Tyler & Napoli, 2019, p. 670).

TABLE 29.1 Structured Communication Processes

SBAR (situation, background, assessment, recommendation)	Provides a framework for communicating information that requires a clinician's immediate attention and action in a specific, structured format
DESC	A method of conflict resolution
"Two-challenge rule"	A patient safety concern must be raised a second time if it has gone unacknowledged and/or uncorrected. A quick conflict-resolution technique by which a team member may question an action two times and, if a sufficient answer is not provided, may halt that action
"Check backs"	Require the receiver of an order or instruction to repeat it back to the sender to ensure it was clearly transmitted and understood
"Callouts"	Critical steps in a procedure are announced to team members so everyone is clear where they are in a given situation and so the next step can be anticipated, and it identifies who is in charge
"Stop the line"	In which a coded expression is chosen by the team to be used in front of a patient and understood by all team members to indicate a patient safety concern

DESC, describe, express, specify, consequences.

Sources: Data from Pettker, C., & Grobman, W. (2019). Patient safety and quality improvement in obstetrics. In R. Resnik, C. Lockwood, T. Moore, M. Greene, J. Copel, & R. Silver (Eds.), *Creasy and Resnik's maternal–fetal medicine: Principles and practice* (8th ed., p. 842). Philadelphia, PA: Elsevier; Simpson, K. (2014). Perinatal patient safety and professional liability issues. In K. Simpson & P. Creehan (Eds.), *Perinatal nursing* (4th ed., p. 21). St. Louis, MO: Lippincott Williams & Wilkins.

Factors That Increase Risk of Adverse Reactions in Neonatal Patients

- Greater pharmacokinetic variability
- Dependence on individualized dosage calculations
- Lack of appropriate pediatric dosage forms
- Lack of Food and Drug Administration-approved pediatric labeling
- Dependence on precise measurement and delivery devices
- Inability of neonatal patients to communicate adverse drug effects directly to providers (Pettker & Grobman, 2019, p. 848; Profit et al., 2015, p. 60)

Select Types of Common Errors

- Medication errors are those that occur during the process of administrating medication. Approximately 47% of medical errors in the hospital are related to medication. Although establishing the frequency of medication errors in the NICU is difficult, published studies indicate that medication errors in the NICU are common, ranging from 13 to 91 medication errors per 100 NICU admissions (Profit et al., 2015, p. 60).
  - Five steps in the process for medication use where medication errors may occur are prescription, transcription, preparation/dispensing, administration, and effects. Incorrect dosing prescription is the most common medication error (Smith & Donze, 2015, p. 361).
  - NICU patients are more likely to experience a medication error than other hospital patients and to experience more harm when a medication error occurs (Profit et al., 2015, p. 60).
- Patient misidentification can happen more easily in the NICU since the patients cannot self-identify. In order to avoid this, patient bar-code identifiers, and a time-out prior to procedures are encouraged to avoid patient misidentification (Smith & Donze, 2015, p. 361).
- Error in administration of breastmilk or blood products. Multiple steps are involved with both processes and therefore there are multiple places in which the process can go badly. The wrong patient may receive the wrong product, or, in cases of blood products, incompatibility errors may be overlooked. Either substance may inadvertently mishandled or incorrectly stored (Smith & Donze, 2015, p. 361).
- Healthcare-associated infections occur in patients during the course of receiving treatment in a healthcare setting. Of particular concern are central line-associated bloodstream infections (CLABSIs) and ventilator-associated pneumonias (VAPs). The risk of either or both can be minimized through the use of standardized guidelines and practice bundles (Smith & Donze, 2015, pp. 365–366).
- Unplanned extubations may be accidental or caused by the patient. Unplanned endotracheal extubations requiring re-intubation generally rank within the top five adverse events in the NICU (Smith & Donze, 2015, p. 366).

CONCLUSION

Due to the emphasis on creating a culture of safety and transparency, neonatal units across the country are making progress to provide consist, safe, and evidence-based care. The goal remains to identify, report, and learn from near misses, precursor events, and serious safety issues. This will permit healthcare systems to evolve into HROs with patient safety being at the forefront. The Joint Commission stresses new patient safety goals each year for which healthcare organizations strive toward to provide the safest care to our patients.

REVIEW QUESTIONS

1. Team Strategies and Tools to Enhance Performance and Patient Safety (TeamSTEPPS) is a process designed to improve a team's
   A. communication
   B. division of labor
   C. goal orientation

2. One of the descriptors of a high-reliability organization (HRO) is the organization's
   A. preoccupation with failure
   B. commitment to complexity
   C. patient-centeredness care

3. Errors that reach the patient but cause only minimal or no detectable harm are termed
   A. near-miss events
   B. precursor events
   C. serious safety events

4. SBAR is a tool used to help prevent omission of information through standardization of presentation and to ensure consistency in methods of communication between team members. The acronym SBAR stands for
   A. setting, background, appraisal, and resources
   B. situation, background, assessment, and recommendation
   C. status, backdrop, assessment, and planned recourse

5. The NNP is called into an administrator's office to discuss a medical error. The administrator focuses on the NNP's role in the error and questions the thinking process at the time. This method of dealing with errors is known as a
   A. just-culture system's approach
   B. person-centered approach
   C. systems-centered approach

REFERENCES

Pettker, C., & Grobman, W. (2019). Patient safety and quality improvement in obstetrics. In R. Resnik, C. Lockwood, T. Moore, M. Greene, J. Copel, & R. Silver (Eds.), *Creasy and Resnik's maternal–fetal medicine: Principles and practice* (8th ed., pp. 841–851.e3). Philadelphia, PA: Elsevier.

Profit, J., Lee, H., Gould, J., & Horbar, J. (2015). Evaluating and improving the quality and safety of neonatal intensive care. In R. J. Martin, A. A. Fanaroff, & M. C. Walsh (Eds.), *Neonatal–perinatal medicine: Diseases of the fetus and infant* (10th ed., pp. 59–88). Philadelphia, PA: Elsevier Saunders.

Simpson, K. (2014). Perinatal patient safety and professional liability issues. In K. Simpson & P. Creehan (Eds.), *Perinatal nursing* (4th ed., pp. 1–40). St. Louis, MO: Lippincott Williams & Wilkins.

Smith, J., & Donze, A., (2015). Patient safety. In M. T. Verklan & M. Walden (Eds.), *Core curriculum for neonatal intensive care nursing* (5th ed., pp. 348–372). St. Louis, MO: Elsevier Saunders.

Suresh, G., & Raghavan, A. (2017). Quality and safety in respiratory care. In J. Goldsmith, E. Karotkin, M. Meszler, & G. Suresh (Eds.), *Assisted ventilation of the neonate* (6th ed., pp. 49–55.e2). Philadelphia, PA: Elsevier.

Tyler, L., & Napoli, L. (2019). Quality and safety. In B. Walsh (Ed.), *Neonatal and pediatric respiratory care* (5th ed., pp. 669–687). St. Louis, MO: Elsevier.

30 NURSING RESEARCH

Kimberly Horns LaBronte
Kim Friddle
Amy Koehn

INTRODUCTION

Advance practice requires good use of data obtained through research in nursing and other disciplines. Nursing research has had a pivotal role in shaping the decisions in best practices throughout decades of systematic inquiry. Research is disciplined, systematic, and original in its pretense, allowing for specific questions to be answered with descriptive and measurable outcomes.

PRINCIPLES OF RESEARCH

- The formal definition of nursing research is a systematic inquiry designed to generate trustworthy evidence about issues of importance to the nursing profession and its clients, including nursing practice, education, administration, and informatics. The advent of nursing research has brought systematic query to innovative nursing knowledge (Polit & Beck, 2018, p. 2).
- Within the nursing profession, research promotes health and well-being of patient populations through a variety of applications. Research improves practice by providing answers to clinical questions, evaluating the effectiveness of nursing interventions and programs of care, and expanding the body of nursing knowledge (Thomas, 2015, p. 832).
- The fundamental goal of clinical research is to obtain an unbiased answer to the question posed. The structure of a typical study that assesses the effectiveness of a treatment (Lopez & Tyson, 2020, pp. 115–116).

Sources of Research Problems

- Tradition and authority
  - These may encompass unit culture, untested traditions, and "sacred cows" of practice. A person with specialized expertise, an authority, is a valuable source, provided that the "expertise" is not based on personal experience (Polit & Beck, 2018, p. 5).
- Clinical experience and "trial and error"
  - Personal experiences can limit the search for knowledge because the knowledge is too narrow to be useful or is colored by personal views or biases (Polit & Beck, 2018, p. 6).
- Assembled information—often garnered from benchmarking data or quality improvement or risk data (Polit & Beck, 2018, p. 6).
  - An assembled database is an organized, structured collection of data designed for a particular purpose.

Most frequently, the term database is used to refer to a structured electronic collection of information, such as a database of clinical trial data. Databases come in a variety of fundamental types, such as single-table, relational, and object-oriented (Palma & Tarczy-Hornock, 2018, p. 13).
  - Clinical evidence that is relevant to problems in neonatal–perinatal medicine is appearing at an accelerating rate and can be found in journals, conference proceedings, online databases, and other sources. Many published reports provide only weak evidence because strong research designs were not used (Lopez & Tyson, 2020, p. 114).
- The Internet has permitted ready access and sharing of this information between professionals and organizations. The clinician must realize that, unlike journals, textbooks, and guidelines, material on the World Wide Web is not necessarily subject to any editorial or other oversight; therefore "caveat lector" (reader beware; Palma & Tarczy-Hornock, 2018, p. 17).
  - With caution in mind, a search of the World Wide Web using a sophisticated search engine (e.g., Google, Google Scholar) can yield valuable information, though search results typically include a lower proportion of quality resources compared with curated resources.
  - For accessing the primary literature, the most valuable resource is the National Library of Medicine's database of the published medical literature accessible (PubMed; www.ncbi.nlm.nih.gov/pubmed).
    - An underused tool is the Similar Articles tool that is available as a link below each article listed on PubMed. The PubMed system applies a powerful statistical algorithm in order to find similar articles in the database.
  - Another powerful search tool within PubMed is the Clinical Query (www.ncbi.nlm.nih.gov/pubmed/clinical). This tool facilitates searches for papers by clinical study category (e.g., etiology, diagnosis, therapy, prognosis), focuses on systematic reviews, and performs Medical Genetics searches (Palma & Tarczy-Hornock, 2018, p. 17, 19).

Relationships

- Researchers often study phenomena in relation to another phenomena. These can be described in two ways:
  - If more of (or less of) Variable X, then more of (or less of) Variable Y.
  - Relationships expressed as group differences (Polit & Beck, 2018, p. 46)

Data

- The actual values of the research variables constitute the data, or pieces of information gathered during the research process.
  - Quantitative data are information gathered in numeric form.
  - Qualitative data are generally comprised of narrative descriptions (Polit & Beck, 2018, p. 45).

Variables

- A variable is, as the name implies, something that varies or changes between study subjects or conditions. It is these variances which drive research questions.
  - Researchers may also create variables, such as the comparisons of effectiveness between two intervention (Polit & Beck, 2018, p. 43).
- *Independent variable* is believed to cause of influence the dependent variable; in experimental research, the manipulated (treatment) variable.
- *Dependent variable* is the variable hypothesized to depend on or to be caused by another (Polit & Beck, 2018, p. 43).
- Variables are the attributes or properties measured in a research study and are defined both conceptually and operationally.
  - A conceptual definition is described in the abstract.
  - An operational definition defines the variable in measurable terms (Polit & Beck, 2018, p. 45; Thomas, 2015, p. 836).

Instruments and Tools

- These are terms used interchangeably to indicate operational measures. The quality of measurement is critical to research. Validity and reliability describe instrument measurement characteristics.
  - Validity is the degree to which an instrument measures what it is purported to measure. The instrument measures truly the variable.
  - Reliability refers to ability of the instrument to obtain consistent results (i.e., reproducibility) over time or across administrators (Thomas, 2015, p. 836).

Types of Research

- Scientific method describes prescribed rules of logic and imposed controls, ensuring that the knowledge generated is truthful. Research generates empirical (i.e., experienced) knowledge (Thomas, 2015, p. 832).
- The research process describes a logical and orderly progression from development of a question through the conduct of a study, analysis of resultant findings, dissemination of conclusions, translation into practice, and implementation (Thomas, 2015, p. 832).

QUANTITATIVE RESEARCH

- Numeric data are analyzed using a statistical approach specified as part of the planning for the research project.
- Descriptive statistics include measures of central tendency (mean, median, mode) and dispersion (standard deviation, variance, range).
- Inferential statistics are based on probability and allow judgments to be made about the population, and hypotheses to be tested. In general, inferential statistics test either how things differ or how things are related.

- Statistical significance means that the particular finding is not likely due to chance alone.
- Statistical significance is not always consistent with clinical significance, meaning that the magnitude of the effect is not relevant or important in clinical practice (Thomas, 2015, p. 836).

QUALITATIVE RESEARCH

- The focus is in-depth understanding of a phenomenon, with particular emphasis on the subject's reports of personal experience, used to increase understanding of phenomena perceived by individuals, groups, and cultures.
- Participant observation, focus groups, and interviews are methods frequently employed in qualitative research. Maintains the same rigor as quantitative research (Thomas, 2015, p. 836)

"Doing" Versus "Using" Research in Nursing

- Put simply, nurses "do" and/or "use" research. While not all nurses do research, every nurse is a consumer of research. Research findings are an essential component of evidence-based practice (EBP; Thomas, 2015, p. 832). The principles and process of EBP are discussed in Chapter 27. However, a brief description of the contrast between research and EBP is given in Table 30.1.

TABLE 30.1 "Doing" Versus "Using" Research

Research	Evidence-Based Practice
• Originates a research question or hypothesis • Designs an original study • Constructs a study method and involved procedures • Collects and analyzes data • Generates new findings to add to the body of knowledge with the literature • Translates findings into practice	• Identifies a clinical/practice-based question or concern • Gathers evidence • Critically appraises extant knowledge within the body of literature • Develops a practice guideline • Applies the practice change • Evaluates patients' outcomes compared to pre-implementation data

Source: Thomas, K. (2015). Foundations of neonatal research. In T. Verklan & M. Walden (Eds.), *Core curriculum for neonatal intensive care nursing* (5th ed., pp. 832–865). St. Louis, MO: Elsevier.

THE QUANTITATIVE RESEARCH PROCESS

- A thorough review and elaboration of all details of quantitative research program is beyond the scope of this chapter; however, the major points will be discussed in this section. Table 30.2 provides a detailed outline of all components of a quantitative research program.

Research Question

- There are several forms of research questions, and they are guided by the quantifiable concepts; for example, they may be descriptive, measurable, or prognostic (predictive) outcomes (Polit & Beck, 2018, p. 140). All research derives from a purpose and begins with a problem or general question, which is refined to form specific research aims,

TABLE 30.2 Flow Steps in a Quantitative Study

Phases of Research	Activities
Conceptual phase	• Formulating and delimiting the problem • Reviewing the related literature • Undertaking the clinical fieldwork • Defining the framework/developing conceptual definitions • Formulating hypotheses
Design and planning phase	• Selecting a research design • Developing intervention protocols • Identifying the population • Designing the sampling plan • Specifying methods to measure research variables • Developing methods to safeguard subjects • Finalizing the research plan
Empirical phase	• Collecting the data • Preparing the data for analysis
Analytic phase	• Analyzing the data • Interpreting the results
Dissemination phase	• Communicating the findings • Utilizing the findings in practice

Source: Data from Polit, D., & Beck, C. (2018). *Essentials of nursing research* (9th ed.). Philadelphia, PA: Wolters Kluwer.

questions, or hypotheses. These questions or hypotheses are the focal point of a research study, piloting all other aspects of the research (Thomas, 2015, p. 834).
- Throughout the evolution of developing the research purpose statement and problem identification, the investigator proceeds from broad or general topics of interest to more specific ideas. The problems then are evaluated for significance, research ability, and feasibility.

Literature Review

- Quantitative researchers strive to understand what is already known about a topic by undertaking a thorough literature review before any data are collected (Polit & Beck, 2018, p. 49).
- A literature review is a critical summary of the available research on the topic of interest, or a compilation of current known data or theories on the topic. It identifies relationships between concepts, denotes flaws or gaps in the current knowledge base, and aids in formulating the research question or hypothesis (National Association of Neonatal Nurse Practitioners [NANNP], 2010, p. 4).

Framework

- Framework is derived from a review of the literature that establishes what is currently known regarding the study topic and identifies the gaps in knowledge that the study will address (Thomas, 2015, p. 835).
- Studying the research question within the context of a theoretical framework allows the findings to potentially have broader significance and utility. Even without a specific

theory to guide the research, there should be clear conceptual and rational visions as to the concepts under study (Polit & Beck, 2018, p. 50).

Hypotheses

- A research hypothesis is a prediction about the relationship between the independent variable (the presumed cause or intervention) and the dependent variable (the presumed effect or outcome) within a population. They are derived from theory, which in turn develops the questions.
- Put in another way, a hypothesis is a formal statement of expected or predicted relationships between two or more variables in a specified population or group (NANNP, 2010, p. 5).

TYPES OF HYPOTHESES

- *Inductive hypotheses* are inferred from observations (patterns and associations) and predictions are made from those observations.
- *Deductive hypotheses* start with a theory, then predict (deduce) that certain outcomes will be expected.
- *Nondirectional hypothesis* does not state the direction of the expected outcome; rather, the outcome could go either way.
- *Null hypothesis* states there is no relationship between the independent and dependent variables.
  ○ In a type I error, the researcher rejects the null hypothesis when it is true.
  ○ In a type II error, the researcher accepts the null hypothesis as true when it is false (NANNP, 2010, p. 5).
- *Directional hypothesis* specifies the expected direction and the relationship (outcomes) between the variables.
- *One-way hypothesis* states the expected (predicted) direction of the relationship (outcomes) between the independent and dependent variables (Polit & Beck, 2018, pp. 100–101).

Research Design

- The *research design* is the architectural backbone of the research. It is an overall plan for obtaining answers to the research questions. In quantitative research, designs tend to be structured and controlled with the goal to minimize bias. Included is how often data will be collected and what types of comparisons will be made (Polit & Beck, 2018, p. 51).

Identifying the Population and Sampling Plan

- The *population* of a research study is made up of the individuals or objects with similar, defining, and shared characteristics (Polit & Beck, 2018, p. 51). It is an entire group of objects, individuals, events, and substances having common characteristics selected for study
  ○ Inclusion criteria are characteristics that the researcher has determined **must** be present in study participants.
  ○ Exclusion criteria are characteristics that the researcher has determined **must not** be present in study participants (NANNP, 2010, p. 5).
- A *sampling plan* is developed before the data are collected (*a priori*) and optimizes the ability to generalize attributes about the population of interest. Probability sampling is the best method of obtaining representative samples and ensures statistical conclusion validity.

○ Representative sample is one whose characteristics closely resemble those of the population.

○ Nonprobability samples are selected by nonrandom methods.

• Sampling bias refers to the systematic error of over- or under-representation of a population segment (Polit & Beck, 2018, p. 162).

NONPROBABILITY SAMPLING

• *Convenience sampling* is when the inclusion criteria involve using the most conveniently available participants.

• *Snowball sampling (network sampling)* is similar to convenience sampling, where the researcher begins with a convenience sample and then asks those participants to refer others for the study.

• *Quota sampling* occurs when the researcher determines a priori a population and then determines how many participants are needed from each stratum for statistical conclusion validity.

• *Consecutive sampling* involves recruiting all the people from an accessible population who meet the inclusion criteria over a specific time period.

• *Purposive sampling* uses researcher's knowledge about the population to make informed selection of the participants (Polit & Beck, 2018, pp. 163–164).

PROBABILITY SAMPLING

• Probability sampling involves random selection of elements that are proportional within the population, or, in other words, researchers can specify the probability that an element of the population will be included in the sample

○ *Simple random sampling* employs using a simple random sampling plan (either by randomly selecting numbers by computer or the card method).

○ *Stratified random sampling* partitions the sample into subgroups (homogeneous subsets) and the randomized the selection from each of those subgroups.

○ *Multistaged cluster sampling* involves selecting broad groups where all the characteristics of the group may not be known and then randomly selecting from the clusters.

○ *Systematic sampling* employs selecting every kth case from a list, such as every 10th person on a student roster.

○ *Sampling strata* is directed toward subpopulations of the whole or divisions (e.g., premature infants with respiratory distress syndrome).

○ *Staged sampling* occurs when sampling is selected in multiple phases, generally from large groups to more specific characteristics within a group (Polit & Beck, 2018, pp. 164–165).

Safeguard of Human Subjects

• The Institutional Review Board (IRB) is an administrative body established to protect the rights and welfare of human research subjects recruited to participate in research activities conducted under the auspices of the institution with which it is affiliated. Its responsibilities include:

○ The review, prior to its initiation, all research (whether funded or not) involving human participants.

○ Protecting the welfare, rights, and privacy of human subjects.

○ To approve, disapprove, monitor, and require modifications in all research activities that fall within its

jurisdiction as specified by both the federal regulations and institutional policy.

• The IRB is composed of at least five members of varying backgrounds in order to provide complete and adequate review of human research and its institutional, legal, scientific, and social implications. It will also include at least one member who is not affiliated with the institution and one member who is not a scientist. Finally, the IRB has several consultants who advise the board and are periodically involved in protocol review (Polit & Beck, 2018, pp. 85–86).

• A guiding principle of research is that participation should be uncoerced. Informed consent is obtained when participants are told about the study and the treatment to be given is described, including possible effects. Participants should also be told they have the right to withdraw at any time without fear of harm or limits to their continued care (NANNP, 2010, p. 5).

Data Collection

• The process of data collection is rigorous and carefully planned a priori. The process prescribes what data are needed and how data are to be collected. The process is driven by how the data are asked, final analysis of the data, and how the findings are disseminated (Polit & Beck, 2018, p. 52).

Data Analysis

• Analysis uses statistical or analytic techniques on the data collected to answer the research questions or compare findings with stated hypotheses (Thomas, 2015, p. 836).

• The data must be collected in the proper form for collecting and coding. Many issues with minor coding and ultimate analysis steps may be avoided by planning and performing a preliminary analysis; therefore, a solid plan for the data analysis phase should be done prior to the data collection.

STATISTICS

• *Univariate statistics* are one-variable, or descriptive statistics used to synthesize and describe data. A summary of univariate statistics is given in Table 30.3.

• *Bivariate statistics* describe the relationships between two variables (Polit & Beck, 2018, pp. 229, 234). A summary of bivariate statistics is given in Table 30.4.

STATISTICAL RELIABILITY AND VALIDITY

• *Reliability* of a quantitative measure is a major criterion for assessing its quality. Reliability is the extent to which scores for people who have not changed are the same for repeated measures, under several situations. Included within this concept is measurement error (Polit & Beck, 2018, p. 175)

• *Validity* is defined as the degree to which an instrument is measuring the construct it purports to measure (Polit & Beck, 2018, p. 176).

Results

• The start of the result section delineates the sample with descriptive statistics and then follows with results from the original research questions (Polit & Beck, 2018, p. 62). Results include a description of the study sample as well as findings from the analysis based on stated aims, questions, or hypotheses (Thomas, 2015, p. 836).

TABLE 30.3 Univariate/Descriptive Statistics

UNIVARIATE	
Frequency distributions	Arrangement of values from lowest to highest and a count of percentage of how many times each value occurred.
Central tendency	Indexes of central tendency indicate what is "typical." These include the **mode** (most frequent), **median** (point that divides the distribution of scores), and **mean** (sum of values divided by number of participants).
Variability	How individuals differ from each other over the attribute. This includes **range** (highest minus lowest value) and **standard deviation** (the average amount of variation).
Bivariate	
Cross-tabulations	The frequencies of two variables are cross-tabulated to identify relationships.
Correlation	The extent two variables are related to each other.
Describing Risk	
Absolute Risk (AR)	The proportion of people who experienced undesirable outcomes.
Absolute Risk Reduction (ARR)	Estimated proportion of people who would be spared the undesirable outcome through exposure to the intervention.
Odds Ratio (OR)	The proportion of people with the adverse outcome relative to those without it.
Number Needed to Treat (NNT)	Estimates how many people would need to receive an intervention to prevent one undesirable outcome.

Source: Data from Polit, D., & Beck, C. (2018). *Essentials of nursing research* (9th ed.). Philadelphia, PA: Wolters Kluwer.

TABLE 30.4 Bivariate Statistics

t-Tests	Testing differences in two group means
ANOVA	Used to test mean group differences of three of more groups.
Chi-squared test	Used to test hypotheses about differences in proportions, as in a crosstab.
Pearson's *r*	Both descriptive (summarizes the direction of relationship between variables) and inferential (tests hypotheses about population correlations).
Effect size indexes	Estimates of the magnitude of effects of an intervention on an outcome.

ANOVA, analysis of variance.

Source: Data from Polit, D., & Beck, C. (2018). *Essentials of nursing research* (9th ed.). Philadelphia, PA: Wolters Kluwer.

Conclusion

- Conclusion: Includes discussion of study findings, implications, limitations, and recommendations for future research. Practice recommendations are supported by the study results (Thomas, 2015, p. 836).

THE QUALITATIVE RESEARCH PROCESS

- Rather than numbers, the focus of qualitative research is an in-depth understanding of a phenomenon, with particular emphasis on the subject's reports of personal experience. This is used to increase understanding of how phenomena are perceived from individuals', groups', and cultures' point of view (Thomas, 2015, pp. 836–837).
- Qualitative research identifies the complexity of human experience with the "lived experience" and offers rich, in-depth information about human and caregiving phenomena (Polit & Beck, 2018, p. 54).
- Although the approach to qualitative research is more flexible than quantitative methodology, qualitative research still entails defined specifying aims, defined approach, description of sampling and data collection procedures, and a plan for analysis consistent. The approach and aims and actions to assure validity are in place to maintain the same rigor as quantitative research (Thomas, 2015, p. 837).
- The baseline difference is the two methodologies is approach is qualitative study is more circular than the linear quantitative approach. Qualitative study continuously examines and interprets data to make decisions about how to proceed based on what has been discovered. Researchers themselves may not know how the study the study will unfold (Polit & Beck, 2018, p. 53).

Research Problem

- Qualitative researchers generally begin with a broad topic, seeking answers to something about which little or nothing is known. The focus of the study becomes more delineated as the study progresses (Polit & Beck, 2018, p. 54).
- Qualitative research may contribute to neonatal practice in several areas: (1) descriptions of patient needs and experiences; (2) providing the groundwork for instrument development and evaluation; and (3) elaborating on concepts relative to theory development (Pantoja & Hines, 2016, p. 7).

Literature Review

- Whether the literature is reviewed prior to, during, or after data collection depends on the qualitative methodology chosen. Some believe reviewing literature prior to the study could potentially introduce bias into the researchers' understanding of what study participants tell them. Other believe the researchers should have a working knowledge of the topic prior to interviewing participants in order to facilitate communication (Polit & Beck, 2018, p. 54).

Gaining Entrée

- Gaining entrée is more than determining a site at which to perform the research; it may also involve negotiating and gaining permission from gatekeepers of the community to which the research wishes to access. Due to the often personal nature of the qualitative research, this can be an important step in assuring the data are collected is a true reflection of the phenomena of interest (Polit & Beck, 2018, p. 54).

Approach

- The specific research approach stems from an underlying philosophical perspective (Thomas, 2015, p. 837). While certain design features are guided by tradition, qualitative researchers employ an emergent design that materializes during data collection. Analysis and interpretations are ongoing activities which guide subsequent choices (Polit & Beck, 2018, p. 55).
- Types of perspectives commonly used in nursing qualitative research include:
  - Phenomenology: seeks to understand the lived experience of individuals.
  - Grounded theory: symbolic interaction forms the basis for understanding social processes and behavior.
  - Ethnography: describes a cultural group (Thomas, 2015, p. 837).
  - Table 30.5 provides a more detailed list and description of qualitative study methods.

SATURATION

- Many qualitative researchers use the principle of saturation to determine when the study is complete. Rather than a calculated *n* of a quantitative study, the research continues until the researcher determines saturation of the data have occurred. Saturation occurs when participants' accounts become redundant, and that no new information is emerging from continued study (Polit & Beck, 2018, p. 55).

Rigor and Validity

- Defining high-quality qualitative research is controversial, and several frameworks for qualitative study evaluation have been developed. Regardless of specifics of a framework, there are enhancement strategies qualitative researchers can use to argue the rigor of the studies
  - *Prolonged engagement:* Researchers must demonstrate an investment of sufficient time both for building trust with participants and collecting data.
  - *Persistent observation* concerns the salience of the data gathered; that is, did the researcher stay focused on the phenomena of interest or were extraneous data included that diluted study findings.
  - *Reflexivity strategies* involve awareness of the researcher "self" as an individual and the role of the researcher's own world view plays in the collection and interpretation of qualitative data.
  - *Triangulation* is demonstrated by using multiple references to draw conclusions from the information. This leads to a completer and more contextual picture of the phenomenon.
  - *Audit trails* are created by researchers to demonstrate to an independent auditor how conclusions were drawn. Items collected may include raw data (interview transcripts), reflexive notes, memos, and drafts (Polit & Beck, 2018, pp. 298–300).

Interpretation of Qualitative Results

- Qualitative research is productive when it is used to describe a poorly understand phenomena; however, the phenomenon must be one which merits scrutiny, and one for which elucidation will be transferrable and/or applicable to others. Qualitative researchers strive for transferability of results in order to improve circumstances for larger areas of population than the ones studied (Polit & Beck, 2018, p. 304).

TABLE 30.5 Qualitative Study Methods

Ethnography	Involves the description and interpretation of a culture and cultural behavior. Typically involves extensive fieldwork in which the researcher immerses himself or herself into the culture.
Phenomenology	An approach to understanding people's everyday life experiences. Researchers seek out the "essence" of the phenomenon as experiences by someone living it.
Grounded theory	Tries to account for people's actions from the perspective of those involved. Its theoretical roots are in symbolic interaction, which focuses on the manner in which people make sense of social interactions.
Case studies	In-depth investigations of a single entity or small number of entities in an attempt to understand issues that are important to the circumstances of the focal entity.
Narrative analyses	Focuses on story as the object of inquiry to understand how individuals make sense of events in their lives.

Source: Data from Polit, D., & Beck, C. (2018). *Essentials of nursing research* (9th ed.). Philadelphia, PA: Wolters Kluwer.

CONCLUSION

Ultimately, original research topics are evaluated for their merit in adding knowledge or filling gaps in knowledge. By understanding individual research projects, new knowledge is gained to help guide best practices and develop and evolve clinical practice. By understanding the components of nursing research both in the quantitative and qualitative realms, the advanced practice nurse is better prepared to lead healthcare teams and improve patient care practices.

REVIEW QUESTIONS

1. Systematic inquiry designed to generate trustworthy evidence about issues of importance to the nursing profession and their clients, including nursing practice, education, administration, and informatics is nursing
   A. Evidence.
   B. Inquiry.
   C. Research.

2. The variable which is manipulated in experimental research is the
   A. Dependent variable.
   B. Independent variable.
   C. Randomized variable.

3. Measures of central tendency (mean, median, mode) and dispersion (standard deviation, variance, range) are examples of
   A. Descriptive statistics.
   B. Inferential statistics.
   C. Magnitudinal statistics.

4. A process which involves negotiating and gaining permission from gatekeepers of the community to which the researcher wishes to access is called gaining
   A. Access.
   B. Course.
   C. Entrée.

5. The NNP is interested in doing research regarding the level of a mother's reading comprehension compared to comfort with discharge teaching. This is an example of a study in which results would be analyzed using
   A. Bivariate statistics.
   B. Duovariate statistics.
   C. Univariate statistics.

REFERENCES

Lopez, S., & Tyson, J., (2020). Practicing evidenced-based neonatal–prenatal medicine. In R. Martin, A. Fanaroff, & M. Walsh (Eds.), *Fanaroff and Martin's neonatal–perinatal medicine: Diseases of the fetus and infant* (11th ed., pp. 113–119). Philadelphia, PA: Elsevier.

National Association of Neonatal Nurse Practitioners. (2010). *Understanding clinical research: A practical guide.* Glenview, IL: NANN.

Palma, J., & Tarczy-Hornoch, P. (2018). Biomedical informatics in neonatology. In C. Gleason & S. Juul (Eds.), *Avery's diseases of the newborn* (10th ed., pp. 11–19.e2). Philadelphia, PA: Elsevier.

Pantoja, A., & Hines, M. (2016). Evidence-based clinical practice. In S. Gardner, B. Carter, M. Hines, & J. Hernandez (Eds.), *Merenstein & Gardner's handbook of neonatal intensive care* (8th ed., pp. 1–10.e4). St. Louis, MO: Elsevier.

Polit, D., & Beck, C. (2018). *Essentials of nursing research* (9th ed.). Philadelphia, PA: Wolters Kluwer.

Thomas, K. (2015). Foundations of neonatal research. In T. Verklan & M. Walden (Eds.), *Core curriculum for neonatal intensive care nursing* (5th ed., pp. 832–865). St. Louis, MO: Elsevier.

31 ANSWERS WITH RATIONALES

CHAPTER 1

1. **C.** Hypertension is the most common complication in pregnancy and cause of most of the morbidity/mortality in both maternal and neonatal cases. Hypertension-related complications are a leading cause of maternal death in the United States (Jeyabalan, 2015, p. 250; Moore, 2018, p. 119; Poole, 2014, p. 124).

2. **B.** Pulmonary changes in pregnancy include an increase in minute ventilation, alveolar ventilation, tidal volume, oxygen consumption, PaO_2, and arterial pH; a decrease in functional residual capacity, residual volume, and $PaCO_2$. Respiratory rate remains unchanged (Arafeh, 2013, p. 226; Whitty & Dombrowski, 2019, p. 1043).

3. **C.** Varicella vaccine is not indicated in pregnancy; however, knowing maternal antibody status aids in identifying women most at risk for infection during pregnancy. Administration of varicella vaccine in pregnancy or within 3 months of conception has been associated with increased risk of birth defects (Whitty & Dombrowski, 2019, p. 1050).

4. **A.** Gonorrhea is the oldest known sexually transmitted infection (STI), is caused by *N. gonorrhoeae*, and may cause gonococcal ophthalmia neonatorum, disseminated gonococcal infection, preterm premature rupture of membranes, chorioamnionitis, preterm delivery, intrauterine growth restriction (IUGR), and fetal/neonatal septicemia (Duff, 2019, pp. 866–868).

5. **B.** The BPP combines an NST with amniotic fluid volume (vertical fluid pocket >2 cm), fetal breathing movements, fetal activity, and normal fetal musculoskeletal tone. A score of 0 to 2 is assigned to each category (Barron, 2014, p. 114; Cypher, 2016, p. 143; Dukhivny & Wilkins-Haug, 2017, pp. 9–10; Hackney, 2015, p. 183; Kaimal, 2014, p. 551).

CHAPTER 2

1. **A.** The etiology of an increased amniotic fluid level falls into three categories: decreased absorption, overproduction, or idiopathic. Fetal swallowing is the predominant mechanism of amniotic fluid removal, so congenital abnormalities associated with the gastrointestinal tract (tracheal atresia, duodenal atresia, tracheal or bowel obstruction) or the neurologic system (anencephaly, trisomy 18, trisomy 21) are often present (Dubil & Magin, 2015).

2. **C.** In vasa previa, the insertion of the umbilical cord into the placenta is velamentous, with the umbilical vessels

coursing through the fetal membranes before inserting into the placental disk and the unsupported vessels then overlying the cervix (Hull, Resnik, & Silver, 2019, p. 791).

3. **B.** Since fetal skin remains nonkeratinized until week 22 to 25, surface exchange is a main factor contributing to fluid dynamics in early pregnancy (Dubil & Magann, 2015, p. 340).

4. **A.** The etiology of an increased amniotic fluid level falls into three categories: decreased absorption, overproduction, or idiopathic (Dubil & Magin, 2015).

5. **C.** If oligohydramnios is prolonged and occurs during the canalicular phase of alveolar proliferation (16–18 weeks' gestation), severe pulmonary hypoplasia associated with a high perinatal mortality can occur. Although the exact physiologic cause of pulmonary hypoplasia is unclear, any maternal or fetal complication leading to the inhibition of fetal breathing, any lack of a trophic function of amniotic fluid within the airways, or any simple mechanical compression of the chest are proposed as causes (Dubil & Magann, 2015, p. 348).

CHAPTER 3

1. **A.** Caput succedaneum is caused by edema (subcutaneous, extraperiosteal fluid) from the birth process. Findings include maximum swelling noted at birth, which may include ecchymosis, petechiae, or purpura; poorly defined edges; crosses suture lines; occurs over presenting portion of scalp; and usually present with molding. There is usually spontaneous resolution, within days (24–48 hours) of birth (Abdulhayoglu, 2017, p. 64; Benjamin & Furdon, 2015, p 127; Johnson, 2016, p. 65; Vargo, 2014, p. 602).

2. **B.** Abdulhayoglu, 2017, pp. 68–69; Benjamin & Furdon, 2015, p. 139; Tappero, 2016, pp. 153–154, 183–187; Vargo, 2014, p. 619

3. **A.** PMA is the age from first day of LMP to day of assessment (Trotter, 2016, p. 23).

4. **C.** Findings can be normal variants or associated with syndromes or chromosomal abnormalities. Ninety percent of all visible anomalies at birth are found in the head area (Benjamin & Furdon, 2015, p. 116; Johnson, 2016, p. 97; Vargo, 2014, p. 602).

5. **A.** If central cyanosis is present and there is no evidence of respiratory distress and/or it worsens with crying, the cause is likely congenital heart defect (CHD). It can be

assessed by the oxygen challenge test (administration of 100% oxygen). If no improvement in saturations, etiology is likely CHD disease (Benjamin & Furdon, 2015, pp. 128–129; Vargo, 2014, pp. 603–604).

CHAPTER 4

1. **C.** Antibiotics levels are gauged through TDM. This uses plasma medication concentrations to determine and optimize medication therapy (Domonoske, 2015, p. 217).

2. **C.** Immature/total neutrophil (I/T) ratio = (% bands + % immature forms) ÷ (% mature + % bands + % immature forms)
   I/T = (0 + 8 + 6 + 4) divided by (32 + 0 + 8 + 6 + 4) or 18/50= 0.36

3. **B.** ANC = WBC × (% immature neutrophils + % mature neutrophils) × 10 (Diab & Luchtman-Jones, 2015, pp. 1319–1324)
   4 × [(4+2) × 10] =
   4 × [6 × 10]
   4 × 60 = 240 (severe neurtrophenia)

4. **A.** Lateral decubitus view is obtained with the infant lying on the side and shot back to front. A right or left lateral decubitus indicates on which side the infant is lying. The most common example in the NICU is to obtain a left lateral decubitus (lie on left side, right side up) view to assess for free abdominal air, which will layer out over the liver taking advantage of the contrast in densities to increase visibility (Jensen et al., 2017, p. 67).

5. **B.** Findings on an EEG are considered best in terms of the continuity of background activity, the synchrony of this activity, and the appearance and disappearance of specific waveforms and patterns (Neil & Volpe, 2018, p. 227)

CHAPTER 5

1. **C.** The problem or malformation of the baby can immediately cause a lowering of self-esteem and the parents may view this as a failure. Guilt is one of the overwhelming emotions that plague these parents (Ballard, 2015, p. 632; Gardner, Voos, & Hills, 2016, p. 827).

2. **C.** Parental perception of support by the medical team has been shown to be inversely correlated with maternal depressive symptoms. The more support the parents feel is being given by the medical team, the fewer depressive symptoms are manifested. (Gardner et al., 2016, p. 828).

3. **B.** During medically necessary interventions, it is important to give parents as much interaction (or at least visual contact) with their infant as is possible (Gardner et al., 2016, p. 822, 827; Kenner & Boykova, 2015, p. 342).
   Facilitate opportunities for parents to be involved in their baby's care (Gardner et al., 2016, p. 832; Kenner & Boykova, 2015, p. 333).

4. **A.** Family-centered care has been shown to have a significant positive influence on the family's ability to cope with the NICU stress. The use of FCC has been shown to enhance the likelihood of successful parent–child relationships (Gardner et al., 2016, p. 828).

5. **B.** Klaus and Klaus suggest that at least 60 minutes of uninterrupted private time for parents and infants to encourage and enhance the bonding experience (Klaus, Kennell, & Fanaroff, 2013, p. 209).

CHAPTER 6

1. **B.** Create an environment that will facilitate a safe, quiet environment to have these discussions. Introduce everyone from the medical team present, with their respective role. Discuss with the family their understanding of the presenting issue, then state the purpose of the meeting. Identify decision-makers if necessary. Explore options with the family. Provide moments of silence intermittently to allow the family to process the information discussed. Review relevant data and decisions (Fanaroff, 2015, pp. 31–33).

2. **C.** End-of-life discussions should be family-centered, with an interdisciplinary team to promote clear communication, identify family goals, and assess cultural, spiritual, and religious concerns that will need to be honored (Fanaroff, 2015, pp. 31–33).

3. **B.** Use of consistent information from all health care providers is important to minimize anxiety (Kenner, 2015, p. 339). The overall goals with these conversations are to assess and develop the goals of care for their child. (Cortezzo & Carter, 2018 p. 447; Fanaroff, 2015, p. 33).

4. **A.** The more complex the medical situation, the more crucial it is that parents receive consistent information, perhaps from a single designated person on the healthcare team (Swaney, English, & Carter, 2016, p. 938).

5. **B.** Criteria for considering withholding or withdrawing life-sustaining medical treatment are inevitability of death, ineffective treatment, and poor quality of life (Cortezzo & Carter, 2018, p. 447; Fanaroff, 2015, p. 33).

CHAPTER 7

1. **A.** The AAP recommends that all preterm infants receive routine immunizations at their chronologic age, rather than their corrected age (Carter, Gratney, & Carter, 2016, p. 908; Demauro & Hintz, 2018, p. 988; Hummel, 2014, p. 386; Smith & Andrews, 2017, p. 291; Stewart, Bentley, & Knorr, 2017, p. 262).

2. **A.** Auditory dyssynchrony or auditory neuropathy accounts for 10% of all infants diagnosed with severe permanent hearing loss. The function of the outer hair cells remains intact; however, a pathology of the inner hair cells or the myelinated fibers of cranial nerve VIII impairs neuroconduction of sound energy to the brainstem. The electric signals to the brain have responses that are dyssynchronous, so information is not relayed in a consistent

manner (Stewart et al., 2017, p. 994; Vohr, 2015, p. 994; Vohr, 2018, p. 1559).

3. **B.** The ABR uses surface electrodes to record neural activity in the cochleae, outer and inner hair cells, auditory nerve (VIII), and brainstem. It detects auditory neuropathy where the EOAE does not (Stewart et al., 2017, p. 996; Vohr, 2015, pp. 994–995; Vohr, 2018, p. 1560).

4. **A.** Infants who are born after 30 weeks' gestational age or born at 1,500 to 2,000 g may be considered for screening if they have had a medically unstable course (e.g., severe respiratory distress syndrome, hypotension requiring pressor support, or surgery in the first several weeks of age). Some recommend infants who are born at >30 weeks are screened at the postnatal age of 3 weeks (Campomanes & Binenbaum, 2018, p. 1553; Carter et al., 2016, p. 907; De Alba; Hummel, 2014, p. 376; Leeman & VanderVeen, 2017, p. 987; Martin & Crowley, 2013, p. 247; Sun et al., 2015, p. 1772).

5. **B.** Specialized feedings for the first 6 to 9 months post discharge are needed in infants with ongoing and catch-up requirements not met by term infant formulas. Increased calorie post-discharge formulas with increased protein, minerals, and long-chain polyunsaturated fatty acids are necessary to aid catch-up growth (Abrams, 2017, p. 857; Adamkin, Radmacher, & Lewis, 2013, pp. 179–180; Anderson, Poindexter, & Martin, 2017, p. 282; Carter et al., 2016, pp. 922–923; Colaizy, Demauro, Mcnelis, & Poindexter, 2018, p. 1021; Demauro & Hintz, 2018, p. 985; Hack, 2013, p. 529; Poindexter & Ehrenkranz, 2015, pp. 608–609; Stark et al., 2017, p. 213; Stewart et al., 2017, p. 63).

CHAPTER 8

1. **B.** In the case of premature infants with thin permeable skin, evaporative heat loss occurs through transepidermal water loss (TEWL). The more immature the newborn, the larger the relative surface area (Hodson, 2018, p. 362). Evaporative heat losses are inversely related to ambient humidity and measures to increase the vapor pressure close to the skin simplify fluid and thermal management of extremely preterm infants (Agren, 2015, p. 502).

2. **B.** Production of brown fat begins around 26 to 28 weeks' gestation and continues for 3 to 5 weeks after birth (Fraser, 2016, p. 586).

3. **A.** Sepsis in infants may present with hypothermia or hyperthermia (Gardner & Hernandez, 2016, p. 112). Hypothermia is more likely to occur in premature infants with bacterial sepsis. Term infants are more likely to present with hyperthermia as a sign of infection (Wilson & Tyner, 2014, p. 699).

4. **A.** After the immediate newborn period, the more common and chronic problem facing premature infants than actual hypothermia is caloric loss from unrecognized chronic cold stress that results in excess oxygen consumption and slow weight gain (Chatson, 2017, p. 186).

5. **C.** An increased risk of Pseudomonas infections has been demonstrated with the use of incubator humidification when condensation of vapor on the inner incubator walls occurs which, therefore, should be avoided (Agren, 2015, p. 507).

CHAPTER 9

1. **A.** Cord blood samples are performed when events of pregnancy or labor are connected to adverse outcomes in the neonate. This may include a low five minute Apgar score (Barry, Deacon, Hernandez, & Jones, 2016, pp. 154–155).

2. **A.** Delayed cord clamping (DCC) is especially beneficial to premature infants but is also recommended for full-term infants. It decreases the need for transfusions, increases hemoglobin and iron stores in early infancy, reduces anemia during the first 6 months of life, increases cardiac output, and increases circulatory stability (Katheria & Finer, 2018, pp. 277–279; Niermeyer, Clarke, & Hernandez, 2016, p. 50).

3. **B.** Epinephrine is indicated if heart rate is less than 60 beats a minute despite 60 seconds of adequate coordinated ventilation and compressions. The heart is now without energy (adenosine triphosphate or ATP) and will no longer beat adequately (Wyckoff & Goldsmith, 2015, pp. 491–492).

4. **C.** EKG leads should be placed when compressions are anticipated/begun (Katherina & Finer, 2018, p. 279).

5. **C.** The American Academy of Pediatrics and the American College of Obstetricians and gynecologists in their Guidelines for Perinatal Care established classifications of perinatal resources according to different levels of care. Level IV NICUs provide level III care, plus provide surgery and facilitate outreach (Rojas, 2016, pp. 33–34).

CHAPTER 10

1. **C.** 3,620 g – 3,500 g = 120 g/wk
120 g/wk ÷ 7 days = 17.14 g/d
17.14 g/d ÷ 3.62 kg = 4.73 g/kg/d

2. **B.** 20 kcal/oz ÷ 30 mL/oz = 0.67 kcal/mL
75 mL × 8 feeds/d = 600 mL/d
600 mL/d × 0.67 kcal/mL = 402 kcal/d
402 kcal/d ÷ 3.620 kg = 111 kcal/kg/d
or
75 mL/feed × 8 feeds/d = 600 mL/d
600 mL/d ÷ 3.62 kg = 166 mL/kg/d
166 mL/kg/d × 0.67 kcal/mL = 111 kcal/kg/d

3. **A.** Infants with NEC are at higher risk for malnutrition secondary to increased nutrient losses and malabsorption, therefore it is imperative to support the infants' nutritional needs with PN specifically through the acute phase (Brown et al., 2016, p. 416).

4. **B.** It is recommended to reduce or omit copper and manganese from PN in patients with impaired biliary excretion and/or liver disease because they are excreted in the bile (Anderson, Poindexter, & Martin, 2017, p. 263).

5. B. Infants with galactosemia are unable to receive maternal human milk or donated human milk (Furman & Schanler, 2018, p. 1001; Hurst & Puopolo, 2017, p. 291).

CHAPTER 11

1. A. The total body water (TBW) varies from 85% to 90% in the ELBW infant to 75% in the term newborn infant (Halbardier, 2015, p. 146).

2. A. Edema results when there is an abnormal accumulation of fluid in the IS. Etiology of edema can include decreased capillary oncotic pressure from inadequate protein intake or kidney glomerular disease, increased capillary hydrostatic pressure, increased capillary wall permeability from infection affecting the integrity of the capillary wall, or hypertension from venous obstruction (Wright, Posencheg, Seri, & Evans, 2018, pp. 370–371).

3. C. Insensible water loss can be calculated using the formula IWL = fluid intake − urine output + weight change (Doherty, 2017, p. 296)
U.O. = 3 mL/kg/hr × 1.5 kg × 24 hr/d = 108 mL/d
Intake = 150 mL/kg/d × 1.5 kg = 225 mL/d
IWL = 225 mL − (108 + 200) = −83 mL

4. C. Initially Na$^+$ and K$^+$ supplementation are not required in the first 24 hours in newborn infants (Doherty, 2017, p. 299; Nyp, Brunkhorst, Reavy, & Pallotto, 2016, p. 325).

5. B. Excessive intake of isotonic fluids will precipitate edema and signs of fluid overload. Development of edema can also occur under conditions such as heart failure, sepsis, and long-term use of paralytics (Doherty, 2017, p. 300).

CHAPTER 12

1. B. The amount of drug administered equals the amount of drug eliminated and occurs after the fourth dose of drug given; however, the time it takes to reach steady-state concentration is mostly dependent on drug half-life and can be reached sooner if the dosing interval is shorter than the drug half-life (Allegaert, Ward, & Van Den Anker, 2018, p. 426; Holford, 2018, pp. 49–54).

2. C. Mathematically described as the equation of a straight line, first-order pharmacokinetics is also called single-compartment first-order kinetics (Allegaert et al., 2018, p. 423). A constant percentage of drug is eliminated over time; it is a proportional rate of elimination (Allegaert et al., 2018, p. 423; Wade, 2015, pp. 667–668).

3. C. Concepts relative to zero-order pharmacokinetics include enzyme/transport systems and drug dose. Enzymes or transport-system receptors are saturated with drugm thereby preventing proportional drug elimination (Allegaert et al., 2018, p. 424).
Small dose increases result in large serum concentration changes until receptors are free from drug (Allegaert et al., 2018, p. 424). Examples of drugs with zero-order kinetics: caffeine, diazepam, furosemide, indomethacin, phenytoin (Allegaert et al., 2018, p. 424; Wade, 2015, p. 668).

4. B. Drug metabolism is the biotransformation of drug into inactive and active metabolites; occurs in the liver, kidney, intestinal mucosa, and lungs; and is generally classified as Phase I or Phase II metabolism (Allegaert et al., 2018, p. 420; Blackburn, 2018, p. 201; Domonoske, 2015, p. 224; McClary, 2015b, pp. 655–657; Wade, 2015, p. 666). Phase I metabolism: enzymatic drug conversion to metabolites via oxidation, reduction, and hydrolysis (Blackburn, 2018, p. 181; Domonoske, 2015, p. 224).
Cytochrome P450 (CYP450) enzymes mediate Phase I metabolism and are present in many tissues, but they are most highly concentrated in hepatic tissues (Allegaert et al., 2018, pp. 655–657; McClary, 2015b, pp. 420–421).

5. A. Poor perfusion to the muscle limits absorption with the intramuscular route; the drug may deposit and remain at the injection site for a prolonged period, and neonates are at risk for sclerosis at the injection site or abscess development (Allegaert et al., 2018, p. 420). Muscle and subcutaneous tissues are limited in the preterm and low birth weight infant, limiting the use of these sites for drug therapy (Blackburn, 2018, p. 198; Domonoske, 2015, p. 221). Gestational age and health status of the neonate may result in delayed or erratic absorption from the muscle (Blackburn, 2018, p. 198).

CHAPTER 13

1. A. Digoxin has narrow therapeutic window; dosage must be individualized considering renal function. Sinus bradycardia is a sign of toxicity (Taketomo, Hodding, & Kraus, 2018, pp. 636–640).

2. C. Prednisolone (Pediapred) dose depends on the condition being treated and response of patient. Dosage for infants should be based on disease severity and patient response rather than rigid adherence to dosing guidelines. Consider alternate day therapy for long-term therapy (Taketomo et al., 2018, pp. 1668–1670).

3. A. Surfactant prevents the alveoli from collapsing during expiration by lowering surface tension between air and alveolar surfaces. Produces rapid improvements in lung oxygenation and compliance may require frequent adjustments to oxygen and ventilator settings (Taketomo et al., pp. 264–265).

4. B. Indomethacin (Indocin) may be given at 12-hour intervals if urine output (UOP) is ≥1 mL/kg/hr after first dose; use 24-hour interval if <1 mL/kg/hr after first dose. Dose should be held if UOP <0.6 mL/kg/hr or anuria is noted (Taketomo et al., 2018, pp. 1066–1069).

5. A. With fentanyl (Duragesic), give intermittent IV doses slowly: rapid infusion may cause chest wall rigidity (Taketomo et al., 2018, pp. 837–849).

CHAPTER 14

1. A. Anomalous external physical features are called dysmorphisms (Parikh & Mitchell, 2015, p. 436).

2. B. Trisomy 18 Phenotypic features which are notable at birth include intrauterine growth restriction (IUGR) with a small narrow cranium with prominent occiput, open metopic suture, low-set and posteriorly rotated ears, and micrognathia. Characteristic are clenched hands with overlapping fingers, hypoplastic nails, and rocker bottom feet (Haldeman-Englert, Saitta, & Zackai, 2018, p. 215; Schiefelbein, 2015, p. 404; Sterk, 2015, p. 774).

3. **B.** Trisomy 13 is associated with midline malformations including congenital heart disease, cleft palate, holoprosencephaly, renal anomalies, and postaxial polydactyly. Eye anomalies and scalp defects can suggest the diagnosis. Aplasia cutis congenita is a congenital absence of skin involving the scalp. Lesions have sharp margins and may present as ulcers, bullae, or scars. Most defects are small and superficial (Skert, 2015, p. 777).

4. **C.** Most patients with a deletion receive the diagnosis (of DiGeorge syndrome) following identification of significant cardiovascular malformations, conotruncal cardiac anomaly including interrupted aortic arch type B, truncus arteriosus, or tetralogy of Fallot. With further evaluation, often aplasia or hypoplasia of the thymus and parathyroid glands are noted, along with functional T-cell abnormalities and hypocalcemia (Haldeman-Englert et al., 2018, p. 218). Hypocalcemia occurs in 60% of neonates, severe cases will cause seizures (Sterk, 2015, p. 778).

5. **C.** Inborn errors of metabolism are genetic biochemical disorders in which the function of a protein is compromised, resulting in alteration of the structure or amount of the protein synthesized (Sterk, 2015, p. 789).

CHAPTER 15

1. **A.** Holoprosencephaly refers to an entire spectrum of cleavage disorders sharing a common embryologic origin. The essential abnormality is the incomplete separation of the prosencephalon along one or more of its three major planes: horizontal, transverse, and sagittal (Du Plessis & Volpe, 2018, p. 37; Gressens & Hüppi, 2015, p. 855).

2. **B.** A major category of ventriculomegaly that results in ventricular dilation by an accumulation of CSF. This is due to the fact that CSF production exceeds CSF absorption. The majority is caused by decreased absorption due to an obstruction.
   ○ Can result from abnormalities anywhere in the CSF pathway.
   ○ Enlargement of any or all ventricles due to an obstruction of CSF flow upstream or at the fourth ventricle foramina is called noncommunicating hydrocephalus.
   ○ Impaired CSF flow distal to the fourth ventricle foramina results in communicating hydrocephalus (Volpe et al., 2018, p. 58–72).

3. **B.** Myotonic dystrophy is the most common disorder affecting musculature (Darras & Volpe, 2018, p. 927). Clinical presentation: Facial paralysis.
   Respiratory distress related to diaphragmatic weakness. Hypotonia arthrogryposis—mostly lower extremities, feeding difficulties, aspiration tent-shaped upper lip cardiomyopathy (Darras & Volpe, 2018, pp. 922–923).

4. **C.** IVH Grade III—Blood fills more than 50% of the ventricle; ventricles begin to dilate and affect the brain material (Volpe et al., 2018, p. 637).

5. **A.** The following decreases the risk of IVH: delayed cord clamping, antenatal steroids, gentle handling, closer attention to blood pressures, synchronous ventilation, postnatal surfactant administration (De Vries, 2015, p. 890; Volpe et al., 2018, pp. 649–662).

CHAPTER 16

1. **B.** TOF is the most common cyanotic congenital heart defect, occurring in about 3 in 10,000 live births and causes 7% to 10% of all congenital cardiac malformations. TOF presentation relates to the degree of pulmonary stenosis (Swanson & Ericson, 2016, p. 674).

2. **A.** Cyanosis is a bluish color of the lips, tongue, mucous membranes, skin, ear lobes, and nail beds due to deoxygenated blood venous blood (Vargo, 2018, p. 96).

3. **C.** Tachyarrhythmias originate from areas other than the sinus node, such as conduction via the conduct through the AV node, bundle of His and right and left bundle branches, and result in P wave changes. Prolonged arrhythmias may result in cardiac failure or sudden death (Ashwath & Snyder, 2013, pp. 1261–1262).

4. **A.** Persistent PDA clinical presentation stems from left-to-right shunting which may also decrease cardiac output and increase the workload of the left side of the heart and result in decreased blood flow to vital organs (Beniz, 2013, p. 1225), and presents as an LUQ systolic "machinery" murmur, bounding pulses, visible precordium, widened pulse pressure, worsening respiratory status due to pulmonary edema (Beniz, 2013, p. 1224), and wide pulse pressure (Scholz & Reinking, 2017, p. 806; Swanson & Ericson, 2016, p. 658).

5. **A.** Maternal presence of anti-Ro or anti-La antibodies related to maternal systemic lupus erythematosus results in placental passage of immunoglobulin C antibody which deposits compliment near the AV node, resulting in fetal heart block or possible hydrops. (Martin, Fanaroff, & Walsh, 2015, p. 1212). Maternal lupus disease is associated with fetal and neonatal complete congenital heart block and dilated cardiomyopathy (Sadowski, 2015, p. 537).

CHAPTER 17

1. **B.** Surfactant is produced in type II alveolar cells. It is packaged and stored in the lamellar bodies. Lamellar bodies are extruded into the alveoli by exocytosis forming tubular myelin. Tubular myelin is a lattice-like structure with the hydrophobic ends of the phospholipid extending into the alveolar air and the hydrophilic end binding with water at the air–liquid interface. This process reduces surface tension Surfactant components are also "recycled" by the lamellar bodies or broken down by lysosomes (Fraser, 2015, p. 448; Suresh, Soll, & Mandy, 2017, pp. 338–339).

2. B. The most common precipitating factor for PPHN is intrauterine asphyxia (Fraser, 2015, p. 458).

3. A. Symptoms of RDS present soon after delivery, and respiratory difficulty increases within the first few hours of life (Blackburn, 2013, p. 343; Fraser, 2015, pp. 449–451; Hansen & Levin, 2019, p. 411; Shepherd & Nelin, 2017, pp. 62–63, 71–72; Wambach & Hamvas, 2015, p. 1078).

4. B. Mean airway pressure (P_{aw}) the average pressure applied to the lungs during the respiratory cycle. Mean airway pressure is affected by PEEP, PIP, inspiratory time, frequency, and gas flow. Excessive P_{aw} can contribute to barotrauma and lung damage (Donn & Sinha, 2015, p. 1091).

5. C. With lung expansion, surfactant is released which helps maintain FRC by homogeneously decreasing surface tension and creating a pressure gradient for lung fluid removal through the alveoli (Keszler & Chatburn, 2017, p. 140).

CHAPTER 18

1. A. Clinical presentation includes bilious emesis (obstruction usually distal to the ampulla of Vater) within a few hours to 24 hours after birth, minimal abdominal distention limited to the upper abdomen, and failure to pass meconium (Bradshaw, 2015, pp. 597–598; Ringer & Hansen, 2017, p. 954). Radiography that demonstrates the classic "double bubble," air in the stomach, and upper duodenum but no air distally in the small or large intestine is diagnostic; "double bubble" with air present distally suggests duodenal stenosis (Bradshaw, 2015, p. 598; Bucher, Pocatti, Lauvorn, & Carter, 2016, p. 799; Ringer & Hansen, 2017, p. 954).

2. B. A subtle presentation (of NEC) may include general systemic signs mistaken for sepsis including lethargy, temperature instability, increased apnea and bradycardia events, poor feeding, in addition to GI symptoms including feeding intolerance (emesis, increased gastric aspirates), abdominal distention with or without tenderness, abdominal wall erythema, and bloody stools. Radiological findings are diagnostic with presence of pneumatosis intestinalis (hallmark finding of hydrogen gas in the bowel wall), portal venous gas, and/or pneumoperitoneum (Bradshaw, 2015, p. 608; Bucher et al., 2016, p. 802; Weitkamp, Premkumar & Martin, 2017, pp. 342–343). A fixed bowel loop on serial studies and stacking of intestinal loops supports the concern for NEC. Presence of periumbilical air collection noted in an anterior–posterior x-ray is referred to as the "football sign" (Javid, Riggle, & Smith, pp. 1092–1093; Weitkamp et al., 2017, p. 357).

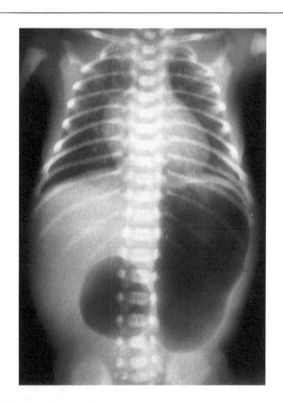

FIGURE 1 Duodenal atresia

Source: Reproduced with permission from Ehret, L. (2015). Radiologic evaluation. In T. Verklan & M. Walden (Eds.), *Core curriculum for neonatal intensive care nursing* (5th ed., pp. 253–281). St. Louis, MO: Elsevier.

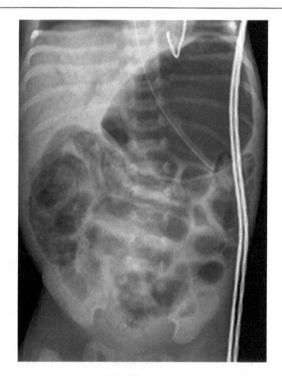

FIGURE 2 Necrotizing enterocolitis

Source: Reproduced with permission from Ehret, L. (2015). Radiologic evaluation. In T. Verklan & M. Walden (Eds.), *Core curriculum for neonatal intensive care nursing* (5th ed., pp. 253–281). St. Louis, MO: Elsevier.

3. B. Clinical presentation of malrotation with volvulus is sudden onset of bilious emesis in an otherwise healthy infant who has been stooling and feeding normally. Majority of infants will become symptomatic within the first week of life, the remaining present within the first month of life; presentation after 1 month of age is less common (Bradshaw, 2015, p. 600; Bucher et al., 2016, p. 797; Ringer & Hansen, 2017, p. 955).

4. A. Medical management (of Hirschsprung disease) includes gentle rectal irrigations with warm saline solution twice a day to empty the colon and minimize the risk for enterocolitis until surgery (Bradshaw, 2015, p. 605; Bucher et al., 2016, pp. 807–808; Ringer & Hansen, 2017, p. 952).

5. B. Adaptation occurs less in the jejunum compared to the ileum, however, other areas of the intestine can perform the functions lost by the jejunum therefore, these infants tend to do better than infants with loss of the ileum (Bradshaw, 2015, p. 610; Javid et al., 2018, p. 1096).

CHAPTER 19

1. A. FEN reflects the balance between glomerular filtration and tubular reabsorption of sodium. A level of <1% indicates prerenal factors that may decrease renal blood flow leading to prerenal azotemia. Level of 2.5% seen with intrinsic cause of acute kidney injury (AKI). Not useful diagnostic test in preterm infants <32 weeks' gestation due to renal immaturity (Doherty, 2017, p. 299).

2. B. Indomethacin is a nonsteroidal anti-inflammatory drug if taken during pregnancy has been associated with both structural and/or functional alterations in the newborn kidney due to decreased glomerular capillary pressure and glomerular filtration rate (GFR) that can lead to AKI (Samuels, Munoz, & Swinford, 2017, p 371; Vogt & Dell, 2015, p. 1680).

3. C. Eagle–Barrett syndrome or prune belly syndrome results in a lack of abdominal musculature, hydronephrosis (dilated but unobstructed urinary tract) with dilated bladder, and bilateral cryptorchidism (Sherman, 2015, p. 731).

4. C. Testicular torsion is a surgical emergency and can result in loss of testicular function and/or fertility if untreated. The surgery is needed to assess the viability of the testis that is twisted, but also to ensure that the second testis does not become twisted also (Merguerian & Rowe, 2018, p. 1271).

5. C. Gentamicin, an aminoglycoside, is the one antibiotic frequently given to infants that can cause kidney damage in high doses (Askenazi, 2018, p. 1285).

CHAPTER 20

1. B. Metabolic or endocrine disorders of the newborn include problems known as inborn errors of metabolism and encompass both metabolic and biochemical genetic disease. Most conditions involve gene mutation, which causes an absent or defective enzyme, or over- or under-production of hormones, with life-threatening physiological or biochemical system regulation dysfunction (Cederbaum, 2018, p. 224).

2. B. Since tyrosine is elemental to the production of dopamine and other essential neurotransmitters, infants with this disorder experience developmental and intellectual disabilities, skin problems, and epilepsy (Merritt & Gallagher, 2018, pp. 241–242). Treatment for PKU is life-long dietary therapy.

3. A. Infants with galactosemia often present with severe jaundice and coagulopathy while infants with other disorders of carbohydrate metabolism may present with hypoglycemia, lactic acidosis, infection, or intestinal problems (Merritt & Gallagher, 2018, p. 236).

4. C. Persistent hypoglycemia is the product of intrinsic metabolic problems of the infant, such as hyperinsulinism, congenital disorders, endocrine disorders, or inborn errors of metabolism (Devaskar & Garg, 2015, p. 1439; Werny, Taplin, Bennett, Pihoker, 2018, p. 1410).

5. A. The infant may be symptom-free initially; then demonstrate acute or progressive intoxication. The infant presents with increased drowsiness and poor feeding after the metabolite accumulates, with stress, or when feeds are introduced (Merritt & Gallagher, 2018, p. 243).

CHAPTER 21

1. B. Hematopoiesis is responsible for the formation, production, and maintenance of blood cells. It is the process of pluripotent, stem cells delineation into segregated blood cells (Blackburn, 2013a, p. 229; Diab & Luchtman-Jones, 2015, p. 1294; Diehl-Jones & Fraser, 2015, p. 662; Juul & Christensen, 2018, p. 1113, 1116).

2. A. It is important to recognize that polycythemia is not synonymous with hyperviscosity and that not every neonate with polycythemia also has hyperviscosity (Christensen, 2018, p. 1176). The viscosity of blood increases linearly with hematocrit up to 60% then increases exponentially. Viscosity cannot easily be measured directly, so hematocrit is often used as a surrogate for viscosity (Manco-Johnson, et al., 2016, p. 492).

3. C. The enzyme heme oxygenase acts on heme to produce biliverdin. Biliverdin reductase will then convert biliverdin into bilirubin (Kamath-Rayne et al., p. 511).

4. A. The hallmark of isoimmunization is a positive DAT (also known as the Coombs test). This is indicative of maternally produced antibody that has traversed the placenta and is now found within the fetus.
The test is termed direct if the antiglobulin is adhered to the red blood cells (RBCs).
An indirect test refers to the antibody being detected in the serum (Kaplan, 2015, p. 1630).

5. A. There is no single serum bilirubin level at which phototherapy should be initiated. Instead, each infant needs to be evaluated individually with consideration to the bilirubin level and the infant's level of risk for hyperbilirubinemia (Kaplan et al., 2015, pp. 1651–1652; Snell & Gardner, 2016, p. 265).

CHAPTER 22

1. **C.** Lethargy or poor feeding may be the only symptoms, initially, for sepsis, although the most common clinical sign is respiratory distress (Wilson & Tyner, 2015, p. 690; Leonard & Dobbs, 2015, p. 735). Definitive diagnosis is the isolation of an organism from a sterile body site, such as blood, cerebrospinal fluid (CSF), or urine (Bailey & Leonard, 2013, p. 347; Leonard & Dobbs, 2015, p. 735; Wilson & Tyner, 2015, p. 694).

   Blood culture volume should be at least 1 mL for improved recovery, particularly, in low colony count bacteremia (Leonard & Dobbs., 2015, p. 735; Wilson & Tyner, 2015, p. 694). Indirect indices of infection include the following: white blood cells (WBC), absolute neutrophil count (ANC), CRP, procalcitonin level, and various cytokines; none are specific or sensitive enough to confirm or exclude sepsis (Bailey & Leonard, 2013, p. 347). These indices can be used to help identify infected infants and guide decisions on antimicrobial therapy (Leonard & Dobbs, 2015, p. 736).

2. **B.** Detection of neonatal sepsis requires a high index of suspicion as clinical signs may be nonspecific and nonlocalizing (Leonard & Dobbs, 2015, p. 735; Pammi, Brand & Weisman, 2016, p. 537; Wilson & Tyner, 2015, p. 690).

3. **A.** Preventative efforts to reduce the risk of HAIs focus on infection control-hand hygiene, proper management of central venous catheters, appropriate use of antibiotics, limited use of H-2 blockers and proton pump inhibitors (Leonard & Dobbs, 2015, p. 737; Pammi, Brand & Weisman, 2016, p. 537; Wilson & Tyner, 2015, p. 715).

4. **A.** Symptoms at birth for fulminant CMV infection are: intrauterine growth restriction, hepatosplenomegaly with jaundice, abnormal LFTs, thrombocytopenia with or without purpura, severe central nervous system involvement (Permar, 2017, p. 644–645). Testing using polymerase reaction (PCR), can be done on blood, urine, or saliva by viral isolation in tissue culture from the infant's urine or saliva, and by spin-enhanced urine culture (Baley & Leonard, 2013; Greenberg et al., 2014, p. 1236; Wilson & Tyner, 2014, p. 708).

5. **C.** Most mothers of severely affected infants have no known history of HSV or lesion present at the time of delivery (Greenberg et al., 2014, p. 1237), therefore a negative maternal history should not deter the practitioner from evaluating the infant with HSV symptoms (Schleis & Marsh, 2018, p. 485). Symptoms present by 7 to 14 days of life with skin lesions (in <30%). Lesions are localized to skin, eyes, and mouth (SEM). Culture of vesicular fluid, blood (CSF culture yield is less than 50%) and surface cultures from mouth, nasopharynx, conjunctiva, and anus after 24 hours from birth and after initial bath (Baley & Leonard, 2015, p. 359; Greenberg et al., 2014, p. 123; Pammi, Brand, & Weisman, 2016, p. 548; Schleis & Marsh, 2018, p. 485; Wilson & Tyner, 2015, p. 709).

CHAPTER 23

1. **C.** Developmental dysplasia of the hip (DDH) diagnosis is highly suspected when Barlow and Ortolani tests are positive, and with asymmetric thigh and gluteal skin folds, uneven knee levels (Allis or Galeazzi sign), and the absence of normal knee flexion (Son-Hing & Thompson, 2015, p. 1796; Sterk, 2015, p. 783; Tappero, 2019, p. 157).

2. **C.** Both scoliosis and kyphosis may be difficult to detect at birth, however, early detection is critical to prevent severe deformities and maintain neurologic function (Kasser, 2017, p. 847; Son-Hing & Thompson, 2015, p. 1793; Tappero, 2019, p. 153; White, Bouchard, & Goldberg, 2018, p. 1446). Congenital scoliosis is a lateral curvature of the spine resulting from an embryologic failure of spinal formation or segmentation. Congenital kyphosis is the failure of formation of all or part of the vertebral body with preservation of the posterior elements as well as the failure of anterior segmentation of the spine (Kasser, 2017, p. 847; Son-Hing & Thompson, 2015, p. 1793; Tappero, 2019, p. 153; White et al., 2018, p. 1358).

3. **C.** Syndactyly, or fusion of digits, is likely a normal variant but can be associated with genetic syndromes (Son-Hing & Thompson, 2015, p. 1790; Tappero, 2019, p. 162). Intervention of syndactyly is not routine but may be requested by parents, and treatment depends on the severity of the webbing, bony structure, and vascular involvement (Son-Hing & Thompson, 2015, p. 1790).

4. **B.** Talipes equinovarus (TE) is characterized as adduction of forefoot; pronounced varus, foot, and toes in downward pointing position; equinus position; and atrophy of the affected lower extremity. TE may be unilateral or bilateral (Kasser, 2017, p. 851; Son-Hing & Thompson, 2015, p. 1802; Tappero, 2019, pp. 160–116, 226; White & Goldberg, 2018, p. 1354).

5. **A.** Clavicle fractures are one of the most common birth injuries, and associated with shoulder dystocia and difficult delivery. Intervention includes pinning the sleeve of the infant's shirt to the front as a means to immobilize the extremity for 7 to 10 days (Abdulhayoglu, 2017, p. 64 & 73; Song-Hing & Thompson, 2015, p. 1779; Tappero, 2019, p. 145; White et al., 2018, p. 1359).

CHAPTER 24

1. **B.** Immersion bathing for stable term and preterm infants have been shown to be beneficial; it can be more soothing and less stressful. However, bathing can alter the skin pH, so baths should be done every 4 days or less (Lund & Durand, 2016, p. 469).

2. **A.** Most infantile hemangiomas (his) (80%) have completed their growth by 3 months of age and 90% regress by 4 years of age (Gupta & Sidbury, 2018, p. 1512).

3. **C.** Treatment aims [for EB] are preventing trauma to skin, providing wound healing dressings, maximizing nutrition, and preventing secondary infections (Witt, 2015, p. 809).

4. B. Milia are common in newborns. They present as tiny, white monomorphic papules with a smooth surface and are commonly seen on the forehead, cheeks, and chin. No treatment is necessary, and they will resolve spontaneously over several months (Khorsand & Sidbury, 2018, p. 1505).

5. C. Accessory tragus (preauricular tags) are relatively common congenital malformations of the external ear (Gupta & Sidbury, 2018, p. 1534).

CHAPTER 25

1. B. ROP develops because of poor retinal vascularization resulting in retinal hypoxia and pathologic neovascularization (Campomanes & Binenbaum, 2018, p. 1552; Sun et al., 2015, p. 1769).

2. A. As infants are preferential nose breathers for the first 4 to 6 weeks of life, symptoms of bilateral choanal atresia can be severe and depends on the severity of the lesion (Otteson & Arnold, 2015, p. 1147). Choanal atresia presents with noisy breathing, cyanosis that resolves during crying, and apnea of the quiet infant (Benjamin & Furdon, 2015, p. 129; Gardner & Hernandez, 2016, p. 94; Walker, 2018, p. 304).

3. C. Normal ear placement is considered to be above the imaginary line drawn from the inner to outer canthus of the eye toward the ear. If the insertion of the ear is lower than this point, the ear is considered low set. Both ears should be examined for insertion and rotation as one ear may be posteriorly rotated and appear low set, while the other ear appears in normal position (Bennett & Meier, 2019, p. 221; Johnson, 2019, p. 69; Lissaur, 2015, p. 394).

4. C. Cleft lip/palate is not an automatic ICU admission. A multidisciplinary approach to management and early intervention follow-up is recommended. Nutritionist consult should be considered as cleft lip and palate infants may have higher caloric requirements and are at higher risk for failure-to-thrive (Evans et al., 2012, p. 1335).

5. A. Incidence of macroglossia is unknown, however, it is commonly seen in genetic disorders such as Beckwith–Wiedemann syndrome and Down syndrome. It may also be associated with hypothyroidism and mucopolysaccharidosis (Bennett & Meier, 2019, p. 222; Johnson, 2019, p. 74).

CHAPTER 26

1. B. Women who are compliant in opioid agonist treatment with methadone (Dolophine) or buprenorphine (Subutex) should be encouraged to breastfeed because drug concentrations in breastmilk are low (Hudak, 2015, p. 687; Patrick, 2017, p. 149; Prasad & Jones, 2019, p. 1251; Sherman, 2015, p. 54).

2. A. Maternal drinking during pregnancy can lead to fetal alcohol spectrum disorder, which shows fetal growth problems and facial dysmorphia (e.g., smooth philtrum, midface hypoplasia, broad flat nasal bridge, thin vermilion border, short palpebral fissures); (Barron, 2014, p. 103; Prasad & Jones, 2019, p. 1248; Sullivan, 2016, p. 573;

Wallen & Gleason, 2018, p. 129; Wallman, 2018, p. 257; Weiner & Finnegan, 2016, p. 202).

3. A. The goal of medication to treat neonatal abstinence syndrome (NAS) is to relieve severe signs and symptoms and prevent complications such as fever, weight loss, and seizures if nonpharmacologic care is not able to manage the symptoms. The reduction of symptoms is the only clear benefit of drug therapy (Hudak, 2015, p. 688; Sherman, 2015, p. 53).

4. B. Symptoms of neonatal abstinence syndrome (NAS) l may present as late as 7 to 14 days after birth (Hudak, 2015, p. 686; Smith & Carley, 2014, p. 681; Weiner & Finnegan, 2016, p. 207).

5. C. Preconception education of women of childbearing age, families, and physicians is key to prevention of drug effects on the fetus and newborn. Early education about drug effects on a fetus and newborn that begins at home and is reinforced in elementary and middle school is optimal. Teenagers who become pregnant are more likely to engage in substance use than their nonpregnant peers (Hudak, 2015, p. 682).

CHAPTER 27

1. A. The process of EBP is the utilization of the best available evidence for care with the integration of nursing expertise and consideration of the individual needs and values of each patient (Polit & Beck, 2018, p. 21; Thomas, 2015, p. 840). In the medical literature, EBP may be referred to as evidence-based medicine (Walsh & Higgins, 2013, p. 1).

2. B. With their nursing expertise and educational preparation, nurse practitioners are in an excellent position to lead and participate in EBP projects.
Graduate nursing programs incorporate the Essentials for MSN Education from the American Association of Colleges of Nursing (AACN) into their curricula and the MSN Essential IV is "Translating and Integrating Knowledge into Practice" (Thomas, 2015, p. 834).

3. A. Research is the generation of new knowledge. This new knowledge can be used to guide EBP. The EBP process includes taking knowledge gleaned from research and incorporating nursing expertise and patient values to establish best practices (Thomas, 2015, p. 840).

CHAPTER 28

1. B. Consent has two key components:
- The prevention of a battery (nonconsensual touching) and
- a person's right to control what is done to his or her body body (Guido, 2013, p. 118).

2. C. To be successful in a court case involving malpractice or negligence, the plaintiff (injured party) must prove the following four elements in a malpractice case.
- ○ A duty was owed to the patient.
- ○ There was a breach of that duty.
- ○ Harm or damage occurred to the patient.
- ○ Breach of the duty resulted in harm (proximal cause) (Guido, 2013, p. 70; Verklan, 2015, p. 853).

3. B. This ethical principle [justice] is derived from Aristotle. It is the obligation to treat individuals equally or comparably and to distribute benefits and burdens equally throughout society (Verklan, 2015, pp. 844–845).

CHAPTER 29

1. A. The three-step process developed by the Agency for Healthcare Research and Quality (AHRQ) is founded on four core competencies: leadership, situation monitoring, mutual support, and communication. TeamSTEPPS is designed to provide hospitals a systematic approach to integrating teamwork into everyday practices of healthcare workers to improve quality, safety, and efficiency of care (Tyler & Napoli, 2019, pp. 671–672).

2. A. HROs share similar characteristics, such as a preoccupation with failure, a reluctance to simplify interpretations, a sensitivity to operations, commitment to resilience, and deference to expertise (Simpson, 2014, p. 3; Suresh & Raghavan, 2017, p. 59).

3. B. Precursor events are errors that reach the patient but result in no detectable or only minimal harm. Near misses are errors detected before they reach the patient, usually through skillful nursing assessment and intervention. Serious safety issues are any error that reaches the patient and results in moderate to severe harm, including death. May also be called a "sentinel" event (Simpson, 2014, p. 27).

4. B. Situation, Background, Assessment, and Recommendation (SBAR) (Simpson, 2014, p. 21; Smith & Donze, 2015, p. 353).

5. B. Traditional practice is for organizations to respond to errors by naming and blaming individuals. This is known as a person-centered approach.

A systems approach recognizes the complexity of a system and that most errors are based in flawed systems in which the individuals work (Smith & Donze, 2015, p. 350).

CHAPTER 30

1. C. The formal definition of nursing research is a systematic inquiry designed to generate trustworthy evidence about issues of importance to the nursing profession and its clients, including nursing practice, education, administration, and informatics. The advent of nursing research has brought systematic query to innovative nursing knowledge (Polit & Beck, 2018, p. 2).

2. B. The independent variable is believed to influence the dependent variable; in experimental research, it is the manipulated (treatment) variable.
The dependent variable is the variable hypothesized to depend on or to be caused by another (Polit & Beck, 2018, p. 43).

3. A. Descriptive statistics include measures of central tendency (mean, median, mode) and dispersion (standard deviation, variance, range). Inferential statistics are based on probability and allow judgments to be made about the population and hypotheses to be tested. In general, inferential statistics test either how things differ or how things are related (Thomas, 2015, p. 836).

4. C. Gaining entrée is more than determining a site at which to perform the research; it may also involve negotiating and gaining permission from gatekeepers of the community that the researcher wishes to access (Polit & Beck, 2018, p. 54).

5. A. Bivariate statistics describe the relationships between two variables.
Univariate statistics are one-variable or descriptive statistics used to synthesize and describe data (Polit & Beck, 2018, pp. 229, 234).

INDEX